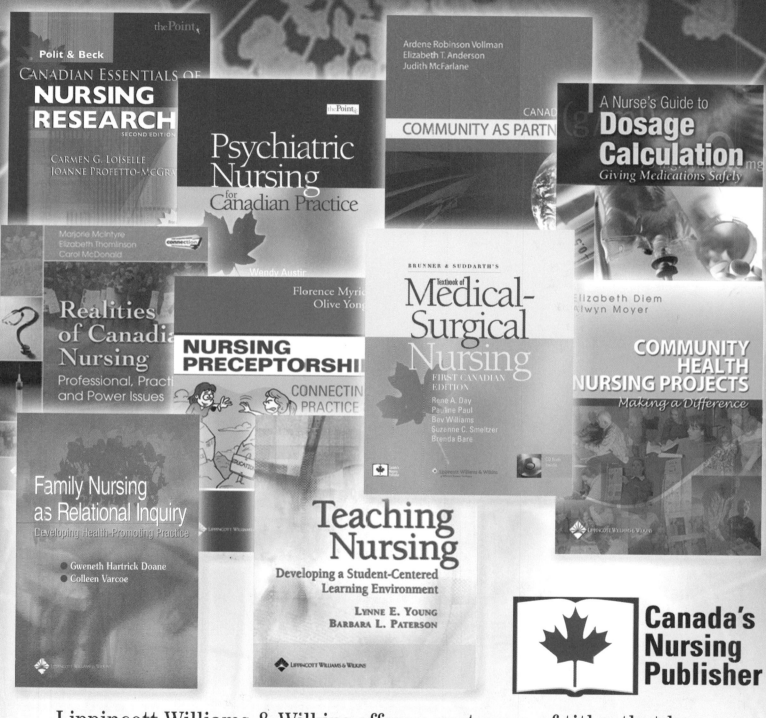

Psychiatric Nursing
for Canadian Practice

Wendy Austin, RN, MEd (Counselling), PhD
Professor and Canada Research Chair (Relational Ethics in Health Care)
Faculty of Nursing and the Dossetor Health Ethics Centre
University of Alberta
Edmonton, Alberta, Canada

Mary Ann Boyd, PhD, DNS, APRN, BC
Professor and Associate Dean
Southern Illinois University Edwardsville
Edwardsville, Illinois

Lippincott Williams & Wilkins
a Wolters Kluwer business

Philadelphia · Baltimore · New York · London
Buenos Aires · Hong Kong · Sydney · Tokyo

Senior Acquisitions Editor: Margaret Zuccarini
Development Editor: Helen Kogut
Senior Production Editor: Marian A. Bellus
Director of Nursing Production: Helen Ewan
Managing Editor/Production: Erika Kors
Art Director,Design: Joan Wendt
Art Director, Illustration: Brett MacNaughton
Manufacturing Manager: William Alberti
Indexer: Ann Cassar
Compositor: TechBooks
Printer: Courier

9 8 7 6 5 4

Library of Congress Cataloging-in-Publication Data

Austin, Wendy, 1947-
    Psychiatric nursing for Canadian practice / Wendy Austin, Mary Ann Boyd.
      p. ; cm.
    Includes bibliographical references and index.
    ISBN-13: 978-0-7817-9608-8
    ISBN-10: 0-7817-9608-3
  1. Psychiatric nursing—Canada.   I. Boyd, M. (Mary Ann)   II. Title.
    [DNLM: 1. Mental Disorders—nursing—Canada.   2. Nursing Care—methods—Canada.
3. Psychiatric Nursing—methods—Canada.   WY 160 A9375p 2008]
RC440.A87 2008
616.89'0231—dc22

                                                              2006009361

Care has been taken to confirm the accuracy of the information presented and to describe generally accepted practices. However, the author, editors, and publisher are not responsible for errors or omissions or for any consequences from application of the infor-mation in this book and make no warranty, express or implied, with respect to the content of the publication.

The author, editors, and publisher have exerted every effort to ensure that drug selectin and dosage set forth in this text are in accordance with the current recommenda-tions and practice at the time of publication. However, in view of ongoing research, changes in government regulations, and the constant flow of information relating to drug therapy and drug reactions, the reader is urged to check the package insert for each drug for any change in indications and dosage and for added warnings and precautions This is particularly important when the recommended agent is a new or infrequently employed drug.

Some drugs and medical devices presented in this publication have Food and Drug Administration (FDA) clearance for limited use in restricted research settings. It is the responsibility of the health care provider to ascertain the FDA status of each drug or device planned for use in his or her clinical practice.

LWW.com

This book is dedicated to my children, Mark and
Kara Hurtig, in gratitude for their loving presence in
my life.

In Memorium
Marlene Reimer

Canadian Contributors

Geertje Boschma, RN, PhD
Assistant Professor
School of Nursing
University of British Columbia
Vancouver, British Columbia, Canada

Freida S. Chavez, RN, BScN, MHSc, CHE
Lecturer
Faculty of Nursing
University of Toronto
Toronto Ontario, Canada

Diana Clarke, RN, PhD
Assistant Professor
Faculty of Nursing
University of Manitoba
Winnipeg, Manitoba, Canada

Anne Marie Creamer, RN, MSN
Nurse Practitioner Primary Health care
Saint Joseph's Community Health Centre
Atlantic Health Sciences Corporation
Saint John, New Brunswick, Canada

Christine Davis RN, MEd, MN(c), CPMHN(C)
Coordinator
Laurentian University St Lawrence College
Collaborative BScN Program
Brockville, Ontario, Canada

Carol Ewashen, PhD, RN
Associate Professor, Faculty of Nursing
University of Calgary
Calgary, Alberta, Canada

Cheryl Forchuk, RN, PhD
Professor
Faculty of Health Sciences
University of Western Ontario
London, Ontario, Canada

Ruth Gallop, RN, PhD
Professor Emerita
Faculty of Nursing
University of Toronto
Toronto, Ontario, Canada

Marlee Groening, RN, MSN
Lecturer
School of Nursing
University of British Columbia
Vancouver, British Columbia, Canada

Sandy Harper-Jaques, RN, MN
Clinical Nurse Specialist
Adult Mental Health
Calgary Health Region
Calgary, Alberta, Canada

Yvonne Hayne, RN, PhD
Psychiatric and Mental Health Nursing
Mount Royal College
Calgary, Alberta, Canada

Marion Healey-Ogdon, RN, PhD(c)
Nursing Instructor
College of New Caledonia
Prince George, British Columbia, Canada

Kathy Hegadoren, RN, BScN, MSc, PhD
Associate Professor
Canada Research Chair in Stress Disorders in Women
Faculty of Nursing
University of Alberta
Edmonton, Alberta, Canada

L. Elizabeth Hood, RN, MSN, PhD
Clinical Nurse Specialist (Mental Health)
Regional Mental Health Program, Alberta
   Hospital Edmonton
Edmonton, Alberta, Canada

Jean Hughes, RN, PhD
Associate Professor
School of Nursing
Dalhousie University
Halifax, Nova Scotia

Arlene Kent-Wilkinson, RN, MN, PhD(c)
Assistant Professor
College of Nursing
Univeristy of Saskatchewan
Saskatoon, Saskatchewan, Canada

Nazilla Kahnlou, RN, PhD
Associate Professor
Faculty of Nursing
University of Toronto
Toronto, Ontario, Canada

Annette Lane, RN, PhD(c)
Instructor
Faculty of Nursing
University of Calgary
Calgary, Alberta, Canada

Jan Landeen, RN, MEd, PhD
Associate Professor, Assistant Dean
School of Nursing
McMaster University
Hamilton Ontario, Canada

Gerri Lasiuk, RN, BA, PhD(c), CPMHN(c)
Faculty of Nursing
University of Alberta
Edmonton, Alberta, Canada

Lori Limacher, RN, PhD
Assistant Professor
Faculty of Nursing
University of Calgary
Calgary, Alberta, Canada

Elizabeth McCay, RN, PhD
Professor
School of Nursing
Ryerson University
Toronto, Ontario, Canada

Sharon Moore, RN, BA, MEd, PhD
Associate Professor
Centre for Nursing and Health Studies
Athabasca University
Athabasca, Alberta, Canada

B. Lee Murray, RN, PhD(c)
Clinical Nurse Specialist
Assistant Professor
College of Nursing
University of Saskatchewan
Saskatoon, Saskatchewan, Canada

Julia Noel, RN, BA, MN
Certificate in Mental Health Nursing
Senior Teaching Associate
Faculty of Nursing
University of New Brunswick
Fredrickton, New Brunswick, Canada

Ginette Pagé, RN, PhD
Clinical Nurse Specialist, Consultant in Nursing
Private Practice
Dunham, Québec, Canada

Hélène Provencher, RN, PhD
Professor
Faculty of Nursing
Laval University
Quebec, Canada

Marlene Reimer, RN, PhD, (NNCC)
Professor and Dean
Faculty of Nursing
University of Manitoba
Winnipeg, Manitoba, Canada

Michel Tarko, RPN, PhD
Instructor
Department of Psychiatric Nursing
Douglas College
New Westminster, British Columbia, Canada

Cindy Peternelj-Taylor, RN, MSc (PhD Student)
Professor
College of Nursing
University of Saskatchewan
Saskatoon, Saskatchewan, Canada

Tracey Tully, RN, PhD
Clinical Nurse Specialist
Sunnybrook and Women's College Health
    Sciences Centre
Toronto, Ontario, Canada

Stephen Vanslyke, RN, MN
Senior Instructor
Faculty of Nursing
University of New Brunswick
Fredrickton, New Brunswick, Canada

Kathryn Weaver, RN, PhD
Assistant Professor
University of New Brunswick
Fredericton, New Brunswick, Canada

Olive Yonge, RN, PhD, C Psych
Professor
Faculty of Nursing
University of Alberta
Edmonton, Alberta, Canada

American Contributors

Marjorie Baier, PhD, APRN, BC
Associate Professor of Nursing
Southern Illinois University School of Nursing
  Edwardsville
Edwardsville, IL

Doris E. Bell, PhD, APRN, BC
Professor of Nursing
Southern Illinois University Edwardsville
Edwardsville, IL

Andrea C. Bostrom, PhD, RN, APRN, BC
Associate Professor & Associate Dean for
  Academic Programs
Kirkhof College of Nursing
Grand Valley State University
Allendale, MI

Mary R. Boyd, PhD, RN
Associate Professor
College of Nursing
University of South Carolina
Columbia, SC

Kathleen C. Buckwalter, PhD, RN, FAAN
Associate Provost for the Health Sciences &
  University of Iowa Foundation Distinguished
  Professor of Nursing
University of Iowa, College of Nursing
  Iowa City, Iowa

Catherine Gray Deering, PhD, RN, APRN, BC
Professor
Clayton College & State University
Morrow, GA

Barbara G. Faltz, MS, RN
Clinical Nurse Specialist, Addiction Treatment Services
Veterans Administration Palo Alto Health Care System
Palo Alto, CA

Cheryl Forchuk, PhD, RN
Professor
Nursing, Faculty of Health Sciences
University of Western Ontario
Lawson Health Research Institute
London, Ontario
Canada

Linda Garand, PhD, RN, CS
Post Doctoral Fellow,
Western Psychiatric Institute and Clinic
Assistant Professor, University of
  Pittsburgh School of Nursing
Pittsburgh, Pennsylvania

Linda A. Gerdner, PhD, RN
Assistant Professor
College of Nursing
University of Minnesota
Minneapolis, Minnesota

Denise M. Gibson, MSN, APRN, BC
Instructor
Southern Illinois University School of
  Nursing Edwardsville
Edwardsville, IL

Vanya L. Hamrin, MS, APRN, BC
Assistant Professor
School of Nursing
Yale University
New Haven, CT

Sandy Harper-Jaques, MN, RN
Clinical Counselor
Dominican Sisters Family Service
Bronx, NY

Emily J. Hauenstein, PhD, APRN, LCP, BC
Associate Professor
University of Virginia
Charlottesville, VA

Nancy Anne Hilliker, MA, RN, ANP, CS
Nurse Practitioner
Washington University School of Medicine
St. Louis, MO

Gail L. Kongable, MSN, RN, FNP
Associate Professor
Neurological Surgery
University of Virginia Health Systems
Charlottesville, VA

Ronna E. Krozy, EdD, RN
Associate Professor of Nursing
Boston College, School of Nursing
Chestnut Hill, MA

Kathy Lee, MS, RN, APRN, BS
Director
Memorial Behavioral Health Group
Memorial Medical Centre
Springfield, Illinois

Barbara J. Limandri, DNSc, APRN, BC
Associate Professor & Psychiatric Mental Health
   Nurse Practitioner
School of Nursing - SNSN
Oregon Health & Science University
Centre for Women's Health
Portland, OR

Susan McCabe, EdD, APRN, BC
Associate Professor
College of Nursing
East Tennessee State University
Johnson City, TN

Mark J. Muehlbach, PhD
Diplomate of the American Board of Sleep Medicine
Associate Director
Sleep Disorders and Research Centre
Forest Park Hospital
St. Louis, Missouri
   and
Adjunct Faculty
Webster University
Webster Groves, Missouri

Ruth Beckmann Murray, EdD, APRN, BC, N-NAP, FAAN
Professor & Coordinator
Psychiatric Mental Health Nursing Graduate
   Specialty
Saint Louis University School of Nursing
St. Louis, MO

Robert B. Noud, MS, APRN, BC
Adjunct Faculty
University of Missouri St. Louis
Staff
St. Louis University Hospital
   St. Louis

Marlene Reimer, PhD, RN, CNN(C)
Professor
Faculty of Nursing
University of Calgary
Calgary, Alberta
Canada

Nan Roberts, MS, APRN, BC
Advanced Practice Nurse
Saaid Khojasten & Associates, Inc.
St. Charles, MO

Roberta Stock, MS, APRN, BC
Advanced Practice Nurse
Saaid Khojastek & Associates, Inc.
St. Charles, MO

Lawrence Scahill, PhD, APRN, BC, FAAN
Associate Professor
Yale University
School of Nursing & Child Study Centre
New Haven, CT

Sandra Sellin DNSc, RN
Lecturer, Psychiatric Nursing
California State University – San Francisco
Clinical Professor
City College of San Francisco
   and
University of San Francisco

Mickey Stanley, PhD, RN
Associate Professor
Southern Illinois University School of Nursing
   Edwardsville
Edwardsville, IL

Bonnie J. Wakefield, PhD, RN
Research Scientist
Iowa City VA Medical Centre
Clinical Associate Professor
College of Nursing
University of Iowa
Iowa City, Iowa

Jane H. White, DNSc, APRN, BC
Executive Director APNA
Adjunct Professor
The Catholic University of America
School of Nursing
Arlington, VA
Private Practice
Washington, DC

Lorraine D. Williams, PhD, APRN, BC
Associate Professor
School of Nursing
Southern Illinois University Edwardsville
Edwardsville, IL

Richard V. Wing, BSN, MS
Program Manager Inpatient Addiction Treatment
Nurse Manager Addiction Treatment Services
Department of Veterans Affairs
VA Palo Alto Health Care System
Menlo Park, CA

Sandra Jean Wood, MSN, RN, APRN, BC
Clinical Assistant Professor
Indiana University School of Nursing
Indianapolis, IN

Reviewers

Wendy Azzopardi, BScN, MSc(N), CPMHN
Professor
Conestoga College
Kitchener, Ontario, Canada

Leigh Blaney, RN, BScN, MA
Professor – Faculty of Nursing
Malaspina University-College
Nanaimo, British Columbia, Canada

Freida S. Chavez, RN, MHSc, CHE
Lecturer, Fleming School of Nursing
University of Toronto
Toronto, Ontario, Canada

Cathy Graham, RN, BScN, MSc
Lecturer – Trent/Fleming School of Nursing
Trent University
Peterborough, Ontario, Canada

Dianne Groll, RN, PhD, BA, BSc, MSc
Assistant Professor
University of Ottawa
Ottawa, Canada

L. Elizabeth Hood, RN, PhD, MSN, BScN
Instructor
Grande Prairie Regional College
Grande Prairie, Alberta, Canada

Sonya Jakubec, RN, PhD, BHScN, MN
Faculty, Department of Undergraduate Nursing
Faculty of Health and Community Studies, Mount
   Royal College
Calgary, Alberta, Canada

Nela Karagach, RN, BScN, CPMHN
Registered Nurse
Baycrest Centre for Geriatric Care
Toronto, Ontario, Canada

Annette M. Lane, RN, PhD
Instructor – Faculty of Nursing
University of Calgary
Calgary, Alberta, Canada

Barbara Maxwell, MSN, CNS, RNC
Assistant Professor of Nursing
SUNY Ulster County Community College
Stone Ridge, New York

Marilyn Merritt-Gray, MN, BN
Professor, Faculty of Nursing
University of New Brunswick
Fredericton, New Brunswick, Canada

Judy Osborne, RN
Clinical Instructor Mental Health
Fleming College
Peterborough, Ontario, Canada

Kathy Quee, MScN
Instructor
British Columbia Institute of Technology
Burnaby, British Columbia, Canada

Lori Shortridge, RN, MSN
Coordinator Graduate Nurse Programs
Kwantlen University College
Surrey, British Columbia, Canada

Nicole Snow, RN, BN, MN
Nurse Educator
Centre for Nursing Studies
St. John's, Newfoundland and Labrador, Canada

Wendy Stanyon, RN, BN, MA, ED, EdD
Assistant Nursing Professor
University of Ontario Institute of Technology
Oshawa, Ontario, Canada

John Stone, RN, BA, BScN, CPMHN
Professor
Humber Institute of Training & Advanced Learning
Toronto, Ontario, Canada

Landa Terblanche, PhD
Associate Professor
Trinity Western University
Langley, British Columbia, Canada

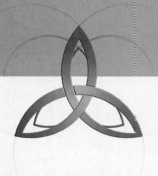

Preface

As the first Canadian psychiatric and mental health (PMH) nursing text, this book, *Psychiatric Nursing for Canadian Practice*, fulfills an aspiration of many Canadian PMH nurses and nurse educators. Our students now have a reference that reflects contemporary Canadian practice, its standards, its context, and its issues. An adaptation of the award-winning text, *Psychiatric Nursing: Contemporary Practice (3rd Edition)*, by Mary Ann Boyd, this Canadian edition was made possible by the contributions of experts in PMH nursing from across our country.

There are three completely new chapters in this Canadian edition, *Ethical Psychiatric and Mental Health Nursing Practice*, *Cognitive Behavioural Therapy*, and *Forensic Psychiatric and Mental Health Nursing*. Many other chapters consist of primarily new Canadian content, particularly those of Unit I in which our understanding of the nature of mental health and mental illness is addressed. In other chapters, for instance those focussed on specific disorders, Canadian statistics, research, and resources are highlighted. The Canadian landscape of PMH practice informs the text's content: Canada's multiculturalism, its mental health legislation and its publicly-funded healthcare system. Although the values of the *Canadian Nurses Association Code of Ethics for Registered Nurses* and the *Canadian Standards of Psychiatric and Mental Health Nursing* were included in the 3rd edition of the Boyd text, they are central to this edition. There are brief "CRNE Notes" throughout the text to help students prepare for the Canadian Registered Nurse Examination. Whenever appropriate, it is Canadians that are described in the "In a Life" feature and Canadian films are recommended in the "Movies" section of each chapter. That this is a Canadian text is apparent also in small ways, such as spelling and the use of metric measurements.

Although the unique characteristic of this book is its Canadian perspective, the fact that Canada is part of a global community is recognized. Mental illness affects the lives of individuals, families, and communities across the world. Nurses can contribute significantly to addressing the impact of mental illness on human life and promote mental health worldwide. Like other nurses around the globe, Canadian nurses are actively seeking to do this. The Faculty of Nursing at the University of Alberta, for instance, is currently a World Health Collaborating Centre in Nursing and Mental Health. This book is intended as a resource to prepare nurses to practice PMH nursing both at home and abroad.

TEXT ORGANIZATION

This edition follows the organization of previous editions of *Psychiatric Nursing: Contemporary Practice*, employing the biopsychosocial model of mental illness. In this Canadian edition, the spiritual dimension is explicitly included under the psychological domain. Spirituality is an area of human existence that is important to all aspects of health care, and certainly to PMH nursing. We are continually learning how to better enact the spiritual aspects of care.

In Canadian nursing practice, we are in a stage of transition regarding the terminology used to identify the recipients of nursing care—patient, client, consumer, user, person—these are all used in the contemporary literature. For this edition, the decision was made to allow the Canadian authors to use whichever term they prefer. It will be interesting to see which term, if any, will predominate in future editions.

FEATURES

There are many pedagogical features to the text, all retained from the Boyd 3rd edition.

- Chapters open with **Learning Objectives, Key Terms,** and **Key Concepts** that cue students to the material they will encounter.
- **Summary of Key Points** encapsulates core chapter content to facilitate assimilation and review.
- **Critical Thinking Challenges** are grounded in chapter content and aimed at stimulating both

analytical and reflective thinking on the part of readers.

- Selected films are described and viewing points identified in the **Movies** feature. Movies are a rich, evocative means to raising and exploring complex ideas. Students can use the suggested works to stimulate discussion with their family and friends, as well as their classmates and teachers.
- **Web Links** are listed to direct students to excellent sources of supplemental information.
- **CRNE Notes** are the Canadian authors' suggestions regarding important areas of preparation for the national registration examination.
- The **In a Life** feature (termed "Fame and Fortune in the 3ʳᵈ edition) illustrates the way the topic of the chapter has shaped or been played out in a particular person's life.
- **Research Boxes** focus on specific studies that contribute to improving PMH nursing practice. Most are recent Canadian nursing research projects and many may reflect the work of the chapter's author(s). When a less recent study is highlighted, it is because of its significance to the topic.
- **Therapeutic Dialogue Boxes** encourage the comparison of therapeutic and nontherapeutic communication by giving relevant examples of both.
- **Clinical Vignette Boxes** present reality-based clinical portraits of persons with symptoms of interest to the chapter topic. Questions are posed to help students consider solutions to issues presented.
- **Drug Profile Boxes** present a profile of specific psychotropic medication, commonly prescribed in the treatment of mental disorders.
- **Psychoeducation Checklists** identify content areas for the education of persons with specific disorders and their families.
- **Key Diagnostic Characteristics** tables and summaries outline diagnostic criteria for disorders as standardized in the *Diagnostic and Statistical Manual of Mental Disorders*, 4ᵗʰ edition, text revision, (DSM-IV-TR) authored by the American Psychiatric Association.
- **Line art, photos, scan images, and flow charts** illustrate the interrelationship of the biologic, psychological and social domains of mental health and illness.

TEACHING-LEARNING PACKAGE
thePoint

Students can find rich online multimedia resources at thePoint.lww.com.

Student Resource CD-ROM:

The CD-ROM includes
- NCLEX-Style Questions
- Clinical Simulations
- Movie Viewing Guides
- Monographs of Psychotropic Guides

Th CD-ROM included with this book is designed to accompany the US edition of *Psychiatric Nursing*. As such, there may be slight differences between the materials provided here and the Canadian edition of the textbook.

INSTRUCTOR'S RESOURCE CD-ROM

The Instructor's Resource CD-ROM includes
- Instructor's Manual
- Answers to Movie Viewing Guides
- Test Generator
- PowerPoint Presentations
- Image Bank
- WebCT and Blackboard-Ready Material

This CD-ROM is designed to accompany the US edition of *Psychiatric Nursing*. As such, there may be slight differences between the materials provided here and the Canadian edition of the textbook.

This text is a first attempt to provide Canadian students with a resource that directs and supports their study of PMH nursing. This is an important area of all nursing practice: every registered nurse in Canada is expected to be able to provide competent and ethical PMH care whenever necessary. PMH nursing is also a designated specialty area for which there is a Canadian credentialing examination. It is hoped that this book may contribute to nurses' interest in pursuing such specialty practice. Nurses can make a significant, positive difference in mental health promotion, the prevention of mental illness and the care of persons living with mental illness. It is the ultimate aim of this work to support them in doing so.

Wendy Austin
RN, MEd (Counselling), PhD

Contents

HOW TO USE
Psychiatric Nursing for Canadian Practice

LEARNING OBJECTIVES let students know what they'll learn upon chapter completion.

KEY CONCEPTS boxes highlight critical terminology.

CRNE NOTES highlight pertinent information to help students enhance exam performance.

THERAPEUTIC DIALOGUES juxtapose effective and ineffective approaches to client communication.

---

720 UNIT VI — Older Adults

Cognition and memory are important in many psychiatric disorders, but in this chapter, they are the key concepts. Cognition is the ability to think and know. Now the definition is further refined to be understood as a relatively high level of intellectual processing in which perceptions and information are acquired, used, or manipulated.

> **KEY CONCEPT Cognition** is based on a system of interrelated abilities, such as perception, reasoning, judgment, intuition, and memory, that allow one to be aware of oneself and one's surroundings. Impairments in these abilities can result in a failure of the afflicted person to recognize that he or she is ill and in need of treatment.

Cognition involves both how reality is perceived and how those perceptions are understood in relation to internal representations of reality previously acquired. In the broadest sense, cognition denotes how the brain processes information. Cognition includes a number of specific functions, such as the acquisition and use of language, the ability to be oriented in time and space, and the ability to learn and solve problems. It includes judgment, reasoning, attention, comprehension, concept formation, planning, and the use of symbols, such as numbers and letters used in mathematics and writing.

Memory, a facet of cognition, refers to the ability to recall or reproduce what has been learned or experienced. It is more than simple storage that includes more a complex cognitive mental function that includes most areas of the brain, especially the hippocampus, which is believed to be essential to the transfer of some memories from short-term to long-term storage. Defects of memory are an essential feature of many cognitive disorders, particularly dementia.

> **KEY CONCEPT Memory** is a facet of cognition concerned with retaining and recalling past experiences, whether they occurred in the physical environment or internally as cognitive events.

The disorders discussed in this chapter—delirium, dementia, and related cognitive disorders—are characterized by deficits in cognition or memory that represent a clear-cut deterioration from a previous level of functioning. Delirium is a disorder of acute cognitive impairment and can be caused by a medical condition (eg, infection) or substance abuse, or it may have multiple etiologies. Dementia is characterized by underlying cognitive impairments and is differentiated by chronic cause, not by symptom patterns, which are often similar. Some dementias are irreversible and dementias are sive, such as Alzheimer type, but not all dementias are irreversible. For example, some organic compounds and

---

Table 30.1	Selected Chemical Produce
Substance	**Re**
Arsenic	
Mercury	
Lead	
Manganese	
Aluminum	
Toluene (m benzene)	

22

Eating Disorders
Kate Weaver

LEARNING OBJECTIVES
After studying this chapter, you will be able to:
- Distinguish the signs and symptoms of anorexia nervosa from those of bulimia nervosa.
- Describe two etiologic theories of both anorexia nervosa and bulimia nervosa.
- Explain the importance of body image, body dissatisfaction, and gender identity in developmental theories that explain etiology of eating disorders.
- Describe the neurobiology and neurochemistry in both anorexia nervosa and bulimia nervosa.
- Explain the impact of sociocultural norms on the development of eating disorders.
- Describe the risk factors and protective factors associated with the development of eating disorders.
- Formulate nursing diagnoses for individuals with eating disorders.
- Describe nursing interventions for individuals with anorexia nervosa and bulimia nervosa.
- Differentiate binge eating disorder from bulimia nervosa.
- Analyze special concerns within the nurse–client relationship for the nursing care of individuals with eating disorders.
- Identify strategies for prevention and early detection of eating disorders.

---

populations (Eckert, Halmi, Marchi, Grove, & Crosby, 1995; Sullivan, 1995). Factors that correlate with death are illness of long duration, bingeing and purging, and comorbid illnesses (Herzog et al., 2000). Substance abuse, particularly severe alcohol use, predicts mortality in patients with anorexia nervosa (Keel et al., 2003; Korndorfer et al., 2003).

Another issue to consider with this population is stigma. Many young girls are avoided, especially in their emaciated state. Peers do not know how to approach them because they may appear both frightening and fragile (Gowers & Shore, 1999). A recent university study supported this theory and found that most men would feel uncomfortable dating a woman with an eating disorder. Males in the study who had experienced dating someone with an eating disorder expressed even stronger uncomfortable feelings, stating that conflict was the predominant issue in the relationship (Sobol & Bursztyn, 1998).

NURSING MANAGEMENT: HUMAN RESPONSE TO DISORDER
Therapeutic Relationship

Establishing a therapeutic relationship with individuals with anorexia nervosa may be difficult initially because they are suspicious and mistrustful. They often express fear of adults, especially health care professionals, whom they believe want to "make them fat." By the time they are hospitalized, mistrust can almost reach a state of paranoia. Because of their low body weight and starvation, they are often impatient and irritable. A firm, accepting, and patient approach is important in

---

CHAPTER 22 — Eating Disorders **485**

working with these individuals. Providing a rationale for all interventions helps build trust, as does a consistently nonreactive approach. Power struggles over eating are common, and remaining nonreactive is a challenge. During such power struggles, the nurse should always think about his or her own feelings of frustration and need for control (see Box 22-6).

Biologic Domain
Assessment

A thorough evaluation of body systems is important because many systems can be compromised by starvation. A careful history from both the individual with anorexia nervosa and the family, including the length and duration of symptoms, such as fasting, avoiding meals, and overexercising, is necessary to assess altered nutrition. The longer the duration of these behaviours typically means more difficult and prolonged recovery periods. Nursing management involves various biopsychosocial assessment and interventions (see Nursing Care Plan 22-1).

> **CRNE Note**
> Eating disorders are serious psychiatric disorders that threaten life. Careful assessment and referral for treatment are important nursing interventions.

The individual's weight is determined using the BMI and a scale. Currently, criteria for discharge require

---

BOX 22.6

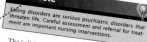

Therapeutic Dialogue: The Client With an Eating Disorder

Ineffective Approach
NURSE: You haven't eaten your lunch yet.
CLIENT: I can't. I'm already fat.
NURSE: Look at you, you're skin and bones.
CLIENT: I'll eat when I go out this afternoon on pass.
NURSE: You can't go on pass. You have to start realizing that you are sick. Because you can't take care of yourself, we are in charge.
CLIENT: You're trying to control me.
NURSE: We are trying to be responsible.
CLIENT: I won't eat!
NURSE: We have set up punishments for not eating.
CLIENT: Then I won't go out! At least I won't get fatter.

Effective Approach
NURSE: You haven't eaten your lunch.
CLIENT: I can't. I'm already fat.
NURSE: You're uncomfortable with how you see yourself and with eating?
CLIENT: I'll eat when I go out on pass.
NURSE: You and I, and the other members who are part of your treatment team, wrote your behavioural plan

together, and you know you will not be able to go out because your pass is dependent on eating both breakfast and lunch. Here!
CLIENT: You're trying to control me.
NURSE: The intent of the plan is to help you learn to take control over the eating disorder. It sure does mean a lot of hard work for you. How can I help you now with this meal?
CLIENT: What if I eat half?
NURSE: No, you must eat all of it. Why don't I sit here while you eat? Eating is scary for you. We can talk about other choices you have on the unit; tonight, you can choose the movie or board games.
CLIENT: Okay, at least I have some choices.

Critical Thinking Challenge
- What effect did the first interaction have on the client's behaviour? Why?
- In the second interaction, what theories and interventions regarding eating disorders did the nurse use in her approach to the client?

BIOPSYCHOSOCIAL model provides students with a strong knowledge base grounded in theory and research.

RESEARCH BOXES emphasize nursing implications of recent findings.

CLINICAL VIGNETTES engage students through real-world examples.

NURSING CARE PLANS present case scenarios followed by appropriate diagnoses and actions.

CHAPTER 22

anorexia nervosa have been ... of starvation and are consid... or causative, factors. Little ... ate that dysregulations in ... anorexia nervosa, as some... with early-stage dementia.

BOX 30.6   RESEARCH FOR BEST PRACTICE

Learning to Live With Early Dementia

THE QUESTION: Few studies address the needs and concerns of dementia patients from their own perspective. To address this gap, research was undertaken to explore and conceptualize the process of learning to live with memory loss in older adults with early-stage dementia.

METHODS: A qualitative grounded theory approach was used to explore the subjective experience of people with early-stage dementia. Theoretical sampling was carried out to obtain six participants who were interviewed twice. Data from the first interviews were coded and analyzed, and a preliminary theory was developed. The second interview, which was less structured, was used to verify and clarify the emerging theory.

FINDINGS: The theory that emerged can best be described as a *continuous process of adjusting to early-stage dementia*. The process consists of five core categories or stages: antecedents, anticipation, appearance, assimilation, and acceptance.

IMPLICATIONS FOR NURSING: The proposed framework offers a base of valuable information to nurses working with people who have early-stage dementia, whereas the core concepts provide a foundation for future research to test the applicability of the model in the larger population of people with dementia.

From Werezak, L., & Stewart, N. (2002). Learning to live with early dementia. *Canadian Journal of Nursing Research, 34*(1), 67–85.

Neuropathologic ...

Magnetic resonan... tomography (CT) ... viduals with an... weight loss (eg, ... enlargement, in... eral ventricles, ... and the inter...

This neuropa... with weight ... from starva... months of ... Lambe, & ... Kennedy, ... ports tha... cause an...

Gene...

Gene... The... influ... Ke... m... o... e...

FIGURE 22.2 Biopsychosocial etiologies for patients with anorexia nervosa. OCD, obsessive-compulsive disorder.

Biologic
Increased genetic vulnerability
Dieting → starving
Overexercising
Decreased awareness of hunger
OCD
Decreased serotonin activity

Social
Idealization of thinness-media
Pursuit of thinness
Enmeshment with family
Overprotective family

Psychological
Separation–individuation struggle
Sexuality conflicts
Decreased awareness of emotional cue
Feminist view → Role pressures
Negative body image–body dissatisfaction

CHAPTER 30 — Delirium, Dementias, and Related Disorders   743

misleading or disturbing stimuli, such as mirrors or art work, can be easily covered or removed from the environment.

MANAGING HALLUCINATIONS. Reassurance and distraction may be helpful for the hallucinating patient. For example, an 89-year-old patient with AD in a residential care facility would get up each night, walk to the nursing station, and whisper to the nurses, "There's a man in my bed who won't let me sleep. You should patrol this place better!" If the hallucination is not too disturbing for the patient, it can often be dismissed calmly with diversion or distraction. Because this patient did not seem too concerned by the man in her bed, the nurse may gently respond by saying, "I'm sorry you have to put up with so much. Just wait here (or come with me) and I'll make sure your room is ready for you." The nurse should then take the patient back to her room and help her into bed.

Frightening hallucinations and delusions usually require antipsychotic medications to dampen the patient's emotional reactions, but they can also be dealt with by optimizing perceptual cues (cover mirrors or turn off the television) and by encouraging patients to stay physically close to their caregivers. For example, one patient complained to her visiting nurse that she was being poisoned by deadly bugs that crawled up and down her arms and legs while she tried to sleep at night. Antipsychotic medication may help this patient sleep at night, and she would also likely benefit from reassurance and protection. Patients benefit more if nurses give them a specific intervention to help the hallucination, such as applying moisturizing lotion to her legs and arms to repel the bugs at night. The nurse does not have to agree with the patient's hallucination or delusion but should let the patient know that the feelings are justified based on the patient's perception of the threat.

BOX 30.10

Clinical Vignette: A Nurse's Dilemma

It is 8 o'clock and you are working as a nurse on an inpatient general medical unit of a large urban hospital. A 72-year-old man is admitted to your unit with symptoms of disorientation to time and place, and he is intermittently exhibiting signs of agitation. He thinks you are his child, and he falls asleep while you ask him questions about his symptoms. When you ask him to sign a consent form and hand him a pen, he looks at you as if he didn't understand your request.

The patient's wife tells you that he has had trouble with his memory for the past 3 or 4 years but that her husband has been "acting strange for the past 4 days." The patient's wife denies any history of substance abuse or head injury, but states that her husband has been recently diagnosed as having dementia of the Alzheimer's type.

The patient's physician gives a verbal order to restrain the patient "as needed" while writing orders for lab work.

What Do You Think?

• What assessment techniques would you use to determine whether this patient has dementia, delirium, or both?
• What nursing diagnosis would be included in the patient's plan of care?
• What nursing interventions would promote comfort and safety for this patient?
• Is this patient able to give consent?
• What would be the possible outcomes of physically restraining this patient (eg, would restraints be helpful or harmful for the patient)?

project (such as folding linens or setting the table), especially one that involves helping someone else. Assist the patient to meet self-care needs while encouraging independence when possible.

MANAGING ANXIETY. Cognitively impaired patients are particularly vulnerable to anxiety. As patients with dementia become more unsure of their surroundings or ... of them, they tend to react with fear

---

486   UNIT IV — Care of Persons with Psychiatric Disorders

NURSING CARE PLAN 22.1

Nursing Care Plan for a Patient With Anorexia Nervosa

JS is a 16-year-old female adolescent who appears much younger. She is 165 cm (5'5") and weighs 42 kilograms (92 pounds). She has been treated unsuccessfully in an outpatient clinic and now is being admitted to stabilize her weight. She does not believe that she is too thin and resents being forced to be hospitalized. Hospitalization was precipitated by being asked to leave the gymnastics team because of low body weight.

SETTING: INPATIENT PSYCHIATRIC UNIT

Baseline assessment: JS appears frail, pale, and dressed in oversized clothes. She is tearful, states that she is depressed and angry and that she has no friends. Physical examination results: bradycardia—pulse = 58, hypotension (98/60), constipation, amenorrhea, dry skin patches, and cold intolerance. BMI = 15.3. Hypokalemia (K+, ≤ 3.5); leukopenia (WBCs <5,000). Dehydration, temperature elevation, 99°F, elevated BUN, abnormal thyroid functioning, bone density of one standard deviation below mean age-adjusted scores.

Associated Psychiatric Diagnosis

Axis I: Anorexia nervosa
Binge-eating/purging type
Axis II: None
Axis III: None
Axis IV: Social support (social withdrawal)
GAF = Current 55
Potential 75

Medications

Fluoxetine (Prozac), 20 mg in AM

NURSING DIAGNOSIS 1: IMBALANCED NUTRITION: LESS THAN BODY REQUIREMENTS

Defining Characteristics

Unable to increase food intake
Weight more than 20% below ideal weight

Related Factors

Believes she cannot eat most foods
Purges by vomiting "occasionally"
Exercises 6–8 h daily
Sleep pattern disturbed by exercise

Outcomes

Initial

Maintains daily intake of 1,500 calories
Eliminates exercising while in hospital
Ceases purging for 1 week

Long-term

Gains .5–1.5 kg (1–3 pounds) per week until weight is at least 85% of ideal weight.
Develops strategies to maintain weight.

Interventions

Interventions

Allow JS to verbalize feelings such as anxiety related to food and weight gain—develop a therapeutic relationship.

Monitor meals and snacks, record amount eaten.

Do not substitute other foods for food on meal trays. Limit caffeine intake to 1 cup coffee (soda) daily.

Monitor 1 h after meals for purging. Weigh daily in hospital gown after she has voided. Monitor vital signs daily, electrolytes.

Provide psychoeducational inter-

Rationale

Through a relationship and examining her feelings, she may be more likely to cooperate with nutritional regimen.

Severe anorexia is life threatening. Aggressive interventions are needed to ensure adequate intake. People with anorexia usually "play games" with food. By prohibiting substitution, a more positive approach is encouraged. Caffeine is an appetite suppressant and has a diuretic effect.

Physical signs of impending complications include evidence of purging, decreasing body weight, hypotension, hyperthermia, and hypokalemia.

Increase awareness.

Ongoing Assessment

Determine anxiety level when discussing food and weight gain.

Monitor intake. Assess JS's ability to complete meals on time and without supplements.

Determine how willing JS is to follow nutritional regimen.

Monitor vital signs, weight, and electrolytes, especially potassium.

Observe comprehension of material.

DRUG PROFILES Present psychopharmacologic content with an emphasis on patient
and family education.

IN A LIFE highlights nursing of
famous persons who dealt with
mental health issues.

MOVIE VIEWING POINTS highlight films
that depict various mental health disorders.

CHAPTER 22 — Eating Disorders   **499**

Interventions for Biologic Domain

social or unrelated issues in an attempt to engage the nurse. A nonjudgmental, accepting approach, stressing the importance of the relationship and outlining its purpose, are important at the outset. Explaining the nature of the relationship and the goals of therapy will help clarify the boundaries.

Biologic Domain

Despite that most individuals with bulimia nervosa maintain normal weights, the physical ramifications of this disorder may be similar to those of anorexia nervosa. Hypokalemia can contribute to muscle weakness and fatigability, as well as to the development of cardiac arrhythmias, palpitations, and cardiac conduction defects. Patients who purge risk fluid and electrolyte abnormalities that can further compromise cardiac status. Neuropsychiatric disturbances, such as poor concentration and attention, and sleep disturbances are common.

Assessment

The nurse should assess current eating patterns, determine the number of times a day the individual binges and purges, and note dietary restraint practices. Sleep patterns and exercise habits are also important.

Nursing Diagnoses for Biologic Domain

Imbalanced Nutrition: Less Than Body Requirements and Disturbed Sleep Pattern are typical nursing diagnoses for the biologic domain.

If the patient is admitted to the hospital, meals and all food intake must be strictly monitored to normalize eating. Bathroom visits should also be supervised to prevent purging. Outpatients are asked to form a intake binges, and purges to form a changing behaviours with CBT (see description of CBT). Because individual nervosa have chaotic lifestyles and a mitted, sleep may be a low prior individuals may assume that food w they begin to eat, triggering a bing ula sleep patterns, individuals sho at about the same time every day

Pharmacologic Intervention

Whereas pharmacologic inter symptom remission in bulimi that the combination of CBT the best results (Wilson (Prozac) has been the most in clinical trials (see Box usually 60 mg per day, a h to treat depression. Sertr used effectively. These binge eating and purg depression is not present & Al-Banna, 1999). T using these medicati weight loss during t tion. Weight shoul this period.

BOX 22.13
Drug Profile: Fluoxetine Hydrochloride (Prozac)

DRUG CLASS: Selective serotonin reuptake inhibitor
RECEPTOR AFFINITY: Inhibits central nervous system neuronal uptake of serotonin with little effect on norepinephrine; thought to antagonize muscarinic, histaminergic, and α adrenergic receptors.
INDICATIONS: Treatment of depressive disorders, most effective in major depression, obesity, bulimia, and obsessive-compulsive disorder
ROUTES AND DOSAGE: Available in 10- and 20-mg pulvules and 20 mg/5 mL oral solution
Adults: 20 mg/d in the morning, not to exceed 80 mg/d. Full antidepressant effect may not be seen for up to 4 weeks. If no improvement, dosage is increased after several weeks. Dosages >20 mg/d are administered twice daily. For eating disorders: typically 40 mg to 60 mg/d recommended.
Geriatric: Administer at lower or less-frequent doses; monitor responses to guide dosage.
Children: Safety and efficacy have not been established.

SELECTED ADV
insomnia, dr
headedness
anorexia, d
respiratory
sexual dy
pruritus,
WARNINGS
Use wit
renal f
toxicit
SPECIAL
• Be av
antic
• Take
• Rep
• A
b
• E

---

474   UNIT IV — Care of Persons with Psychiatric Disorders

The first Canadian publication about eating disorders was a detailed clinical case report in the *Maritime Medical News* of April 1895 by Dr. Peter Inches, a registered physician in the province of New Brunswick. Inches described the following characteristics that he observed in a 17-year-old patient separated from her family while attending boarding school: low weight, loss of menses, and "almost complete refusal of food of any kind" (p. 74). This 19th century publication was for the most part ignored in subsequent reviews.

Only since the 1970s have eating disorders received national attention because several high-profile personalities and athletes with these disorders have received front-page news coverage and because increasingly more individuals, families, and communities were affected. The increased incidence of anorexia nervosa and bulimia nervosa has prompted mental health professionals to understand their causes and devise effective treatments. Moreover, there has been a concomitant increase in research studies addressing the intense obsession with being thin and the dissatisfaction with one's body that underlie these potentially life-threatening disorders. Thus, mental health professionals are crucial to prevention, early diagnosis, and treatment of both anorexia nervosa and bulimia nervosa.

This chapter focuses on anorexia nervosa and bulimia nervosa. In addition, binge eating disorder (BED), a newly identified eating disorder in its infancy relative to research, is briefly considered. Symptoms of these disorders, such as dieting, binge eating, and preoccupation with weight and shape, overlap significantly. Experts view these symptoms along a continuum of normal to pathologic eating behaviours (White, 2000a) (Fig. 22-1), an approach that helps to id

IN A LIFE

GETTING THE MESSAGE OUT
Sheena Carpenter (1971–1993):
A Canadian Daughter

Sheena Carpenter wanted to be a model. She had long blond hair and never weighed much over 45.5 kg (100 pounds). At 17, her mother found Sheena purging in the bathroom. A spiral of doctors, clinics, bingeing, and purging followed. Sheena's weight plummeted. Her organs shrank to one half of their normal size. Sheena had seizures. She weighed 22.75 kg (50 pounds) when she died at the age of 22.

Sheena's Place, Toronto, was founded in 1996. It has support programs and group sessions for people like Sheena. It helps some 300 people a week, nearly all women. If Sheena's Place had existed, Sheena's mother believes "It might have saved her." In life, Sheena wanted people to know her name as a model. Her death imprinted on public consciousness the acuity of having an eating disorder.

From Lynn Carpenter (personal communication), August 15, 2005; Strobel, 2002; Tranquada, 2000/1995.

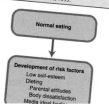

Normal eating

Development of risk factors
Low self-esteem
Dieting
Parental attitudes
Body dissatisfaction
Media ideal bodies

CHAPTER 30 — Delirium, Dementias, and Related Disorders   **755**

some environmental factors (ie, aluminum and other heavy metals).

■ Some of the psychosocial stressors known to precipitate delirium and contribute to worsening dementia include sensory overload or underload, immobilization, sleep deprivation, fatigue, pain or hunger, change in routine (pace or caregiver), or demands beyond the patient's ability. Nursing interventions should include reducing the impact of these stressors on patients and educating their families or caregivers.

■ Educating families and caregivers about what to expect, progressive cognitive decline and behaviour changes, environment safety, and community resources for patients with dementia is essential to ensuring proper care.

■ Symptoms of dementia may occur as a result of a number of disorders, including vascular and amnestic disorders, head trauma, AIDS, and substance abuse and as a symptom of Parkinson's, Huntington's, Pick's, and Creutzfeldt-Jakob diseases.

CRITICAL THINKING CHALLENGES

1 What factors should the nurse consider in differentiating Alzheimer's disease from vascular dementia?
2 Compare the defining characteristics and related risk factors of acute confusion with those for the NANDA diagnoses of Impaired Thought Processes and Sensory/Perceptual Disturbances. What are the differences and similarities between the recommended nursing interventions for delirium and dementia? What is the theoretic base for these similarities and differences?
3 Describe three ways in which medical disease can disrupt brain functioning, and relate these mechanisms to the neuropsychiatric disorders presented in this chapter.
4 Suggest reasons that older adults are particularly vulnerable to the development of neuropsychiatric disorders.
5 In what ways can culture and education influence mental status test scores?
6 The physical environment is particularly important to the patient with dementia. Every effort should be made to modify the physical environment to compensate for the cognitive and functional impairment associated with AD and related disorders, including safety measures and the avoidance of misleading stimuli. Visualize your last experience in a health care setting (hospital, nursing home, day care program, or home care setting). Identify environmental factors that could be misleading or stress producing to a person with impaired cognition (dementia), and identify ways to modify this environment to alleviate some of the stressors or misleading stimuli.

WEB LINKS

www.alz.org This Alzheimer's Association website provides information, resources, and consumer and caregiver support.
www.rnao.org/bestpractices Screening & Selecting Care Strategies for Delerium, Dementia & Depression in Older Adults.
www.pdsg.org.uk This website of the Pick's Disease Support Group provides information on Pick's disease, Lewy bodies, and other dementias.
www.alzheimer.ca/english/misc/redirect.htm This site of the Alzheimer's Association of Canada provides information and resources related to the disease.
www.pieces.cabhru.com/prc/videos.htm A. Tassonyi. Recognizing Delirium in the Elderly.

MOVIES

Iris: 2001. Based on the book by her husband, John Bayley, this movie (directed by Richard Eyre) tells the story of an influential British woman of letters, Dame Iris Murdoch. Young Iris is played by Kate Winslet, and the older Iris by Dame Judi Dench, in the unfolding of her rich and interesting life. The story reveals the couple's struggle with Iris's Alzheimer disease as her exceptional capabilities are increasingly diminished.
VIEWING POINTS: Consider how the love and friendship of the couple is both strengthened and challenged by AD. Are there any external supports and resources that might have made their situation in living with AD less difficult?

The Notebook: 2004. Every day an elderly man reads to a woman from his faded notebook. They are in a nursing home, and it is their own love story that he is reading. It is a story about how they met, fell in love, and then spent their lives together. Based on a novel by Nicholas Sparks, the movie reveals the fleeting moments of clarity that Noah's story brings to Allie, his wife, who is suffering from dementia. It shows the hope that keeps him trying to reach her.
VIEWING POINTS: Consider what it might be like to hear your own life story and to recognize it only momentarily and vaguely. Can you think of other ways people cope with the loss of a loved one who remains, at least physically, before them?

REFERENCES

Alexopoulos, G. S. (1991). Anxiety and depression in the elderly. In C. Salzman & B. D. Lebowitz (Eds.), *Anxiety in the elderly.* New York: Springer.
American Psychiatric Association. (2000). *Diagnostic and statistical manual of mental disorders* (4th ed., Text revision). Washington, DC: Author.

The Nature of Mental Health and Mental Illness

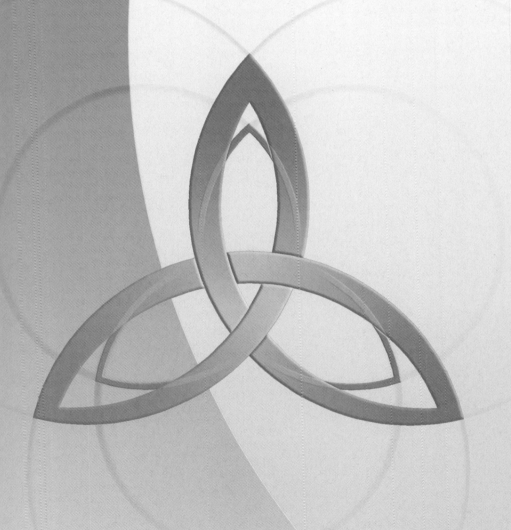

CHAPTER 1

Psychiatric and Mental Health Nursing From Past to Present

Geertje Boschma, Marlee Groening,
and Mary Ann Boyd

LEARNING OBJECTIVES

After studying this chapter, you will be able to:

- Identify historical influences and social changes that affect the delivery of mental health care.
- Relate the concept of social change to the history of psychiatric and mental health care.
- Discuss the history of psychiatric and mental health (PMH) nursing and its place within nursing history.
- Analyze the theoretical arguments that shaped the development of contemporary scientific thought about PMH nursing practice.
- Summarize the impact of current social, economic, and political forces on the delivery of mental health services.

KEY TERMS

- biologic view - deinstitutionalization - moral treatment - psychiatric hospitals - psychiatric and mental health nursing education - psychiatric pluralism - psychoanalytic movement - psychosocial theory

KEY CONCEPT

- social change

Until the 19th century, mentally ill people were kept mostly at home, cared for by their families. Sometimes, their legal guardians boarded them with other families for a fee, as part of a broader poor relief system. Only the most seriously afflicted people whose behaviour was severely disturbing or dangerous, to either themselves, their families, or other citizens, were locked in, often in prisons or a separate wing of a local poor house. Indigent mentally ill people were grouped with other old, sick, orphaned, or convicted people, and the circumstances in these scanty public facilities were most basic and often harsh. (Boschma, 2003; Shorter, 1997). For those who could afford it, privately maintained institutions emerged as well (McKenzie, 1992; Warsh, 1989).

EARLY FORMS OF INSTITUTIONAL CARE

As of the 1400s, the beginning of the Renaissance, some European towns established small-scale asylums as charitable enterprises, initially housing about 10 people. Most often they were civilian, charitable initiatives in which neither the church nor doctors were involved. Bedlam in London, Britain, founded in 1371, and the Reinier van Arkel asylum, founded in 1442, in the Dutch town of Den Bosch, are early examples of insane asylums or "mad houses" spreading throughout Europe, and, in the wake of colonialism, in other parts of the world over the next centuries. These asylums were managed as a large household, like other guest houses or poor houses, administered by a board of noted citizens, with a steward and matron, often a married couple, taking charge of the day-to-day management, assisted by a few servants. In the changing social and economic context of the 18th and 19th century, these homes grew into larger institutions (Boschma, 2003) (Fig. 1-1).

Religious orders, often under the protection or authority of the church, also involved themselves with charitable work and poor relief. Roman Catholic orders, for example, reemerged in 17th-century France during the Counter Reformation, and many of them managed the care in small-scale, premodern hospitals. Sometimes, the orders themselves owned the houses. Influential cases in point were the male order of the Congregation of Lazarists and the female congregation of the Sisters of Mercy (or Daughters of Charity), founded by Vincent the Paul in 1625 and 1633, respectively (Jones, 1989). These orders generated the early models for nursing work as a socially respectable endeavour at a time when medical care was hardly available nor developed (Nelson, 1999, 2001; Porter, 1993). In the Americas, one of the first institutions that took in mentally ill people was San Hipólito in Mexico City, which opened as a hospital for the insane in 1589, under the auspices of the Roman Catholic Church. It was run

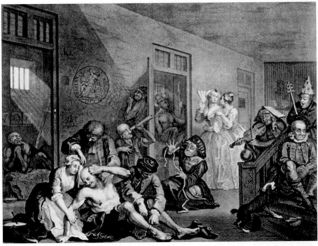

FIGURE 1.1   Interior of Bethlehem Asylum, London. (From U.S. National Library of Medicine. *Images from the history of medicine.* National Institutes of Health, Department of Health and Human Services.)

by the brothers of the order of La Caridad y San Hipólito, founded a few decades earlier in 1566. Living by the vows of poverty and charity, the brothers relied on alms to support themselves, and working as attendants in the institution was one of their activities (Leiby, 1992).

Diverse approaches to deal with mental illness or attempts to treat it have been employed throughout history and reflect the beliefs of the time. Spiritual, biologic, and social explanations commonly were intertwined in popular perceptions of causes of mental illness. Evil spirits, sin, demonic possession, contagious environments, or brain disturbances figured in explanations of mental disorders and shaped people's responses and medical treatments accordingly. The various ways of caring for mentally ill people typically depended on a community's perceived notions and fears of those with mental disorders as well as communities' resources.

History reflects that, generally, in periods of relative social stability, there are fewer fears and more tolerances for deviant behaviour, and it is easier for individuals with mental disorders to live safely within their communities. During periods of rapid **social change** and instability, there are more general anxieties and fears and, subsequently, more intolerances and ill treatments of people with mental disorders. As industrialization and urbanization increased during the 18th and 19th century, the rising middle class became concerned about a growing number of poor and deviant people who were not able to work and sustain themselves. Moreover, under the influence of the Enlightenment, medical and social ideas about mental illness changed during this time, and medical concern with the treatment of mental illness increased. Insight gained ground so that, rather than being afflicted by a loss of reason, the mentally ill were perceived as rational beings with a human nature just like all human beings. The idea that spirits or demons kept the insane in a bestial stage and, therefore, that restraints or enchainment seemed a reasonable approach, was rejected in favour of the view that mentally afflicted people should be treated humanely. Hence, the idea of a moral, pedagogical treatment emerged that would help these sufferers to restore their innate capacity for self-control (Boschma, 2003; Shorter, 1997; Tomes, 1994).

> ⬟ **KEY CONCEPT Social change,** the structural and cultural evolution of society, is constant and, at times, erratic. Psychiatric and mental health care has evolved within the social framework and cannot be separated from economic, sociocultural, and political realities.

IN A LIFE

Boarding Mentally Ill People With Families (12th– 19th Centuries)
The Geel Lunatic Colony, Belgium

The Legend of Saint Dymphna
According to the legend, Dymphna, an Irish princess, came to Geel in the 6th century. Disappointed that she was not a son, her father, king of Ireland, had left her and her mother in the care of a priest who converted them to Christianity. After Dymphna's mother died, the king became filled with grief and wanted another woman, just like his former wife. His advisors decided that only his own daughter could match the queen. However, when her pagan father wanted to marry Dymphna, she fled out of fear with her priest and came to Geel. When the Irish king eventually found Dymphna and the priest, he beheaded both. In some sources, the legend tells that several lunatics witnessing this frightful scene suddenly became cured. Symbolic for her resistance to the spirit of evil, Dymphna became patron of lunatics, and the site of her death, a place of miraculous healing. Some sources tell how the Saint Dymphna Guesthouse and chapel were built at this place, evolving into a place of pilgrimage.

A Powerful Example of Family Care in Geel, Belgium
Since the Middle Ages (1286), the Saint Dymphna Guesthouse and chapel have existed in Geel, Belgium, eventually with a separate sick room for lunatic pilgrims. Chronically mentally ill patients who came to the Guesthouse as pilgrims seeking healing were often boarded out to families, and the Geel Lunatic Colony came into being. In the 19th century, the place evolved into a formal institution with a strong emphasis on boarding out patients with foster families, which became a model for many countries to follow. The legend of Saint Dymphna illustrates mythical and religious beliefs, explanations, and practices that have lost their meaning today. However, the cultural heritage of the Geel Colony demonstrates how powerful

past ideas and beliefs can be in structuring creative and humane solutions to the care of mentally ill people.

From Parry-Jones, 1981; Boschma, 2003, pp.182–183, 277–278; and Goldstein & Godemont, 2003.

A REVOLUTIONARY IDEA: HUMANE TREATMENT

By the height of the French Revolution in 1792, **moral treatment** became a most influential idea, dramatically altering the care of the mentally ill and generating important reform initiatives in which reform-minded physicians had an influential role. It was during this time that Philippe Pinel (1745–1826) was appointed physician to Bicêtre, a hospital for men, which had a very poor reputation. Pinel, influenced by enlightened ideas, believed that the insane were sick patients who needed special treatment, and, once installed in his position, ordered the removal of the chains, stopped the abuses of drugging and bloodletting, and placed the patients under the care of more adequately prepared physicians. Three years later, the same standards were extended to Salpetrière, the asylum for female patients. At about the same time in England, William Tuke (1732–1822), a Quaker tea-merchant in York and a member of the Society of Friends, raised funds for a retreat for members of his Quaker community who had mental disorders. The York Retreat, which opened in 1796, became an evenly influential example for reform initiatives (Fig. 1-2). Tuke introduced a regimen of moral treatment, a humane, pedagogical approach of kind supervision, proper medical treatment, and meaningful distractions. Reform-minded physicians believed that such a purposefully designed asylum provided the

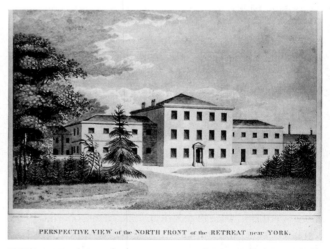

PERSPECTIVE VIEW of the NORTH FRONT of the RETREAT near YORK.

FIGURE 1.2   The perspective view of the north front of the retreat near York. (From U.S. National Library of Medicine. *Images from the history of medicine.* National Institutes of Health, Department of Health and Human Services.)

proper environment to indeed cure the mentally ill (D'Antonio, 2001; Shorter, 1997; Tomes, 1994).

Based on these influential examples, initiatives emerged throughout the Western world to establish purposefully designed asylums that provided sympathetic care in quiet, pleasant surroundings with some form of industrial occupation such as weaving or farming. In the United States, the Quaker Friends Asylum was proposed in 1811 and opened 6 years later in Frankford, Pennsylvania (now Philadelphia) to become the second asylum in the United States. The humane and supportive rehabilitative attitude of the Quakers was seen as an extremely important influence in changing techniques of caring for those with mental disorders (D'Antonio, 2001).

THE 19TH AND EARLY 20TH CENTURIES: AN ERA OF ASYLUM BUILDING

In Canada, New Brunswick was the first of the old British North American provinces to open a mental institution. In 1835, a committee was appointed to prepare a petition to the provincial legislature proposing the establishment of a provincial lunatic asylum. Until that time, counties had carried the responsibility under the Poor Laws system to confine indigent insane who could no longer be managed within the family, in local jails, or in poor houses. Yet, as the population rapidly increased in the early 1800s, the number of mentally ill in the need of publicly provided care grew. In 1835, the provincial government approved the conversion of a building in St. John, formerly a hospital for cholera patients a few years prior, in 1832, to a Provincial Lunatic Asylum until a new facility could be built. By 1848, this new facility was ready for use (Fig. 1-3) (Heritage Resources Saint John, 2000; Hurd, 1973/1916–17; Sussman, 1998).

The Legal Basis for Mental Health Care

Following the terms established by the British North America Act of 1867, the organization of mental health care became provincially based in Canada. In the late 19th century, all provinces passed legislation, most often called an Insanity Act, to provide a legal basis to publicly supported confinement of the mentally ill. All provinces, beginning with New Brunswick in 1835, established an asylum (Table 1-1). In the course of the 20th century, the legislation has been changed and updated several times and eventually renamed into a provincial Mental Health Act, reflecting changing views and a stronger medical influence on the care and treatment of the mentally ill. In the beginning of institutional psychiatric care in Canada, all patients admitted

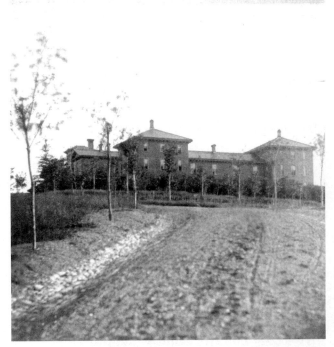

FIGURE 1.3   Canada's first hospital for the mentally ill, Saint John, New Brunswick, ca. 1885. (From Provincial Archives of New Brunswick, Saint John Stereographs—P86–67.)

to public institutions were certified patients. Today, patients are being admitted to an institutional facility on either a voluntary or a certified basis. A carefully designed legal process has to be followed for patients admitted as certified patients under the terms of a mental health act.

A Social Reformer: Dorothea Lynde Dix

An ardent advocate for establishing state-supported, public care of the mentally ill was Dorothea Lynde Dix (1802–1887). Responsible for much of the reform of the mental health care system in North America in the 19th century (Fig. 1-4), she extended her influence to the United States and Canadian state and provincial governments in her crusade for a more humane treatment of patients with mental illness. Almost 40 years of age, Dix, a retired school teacher living in Massachusetts, was solicited by a young theology student to help in preparing a Sunday School class for women inmates at the East Cambridge jail. Dix herself led the class and was shocked by the filth and dirt in the jail. She was particularly struck by the treatment of inmates with mental disorders. It was the dead of winter, and the jail provided no heat. When she questioned the jailer about the lack of heat, his answer was that "the insane need no heat." The prevailing myth was that the insane were insensible to extremes of temperature. Dix's outrage initiated a long struggle in the reform of care (Lightner, 1999).

Table 1.1	The First Asylums in British North America and Canada	
Province	**Date**	**Notes**
Quebec	1845	• Beauport, or the Quebec Lunatic Asylum, was opened.
		• A small dwelling for 12 mentally ill women was erected by Bishop St. Vallier.
	1714	• The Hotel Dieu cared for indigents, the crippled, and "idiots."
New Brunswick	1848	• The Provincial Lunatic Asylum was erected.
	1835	• Canada's first mental hospital opened in a small wooden building, a former cholera hospital, and was used as a temporary asylum.
Ontario	1850	• The Provincial Lunatic Asylum in Toronto admitted patients.
	1841	• Mentally ill people were placed in county jails until 1841 after which the Old York Jail served as a temporary asylum.
Newfoundland	1854	• An asylum for mentally ill patients was erected and admitted its first patients.
Nova Scotia	1857	• The first patients were admitted to the Provincial Hospital for the Insane.
British Columbia	1872	• A remodelled provincial general hospital (the old Royal Hospital) was opened as the Asylum for the Insane in British Columbia.
Prince Edward Island	1877	• The Prince Edward Island Hospital for the Insane was built.
Manitoba	1886	• The Selkirk Lunatic Asylum was opened.
Saskatchewan	1914	• The Saskatchewan Provincial Hospital admitted the first patients.
Alberta	1911	• The Provincial Asylum for the Insane opened in Ponoka.
Yukon and North West Territories		• These districts had no asylums in the early 20th century. The Royal North West Mounted Police assisted in transporting mentally ill patients to asylums in neighbouring provinces.

Adapted from Sussman, 1998; and Hurd, 1973/1916–17.

Influenced by a wider social reform movement that had a strong cultural influence throughout the Western world, drawing men and women into a wide range of reform activities, Dix disregarded the New England role of a Puritan woman and diligently investigated the conditions of jails and the plight of the mentally ill. She followed patterns of new women's activism, also employed by social reformers such as Elizabeth Fry in prison reform and Josephine Butler in protecting women against prostitution (Van Drenth & De Haan,

1999). Dix's solution to the quandary of the mentally ill was the building of more state hospitals. She first influenced the Massachusetts legislature to expand the Massachusetts State Hospital. Then, through public awareness campaigns and lobbying efforts, she managed to persuade state after state to build hospitals. She also turned her attention to the plight of the mentally ill in Canada, where she was instrumental in advocating for mental institutions in Halifax, Nova Scotia, and St. John, Newfoundland (Hurd, 1973/1916–17; Lightner, 1999). Eventually, Dix expanded her work into Great Britain and other parts of Europe. During the Civil War, she was appointed Superintendent of Women Nurses, the highest position held by a woman during the war.

Life Within Early Institutions

Despite the good intentions of early reformers, the approach inside the institution was one of custodial care and practical management, and treatment hardly occurred. The major concern was the management of a large number of people, often with disruptive behaviours. Patient numbers rapidly grew from the time provinces became legally responsible for financing care of the mentally ill. Soon, institutions experienced severe overcrowding and had little more than food, clothing, pleasant surroundings, and perhaps some means of employment and exercise to offer. Although a medical superintendent usually directed the institutions,

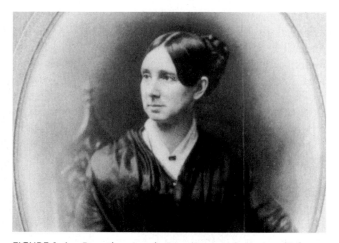

FIGURE 1.4   Dorothea Lynde Dix. (From U.S. National Library of Medicine. *Images from the history of medicine.* National Institutes of Health, Department of Health and Human Services.)

management of such large numbers of patients with limited resources made life in the institutions difficult. Overcrowded wards and few resources created rowdy, dangerous, and unbearable situations. Quiet patients were involved in work as institutions grew into self-contained communities that produced their own food and made their own clothing. Day-to-day care was in the hands of lay personnel who shared with the patients the same routines of eating, sleeping, and working. Once admitted, many patients had little hope of re-entering society.

Ontario psychiatrist Charles K. Clarke (1857–1924) had an influential role in bringing about new models of care that would influence change of this situation. As superintendent of various Ontario provincial psychiatric hospitals, he was aware of the enormous problems that asylums experienced. He continuously brought improvement to the asylums that he directed, including the introduction of nurse training for asylum personnel. To find better treatments and approaches, he sought to start an urban centre for the treatment of acute mental illness under the best possible conditions and supported by university-based scientific research. Eventually, his dream came through in the establishment of the Toronto Psychiatric Hospital (TPH), which opened in 1925. Clarke's name was commemorated in Toronto's Clarke Institute of Psychiatry, the 1966 successor of TPH (Greenland, 1996).

Soon, wider public commotion arose over the deplorable state of large mental institutions. In 1908, Clifford Beers (1876–1943) published an autobiography, *A Mind That Found Itself*, depicting his 3-year experience in three different types of hospitals: a private for-profit hospital, a private nonprofit hospital, and a state institution. In all these facilities, he reported that he was beaten, choked, imprisoned for long periods in dark, dank, padded cells, and confined for many days in a straight jacket. At the end of his book, he recommended that a national society be established for the purpose of reforming care and treatment, disseminating information, and encouraging and conducting research. Beers' cause was supported by a prominent neuropathologist, Adolf Meyer (1866–1950), who suggested the term "mental hygiene" for bringing about improvement of people's mental health similar to public health initiatives. By 1909, Beers formed a National Committee for Mental Hygiene. Through the committee's efforts, child guidance clinics, prison clinics, and industrial mental health approaches were developed. In Canada, Beers and Meyer found a close ally in Clarence Hincks, a leading Toronto psychiatrist, who was instrumental in founding the Canadian National Committee for Mental Hygiene (CNCMH) in 1918, together with his colleague Charles Clarke.

The appalling situation of Canadian provincial mental hospitals triggered particular political concern when returning veterans suffering from shell shock had to rely on existing psychiatric facilities in their home provinces. The new CNCMH obtained an instrumental role in asylum inspection. The broader goal of the committee was not only to improve existing facilities, but also to prevent mental illness. A new belief in scientific approaches and reliance on expert knowledge in the prevention of mental illness and so-called weak-mindedness gained ground. These views were intertwined with class-based concern about the alleged excessive growth of the weak-minded and betterment of the human race, influenced by eugenic ideas of the time. This context of change provided a climate for expanding professionalism of many professional groups, including psychiatrists, psychologists, and nurses. The CNCMH clearly promoted the transformation of asylums in mental hospitals, and introducing a trained nursing staff was part of its strategy. The CNCMH strongly promoted voluntary admission controlled by physicians, thus supporting the view that mental illness was similar to any physical illness. In its many surveys of institutional facilities, the CNCMH recommended the enhancement of asylum personnel and suggested the introduction of training schools for mental nurses, later called psychiatric nurses, similar to nurse training schools in general hospitals (Boschma, Yonge, & Mychajlunow, 2005; MacLennan, 1987).

Development of Psychiatric and Mental Health Nursing

Early Developments

One of the first initiatives to implement nurse training in Ontario mental hospitals came from Charles K. Clarke, superintendent of Rockwood Hospital (1881–1905) and later of the Provincial Hospital in Toronto (Brown, 2000). In both mental hospitals, he established a Training School for Nurses, open to female nurses. The promise of hospital reform brought about by the sense for order and compassion of well-educated women had been essential in the introduction of training schools in general hospitals. In their efforts to model psychiatric asylums after the general hospitals, psychiatrists took that ideal and geared the training of mental nurses toward women, thus creating a gendered hierarchical structure that would bring them assistance as well as the outlook of a hospital (Brown, 2000; Connor, 1996). It was thought that women had the right moral, feminine characteristics for good patient care. Whereas in general hospitals early on, the care of male patients was put in the hands of female nurses assisted by male orderlies, in psychiatry, this shift was less easily made, owing to the nature of difficult patient behaviour. Male attendants retained a prominent place in the care of the mentally ill, but their training obtained a lower status, or, in the Ontario mental hospitals, they initially did not receive any training at all (Tipliski, 2002). See Box 1-1 for historical highlights.

Highlights From Psychiatric and Mental Health Nursing History

1888   The first mental nurse training school established at Kingston's Rockwood Asylum

1918   Foundation of the Canadian National Committee of Mental Hygiene

1920   First psychiatric nursing text published, *Nursing Mental Disease,* by Harriet Bailey

1922   First Registration of Nurses Act passed in Ontario including nurse training schools at the mental hospitals

1930s Mental hospitals in western Canada established schools for mental nurses and attendants

1950   Psychiatric Nurses Association of Canada (PNAC) founded

1952   Publication of Hildegard E. Peplau's *Interpersonal Relations in Nursing*

1963   *Perspectives in Psychiatric Care* and *Journal of Psychiatric Nursing* published

1979   PNAC *Working paper on Standards of Practice for Psychiatric Nurses* published

1986   The Canadian Nurses Association establishes a national certification program for specialty nursing practice

1988   Canadian Federation of Mental Health Nurses (CFMHN) founded

1995   CFMHN *Standards of Psychiatric and Mental Health Nursing Practice* published

Regional Influences

In western Canada, which had a stronger orientation to British traditions of institutional care, the introduction of mental nurse training also followed the Training School model, yet had a slightly different pattern, in the sense that men were trained as well. In Alberta, for example, in 1932, the Alberta Department of Health hired psychiatrist Charles A. Barager, initially as acting superintendent and soon as commissioner of mental health service, to implement reform. Barager came from Manitoba, where he had introduced a nurse training school as superintendent at the Brandon Asylum. He had a strong belief in the ability of female compassion: "The nursing of mental patients requires women of finer personality, of wider sympathies, greater self-control and higher intelligence than even the nursing of those who are physically ill" (Boschma et al., 2005; Dooley, 2004; Tipliski, 2002, p. 95).

Barager's term in Alberta was short-lived; he died suddenly in 1936. However, the training for nurses and attendants that he initiated in the Alberta Hospital at Ponoka had a lasting influence. Despite opposition to his ideas from the Registered Nurses Association in Alberta, which had controlled registration of nurses since 1916, he was able to secure approval for a new diploma in mental nursing through the Alberta Department of Health. Creatively, he established arrange-

ments with general hospitals in the province, so that, after 2 years of training in the mental hospital, female nurse students could undertake an additional 18 months of training to the general hospital and take licensing exams for registered nurses, after which they would return to the mental hospital. For male attendants, a 3-year certificate course was implemented, leading to a diploma in mental nursing. Male graduates did not obtain registered nursing status, reflective of the gendered context in which mental nurse training emerged. Skilled nursing was essential for new therapies, such as electroshock and insulin coma therapy introduced in the 1930s and 1940s. Alberta Hospital at Ponoka, for example, had a large infirmary with many frail and sick patients (Boschma et al., 2005).

This climate of change created many new opportunities for working and middle-class women to pursue a career as psychiatric nurses, and nursing thought continued to develop. The first PMH nursing textbook that appeared in North America, *Nursing Mental Disease*, was written by Harriet Bailey in 1920. The content of the book reflected an understanding of mental disorders of the times and set forth nursing care in terms of appropriate procedures.

MODERN THINKING

Evolution of Scientific Thought

As PMH nursing began to develop as a profession in the early part of the 20th century, modern perspectives on mental illness were emerging. These new theories would profoundly shape the future of mental health care for all practitioners. Chapter 7 examines the underlying ideologies, but it is important to understand their development within the social and historical context to appreciate fully their impact on treatment approaches.

In the early 1900s, two opposing views were held regarding mental illnesses: the belief that mental disorders had biologic origins and the belief that the problems were attributed to environmental and social stresses. **Psychosocially oriented ideas** proposed that mental disorders resulted from environmental and social deprivation. Moral treatment grew out of this idea, and the notion of prevention advocated by the mental hygiene movement also reflected a psychosocial orientation. The **biologic view** held that mental illnesses had a biologic cause and could be treated with physical interventions. However, biologic approaches and physical treatments such as bed rest; wet packs, which entailed wrapping patients in wet sheets; and prolonged baths became popular as new treatments around 1900 as part of the rise of scientific psychiatry. They were grounded in the idea that overstrained nerves should obtain rest. This turned out to be largely ineffective.

Meyer and Psychiatric Pluralism

Adolf Meyer attempted to bridge the ideologic gap between the two approaches by introducing the concept of **psychiatric pluralism**, an integration of human biologic functions with the environment. His approach focussed on investigating how the organs related to the person and how the person, constituted of these organs, related to the environment (Neill, 1980). However, the ideas that Meyer promoted had little chance to flourish as the emerging psychoanalytic theories soon dominated the psychiatric world in North America for a long time to come.

Freud and the Psychoanalytic Theory

Sigmund Freud (1856–1939) and the **psychoanalytic movement** of the early 1900s promised a radically new approach to PMH care. Freud, trained as a neuropathologist, developed a personality theory based on unconscious motivations for behaviour, or drives. Using a new technique, psychoanalysis, he delved into the patient's feelings and emotions regarding past experiences, particularly early childhood and adolescent memories, to explain the basis of aberrant behaviour. He showed that symptoms of hysteria could be produced and made to disappear while patients were in a subconscious state of hypnosis.

As psychoanalytic theory gained in popularity, ideas of the mind–body relationship were lost. According to the Freudian model, normal development occurred in stages, with the first three—oral, anal, and genital—being the most important. The infant progressed through the oral stage, experiencing the world through symbolic oral ingestion; into the anal stage, in which the toddler developed a sense of autonomy through withholding; and on to the genital stage, in which a beginning sense of sexuality emerged within the framework of the Oedipal relationship. If there was any interference in normal development, such as psychological trauma, psychosis or neurosis would develop.

Primary causes of mental illnesses were now viewed as psychological, and any physical manifestations or social influences were considered secondary (Malamud, 1944). The psychiatric community generally believed that mental illnesses were a result of disturbed personality development and faulty parenting. Mental illnesses were categorized either as a psychosis (severe) or neurosis (less severe). A psychosis impaired daily functioning because of breaks in contact with reality. A neurosis was less severe, but individuals were often distressed about their problems. The terms *psychosis* and *neurosis* entered common, everyday language and added credibility to Freud's conceptualization of mental disorders. Soon, Freud's ideas represented the forefront of psychiatric thought and began to shape society's view of mental health care. Freudian ideology dominated psychiatric thought well into the 1970s.

Intensive psychoanalysis, which focussed on repairing the trauma of the original psychological injury, was the treatment of choice. Psychoanalysis was costly and time-consuming and required lengthy training. Few could perform it. Thus, thousands of patients in state institutions with severe mental illnesses were essentially ignored.

Integration of Biologic Theories into Psychosocial Treatment

Until the 1940s, the biologic understanding of mental illness was unsophisticated and misguided. Biologic treatments during this century often were unsuccessful because of the lack of understanding and knowledge of the biologic basis of mental disorders. For example, the use of hydrotherapy, or baths, was an established procedure in mental institutions. The use of warm baths and, in some instances, ice cold baths were thought to produce calming effects for patients with mental disorders. However, the treatment's success was ascribed to its effectiveness as a form of restraint because the physiologic responses that hydrotherapy produced were not understood. Baths were applied indiscriminately and used as a form of restraint, rather than as a therapeutic practice. Other examples of biologic procedures applied either indiscriminately or inappropriately included psychosurgery and electroconvulsive therapy (see Chapters 13 and 20). Thanks to modern technology, neurosurgical techniques and electroconvulsive therapy can now be applied more humanely with positive therapeutic outcomes for some psychiatric disorders.

Support for the biologic approaches received an important boost as successful symptom management with psychopharmacologic agents became a more widespread possibility in the early 1950s. Psychopharmacology revolutionized the treatment of mental illness and led to an increased number of patients discharged into the community, and the eventual focus on the brain became a key to understanding psychiatric disorders.

Chlorpromazine was an early neuroleptic drug that became widely used. Profound behavioural changes, observed as a result of this medication in long-term mentally ill patients, created an enormous enthusiasm about the potential of new medications. However, the knowledge about the working of the drugs was in infancy, and side effects of the new medications soon became serious drawbacks. As knowledge increased, and the management of side effects improved, psychopharmacotherapeutics obtained a central place in the treatment of mental illness. The introduction of lithium in the early 1970s brought a lasting change in the treatment of bipolar disorder, as did antidepressants in the treatment of mood disorders (LaJeunesse, 2000).

Nurses obtained an essential role in administering medication, in monitoring its effect, and in teaching clients about their working.

New Trends in Post–World War II Mental Health Care

Following the experiences of World War II, insight grew among governments, as well as health professionals, that psychiatric services had to be placed on a new footing. By the end of the 1940s, patients in overcrowded, isolated psychiatric hospitals outnumbered the number of patients in other health care facilities, including general hospitals. Increased federal funding for health services and training of health care personnel created new opportunities. The implementation of universal health insurance for hospital care and medical services during the 1950s and 1960s, based on a 50%/50% cost-sharing between federal and provincial governments, generated funding for the establishment of psychiatric departments in general hospitals, shifting the focus of services away from large provincial institutions. The Canadian Mental Health Association (CMHA), renamed from the earlier CNCMH, had an instrumental role in policy development for integrated services in general hospitals and the community. In its influential 1963 report, *More for the Mind*, the CMHA argued that mental illness had to be dealt with in similar ways to physical illness, and it argued for the application of multiple perspectives—medical, social, and familial—in multidisciplinary services and community treatment. A shift in mental health policy resulted in deinstitutionalization, the downsizing of the large provincial psychiatric hospitals, and a new orientation on community-based services. Biologic approaches such as use of psychopharmacology and safer application of electroconvulsive therapy were complemented by new rehabilitative services, the use of group therapy and other psychotherapies, as well as the provision of day treatment (Greenland et al., 2001; Shorter, 1997).

Because of these policies and trends, Canadian developments in psychiatric care differed substantially from post–World War II changes in the United States, where after the passage of the 1946 National Mental Health Act and the subsequent 1963 Mental Retardation Facilities and Community Mental Health Centres Construction Act, the emphasis was placed on newly built community mental health centres. In Canada, funding for mental health care became part of the larger health care system, with a strong emphasis on general hospital-based psychiatric care. Although the services in the new general hospital units improved treatment opportunities, the needs of the former provincial hospital population were not always adequately met, and it became apparent that problems created by persistent and severe mental illness were not resolved (Hector, 2001; Shorter 1997).

In the late 1970s, the federal government shifted to a new funding structure for health care, reducing its share in the cost. Provinces developed different models and strategies to fund specialized services, for example, alcohol and substance abuse treatment programs, a pressing post–World War II mental health care need. To address the needs of different population groups, subspecialties such as child psychiatry, forensic, and geriatric services also emerged. The perception of health care as a right enhanced consumer and volunteer involvement, as well as public education on mental illness, and it increased the demand for patient autonomy. The 1981 Charter of Rights and Freedoms was a reflection of this social change (Greenland et al., 2001).

Continued Evolution of Psychiatric and Mental Health Nursing

The new multidisciplinary services generated an enormous need for more and better trained mental health care personnel, including nurses. The changes created a context for new developments in PMH nursing education. Organized responses of provincial professional nurses organizations, as well as efforts of hospital administrators and psychiatrists, who traditionally had a central role in hospital-based nurse training programs to staff the psychiatric hospitals and new health care facilities, resulted in a diverse pattern of psychiatric and mental health nurse education. As of the 1950s, Canada entertained two models of education for PMH nursing, resulting in the preparation of two different professional nursing groups for nursing care in mental health services. Regional influences played a large role in the generation of the two models. On the one hand, general hospital-based schools of nursing, especially in eastern Canada, began to integrate psychiatric nursing into their curriculum. In Ontario, for example, under the influence of the mental hygiene movement, as of the 1930s, general hospital training schools began to include care of mentally ill patients into their training. Student nurses attended the provincial psychiatric hospitals for a brief period of training, called an *affiliation program*. Conversely, mental nurse trainees, mostly women, from the psychiatric hospital-based nurse training programs opted for an affiliation to the general hospital, resulting in both groups' obtaining the title of registered nurse. After World War II, the provincial government and the provincial association of registered nurses in Ontario formalized this pattern into a permanent structure. Gradually, the psychiatric hospital-based programs decreased in number and size, and the registered nurse became the main nursing care provider in mental health services (Tipliski, 2004).

In the less densely populated western Canadian provinces, the pattern that general hospital nurse trainees chose affiliation experiences at the psychiatric

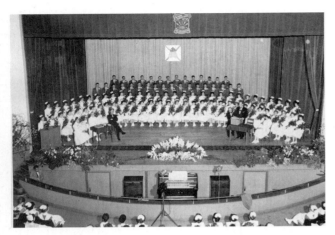

FIGURE 1.5 Graduation ceremony, School of Psychiatric Nursing, Essondale (Riverview Hospital), ca. 1950s. (From Historical collection, Riverview Hospital Historical Society, Coquitlam, B.C.)

hospitals also emerged, but the bulk of nursing care in the provincial hospitals continued to be provided by nurses and attendants graduated from psychiatric hospital-based training programs. As noted previously, some western provinces, such as Alberta Hospital in Ponoka, established an affiliation program for female mental nurse trainees, and its graduates obtained the title of registered nurse. Yet, the program was limited in size, and many women worked in the institution as untrained attendants until the 1960s. Male trainees received a diploma in mental nursing. In British Columbia a training school for mental nurses, later called psychiatric nurses, was established in 1930 at Essondale, which eventually became Riverview Hospital (Fig. 1-5). In the western provinces, the government had less control over nurse training than in neighbouring Ontario. Provincial associations of registered nurses in western provinces failed to support affiliation for psychiatric hospital-based nurse trainees, while medical superintendents of psychiatric hospitals retained much of their influence over psychiatric nurse education (Boschma et al., 2005; Tipliski, 2004).

In the late 1940s, attendants in the province of Saskatchewan took the lead in obtaining political support for a different pattern of nurse education that would lead to a separate Psychiatric Nurses Act and subsequent training acts, independent of provincial registered nurse practice acts. Their action resulted in a distinct professional group of psychiatric nurses. During the 1950s, all four western Canadian provinces passed such acts, which entitled graduates of psychiatric hospital-based nurse training programs in the West to receive the title of psychiatric nurse. In Saskatchewan, registered nurses had never successfully integrated into the mental hospitals. The very dominant medical superintendent, James Mac-Neill, who held sway over North Battleford hospital until the 1940s, strongly believed that general hospital training had little relevance for mental hospitals. In the 1930s, a

psychiatric training program emerged for Saskatchewan asylum attendants, which was expanded after World War II to address the new need for psychiatric expertise, but it never resulted in registration as a nurse. Dissatisfied with their exclusion from any professionally recognized nursing title, provincial hospital attendants, who in Saskatchewan had obtained the right to unionize after the election of the new Co-operative Commonwealth Federation government in 1944, became instrumental in generating union support, as well as backing from the new government, for legislation of a separate psychiatric nurses act, which passed Parliament in 1948. Soon, the other western provinces followed suit, and in 1950, the Psychiatric Nurses Association of Canada was formed (Dickinson, 1989; Tipliski, 2002, 2004). The two separate models of psychiatric nursing education exist until today and have been integrated into the regular education system over the past decades.

THE LATE 20TH CENTURY

In the post–World War II era, nurses continued their central role in facilitating the therapeutic climate within psychiatric hospitals (Fig. 1-6). The community mental health movement and deinstitutionalization advocated with much enthusiasm during the 1960s and 1970s generated many new functions for psychiatric and mental health nurses (Boschma et al., 2005; Church, 1987). Nurses became involved in preparing and guiding persons with chronic, yet stabilized mental illness for discharge and living into the community. In the psychiatric hospitals and general hospital units, nurses obtained new therapeutic roles in group therapies, and their work in community mental health services expanded. New theoretical models became available that emphasized building therapeutic nurse–patient relationships and holistic nursing approaches. Hildegard Peplau, in recent scholarship recognized as "Psychiatric Nurse of

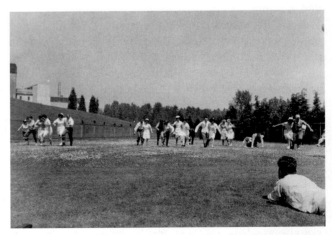

FIGURE 1.6 Sports Day on Riverview Hospital grounds, nurses and patients, 1966. (From Historical collection, Riverview Hospital Historical Society, Coquitlam, B.C.)

the Century," proved to be a strong leader in the field (Boschma et al., in press; Calaway, 2002).

Expansion of Holistic Nursing Care

In 1952, Peplau published the landmark work, *Interpersonal Relations in Nursing*. It introduced psychiatric and mental health nursing practice to the concepts of interpersonal relations and the importance of the therapeutic relationship. In fact, the nurse–patient relationship was defined as the very essence of psychiatric and mental health nursing and supported a holistic perspective on patient care (see Chapters 6 and 8). Peplau's view was also important in its conceptualization of nursing care as truly independent of physicians. The nurse's use of self as a nursing tool was outside the dominance of both hospital administrators and physicians.

By 1963, two U.S.-based nursing journals, the *Journal of Psychiatric Nursing* (now the *Journal of Psychosocial Nursing and Mental Health Services*) and *Perspectives in Psychiatric Care*, focussed on psychiatric nursing. Also, the *Canadian Journal for Nursing Research* began to publish psychiatric and mental health nursing research. During the 1980s, the Canadian Federation of Mental Health Nurses (CFMHN) formed as an interest group of the Canadian Nurses Association with the view to promote the interests of mental health nurses and to bring matters of mental health nursing interest and psychiatric patient care to the attention of the public at large. In 1995, this group published the *Canadian Standards of Psychiatric and Mental Health Nursing Practice*. Based on the influential work of Patricia Benner (1984), the standards were written within a "domains of practice" framework. It promoted a holistic perspective on nursing care, with psychiatric and mental health nurses practicing in a variety of settings with a variety of clientele. The emphasis was on activities ranging from health promotion to health restoration. The standards reflected the belief that psychiatric and mental health nursing should be research driven, continually incorporating new findings into nursing practice. Relying on these standards, the Canadian Nurses Association created the opportunity to become certified in mental health nursing as part of their larger certification program of specialty nursing areas established during the 1980s. Currently, the CFMHN is in the process of revising and incorporating the most recent perspectives on psychiatric care into the standards (Canadian Federation of Mental Health Nurses, 1995).

Contemporary Issues

During the 1980s, wrinkles in the social fabric of mental health care emerged. The mixed results of deinstitutionalization became apparent and generated a series of government-commissioned reports in all provinces to improve mental health services. Enormous variation existed among provinces in the extent and timing in which they implemented deinstitutionalization policies. People with mental disorders were discharged into communities that were often ill prepared to offer sufficient support in the way of community support programs, housing, or vocational opportunities. These communities were also sometimes hesitant in accepting people with persistent mental illness in their midst, and stigma remained attached to mental health services (Hector, 2001; Sealy & Whitehead, 2004).

Self-help groups and family and consumer organizations, such as the Schizophrenia Society of Canada and the Mood Disorder Society of Canada, have become active participants in mental health care services during the past decades. Outreach and mobile crisis response teams emerged to address problems created by severe mental illness in the community. A new category of "revolving door" patients signified that long-term, severe mental illness remained a persistent problem, with patients continuously moving in and out of the acute care system. Also, the interconnected issues of severe mental illness, substance dependency, and inadequate community resources and housing have resulted in a growing number of homeless people with mental illness, as well as a large population of mentally ill winding up in the criminal justice systems. Within these groups, the specific mental health needs of women remain poorly addressed. Moreover, there exists a growing awareness that diverse cultural populations have distinctive mental health needs. Aboriginal mental health is a pressing issue in Canada because Aboriginal communities experience disproportionate rates of both physical and mental illness due to an unbalanced health care system that has not been adaptive to the specific health needs of Aboriginal peoples.

Today mental health services are still inadequate and fragmented. Millions of adults and children are disabled by mental illness every year. When compared with all other diseases, mental illness ranks first in terms of causing disability in North America and Western Europe (Greenland et al, 2001; Hart Wasakeesikaw, 2006; Hector, 2001; Morrow, 2002; World Health Organization [WHO], 2001).

The New Era of Health Care Reform

Both public and private expenditures for health care services have increased in North America. Financial and social barriers continue to affect the overall funding for mental health. Now, large networks of public and private organizations share responsibility for mental health care, with the state remaining as the major decision maker for resource allocation. Emphasis is on reducing expensive institutional care and increasing the resources devoted to community-based care for the mentally ill, such as those in clinics, homes, schools, and treatment centres. With so many organizations involved in mental health services,

BOX 1.2

The CAMIMH Presents Four Sets of Goals in "A Call for Action: Building Consensus for a National Action Plan on Mental Illness and Mental Health" (2002)

Set 1 Public education and awareness
Set 2 Development of a national policy framework
Set 3 Generating a national research agenda with input from new researchers, consumers, and other stakeholders and their organizations
Set 4 Creating a national data/information system to more carefully monitor mental illness

From Health Canada (2002). *A report on mental illnesses in Canada* (appendix B). Ottawa: Author.

the voice of mental health care has become fragmented. It became clear during the 1990s that new federal initiatives in mental health policy were urgently needed. In 1998 the Canadian Alliance on Mental Illness and Mental Health (CAMIMH) was formed as a conjoint initiative of the Canadian Psychiatric Association, the Canadian Mental Health Association, the Mood Disorder Association of Canada, the National Network for Mental Health, and the Schizophrenia Society of Canada. Jointly, consumers and service providers began to lobby the federal government to come to an action plan and a new national agenda for mental health care (Beauséjour, 2001). Two years later, the CAMIMH presented its framework for action (Box 1-2).

In 2002, the CAMIMH published its first report, a collation of the latest Canadian data on mental illness, with assistance from Health Canada. The report revealed that currently 86% of hospitalizations for mental illness in Canada occur in general hospitals. Twenty percent of Canadians will personally experience mental illness over their lifetime. Approximately 8% of adults will experience major depression. Bipolar disorder and schizophrenia each affect 1% of the Canadian population. The hospitalization rates in general hospitals of anxiety disorders, affecting 12% of the population, are twice as high among women as men. Suicide accounts for 24% of all deaths among 15- to 24-year-olds and for 16% among 25- to 44-year-olds. Although the report also found that mental illness can be treated more effectively, the data clearly reveal the need for continued, integrated mental health policy development (Health Canada, 2002). In 2001, the World Health Organization focussed its annual *World Health Report* on mental health, also emphasizing the importance of mental health to the well-being of individuals (WHO, 2001)

National Mental Health Objectives

In 2003, seeking to address the significant and universal service gaps identified in the mental health care system,

the Senate Standing Committee on Social Affairs, Science and Technology, with Senator Michael Kirby as a chairperson, began a national review of the Canadian mental health system. In 2004, the review has published three of the expected four reports (Kirby, 2004). The first report detailed the personal stories of individuals and families afflicted by mental illness, which highlighted the fragmented mental health and addiction services. The second report drew attention to Canada's lack of a national mental health strategy through the examination and comparison of the mental health services of four G8 countries (New Zealand, Australia, England, and the United States). The third report summarized and set options for mental health and addiction services in Canada (Box 1-3). The fourth report with recommendations appeared in the fall of 2005 (Kirby, 2005b).

Woven throughout the first three reports, the complex issue of stigmatization and discrimination is clearly apparent for those individuals and families suffering from mental illness, as well as for the health care professionals working in the field. Stigmatization and discrimination of the mentally ill still have far-reaching social and economic effects for Canadians related to housing, employment, social welfare, and the justice system, Kirby noted. He found this exemplified by the "national health policy in Canada, the *Canada Health Act* (CHA), [which] explicitly excludes coverage for treatment in psychiatric hospitals" (Kirby, 2005a, p. 9).

The Kirby report also highlights disparities in access to care between urban and rural Canada, which are further complicated by unique regional multicultural needs. Much of this regional discrepancy is blamed on the lack of a nationwide mental health strategy and the inconsistent provincial jurisdictions that determine mental health policies and resource allocation of service and delivery (Kirby, 2004).

The report has not been received without its critics. Some of these are related to being "prevalence focused," with not enough emphasis on "preventative determinants," as well as the lack of recognition of the depth of disability caused by mental illness (Arboleda-Flórez, 2005). Overall, however, the report has been well received by mental health care consumers and caregivers. The fourth and final "recommendation" report addresses many options for mental health care reform. To that end the report recommends a national (not federal) initiative in the form of a Canadian mental health commission that will direct policy on mental health and addiction services across Canada. The goals of this initiative are to provide leadership, minimize fragmentation of mental health services, and develop research and strategies around best practices in order to achieve equitable physical and mental health care in Canada (Kirby, 2005b).

The challenge before nurses is to strive to address these findings while working within the constraints to provide cost-effective services. To address the pressing

BOX 1.3

Issues and Options for Canadian Mental Health Care: Kirby Report 3, November 2004

Delivery of Services and Supports

- A patient/client-centred system oriented toward recovery and with personalized care plans; culturally appropriate delivery of services and supports; system coordination and integration with strong focus on community-based delivery; early detection and intervention; enhancing access

Specific Population Groups

- Children and adolescents; Aboriginal peoples; seniors; individuals with complex needs

The Workplace

- Employers; workers' compensation boards; federal income security programs; the federal government as an employer

Specific Issues

- Combating stigma and discrimination; suicide prevention

Human Resources

- Supply of mental health and addiction human resources; primary health care sector; community support workers and police officers; support caregivers

National Informational Database, Research and Technology

- Canadian community health survey; national information database; research; information and communications technology; privacy

The Role of the Federal Government

- Direct and indirect role; intergovernmental collaboration; national Action plan

Financing Reform and Fostering Performance and Accountability

- Level of funding; dedicated funding; performance and accountability

mental health care needs in the 21st century, nurses must continue to participate in devising and implementing a continuum of mental health services that provides access for all and to develop appropriate partnerships with other health professionals and consumer groups.

SUMMARY OF KEY POINTS

- Throughout history, attitudes and treatment toward those with mental disorders have drastically changed as a result of the changing socioeconomic backdrop of our society and the development of new theories and study by key individuals and groups.
- During the 1800s, as mental illness began to be viewed as an illness, more humane and moral treatments began to develop.
- Social reformers, such as Dorothea Dix, C. K. Clarke, Clifford Beers, and C. Hincks, dedicated their efforts to raising society's awareness and to advocating public responsibility for proper treatment of persons with mental illness.
- Theoretic arguments characterized the evolution of scientific thought and psychiatric practice. Gradually, the importance of the biologic aspect of mental disorders has been recognized while psychosocial approaches were also developed.
- Although the need for PMH nursing was recognized near the end of the 19th century, initially there was resistance to training attendants for the care of the insane. At the initiative of C. K. Clarke, medical superintendent of Rockwood Hospital (1881–1905), the first Training School for Mental Nurses was established in 1888.
- Gradually, all provinces adapted to education for PMH nurses. By the 1930s, all provinces had estab-

lished training schools for asylum attendants and nurses. In the post–World War II era, two models of education for psychiatric nurses emerged, leading to two distinct professional groups.

- Through key federal and state legislative initiatives, mental health services were funded, but remain inadequate in meeting the needs.
- Recent reports, such as Health Canada's *A Report on Mental Illnesses in Canada*, 2002 and the 2004 Kirby report highlight the continued need for resource planning and mental health policy specifically devoted to the care of persons with mental illness and their families.

CRITICAL THINKING CHALLENGES

1 Compare the ideas of psychiatric care during the 1800s with those of the 1990s and 2000s and identify some major political and economic forces that influenced care.

2 Analyze the social, political, and economic changes that influenced the transition to community mental health.

3 Explain how training and education of nurses became essential in psychiatric care.

4 Present an argument for the moral treatment of people with mental disorders.

5 Trace the history of biologic psychiatry and highlight major ideas and treatments.

WEB LINKS

www.saintjohn.nbcc.nb.ca/Heritage/LunaticAsylum/index.htm   This website provides interesting historical information about Canada's first asylum for the mentally ill. The website also includes a personal account of a staff member who worked in the asylum in the 20th century and a story about a day in the life of a patient.

www.cpa-apc.org/Publications/Position Papers /Position Papers.asp This is the website of the Canadian Psychiatric Association and houses clinical practice guidelines and position papers.

www.phac-aspc.gc.ca/mh-sm/mentalhalth/index. html This mental health website at the Public Health Agency of Canada has information on mental disorders and mental health promotion. The website also includes links.

www.hc-sc.gc.ca/ahc-asc/pubs/drugs-drouges/ mental-mentale discussion/index e.html This government site outlines the history of substance abuse and makes recommendations regarding the management of substance abuse issues.

www.parl.gc.ca/37/2/parlbus/commbus/senate/com -e/ soci-e/rep-e/repoct02vol6-e.htm This website has the Kirby report (2002).

www.mentalhealth.com This website has information on disorders and diagnoses and provides links to other sites.

www.cna-nurses.ca/CNA/documents/pdf/ publications The website of the Canadian Nurses Association offers a listing of CNA publications, including the 1992 report on mental health care reform.

www.cfmhn.org This is the website of the Canadian Federation of Mental Health Nurses.

www.cmha.com The website of the Canadian Mental Health Association has information on mental health and resources.

www.samhsa.gov/oas/oasftp.htm This Substance Abuse and Mental Health Statistics website provides national statistics on alcohol, tobacco, and illegal drug use, substance abuse treatment, and mental health.

www.who.org The website of the World Health Organization has information on mental health disability and programs.

MOVIES

One Flew Over the Cuckoo's Nest: 1975. This classic film, starring Jack Nicholson as Randle P. McMurphy, who challenges the state hospital establishment, won all five of the top Academy Awards: Best Picture, Best Actor, Best Actress, Best Director, and Best Adapted Screenplay. The film depicts life in an inpatient psychiatric ward of the late 1960s and offers increased public awareness of the potential human rights violations inherent in a large, public mental system. However, the portrayal of electroconvulsive therapy is stereotyped and inaccurate, and the suicide of Billy appears to be linked simplistically to his domineering mother. You might want to discuss whether this film probably contributes to the stigma of mental illness.

VIEWING POINTS: This film should be viewed from several different perspectives: What is the basis of McMurphy's admission? How does Nurse Ratchet interact with the patients? What is missing? What is different in today's public mental health systems?

An Angel at My Table: 1989. This thought-provoking, three-part television mini-series from New Zealand, based on Janet Frame's autobiography, traces her life from a shy, socially inept little girl to New Zealand's most famous writer/poet. Produced by Jane Campion and starring Kerry Fox, the story is told in three stages of the main character's life: childhood, young adulthood, and adulthood. During the second period, Janet Frame receives an inaccurate diagnosis of schizophrenia and is hospitalized for 8 years. She barely avoids a leukotomy.

VIEWING POINTS: Observe how the role of the woman in society influenced Janet Frame's admission to the hospital. Do you observe any changes in the perspective on women by today's standards?

Beautiful Dreamers: 1992. This Canadian film is based on a true story about poet Walt Whitman's visit to an asylum in London, Ontario. Whitman, played by Rip Torn, is shocked by what he sees and persuades the hospital director to offer humane treatment. Eventually, the patients wind up playing the townspeople in a game of cricket.

VIEWING POINTS: Observe the stigma that is associated with having a mental illness.

REFERENCES

Arboleda-Flórez, J. (2005). The epidemiology of mental illness in Canada. *Canadian Public Policy: Analyse de Politique, 31*(s1),13–16.

Bailey, H. (1920). *Nursing mental diseases.* New York: Macmillan.

Beauséjour, P. (2001). Advocacy and misadventures in Canadian Psychiatry. In: Q. Rae-Grant (Ed.), *Psychiatry in Canada: 50 years, 1951–2000* (pp. 137–148). Ottawa: Canadian Psychiatric Association.

Beers, C. (1908). *A mind that found itself.* New York: Longmans, Green, & Co.

Benner, P. (1984). *From novice to expert: Excellence and power in clinical nursing practice.* Menlo-Park, CA: Addison-Wesley.

Boschma, G. (2003). *The rise of mental health nursing: A history of psychiatric care in Dutch asylum, 1890–1920.* Amsterdam: Amsterdam University Press.

Boschma, G., Yonge, O., & Mychajlunow, L. (2005). Gender and professional identity in psychiatric nursing practice in Alberta, Canada, 1930–1975. *Nursing Inquiry, 12*(4), 243–255.

Brown, W. H. (2000). Dr. C. K. Clarke and the Training School for Nurses. In: E. Hudson (Ed.), *The provincial asylum in Toronto: Reflections on social and architectural history* (pp. 167–180). Toronto: Toronto Region Architectural Conservancy.

Calaway, B. J. (2002). *Hildegard Peplau: Psychiatric nurse of the century.* New York: Springer.

Canadian Federation of the Mental Health Nurses. (1995). *Canadian standards of psychiatric and mental health nursing practice.* Standards Committee of the Canadian Federation of Mental Health Nurses. Canada: Author.

Church, O. (1987). From custody to community in psychiatric nursing. *Nursing Research, 36*(1), 48–55.

Connor, P. J. (1996). "Neither courage nor perseverance enough": Attendants at the Asylum for the Insane, Kingston, 1877–1905. *Ontario History, 88*(4), 251–272.

D'Antonio, P. (2001). Founding friends: Families and institution building in early nineteenth century Philadelphia: *Nursing Research, 50*, 260–266.

Dickenson, H. D. (1989). *The two psychiatries: The transformation of psychiatric work in Saskatchewan, 1905–1984.* Regina: University of Regina Canadian Plains Research Centre.

Dooley, C. (2004). "The gave their care, but we gave loving care": Defining and defending boundaries of skill and craft in the nursing service of a Manitoba Mental Hospital during the Great Depression. *Canadian Bulletin of Medical History. 21*(2), 229–251.

Goldstein, J. L., & Godemont, M. M. L. (2003). The legend and lessons of Geel, Belgium: A 1500-year-old legend, a 21st century model. *Community Mental Health Journal, 39*(5), 441–458.

Greenland, C. (1996). Origins of the Toronto Psychiatric Hospital. In: Shorter, E. (Ed.). *TPH: History and memories of the Toronto Psychiatric Hospital, 1925–1966.* Toronto: Wall & Emerson.

Greenland, C., Griffin, J., & Hoffman, B. F. (2001). Psychiatry in Canada from 1951–2000. In: Q. Rae-Grant (Ed.), *Psychiatry in Canada: 50 years, 1951–2001* (pp. 1–16). Ottawa: Canadian Psychiatric Association.

Hart Wasekeesikaw, F. (2006). Challenges for the new millennium: Nursing in First Nations. In M. McIntyre, E. Thomlinson, & C. McDonald (Eds.), *Realities of Canadian nursing: Professional, practice and power issues* (pp. 415–433). Philadelphia: Lippincott Williams & Wilkins.

Health Canada. (2002) *A report on mental illnesses in Canada.* Ottawa: Author.

Hector, I. (2001). Changing funding patterns and the effect on mental health care in Canada. In: Q. Rae-Grant (Ed.), *Psychiatry in Canada: 50 years, 1951–2001* (pp. 59–76). Ottawa: Canadian Psychiatric Association.

Heritage Resources Saint John. Updated 2000. Retrieved August 22, 2005, from http://www.saintjohn.nbcc.nb.ca/Heritage/LunaticAsylum/index.htm.

Hurd, H. M. (Ed.). (1973, originally printed 1916–17). *The institutional care of the insane in the United States and Canada* (vol. IV). New York: Arno Press.

Jones, C. (1989). *The charitable imperative: Hospital and nursing in ancient régime and revolutionary France.* London: Routledge.

Kirby, M. J. L. (2005). Mental health reform for Canada in the 21st century: Getting there from here. *Canadian Public Policy: Analyse de Politique, 31*(s1), 5–12.

Kirby, M. J. (2005b). A proposal to establish a Canadian mental health commission: Report 4. Interim Report of the Standing Senate Committee on Social Affairs, Science and Technology. Retrieved March 16, 2006, from http://www.parl.gc.ca/38/1/parlbus/commbus/senate/com-e/SOCI-E/rep-e/rep16nov05-e.pdf.

Kirby, M. J. L. (2004). *Mental health, mental illness and addiction: Reports 1, 2, & 3.* Interim Report of the Standing Committee on Social Affairs, Science and Technology. Retrieved September 29, 2005, from http://www.parl.gc.ca/38/1/parlbus/commbus/senate/com-e/soci-e/rep-e/repintnov04-e.htm.

LaJeunesse, R. A. (2000). *Political asylums.* Edmonton: Muttart Foundation.

Leiby, J. S. (1992). San Hipólito's treatment of the mentally ill in Mexico City, 1589–1650. *The Historian, 54*(3), 491–498.

Lightner, D. L. (1999). *Asylum prison and poorhouse: The writings and reform work of Dorothea Dix in Illinois.* Carbondale and Edwardsville, IL: Southern Illinois University Press.

MacLennan, D. (1987). Beyond the asylum: Professionalization and the Mental Hygiene Movement in Canada, 1914–1928. *Canadian Bulletin of Medical History, 4*, 7–23.

Malamud, W. (1944). The history of psychiatric therapies. In J. K. Hall, G. Zilboorg, & H. Bunker (Eds.), *One hundred years of American psychiatry*, 273–323. New York: Columbia University Press.

McKenzie, C. (1992). *Psychiatry for the rich: A history of Ticehurst Private Asylum, 1792–1917.* London: Routledge.

Morrow, M. (2002). *Violence and trauma in the lives of women with serious mental illness: Current practices in service provision in British Columbia.* Vancouver: Centre of Excellence for Women's Health.

Neill, J. (1980). Adolf Meyer and American psychiatry today. *American Journal of Psychiatry, 137*(4), 460–464.

Nelson, S. (1999). Entering the professional domain: The making of the modern nurse in 17th century France. *Nursing History Review, 7*, 171–187.

Nelson, S. (2001). *Say little, do much: Nursing, nuns, and hospitals in the nineteenth century.* Philadelphia: University of Pennsylvania Press.

Parry-Jones, W. L. L. (1981). The model of the Geel Lunatic Colony and its influence on the nineteenth-century asylum system in Britain. In: Scull, A. (Ed.), *Madhouses, mad-doctors, and madmen. The social history of psychiatry in the Victorian Era* (pp. 201–217) London: The Athlone Press.

Peplau, H. (1952). *Interpersonal relations in nursing.* New York: Putnam.

Porter, R. (1993). Disease, medicine and society in England 1550–1860. Houndmills: Macmillan Education.

Sealy, P., & Whitehead, P. C. (2004). Forty years of deinstitutionalization of psychiatric services in Canada: An empirical assessment. *Canadian Journal of Psychiatry, 49*, 249–257.

Shorter, E. (1997). *A history of psychiatry: From the era of the asylum to the age of Prozac.* New York: John Wiley & Sons.

Sussman, S. (1998). The first asylums in Canada: A response to neglectful community care and current trends. *Canadian Journal of Psychiatry, 43*, 260–264.

Tiplisky, V. M. (2002). Parting at the crossroads: The development of education for psychiatric nursing in three Canadian provinces, 1909–1955. Ph.D. thesis, University of Manitoba.

Tipliski, V. M. (2004). Parting at the crossroads: The emergence of education for psychiatric nursing in three Canadian provinces, 1909–1955. *Canadian Bulletin of Medical History 21*(2), 253–279.

Tomes, N. (1994). *The art of asylum-keeping: Thomas Story Kirkbride and the origins of American psychiatry.* Philadelphia: University of Pennsylvania Press.

Van Drent, A., & De Haan, F. (1999). *The rise of caring power: Elizabeth Fry and Josephine Butler in Britain and the Netherlands.* Amsterdam: Amsterdam University Press.

Warsh, C. K. (1989). *Moments of unreason: The practice of Canadian psychiatry and the Homewood Retreat, 1883–1923.* Montreal and Kingston: McGill-Queens University Press.

World Health Organization. (2001). *The world health report: Mental health 2001. Mental health: New understanding, new hope.* Geneva: Author.

For challenges, please refer to the **CD-ROM** in this book.

CHAPTER 2

Health and Mental Illness

Marion Healey-Ogden

Mental health and mental illness are not polar opposites; rather, they can be viewed as separate concepts on two separate and simultaneously occurring continua. According to a Canadian government document, *Mental Health for Canadians: Striking a Balance* (Epp, 1988), optimal mental health and minimal mental health represent the extremes on one continuum, whereas maximal **mental disorder** and absence of mental disorder represent the extremes on the other continuum (Figure 2-1). Optimal mental health involves "individual, group and environmental factors [that] work together effectively, ensuring subjective well-being; optimal development and use of mental abilities; achievements of goals consistent with justice; and conditions of fundamental equality" (Epp, p. 9). In contrast, minimal mental health is defined as "individual, group, and environmental factors [that] conflict, producing subjective distress; impairment or underdevelopment of mental abilities; failure to achieve goals; destructive behaviours; and entrenchment of inequalities" (Epp, 1988, p. 9). A person's mental health experiences can vary throughout his or her life.

Maximal mental disorder on the mental illness continuum includes the "greatest severity; frequency and range of psychiatric symptoms" (Epp, 1988, p. 9). Absence of mental disorder on the other end of this continuum includes "freedom from psychiatric symptoms; effective prevention or cure" (Epp, 1988, p. 9). Mental illness refers to mental disorders that are diagnosable when they follow most recently established criteria based on the American Psychiatric Association's (2002) *Diagnostic and Statistical Manual of Mental Disorders*, 4th edition, text revision *(DSM-IV-TR)* discussed later in this chapter. Like the mental health continuum, a person's experiences of mental disorders can vary throughout his or her life.

UNIVERSALITY OF MENTAL HEALTH

A person who is mentally healthy is able to deal effectively with human emotions, is productive, has successful relationships with others, can adapt to change, and can positively cope with adversity. Everyone has the potential to be mentally healthy. Mental health is a universal condition that shapes the way we think, feel, and communicate. A person can be physically ill yet be mentally healthy. In contrast, it is possible for a person with a mental illness to learn to cope with the symptoms and treatment of a disorder in order to live a life that includes mentally healthy responses and achievements.

Included within mental health is the concept of **well-being** that is not well defined in the health-related literature. A dictionary definition (Cayne, 1988) states that well-being is "the state of being healthy, happy, and free from want" (p. 1117). Similarly, the World Health Organization (WHO, 2001) defines mental health as "a state of well-being in which the individual realizes his or her own abilities, can cope with the normal stresses of life, can work productively and fruitfully, and is able to make a contribution to his or her community" (How does one define mental health? section, para. 1). Both definitions refer to well-being as existing within health and illness and without the extreme of prosperity.

Health of Canadians

This Canadian text is built on a foundation of understanding derived from the definition of health clarified within the Epp (1986/2001) report. Specifically, this report states that "health is a basic and dynamic force in our daily lives, influenced by our circumstances, our beliefs, our culture and our social, economic and physical environments" (p. 2). The breadth of this definition means that health is considered to extend beyond a limited perspective of physical, mental, and social well-being. In particular, the Epp report identified three challenges in maintaining the health of Canadians: reducing inequalities, increasing the prevention effort, and enhancing people's capacity to cope. The unequivocal link between mental health and mental illness that is brought to attention in the Epp report gives equal weight to assisting people who are mentally ill and to working to assist people to maintain their mental health.

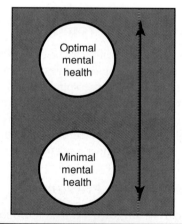

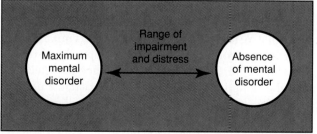

FIGURE 2.1 *Diagrams of the mental health and mental disorder continua. (Adapted from* Epp, J. [1988]. *Mental health for Canadians: Striking a balance* [Cat. H39-128/1988E]. Ottawa: Supply and Service Canada [p. 9]).

Margot Kidder (1948–)
Actress

Public Persona
Margot Kidder is a Canadian actress who has starred in many movies and television shows. The Superman series in which she played Lois Lane stands out among her most well-known movies. Kidder's ongoing accomplishments extend to her far-reaching advocacy work.

Personal Realities
Kidder documented her experiences with bipolar disorder in her autobiography, *Calamities*. In the midst of writing that book in 1996, her bipolar disorder swung out of control. In the 1990s she had been experiencing an overwhelming amount of stress that was coupled with the near loss of her autobiographical documents from her computer. This loss was the ultimate catalyst that sent Kidder into a psychotic break, with extreme paranoia, leading her into a brief period of homelessness.

Kidder was born in Yellowknife, Northwest Territories (NWT). During her childhood and adolescence, she lived with her parents and four siblings in various mining towns in the NWT and in Newfoundland. Her experiences with bipolar disorder began when she attempted suicide during her adolescence.

Mental illness awareness groups benefit from Kidder's ongoing support. Often she is the keynote speaker at mental health conferences. She attributes her recovery and mental health to holistic treatment and to a balanced lifestyle.

From Carlson, 2000; January; CMHA Newsletter, 1999; and Nunes & Simmie, 2002.

Health Promotion

The Ottawa Charter for Health Promotion (1986), a WHO document, states, **"health promotion** is the process of enabling people to increase control over, and to improve, their health" (Health promotion section, para. 1). Rather than being a goal toward which a person strives, the Ottawa Charter states that health is "a resource for everyday life . . . [that] goes beyond healthy lifestyles to wellbeing" (Ottawa Charter, Health promotion section, para. 1). This WHO statement is reflected in the health promotion framework advocated in the Epp report. Health promotion is built on the concept of **primary health care** outlined in the Alma-Ata Declaration (WHO, 1978) that says that primary health care includes the main concepts of "equity, community involvement/participation, intersectorality, appropriateness of techniques and affordable costs" (p. 3). Although the concept of primary health care is well defined, it is apparent that much work remains to improve primary care and thereby improve the mental health needs of

Canadians (Kirby, 2004). The global nature of mental illness means that it is important for primary health care practitioners, such as nurses, to honour and develop local cultural responses (Desjarlais, Eisenberg, Good, & Kleinman, 1995). Health education is one of the key primary health care activities that, when applied to mental health, can become a catalyst for each person to work toward experiencing optimal mental health. The Canadian Registered Nurse Examination (CRNE) is based on a primary health care framework (Canadian Nurses Association [CNA], n. d.). Therefore, the nursing care in this book reflects primary health care and health promotion.

Social Determinants of Health

The **social determinants of health** lie at the forefront of health promotion. In a 2002 conference at York University, a broad spectrum of social determinants of health were discussed in view of developing policies to address the following key social determinants in Canada: income inequality, social inclusion and exclusion, employment and job security, working conditions, contributions of the social economy, early childhood care, education, food security, and housing. Mental health is contingent on policies and action that support and promote these social determinants of health across all sectors within Canada (Social Determinants of Health, 2004, p. 1).

Mental Health Promotion

A person's mental health can be challenged by a variety of factors such as biologic changes or illnesses, psychological pressures, and interpersonal tension. Healthy life span development includes formulating strategies to eliminate or reduce the impact of these destructive factors on one's life. Relaxation, proper nutrition, sleep, and a trusting relationship can support a person's mental health.

Mental Illness Prevention

Specific **risk factors**, or characteristics that increase the likelihood of developing a disorder, can contribute to minimal mental health and influence the development of a mental disorder. Risk factors do not cause the disorder or problem and are not symptoms of the illness, but rather are factors that influence the likelihood that the symptoms will appear. The existence of a risk factor does not always mean the person will get the disorder; it increases the person's chances. There are many different kinds of risk factors, including genetic, biologic, environmental, cultural, and occupational. Gender, too, is a risk factor for some disorders. For example, more women experience depression than men

(Gender and Women's Mental Health, n. d.; Health Canada, 2002).

Some risk factors can be controlled or changed through mental health promotion activities, whereas others cannot. For example, genetic predisposition cannot be changed because individuals cannot change the genetic makeup with which they are born. Risk factors that can be changed include those related to lifestyle behaviours or environment. Someone who is genetically at high risk for bipolar disorder (i.e., one or more family members have the disorder) can modify his or her lifestyle and environment to decrease the impact of these factors. Selecting a job with minimal stress can reduce the likelihood of manifestations related to some of the anxiety disorders. However, even if it is possible to change behaviours, occupations, and environmental conditions, the actual change can be difficult. Many risky behaviours are physically, psychologically, or socially rewarding and pleasurable, such as eating a high-calorie meal, engaging in unprotected sexual intercourse, or sustaining an interpersonal relationship with someone who is abusive. One of the challenges of nursing is helping people identify and monitor their own risk factors.

Homelessness

Mental illness and homelessness are not necessarily linked; however, it is becoming increasingly apparent, when homelessness is explored, that mental illness is related to many people's homeless lifestyles in Canada (Government of Canada, 2004b). Until this decade, little attention was paid to the impact of homelessness on a person's mental health. By focusing on the social determinants of health, it is not surprising to note that when a person is homeless, his or her mental health is at risk. In 1999, the Canadian government announced a 3-year National Homelessness Initiative (NHI) to take place between 2003 to 2006 that would identify key areas of research and consultation needed to address homelessness across Canada (Government of Canada, 2004a). The National Research Group (NRG) that grew out of the NHI is focussing on six areas of research: health; education, employment, and income; justice; cycles of homelessness; immigration; and the north (Government of Canada, 2004b). The NRG identified mental illness as a main health concern. Much work is needed in the near future to understand all aspects of homelessness within all sectors of Canada.

Culture and Mental Health

Mental health and mental illness are often defined by cultural norms and beliefs that identify mentally healthy behaviour. Canadians represent a blend of people from a vast array of cultures. Some people strictly maintain their cultural practices when living in Canada, whereas other people adapt to the general Canadian culture. Cultural practices can be in conflict with individuals' needs and, therefore, can present a challenge for the acculturation of, in particular, adolescents and elderly people. The resultant conflict and stress places the immigrant and refugee population at risk for mental illness and less than optimum mental health (Kinnon, 1999). Aboriginal people in Canada experience many cultural factors that contribute to mental illness and related concerns such as addictions. Their marginalization, as well as their historical treatment in residential schools, are examples of cultural factors that negatively affect the mental health of Aboriginal people (Kinnon, 1999).

MENTAL ILLNESS

Mental illnesses, in other words, diagnosable mental disorders, are considered syndromes or clusters of symptoms that occur together and that could have multiple causes.

Importance of Epidemiology

The occurrence of mental disorders is studied through epidemiological research, just like any other disorder. **Epidemiology** is the study of patterns of disease distribution in time and space. It focuses on the health status of population groups, or aggregates, rather than individuals, and it involves quantitative analysis of the occurrence of illnesses in population groups. Epidemiologic approaches are useful in understanding the occurrences of mental disorders. Throughout this book, mental disorders are described using epidemiologic data. See Box 2-1 for an explanation of terms.

Mental Disorders Overview

> **KEY CONCEPT Mental disorders** are health conditions characterized by alterations in thinking, mood, or behaviour. They are associated with distress or impaired functioning.

These alterations are unexpected and are outside the limits of expected psychological states, such as sadness, grief, and mild depression normally associated with the death of a spouse. Cultural definitions of "normal" responses are also taken into consideration. If a behaviour is considered normal within a specific culture, it is not viewed as a symptom by members of that group. For example, it is common in some religious groups to "speak in tongues." To an observer, it appears that the individuals are experiencing hallucinations (see Chapter 10), a psychiatric symptom, but this behaviour is normal for this group within a particular setting.

BOX 2.1

Epidemiologic Terms

In epidemiology, certain terms have specific meanings relative to what they measure. When expressing the number of cases of a disorder, population rates, rather than raw numbers, are used.

Rate is a proportion of the cases in the population when compared with the total population. It is expressed as a fraction, in which the numerator is the number of cases and the denominator is the total number in the population, including the cases and noncases. The term *average rate* is used for measures that involve rates over specified time periods:

$$Rate = \frac{Cases\ in\ the\ population}{Total\ population}$$
$$(includes\ cases\ and\ noncases)$$

Prevalence refers to the total number of people who have the disorder within a given population at a specified time, regardless of how long ago the disorder started.

Point prevalence is the basic measure that refers to the proportion of individuals in the population who have the disorder at a specified point in time. This point can be a day on the calender, such as April 1, 2010, or a point defined in relation to the study assessment, such as the day of the interview. This is also expressed as a fraction:

$$Point\ prevalence\ rate = \frac{Cases\ at\ t}{Population\ at\ t}$$

Incidence refers to a rate that includes only *new* cases that have occurred within a clearly defined time period, most commonly 1 year. The study of incidence cases is more difficult than a study of prevalent cases. The study of incidence cases requires at least two measurements to be taken, one at the start of the prescribed time period and another at the end of it.

BOX 2.2

Selected Culture-Bound Syndromes

DEFINITION: Behaviours limited to specific cultures that have meaning within that culture

BRAIN FAG: Condition experienced by high school or university students in response to the challenges of schooling. Symptoms include difficulties in concentrating, remembering, and thinking. A term originally used in West Africa.

FALLING-OUT OR BLACKING OUT: An episode of sudden collapse that is sometimes preceded by feelings of dizziness. Individuals' eyes are usually open, but the person claims an inability to see. Occurs primarily in southern United States and Caribbean groups.

MAL DE OJO: Known as the "evil eye" in Mediterranean cultures and elsewhere in the world. Symptoms include fitful sleep, crying without apparent cause, diarrhea, vomiting, and fever in a child or infants.

Adapted from American Psychiatric Association. (2000). *Diagnostic and statistical manual of mental disorders*, 4th ed, text revision (pp. 898–903). Washington, DC: Author.

Diagnosis of Mental Disorders

The *DSM-IV-TR* system contains subtypes and other specifiers to describe further the characteristics of the diagnosis as exhibited in a given individual. Some disorders are influenced by cultural factors, and others are culture-bound syndromes that are present only in a particular setting (Box 2-2). Although the *DSM-IV-TR* provides criteria for diagnosing mental disorders, there are no absolute boundaries separating one disorder from another, and similar disorders may have different manifestations at different points in time.

The *DSM-IV-TR* diagnostic criteria are based on a **multiaxial diagnostic system** that includes five axes, or domains of information. Axis I includes most *clinical disorders* and other conditions that may be the focus of clinical attention, and Axis II contains *personality disorders* and *mental retardation*. Axis III includes the *general medical conditions* that must be considered in the diagnosis and treatment of the primary psychiatric disorders. Each axis is essential to the complete understanding and treatment of an individual with psychiatric concerns. For example, a person with a major depression (Axis I) may meet the criteria for having a dependent personality disorder (Axis II) and may also have diabetes (Axis III). See Table 2-1 for a listing of disorders and conditions that might be considered under each axis and Box 2-3 for a clinical example.

Although the first three axes appear to contain all of the diagnostic information, a truly accurate picture of the individual is incomplete without considering other factors, such as life stressors and current level of functioning. Axis IV relates to any psychosocial or environmental situation that may produce added stress, confound the diagnosis, or must be considered in the treatment of the primary psychiatric problem. Life stressors may be negative or positive. On the one hand, a negative life event, such as the death of a spouse, a recent divorce, or job discrimination, may exacerbate symptoms of depression. On the other hand, positive stressors, such as starting a new job, getting married, or having a baby, may also prompt the symptoms to emerge. Using the *DSM-IV-TR* suggestions for identifying areas of concern, the prudent clinician making the diagnosis would clearly describe the individual's specific response on this axis.

Ratings given on Axis V provide an estimate of *overall functioning* in psychological, social, and occupational spheres of life. These data are useful in planning treatment and measuring its impact. The Global Assessment of Functioning (GAF) scale usually is used and is scored from low functioning of 0 to 10, to high functioning of 91 to 100 (see Table 2-1). This rating may be made at the beginning of treatment, at discharge from the hospital,

Table 2.1   *DSM-IV* Multiaxial Diagnoses for Persons With Mental Disorders

Diagnostic Axes and Their Disorders and Conditions

Axis I: Clinical Disorders and Other Conditions That May Be a Focus of Clinical Attention

Disorders Usually First Diagnosed During Infancy, Childhood, or Adolescence
Delirium, Dementia, Amnestic Disorder, and Other Cognitive Disorders
Mental Disorders Due to General Medical Conditions
Substance-Related Disorders
Schizophrenia and Other Psychotic Disorders
Mood Disorders
Anxiety Disorders
Somatoform Disorders
Factitious Disorders
Dissociative Disorders
Sexual and Gender Identity Disorders
Eating Disorders
Sleep Disorders
Impulse Control Disorders (Not Elsewhere Classified)
Adjustment Disorders
Other Conditions That May Be a Focus of Clinical Attention

Axis II: Personality Disorders and Mental Retardation

Personality Disorders:
  Paranoid Personality Disorder
  Schizoid Personality Disorder
  Schizotypal Personality Disorder
  Antisocial Personality Disorder
  Borderline Personality Disorder
  Histrionic Personality Disorder
  Narcissistic Personality Disorder
  Avoidant Personality Disorder
  Dependent Personality Disorder
  Obsessive-Compulsive Personality Disorder
  Personality Disorder Not Otherwise Specified
  Mental Retardation

Axis III: General Medical Conditions

Infectious and Parasitic Diseases
Neoplasms
Endocrine, Nutritional, and Metabolic Diseases and Immunity Disorders
Diseases of the Blood and Blood-Forming Organs
Diseases of the Nervous and Sense Organs
Diseases of the Circulatory System
Diseases of the Respiratory System
Diseases of the Digestive System
Diseases of the Genitourinary System
Complications of Pregnancy, Childbirth, and the Puerperium
Diseases of the Skin and Subcutaneous Tissue
Diseases of the Musculoskeletal System and Connective Tissue

Congenital Anomalies
Certain Conditions Originating in the Perinatal Period
Symptoms, Signs, and Ill-Defined Conditions
Injury and Poisoning

Axis IV: Psychosocial and Environmental Problems

Problems with primary support group
Problems related to the social environment
Educational problems
Occupational problems
Housing problems
Economic problems
Problems with access to health care services
Problems related to interaction with the legal system/crime
Other psychosocial and environmental problems

Axis V: Global Assessment of Functioning*

  Current =
  Potential =

Psychological, social, and occupational functioning on a hypothetical continuum of mental health–illness.

Scores	
91–100	Superior functioning, no symptoms
81–90	Absent or minimal symptoms, good functioning in all areas
71–80	If symptoms are present, they are transient and expectable reactions to psychosocial stressors; no more than slight impairment in social, occupational, or school functioning
61–70	Some mild symptoms or some difficulty in social, occupational, or school functioning, but generally functioning well; has some meaningful interpersonal relationships
51–60	Moderate symptoms or moderate difficulty in social, occupational, or school functioning
41–50	Serious symptoms or any serious impairment in social, occupational, or school functioning
31–40	Some impairment in reality testing or communication or major impairment in several areas, such as work or school, family relations, judgment, thinking, or mood
21–30	Behaviour is considerably influenced by delusions or hallucinations or serious impairment in communication or judgment or inability to function in almost all areas
11–20	Some danger of hurting self or others or occasionally fails to maintain minimal personal hygiene or gross impairment in communication
1–10	Persistent danger of severely hurting self or others or persistent inability to maintain minimal personal hygiene or serious suicidal act with clear expectation of death

*The person's current GAF score represents his or her lowest level of functioning or symptoms.

BOX 2.3

Diagnostic Axes and Their Disorders and Conditions

Clinical Example

Axis I: 300.21* Panic Disorder With Agoraphobia
Axis II: 301.4 Obsessive-Compulsive Personality Disorder
Axis III: 250.00† Diabetes Mellitus
Axis IV: Occupational Problems: Frequent Absences From Work
Axis V: Global Assessment of Function
      GAF = 55 (current)
             90 (potential)

---

*In this example, code numbers are used and can be found in the *Diagnostic and Statistical Manual of Mental Disorders*, 4th ed, text revision *(DSM-IV-TR)*. To improve readability, these code numbers are not used when discussing the various disorders. The student will see them used in the clinical setting.
†The medical conditions in Axis III are coded according to the *International Classification of Diseases (ICD)*.

or at any point thereafter. When including this rating, the point of time should also be indicated, such as "current," or "at discharge from the hospital."

Consequences of Labelling

A diagnosis becomes a way of labelling a particular patient problem. However, negative consequences of a label include, for example, loss of personal identity when the labelled person becomes a disease and experiences stigma associated with mental illness. To avoid labelling, a person with diabetes mellitus would be referred to as a "person with diabetes" rather than as a "diabetic." Likewise, a person with a mental disorder would be referred to as a "person with schizophrenia" or as a "person with bipolar disorder" rather than as a "schizophrenic" or as a "bipolar." It is important for nurses and other health care professionals to avoid the pitfalls of negative labelling and stigmatization (Austin, 2000; Kirby, 2004).

Individualizing Diagnoses and Care

DSM-IV-TR diagnosis is useful in identifying a disorder but is limited in that it does not provide information regarding individual responses to the disorder and specific patient needs. For example, two individuals may acquire the same flu virus, but one may experience a high fever, an upset stomach, and a dry, harsh cough, whereas the other may have only a mild fever, a slight cough, and no nausea. Alternately, of two individuals who are diagnosed with clinical depression, one person may be unable to carry on with day-to-day activities and

be hospitalized because of a suicide attempt, whereas the other person may continue to maintain home and family responsibilities. A person's response to a mental disorder also ranges in degree. For example, aggression can range from verbal anger to physical assault; anxiety, from mild to panic; self-destruction, from indirect to direct; or depression, from grief to major depression. Human responses to illness provide direction for the health care team to guide people toward mental health or successful coping with mental disorders.

EVIDENCE-BASED CARE

One of the challenges in the psychiatric–mental health field is to generate interventions for **evidence-based care**. Traditionally, interventions have been developed by clinicians' own experiences and have not necessarily been subjected to rigorous testing. Today, the focus is on developing evidenced-based care that involves defining clinical questions and finding evidence that serves as a basis of practice (CNA, 2002). Throughout this book, research-supported interventions are highlighted.

From the evidence, treatment guidelines can be developed. There is general agreement in the psychiatric community that treatment guidelines are useful. These guidelines usually include algorithms (or decision trees) that can be used in making treatment decisions. The best guidelines are evidence based and combined with an individualized approach to health care. Most of the disorders discussed in this book have several treatment guidelines.

SUMMARY OF KEY POINTS

- Mental health and mental illness can be viewed as separate concepts on two separate and simultaneously occurring continua.
- Mentally healthy people are able to deal effectively with normal human emotions. Mental illnesses are diagnosable mental disorders that follow the *DSM-IV-TR* criteria.
- The use of diagnosis in mental health can be problematic because of the negative association of the label, *mental illness*, or of the name of a specific mental disorder. The diagnoses outlined in the *DSM-IV-TR* are the standardized, accepted language in the mental health field. There are five diagnostic axes: clinical disorders; personality disorders and mental retardation; general medical problems; psychosocial or environmental problems; and overall functioning.
- Epidemiology is important in understanding the distribution of mental illness within a given population. The rate of occurrence refers to the proportion

of the population that has the disorder. The prevalence is the rate of occurrence of all cases at a specified time, whereas point prevalence refers to the proportion of individuals in the population who have the disorder at a specified point in time. The incidence is the rate of new cases within a specified time.

☐ Risk factors include factors that can and cannot be changed. Genetic predisposition cannot be changed, although lifestyle and behaviour are amenable to change.

☐ Cultural norms and beliefs contribute to the identification of mentally healthy behaviour.

☐ Health promotion is built on the concept of primary health care that forms the basis for mental health nursing. A focus on social determinants of health and on health education promotes optimal mental health.

☐ The Canadian Epp (1988) report gives equal weight to assisting people who are mentally ill and to working to assist people to maintain their mental health.

CRITICAL THINKING CHALLENGES

1 Distinguish between the terms mental health, mental illness, and mental disorder.
2 Describe the framework on which the Canadian approach to mental health is based.
3 Relate homelessness to mental health and mental illness.
4 Define the epidemiologic terms *prevalence*, *incidence*, and *rate*.
5 Define risk factors and identify the various types of risk factors related to mental illness.
6 State the differences between the five axes of the *DSM-IV-TR* and explain the importance of considering all five axes as they apply to each person.
7 Discuss the negative impact of labelling someone with a psychiatric diagnosis.
8 Discuss the value of evidence-based care.

WEB LINKS

www.bcmhs.bc.ca/library This is the site of the Riverview Hospital for Mental Health Services library.

www.cna-nurses.ca This site provides the Canadian Nurses Association Policy Statement.

www.gov.ns.ca/health/policywatch This Nova Scotia government site includes links to Canadian Mental Health resources.

www.hc-sc.gc.ca Information on the Canadian Health Care System and Primary Health Care can be found at this Health Canada site.

www.phac-aspc.gc.ca This site of the Public Health Agency of Canada, under the Mental Health category, provides various links, including those to best practices.

www.pharmacists.ca This site includes the report, "Mental Health in a Primary Care Context: Collaboration is the Key."

www.who.int This site of the World Health Organization, under the topic of Mental Health, includes links to related sites. It also includes documents related to the "World Health Report 2001—Mental Health: New Understandings, New Hope."

REFERENCES

American Psychiatric Association. (2000). *Diagnostic and statistical manual of mental disorders* (4th edition, text revision). Washington, DC: Author.

Austin, W. (2000, Feb.). Ethics and the stigma of mental illness. *Health Ethics Today, 2*(12). Retrieved August 8, 2005, from http://www.phen.ab.ca/materials/intouch/vol2/intouch2-12.html

Canadian Nurses Association. (n.d.). *CRNE readiness test.* Ottawa: Author. Retrieved August 12, 2005, from http://readiness.cna-aiic. ca//english/crne.aspx.

Canadian Nurses Association. (2002). *Position statement: Evidence-based decision-making and nursing practice.* Retrieved August 11, 2005, from http://cna-aiic.ca/CNA/documents/pdf/publications/PS63_ Evidence_based_Decision_making_Nursing_Practice_e.pdf.

Carlson, J. (2000, Jan.). Margot Kidder: Speaks up for mental health. Retrieved August 2, 2005, from *Networking Newspaper for Women,* http://www.networkwomen.com/archives/coverstory01_00.html.

Cayne, B. (Ed.). (1988). *The new lexicon Webster's encyclopedic dictionary of the English language* (Canadian edition). New York: Lexicon Publications.

Canadian Mental Health Association (CMHA). (1999, July). *CMHA Newsletter—Mental Health Matters, 2*(2). Retrieved August 12, 2005, from http://www.cmha.ca/english/info_centre/mhm_ newsletter/mhm_july99_v2i2.htm.

Desjarlais, R., Eisenberg, L., Good, B., & Kleinman, A. (1995). *World mental health: Problems and priorities in low-income countries.* New York: Oxford University Press.

Epp, J. (1986/2001). *Achieving health for all: A framework for health promotion* (Cat. H39- 102/1986E), Ottawa: Supply and Services Canada.

Epp. J. (1988). *Mental health for Canadians: Striking a balance* (Cat. H39-128/1988E). Ottawa: Supply and Services Canada.

Gender and Women's Mental Health. (n. d.). Retrieved August 13, 2005, from the World Health Organization site, http://www.who. int/mental_health/prevention/genderwomen/en/.

Government of Canada. (2004a). *About the initiative.* Retrieved August 12, 2005, from http://www.homelessness.gc.ca/initiative/ index_e.asp.

Government of Canada. (2004b). *Summary of conclusions of consultations on national research program on homelessness.* Retrieved August 12, 2005, from http://www.homelessness.gc.ca/research/consultations2003/ index_e.asp.

Health Canada. (2002). *A report on mental illnesses in Canada.* Retrieved August 12, 2005, from Government of Canada: http:// www.phac-aspc.gc.ca/publicat/miic-mmac/.

Kinnon, D. (1999). *Canadian research on immigration and health: An overview* (Cat. J21-149/1999E). Retrieved August 12, 2005, from the Health Canada site, http://dsp-psd.communication.gc.ca/ Collection/H21-149-1999E.pdf.

Kirby, M. (2004). *Report 3. Mental health, mental illness and addiction: Issues and options for Canada.* Retrieved August 12, 2005, from the Health Canada site, http://www.parl.gc.ca/38/1/parlbus/commbus/ senate/com-e/soci-e/rep-e/report3/repintnov04vol3-e.pdf.

Nunes, J. & Simmie, S. (2002). *Beyond crazy*. Toronto, ON: McClelland & Stewart.

Ottawa Charter for Health Promotion. (1986). Retrieved August 13, 2005, from the World Health Organization site, http://www.euro.who.int/AboutWHO/Policy/20010827_2.

Social Determinants of Health. (2004). Retrieved August 13, 2005, from the Public Health Agency of Canada site, http://www.phac-aspc.gc.ca/ph-sp/phdd/overview_implications/01_overview.html.

World Health Organization. (1978). *Primary health care: Report of the international conference on primary health care*. Alma Ata, USSR. Geneva: Author.

World Health Organization. (1998). *Health promotion glossary* (document WHO/HPR/HEP/98.1). Geneva: Author.

World Health Organization (2001). *Mental health: Strengthening mental health promotion*. Retrieved August 11, 2005, from http://www.who.int/mediacentre/factsheets/fs220/en/ print.html.

For challenges, please refer to the **CD-ROM** in this book.

CHAPTER 3

The Context of Mental Health Care

Arlene Kent-Wilkinson and Mary Ann Boyd

LEARNING OBJECTIVES

After studying this chapter, you will be able to:

- Explore the cultural roots of mental illness and its relationship to beliefs of religion and spirituality.
- Relate the concept of cultural competence to the role of the psychiatric and mental health (PMH) nurse.
- Consider the unique culture of Aboriginal peoples in Canada and their mental health beliefs.
- Identify the influence of socioeconomic factors (poverty, geographic) on the mental health of Canadians.
- Describe the mental health care delivery issues related to providing services to culturally diverse populations in Canada's many geographic areas.
- Identify and explain the mental health legislation enacted to help protect, promote, and improve the lives and mental well-being of Canadians.

KEY TERMS

- assimilation - best interests - colonialism - community treatment order - competence - cultural safety - discrimination - displacement - ethnocentrism - mandatory outpatient treatment - prejudice - spirituality - stereotyping - stigma - substitute decision maker - telehealth

KEY CONCEPTS

- culture - cultural competence - poverty - Mental Health Act

The health, including the mental health, of any human population is the product of a complex web of cultural, environmental, historical, physiologic, psychological, spiritual, socioeconomic, and legislative factors. This chapter examines three contexts of mental health and illness in Canada: *cultural*, *socioeconomic*, and *legal*. Culture will be examined with regard to cultural roots, spirituality, and religion. Then, socioeconomic factors that influence mental health (poverty, geographic access to services) will be explored. Finally, international agreements and Canadian legislation enacted to protect, promote, and improve the lives and mental well-being of citizens will be discussed.

CULTURAL CONTEXT OF MENTAL HEALTH CARE

All people have a culture. It reflects the basic values and biases through which we interpret the world around us and make decisions about our own behaviour and our relationships with others. Our culture shapes our perceptions and attitudes, from our personal-space comfort zones to our attitudes toward mental health and mental illness.

Culture

Geertz (1973) described humans as animals who have spun "webs of significance" for themselves. These webs are culture. Understanding mental health and culture is not about finding its "laws" but about interpreting its meaning. The metaphor of a complex web is strong as webs show intricacy and interconnectedness, creativity and skill that can only be seen close up. Each individual thread contributes to the strength of the web.

> **KEY CONCEPT Culture** is not only a way of life for people who identify or associate with one another on the basis of some common purpose, need, or similarity of background, but also the totality of learned, socially transmitted beliefs, values, and behaviours that emerge from its members' interpersonal transactions.

Cultural Diversity in Canada

Canada was the first country to develop a multiculturalism policy (in 1971), a policy that states that Canadians should "be able to maintain and develop their own cultural identities if they so wish, be willing to share their cultures with other Canadians, and be free from prejudice and discrimination" (Canadian Health Network, 1997). This policy challenges Canadians to accept cultural pluralism, while encouraging them to participate fully and equally in Canadian society.

Culture is one of the 12 key determinants of health (Canadian Nurses Association [CNA], 2004), and nurses are responsible to provide culturally competent care (some nurses prefer the term *culturally sensitive care*) to diverse populations with different cultural beliefs. Nurses must strive to understand the way people of various cultures think, feel, behave, and respond when it comes to matters of health. This can be especially difficult because the cultural face of Canada has changed over the past 15 years, and we have a larger range of ethnicity, language, and country-of-origin than ever before. The culture of Aboriginal peoples has been chosen as a focus in this discussion on culture as Canadian psychiatric and mental health (PMH) nurses have identified a pressing need for such knowledge and understanding (Austin, Gallop, McCay, Peternelj-Taylor, & Bayer, 1999).

Aboriginal Peoples

More than 1.3 million people in Canada report having at least some Aboriginal ancestry, representing 4.4% of the total population (Statistics Canada, 2003). Aboriginal peoples in Canada are the descendants of the original inhabitants of North America. The Canadian Constitution under section 35(2) recognizes three groups of Aboriginal peoples: Indians (First Nations), Métis people, and Inuit. These represent three separate peoples with unique heritages, languages, multiple cultural practices, and spiritual beliefs (Aboriginal Health Glossary, 2004). See Box 3-1 for definitions of the three groups of Aboriginal peoples in Canada.

Cultural Diversity Within Aboriginal Peoples in Canada

There is great diversity among Aboriginal peoples in our country, with 11 major language groups and more than 58 dialects, 596 First Nations bands, and 2284 reserves. Although many live on reserves, 41% reside in nonreserve areas (36% urban, 5% rural) (Frideres, 1998; Morrison & Wilson, 1988). The cultural and linguistic differences among the groups are greater than the differences that divide European nations. In addition to intergroup social, cultural, and environmental differences, there is an enormous diversity of values, lifestyles, and perspectives within any community or urban Aboriginal population (Kirmayer, Brass, & Tait, 2000).

Cultural Roots of Mental Health and Illness

Members of a culture rarely have insight into their own culturally learned ideas and values regarding normal and abnormal behaviour; typically these values are seen as correct and proper for everyone (ethnocentrism). The expression of mental illness is heavily determined by culture. Symptoms of a disorder that are prominent in one culture may be insignificant or absent in another

BOX 3.1

Aboriginal Peoples

First Nations

The term *First Nation* replaces the term *Indian* (Royal Commission on Aboriginal Peoples, 1996). This term began to be used in the 1970s as a substitute for Indians, a term that has fallen into disfavour with Aboriginal people. The term does not mean the same as *Aboriginal people* or *First Peoples* because it does not include Inuit and Métis (Public Health Agency of Canada, 2005). *Indian Band Member* or *First Nation* refers to those people who reported being a member of an Indian band or a First Nation of Canada. Band membership is 554,860 (Statistics Canada, 2003).

Inuit

The term *Inuit* replaces the term *Eskimo* (Royal Commission on Aboriginal Peoples, 1996). The Inuit are an Aboriginal people in northern Canada, who live above the tree line in Nunavut, the Northwest Territories, Northern Quebec, and Labrador. The word means "people" in the Inuit language—*Inuktitut*. The singular of Inuit is Inuk (Aboriginal Health Glossary, 2004).

Métis

The term *Métis* refers to Aboriginal people of mixed First Nation and European ancestry who identify themselves as Métis people, as distinct from First Nations people, Inuit, or non-Aboriginal people. The Métis have a unique culture that draws on their diverse ancestral origins, such as Scottish, French, Ojibway, and Cree (Government of Saskatchewan, 2003).

and may even be interpreted as normal in a third (Health Canada, 2003c). Some disorders may be exotic and specific to a particular culture (eg, Windigo among the Cree and Ojibwa; Pibloktog among the Inuit).

Diagnostic Cultural Formulations

The American Psychiatric Association (APA) *Diagnostic and Statistical Manual of Mental Disorders* is used to set the boundaries, conditions, and criteria for psychiatric diagnosis throughout North America. Culture was not specifically addressed until the fourth edition of the manual (DSM-IV) (APA, 1994). After exploring different ways of facilitating the application of a cultural perspective to the process of clinical interviewing, a cultural formulation outline was adopted for use in the fourth edition. However, it was relegated to the back of the book, in the ninth appendix along with a glossary of cultural terms and idioms of distress. This was a problematic solution for many, who believe that culture must be more central to the process of clinical evaluation and treatment (Austin et al., 1999). It has been argued that psychiatric researchers, focussed on a biologic model of mental disorders, tend to ignore cultural factors. For instance, in a review of psychiatric drug studies, it was found that only 8% of patient subjects were from minority groups (Vedantam, 2005).

Some new disorders may be a recent development in response to cultural change. The "totally discouraged syndrome" (depression, alcoholism, lack of social responsibility, neglect of family, suicidal behaviour), described for the Sioux, may be such a disorder (Health Canada, 2003c). (See Chapter 2 for further information on the *Diagnostic and Statistical Manual of Mental Disorders (DSM-IV-TR)*).

Aboriginal Mental Health

Aboriginal health is influenced by the rich diversity of social, economic, and political circumstances that give rise to a variety of health problems and healing strategies in Aboriginal communities (Waldram, Herring, & Young, 1995). Many Aboriginal people are raised to believe the body is affected by four elements comprising the spiritual, emotional, mental, and physical. Aboriginal peoples have adopted a holistic view of mental health with mental health seen as part of full health.

The traditional Aboriginal healing system encompasses a holistic view of manifestations of illness in an individual. There is little evidence of a clear distinction between what science would call somatic disorders and disorders of the psyche. The mind, body, and spirit are seen as an integrated whole. Notions of "sanity" and "insanity" and of personality disorders are not strictly defined, as in the case of the biomedical tradition. The Western approach, in contrast, separates the body from the mind and spirit, and the emphasis is on disease and treatment (Waldram, 2004). It is necessary to recognize the historical, socioeconomic, and political circumstances of Aboriginal people in Canada in order to understand the mental health problems or disorders of a person from this culture because they may be related to factors that have historically confronted them.

Colonialism, Assimilation, and Displacement
Colonialism, according to the Public Health Agency of Canada (2004), is the institutionalized political domination of one nation over another. There is direct political administration by the colonial power, control of all economic relationships, and a systematic attempt to transform the culture. Before Confederation and up through the first half of the 20th century, the strategy of the Government of Canada toward First Nations was a colonial one. Government policy was to "Canadianize" Aboriginal people and assimilate them into the majority culture.

Part of making Native peoples into "Canadians" was to convert them to Christianity: government and several churches and religious orders cooperated to run residential schools. As a result of this residential school policy, Aboriginal children, often as young as 6 years of age, were displaced from their parental homes, families, culture, language, and traditions and placed into boarding schools for 10 months of the year (Industry Canada, 2003). This displacement has had long-lasting effects on Aboriginal peoples, such as an array of psychosocial problems. In two recent surveys, 6 of 10 First Nations and Métis respondents identified residential schools as a significant contributor to poorer health status (Canadian Institute for Health Information, 2004). In 2001, the Canadian government, after deeply apologizing for this past policy, established the Indian Residential Schools Resolution Canada, a department dedicated to working with First Nations, Inuit, and Métis peoples to address and resolve issues arising from the legacy of residential schools (Indian Residential Schools Resolution Canada, 2005).

Religion as a Culture System

Religion can be seen as a cultural system, in that it is a system of meanings that shapes our experience. People who have shared common experiences over time develop commonalities of culture. (*Religion* comes from *re-ligare*: to bind together.) Family traditions are a commonality that develops over a generation or two. Religion is a commonality that develops over a longer time in groups of peoples.

Religious Beliefs and Approaches to Mental Illness

Religious beliefs often define an individual's relationship within a family and community. Many different religions are practiced throughout the world. Although Judeo-Christian beliefs tend to dominate Western societies and other religions, such as Islam, Hinduism, and Buddhism, to dominate Eastern and Middle Eastern cultures, it is likely that all religions are represented among Canadians. (See Connection Website for the Table: *World's Major Religions or Belief Forms.*)

Beliefs about mental illness are intimately linked with concepts of religion, social values, norms, and ideals of human relationships. These shared beliefs determine the nature of traditional medicine and provide the framework for interpreting symptoms and guiding action in response to them. Western medicine and psychiatry are premised on the belief that mental illness is caused by biologic and experiential events; many other cultures ascribe a metaphysical or spiritual cause as well (Health Canada, 2003c).

Aboriginal Spirituality and Culture

Aboriginal culture advocates that spiritual needs are as important as hunger and thirst (Scott, 1994). Getting in touch with one's own spirituality is identified as a key to recovery or healing. Spirituality is linked to a sense of life purpose and personal identity, and is seen as a key element for individuals to find their place in the world. To most Aboriginal people, the concept of spirituality refers to a sense of direction: it is not a religion, but a way of life.

Prejudice, Discrimination, Stereotyping, and Stigma

It is often difficult for one cultural group to understand the values, beliefs, and patterns of accepted behaviour of a different cultural group. This is especially true in regard to mental illness—some cultures view it as a condition for which the ill person must be punished and ostracized from society, whereas other cultures are more tolerant and believe that family and community members are key to the care and treatment of the mentally ill. In some cultures and with some disorders, the individual is not held responsible, and the family and community provide support. In others, particularly when the person has been violent or has caused others to suffer, the disruption to community well-being may lead to rejection, including subtle forms of banishment (Health Canada, 2003c). Mental illness indirectly affects all Canadians through a family member, friend, or colleague. Arboleda-Florez (2005) notes that families may also become casualties under the stress of caring for acutely mentally ill relatives, especially within a rejecting community.

The concepts of stereotyping, prejudice, discrimination, and stigma are important in understanding the life of people with mental disorders. **Stereotyping** is expecting individuals to act in a characteristic manner that conforms to a usually negative perception of their cultural group. Individual characteristics are not considered. Stereotyping occurs because of lack of exposure to enough people in a particular group. **Prejudice** is a hostile attitude toward others simply because they belong to a particular group that is considered to have objectionable characteristics. **Discrimination** is the differential treatment of others because they are members of a particular group or identified as being negatively different. It can include ignoring, derogatory name calling, denying services, and threatening. Prejudice, discrimination, and stereotyping lead to a lack of understanding and appreciation of differences among people. **Stigma** is the mark of a spoiled identity. In Ancient Greece, stigma was literally a sign cut or burnt into a person's body to indicate low moral status (Goffman, 1963). Stigma prevents a person, and often those with whom that person are connected, from being fully accepted within their society and leaves them feeling unaccepted, devalued, ostracized, and isolated (Jones et al., 1984). Even large groups within a society can become victims of stigma, such as those of certain ethnic or cultural groups, those of certain socioeconomic status, and certainly those with a mental handicap or illness. The presentation of mental disorders as unique to particular cultures can lead to stereotyping and increased stigmatization (Austin et al., 1999).

The Stigma of Mental Illness

People with mental illnesses or mental health problems often are stigmatized by the society in which they live, a phenomenon that has occurred across history (see Chapter 1). In his work, *Madness and Civilization*, Foucault (1967) argues that in the Middle Ages, madness came to occupy the position leprosy once held. Individuals deemed mad were excluded from society as lepers had been. Even with today's more enlightened view of mental illness, a stigma remains attached to those with mental disorders or those who seek help for mental illness. Individuals with mental illnesses typically are characterized in today's society as "crazy" or "nuts."

Despite the fact that 95% to 97% of violent crimes are committed by individuals without a mental illness (Monahan, 1996), mental illness is associated with violence in the public mind. Representations of people with mental illness in the media (eg, movies, television, magazines, and newspapers) can perpetuate this negative stereotype. Webster (2005) compared Canadian media coverage of a death due to domestic violence with that of the killing of an RCMP officer by a man with schizophrenia. She found the latter act received much greater coverage. As well, terms or phrases such as "crazies on the streets," "unpredictable," "off the wall," "uncontrollable," "monster," "tortured" and "a schizophrenic with a fondness for guns" were used.

Stigmatization is a great obstacle to progress in mental health care and a powerful force in influencing the treatment and rehabilitation of people with a mental disorder. It is a barrier to seeking help. Despite availability of treatment, nearly two thirds of people with a known mental disorder never seek help from a health professional (World Health Organization [WHO, 2001]). When people are subjected to stigmatization, they become discouraged, hurt, and angry and develop low self-esteem.

They may try to conceal their disorder and worry that others may discover their illness (Wahl, 1999).

Cultural Competence

Health care professionals at every level need to add **cultural competence** to their repertoire of skills (Kent-Wilkinson, 2005). The CNA's (2004) position paper, *Promoting Culturally Competent Care*, outlines this obligation in relation to nursing.

> ◤ **KEY CONCEPT Cultural competence** is the application of knowledge, skill, attitudes and personal attributes required by nurses to provide appropriate care and services in relation to cultural characteristics of their clients (CNA, 2004).

Cultural competence includes valuing diversity, knowing about cultural mores and traditions of the populations being served, and being sensitive to these while caring for the individual. Nurses are responsible for acquiring, maintaining, and continually enhancing cultural competencies in relation to their clients. They are responsible for incorporating culture into all phases of the nursing process and in all domains of nursing practice (CNA, 2004).

To be culturally competent according to Browne and Fiske (2001), one does not have to have extensive knowledge of all cultures—this would be impossible. Rather, one must be aware that cultural differences exist; be aware that one's own culture is not superior to that of others; be careful to avoid imposing one's cultural beliefs on others; be willing to learn about and understand other people's cultures; and be willing to incorporate that knowledge into practice and educational curricula. An important first step is to recognize the influence of one's own culture on one's belief system and practice. See Box 3-2 for a research study on culturally competent care.

BOX 3.2 RESEARCH FOR BEST PRACTICE CULTURAL COMPETENCE

Culturally Competent Care for Psychiatric Clients Who Have a History of Sexual Abuse

THE QUESTION: What are nurses' perceptions of their ability to nurse clients with a history of sexual abuse when cultural differences are present?

METHOD: Survey of Canadian PMH nurses (N = 1,701)

FINDINGS: Cultural aspects of PMH nurses' attitudes, knowledge, and competencies regarding working with clients who have a history of sexual abuse were self-reported in the survey. Thirty-nine percent of the respondents worked at a facility having a significant number of clients from a different culture. Only 4.6% rated themselves as "very

competent." One cultural group, First Nations, was identified by sufficient numbers of nurses to generate themes concerning the challenge of working with clients from a particular culture. These themes included abuse as a cultural norm, concurrent and related health and social problems, reluctance to talk about problems, a need to learn about First Nations culture, and developing culturally competent nurses. PMH nurses indicated that they need further knowledge and understanding of cultural norms and practices if they are to provide appropriate care to clients with histories of sexual abuse.

Austin, W., Gallop, R., McCay, E. Peternelj-Taylor, C., & Bayer, M. (1999). Culturally competent care for psychiatric clients who have a history of sexual abuse. *Clinical Nursing Research, 8*(1), 5–25.

SOCIOECONOMIC CONTEXT OF MENTAL HEALTH CARE

The determinants of health, factors that influence our health status, are greatly affected by social and socioeconomic circumstances. Factors such as income and social status, social support networks, education, employment and working conditions, physical environment, and health services affect one's well-being. In 2000, the United Nations rated Canada the best country in the world in which to live. In subsequent years, it remained consistently in the top five. This assessment is based on a country's Human Development Index. Not everyone in Canada, however, enjoys the advantages of living in a highly developed country (Kendall, 2001).

Poverty in Canada

In Canada, 15% of all people were living in poverty in 1990. By 1999, this proportion had increased to 16.2%, an estimated 4,886,000 people, of whom 1,298,000 were children under the age of 18 years (Canadian Council on Social Development, 1999). Poverty changes a population's ability to make choices. Poverty chooses your life for you. Poverty in the North American context is primarily relative rather than absolute.

> ◆ **KEY CONCEPT Poverty** can be measured as absolute or relative. *Absolute poverty* is calculated by comparing a person's total income against the cost of goods and services essential to daily life. *Relative poverty* is measured by comparing total income and spending with those of the general population. (See http://canadianeconomy.gc.ca.)

Poverty and Mental Illness

Families living in poverty are under tremendous financial and emotional stress, which may trigger or exacerbate mental problems. Along with the daily stressors of trying to provide food and shelter for themselves and their families, lack of time, energy, and money prevents them from attending to their psychological needs. Often, these families become trapped in a downward economic spiral, as tension and stress mount. The inability to gain employment and the lack of financial independence only add to the feelings of powerlessness and low self-esteem. Being self-supporting gives one a feeling of control over life and bolsters self-esteem. Dependence on others or the government causes frustration, anger, apathy, and feelings of depression and meaninglessness (Axelson, 1999). Alcoholism, depression, and child and partner abuse may become a means of coping with such hopelessness and despair. The homeless population is the group most at risk for being unable to escape this spiral of poverty. The number of homeless people with mental illness in Canada is causing great concern, and adequate societal responses are being sought (see Chapter 2).

The chances of becoming poor are greater if someone is mentally ill. Three percent of Canadians suffer from severe and chronic mental disorders that can cause serious functional limitations and social and economic impairment (Kirby Report, 2002). Still, many people with mental illness hold down well-paid jobs. A key factor for many of these people is a strong support network of family and friends. The World Health Organization (WHO), in a three decade study, found that people with schizophrenia living in less-developed nations typically do better than those in industrialized countries like Canada. The reason may be that people with schizophrenia in those countries are included in social events, family obligations, and work (WHO, 2001).

Socioeconomic Influences on Aboriginal Mental Health

Although Canada is considered to have one of the finest publicly funded health care systems, Aboriginal populations continue to exhibit morbidity and mortality rates in some dimensions in excess of some Third World countries. Shamefully, the gap in life expectancy between First Nations individuals and other Canadians is 7 years. Approximately half of the children in our Aboriginal communities live in poverty (Canadian Criminal Justice Association, 2000). Aboriginal peoples experience lower education levels and are seriously underrepresented in the labour force (Health Canada, 2003a). Those living in rural areas also contend with inadequate housing. Many Aboriginals homes do not have a telephone, computer, or Internet access. Aboriginal peoples, according to Health Canada (2003b) experience higher rates of suicide, infant mortality, and incarceration.

There is a connection between socioeconomic status and involvement with the criminal justice system, and Aboriginal peoples are overrepresented in that system. Although they represent about 3% of the population, they form about 16% of the offender population (Canadian Criminal Justice Association, 2000). Social and health problems, along with the effects of rapid culture change, cultural oppression, and marginalization (Kirmayer, Simpson, & Cargo, 2003), are reflected in high rates of mental health problems (Kirmayer, Brass, & Tait, 2000; Petawabano, Gourdeau, Jourdain, Palliser-Tulugak, & Cossette, 1994; Waldram, 1997).

Epidemiologic studies have documented high levels of mental health problems in many Canadian Aboriginal communities (Waldram, Herring, & Young, 1995; Kirmayer, 1994; Kirmayer, Gill, Fletcher, Ternar, Quesney, & Smith, 1993; Royal Commission on Aboriginal Peoples, 1995). These studies indicate rates of psychiatric disorders varying from levels comparable to those found in the general population to up to twice those of neighbouring non-Aboriginal communities (Kirmayer, Brass, & Tait, 2000). Most estimates of the prevalence of psychiatric disorders are based on service utilization records, but because many Aboriginal people never come for treatment, service utilization is at best only a lower estimate of the true prevalence of distress in the community.

There is a tendency of First Nations individuals not to use the mental health services provided by the dominant culture. If services are accessed, approximately 50% drop out, and for many, treatments are not effective (Smye & Browne, 2002), partly because mental health services ignore the unique cultural identities, histories, and sociopolitical contexts of the everyday lives of Aboriginal peoples. Many indigenous communities are doing well despite the challenges they face. Transforming attitudes, policies, and practice principles by gaining an awareness of the political and historical forces shaping the health and social status of indigenous peoples is vital (Browne & Fiske, 2001). Culturally sensitive mental health services and health promotion could contribute to greater well-being.

Geographic Location and Access to Mental Health Services

Most mental health services are located in urban areas, with access for people in the far North being very different from that of people living in the more highly populated areas of Canada. All age groups in rural areas have limited access to health care, but the lack of resources is particularly problematic for children and elderly people, who have specialized needs.

Treatment approaches may be effective in one part of the country but not in another. Haddon, Merritt-Gray, and Wuest (2004) have noted that "historically it has been assumed that urban social service models will work well in rural communities" (p. 249). This, however, is not always the case. The way in which a rural environment influences social and health needs, as well as help-seeking behaviours, is only beginning to be explored. Yet more than 22% of Canadians and 50% of Atlantic Canadians live in rural areas (Statistics Canada, 1997).

Transportation is a major barrier to the receipt of health services in rural areas. Costs of travel and accommodation for patients and families can be high, in dollars and energy. Services should be delivered in communities where possible. Mobile service delivery and specialist circuits are one option. **Telehealth** also holds promise. Telehealth is the use of electronic information and communication technologies to support health care services over distance. It ranges from the retrieval of laboratory results or other health records posted on a network to the assessment of a person by a psychiatrist through videoconferencing.

Role of Psychiatric and Mental Health Nurses in Rural and Remote Areas and in the North

The role of nurses takes on new dimensions in rural and remote areas or in Canada's north, where they are often the only health care professional. Nurses in these regions often practice in expanded roles, acting as the first point of contact within the health system. Delivering health services to First Nations people is challenged by this population's geographic dispersion. According to the Auditor General, in 1997, there were 121 First Nations communities with no road access, and an additional 75 communities that had road access but were more than 90 kilometres from the nearest physician. About 75% of the communities had fewer than 1,000 members (Health Canada, 1997).

LEGAL CONTEXT OF MENTAL HEALTH CARE

Every society needs laws to achieve its objectives. According to WHO (2005b), the fundamental aim of mental health legislation is to protect, promote, and improve the lives and mental well-being of citizens.

Human Rights and Mental Illness

In accordance with the objectives of the United Nations (UN) Charter and international agreements, a fundamental basis for mental health legislation is human rights. Key rights and principles include equality and nondiscrimination, the right to privacy and individual autonomy, freedom from inhuman and degrading treatment, the principle of the least restrictive environment, and the rights to information and participation.

In most parts of the world, according to the Romanow Report in 2002, mental health and mental illness are not given the same degree of importance as physical health (Health Canada, 2002). Global resources for people suffering from mental and neurologic disorders are grossly insufficient to address the growing burden of mental health needs (WHO, 2005b). The WHO (2005a) *Mental Health Atlas—2005* shows no substantial change in global mental health resources since 2001 and a growing gap between allocations in high and low-income countries (CNA, 2005). Currently, more than 40% of countries have no mental health policy and more than 30% have no mental health program. About 25% of countries have no mental health legislation (WHO, 2001). Canada is one of the few industrialized countries without a national mental health strategy. The Canadian Minister of Health announced at the end of 2005 that a Commission on Mental Health and Mental Illness will be established (Canadian Mental Health Association, 2005c).

BOX 3.3

International Agreements Relevant to Culture and to Mental Health

1948   Universal Declaration of Human Rights
1957   The Indigenous and Tribal Populations Convention, 1957 (No. 107)
1976   International Covenant on Economic, Social, and Cultural Rights (ICESCR)
1989   Indigenous and Tribal (Peoples Populations) Convention (Revised)
1990   Declaration of Caracas (WHO, 1990)
1991   Principles of Protection of Persons With Mental Illness (United Nations, 1991)

International Agreements

There are many significant international agreements to help protect people with mental illness. The most significant are listed in Box 3-3. Mental health principles, adopted by the UN in 1991, are outlined in Box 3-4. See Web Links at the end of the chapter for Internet access information regarding national and international advocacy organizations.

Mental Health Legislation

Mental health legislation is a powerful tool for codifying and consolidating these fundamental values and principles, for protecting the rights of people with mental disorders, and for promoting the mental health of populations. It offers an important mechanism to ensure adequate and appropriate care and treatment. Being unable to access treatment and care is an infringement of a person's right to health and right to access can be included in legislation (WHO, 2005c).

BOX 3.4

Rights of Persons With Mental Illness

- Right to medical care (Principle 1.1)
- Right to be treated with humanity and respect (Principle 1.2)
- Equal protection right (Principle 1.4)
- Right to be cared for in the community (Principle 7)
- Right to provide informed consent before receiving any treatment (Principle 11)
- Right to privacy (Principle 13)
- Freedom of communication (Principle 13)
- Freedom of religion (Principle 13)
- Right to voluntary admission (Principles 15 and 16)
- Right to judicial guarantees (Principle 17)

From United Nations. (1991). Principles for the protection of persons with mental illness and the improvement of mental health care. Adopted by General Assembly resolution 46/119 of 17 December 1991, Office of the United Nations High Commissioner for Human Rights. Retrieved October 15, 2005, from http://www.unhchr.ch/html/menu3/b/68.htm.

BOX 3.5

Provincial Mental Health Care Acts

PROVINCE	WEBSITE ADDRESS
Alberta	www.canlii.org
British Columbia	www.qp.gov.bc.ca
Manitoba	http://web2.gov.mb.ca
New Brunswick	www.gnb.ca
Nfld. & Labrador	www.canlii.org
Northwest Territories	http://www.canlii.org
Nova Scotia	http://www.gov.ns.ca
Nunavut	www.nunavutcourtofjustice.ca
Ontario	www.mhcva.on.ca
	www.ontario.cmha.ca
	Note: The Act must be purchased.
Prince Edward Island	www.canlii.org
Quebec	www2.publicationsduquebec.gouv.qc.ca
	Note: The Act must be purchased.
Saskatchewan	www.qp.gov.sk.ca
Yukon	www.canlii.org

Canadian Mental Health Acts

Legislation in Canada strongly influences the context of our mental health care. Each province and territory is guided by its own Mental Health Care Acts. These acts must be congruent with the rights stipulated under the *1982 Charter of Rights and Freedoms* (Department of Justice Canada, 2005) and the resources to enforce the acts must be in place. See Box 3-5 for Internet access information on the various mental health acts.

> **KEY CONCEPT A Mental Health Act** is a law that gives certain powers, and sets the conditions (including time limits) for those powers, to stipulated health care professionals and designated institutions regarding the admission and treatment of individuals with a mental disorder.

Gray and O'Reilly (2001) reviewed the mental health act provisions in all Canadian jurisdictions. They found significant differences among the provinces and territories and raised a concern that some provisions might prevent people from receiving appropriate care. See Box 3-6 for an overview, based on their work, of basic criteria for involuntary admission in the various jurisdictions. It is the responsibility of PMH nurses to understand the Mental Health Act of their province or territory. Nurses need to be able to explain the Act's basic provisions to people with mental illness and their families.

Canadian mental health acts may allow involuntary treatment of a person admitted under such an act if the person is not considered **competent** to make decisions regarding treatment. Competence, in this respect, means being able to understand (at a basic level) matters relevant to the decision and to understand the consequences of the decision. Competence is not a fixed

BOX 3.6

Involuntary Admission Criteria in Provincial and Territorial Mental Health Acts

Is not suitable as a voluntary inpatient: A person who is willing and capable of consenting to a voluntary admission cannot be admitted with an involuntary status anywhere in Canada.

Meets the definition of mental disorder: The person must have a mental disorder. In many, but not all, of the jurisdictions, it is specified that the disorder must seriously impair the person's functioning.

Meets the criteria for harm: In most jurisdictions, this is not limited to serious bodily harm; nonbodily harms are acceptable. The criterion of "danger" stipulated in some acts, however, has been interpreted by the courts to mean bodily harm.

Likely to suffer substantial mental or physical deterioration: This is included in some provinces (British Columbia, Saskatchewan, Manitoba, and Ontario) as an alternative to the harm criterion.

In need of psychiatric treatment: This is a criterion in British Columbia, Saskatchewan, and Ontario. It is possible in other jurisdictions to commit a person with a mental disorder who is dangerous, but for whom there is no treatment (e.g., antisocial personality disorder) for the purpose of preventative detention.

Refusal of treatment: by the person after admission: This is allowed in some jurisdictions but not others. In some jurisdictions, a refusal can be overruled in the person's best interests.

Review and appeal procedures regarding the validity of involuntary hospitalization: These are found in all jurisdictions.

From Gray, J., & O'Reilly, R. (2001). Clinically significant differences among Canadian Mental Health Acts. *Canadian Journal of Psychiatry, 46*, 315–321.

capacity; it changes over time. There are specific provisions within mental health acts regarding the evaluation of competency and what action may be taken if a person is deemed not competent.

When a person is unable to consent to treatment, consent from a **substitute decision maker** may be sought. Depending on the jurisdiction, these substitute decision makers can be state appointed, appointed by the person when competent, or be a guardian or relative. There are different criteria to guide substitute decision making: *best interests* (eg, treatment will make the person less ill; the person will get more ill without treatment; the benefits outweigh any risks), *capable wishes* (what the person expressed while capable, even if not in current best interests), and *modified best interests* (follow expressed wishes except if they would endanger the person or others).

Mandatory Outpatient Treatment

In some jurisdictions, an involuntary patient may return to the community on a *conditional leave* if the admission criteria are still met and if stipulations for treatment are followed. If the stipulations (eg, taking medication and meeting with a physician) are not followed, the person can be returned to the hospital. **Mandatory outpatient treatment** (MOT) involves legal provisions requiring people with a mental illness to comply with a treatment plan while living in the community (O'Reilly et al., 2003). **Community treatment orders** (CTOs) are a type of MOT, existing in Saskatchewan and Ontario, that are usually initiated by a physician. People who do not meet involuntary admission criteria and who are not necessarily in a hospital at the time of the CTO can be required to comply with the stipulated treatment.

CTOs are meant to ensure that people with serious mental illness get the care and treatment they need in a community-based system. The intent is to remove barriers to help from families, police, and health care professionals in getting people at risk for harm to self or others the care and treatment they need (CMHA, 2005a, 2005b; Government of Ontario, 2005). It is, perhaps, unfortunate that there is a tendency to name MOT legislation, such as Brian's Law in Ontario, after an individual killed by a person who acted on the basis of psychotic delusions. This emphasizes protection of society, rather than the health of the ill person.

MOT remains a somewhat controversial concept in Canada, although it has existed for more than 20 years in some states in the United States. The concern is that a person's right to autonomy should not be infringed on unless absolutely necessary. Szasz (1961, 2005), who challenges the legitimacy of any psychiatric treatment, argues that CTOs have "turned all of society into a kind of mental hospital" (2005, p. 81).

Separate from mental health legislation are the legal provisions that can require people to follow treatment as a condition of probation. People who have been found not criminally responsible for a crime may need to comply with treatment monitored by Criminal Code Review Boards (O'Reilly et al., 2003) (see Chapter 33).

RESEARCH AND THE CONTEXT OF MENTAL HEALTH CARE

Many health professionals, advocacy groups, and policy analysts believe that greater support for research on the context of mental health issues is urgently required. Unresolved, these issues pose a serious threat to the survival and health of Canadian communities. Such research should include studies on methodologies to identify the determinants of mental health disorders; to explore the prevalence of preventable causative factors related to mental illness; to determine the nature and extent of barriers to access to mental health treatment and care; and to determine whether mental health legislation is effective (Arboleda-Florez, 2005).

SUMMARY OF KEY POINTS

- The term *culture* is defined as a way of life that manifests the learned beliefs, values, and accepted behaviours that are transmitted socially within a specific group.
- Cultural competence consists of cultural awareness, cultural knowledge, cultural skills, and cultural encounters. It is an obligation of all Canadian nurses.
- Aboriginal mental illness and disorders encompass the recognition of the historical, socioeconomic, and political circumstances of Aboriginal people in Canada. Mental imbalance as experienced by Aboriginal peoples may be related to one or all of the life experiences historically confronting Aboriginal people.
- Stigmatization occurs as a result of prejudice, discrimination, and stereotyping. Cultural groups and people with mental illness are stigmatized.
- Religious beliefs are closely intertwined with beliefs about health and mental illness.
- Mental health services should be integrated as completely as possible into the helping systems currently accepted by the culture.
- Access to mental health treatment is particularly limited for those living in rural, remote, and northern areas or those living in poverty.
- Progressive legislation can be an effective tool to promote access to mental health care as well as to promote and protect the rights of people with mental disorders.

CRITICAL THINKING CHALLENGES

1 Discuss to what extent culture matters in the treatment of mental illness and Aboriginal health in Canada.
2 Explore the Aboriginal understanding of mental health through conversations with people of the Aboriginal culture or by reading books such as Waldram's *Revenge of the Windigo: The Construction of the Mind and Mental Health of North American Aboriginal Peoples (Waldram, 2004).*
3 Compare the access to mental health services between rural areas to urban areas in your province or territory.
4 What does poverty look like in your local community?
5 Discuss how socioeconomics factors influence the mental health of Canadians.
6 Compare Canada's mental health legislation to international initiatives.
7 Outline the basic tenets of the mental health act of your province or territory.
8 Identify the research needed to improve the context of Canadian mental health care.

WEB LINKS

www.camimh.ca The Canadian Alliance on Mental Illness and Mental Health (CAMIMH) is the largest mental health advocacy group in Canada. It is an alliance of mental health organizations comprised of health care providers as well as of the mentally ill and their families.

www.cmha.ca The Canadian Mental Health Association (CMHA) is a national, voluntary organization that promotes mental health and serves consumers and others through education, public awareness, research, advocacy, and direct services.

www.mdri.org Mental Disability Rights International (MDRI) is an advocacy organization dedicated to the recognition and enforcement of rights of people with mental disabilities.

www.who.int/about/en The World Health Organization (WHO) is the United Nations agency for health. The WHO objective is, as set out in its Constitution, the attainment by all peoples of the highest possible level of health.

www.wfmh.org The World Federation for Mental Health (WFMH) is the only international, multidisciplinary, grassroots advocacy and education mental health organization.

MOVIES

Saint Monica: 2002. Set in Toronto's Portuguese-Canadian community, this film tells the story of Monica, a lonely ten-year-old girl fixated on things spiritual: she plays with toy angels and Blessed Virgin Mary figurines the way other kids play at Harry Potter. When Monica is denied the role of an angel in her church's holy day procession because her family moves to a new neighbourhood, she steals the angel wings, only to lose them. The wings are found by a mentally ill, homeless woman, Mary. The story evolves as Monica attempts to recover the wings and develops a unique relationship with Mary.

VIEWING POINTS: Consider how the religious beliefs of others may be difficult to understand at first glance. Did Monica's and Mary's behaviours gain meaning for you by the end of the film? Note the settings of the drop inn center and the psychiatric hospital.

Where the Spirit Lives: 1989. This Canadian movie reveals the oppression of Aboriginal culture in residential schools through the story of a young girl, Komi. It is 1937 and Komi, along with others, is abducted to a Catholic residential school (based on Shubenacadie

Indian Residential School in Nova Scotia). This movie captures, in a thoughtful way, the experience of the children and their families. It shows the complex motivations of those enacting this coercive policy.

VIEWING POINTS: Reflect on what is revealed about self-identity and the role culture plays within its development. How does the film reveal the "the tyranny of the majority?"

Nuts: 1987. A strong willed, high-priced prostitute, played by Barbra Streisand, is accused of manslaughter. Her family and attorney want her to plead guilty by reason of insanity. The movie revolves around their attempts to have her declared incompetent to stand trial, which would commit her to a mental health facility and deny her a trial, and her anger and rebellion against this type of plea.

VIEWING POINTS: Consider the complexities of the concept of "competence" and "incompetence" as illustrated in this film.

REFERENCES

Aboriginal Health Glossary. (2004). *Aboriginal health and cultural diversity online glossary.* Compiled by A. Kent-Wilkinson (assistant professor) & technology by M. Tomtene (programmer analyst). College of Nursing, University of Saskatchewan, Saskatoon, SK. Retrieved January 2, 2005, from http://www.usask.ca/nursing/aboriginalglossary.

American Psychiatric Association. (1994). *Diagnostic and statistical manual of mental disorders* [DSM IV] (4th ed.). Washington, DC: Author.

American Association. (2000). (4th ed., text revision). Washington, DC: Author.

American Psychiatric Association. (2000). *Diagnostic and statistical manual of mental disorders* [DSM IV-TR] (4th ed., text revision). Washington, DC: Author.

Arboleda-Florez, J. (2005). The epidemiology of mental illness in Canada. *Canadian Public Policy-Analyse de Politiques, 31,* S13–S16. Retrieved December 6, 2005, from Special Electronic Supplement on Mental Health Reform for the 21st Century: http://economics.ca/cgi/jab?journal=cpp&view=v31s1/CPPv31s1p013.pdf\.http://www.afn.ca/Programs/Health%20Secretariat/health.htm.

Austin, W., Gallop, R., McCay, E. Peternelj-Taylor, C., & Bayer, M. (1999). Culturally competent care for psychiatric clients who have a history of sexual abuse. *Clinical Nursing Research, 8*(1), 5–25.

Axelson, J. (1999). *Counseling and development in a multicultural society.* Belmont, CA: Wadsworth, Brooks/Cole.

Browne, A. J., & Fiske, J. (2001). First Nations women's encounters with mainstream health care services. *Western Journal of Nursing Research, 23*(2), 126–147. Retrieved May 9, 2003 from EBSCO database, http://content.ebsco.com/fulltext.asp?wasp=1b22a8wryn2ywvuhugdh&ext=.pdf.

Canadian Council on Social Development. (1999). *Poverty statistics.* Retrieved November 13, 2005, from http://www.ccsd.ca/factsheets/fs_pov9099.htm.

Canadian Criminal Justice Association. (2000, May 15). *Aboriginal people and the criminal justice system.* Retrieved February 5, 2005, from http://www.ccja-acjp.ca/en/abori.html.

Canadian Health Network. (1997). *Facts about multiculturalism.* Retrieved May 13, 2004, from http://www.canadian-health-network.ca/english/multicul/facts_issues.html.

Canadian Institute for Health Information. (2004). *Aboriginal peoples health: Improving the health of Canadians.* Chapter 4 Report by the Canadian Population Health Initiative (CPHI) of the Canadian Institute for Health Information. Retrieved August 26, 2004, from http://secure.cihi.ca/cihiweb/dispPage.jsp?cw_page=media_25feb2004_b3_e.

Canadian Mental Health Association. (2005a). *CMHA community treatment orders.* Retrieved November 21, 2005, from http://www.ontario.cmha.ca/content/mental_health_system/legislation/community_treatment_orders.asp.

Canadian Mental Health Association. (2005b). *CMHA Mental Health Act.* Retrieved November 21, 2005, from http://www.ontario.cmha.ca/content/mental_health_system/legislation/mental_health_act.asp.

Canadian Mental Health Association. (2005c, Nov. 24). *Commission established to serve country's mental health needs.* Ottawa: Author. Retrieved December 7, 2005, from http://www.cmha.ca/bins/content_page.asp?cid=6-20-21-809.

Canadian Nurses Association. (2004). *Promoting culturally competent care* [Position Statement]. Retrieved January 31, 2005, from http://cna-aiic.ca/CNA/documents/pdf/publications/PS73_Promoting_Culturally_Competent_Care_March_2004_e.pdf.

Canadian Nurses Association. (2005). Global mental health care. *CNA Review,* October 10–23.

Department of Justice Canada. (2005). *Canadian Charter of Rights and Freedoms.* Constitution Act, 1982(79). Constitution Acts 1967–1982. Retrieved November 21, 2005, from http://canada.justice.gc.ca/Loireg/charte/const_en.html.

Foucault, M. (1967). *Madness and civilization: A history of insanity in the age of reason.* (R. Howard, Trans.). London: Tavistock Publications. (Original work published 1961.)

Frideres, J. S. (1998). *Aboriginal peoples in Canada: Contemporary conflicts* (5th ed.). Scarborough, Ontario: Prentice Hall, Allyn & Bacon.

Geertz, C. (1973). *The interpretation of cultures: Selected essays.* New York: Basic Books.

Goffman, I. (1963). *Stigma: Notes on the management of spoiled identity.* Englewood Cliffs, NJ: Prentice Hall.

Government of Ontario. (2005). *Community treatment orders.* Ministry of Health & Long Term Care. Retrieved November 21, 2005, from http://www.health.gov.on.ca/english/public/pub/mental/treatment_order.html.

Government of Saskatchewan. (2003). *Glossary.* Government Relations and Aboriginal Affairs (GS-GRAA). Regina: Author.

Gray, J. & O'Reilly, R. (2001). Clinically significant differences among Canadian Mental Health Acts. *Canadian Journal of Psychiatry, 46,* 315–321.

Haddon, A., Merritt-Gray, M., & Wuest, J. (2004). Private matters and public knowledge in rural communities: The paradox. In M. L. Stirling, C. A. Cameron, N. Nason-Clark, & B. Miedema (Eds.), *Understanding abuse: Partnering for change* (pp. 249–266). Toronto: University of Toronto Press.

Health Canada. (1997, Oct.). *Report of the Auditor General of Canada to the House of Commons.* Chapter 13, Health Canada—First Nations Health. Retrieved October 10, 2005, from http://www.oag-bvg.gc.ca/domino/reports.nsf/html/ch9713e.html.

Health Canada. (2002, November 28). *Romanow Report.* Final report. Commission on the Future of Health Care in Canada. Retrieved October 14, 2005, from http://www.hc-sc.gc.ca/english/care/romanow/hcc0086.html.

Health Canada. (2003a, July 8). *First Nations and Inuit regional health survey.* Retrieved March 7, 2005, from http://www.hc-sc.gc.ca/fnihb-dgspni/fnihb/aboriginalhealth/reports_summaries/regional_survey.htm.

Health Canada. (2003b). Suicidal behaviour. In *Clinical guidelines for nurses in primary care, Chapter 15, Mental health.* Nursing in First Nations Communities. Retrieved February 21, 2005, from http://www.hc-c.gc.ca/fnihb/ons/nursing/resources/clinical_guidelines/chapter_15.htm#15-35.

Health Canada. (2003c). *What determines health? Sante de la population health?* Retrieved January 6, 2005, from http://www.hcsc.gc.ca/hppb/phdd/determinants/determinants.html.

Indian Residential Schools Resolution Canada. (2005). *Government of Canada reaches historic Agreement in Principle—November 23, 2005.* Retrieved January 15, 2005, from http://www.irsr-rqpi.gc.ca/english/index.html.

Industry Canada. (2003). *Residential schools. Contemporary Aboriginal Issues. Canada's SchoolNet.* Retrieved November 6, 2005, from http://www.schoolnet.ca/aboriginal/issues/schools-e.html.

Jones, E. E., Farina, A., Hastorf, A. H., Markus, H., Miller, D. T., & Scott, R. (1984). *Social stigma: The psychology of marked relationships.* New York: Freeman.

Kendall, J. (2001). Circles of disadvantage: Aboriginal poverty and underdevelopment in Canada. *American Review of Canadian Studies* (p. 43). Retrieved January 17, 2003, from Expanded Academic ASAP database.

Kent-Wilknson, A. (2005). *Aboriginal health and cultural diversity: Educational resources for teachers.* Paper included in Conference Proceedings. Creating the Future, WestCAST 2005, University of Saskatchewan, Saskatoon, SK. February 16–19, 2005.

Kirby Report. (2002). *The health of Canadians—The federal role: Final report. Volume Six: Recommendations for reform.* The Standing Senate Committee on Social Affairs, Science and Technology. Retrieved October 15, 2005, from http://www.parl.gc.ca/37/2/parlbus/commbus/senate/com-e/soci-e/rep-e/repoct02vol6-e.htm.

Kirmayer, L. J. (1994). Is the concept of *mental* disorder culturally relative? In S. A. Kirk & S. Einbinder (Eds.), *Controversial issues in mental health* (p 1–20). Boston: Allyn & Bacon.

Kirmayer, L. J., Brass, G. M., & Tait, C. L. (2000). The *mental health of Aboriginal* peoples: Transformations of identity and community. *Canadian Journal of Psychiatry, 45*(7), 607–616.

Kirmayer, L. J., Gill, K. Fletcher, C., Ternar, Y., Quesney, C., Ferrara, N., & Smith, A. (1993). *Emerging trends in mental health research among Canadian Aboriginal peoples.* Culture & Mental Health Research Unit Report No. 2, prepared for the Royal Commission on Aboriginal Peoples, Montreal.

Kirmayer, L., Simpson, C., & Cargo, M. (2003). Indigenous populations healing traditions: Culture, community and *mental health* promotion with Canadian Aboriginal peoples. *Australasian Psychiatry, 11*(Suppl.), S15.

Monahan, J. (1996, Oct.). Mental illness and violent crime. *Research preview: National Institute of Justice.* Retrieved January 25, 2006 from http://www.ncjrs.gov/pdffiles/mentiln.pdf.

Morrison, R. B., & Wilson, C. R. (Eds.). (1988). *Native peoples: The Canadian experience.* Toronto: McClelland and Stewart.

O'Reilly, R., Brooks, S., Chaimowitz, G., Neilson, G., Carr, P., Zikos, E., Leichner, P., & Beck, P. (2003, Jan.). Mandatory outpatient treatment. *Canadian Psychiatric Association Position Paper.* Retrieved February 1, 2006, from http://www.psychdirect.com/forensic/PsychLaw/cto/pos_paper_mandatory_treat.htm

Petawabano, B., Gourdeau, E., Jourdain, F., Palliser-Tulugak, A., & Cossette, J. (1994). *Mental health and Aboriginal people of Québec.* Montréal: Gaëtan Morin Éditeur.

Public Health Agency of Canada. (2004). *Is mental illness related to poverty?* Canadian Health Network. Retrieved February 21, 2005, from http://www.canadian-health network.ca/servlet/ContentServer?cid=1001871&pagename=CHNRCS%2FCHNResource%2FFAQCHNResourceTemplate&c=CHNResource&lang=En.

Public Health Agency of Canada. (2005). *Appendix 1: Using the right terms.* Division of Aging and Seniors. Retrieved January 21, 2005, from http://www.phac-aspc.gc.ca/seniors-aines/pubs/communicating_aboriginal/appendix_e.htm#ab.

Royal Commission on Aboriginal Peoples. (1995). *Choosing life: Special report on suicide among Aboriginal people.* Ottawa: Supply and Services.

Royal Commission on Aboriginal Peoples. (1996). *Final report.* Ottawa: Communication Group.

Scott, K. (1994). Substance use among Indigenous Canadians. National Native Alcohol and Drug Addiction Program, Health and Welfare Canada In: McKenzie, D. (Ed.), *Aboriginal substance use: Research issues.* Ottawa: Canadian Centre on Substance Abuse.

Smye, V., & Browne, A. (2002). "Cultural safety" and the analysis of health *policy affecting* Aboriginal people. *Nurse Researcher, 9*(3), 42–56.

Statistics Canada. (1997). *A statistical comparison of women's experience of violence in urban and rural areas.* Ottawa: Canadian Centre for Justice Statistics.

Statistics Canada. (2003, Jan. 21). *Aboriginal peoples of Canada: A demographic profile.* 2001 Census: Analysis series. Report no. 96F0030XIE2001007. Ottawa: Author. Retrieved October 21, 2005, from http://www12.statcan.ca/english/census01/products/analytic/companion/abor/pdf/96F0030XIE2001007.pdf.

Szasz, T. (1961). *The myth of mental illness: Foundations of a theory of personal conduct.* New York: Hoeber-Harper.

Szasz, T. (2005). "Idiots, infants, and the insane": Mental illness and legal incompetence. *Journal of Medical Ethics 31*(2), 78–81.

United Nations. (1991). Principles for the protection of persons with mental illness and the improvement of mental health care. Adopted by General Assembly resolution 46/119 of 17 December 1991, Office of the United Nations High Commissioner for Human Rights. Retrieved October 15, 2005, from http://www.unhchr.ch/html/menu3/68.htm.

Vedantam, S. (2005, June 26). Patients' diversity is often discounted: Alternatives to mainstream medical treatment call for recognizing ethnic, social differences. Mind and Culture: Psychiatry's Missing Diagnosis. *Washington Post,* A01. Retrieved October 22, 2005, from http://www.washingtonpost.com/wp-dyn/content/article/2005/06/25/AR2005062500982.html.

Wahl, O. F. (1999). Mental health consumers' experience of stigma. *Schizophrenia Bulletin, 25*(3), 467–478.

Waldram, J. B. (1997). The Aboriginal people of Canada: Colonialism and mental health. In I. Al-Issa, & M. Tousignant (Eds.), *Ethnicity, immigration, and psychopathology.* New York: Plenum Press.

Waldram, J. B. (2004). *Revenge of the Windigo: The construction of the mind and mental health of North American Aboriginal peoples.* Toronto: University of Toronto Press.

Waldram, J. B., Herring, D. A., & Young, T. K. (1995). *Aboriginal health in Canada: Historical, cultural, and epidemiological perspectives.* Toronto: University of Toronto Press.

Webster, C. (2005, Nov.). News media critique: "Crazies in the Streets." *International Journal of Mental Health & Addiction, 3*(2), 64–68.

World Health Organization. (1990). *Declaration of Caracas.* Adopted by WHO in 1990. Geneva: Author.

World Health Organization. (2001, Oct. 4). *The world health report 2001. Mental health: New understanding, new hope.* Geneva: Author. Retrieved October 13, 2005, from http://www.who.int/whr/2001/en/.

World Health Organization. (2005a). *Mental Health Atlas—2005.* A project of the Department of Mental Health and Substance Abuse, Geneva: Author. Retrieved October 31, 2005, from http://www.who.int/mental_health/evidence/atlas/.

World Health Organization. (2005b, Oct. 7). *New WHO mental health atlas shows global mental health resources remain inadequate.* Geneva: Author. Retrieved October 31, 2005, from http://www.who.int/mediacentre/news/notes/2005/np21/en/index.html.

World Health Organization. (2005c). *WHO Resource book on mental health, human rights and legislation.* Geneva: Author. Retrieved October 15, 2005, from http://whqlibdoc.who.int/publications/2005/924156282X.pdf.

CHAPTER

4

The Continuum of Psychiatric and Mental Health Care

Freida Chavez, Denise M. Gibson, and
Robert B. Noud

LEARNING OBJECTIVES

After studying this chapter, you will be able to:

- Identify the different treatment settings and associated programs along the continuum of care.
- Discuss the role of the nurse at different points along the continuum of care.
- Describe current health care trends in psychiatric services.
- Explain how the concept of the least restrictive environment influences the assessment of patients for placement in different treatment settings.
- Discuss the Tidal Model and person-centred care in psychiatric and mental health nursing.

KEY TERMS

assertive community treatment ▪ case management ▪ clubhouse model ▪ continuum of care ▪ coordination of care ▪ crisis intervention ▪ empowerment ▪ in-home mental health care ▪ intensive case management ▪ intensive residential services ▪ intensive outpatient program ▪ least restrictive environment ▪ outpatient detoxification ▪ partial hospitalization ▪ psychiatric rehabilitation programs ▪ referral ▪ reintegration ▪ relapse ▪ residential services ▪ stabilization ▪ tidal model

⬟ KEY CONCEPT

- continuum of care

The evolution of a behavioural health care system is affected by scientific advances and social factors. The nature of mental illnesses requires varying levels of support and intervention at different times of the disorders, as well as family, peer, and community support. A demand exists for a comprehensive, holistic and person-centred approach to care that encompasses all levels of need. Consumers, families, providers, advocacy groups, and policy makers no longer accept long-term institutionalization, once the hallmark of psychiatric care. Instead, they advocate for short-term treatment in an environment that promotes dignity and well-being while meeting the patient's biologic, psychological, and social needs.

The mental health system within the framework of national health care in Canada consists of provincial psychiatric hospitals, general hospital psychiatric units, reimbursements to physicians (including psychiatrists), and community mental health programs. These services are under the provincial health ministries and operate under a single-payer health care system (Goering et al., 2000).

DEFINING THE CONTINUUM OF CARE

An individual's needs for ongoing clinical treatment and care are matched with the different services and programs and intensity of professional health services. The **continuum of care** for mental health services can be viewed from various perspectives and ranges from intense treatment (hospitalization) to supportive interventions (community).

> ⬟ **KEY CONCEPT** A **continuum of care** consists of an integrated system of settings, services, health care clinicians, and care levels, spanning illness-to-wellness states.

In a continuum, continuity of care is provided over an extended time. The appropriate medical, nursing, psychological, or social services may be delivered within one organization or across multiple organizations. The continuum facilitates the stability, continuity, and comprehensiveness of service to an individual and maximizes the **coordination of care** and services.

Least Restrictive Environment

The primary goal of the continuum of care is to provide treatment that allows the patient to achieve the highest level of functioning in the **least restrictive environment**. Treatment is delivered in the community, unless the acuity of the patient's illness requires hospitalization, and includes the use of outpatient settings (Wasylenki et al., 2000) and home care.

Coordination of Care

Coordination of care is the integration of appropriate services so that individualized person-centred care is provided. Appropriate services are those that are tailored to address a patient's strengths and weaknesses, cultural context, service preferences, and recovery goals, including **referral** to community resources and liaisons with others (e.g., physician, health care organizations, community services). Several agencies could be involved, but when care is coordinated, a person's needs are met in various flexible settings. Coordination of care requires collaborative and cooperative relationships among many services, including primary care, public health, mental health, social services, housing, education, the workplace, and criminal justice, to name a few.

In some instances, a whole array of integrated services is needed. For example, children can benefit from treatment and specialized support at home and school. These wraparound services represent a unique set of community services and natural supports individualized for the child or adult and family to achieve a positive set of outcomes.

COMPREHENSIVE MENTAL HEALTH SYSTEM: CORE PROGRAMS AND SERVICES

Case Management

Although there is no standardized definition of **case management**, coordinated care is often accomplished through this service model. (There is some controversy regarding the term "case management" in that consumers of services dislike being referred to as "cases to be managed." For this reason, the term "care coordinator" may be used.) There are different models of case management in Canada and the United States that differ in the basic philosophy of approaches and the emphasis on the different functions. Some programs use the "broker" model, in which the case manager locates services, links the patient with these services, and then monitors the patient's receipt of these services. "Clinical" case management is the model often referred to for the seriously mentally ill, which focuses on patients' needs and employs a therapeutic relationship.

Intensive case management is targeted for adults with serious mental illnesses or children with serious emotional disturbances. Managers of such cases have 24-hour availability, frequency of contact, proactive outreach, community-based practice, and fewer caseloads.

Case management is an integral part of mental health services and is organized around fundamental elements, including a comprehensive needs assessment, development of a plan of care to meet those needs, a method of ensuring the individual has access to care, and a method of monitoring the care provided. Case

---

BOX 4.1

Best Practices: Case Management and Assertive Community Treatment

Research Evidence

A wide array of rigorous trials have accumulated evidence demonstrating that Assertive Community Treatment (ACT) programs are superior for improving clinical status and reducing hospitalization. Studies generally support that ACT

- is a cost-effective alternative to hospitalization with standard after-care
- is for people at risk for repeated hospitalization
- produces high rates of patient and family satisfaction
- places no increased burden on families

A smaller body of controlled and uncontrolled studies shows that rehabilitation and personal strengths models are effective in improving social and vocational functioning and promoting residential stability and independence.

Key Elements of Best Practice

ACT programs include the following components:

- assertive outreach
- continuous, around-the-clock, time-unlimited, individual support to people with serious mental illness

- services that are predominantly provided in the community, as opposed to office based
- provision of flexible support specifically tailored to meet the needs of each individual
- involvement of consumers and their families in all aspects of service delivery, including design, implementation, monitoring, and evaluation
- provision of programs to serve special needs groups such as those with dual disorders

Other clinical case management programs based on different models are provided to serve patients with less intensive needs. Examples include

- rehabilitation model that focusses on improving living skills, is individually tailored to patient needs, and provides continuous interpersonal support
- personal strengths model which focuses on patient strengths and identifies or develops community resources and environments where patients can achieve success.

From Health Canada. (1998). *Review of best practices in mental health reform.* Prepared for the Federal/Provincial/Territorial Advisory Network on Mental Health.

---

managers collect a large amount of patient information and are confronted with coordinating multiple health care clinicians. One of the most valuable assets case managers possess is their ability to synthesize patient data and act as conduits between patients and the health care system (Williams, 2001).

Assertive Community Treatment

The **assertive community treatment** (ACT) model is a multidisciplinary clinical team approach providing 24-hour, intensive community services in the individual's natural setting that helps individuals with serious mental illness live in the community. The ACT approach provides a comprehensive range of treatment, rehabilitation, and supportive services to help patients meet the requirements of community living. One goal of ACT is to reduce recurrences of hospitalization. The rationale for ACT is that concentrating services for high-risk patients within a single multiservice team enhances continuity and coordination of care, improving both the quality of care and its cost-effectiveness (Bustillo et al., 2001). Initially, patients receive frequent direct assistance while reintegrating into the community. Emergency telephone numbers, or crisis numbers, are shared with patients and their families in the event that immediate assistance is needed. The ACT program is staffed 24 hours a day for emergency referral. Mobile treatment teams often are a part of the ACT model and provide assertive outreach, crisis intervention, and independent-living assistance with linkage to necessary sup-

port services. See Box 4-1 for a summary of Best Practices related to case management and assertive community treatment.

The Nurse as Case Manager

Because of the often cyclical nature of serious mental illness, psychiatric and mental health nurses serve in various pivotal functions across the continuum of care. These functions can involve both direct care and coordination of the care delivered by others. The case manager role is one in which the nurse must have commanding knowledge and special training in individual and group psychotherapy, psychopharmacology, and psychosocial rehabilitation. The nurse must have expertise not only in psychopathology and up-to-date treatment modalities, but also in treating the family as a unit. Modalities include the therapeutic use of self, networking and social systems, **crisis intervention**, pharmacology, physical assessment, psychosocial and functional assessment, and psychiatric rehabilitation. The repertoire of required skills includes collaborative, teaching, management, leadership, group, and research skills. The nurse as case manager probably is the most diverse role within the psychiatric continuum.

Crisis Response Systems and Psychiatric Emergency Services

An organized approach is required to treat individuals in crisis, including a mechanism for rapid access to care

(24/7), telephone crisis services, mobile crisis response, access to crisis emergency residential services, or psychiatric emergency services in hospitals. Crisis response systems emphasize crisis supports that are flexible, portable, and person centred. This type of short-term intervention care focusses on de-escalation, **stabilization**, symptom reduction, and prevention of **relapse** requiring inpatient services.

Crisis intervention units can be found in the emergency department of a general or psychiatric hospital or in crisis centres within a community mental health centre. Patients in crisis demonstrate severe symptoms of acute mental illness, including labile mood swings, suicidal ideation, or self-injurious behaviours. Therefore, this treatment option commands a high degree of nursing expertise. Patients in crisis usually require medications such as anxiolytics or benzodiazepines for symptom management. Key nursing roles include assessment of short-term therapeutic interventions and medication administration. Nurses also facilitate referrals for admission to the hospital or for outpatient services.

Crisis Stabilization

When the immediate crisis does not resolve quickly, crisis stabilization is the next step. The primary purpose of stabilization is control of precipitating symptoms through medications, behavioural interventions, and coordination with other agencies for appropriate aftercare. The major focus of nursing care in a short-term inpatient setting is symptom management. Ongoing assessment; short-term, focussed interventions; and medication administration and monitoring of efficacy and side effects are major components of nursing care during stabilization. Nurses also may provide focussed group psychotherapy designed to develop and strengthen the personal management strategies of patients. When treating aggressive or violent patients, the nurse monitors the appropriate use of seclusion and restraints. See Box 4-2 for a summary of Best Practices related to crisis response systems and psychiatric emergency services.

Acute Inpatient Care

Acute inpatient hospitalization involves the most intensive treatment and is considered the most restrictive setting in the continuum. Inpatient treatment is reserved for acutely ill patients who, because of a mental illness, meet one or more of three criteria: high risk for harming oneself, high risk for harming others, or inability to care for one's basic needs. Delivery of inpatient care can occur in a psychiatric hospital or psychiatric unit within a general hospital. Admission to inpatient environments can be voluntary or involuntary (see Chapter 3). Provincial legislation mental health acts describe conditions that warrant hospitalization. Length of inpatient stay is

---

BOX 4.2

Best Practices: Crisis Response Systems and Psychiatric Emergency Services

Research Evidence

Nonexperimental and descriptive studies suggest that
- crisis housing provides a viable alternative to hospitalization for people with serious mental illness
- diversion programs are effective
- crisis centres can serve people with psychosocial problems

Key Elements of Best Practice

Services are established that resolve crises for people with serious mental illness using minimally intrusive options. Crisis programs are in place to divert people from inpatient hospitalization. Evaluation and research protocols are incorporated into crisis programs. Examples of crisis programs are
- telephone crisis services
- mobile crisis units
- crisis residential services (eg, supervised apartments/houses, foster homes)
- psychiatric emergency/medical crisis services in hospitals

From Health Canada. (1998). *Review of best practices in mental health reform.* Prepared for the Federal/Provincial/Territorial Advisory Network on Mental Health.

---

kept as short as possible without harmful effects on patient outcomes.

Partial Hospitalization

During the 1980s, the costs associated with inpatient adult psychiatric and substance abuse treatment exceeded the clinical benefits when compared with outpatient care (Wise, 2000). **Partial hospitalization** programs ("Phips") or "day hospital care" were developed. Day hospital services complement inpatient mental health care and outpatient services and provide treatment to patients with acute psychiatric symptoms who are experiencing a decline in social or occupational functioning, who cannot function autonomously on a daily basis, or who do not pose imminent danger to themselves or others. It is a time-limited, ambulatory, active treatment program that offers therapeutically intensive, coordinated, and structured clinical services within a stable milieu. The aim of PHPs is patient stabilization without hospitalization or reduced length of inpatient care. An alternative to inpatient treatment, PHP, usually provides the resources to support therapeutic activities both for full-day and half-day programs.

In partial hospitalization, the interdisciplinary treatment team devises and executes a comprehensive plan of care encompassing behavioural therapy, social skills training, basic living skills training, education regarding illness and symptom identification and relapse prevention, community survival skills training, relaxation training, nutrition and exercise counselling, and other forms of expressive therapy. Compared with other outpatient programs, PHPs offer more intensive nursing care.

Outpatient Care

Outpatient care is a level of care that occurs outside of a hospital or institution. Outpatient services usually are less intensive and are provided to patients who do not require inpatient, residential, or home care environments. Many patients enrol in outpatient services immediately upon discharge from an inpatient setting. This promotes community **reintegration**, medication management and monitoring, and symptom management. Patients gain the right to choose home as a placement option, become more involved in after-care support services individualized to the care they need, and become more socially integrated into society (Friedrich et al., 1999). Outpatient services are provided by private practices, clinics, and community mental health centres.

Intensive Outpatient Programs

The primary focus of **intensive outpatient programs** is on stabilization and relapse prevention for highly vulnerable individuals who function autonomously on a daily basis. People who meet these criteria have returned to their previous lifestyle (e.g., interacting with family, resuming work, or returning to school). Attendance in this type of program benefits individuals who still require frequent monitoring and support within a therapeutic milieu that enables them to remain connected to the community. The duration of treatment and level of services rendered are based on the patient's immediate needs. Treatment duration usually is time limited, with sessions offered 3 to 4 hours per day and 2 to 3 days per week. The treatment activities of the intensive outpatient program are similar to those offered in PHPs, but PHPs emphasize social skills training, whereas intensive outpatient programs teach patients about stress management, illness, medication, and relapse prevention. See Box 4-3 for Best Practices related to inpatient and outpatient care.

Housing and Community Support

With the focus on community-based care, there has been increasing attention to housing and community support. New approaches and philosophies about housing have emerged for those with serious mental illness. Patients with psychiatric disabilities who are homeless are a vulnerable population. One of the largest hurdles to overcome in treating the severely mentally ill patient is finding appropriate housing that will meet the patient's immediate social, financial, and safety needs. The course of chronic mental illness, as symptoms wax and wane, preys on the stamina of families and

---

BOX 4.3

Best Practices: Inpatient and Outpatient Care

Research Evidence
Well-designed follow-up studies show that
- discharge of long-stay patients is associated with improved social functioning over time
- individuals and families prefer community care to hospitalization
- clinical and social outcomes are at least as good for discharged patients receiving community care as for matched counterparts remaining in hospital

Numerous controlled trials show that
- day hospitalization is less costly than inpatient care with comparable outcomes
- day hospitalization offers more intensive treatment in a less restrictive and more homelike environment
- shorter length of stay is generally not associated with increased readmission and achieves similar outcomes to longer-stay admissions
- home-based treatment is an effective alternative to admission for many patients

Preliminary descriptive studies show that integrating mental health professionals in primary care settings can
- enhance continuity of care

- increase accessibility to mental health services
- lead to more efficient use of mental health services
- provide new opportunities for continuing education for physicians
- improve communication between mental health services and family practitioners

Key Elements of Best Practice
- Long-stay patients in provincial psychiatric hospitals are moved into the community with carefully planned transitions to alternative care models.
- Inpatient stays are kept as short as possible without harmful effects on patient outcomes.
- Partial hospitalization programs are available as an alternative to inpatient admission.
- Day treatment is an option for those with nonpsychotic diagnosis.
- Home treatment programs (that are either assertive community treatment teams or adjuncts to intensive case management) are available as an alternative for inpatient admission.
- New service delivery models that link family physicians with mental health specialists are in place.

From Health Canada. (1998). *Review of best practices in mental health reform.* Prepared for the Federal/Provincial/Territorial Advisory Network on Mental Health.

caregivers. The prevalence of mental illness among homeless people may range as high as 35% (Tsemberis & Eisenberg, 2000). Most individuals live in some form of supervised or supported community living situation, which ranges from highly supervised congregate settings to independent apartments. Those who lack the resources to find housing suffer higher rates of substance abuse, physical illness, incarceration, and victimization (Tsemberis & Eisenberg, 2000).

Supported Housing

There has been a paradigm shift from a reliance on the residential continuum to what is now known as supported housing. This model incorporates use of generic housing in the community, provision of individualized support at varying degrees at different times, consumers' choice, and assistance in finding and maintaining their homes (Health Canada, 1998).

Residential Services/Housing

Community-based residential services provide a place for people to reside during a 24-hour period or any portion of the day, on an ongoing basis. A residential facility can be publicly or privately owned. **Intensive residential services** are intensively staffed for patient treatment. These services may include medical, nursing, psychosocial, vocational, recreational, or other support services. Combining residential care and mental health services, this treatment form offers rehabilitation and therapy to people with serious and persistent mental illnesses, including chronic schizophrenia, bipolar disorder, and unrelenting depression. These services may provide short-term treatment for stays from 24 hours to 3 or 6 months or long-term treatment for several months to years.

As a result of deinstitutionalization, there has been increasing attention on housing and community support for those with serious and persistent mental illness. Many patients who were unable to live independently were placed in nursing homes and other types of privately operated boarding homes. Over time, a number of residential and housing services evolved.

Nursing plays an important role in the care of people who have severe and persistent mental illnesses and who require long-term stays at residential treatment facilities. Nurses provide basic psychiatric nursing care with a focus on psychoeducation, basic social skills training, aggression management, activities of daily living (ADLs) training, and group living. Education on symptom management, understanding mental illnesses, and medication is essential to recovery. *The Scope and Standards of Psychiatric–Mental Health Nursing Practice* guides the nurse in delivering patient care (Canadian Federation of Mental Health Nurses, 2005). See Chapter 6.

Respite Residential Care

Sometimes families of a person with mental illness who lives at home may be unable to provide care continuously. In such cases, respite residential care can provide short-term necessary housing for the patient and periodic relief for the caregivers. Community-based emergency respite also provides immediate support and shelter needs for those experiencing crisis. See Box 4-4 for Best Practices related to housing and community support.

In-Home Mental Health Care

If at all possible, a person with a mental illness lives at home, not at a residential treatment setting. Choices, not placement; physical and social integration, not segregated and congregate grouping by disability; and individualized flexible services and support, not standardized levels of service, are the goals. When a person can live at home, but outpatient care does not meet the treatment needs, **in-home mental health care** may be provided. Many people prefer home care treatment (Wise, 2000). In this setting, direct patient care and case management skills are used to decrease hospital stays and increase the functionality of the patient within the home. Individuals who most benefit from in-home mental health care include patients with serious, persistent mental illness and patients with mental illness and comorbid medical conditions that require ongoing monitoring.

In-home mental health care services rely on the skills of the mental health nurse in providing ongoing assessment and implementing a comprehensive, individualized treatment plan of care. Components of the care plan and the ongoing assessment include data on mental health status, the environment, medication administration and monitoring, family dynamics and home safety, supportive psychotherapy, psychoeducation, coordination of services delivered by other home care staff, and communication of clinical issues to the patient's psychiatrist. In addition, the plan should address care related to collecting laboratory specimens (blood tests) and crisis intervention to reduce rehospitalization.

Supportive Employment

Supportive employment services assist individuals to find work; assess individuals' skills, attitudes, behaviours, and interest relevant to work; offer vocational rehabilitation or other training; and provide work opportunities. Supportive employment programs are new, highly individualized, and competitive. They provide on-site support and job-coaching services on a one-to-one basis. They occur in real work settings and are used for patients with severe mental illnesses. The primary focus is to maintain attachment between the

BOX 4.4

Best Practices: Housing and Community Support

Research Evidence

Quasi-experimental and longitudinal studies show that
- community residential programs can successfully substitute for long-term inpatient care
- supported housing can successfully serve a diverse population of persons with psychiatric disabilities but support networks need to be monitored
- consumer choice is associated with housing satisfaction, residential stability, and emotional well-being

Cross-sectional studies show that
- consumers prefer single occupancy, choice, and supports when requested

Controlled and noncontrolled trials have demonstrated that
- individuals with severe mental illness, including homeless people, can be housed when provided with assertive case management services

Key Elements of Best Practice
- A range of different housing alternatives (eg, supervised group homes or other residential settings) is provided.

- There is a shift of resources to sustain an emphasis on supported housing.

Supported housing incorporates the following critical elements:
- use of generic housing dispersed widely in the community
- provision of flexible individualized supports that vary in intensity
- consumer choice
- assistance in locating and maintaining housing
- no restrictions on length of time patient can remain in the residence
- case management services not tied to particular residential settings but available to the patient regardless of whether the patient moves or is hospitalized
- community residential housing that is provided as a substitute for long-term inpatient care
- housing needs of the homeless mentally ill addressed, which include an assertive outreach component
- evaluation/research protocols incorporated into housing programs

From Health Canada. (1998). *Review of best practices in mental health reform.* Prepared for the Federal/Provincial/Territorial Advisory Network on Mental Health.

---

mentally ill person and the work force. Transitional employment programs offer the same support as supported employment programs, but the employment is temporary. This type of work has a time frame agreed on by the employer and the participant. The person works at the temporary position until he or she can find permanent, competitive employment (Bustillo, Laurello, Horan, & Keith, 2001).

Other Services Integrated Into a Continuum of Care

Within the continuum of care, other outpatient services may be received separately or simultaneously within various settings. They involve discrete services and patient variables.

Outpatient Detoxification

Except for situations involving severe or complicated withdrawal, alcohol and drug rehabilitation is now almost exclusively outpatient based. Community- and domiciliary-based substance detoxification services have proved effective in providing accessible and convenient treatment options, with only a few severely alcohol-dependent patients requiring hospitalized detoxification (Bennie, 1998). **Outpatient detoxification** is a specialized form of partial hospitalization for patients requiring medical supervision. During the initial withdrawal phase, use of a 23-hour bed may be

a treatment option, depending on the stage of withdrawal and the type of addictive substance used. Or the patient may be required to attend a detoxification program 4 to 5 days per week until symptoms resolve. The length of participation depends on the severity of addiction.

Outpatient detoxification includes the 12-step recovery model, such as Alcoholics Anonymous (AA) and Narcotics Anonymous (NA), which provides outpatient involvement with professionals experienced in addiction counselling. It encourages abstinence and provides training in stress management and relapse prevention. Ala-Non and Ala-Teen rely on 12-step support for families, who are usually included in the treatment program (Enoch & Goldman, 2002).

In-Home Detoxification

It is estimated that 1 in 10 Canadians engage in heavy drinking (Canadian Addiction Survey, 2004). There is an increasing shift toward outpatient detoxification of patients with alcohol addiction. Except for situations involving severe or complicated withdrawal or for adolescents, alcohol detoxification may be implemented on an outpatient basis. In such cases, the nurse is required to visit the patient daily for medication monitoring during the patient's first week of sobriety. Daily visits are necessary until the patient is in medically stable condition. Referrals may come from primary care physicians, court mandates, or employee assistance programs.

Psychiatric Rehabilitation and the Nurse's Role

Psychiatric rehabilitation programs, also termed psychosocial rehabilitation, focus on the reintegration of people with psychiatric disabilities into the community through work, education, and social avenues while addressing their medical and residential needs. The goal is to empower patients to achieve the highest level of functioning possible. Therapeutic activities or interventions are provided individually or in groups. They may include development and maintenance of daily and community-living skills, such as communication (basic language), vocational, self-care (grooming, bodily care, feeding), and social skills that help patients function in the community. These programs promote increased functioning with the least necessary ongoing professional intervention. Psychiatric rehabilitation provides a highly structured environment, similar to a PHP, in a variety of settings, such as office buildings, hospital outpatient units, and freestanding structures.

The psychiatric and mental health nurse's role continues to adapt to the changing needs of people with mental illness. As behavioural health care delivery occurs more in outpatient settings, so does the work of the nurse. Most rehabilitation programs have a full-time nurse who functions as part of the multidisciplinary team.

The psychiatric–rehabilitation nurse is concerned with the holistic evaluation of the person and with assessing and educating the patient on compliance issues, necessary laboratory work, and environmental and lifestyle issues. This evaluation assesses the five dimensions of a person—physical, emotional, intellectual, social, and spiritual—and emphasizes psychiatric rehabilitation. Issues of psychotropic medication—evaluation of response, monitoring of side effects, and connection with pharmacy services—also fall to the nurse.

Clubhouse Model

The **clubhouse model** is a form of psychosocial rehabilitation that aims to reintegrate a person with mental illness into the community. Fountain House in New York City developed the clubhouse model in the 1940s. Its belief system involves membership and belonging—being wanted, needed, and expected. Additional fundamental beliefs include the following: all members of society can be productive; every human aspires to achieve gainful employment; humans require social contacts; and programs are incomplete if they offer recreational, social, and vocational opportunities but neglect housing needs (Bustillo et al., 2001). Fountain House seeks to improve its members' quality of life by organizing daytime support, providing meaningful daytime activities, and offering opportunities for paid labour.

The clubhouse model can successfully incorporate a number of services and supports, commonly providing employment and support services. Clubhouses are a unique treatment form because they are run entirely by patients with psychiatric illnesses with minimal assistance from mental health professionals. Patients who join a clubhouse are voluntary members, and they are expected to help operate the house. Membership is not time limited. Generally, members do not live in the clubhouse; however, the clubhouse may have formed relationships with providers of low-cost housing. Open 365 days a year, the clubhouse makes services available anytime an individual needs them.

Members of the clubhouse are expected to assist with household chores, follow instructions of others, volunteer for tasks, and be punctual. Most new members begin vocational training by participating in work units at the clubhouse, such as janitorial services, meal preparation, clerical services, public relations, and maintenance services. As members improve, they may move on to transitional employment, which is part-time paid work outside the clubhouse setting. When vocational skills have been acquired, members move into competitive employment.

The role of the staff person in this unique setting is different from other inpatient and outpatient settings. Because a clubhouse is operated by its members, staff roles are limited. The focus of the staff member is to accentuate the skills and performance of the members. The employee works with, rather than for, the member. The clubhouse model requires the employee nurse to function as a member of the clubhouse and be active in all components of the program. Although the nurse has expertise in pathology of mental illness, the focus is strictly on the individual's recovery. Case management in the clubhouse setting requires staff to participate in work units or transitional employment settings with members. More commonly, a nurse plays a pivotal role in urging a patient's participation in a clubhouse program and may actually refer patients to the program.

Consumer Self-Help and Consumer/Survivor Initiatives

During the past two decades, there has been tremendous growth in the number of self-help groups and organizations of people who have experienced mental illness (Segal et al., 1993, 1994, 1995) and who refer to themselves as "consumers." Some consider themselves as "survivors"—not survivors of their illness, but survivors of their health care experience. Consumer/survivor initiatives (CSIs) are self-help organizations that are operated exclusively by and for people with serious mental illness. Self-help groups offer the opportunity to provide support as well as to receive support and develop friendships, which are important for well-being and self-esteem (Constantino & Nelson, 1995)

CSIs are a unique component of the mental health system. Participation in CSIs provides personal empowerment, utilization of mental health care, social support and friendship, community integration, access to valued resources (work, education, finances, housing). In Ontario, there are more than 60 CSIs funded by the Ministry of Health and Long Term Care (Canadian Mental Health Evaluation Initiative, 2002). There is a longitudinal study of CSIs in Ontario, and the preliminary findings indicate that CSI participants felt more supported and more control over their treatment. (IAP-SRS Annual Conference, Toronto, Ontario, June 2002). See Box 4-5 for Best Practices related to consumer self-help initiatives.

Role of the Nurse: The Tidal Model

It is evident from the diverse role of the nurse through the continuum of care that there is emphasis on partnerships and empowerment of patients. The Tidal Model (Barker, 1998) emerged from the Newcastle University study of the "need for nursing" (Barker, 1996; Jackson & Stevenson, 1998). The Tidal Model

has incorporated Barker and colleagues' (2000) Model for Empowering Interactions, which defined caring through interpersonal interactions that are necessary for the empowerment experience. It assumes that nurses need to get close to the people in their care so that they may together explore the meaning of health and illness. The model recognizes that the need for nursing flows with the patients' needs, whether in hospital or community. The nurses' role is focussed on the changing needs of the patients in the continuum of care, thus maintaining a focus on the needs of the patients for critical, transitional, or developmental care and on the necessary interdependence of different services if different needs are to be met (Barker, 2001).

SUMMARY OF KEY POINTS

☑ The continuum of care is a comprehensive system of services and programs designed to match the needs of the individual with the appropriate care and treatment, which vary according to levels of service, structure, and intensity of care.

☑ The psychiatric and mental health nurse's specific responsibilities vary according to the setting. In most settings, nurses function as members of a multidisciplinary team. Consumers of mental health services and their families should be considered as members of that team. The Tidal Model is a new nursing model that emphasizes this assumption.

☑ A review of Best Practices for Canadian mental health services, based on research findings, was completed by Health Canada in 1998 and can be used to guide psychiatric and mental health nurses.

CRITICAL THINKING CHALLENGES

1 Define the continuum of care and discuss the importance of the least restrictive environment.
2 Differentiate the role of the nurse across the continuum of care.
3 Consider, in light of recommended Best Practices, the housing and community support arrangements for people with mental disorders that are available in your community.
4 Envision an integration of services that you believe would best serve patients and their families in your community.

BOX 4.5

Best Practices: Consumer Self-Help and Consumer Initiatives

Research Evidence

Although there is variability in the quality of studies conducted to evaluate self-help and consumer initiatives, there is consistency in findings.
Participation in self-help is associated with
- reduced hospitalization
- reduced use of other services
- increased knowledge, information, and coping skills
- increased self-esteem, confidence, sense of well-being and of being in control
- stronger social networks and support

Compared with professionally led groups, self-help groups emphasize experiential knowledge and social support and tend to be more spontaneous, unstructured, and unconstrained by time.

Key Elements of Best Practice

There are growing numbers of funded organizations that utilize nonservice models to engage in
- mutual support
- advocacy
- cultural activities
- knowledge development and skills training
- public education
- educating professionals
- economic development

Evaluation of the effectiveness of these initiatives that uses appropriate, alternative methods is supported. The general public and mental health professionals are educated about the value of self-help. Steps are taken to attract and train strong leaders for self-help groups.

From Health Canada. (1998). *Review of best practices in mental health reform.* Prepared for the Federal/Provincial/Territorial Advisory Network on Mental Health.

WEB LINKS

www.hc-sc.gc.ca   This is the Health Canada website. Use the "search" feature to explore information on Best Practices.

www.cmha.ca/bins/index.asp   The Canadian Mental Health Association advocates leadership by federal and provincial governments to ensure equitable access to services and treatment across Canada.

www.mentalhealth.samhsa.gov   At this website of the U.S. Substance Abuse and Mental Health Services Administration (SAMHSA), one can find "toolkits" for evidence-based practices, including assertive community treatment.

www.recovery-inc.org   This is the website of Recovery, Inc., a self-help mental health program active since 1937 that is nonprofit, nonsectarian, and completely member-managed. Groups meet every week around the world.

www.mind.org.uk   This is the website of Mind, the leading mental health charity in England and Wales. Among its objectives is to inspire the development of quality services that reflect expressed need and diversity.

MOVIES

Benny and Joon: 1993. This movie with an all-star cast (Johnny Depp, Aidan Quinn, Mary Stuart Masterson, and Julianne Moore) tells the story of Joon, a girl with schizophrenia, and Benny, her loving brother. As Joon comes of age (and falls in love), the decision about where she should live becomes a pressing one. This movie illustrates the concerns that can shape such an important decision.

VIEWING POINTS: Do you think the decision made in the movie was the best for Joon and Benny? Identify the issues that are involved in such a decision.

REFERENCES

Auslander, L., & Jeste, D. (2002). Perceptions of problems and needs for service among middle-aged and elderly outpatients with schizophrenia and related psychotic disorders. *Community Mental Health Journal, 38*(5), 391–402.

Barker, P. (2001). The Tidal Model: The lived-experience in person-centred mental health nursing care. *Nursing Philosophy, 2,* 213–223.

Bartels, S., Levine, K., & Shea, D. (1999). Community-based long-term care for older persons with severe and persistent mental illness in an era of managed care. *Psychiatric Services, 50*(9), 1189–1197.

Bustillo, J. R., Laurillo, J., Horan, W. P., & Keith, S. J. (2001). The psychosocial treatment of schizophrenia. *American Journal of Psychiatry, 158*(2), 163–175.

Clark, C., & Krupa, T. (2000). Reflections on empowerment in community mental health: Giving shape to an elusive idea. *Psychiatric Rehabilitation Journal, 25*(4), 341–349.

Canadian Federation of Mental Health Nurses. (1998). *Canadian Standards of Psychiatric and Mental Health Nursing Practice* (2nd ed.). Ottawa.

Canadian Federation of Mental Health Nurses (2005). *Canadian Standards of Psychiatric and Mental Health Nursing Practice* (3rd ed.). Ottawa.

Centers for Medicaid and Medicare Services. (2002, May 15). *Institutions for mental disease.* Baltimore: Author. Retrieved June 29, 2003, from http://www.cms.hhs.gov/medicaid/services/imd.asp.

Chan, S., Mackenzie, A., Tin-Fu, N. G. D., & Ka-yi Leung, J. (2000). An evaluation of the implementation of case management in the community of psychiatric nursing service. *Journal of Advanced Nursing, 31*(1), 144–156.

Constantino, V., & Nelson, G. (1995) Changing relationships between self-help and mental health professionals: Shifting ideology and power. *Canadian Journal of Community Mental Health, 14*(2), 55–70.

Davison, G. (2000). Stepped care: Doing more with less? *Journal of Consulting and Clinical Psychology, 68*(4), 580–585.

Enoch, M., & Goldman, D. (2002). Problem drinking and alcoholism. *American Family Physician, 65*(3), 441–448; 449–450.

Friedrich, R., Hollingsworth, B., Hradek, E., et al. (1999). Family and client perspectives on alternative residential settings for persons with severe mental illness. *Psychiatric Services, 50*(4), 509–514.

Goering, P., Wasylenki, D., & Durbin, J. (2000). Canada's mental health system. *International Journal of Law and Psychiatry, 23,* 345.

Gold, M., & Mittler, J. (2000). Medicaid-complex goals: Challenges for managed care and behavioral health. *Health Care Financing Review, 22*(2), 85–101.

Health Canada. (1998). *Review of best practices in mental health reform.* Prepared for the Federal/Provincial/Territorial Advisory Network on Mental Health.

Hochberger, J. (1995). A discharge checklist for psychiatric patients. *Journal of Psychosocial Nursing and Mental Health Services, 33*(12), 35–38.

Hughes, W. (1999). Managed care, meet community support: Ten reasons to include direct support services in every behavioral health plan. *Health and Social Work, 24*(2), 103–111.

Jackson, S., & Stevenson, C. (1998) The gift of time from the friendly professional. *Nursing Standard, 12,* 31–33

Lee, G., & Gurney, D. (2002). The legal use of restraints. *Journal of Emergency Nursing, 28*(4), 335–337.

Leslie, D., & Rosenheck, R. (2000). Comparing quality of mental health care for public-sector and privately insured populations. *Psychiatric Services, 51*(5), 650–655.

Martin, A. (2000). Protocol for alcohol outpatient detoxification. *Lippincott's Primary Care Practice, 4*(2), 221–227.

National Association of Psychiatric Health Systems. (2003). *The annual survey report: Trends in behavioral healthcare systems.* Washington, DC: Author.

Rabins, P. V., Black, B. S., Roca, R., German, P., McGuire, M., Robbins, B., Rye, R., & Brant, L. (2000). Effectiveness of a nurse-based outreach program for identifying and treating psychiatric illness in the elderly. *Journal of the American Medical Association, 283*(21), 2802–2809.

Segal, S., Silverman, C., & Temkin, T. (1995) Characteristics and service use of long term members of self-help agencies for mental health clients. *Psychiatric Services, 46*(3), 269–274.

Tsemberis, S., & Eisenberg, R. (2000). Pathways to housing: Supported housing for street-dwelling homeless individuals with psychiatric disabilities. *Psychiatric Services, 51*(4), 487–493.

Ward, M., Armstrong, C., Lelliott, P., & Davies, M. (1999). Training, skills and caseloads of community mental health support workers involved in case management: Evaluation from the initial UK demonstration sites. *Journal of Psychiatric and Mental Health Nursing, 6,* 187–197.

Wasylenki, D., Goering, P., Cochrane, J., Durbin, J., Rogus, J., & Prendergast, P. (2000). Tertiary mental health services. I. Key concepts. *Canadian Journal of Psychiatry, 45*(2), 179–184.

Williams, D. (2001). Connections in case management. *Lippincott's Case Management, 6*(5), 183.

Wise, D. (2000). Mental health intensive outpatient programming: An outcome and satisfaction evaluation of a private practice model. *Professional Psychology: Research and Practice, 31*(4), 412–417.

For challenges, please refer to the **CD-ROM** in this book.

5

Ethical Psychiatric and Mental Health Nursing Practice

Wendy Austin

LEARNING OBJECTIVES

After studying this chapter, you will be able to:

- Define ethics.
- Distinguish between the domains of ethics and law.
- Describe the nurse as a moral agent.
- List and describe the eight values and related responsibilities of the Canadian Nurses Association *Code of Ethics for Registered Nurses.*
- Identify the most common approaches to ethics that inform health ethics.
- Distinguish between a moral dilemma and moral distress.
- Discuss five ethical issues in psychiatric and mental health nursing.
- Identify the ethical responsibilities of nurses related to psychiatric research.

KEY TERMS

beneficence ▪ casuistry ▪ deontology ▪ ethics of care ▪ feminist ethics ▪ human rights ▪ nonmaleficence ▪ practical wisdom ▪ principlism ▪ relational ethics ▪ respect for autonomy ▪ justice ▪ utilitarianism ▪ virtue

◆ KEY CONCEPTS

ethics ▪ everyday ethics ▪ moral dilemma ▪ moral agent ▪ moral distress

WHAT IS ETHICS?

Ethics is about how we should live; it is *"aiming at the 'good life' with and for others in just institutions"* (Ricouer, 1992, p. 172, original italics). Ethics is about learning how to reach our potential as human beings, and so it is about values, relationships, principles, duties, rights, and responsibilities. In writing about ethics in *On Equilibrium*, John Ralston Saul (2001) noted that, although we may think about ethics as something exotic or romantic, for heroes or saints, ethics is actually down to earth and practical: it needs to be an everyday part of our lives and built into our society.

In this chapter, the nurse as a moral agent will be described, common approaches to ethics identified, and moral dilemmas and moral distress defined. Several ethical issues common to psychiatric and mental health (PMH) settings will be discussed. Although some philosophers differentiate ethics from morality, ethics and morals can be used as interchangeable terms (*ethics* comes from *ethos*, Greek for *custom*; morals comes from *mores*, Latin for *custom*) and will be so used here.

> **KEY CONCEPT Ethics** is the consideration of the way a person should act in order to live a good life with and for others.

The Legal Domain as Separate From Ethics

Law and ethics are separate domains. In a perfect world, societal laws would be totally compatible with ethical behaviour in every situation. In the real world, however, this is not always the case. Citizens may need to work to change laws that they believe to be unethical. Nurses need to be vigilant about laws that affect their practice. PMH nurses, for instance, must understand the legal context of mental health care in Canada (see Chapter 3). Nurses in forensic psychiatric settings must understand how the competing demands of the health care and justice systems affect their practice (see Chapter 33).

Health Ethics

Margaret Somerville (2000), at the McGill Centre for Ethics, Medicine and Law, describes Canada as a secular society, with diverse religious groups: we have no common, external, absolute moral authority. She asks, how can we know, as a society, how to respond to new approaches to science, technology, and health care? The landscape of contemporary ethics is shaped by factors such as intense individualism (the individual coming before the common good), corporatism (dominance of business interests), unprecedented advances in science and technology, the power of the media, the increased use of law as a means to resolve disputes that are inherently about values, and a loss of a sense of the sacred. She proposes that two absolute values, *profound respect for life* and *commitment to the human spirit*, will allow us to make ethical societal choices. We need, she argues, to act so as to protect these values.

Somerville uses the metaphor of a canary to signify key issues that "test the ethical air in our societal mineshaft" (2000, p. xii). As canaries once served to detect toxic gas in underground mines (ie, sick or dead canaries warned miners that the air was unsafe), these issues warn us that the ethical tone of our society is putting us at risk. Many of these issues are situated in health care. The way in which Canadians address the well-being of those living with mental illness is recognizable to PMH nurses as an ethical canary.

The Ethical Nurse

For nurses, ethics is foundational: "All nursing practice is ethical practice" (Tschudin, 2003, p. ix). Stating that "I am a nurse" is a type of moral claim. Nurses have a fiduciary relationship with the public. (*Fiducial* comes from the Latin, *fidere*, to trust.) Nurses, as professionals, profess or claim that they will use their specialized knowledge and skills for the benefit of the public in a trustworthy way. Nurses are trusted to be ethical (Austin, 2006). In polls, nurses are consistently rated the most honest and ethical profession (Gallup Brain, 2005). Whenever nurses enact their professional responsibilities, they are active as **moral agents**. Being ethical as a nurse requires more than having moral courage in times of crises (although it may require this); it requires the everyday expression of a commitment to the well-being of those in their care (Levine, 1977; Tschudin, 2003).

> **KEY CONCEPT** A **moral agent** is a person engaged in determining or expressing a moral (ethical) choice.

> **KEY CONCEPT Everyday ethics** is "the way nurses approach their practice and reflect on their ethical commitments to the people they serve. It involves nurses' attention to a common ethical event such as protecting a person's physical privacy" (Canadian Nurses Association [CAN], 2002, p. 5).

The Canadian Nurses Association *Code of Ethics* for Registered Nurses

To guide nurses in enacting their moral agency, codes of ethics have been developed by nursing associations.

BOX 5.1

Canadian Code of Ethics Values

A value is something that is prized or held dear; something that is deeply cared about. This code is organized around eight primary values that are central to ethical nursing practice:

SAFE, COMPETENT AND ETHICAL CARE: Nurses value the ability to provide safe, competent and ethical care that allows them to fulfill their ethical and professional obligations to the people they serve.

HEALTH AND WELL-BEING: Nurses value health promotion and well-being and assisting persons to achieve their optimum level of health in situations of normal health, illness, injury, disability, or at the end of life.

CHOICE: Nurses respect and promote the autonomy of persons and help them to express their health needs and values and also to obtain desired information and services so they can make informed decisions.

DIGNITY: Nurses recognize and respect the inherent worth of each person and advocate for respectful treatment of all persons.

CONFIDENTIALITY: Nurses safeguard information learned in the context of a professional relationship and ensure it is shared outside the health care team only with the person's informed consent, or as may be legally required, or where the failure to disclose would cause significant harm.

JUSTICE: Nurses uphold principles of equity and fairness to assist persons in receiving a share of health services and resources proportionate to their needs and in promoting social justice.

ACCOUNTABILITY: Nurses are answerable for their practice, and they act in a manner consistent with their professional responsibilities and standards of practice.

QUALITY PRACTICE ENVIRONMENTS: Nurses value and advocate for practice environments that have the organizational structures and resources necessary to ensure safety, support, and respect for all persons in the work setting.

Source: Canadian Nurses Association. (2002). *Code of ethics for registered nurses.* Ottawa: Author.

These are statements of the shared values and recognized duties and commitments of the profession. They set the ethical standards for practice and inform other disciplines and the public about the ethical commitments of nurses.

In 1954, CNA adopted the *International Council of Nurses Code of Ethics* (created in 1953; revised in 2002). This code delineates nurses' primary responsibilities to the people they serve, to the profession, and to co-workers (see Web Links for access to the International Council of Nurses code). In 1980, Canadian registered nurses (RNs) created their own code.

The current CNA code (CNA, 2002) is framed by eight values and their related responsibilities (Box 5-1). The code document includes, as well, a statement of the nature of ethics in nursing, a glossary of pertinent terms, and steps for addressing incompetent, unsafe, and unethical care. A code of ethics is an evolving document. It must reflect the new challenges that arise with changes in social values and health care environments. The CNA code has been revised several times and will be again in 2008, under the leadership of Dr. Jan Storch.

Although the CNA code is for RNs, it is expected by the nursing profession that students of nursing comply with the code. Those cared for by students should know the status of the student caregiver, and their care should be congruent with the code. Professional nurses are expected to treat students with respect and honesty (CNA, 2002).

To provide further support for ethical practice, CNA has developed an *Ethics in Practice* resource with topics such as advance directives, whistle-blowing, ethical distress, and public health ethics. (See Web Links for access to CNA.) In 2005, a new CNA interest group, *Canadian Nurses Interested in Ethics*, was formed.

APPROACHES TO ETHICS

There are a number of theoretical approaches to ethical knowledge that inform ethical action in health care. Some

IN A LIFE

Jan Storch (1940–)
Canadian Nurse Ethicist

Public Persona

Dr. Jan Storch's laudatory leadership in nursing ethics in Canada includes helping launch a centre of health ethics (at the University of Alberta), a provincial health ethics network (in Alberta), being the President of the Canadian Bioethics Society and the National Council on Ethics in Human Research, doing research in ethics, publishing widely (a recent work with Rodney and Starzomski is *Toward a Moral Horizon*), and speaking passionately about ethics to diverse audiences. Her guidance of the 2008 revision of CNA's *Code of Ethics* will be the fourth time she has so contributed. She has received awards as an outstanding nurse from the nursing associations of both Alberta and British Columbia and has been recognized as a leading public intellectual.

Personal Realities

Jan Storch is a wife and mother, a nurse, and a professor at the University of Victoria. Her deep commitment to ethical health care and to nurses' role in it is truly inspirational.

Sibbald, B. (2005) Nurse to know: Ethics in action. *Canadian Nurse, 101*(5), 44.

Table 5.1	Approaches to Ethics		
Approach	**Core Elements**	**Proponents**	**Critiques**
Virtue ethics	Character of the moral agent Some virtues: honesty, courage, compassion, practical wisdom	Aristotle Alasdair MacIntyre	Exclusive focus on the agent
Deontology	Duty based Some acts are wrong in themselves Universality Do not treat others as a means to an end (respect)	Immanuel Kant	Disregard of consequences Impartiality over relationship Emotion = irrationality
Utilitarianism	Consequence based Actions are right if they promote the best outcome (happiness, pleasure, satisfaction) for the most people	Jeremy Bentham John Stuart Mill	Utility as the only principle Majority rules
Casuistry	Case based Use of paradigm cases to identify issues and courses of action for a new case	Albert Jonsen Stephen Toulmin	Keeps the status quo Can miss the broad issues
Principlism	Based on a set of principles compatible with most moral theories Nonmaleficence, beneficence, respect for autonomy, justice	Tom Beauchamp James Childress	Too abstract Which principle has priority when they compete?
Ethics of care	Care based Connection/responsibility for others Emotional responsiveness	Carol Gilligan Nel Noddings	Creates a dichotomy between "care" (feminine) and "justice" (masculine) approaches to ethics Valorizes women as caregivers
Feminist ethics	Addresses power inequities, dominance, and oppression	Annette Baier Susan Sherwin	Lacks impartiality Lacks universal norms
Relational ethics	Ethical action involves relationships Context matters; emotion accepted Dialogue is supported Aims for the "fitting" response	Vangie Bergum John Dossetor	Too relativistic Lacks impartiality Lacks universality
Human rights	Rights based (negative and positive) Every person is entitled to certain basic rights	John Locke Thomas Paine United Nations	As a concept is "nonsense" Too legalistic Too individualistic

are based in moral philosophy and others in concepts such as human rights. A brief outline of the most common approaches follows. See Table 5-1 for a summary.

Virtue Ethics

Virtue ethics, emphasizing the character of the moral agent, was the earliest approach to ethics used in nursing (Fowler, 1997). A virtuous person is one whom, without strict reliance on rules, is sensitive and wise enough to perceive how to act well in a particular situation. The virtuous person *wants* to behave well. Lists of the virtues vary, but they can include compassion, courage, tolerance, prudence, honesty, humility, and trustworthiness. Aristotle, the Greek philosopher whose works most inform virtue theory, believed that acquiring the virtues would assist a person to flourish as a human being (Aristotle, 1996). He found our moral upbringing to be important: we learn the virtues through our rela-

tionships. Observing compassion in others, for instance, can help us to develop a compassionate disposition. To acquire a virtue, it must become habitual; it is not enough, for instance, to be occasionally honest. Aristotle's concept of the virtue of *phronesis* or *practical wisdom* seems particularly relevant to nurses. It means having the sensitivity, imagination, and experience to do what is ethically fitting in difficult situations.

Virtue ethics is not as influential as it once was. Research indicates that, for some, the character of a PMH nurse does not matter. Armstrong, Parsons, and Barker (2000) explored moral virtues (especially compassion) and PMH nurses. Nearly half of their sample in a Delphi study did not believe that the moral character of a PMH nurse is important in ethical decision making, and most of their round one sample thought virtues could not be acquired. Lützén and da Silva (1996) used examples of practice situations to discuss the place of virtue ethics in PMH nursing, illustrating that ethical action can mean compassionately transcending the rules in the best interest of the patient. This is one of their examples: a nurse in an emergency may restrain a patient without the necessary physician's order, to protect the patient from harming himself. To stand aside as a confused, acutely ill person injures himself may be correct according to rules or policy, but it does not seem ethical.

Anne Scott (2003), a nurse philosopher who finds virtue ethics relevant to practice and a rationale for good role models in nursing education, also warns that focussing naively on the individual without attending to context and collective responsibility is dangerous. A renewed interest in virtue ethics is occurring, stimulated by the work *After Virtue* by Alasdair MacIntyre (1984). A paraphrase of his question, What would a nurse (person) lack, who lacked the virtues? is worth reflecting on.

Deontology

Deontology (from the Greek *deon* or *duty*) postulates duty or obligation as the basis of doing right. This is not duty as in following external orders, but as self-imposed obligation. This approach is also termed *Kantian ethics* because the work of Immanuel Kant (1996), an 18th century philosopher, laid its foundation. Kant believed we should use reason alone to determine how to act. Reason, unhampered by emotion or desires, allows us to determine the types of acts that are wrong in themselves, no matter how good their consequences might be. Kant stipulated a criterion (a *categorical imperative*) for judging the reason (or "maxim") for one's actions: universality. One should act only on a choice that one can conceive of as a universal law. Is a lie acceptable if it saves someone from danger? No, because lying cannot be willed as a universal principle. If we lie to help a person in trouble, truth will be subverted and society corrupted. In Kantian ethics, the moral worth of a person's action is determined by the intent of the person, not the effects of the action. If you act rightly, you are not responsible for bad effects.

Kant stipulated a second imperative: act so that you treat others always as an end and never as a means. Kant argued that we must treat one another with dignity and respect: it is wrong to use other people for our own purposes. Informed consent is grounded on this belief. For instance, individuals should not be used as research subjects unless they understand what will happen and agree to it. Nor should we, according to Kantian ethics, place individuals at risk in research by depriving them of the best known treatment in order to carry out a placebo-controlled study, even though this would provide the most valid evidence.

Kantian ethics supports the quest for universal ethical principles, such as UNESCO's efforts (see Human Rights). It upholds that, from a moral standpoint, all persons should be treated the same. A major problem, however, is its disregard for the role of consequences in ethical action. Consequences, however, are the sole focus of the next approach.

Utilitarianism

The principle of utility is the foundation of utilitarianism: actions are right in proportion to their tendency to promote happiness. What is right to do is what gives the best consequences (happiness, pleasure, preference, satisfaction) for the greater number of people. Jeremy Bentham (1983) and John Stuart Mill (2002), philosophers of the 18th and 19th centuries, originated this theory that uses a type of cost/benefit analysis to determine the moral worth of an action.

The principle of utility can also be applied to determining which moral rules to follow. This is termed **rule utilitarianism** and holds that once we decide on the best rules we should follow them, even if in some situations happiness is not maximized. A rule utilitarian might determine that a good rule for a PMH nurse is not to go against hospital policy except if it is necessary for the best interests of a patient. Covertly putting antipsychotic medication in an acutely ill person's food, for instance, might be regarded as ethically acceptable in a special circumstance when such action causes the least suffering to the ill person (Ipperciel, 2003; Scott, 1998). A Kantian would never approve, and, despite ethical justification from a utilitarian perspective, such an act can result in disciplinary or legal action (Wong, Poon, & Hui, 2005).

Principlism

In the principles approach, it is believed that a few moral principles (ethical norms) can provide a basis for moral reasoning in health ethics (Beauchamp, 1994). Such a set of principles would be compatible with most moral theories (e.g., deontology, utilitarianism). A widely accepted set of principles is that articulated by Tom Beauchamp and James Childress of the Kennedy Institute of Ethics, Georgetown University. They identified four *prima facie* (at first sight) principles: nonmaleficence, beneficence, respect for autonomy, and justice (Beauchamp & Childress, 2001). Nonmaleficence as a principle means that one should do no harm; beneficence means that one should do, or attempt to do, good and to make things better (promote benefit) for others when one can. Respect for autonomy (also considered as respect for persons) means an obligation to respect a person's right to be self-governing and his or her ability to make decisions. Justice, as conceived by Beauchamp and Childress (2001), is about obligations of fairness in the distribution of benefits and risks. A major criticism of principlism is that, when principles compete, as they will in complex situations, there is no framework for settling the conflict.

The nature of mental illness creates situations in which there is conflict between respect for autonomy and beneficence. How should one act when a person with a mental illness chooses to act in a way that brings harm to himself or herself? For instance, what if a person with schizophrenia is living homeless on the streets? Should respect for autonomy be upheld, or should there be an intervention to bring the person to shelter? Respect for autonomy is dependent on a person's competence to make his or her own informed decisions. Evaluating such competence can be difficult.

Casuistry or Case-Based Ethics

Casuistry (pronounced kăzh' ū-ĭ-strē), from the Latin *casus* for *case*, is the use of case comparisons to facilitate moral reasoning and decision making. It is a bottom-up approach. One starts with the details of the present case and locates that case in a taxonomy of cases as a way to identify the pertinent ethical concerns and responses (Jonsen, 1991: Jonsen & Toulmin, 1988). The focus in casuistry is on agreement about cases, not necessarily principles or theories, and precedents are central to this approach. Past decisions about what was right or wrong in significant cases serve to inform decisions about the new case. (This is similar to what happens in legal judgments). The PMH nurse using this approach will need to decide how the "case" fits and does not fit paradigmatic cases. There are suggested steps to use (Strong, 2000):

1. Identify the main ethical values and concerns relevant to the case.
2. Identify the main alternative courses of action that can be taken.
3. Identify casuistic factors (i.e., the morally relevant ways the cases of this type differ).
4. Compare the case with relevant paradigm cases that have been identified.

Casuistry seems congruent with the way nurses think in practice. When a clinical situation confronts us, we often think of similar situations that we have experienced, or we turn to paradigm cases to guide us. A criticism of casuistry is that there is a risk one will miss the broad issues, and that prevalent beliefs and practices will not be sufficiently questioned.

The Ethics of Care and Feminist Ethics

The ethics of care can be seen as a feminine approach to ethics (Sherwin, 1992). Carol Gilligan (1982), in researching moral development, found that females seemed to differ from males in their approach to ethical decision making. Females focussed on caring, connectedness, and responsibility rather than the deductive reasoning and abstract principles preferred by males. She argued that women are different from men in their

approach to moral decisions, not inferior to them. [Aristotle and Kant both assumed the moral agent was male.] Canadian philosopher, Susan Sherwin (1992), in *No Longer Patient: Feminist Ethics and Health Care*, argues that women's perspective of the world as a web of interdependent relationships in which our responsibility to one another is implicit, needs to be incorporated into contemporary ethical theory. Nel Noddings (1984), author of *Caring: A Feminine Approach to Ethics and Moral Education*, says the ethics of care should be *the* theory. For her, receptivity, relatedness, and responsiveness with values and emotions, like compassion, are the important components of ethical responses.

Feminist ethics differs from an ethic of care in that it comes from a political perspective, offering insight into oppression (unjust, unwarranted use of power) and dominance in individual and societal-level relationships. Using understandings gained in analysis of women's oppression, feminist ethicists illuminate negative power differentials that may be so inherent as to be invisible and remain unquestioned. For instance, some feminist ethicists are concerned that the ethics of care valorizes the caregiving traits of women, even when such traits can be viewed as self-defeating (Sherwin, 1992).

Race, religion, class, and disability are factors other than gender that have affected people's ability to flourish within their society. Such discrimination is morally wrong in a feminist ethic (Liaschenko & Peter, 2003). Annette Baier's (1985; 1994) feminist approach has been proposed as useful for nursing ethics. It combines political dimensions with the core values of care and commitment (Peter & Morgan, 2001). It may offer a constructive framework for challenging the oppression of people with mental illness.

Relational Ethics

Relational ethics is based on the assumption that all ethical action is situated in relationship. Ideas of duty and utility, principles, and the character of the moral agent are accepted as important in informing action, but relationship is taken as foundational. Ethics is about how we treat one another, individually and within society, as well as how we resolve moral problems. Ethical situations are encompassed by complexity and uncertainty, and an understanding of the "messiness" of life needs to be cultivated.

Within this perspective, one strives to be responsive to the situation at hand in such a way that genuine dialogue is opened and mutual respect fostered among those involved. Feelings and emotions are viewed as a component of rational thinking and are explored, not ruled out as too subjective or confusing. Context matters. Not anything goes, but one's actions need not only to be shaped by ethical knowledge but also to be adapted to the specific circumstances of the situation. In relational ethics, one aims for the fitting response (Niebuhr, 1963). Questions can be raised within this approach (eg, issues of power and control) that may not be raised in approaches that focus primarily on moral reasoning.

In Canada, this approach to ethics was developed through research at the University of Alberta. Vangie Bergum (a nurse) and John Dossetor (a physician) questioned the dominance of the principle of autonomy in health care ethics. To explore what a different focus, one of relationship and responsibility, might be like in health care, they brought together an interdisciplinary research team of health professionals and scholars (Bergum & Dossetor, 2005; Austin, Bergum, & Dossetor, 2003). Using interpretive inquiry methods, the team explored existing cases and described each case in terms of a relational ethic. Core elements were identified as mutual respect, engagement, embodied knowledge, attention to the interdependent environment, and uncertainty/vulnerability. Although there is not space to discuss these themes here, this research is described in *Relational Ethics: The Full Meaning of Respect* (Bergum & Dossetor, 2005). An article about relational ethics in forensic psychiatric settings with examples from an undergraduate nursing practicum may be also helpful to students who want to better understand this approach (Austin, 2001a).

Relational ethics seems congruent with PMH nursing practice. In a study of PMH nurses' use of ethical principles, Garritson (1988) found that nurses were greatly influenced by situational variables. Nurses did not act consistently on their stated priority of ethical principles. Their specific concerns about the persons in their care and their obligation to keep them and others safe shaped their ethical decisions (Garritson, 1988).

Human Rights

Using human rights as an approach to health ethics is a fairly recent phenomenon (Austin, 2001b). The idea of human rights, however, goes back to 1215 and Britain's Magna Carta, to the rights language of the philosopher, John Locke (Sumner, 2000) in the 17th century, and to Thomas Paine's *Rights of Man* (1996) in the 18th century. The central assumption of human rights is that every person has certain claims or entitlements because they are human. Rights can be conceived as negative or positive. Negative rights are usually civil or political in nature, with the State or others required to refrain from obstructing these rights (e.g., freedom of speech, freedom to worship). Positive rights are obligations of the state or others to provide a right (eg, right to health, to education). These rights are typically social, cultural, or economic in nature.

Rights relating to health are included in many international documents, beginning with the constitution of the World Health Organization (WHO) in 1946 and the *Universal Declaration of Human Rights (UDHR)* adopted by the General Assembly of the United

Nations in 1948. In 1991, the United Nations declared *Principles for the Protection of Persons With Mental Illness and for the Improvement of Mental Health Care* (see Chapter 3 for Web Links). Human rights law allows for international scrutiny of a nation's health policies and practices (Gostin, 2001).

In October 2005, a *Universal Declaration on Bioethics and Human Rights* was adopted by the United Nations Educational, Scientific, and Cultural Organization (UNESCO). Among other things, the principles uphold respect for autonomy, the solidarity among human beings, and the need for sharing the benefits of scientific research and for protecting future generations and the planet itself.

"Health" as a human right means that every person has a right to the highest attainable level of health (including a standard of living that is adequate for health) and to access to health care and social services as needed. Health conceptualized as a right is very different from health as a commodity for purchase. There are important connections between health and human rights that nurses and other health professionals must consider (Mann, Gostin, Gruskin, Brennan, Lazzarini, & Fineberg, 1999). First, *health policies and practices have an impact on human rights*. For instance, mandatory outpatient treatment for persons with a mental illness is an infringement on individual rights. This infringement can only be justified if it is in the best interests of the person or for the necessary protection of the public. Second, *human rights violations impact health*. Torture, for instance, may have long-lasting effects on an individual's mental health. The International Council of Nurses not only supports the United Nation's UDHR, but also stipulates in *Torture, Death Penalty and Participation by Nurses in Executions* that nurses may not voluntarily participate in any deliberate infliction of physical or mental suffering. The World Psychiatric Association's (1996) *Madrid Declaration on Ethical Standards for Psychiatric Practice* stipulates the same for psychiatrists. Third, *health professionals have a responsibility to protect human rights by helping the public identify rights violations*. Mental Disability Rights International (MDRI), a rights advocacy group, reports that in Kosovo women were raped in psychiatric facilities despite the presence of local staff and international relief workers (MDRI, 2002). Such terrible rights violations must be made public.

Human rights approach to ethics requires action not only to end inhumane treatment and conditions but also to stop discrimination that prevents persons with mental illness from fully participating in their communities. The idea that humans are born with "rights" strikes some philosophers as "nonsense" (Waldron, 1987). There is also an argument that universal rights cannot exist because there is no universal human community, every culture being different. A rights approach has been criticized as too legalistic and the law as a slow, ineffective means of addressing rights violations. A final criticism is that human rights are too individualistic, placing the person in an antagonistic position against his or her community (Austin, 2001b). Nevertheless, human rights as an approach to health ethics underscores the point that health is a social good, not merely a medical issue. It reminds us of the need for human dignity and equality and of our obligations to one another (Leary, 1994).

MORAL DILEMMAS AND MORAL DISTRESS

A **moral dilemma** is a conflict that is morally relevant (Audi, 1995). It may be defined more narrowly as a situation in which one has an obligation to act, but must choose between two incompatible alternatives. In health ethics, frameworks have been developed to facilitate the decision-making process. See Box 5-2 for an example of a framework developed by Michael McDonald at the University of British Columbia. For an illustration of its application, see Cindy Peternelj-Taylor's (2003) analysis of a nurse's decision to whistle-blow on a colleague.

> ⬡ **KEY CONCEPT** A **moral dilemma** is a conflict in which one feels a moral obligation to act but must choose between incompatible alternatives.

Moral distress is the anger, frustration, or anguish we feel when we are unable to fulfill our ethical obligations in the way we believe we should. We feel a sense of responsibility and make a moral judgment about the right response, but some constraint prevents us from enacting that response (Austin, Lemermeyer, Goldberg, Bergum, & Johnson, 2005; CNA, 2002; Nathaniel, 2002). A constraint may be internal (eg, a lack of moral courage) or external (eg, inability to influence the actions of the care team).

Jameton (1993) has identified two types: the *initial distress* when obstacles to right action are first experienced,

BOX 5.2

A Framework for Ethical Decision Making

This is the outline of a guide for making ethical decisions developed by Michael McDonald, W. Maurice Young Centre for Applied Ethics (CAE) at the University of British Columbia. The full framework is much more complex; be certain to access it at the CAE website: http://www.ethics.ubc.ca/people/mcdonald/decisions.htm.

- Collect information and identify the problem(s).
- Specify feasible alternatives for treatment and care.
- Use your ethical resources to evaluate alternatives (principles/concepts, standards, personal judgments and experiences, organized procedures for ethical consultation).
- Propose and test possible resolutions.
- Make your choice.

and *reactive distress* that occurs when we do not act on the initial distress. Reactions include headaches, loss of appetite or sleep, heart palpitations, and loss of confidence (Fry et al., 2002). When we do not act, we may feel like we participated in a moral wrongdoing (Nathaniel, 2002). Action on the issue can reduce moral distress and prevent *moral residue*, what we experience when our integrity feels compromised (Webster & Baylis, 2000).

> ⬡ **KEY CONCEPT Moral distress** occurs when one is unable to act on one's moral choices because of internal or external constraints.

Sources of nurses' moral distress include harm to patients (pain, suffering); treatment of patients as objects; effects of cost containment; policy constraints; and inadequate staffing (Corley, 2002). For many PMH nurses, lack of time to engage with patients (including suicidal patients) appears to be a common source of distress (Box 5-3) (Austin, Bergum, & Goldberg, 2003; Midence, Gregory, & Stanley, 1996; McLaughlin, 1999; Sjöstedt, Dahlstrand, Severinsson, & Lützén, 2001).

It is helpful to identify the source of distress, to refer to the CNA *Code of Ethics* and other documents for guidance, and to seek support. Support may be available from peers, the health care team, or the ethics committee of one's institution or agency. It is available from one's nursing regulatory body, association, or union. For more information, refer to CNA's *Ethical Distress in Health Care Environments* that is part of their *Ethics in Practice* series (CNA, 2003a).

SOME ETHICAL ISSUES IN PSYCHIATRIC AND MENTAL HEALTH SETTINGS

It is not possible to identify in this chapter all the complex ethical issues of PMH settings; rather, a few significant ones are discussed. Although some issues are not unique to this specialty area (eg, confidentiality), all are shaped by the PMH context.

Behaviour Control and Restraint

Some users of mental health care systems call themselves "survivors." They are not saying that they survived their illness, as one might say "I have survived cancer." Rather, they are saying that they survived their treatment and care (Gallop, 1993). "We need to recover from being in hospital" (Roper, 2003, p. 14). Such claims are, and should be, very disturbing to PMH nurses. We need to ask: What is it like to use our mental health services? What is it like to be our patient or our patient's family member?

In PMH settings, some patients may be involuntary, committed to care without their consent. They may be treated against their will, as they have been deemed

---

BOX 5.3 RESEARCH FOR BEST PRACTICE

Unable to Answer the Call of Our Patients: Mental Health Nurses' Experiences of Moral Distress

Source: Austin, W., Bergum, V., & Goldberg, L. (2003). Unable to answer the call of our patients: Mental health nurses' experiences of moral distress. *Nursing Inquiry, 10*(3), 177–183.

QUESTION: What is the lived experience of moral distress of mental health practitioners?

METHOD: Hermeneutic phenomenology was used by the interdisciplinary research team to explore practitioners' experiences. Participants from medicine, nursing, psychology, and social work were asked to discuss morally distressing care situations and to elaborate on how their ethical concerns were addressed. These interviews, as well as explorations of moral distress in literature, art, and the media, contributed to the resulting description of moral distress.

FINDINGS: Nurses found lack of resources (time and staff) seriously diminished their ability to meet their professional commitments to those in their care. Unable to answer the call of their patients, they felt dispirited, disconnected, and abandoned by their administration.

IMPLICATIONS: Being able to understand and name the distress caused by lack of resources as *moral distress* may help nurses become better aware of their situation and to enact a more empowered response to it.

---

unable to make informed treatment decisions due to a mental disorder. A person significantly out of touch with reality can require help to survive and recover. Most societies have legal provisions that allow some form of intervention when this is so or if the person is at risk for harming self or others (see Chapter 3). This type of legitimated coercion must be monitored and used with great care. There is abiding potential for its abuse (subtle or otherwise), and this potential is a major concern of persons living with mental illness (Campbell, 1997).

Thomas Szasz (1961, 1993, 2005), among others, questions any use of this type of power. Szasz argues, in the *Myth of Mental Illness* and other works, that mental illness is not a true illness but a societal label for "deviant" behaviour. To Szasz, psychiatry is merely a means to control that deviance. Involuntary patients may be restrained (physically, chemically, or by being placed "in seclusion") if they put self or others (including staff) at risk for harm. To use restraint is a decision dilemma for nurses (Marangos-Frost & Wells, 2000).

Such measures must be used only when absolutely necessary and then with sensitivity and great caution. They can have serious relational consequences. Holmes, Kennedy, and Perron (2004) found, in a Canadian study of seclusion from the patient's perspective, that seclusion was perceived as punitive and as a method of control. Feelings of exclusion, rejection, abandonment, and isolation were intensified, not from the seclusion per se, but from the lack of contact with nurses. Gallop, McCay, Guha, and Khan (1999), in another Canadian study, explored the experience of restraint of women with histories that included childhood sexual abuse. Many of the restraint situations were triggered by self-harm behaviours, but no participant viewed the restraint as necessary or helpful in keeping her safe. It was traumatic, terrifying, and degrading. They suggested clinical responses that they preferred: empathic engagement rather than aloof professionalism, constant observation, comfort measures (eg, hot milk), and outlets for aggression (eg, punching bag). They suggested an orientation

to the consequences of uncontrolled behaviour to increase awareness of its risks. Other solutions, such as good staffing and better environmental design of PMH settings, can reduce the frequency and extent of restraint interventions (Marangos-Frost & Wells, 2000).

Practitioners justify coercive measures as beneficent, for the protection and welfare of patients, when failing to act would seem unethical. Nevertheless, practitioners find these measures difficult to use (McCain & Kornegay; 2005; Slomka, Agisch, Stango & Smith, 1998; Vuckovich & Artinian, 2005). Psychiatric staff in a Swedish study termed them "unpleasant," "hard," and "detestable" (Eriksson & Kjellin, 1989). In "volatile" rather than "violent" conflict situations with patients (prevention of fights or damage to property, protection of visitors, diffusing demands on nursing time), PMH nurses have been found to use a variety of maneuvers (like body block positions, bear hugs, and a show of force) that were rarely charted or evaluated (Ryan & Bowers, 2005). Nurses seem reluctant to question the use of coercion and, rather than do so, try to be as gentle and humane as possible (Olofsson, Gilje, Jacobsson, & Norberg, 1998) and use coercion only as a last resort (Vuckovich & Artinian, 2005).

Being open to questioning and discussing the use of coercive measures, however, seems important (Austin, Begum, & Nuttgens, 2004; Breggin, 1997; Kjellin et al, 1993). It reduces the risk for becoming desensitized to such measures and allowing them to become "routinized" out of awareness (Brody, 1995). Nurses need to question "taken-for-granted" institutional practices whenever those practices place the rights and dignity of patients in jeopardy (Holmes, 2001). Ethical action in PMH settings can be so complex that the nurse philosopher, Anne Scott (1998) asks if at times as nurses, we must choose to do the "least bad thing" (p. 484). In such situations, she urges nurses to confront the question openly and honestly.

Other types of behavioural control in PMH care can raise ethical concerns, including electroconvulsive therapy, behaviour modification, medication, and

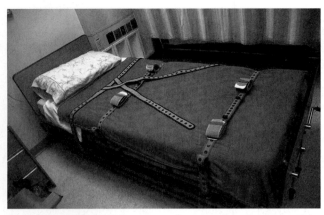

Bed with restraints. (Courtesy of University of Alberta Hospitals, Photographer Pat Marston)

psychosurgery. Discharge from hospital and care centres can also be a form of coercion if premature and unsupported (Eriksson & Westrin, 1995). Psychotherapy, too, can have ramifications for one's autonomy, as when therapists expect their interpretations of clients' experiences to be accepted and acted upon (Austin, Bergum, & Nuttgens, 2004). Research with PMH nurses (Muller & Poggenpoel, 1996) indicates that persons receiving care may encounter a lack of empathy and patronizing and paternalistic attitudes. Some professionals too readily dismiss concerns raised by a person with mental illness as faulty thinking (Davis, Liaschenko, Aroskar, & Drought, 1997). Margot Kidder, Canadian actor and mental health advocate, has described her psychiatric hospitalization as "You're completely invalidated as a human being. You're treated like a naughty child who must be taught a lesson" (Moore, 1999, p. A12). Yet PMH settings should be healing places with sufficient numbers of competent and caring staff who are able to offer respectful, person-centred care. When this is not so, it is an ethical issue that must be addressed.

Relational Engagement

Engagement in therapeutic relationships is an important aspect of most, if not all, PMH care, and complex ethical issues are situated in the boundaries of these relationships (see Chapter 8). Although "boundary," the term that is commonly used to describe the limits of such relationships, implies clear borders that should not be crossed, actual practice can be more complicated. Gift-giving is an example. Although accepting a gift from a person with whom one is in a therapeutic relationship can be seen as an initial step down the "slippery slope" toward a boundary violation and to be always avoided, it may be more complicated than that (Austin, Bergum, Nuttgens, & Peternelj-Taylor, 2006). Ruth Gallop (1997) has shared her experience as a student nurse who received a gift (handmade woolen slippers) from her patient, a young woman with schizophrenia. She kept the gift a secret

from her clinical teacher. "Although we were not permitted to accept gifts, I accepted the slippers, deciding the wrath of my instructor was easier to endure than the injury I would inflict by refusing her gift" (p. 28). Nurses need to be thoughtful about the meaning of a gift and be able to receive knowledgeable advice from members of the team and clinical supervisors.

Campbell (2002) in a survey of Albertan Mental Health nurses, found that nurses did cross boundaries. PMH nurses working in child and adolescent settings or in geriatric settings were more likely to do so than nurses working as group therapists or in forensic settings. The latter were the nurses most likely to have received boundary education. Although some nurses in the study admitted to dating a patient after discharge, it was less than 1% (eight nurses).

One of the most serious types of boundary violation is the sexual harassment and abuse of patients. Despite policies of zero tolerance, abuse occurs and is known to be significantly under-reported (Rodgers, 2004). Professionals who commit serious boundary violations at times argue that it was a mutual decision, made with the patient. Given the power differentials in therapeutic relationships, this "defence" is unacceptable.

Transgressions of boundaries are most often discussed as "over" involvement. "Under" involvement can also be an ethical issue given the definition of a boundary violation as being "any behaviour that infringes upon the primary goal of providing care" (Epstein, 1994, p. 2). There may be times in which a patient evokes a negative response from a nurse, for example, if the patient rejects care, is abusive, or is guilty of a morally reprehensible act, such as child abuse (Liaschenko, 1994). A nurse may, for instance, find engaging with patients with self-harming behaviours more difficult than engaging with other patients (Loughrey, Jackson, Molla, & Wobbleton, 1997). Liaschenko (1994) found that when nurses had difficulty connecting with a patient, they chose among three options: to emotionally distance themselves from the patient, to transfer the patient to another nurse, or to make a conscious effort to be respectful and provide good care. The nurses in this study recognized difficulties in "bridging the gap" to a patient as an ethical issue.

In order to engage ethically with patients, nurses need to attend to their own personal and professional boundaries, as well as to respect those of others. Education about boundaries is helpful, as are strategies such as clinical supervision and resources such as *Professional Boundaries for Registered Nurses: Guidelines for the Nurse–Client Relationship* (Alberta Association of Registered Nurses, 1998).

Confidentiality and Privacy

CNA's *Code of Ethics* defines confidentiality as the duty to preserve a person's privacy. (See CNA's [2003b] "Privacy and Health Information: Challenges for Nurses and for the Nursing Profession" in their *Ethics in Practice* series.) As individuals, there is information about ourselves we do not wish to have disclosed to others, and we may not want others to intrude on our personal space. This may be particularly important in PMH settings, given the stigma attached to mental disorders and to psychiatric care. Consent is a central factor in decisions related to privacy and confidentiality, and this factor becomes more complicated when the person involved has an illness that affects ability to give consent. Overall, nurses safeguard information learned in the context of their professional relationships, sharing it outside the health care team only with the patients' permission or as legally required.

Disclosure of information within the team, however, seems standard, with the team considered as one entity. Nurses should inform persons in their care about this sharing of health information within the team (CNA, 2002). This is particularly important because studies of public perceptions about confidentiality in mental health services reveal the belief that what is said remains in absolute confidence (eg, similar to confession with a priest) (Ormrod & Ambrose, 1999).

In Campbell's survey of Albertan PMH nurses, 94.4% of respondents said that they never kept a confidence regarding the safety of a person in their care from the treatment team at that person's request (Campbell, Yonge, & Austin, 2005). One nurse wrote that if a patient wants to tell him or her something that they don't want disclosed to anyone else, "I decline and state my role and responsibilities." When patients confide information that is peripheral to treatment, however, this type of information is not shared. Nurses have identified "patient privacy" as an ethical issue in PMH home care visits, including the use of various persuasive techniques to gain entrance (Magnusson & Lützén, 1999). Too strict observation of privacy and confidentiality rules can also be problematic (Kirby, 2004). When a person with a mental disorder is not competent to give consent for information to be shared, family members and caregivers may be excluded from knowing what is occurring, and this lack of knowledge can place them and the person at risk.

There are, of course, occasions that legally require the reporting of information received in a patient care situation. Mandatory reporting of child abuse and abuse of adults in care are examples. (Refer to provincial and territorial legislation for reporting requirements.) Nurses are expected to intervene if others within the health care system fail to meet obligations regarding confidentiality and privacy (CNA, 2002).

Advances in Technology as a Threat to Privacy

Electronic health record systems, costing millions of dollars, are being established across Canada in an effort to improve health care services. These information systems require nurses and others to go beyond questioning whether or not to share patient information. Health care staff members need to question their own perusal of information: it must be on a need-to-know basis only (Griener, 2005).

Surveillance devices employed in some mental health care services (eg, closed circuit television) are giving new meaning to patient observation. Nurses need to consider the use of such technology and whether it jeopardizes their patients' rights and dignity, as well as care relationships (Holmes, 2001). Advances in neurotechnology may bring new threats to privacy. Imaging technology may increasingly predict mental events and behaviours with far-reaching ramifications, including such areas as insurance, employment, education, immigration, and counter-terrorism (Kirby, 2004). Illes and Racine (2005), for instance, postulate that brain scans might one day be used to screen passengers at airports for their propensity to violence.

Advances in genetics raise other concerns, some based in past experience (Appelbaum, 2004: Cox, 2005). Eugenics (Greek for "well-born") was once a worldwide movement, beginning at the onset of the 20th century, that aimed at improving the human race. In 1939 in Nazi Germany, a program was initiated that lead to the killing of thousands of "incurable" psychiatric patients ("useless eaters"), who were deemed to have a life "not worth living" and to weaken their society. Nurses actively participated in this program (Aly & Roth, 1984; Benedict & Kuhla, 1999; McFarland-Icke, 1999). For the most part, however, eugenics involved preventing the physically and mentally disabled from reproducing; sterilization was a favoured strategy. Alberta and British Columbia had laws that sanctioned forced sterilization of the mentally ill and the intellectually disabled until the early 1970s (Cox, 2005).

With contemporary advances in genetic engineering, a new eugenics may arise. In the future, genetic testing may allow prenatal selection and termination of a pregnancy when the fetus is at risk for a mental disorder. (Even though it is doubtful that straight linkages between a given gene and a psychiatric disorder exist; see Chapter 7.) Genetic profiles of individuals may lead to discrimination and to "genetic essentialism" (ie, a person is defined by their genes) (Kirby, 2004). In the late 1990s, three applicants for Hong Kong civil service were rejected on the basis that one parent had schizophrenia. Although this decision was challenged in court and overruled, it illustrates the potential risks for misuse of genetic information (Appelbaum, 1994).

Ethical Practice Environments

Ethical practice environments need to be developed and supported. Research has identified nurses' environmental problems to include an inability to engage in ethical deliberations, receive administrative support, and have policies consistent with practice (McDaniel, 1997). Environment is predictive of nurses' moral distress (Corley, Minick, Elswick, & Jacobs, 2005). Relationships (with patients, peers, physicians and administration) are a key issue (Olson, 1998).

Fisher (1995) discovered that when PMH nurses balanced their desire to "do the right thing" with the need to "get along with colleagues," colleagues won out. Carpenter (1991) also found that power structures and concern for relationships were the reasons for PMH nurses' rejection of a first choice of the right thing to do. Forchuk (1991), in her descriptive study of the ethical conflicts of Canadian PMH nurses, learned that staff conflict played a major role in inpatient settings. It must be asked, "In what types of environments can doing the right thing and getting along coexist (Fisher, 1995, p. 203)?"

It should be safe for nurses, including students, to raise their ethical questions and concerns (Dwyer, 1994). Nurses' ethical assertiveness (ie, trying to influence ethical deliberation, even when not invited) is, unfortunately, least likely to occur when nurses do not expect acceptance of their input—exactly when assertiveness is needed (Dodd et al., 2004). For our PMH settings to be morally habitable, a "culture of questioning" must be actively nurtured (Austin, Bergum, & Nuttgens, 2004). CNA, the Canadian Medical Association, and the Boards of Directors of the Canadian Healthcare Association and the Catholic Health Care Association have developed a joint statement on preventing and resolving ethical conflicts involving health care. It is available at the CNA website, as is their position on quality professional practice environments and what is needed for nurses to provide safe, competent, and ethical care to the trusting public (see Web Links).

Research Ethics in Psychiatric and Mental Health Nursing

Psychiatric research in Canada has a tainted history. In the 1950s and early 1960s, the "depatterning" experiments of Dr. Ewen Cameron at the Allen Memorial Institute, McGill University (partially funded by the U.S. Central Intelligence Agency) were an attempt to erase the memories of patients before the insertion of new "positive" ideas. Without their consent, patients were "brainwashed," with many permanently losing their memories. Although Dr. Cameron was an international leader in psychiatric medicine with the reputation of being a humanitarian, his research caused great harm to his patients (Collins, 1988) (see Movies at the end of the chapter). His research is a strong example of the necessity for vigilance regarding the ethics of research.

At the same time, there must be adequate support for mental health and addictions research. Although persons with a mental disorder may be at times more vulnerable because of their illness, they are no more vulnerable than other groups of research participants, as long as the research is conducted in an ethically sensitive way (Usher & Holmes, 1997). DuVal (2004) analyzed study designs in psychiatric research and identified three types that raise particular ethical concerns: (1) placebo-controlled studies may deprive participants in the placebo arm of the research from needed existing treatment; (2) washout studies (in which patients' or subjects' medications are discontinued) can put persons at risk for illness; and (3) challenge studies (a pharmaceutical or psychological challenge is administered under controlled conditions, usually with some deception, and the subject's response observed) may cause adverse effects.

These risks need to be attended to in the planning, conducting, and evaluating of research projects, ensuring that persons with mental illness, addiction, or neurologic impairment are never exploited.

CNA (2003a, 2003b) has developed *Ethical Research Guidelines for Registered Nurses* that speak to nurse researchers and research assistants, to staff nurses who are caring for people who are research subjects or who are collecting research information, to nurses who serve on research ethics committees, to nurse administrators who monitor research activities, and to nurses who are teaching research ethics. The guidelines are in accordance with the *Tri-Council Policy Statement on the Ethical Conduct of Research Involving Humans* (Medical Research Council of Canada, 1998) that delineates the ethics policy of Canada's federal research funding agencies.

Social Justice

Conditions of fundamental equality and justice are seen as important to optimal mental health (Epp, 1988, p. 9; see Chapter 2). Justice, a principle of fair treatment of individuals and groups within society, is a core value underpinning the CNA *Code of Ethics*. "Social justice involves attention to those who are most vulnerable in society, eg, those who have been excluded or forgotten due to handicap, limited education or failing health" (CNA, 2002, p. 20). In Canada, the inequality of resources mandated to mental health care within the overall health care system may be identified as a social justice issue. The stigma and discrimination associated with mental illness negatively affect resource allocation. The nature of mental health problems and mental disorders means that a quality response to them involves more than the health care system itself. Teachers, social workers, clergy, police, and others also contribute to a complex system of supports and services. Unfortunately, this complex system seems to be poorly coordinated—to the extent that it increases the chance for homelessness and incarceration of the mentally ill (Kirby, 2004). To address these and other issues, the government of Canada announced in November 2005

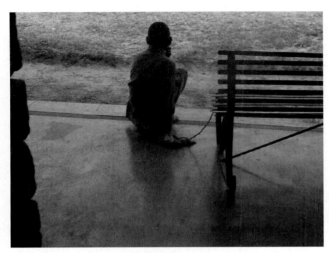

Untitled, Sylvester Kantontoka. (originally published in *Denied Citizens* [2005], World Health Organization.)

the formation of a Canadian Mental Health Commission. Canada is one of the few industrialized nations without a national mental health strategy.

The social injustices related to mental illness exist worldwide (Desjarlais, Isenberg, Good, & Kleinman, 1995). When, in 2001, the WHO report focussed on mental health, its findings were disturbing. Only a small percentage of the 450 million people who suffer from a behavioural disorder receive even minimal treatment; 40% of countries have no mental health policy; 30% have no mental health program; and 90% have no mental health policy that includes children and adolescents. Although mental and behavioural disorders account for 12% of the global burden of disease, mental health receives less than 1% in health spending for most countries (WHO, 2001). In some low-income countries, there are few practitioners trained in PMH care; there is limited access to medications and treatment, and stigma and discrimination against persons with mental illness and their families abound (see Chapter 3). In some communities, people with mental disorders are tied or chained to trees or poles, deprived of clothing, and kept in places that lack clean water and toilet facilities (WHO, 2005).

Canadian nurses have an ethical responsibility to address the social, economic, and political issues that affect health and well-being (CNA, 2002). Their continued contributions to the mental health of Canadians are important. A new ethical question, however, is arising. As members of a global community, what can and should Canadian nurses do to address the inequities and injustices experienced by persons with mental illness living in other parts of the world (Austin, 2001)?

SUMMARY OF KEY POINTS

- Ethics is the consideration of the way a person should act in order to live a good life with and for others.

- Ethics and law are separate domains. Nurses must be vigilant about the laws that affect their practice.
- Key issues can warn us about the ethical tone of our society; many of these issues are situated in health care. The way in which Canadians address the well-being of persons living with mental illness is one of these issues.
- Whenever nurses enact their professional responsibilities, they are active as moral agents. Nursing practice involves "everyday ethics," an attentiveness and responsiveness to their duties and commitments.
- CNA supports ethical practice through the *Code of Ethics for Registered Nurses* and *Ethical Research Guidelines for Registered Nurses*, as well as the development of various position statements (eg, on torture, conflict resolution) and resources such as *Ethics in Practice*.
- There are theoretical approaches to ethical knowledge (based in moral philosophy and concepts such as human rights) that inform health ethics. These include virtue ethics, deontology, utilitarianism, principlism, casuistry, ethics of care, feminist ethics, relational ethics, and human rights.
- A moral dilemma is a morally relevant conflict in which one must choose between incompatible alternatives. Frameworks for ethical decision making are available to assist in such a choice. Moral distress is the anger, frustration, or anguish experienced when one is unable to fulfill one's ethical obligations as one believes one should.
- There are many complex ethical issues in PMH settings. These include issues related to behaviour control and restraint, relational engagement, confidentiality and privacy, ethical practice environments, research ethics, and social justice.

CRITICAL THINKING CHALLENGES

1 Who is your moral hero? What are his or her heroic characteristics? What, for you, constitutes moral courage?
2 In their anthology, *The Moral of the Story*, Peter and Renata Singer (2005) have collected works that raise issues of ethics. Use this resource or select your own stories to help you explore the question of how we should live together.
3 In his "sci-phi" book, *The Philosopher at the End of the Universe*, Mark Rowlands (2004) addresses such issues as good and evil (*Star Wars*), the question of why one should be moral (*Hollow Man*), and the problem of free will (*Minority Report*). View two films in the science fiction genre. Identify the philosophical themes they raise.
4 Identify a PMH nursing situation that involves an ethical dilemma. Use a decision-making model to decide how the nurse should act in the situation.

5 Nurses need to strive to understand the experiences of mental illness and of using the PMH care system. Identify ways to further your own understanding. For instance, you could read autobiographical works by Canadians, such as *Study in Grey* (Edwards & Serviss, 1999) or *Upstairs in the Crazy House* (Capponi, 1992) or attend activities sponsored by mental health advocacy organizations.

6 Recall an experience of moral distress. What were the barriers to doing what you believed was right? Did you discuss your concerns with others? How was the situation resolved? Was it ever resolved for you? Is there anything that you would do differently?

WEB LINKS

www.cna-nurses.ca The website of the Canadian Nurses Association includes the *Code of Ethics*, *Guidelines for Research*, position statements, and the *Ethics in Practice* series.

www.georgetown.edu The National Reference Center for Bioethics Literature (Kennedy Institute of Ethics, United States), on the Georgetown University website, can be accessed to search for articles and books and to request a customized bibliography.

The following are the websites of Canadian health ethics centres:

www.ethics.ubc.ca The W. Maurice Young Centre for Applied Ethics, University of British Columbia

www.ualberta.ca/bioethics Dossetor Health Ethics Centre, University of Alberta

www.utoronto.ca/jcb University of Toronto Joint Centre for Bioethics

www.mcgill.ca/biomedicalethicsunit McGill University Biomedical Ethics Unit

bioethics.medicine.dal.ca Dalhousie University, Department of Bioethics

The following are websites of health ethics organizations:

www.phen.ab.ca The Provincial Health Ethics Network (PHEN) of Alberta is a nonprofit organization that provides resources on addressing ethical issues related to health.

www.bioethics.ca Canadian Bioethics Society

www.msu.edu International Network Feminist Approaches to Bioethics

www.bioethics-international.org International Association of Bioethics

www.unesco.org/shs/bioethics This is the quick link to UNESCO's bioethics page, where the UNESCO Declaration of Bioethics and Human rights can be found.

www.pre.ethics.gc.ca This is the website of the Interagency Advisory Panel on Research Ethics where you can access the *Tri-Council Policy Statement on Ethical Conduct for Research Involving Humans*. Check the "Links" at this site for further research ethics websites.

M O V I E S

The Terminal: 2004. Although it is unlikely that this movie was meant to be an illustration of virtue, it is. The main character, Viktor Navorski, is on a quest to fulfill a promise to his father and arrives in New York from his homeland, Krazkozia. Because a coup occurred in Krazkozia during his journey, Viktor becomes a citizen of nowhere, stranded in the airport. It is during his struggles to survive in the terminal that Viktor reveals what it means to be a virtuous man. Other characters, Gupta (a cleaner), Amelia (a flight attendant), and Frank (the airport manager) are lacking in virtue and act as foils to Viktor's "practical wisdom."

VIEWING POINTS: In one scene, Viktor refuses to lie even though it will help him; yet in another, he does tell a lie. Explain this inconsistency using virtue theory.

Virtue is learned in relationship with others. How is this illustrated in the movie?

The first line of *The Terminal*, "What is the purpose of your visit?" seems to echo a theme of virtue theory, what is the purpose of your life? Imagine how each of the characters might answer such a question. How would you answer it?

The Sleep Room: 1998. This 4-hour CBC miniseries is based on the true story of Dr. Ewen Cameron's CIA-funded "depatterning" experiments in Montreal in the 1950s and early 1960s. It is based on the book, *In the Sleep Room* (Collins, 1988).

VIEWING POINTS: What factors, in your opinion, allowed this research to happen? Could something similar happen today? Imagine that you are a student nurse in the 1950s, assigned to a practicum on Dr Cameron's ward. How might you react? What pressures might shape your reaction to participating in the research?

Wit: 2001. Vivian Bearing, a professor of English literature, learns that she has ovarian cancer with little hope of recovery. She agrees to take part in a research project. Based on a Pulitzer Prize winning play, *Wit* reveals the nuances of relationships between patient/research subject and caregiver/researcher.

VIEWING POINTS: Do you think Professor Bearing gave informed consent for her participation in the research? On what do you base your response? Using the core elements of relational ethics, deconstruct the scene between patient and nurse that occurs in the early hours of the morning.

REFERENCES

Alberta Association of Registered Nurses. (1998). *Professional Boundaries for Registered Nurses: Guidelines for the Nurse–Client Relationship*. Edmonton, AB: Author.

Aly, G., & Roth K. H. (1984). The legalization of mercy killings in medical and nursing institutions in Nazi Germany from 1938 to 1941. *International Journal of Law and Psychiatry, 7*, 145–163.

Appelbaum, P. (2004). Ethical issues in psychiatric genetics. *Journal of Psychiatric Practice, 10*(6), 343–352.

Aristotle. (1996). *Nicomachean ethics*. H. Rackham (Trans.). Ware, UK: Wordsworth Classics.

Armstrong, A., Parsons, S., & Barker, P. (2000). *Journal of Psychiatric and Mental Health Nursing, 7*, 297–306.

Audi, R. (Ed.). (1995). *The Cambridge dictionary of philosophy*. Cambridge, UK: Cambridge University Press.

Austin, W. (2001). Nursing ethics in an era of globalization. *Advances in Nursing Science, 24*(2), 1–18.

Austin, W. (2001a). Relational ethics in forensic settings. *Journal of Psychosocial Nursing, 39*(9), 12–17.

Austin, W. (2001b). Using the human rights paradigm in health ethics: The problems and the possibilities. *Nursing Ethics, 8*(13), 183–195.

Austin, W. (2006). Toward an understanding of trust. In J. Cutcliff & H, McKenna (Eds.), *The essential concepts of nursing* (pp. 317–330). London, UK: Churchill Livingstone.

Austin, W., Bergum, V., & Dossetor, J. (2003). Relational ethics: An action ethic as foundation for health care. In V. Tschudin. (Ed.), *Approaches to ethics* (pp. 45–52). Woburn, MA: Butterworth-Heinemann.

Austin, W., Bergum, V., & Goldberg, L. (2003). Unable to answer the call of our patients: Mental health nurses' experiences of moral distress. *Nursing Inquiry, 10*(3), 177–183.

Austin, W., Bergum, V., & Nuttgens, S. (2004). Addressing oppression in psychiatric care: A relational ethics perspective. *Ethical Human Psychology and Psychiatry, 6*(1), 69–78.

Austin, W., Bergum, V., Nuttgens, S., & Peternelj-Taylor, C. (2006). A re-visioning of boundaries in professional helping relationships: Exploring other metaphors. *Ethics & Behaviour 16*(2).

Austin, W., Lemermeyer, G., Goldberg, L., Bergum, V., & Johnson, M. (2005). Moral distress in healthcare practice: The situation of nurses. *HealthCare Ethics Committee Forum: An Interprofessional Journal on Healthcare Institutions' Ethical and Legal Issues, 17*(1), 33–48.

Baier, A. (1985). "What do women want in a moral theory?" *Noûs, 19*, 53–65.

Baier, A. (1994). *Moral prejudices: Essays on ethics*. Cambridge, MA: Harvard University Press.

Bentham, J. (1983). *Deontology; together with a table on the springs of action; and the article on utilitarianism*. Oxford, UK: Oxford University Press.

Beauchamp, T. (1994). The "four principles" approach. In R. Gillon (Ed.), *Principles of health care ethics* (pp. 3–12). New York: John Wiley & Sons.

Beauchamp, T., & Childress, J. (2001). *Principles of biomedical ethics* (5th ed.). Oxford, UK: Oxford University Press.

Benedict, S., & Kuhla, J. (1999). Nurses' participation in the euthanasia programs of Nazi Germany. *Western Journal of Nursing Research, 21*(2), 246–263.

Bergum, V., & Dossetor, J. (2005). *Relational ethics: The full meaning of respect*. Hagerstown, MD: University Publishing Group.

Breggin, P. (1997). Coercion in voluntary commitment. In Edwards, R. (Ed.), *Ethics of psychiatry*. Amherst, NY: Prometheus Books.

Brody, E. (1995). Editorial: The humanity of psychotic persons and their rights. *Journal of Nervous and Mental Disease, 183*(4), 193–194.

Campbell, J. (1997). How consumer/survivors are evaluating the quality of psychiatric care. *Evaluation Review, 21*(3), 357–363.

Campbell, R. J. (2002). *Attitudes and behaviours of Alberta mental health nurses toward professional boundaries, boundary crossings and boundary violations in patient care*. Unpublished Masters Thesis. University of Alberta.

Campbell, R. J., Yonge, O., & Austin, W. (2005). Intimacy boundaries between mental health nurses and psychiatric patients. *Journal of Psychosocial Nursing and Mental Health Services, 43*(5), 239.

Canadian Nurses Association. (2002). *Code of ethics for registered nurses*. Ottawa, ON: Author.

Canadian Nurses Association. (2003a, Oct.). Ethical distress in health care environments. *Ethics in Practice for Registered Nurses*. Retrieved February 20, 2006, from http://www.cna-nurses.ca/cna/documents/pdf/publications/Ethics_Pract_Ethical_Distress_Oct_2003_e.pdf.

Canadian Nurses Association. (2003b, Oct.). Privacy and health information: Challenges for nurses and for the nursing profession. *Ethics in Practice for Registered Nurses*. Retrieved February 20, 2006, from www.cna-nurses.ca/cna/documents/pdf/publications/Ethics_Pract_Privacy_Health_Nov_2003_e.pdf.

Capponi, P. (1992). *Upstairs in the crazy house: The life of a psychiatric survivor*. Toronto: Viking.

Carpenter, M. (1991). The process of ethical decision making in psychiatric nursing practice. *Issues in Mental Health Nursing, 12*, 179–191.

Collins, A. (1988). *In the sleep room: The story of the CIA brainwashing experiments in Canada*. Toronto: Lester & Orpen Dennys.

Corley, M. (2002). Nurse moral distress: A proposed theory and research agenda. *Nursing Ethics, 9*(6), 636–650.

Corley, M., Minick, R. Elswick, R., & Jacobs, M. (2005). Nurse moral distress and ethical work environment. *Nursing Ethics, 12*(4), 381–390.

Cox, S. (2005). Human genetics, ethics and disability. In J. Storch, P. Rodney, & R. Starzomski (Eds.), *Toward a moral horizon: Nursing ethics for leadership and practice* (pp. 378–395). Toronto: Pearson Education.

Davis, A., Liaschenko, J., Aroskar, M., & Drought, T. (Eds.). (1997). *Ethical dilemmas and nursing practice*. Stamford, CT: Appleton & Lange.

Desjarlais, R., Isenberg, L. Good, B. & Kleinman, A. (1995). *World mental health: Problems and priorities in low-income countries*. Oxford, UK: Oxford University Press.

Dodd, S. J., Jansson, B., Brown-Saltzman, K., Shirk, M., & Wunch, K. (2004). Expanding nurses' participation in ethics: An empirical examination of ethical activism and ethical assertiveness. *Nursing Ethics, 11*(1), 15–27.

DuVal, G. (2004). Ethics in psychiatric research: Study design issues. *Canadian Journal of Psychiatry, 49*(1), 55–59.

Dwyer, J. (1994). Primum non tacere: An ethics of speaking up. *Hastings Center Report, 24*(1), 13–18.

Edwards, W., & Serviss, S. (Eds.) (1999). *Study in grey: Women's writings about depression*. Edmonton, AB: Rowan Books.

Epp, J. (1988). *Mental health for Canadians: Striking a balance* (Cat. H39-128/1988E). Ottawa, ON: Supply and Services Canada.

Epstein, R. (1994). *Keeping boundaries: Maintaining safety and integrity in the psychotherapeutic process*. Washington, DC: American Psychiatric Press.

Eriksson, K., & Kjellin, L. (1989). Study of psychiatric care, especially compulsory care, in two Swedish counties. The psychiatric personnel's attitudes and experience of compulsory care. *Nordic Journal of Psychiatry, 43*, 365–368.

Eriksson, K., & Westrin, C. (1995). Coercive measures in psychiatric care: Reports and reactions of patients and people involved. *Acta Psychiatrica Scandinavica, 92*, 225–230.

Fisher, A. (1995). The ethical problems encountered in psychiatric nursing practice with dangerous mentally ill persons. *Scholarly Inquiry for Nursing Practice: An International Journal, 9*(2), 193–208.

Forchuk, C. (1991). Ethical problems encountered by mental health nurses. *Issues in Mental Health Nursing, 12*, 375–383.

Fowler, M. (1997). Nursing's ethics. In A. Davis, J. Liaschenko, M. Aroskar, & T. Drought (Eds.), *Ethical dilemmas and nursing practice* (pp. 17–34). Stamford, CT: Appleton & Lange.

Fry, S., Harvey, R., Hurley, A., & Foley, B. (2002). Development of a model of moral distress in the military. *Nursing Ethics, 9*(4), 373–387.

Gallop, R. (1993). Balance of power in the provider/client relationship. *College Communiqué, 18*(3), 9–12.

Gallop, R. (1997). Caring about the client: The role of gender, empathy and power in the therapeutic process. In S. Tilley (Ed.), *The mental health nurse: Views from practice and education* (pp. 28–42). Oxford: Blackwell Science.

Gallop, R., McCay, E., Guha, M., & Khan, P. (1999). The experience of hospitalization and restraint of women who have a history of childhood sexual abuse. *Health Care for Women International, 20*(4): 401–416.

Gallup Brain. (2005, Dec.). Nurses remain atop honesty and ethics list. Retrieved January 10, 2006, from http://institution.gallup.com/content/default.aspx.

Garritson, S. (1988). Ethical decision making. *Journal of Psychosocial Nursing and Mental Health Services, 26*(4), 22–24, 25–29, 35.

Gilligan, C. (1982). *In a different voice: Psychological theory and women's development*. Cambridge, MA: Harvard University Press.

Gostin, L. (2001). Beyond moral claims: A human rights approach in mental health. *Cambridge Quarterly of Healthcare Ethics, 10*, 264–274.

Griener, G. (2005). Electronic health records as a threat to privacy. *Health Law Review, 14*(1), 14–17.

Holmes, D. (2001). From iron gaze to nursing care: mental health nursing in the era of panopticism. *Journal of Psychiatric and Mental Health Nursing, 8*, 7–15.

Holmes, D., Kennedy, S., & Perron, A. (2004). The mentally ill and social exclusion: A critical examination of the use of seclusion from the patient's perspective. *Issues of Mental Health Nursing, 25*(6), 559–578.

Illes, J., & Racine, E. (2005). Imaging or imagining? A neuroethics challenge informed by genetics. *American Journal of Bioethics, 5*(2), 5–18.

Ipperciel, D. (2003). Dialogue and discussion in a moral context. *Nursing Philosophy, 4*, 211–224.

Jameton, A. (1993). Dilemmas of moral distress: Moral responsibility and nursing practice. *AWONN's Clinical Issues in Perinatal and Women's Health Nursing, 4*(4), 542–551.

Jonsen, A. (1991). Casuistry as methodology in clinical ethics. *Theoretical Medicine, 12*, 295–307.

Jonsen, A., & Toulmin, S. (1988). *The abuse of casuistry: A history of moral reasoning*. Berkeley, CA: University of California Press.

Kant, I. (1996). *Practical philosophy*. M. Gregor (Trans.). Cambridge, UK: Cambridge University Press.

Kirby, M. (2004, November). *Interim report on mental health, mental illness and addiction of the Standing Senate Committee on Social Affairs, Science and Technology*. Retrieved February 20, 2006, from http://www.parl.gc.ca/38/1/parlbus/commbus/senate/com-e/socie/rep-e/repintnov04-e.htm.

Kjellin, L., Westrin, C-G., Eriksson, K., Axelsson, M., Candefjord, I. L., Ekblom, B., Machl, M., Angfors, G., & Ostman, O. (1993). Coercion in psychiatric care: Problems of medical ethics in a comprehensive-empirical study. *Behavioral Sciences and the Law, 11*, 323–334.

Leary, V. (1994). The right to health in international human rights law. *Health and Human Rights, 1*(1): 25–57.

Levine, M. (1977). Nursing ethics and the ethical nurse. *American Journal of Nursing, 77*(5), 845–849.

Liaschenko, J. (1994). Making a bridge: the moral work with patients we do not like. *Journal of Palliative Care, 10*(3), 83–89.

Liaschenko, J., & Peter, E. (2003). Feminist ethics. In V. Tschudin (Ed.), *Approaches to ethics: Nursing beyond boundaries*. Edinburgh: Butterworth/Heinemann.

Loughrey, L., Jackson, J., Molla, P., & Wobbleton, J. (1997). Patient self-mutilation: When nursing becomes a nightmare. *Journal of Psychosocial Nursing, 35*(4), 30–34.

Lützen, K. & de Silva, A. B. (1996). The role of virtue ethics in psychiatric nursing. *Nursing Ethics, 3*(3), 202–211.

MacIntyre, A. (1984). *After virtue* (2nd ed.). Notre Dame, IN: University of Notre Dame.

Magnusson, A., & Lützen, K. (1999). Intrusion into patient privacy: A moral concern in the home care of persons with chronic mental illness. *Nursing Ethics, 6*(5), 399–410.

Mann, J., Gostin, L., Gruskin, S., Brennan, T., Lazzarini, Z., & Fineberg, H. (1999). Health and human rights. In J. Mann, S. Gruskin, M. Grodin, & G. Annas (Eds.). *Health and Human Rights: A reader* (pp. 7–20). New York: Routledge.

Marangos-Frost, S., & Wells, D. (2000). Psychiatric nurses' thoughts and feelings about restraint use: a decision dilemma. *Journal of Advanced Nursing, 31*(2), 362–369.

McCain, M., & Kornegay, K. (2005). Behavioral health restraint: The experience and beliefs of seasoned psychiatric nurses. *Journal for Nurses in Staff Development, 21*(5), 236–242.

McDaniel, C. (1997). Development and psychometric properties of the Ethics Environment Questionnaire. *Medical Care, 35*, 901–914.

McFarland-Icke, B. R. (1999). *Nurses in Nazi Germany: Moral choice in history*. Princeton, NJ: Princeton University Press.

McLaughlin, C. (1999). An exploration of psychiatric nurses' and patients' opinions regarding in-patient care for suicidal patients. *Journal of Advanced Nursing, 29*(5), 1042–1051.

Medical Research Council of Canada, Natural Sciences and Engineering Research Council of Canada & Social Sciences and Humanities Council of Canada. (1998). *Tri-council policy statement: Ethical conduct for research involving humans*. Ottawa: Authors.

Mental Disability Rights International. (2002). Not on the agenda: Human rights of people with mental disabilities in Kosovo. Retrieved February 19, 2006, from http://www.mdri.org/pdf/KosovoReport.pdf.

Midence, G., Gregory, S., & Stanley, R. (1996). The effects of a patient suicide on nursing staff. *Journal of Clinical Nursing, 5*, 15–20.

Mill, J. S. (2002). *The basic writings of John Stuart Mill: On liberty, the subjection of women and utilitarianism*. New York: Modern Library.

Moore, D. (1999, Aug.). Actor urges people to take control of their mental health. *Edmonton Journal*, A12.

Muller, A., & Poggenpoel, M. (1996). Patients' internal world experience of interacting with psychiatric nurses. *Archives of Psychiatric Nursing, 10*(3), 143–150.

Nathaniel, A. (2002). Ethics and human rights. *American Nurses Association Issues Update, 1*(2), 3–8.

Niebuhr, R. (1963). *The responsible self*. San Francisco, CA: Harper.

Nietzsche, F. (2000). *Basic writings of Nietzsche*. New York: The Modern Library.

Noddings, N. (1984). *Caring: A feminine approach to ethics and moral education*. Berkeley, CA: University of California Press.

Olofsson, B., Gilje, F., Jacobsson, L., & Norberg, A. (1998). Nurses' narratives about using coercion in psychiatric care. *Journal of Advanced Nursing, 28*(1), 45–53.

Olson, L. (1998). Hospital nurses' perceptions of the ethical climate of their work setting. *Image, the Journal of Nursing Science, 30*, 345–349.

Ormrod, J., & Ambrose, L. (1999). Public perceptions about confidentiality in mental health services. *Journal of Mental Health, 8*(4), 413–421.

Paine, T. (1996). *Rights of man*. Ware, UK: Wordsworth Editions.

Peter, E., & Morgan, K. P. (2001). Explorations of a trust approach for nursing ethics. *Nursing Inquiry, 8*(3), 3–10.

Peternelj-Taylor, C. (2003). Whistleblowing and boundary violations: Exposing a colleague in the forensic milieu. *Nursing Ethics, 10*(5), 526–537.

Ricouer, P. (1992). *Oneself as another*. (K. Blamey, Trans.). Chicago: University of Chicago Press. (Original work published 1990.)

Risk, S. (2005). A moment of reflection. *Canadian Nurse, 101*(5), 14–15.

Rodgers, S. (2004). Sexual abuse by health care professionals: The failure of reform in Ontario. *Health Law Journal, 12*, 71–102.

Roper, C. (Ed.). (2003). *Conversations between service receivers: On mental health nursing and the psychiatric service system*. Melbourne, Australia: Centre for Psychiatric Research and Practice.

Rowlands, M. (2004). *The philosopher at the end of the universe: Philosophy explained through science fiction films*. New York: St. Martin's Press.

Ryan, C., & Bowers, L. (2005). Coercive measures in a psychiatric intensive care unit. *Journal of Psychiatric and Mental Health Nursing, 12*, 695–702.

Saul, J. R. (2001). *On equilibrium.* Toronto: Penguin/Viking.

Scott, A. (2003). Virtue, nursing and the moral domain of practice. In V. Tschudin (Ed.), *Approaches to ethics: Nursing beyond boundaries* (pp. 25–32). Edinburgh: Butterworth/Heinemann.

Scott, A. (1998). Professional ethics: Are we on the right track? *Nursing Ethics, 5*(6), 477–496.

Sherwin, S. (1992). *No longer patient: Feminist ethics and health care.* Philadelphia: Temple University Press.

Sibbald, B. (2005) Nurse to know: Ethics in action. *Canadian Nurse, 101*(5), 44.

Singer, P., & Singer, R. (Eds.). (2005). *The moral of the story: An anthology of ethics through literature.* Oxford: Blackwell.

Sjostedt, E., Dahlstrand, A., Severinsson, E., & Lutzén, K. (2001). The first nurse-patient encounter in a psychiatric setting: discovering a moral commitment in nursing. *Nursing Ethics, 8*(4), 313–327.

Slomka, J., Agich, G., Stagno, S., & Smith, M. (1998). Physical restraint elimination in the acute care setting: Ethical considerations. *HEC Forum, 10*(3–4), 244–262.

Somerville, M. (2000). *The ethical canary: Science, society and the human spirit.* Toronto: Penguin Books.

Strong, C. (2000). Specified principlism: What is it and does it really resolve cases better than casuistry? *Journal of Medicine and Philosophy, 25*(3), 323–341.

Sumner, L. (2000). Rights. In H. LaFollette (Ed.), *The Blackwell guide to ethical theory* (pp. 288–305). Oxford, UK: Blackwell.

Szasz, T. (2005). "Idiots, infants, and the insane": Mental illness and legal incompetence. *Journal of the Institute of Medical Ethics, 31*(2), 78–81.

Szasz, T. (1993). *A lexicon of lunacy: Metaphoric madness, moral responsibility and psychiatry.* New Brunswick, NJ: Transaction Publishing.

Szasz, T. (1961). The myth of mental illness: Foundations of a theory of personal conduct. New York: Harper & Row.

Tschudin, V. (2003). Preface. In V. Tschudin (Ed.), *Approaches to ethics: Nursing beyond boundaries.* Edinburgh, UK: Butterworth/Heinemann.

Usher, K., & Holmes, C. (1997). Ethical aspects of phenomenological research with mentally ill people. *Nursing Ethics, 4*(1), 49–56.

Vuckovich, P., & Artinian, B. (2005). Justifying coercion. *Nursing Ethics, 12*(4), 370–380.

Waldron, J. (1987). *"Nonsense upon stilts": Bentham, Burke and Marx on the rights of man.* London: Methuen.

Webster, G., & Baylis, F. (2000). Moral residue. In S. Rubin & L. Zoloth (Eds.), *Margin of error: The ethics of mistakes in the practice of medicine* (pp. 217–232). Hagerstown, MD: University Publishing Group.

Wong, J., Poon, Y., & Hui, E. (2005). "I can put the medicine in his soup." *Journal of Medical Ethics, 31,* 262–265.

World Health Organization. (2005). *Glaring inequalities for people with mental disorders addressed in new WHO effort.* Retrieved February 20, 2006, from http://www.who.int/mediacentre/news/notes/2005/np14/en/print.html.

World Health Organization. (2001). *World Health Report 2001: Mental health: New understandings, new hope.* Geneva: Author.

World Psychiatric Association. (1996). Madrid declaration of ethical standards for psychiatric practice. Retrieved February 20, 2006, from http://www.wpanet.org/generalinfo/ethic1.html.

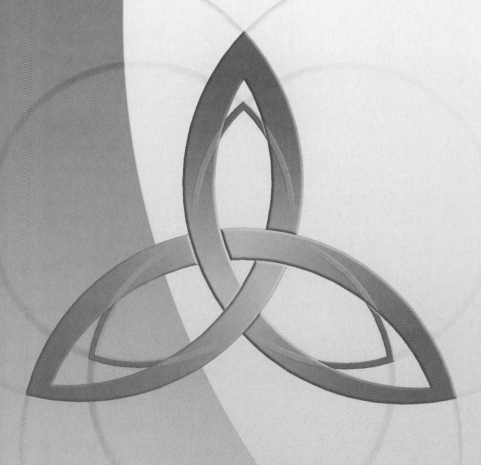

Foundations of Psychiatric and Mental Health Nursing

6

Contemporary Psychiatric and Mental Health Nursing Practice

Olive Yonge, Wendy Austin, and
Mary Ann Boyd

LEARNING OBJECTIVES

After studying this chapter, you will be able to:

- Explain the biopsychosocial model as a conceptual framework for understanding and treating mental health problems and disorders.
- Describe the spiritual dimension of psychiatric and mental health nursing.
- Delineate the scope and standards of psychiatric and mental health nursing practice.
- Identify the seven domains of practice used to structure the *Canadian Standards of Psychiatric and Mental Health Nursing*
- Describe the competencies associated with each domain.
- Discuss the basic tools of psychiatric and mental health nursing.
- Discuss selected challenges of psychiatric and mental health nursing.
- Discuss the impact of professional organizations on psychiatric and mental health nursing.

KEY TERMS

clinical decision making ▪ competencies ▪ critical pathways ▪ domains of practice ▪ interdisciplinary approach ▪ multidisciplinary approach

⬟ KEY CONCEPTS

biopsychosocial model ▪ standards of practice

This chapter introduces the biopsychosocial model as the organizational thread for the rest of the book. The scope of psychiatric and mental health (PMH) nursing is explained, followed by a discussion of the standards of practice expected of Canadian nurses working in psychiatric and mental health care settings. These standards are integral to the understanding of day-to-day practice and should be familiar to all students involved in PMH nursing. The discussion of the challenges of PMH nursing sets the stage for the rest of the text through an overview of the dynamic nature of this specialty.

THE BIOPSYCHOSOCIAL MODEL IN PSYCHIATRIC AND MENTAL HEALTH NURSING

Contemporary PMH nursing uses theories from the biologic, psychological, and social sciences as a basis of practice. This holistic approach, referred to as the biopsychosocial model, is necessary to truly understand the individual who is experiencing mental health problems or a mental disorder. The model is ideal for organizing nursing care and is used throughout this text for organizing theoretic knowledge and the nursing process.

KEY CONCEPT The **biopsychosocial model** consists of separate but interdependent domains: biologic, psychological, social. Each domain has an independent knowledge and treatment focus but can interact and be mutually interdependent with the other domains. The spiritual dimension is subsumed under the psychological domain (Fig. 6-1).

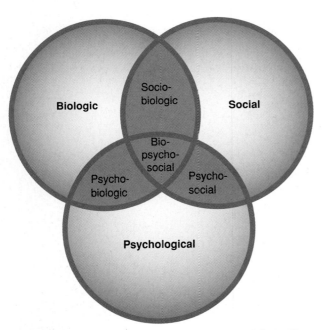

FIGURE 6.1 Biopsychosocial model. (Adapted from Abraham, I., Fox, J., & Cohen, B. [1992]. Integrating the bio into the biopsychosocial: Understanding and treating biological phenomena in psychiatric mental health nursing. *Archives of Psychiatric Nursing, 6*[5], 298.)

Biologic Domain

The *biologic* domain consists of the biologic theories related to mental disorders and problems as well as *all* of the biologic activity related to other health problems. Today, there is evidence of neurobiologic changes in most psychiatric disorders. Within this domain, there are also theories and concepts used as a basis of interventions focussing on the client's physical functioning, such as exercise, sleep, and adequate nutrition. In addition, the neurobiologic theories also serve as a basis for understanding and administering pharmacologic agents (see Chapter 9).

Psychological Domain

The *psychological* domain contains the theoretical basis of the psychological processes—thoughts, feelings, and behaviour (intrapersonal dynamics) that influence one's emotion, cognition, and behaviour. The psychological and nursing sciences generate theories and research that are critical to understanding a client's symptoms and responses to mental disorders. Although mental disorders have a biologic component, they are often manifested in psychological symptoms and physical changes. The person with a thought disorder may have bizarre behaviour that needs to be interpreted within the context of the neurobiologic dysfunction of the mental disorder.

Many PMH nursing interventions are based on knowledge generated within this domain. Cognitive approaches, behaviour therapy, and client education are all based on the use of theories from the psychological domain. These interventions are explained in Unit III. PMH interventions are also based on the use of interpersonal communication techniques, which require nurses to develop awareness of their own, as well as their client's, internal feelings and behaviour. For PMH nurses, understanding their own and their client's intrapersonal dynamics and motivation is critical to developing a therapeutic relationship and motivating clients to learn and understand their disorders and participate in their management. Motivating clients to engage in learning activities best occurs within the context of a therapeutic relationship (see Chapter 8).

The Spiritual Dimension

When clients become ill, there is also the potential for growth and change. One of the processes and product of this change is a client's spirituality. Spirituality is a complex concept and refers to the core of who we are; it involves our feelings and thoughts about what gives us meaning and purpose in our lives. One definition of spirituality is "the unifying force of a person; the essence of being that shapes, gives meaning to, and is aware of one's self-becoming. Spirituality permeates all of life and is manifested in one's being, knowing and doing. It is expressed and experienced uniquely by each individual through and within connection to God, Life Force, the Absolute, the environment, nature, other people, and the self" (Burkhardt & Jackson, 1997, p. 42). People who are spiritual may or may not be religious. Religion involves organized systems of rituals, patterns of beliefs, and groups of people usually congregating around the worship of a deity. A person may be spiritual and not religious; religious and spiritual; or religious and not spiritual (Mauk & Schmidt, 2004).

O'Reilly (2004) notes that mentally ill clients may feel the loss of meaning, which, in turn, could be interpreted as a loss in spirituality and that clients with certain religious beliefs may view mental illness as a form of punishment. Spirituality can also promote healing and give clients comfort. A common example is *The Twelve Steps* program of Alcoholics Anonymous that many people with substance use disorders find central to their healing. A core element of *The Twelve Steps* is turning to a higher spiritual being for strength and courage (O'Reilly, 2004). See Box 6-1.

The biopsychosocial model needs to encompass the spiritual dimension of human life. In its use as a framework for this Canadian text, we place the spiritual dimension within the psychological domain.

BOX 6.1

The Twelve Steps

1. We admitted we were powerless over alcohol, that our lives had become unmanageable.
2. We came to believe that a Power greater than ourselves could restore us to sanity.
3. We made a decision to turn our will and our lives over to the care of God *as we understood Him.*
4. We made a searching and fearless moral inventory of ourselves.
5. We admitted to God, to ourselves, and to another human being the exact nature of our wrongs.
6. We were entirely ready to have God remove all these defects of character.
7. We humbly asked Him to remove our shortcomings.
8. We made a list of all persons we had harmed, and became willing to make amends to them all.
9. We made direct amends to such people wherever possible, except when to do so would injure them or others.
10. We continued to take personal inventory and, when we were wrong, promptly admitted it.
11. We sought through prayer and meditation to improve our conscious contact with God as we understood Him, praying only for knowledge of His will for us and the power to carry that out.
12. Having had a spiritual awakening as a result of these steps, we tried to carry this message to alcoholics and to practice these principles in all our affairs.

From Alcoholics Anonymous World Services, Inc. (1979). *Alcoholics anonymous.* New York: Author.

Social Domain

The *social* domain includes theories that account for the influence of social forces encompassing the client, family, and community within cultural settings. This knowledge base is generated from social and nursing sciences and explains the connections within the family and communities that affect the mental health and treatment of people with mental disorders. Psychiatric disorders are not caused by social factors, but their manifestations and treatment can be significantly affected by the society in which the client lives. Family support can actually improve treatment outcomes. Moreover, family factors, including origin, extended family, and other significant relationships, contribute to the total understanding and treatment of clients. Community forces, including cultural and ethnic groups within larger communities, shape clients' manifestation of disorders, response to treatment, and overall view of mental illness.

STANDARDS OF PROFESSIONAL PRACTICE

As a regulated health profession, nurses are given the authority to practice under provincial or territorial laws that set out governance, registration, and discipline requirements as a means of protecting the public. These laws require the provincial or territorial nursing regulatory bodies to set, monitor, and enforce standards of practice that, along with the Code of Ethics for Registered Nurses (see Chapter 5), articulate the profession's values, knowledge, and skills. Such standards facilitate the profession's self-governance because they make explicit the profession's expectations of its members' competencies and performance. In Canada, specialty areas of nursing practice are designated by the Canadian Nurses Association (CNA). The CNA requires any specialty group desiring designation to establish its own standards of practice. The Canadian Federation of Mental Health Nurses (CFMHN), an Associate group with CNA, created the first Canadian psychiatric and mental health nursing standards and achieved designation in 1995. (See Box 6-2.)

> **KEY CONCEPT** Standards are used by nurses to guide their own actions and to communicate to others the desired and achievable level of performance in providing nursing care (CNA, 1998).

Canadian Standards of Psychiatric and Mental Health Nursing

The *Canadian Standards of Psychiatric and Mental Health Nursing* were developed by expert PMH nurses in 1995 (Austin, Gallop, Harris, & Spencer, 1996), revised in 1998 with a greater community focus, and revised again in 2005. For the 2005 revision, input was sought from

BOX 6.2

Canadian Federation of Mental Health Nurses

Formed in 1988, the Federation's initial endeavour was to achieve national credentialling in psychiatric and mental health nursing. It did so in 1995.

A strong voice for this specialty practice, today the Federation's objectives are to:

- Assure national leadership in the development and application of nursing standards that inform and affect psychiatric and mental health nursing practice.
- Examine and influence government policy and address national issues related to mental health and mental illness.
- Communicate and collaborate with national and international groups that share our professional interests.
- Facilitate excellence in psychiatric and mental health nursing by providing our members with educational and networking resources.

From Canadian Federation of Mental Health Nurses, http://www.cfmhn.org.

consumer groups through focus groups across Canada. The facilitators of the focus groups noted how powerful this experience was for them, and the current standards have been markedly influenced by their input, particularly in the area of forming partnerships.

CRNE Note

Use the Canadian standards of psychiatric and mental health nursing practice as one guide to studying for the CRNE.

Domains of Practice

These standards are organized by a "domains of practice" framework (Benner, 1984), with competencies classified within seven domains. In the standards, each domain is described, and the specific competencies necessary to meet that standard are listed. (See Boxes 6-3 to 6-9.)

Nurses' achievement of competent practice is shaped by the nursing model they utilize, as well as by the social, cultural, economic, and political factors that act on the health care environment (Health and Welfare Canada, 1988). Beliefs underlying the standards include the belief that therapeutic use of self, based on trust and mutual respect, is at the core of PMH nursing practice and that continual advances in knowledge necessitate the incorporation of new research-based findings into practice. Also foundational to the standards is a belief in holistic, reflective ethical practice that includes the protection of human rights and the alleviation of the stigma and discrimination associated with mental illness. The

BOX 6.3

Canadian Standards of Psychiatric and Mental Health Nursing

Standard I: *Provides Competent Professional Care Through the Development of a Therapeutic Relationship*

A primary goal of psychiatric and mental health nursing is the promotion of mental health and the prevention or diminution of mental disorder. The development of a therapeutic relationship is the foundation from where the psychiatric and mental health nurse can "enter into partnerships with clients, and through the use of the human sciences, and the art of caring, develop helping relationships" (CNA, 1997b, p. 43).

The nurse is expected to demonstrate competence in therapeutic relationship by the following:

1. Assesses and clarifies the influences of personal beliefs, values, and life experience on the therapeutic relationship and distinguishes between social and therapeutic relationship.
2. Works in partnership with the client, family, and relevant others to determine goal-directed needs and establishes an environment that is conducive to goal achievement.
3. Uses a range of therapeutic verbal and nonverbal communication skills that include empathy, active listening, observing, genuineness, and curiosity.
4. Recognizes the influence of culture, class, ethnicity, language, stigma, and social exclusion on the therapeutic process and negotiates care that is sensitive to these influences.
5. Mobilizes and advocates for resources that increase clients' and families' access to mental health services and that improve community integration.
6. Understands and responds to human reactions to distress and loss of control that may be expressed as anger, anxiety, fear, grief, helplessness, hopelessness, and humour.
7. Guides the client through behavioural, developmental, emotional, or spiritual change while acknowledging and supporting the client's participation, responsibility, and choices in own care.
8. Supports the client's and family's sense of resiliency, self-esteem, power, and hope through continuity of therapeutic relationship, on a 1:1 basis or within a group context.
9. Fosters mutuality of the relationship by reflectively critiquing therapeutic effectiveness through client and family responses, clinical supervision, and self-evaluation.
10. Understands the nature of chronic illness and applies the principles of health promotion and disease prevention when working with clients and families.

importance of equitable access to culturally competent care is acknowledged. A belief in quality practice environments is also espoused. PMH nurses usually practice in multidisciplinary settings and need to be aware of the impact of team dynamics on care. In interdisciplinary settings, there may be an overlapping of professional

BOX 6.4

Canadian Standards of Psychiatric and Mental Health Nursing

Standard II: *Performs/Refines Client Assessments Through the Diagnostic and Monitoring Function*

Effective assessment, diagnosis, and monitoring is central to the nurse's role and is dependent on theory, as well as on understanding the meaning of the health or illness experience from the perspective of the client. This knowledge, integrated with the nurse's conceptual model of nursing practice, provides a framework for processing client data and for developing client-focussed plans of care. The nurse makes professional judgments regarding the relevance and importance of these data and acknowledges the client as a valued and respected partner throughout the decision-making process.

The nurse is expected to demonstrate competence in the mental health assessment tools in various workplaces, for example, mental status exam and recovery principles.

The nurse explains to the client the assessment process and content and provides feedback for all of the following:

1. Collaborates with clients and with other members of the health care team to gather holistic assessments through observation, examination, interview, and consultation, while being attentive to issues of confidentiality and pertinent legal statutes.
2. Documents and analyzes baseline data to identify health status, potential for wellness, health care deficits, potential for danger to self and others; alterations in thought content or process, affect behaviour, communication and decision-making abilities; substance use and dependency; and history of trauma or abuse (emotional, physical, neglect—sexual or verbal).
3. Formulates and documents a plan of care in collaboration with the client and with the mental health team, recognizing variability in the client's ability to participate in the process.
4. Refines and extends client assessment information by assessing and documenting significant change in the client's status and by comparing new data with the baseline assessment and intermediate client goals.
5. Continuously assesses status and anticipates potential problems and risks. Collaborates with the client to examine his/her environment for risk factors: self-care, housing, and nutrition, economic, psychological, and social. Utilizes assessment data to identify potential risks to client and others. Advocates and practices for interventions that are appropriate to risk type and level.
6. Determines most appropriate and available therapeutic modality that will potentially best meet client's needs, and assists the client to access these resources.

roles, with nurses being accountable for both the discrete and shared functions within their practice. Within the standards, it is acknowledged that supporting these identified beliefs can involve sociopolitical action to promote awareness of issues and to influence health policy (CFMHN, 2005).

TOOLS OF PSYCHIATRIC NURSING PRACTICE

Clinical Decision Making

Decision making involves critical thinking and is at the core of clinical practice. Clinical decision making focuses on the choices made in clinical settings. In addition to the complex decisions, such as collecting, processing, and organizing information and formulating nursing approaches, many moment-to-moment decisions are made, such as deciding whether a client should receive a PRN medication. The development and implementation of efficacious interventions involves critical analysis of client, family, and community data and making decisions about care. Such decision making should involve the client, family, and other significant stakeholders as much as possible. Reflective thinking about the client's illness experience and personal response to the treatment and care situation is an important aspect of choosing interventions as well. The nurse needs to have a thorough understanding of the rationale and the theoretical underpinnings of the client's care plan.

Critical Pathways in Care Planning

Many psychiatric facilities use **critical pathways** to ensure a quality level of care in a cost-effective way. These care paths are similar to individual treatment plans in that all the disciplines' interventions are included on one plan. Critical pathways, however, are designed for a hypothetical client who has typical symptoms and who follows an expected course of treatment. Care paths are not developed for each individual client. This unification of care can be helpful if it means that best practices shape the care received by all clients and if it facilitates the use of expert knowledge by all those providing care. It is not helpful if the unique needs and situation of each client and family are ignored, or if nurses are restrained in their provision of thoughtful, sensitive care.

INTERDISCIPLINARY APPROACH AND THE NURSE'S ROLE

Several professionals other than nurses and physicians provide mental health services. These professionals come from a variety of disciplines and provide services based on their training and licensure, which may vary from province to province. Psychiatric and mental health care has a long tradition of using a **multidisciplinary approach**, with several disciplines providing services to a client. In the hospital, a client may be seeing a psychiatrist for management of the disorder symptoms and for prescribed medications; a psychiatric social worker for individual psychotherapy; a psychiatric nurse for management of responses related to the mental disorder,

BOX 6.5

Canadian Standards of Psychiatric and Mental Health Nursing

Standard III: *Administers and Monitors Therapeutic Interventions*

Due to the nature of mental health problems and mental disorders, there are unique practice issues confronting the psychiatric and mental health nurse in the assessment phase and the administration of therapeutic interventions. Safety in psychiatric and mental health nursing has unique meaning because many clients are at risk for harm to self or others and self-neglect. Clients may not be mentally competent to participate in all aspects of decision making. However, every effort must be made to include the client. In collaboration with the client, the PMH nurse needs to be alert to adverse reactions as clients' ability to self-report may be impaired.

The PMH nurse uses evidence-based and experiential knowledge from nursing, health sciences, and related mental health disciplines to both select and tailor nursing interventions.

The nurse:

1. Utilizes and evaluates evidence-based interventions to provide safe, effective, and efficient nursing care.
2. Provides information to clients and families/significant others, ensuring that the client consents to such information being shared, on an on-going basis about care and treatment.
3. Assists, educates, and empowers clients to select choices that will support positive changes in their affect, cognition, behaviour, and relationships, even when some of these choices may involve a level of risk as assessed by the clinical team (CNA, 1997b, p. 68).
4. Supports clients to draw on own assets and resources for self-care, activities of daily living, mobilizing resources, and mental health promotion (CNA, 1997b, p. 68).
5. Makes discretionary clinical decisions, using knowledge of client's unique responses and paradigm cases as the basis for the decision, eg., frequency of client contact in the community.
6. Uses appropriate technology to perform safe, effective, and efficient nursing intervention (CNA, 1997b, p. 68).
7. Administers medications accurately and safely, monitoring therapeutic responses, reactions, untoward effects, toxicity, and potential incompatibilities with other medications or substances. Provides medication education with appropriate content and in accordance with workplace policies.
8. Assesses client responses to deficits in activities of daily living, mobilizes resources in response to client's capabilities, and offers alternatives when appropriate.
9. Provides support and assists with protection for clients experiencing difficulty with self-protection.
10. Utilizes therapeutic elements of group process.
11. Incorporates knowledge of family dynamics and cultural values and beliefs about families in the provision of care.
12. Collaborates with the client, health care providers, and community to access and coordinate resources and seeks feedback from the client and others regarding interventions.
13. Incorporates knowledge of community needs or responses in the provision of care.
14. Encourages and assists clients to seek out support groups for mutual aid and support.
15. Assesses the client's response to, and perception of, nursing and other therapeutic interventions.

administration of medication, and monitoring side effects; and an occupational therapist for transition into the workplace. In the community clinic, a client may meet weekly with a therapist, monthly with a physician or nurse practitioner who reviews response to prescribed medication, and twice a week with a group leader in a day treatment program. All these professionals bring a specialized skill to the client's care.

However, a multidisciplinary approach may lead to fragmented care when approaches are independent of each other. An **interdisciplinary approach**, in which interventions from the different disciplines are integrated in delivery of care, can be more effective. In this model, a nurse and a psychologist may simultaneously intervene with a client on changing a behaviour related to medication compliance. An interdisciplinary approach requires close collaboration among the care team.

When an interdisciplinary approach is taken, it involves the creation and implementation of an integrated care plan. Nursing care will be a component of the plan, and aspects of collaboration should be outlined. It is often the nurse who coordinates the delivery of care by the various disciplines.

CHALLENGES OF PSYCHIATRIC NURSING

The challenges of psychiatric nursing are increasing in the 21st century. New knowledge is being generated, technology is shaping health care into new dimensions, and nursing practice is becoming more specialized and autonomous. This section discusses a few of the challenges.

Knowledge Development, Dissemination, and Application

Results of new research efforts continually redefine our knowledge base relative to mental disorders and their treatment. For instance, there have been significant advances in neurobiologic knowledge. In the 1900s, the cause of schizophrenia was hypothesized to be overactivity of dopamine. Later, it was discovered that other

BOX 6.6

Canadian Standards of Psychiatric and Mental Health Nursing

Standard IV: *Effectively Manages Rapidly Changing Situations*

The effective management of rapidly changing situations is essential in critical circumstances that may be termed psychiatric emergencies. These situations include self-harm and assaultive behaviours and rapidly changing mental health states. This domain also includes evidence-based assessment and screening for risk factors and referral related to psychiatric illnesses and social problems, ie, substance abuse, violence/abuse, and suicide/homicide (SERPN, 1996, p. 41).

The nurse:

1. Utilizes the therapeutic relationship throughout the management of rapidly changing situations.
2. Assesses the client using a comprehensive holistic approach for actual or potential health problems, issues, risk factors; and crisis/emergency/catastrophic situations. eg, psychotic episode, neuroleptic malignant syndrome, acute onset of extra pyramidal side effects, substance abuse, violence/abuse and suicide/homicide, drug toxicity, and delirium.
3. Knows resources required to manage actual and potential crisis/emergency/catastrophic situations and plans access to these resources.
4. Monitors client safety and utilizes continual assessment to detect early changes in client status, and intervenes accordingly.
5. Implements timely, age-appropriate, client-specific crisis/emergency/catastrophic interventions as necessary.
6. Commences critical procedures: in an institutional setting, ie, suicide precautions, emergency restraint, elopement precautions, infectious disease management, when necessary; in a community setting, uses appropriate community support systems, eg, police, ambulance services, crisis response resources.
7. Coordinates care to prevent errors and duplication of efforts where rapid intervention is imperative.
8. Utilizes a "least restraint" approach to care.
9. Development and adequate documentation of the crisis/emergency/catastrophic intervention/plan.
10. Evaluates the effectiveness of the rapid responses and modifies critical plans as necessary.
11. In collaboration with the client, facilitates the involvement of the family and significant others to assist in the identification of the precipitates of the crisis/emergency event and plan to minimize risk for recurrence.
12. Participates in "debriefing" process with team (including client and family) and other service providers, eg, reviews of critical event and emergency situation.
13. Utilizes safety measures to protect self, colleagues, and clients from potentially abusive situations in the work environment (eg, harassment, psychological abuse, and physical aggression).
14. Implements appropriate protocols for disasters.
15. Participates in educational, organizational, and institutional activities, which improve client safety in the practice setting.

BOX 6.7

Canadian Standards of Psychiatric and Mental Health Nursing

Standard V: *Intervenes Through the Teaching–Coaching Function*

All nurse–client interactions are potentially teaching/learning situations. The PMH nurse attempts to understand the life experience of the client and uses this understanding to support and promote learning related to health and personal development. The nurse provides health promotion information to individual, family, and group populations and communities.

The nurse:

1. In collaboration with the client determines clients' learning needs.
2. Plans and implements, with the client, health promotion education while considering the context of the client's life experiences. Considers: readiness, culture, literacy, language, preferred learning style, and resources available.
3. Engages with the client to explore available options and resources to build knowledge to make informed choices related to health needs and to navigate the system as needed.
4. Facilitates the client's search for ways to find meaning of their experience.
5. Incorporates knowledge of a wide variety of learning models and principles when creating opportunities for clients; for example, health promotion models, adult-learning principles, stages of development, cultural competence, and health beliefs models.
6. Provides relevant information guidance and support to the client's significant others.
7. Documents the teaching/learning process (assessment, plan, implementation, client involvement and evaluation).
8. Determines, with the client, the effectiveness of the educational process and collaboratively develops or adapts the ways to meet learning needs.
9. Engages in teaching/learning opportunities as partners with community agencies and consumer and family groups.

BOX 6.8

Canadian Standards of Psychiatric and Mental Health Nursing

Standard VI: *Monitors and Ensures the Quality of Health Care Practices*

The nurse has a responsibility to advocate for the client's right to receive the least restrictive form of care and to respect and affirm the client's right to self-determination in a safe, fair, and just manner. Mental health care occurs under the provisions of provincial or territorial Mental Health Acts and related legislation. It is essential for the PMH to be informed regarding the interpretation of relevant legislation and its implications for nursing practice.

The nurse:
1. Identifies workplace cultures (philosophy, attitudes, values, and beliefs that affect the nurse's ability to perform with skill, safety, and compassion and takes action as appropriate.
2. Explores how the determinants of health that affect the health of the community, for example, poverty, malnutrition, and unsafe housing, affect mental health nursing practice.
3. Understands current and relevant legislation and the implications for nursing practice, for example, privacy laws.
4. Expands and incorporates knowledge of innovations and changes in mental health and psychiatric nursing practice to ensure safe and effective care.
5. Ensures and documents ongoing review and evaluation of psychiatric and mental health nursing care activities.
6. Understands and questions the interdependent functions of the team within the overall plan of care.
7. Advocates for the client within the context of organizational and professional parameters and family and community interests.
8. Advocates for changes and improvements to the system/organizational structures in keeping with the principles of delivering safe, ethical, and competent care.
9. Recognizes the dynamic changes in health care locally and globally and, in collaboration with stakeholders, develops strategies to manage these changes. For example, considers changes in determinants of health that affect the community, terrorism, decline of industries.

BOX 6.9

Canadian Standards of Psychiatric and Mental Health Nursing

Standard VII: *Practices Within Organizational and Work-Role Structure*

The PMHN role is assumed within organizational structures, in both community and institutional contexts, through the provision of psychiatric/mental health care. For the PMHN, the ethic of care is based on reflective and evidence-based practice judgments within complex and dynamic situations. The increasing move of mental health/psychiatric treatment into the community necessitates the psychiatric and mental health nurse to be knowledgeable and skilful in collaborative care planning and implementation, mental health promotion, social action, and community consultation.

The nurse:
1. Works in collaborative partnerships with clients/families and other stakeholders to facilitate healing environments that ensure the safety, support, and respect of all persons.
2. Understands quality outcome indicators and strives for continuous quality improvement.
3. Actively participates with nurses to sustain and promote a climate that supports ethical practice and the establishment of a moral community (Varcoe, Rodney, & McCormick, 2003).
4. Participates in supporting a climate of trust that sponsors openness, encouraging questioning of the status quo and the reporting of incompetent care (CNA, 2002).
5. Seeks to utilize constructive and collaborative approaches to resolve differences affecting care among members of the health care team (CNA, 2002).
6. Actively participates in developing, implementing, and critiquing mental health policy for community and institutional settings.
7. Supports the contribution of leadership, as it occurs within the advanced practice role, to effective care and treatment.
8. Practices independently within legislated scope of practice.
9. Supports and participates in mentoring and coaching new graduates.
10. Utilizes knowledge of collaborative strategies for social action in working with consumer and advocacy groups.

From Canadian Federation of Mental Health Nurses. (2005). *The Canadian standards of psychiatric and mental health nursing practice* (3rd ed.). Toronto: Author.

neurotransmitters seemed to play a role as well. Such knowledge resulted in new medications with various side-effect profiles becoming available, requiring nurses to redefine their monitoring and interventions related to medication administration.

The presence of comorbid medical disorders is gaining importance in the treatment of mental disorders. For example, hypertension, hypothyroidism, hyperthyroidism, and diabetes mellitus all affect the treatment of psychiatric disorders. In some settings, the nurse may be the only one who has a background in medical disorders, such as human immunodeficiency viral illness, acquired immunodeficiency syndrome, and other somatic health problems.

The challenge for nurses today is to stay abreast of the advances in total health care in order to provide safe, competent care to individuals with mental disorders. Nurses must strive to provide evidence-based nursing care, developing their knowledge on an ongoing basis. Accessing up-to-date information through journals, electronic databases, and continuing education programs is a recognized responsibility.

Not only do nurses need to access current research studies but they also must evaluate the usefulness of the studies. For instance, one research project supporting a particular treatment approach may not be as meaningful as several statistically significant studies. The results of qualitative research studies, although not generalizable, may have important implications for practice, for instance, insights that can deepen our understanding of client experiences. Nurses practicing in psychiatric and mental health settings are challenged to improve care by integrating knowledge into a biopsychosocial model that includes all human responses to potential or actual health problems.

Health Care Delivery System Challenges

Additional continuing challenges for PMH nurses include supporting the integration of mental health care within primary health care and articulating the influence of the determinants of health on mental health. Competent, ethical PMH nursing care provided within integrated hospital and community health services is needed to meet the emerging needs of the Canadian population. Assertive community treatment, for instance, reduces inpatient service use, promotes continuity of outpatient care, and increases the stability and quality of life of clients with serious mental illnesses. Nurses have a role making the Canadian health care system more responsive to the mental health needs of individuals, families, and the community.

Consumers of mental health services are gaining voice and calling for changes in the delivery of services. Inequities in health care for marginalized populations, such as those living with a chronic mental illness, are being challenged. Paternalistic approaches to the delivery of care are being actively rejected, and the use of partnership models is being advocated. Nurses and other health professionals are collaborating with consumers to effect these positive changes.

Impact of Technology

The impact of technologic advances on PMH nursing is unprecedented. Nurses are challenged to gain and develop the skills to use this technology in improving care. Telemedicine, for example, takes many forms, from communicating with remote sites to completing educational programs. Technology can facilitate clients and families in learning about disorders, treatment, and resources. Software programs can make daily functioning easier for some, and electronic mail and the Internet are effective forms of communication. Advocacy groups for consumers of mental health services use these means to organize and lobby for change locally, nationally, and internationally.

A significant challenge related to new technology is maintaining client confidentiality. Client records, once stored in remote areas and rarely viewed, are now readily available and easily accessed. Nurses need to be vigilant in maintaining privacy and confidentiality. Moreover, documentation skills need to be updated continually to reflect quality client care within the changing health care environment.

PSYCHIATRIC AND MENTAL HEALTH NURSING ORGANIZATIONS

Whereas the establishment and reinforcement of standards go a long way toward legitimizing PMH nursing, it is professional organizations that provide leadership in shaping mental health care. They do so by providing a strong voice for meaningful legislation that promotes quality client care and advocates for maximal use of nursing skills.

The CNA is one such organization. Although its focus is on addressing the emergent needs of nursing in general, the CNA supports PMH nursing practice through such activities as advocating for PMH nursing at the national and provincial levels and working closely with PMH nursing organizations. The CNA is a federation of 11 provincial and territorial registered nurses associations. CNA speaks for Canadian registered nurses and represents Canadian nursing to other organizations on national and international levels. The membership of approximately 110,000 registered nurses is broad and diverse and reflects the face of nursing today.

Canadian Certification as a Psychiatric and Mental Health Nurse

Nurses with current registration and licence in Canada who have completed a minimum of 3,900 hours in PMH nursing practice within the past 5 years (Option A) *or* who have a nursing degree or post–basic course/program in the specialty (of at least 300 hours) and have accumulated a minimum of 1,950 hours of PMH nursing practice during the past 3 years (Option B) are eligible to apply for national certification by the CNA, provided they have endorsement by a supervisor or consultant in the specialty. Upon achieving a Pass on the PMHN Certification examination, the nurse is certified for 5 years and can use CPMHN(C) after their name. Recertification is possible if 100 hours of continuous learning activities in the specialty were completed during the 5 years or by retaking the Certification examination.

The Registered Psychiatric Nurse

In the four western provinces of British Columbia, Alberta, Saskatchewan, and Manitoba, PMH nursing is also practiced by registered psychiatric nurses (RPNs). These nurses have provincial regulatory bodies (separate from those of registered nurses) that register graduates from psychiatric nursing programs (ranging from diploma, to postdiploma, to degree). At CNA's 2005 annual meeting, a resolution was carried that the staff of CNA and the Registered Psychiatric Nurses of Canada should begin discussions to consider whether RPN associations should be invited to join CNA and whether RPNs should become eligible for CNA PMHN Certification.

Other Associations

The American Psychiatric Nurses Association (APNA) is the equivalent of the CFMHN in the United States. Its primary mission is advancing the psychiatric and mental health nursing practice; improving mental health care for culturally diverse individuals, families, groups, and communities; and shaping health policy for the delivery of mental health services.

The International Society of Psychiatric–Mental Health Nurses (ISPN) is an organization that works to unite and strengthen the presence and the voice of PMH nurses and to promote quality care for individuals and families with mental health problems. The ISPN consists of three specialist divisions: the Association of Child and Adolescent Psychiatric Nurses, the International Society of Psychiatric Consultation Liaison Nurses, and the Society for Education and Research in Psychiatric–Mental Health Nursing. Student memberships are available.

In Canada, there is a close relationship between mental health providers and those receiving care. One example of this relationship is the Canadian Alliance on Mental Illness and Mental Health (CAMIMH). CAMIMH, created in 1998, consists of consumers, their families, researchers, and care providers from numerous professions. Their mission is to influence national policy, to speak in a unified voice, and to focus strategically on mental health and mental illness. CAMIMH is also a member of the Canadian Collaborative Mental Health Initiative (CCMHI). The CCMHI has received national funding from Health Canada's Primary Health Care Transition Fund. Their prime goal is to improve the mental health of Canadians by strengthening relationships and enhancing collaboration among consumers, families, communities, and health care providers. They believe that consumers require access to services from the appropriate providers, in a timely manner, at an accessible location and with the fewest obstacles. An international advocacy group is Mental Disability Rights International (MDRI), dedicated to the enforcement of rights of people with mental disabilities. They have reports on human rights and mental health in Uruguay (1995), Hungary (1997), Mexico (2000), and Peru (2004).

The World Federation for Mental Health (WFMH) is an international organization whose mission, since 1948 when it was founded, has been to advance mental health promotion and mental disorder prevention and care among all peoples and nations. It works with governments (members are from 112 countries) and non-government groups. The CFMHN joined the WFMH in 1993.

PSYCHIATRIC AND MENTAL HEALTH NURSING IN A GLOBAL COMMUNITY

Professional associations and alliances with advocacy groups can support PMH nurses in responding to their responsibilities as health professionals in a global community. These responsibilities include opposing the stigma and discrimination associated with mental illness around the world and the inequities experienced by people with mental disorders in their daily lives and within the health care systems upon which they rely for treatment and care (Desjarlais, Eisenberg, Good, & Kleinman, 1995).

Capacity building among health care practitioners to enable them to promote mental health, to prevent mental illness, and to provide quality mental health care is a pressing priority for the WHO (2001), as outlined in their report, *Mental Health: New Understanding, New Hope.*

The Faculty of Nursing at the University of Alberta is a WHO Collaborating Centre in Nursing and Mental Health, with capacity building for mental health care being the Centre's prime directive. The Centre's work involves such initiatives as supporting countries in the Caribbean in their move toward community-based care and helping nurses in Latin America to develop research expertise related to mental health and addiction issues. Through such local, national, and international organizations, the individual PMH nurse can make a significant contribution in bringing mental health to all.

SUMMARY OF KEY POINTS

- The biopsychosocial model focuses on the three separate but interdependent dimensions of biologic, psychological, and social factors in the assessment and treatment of mental disorders. The spiritual dimension is also a key factor, encompassed within the psychological dimension. This comprehensive and holistic approach to mental disorders is the foundation for effective PMH nursing practice and is used as the basic organizational framework for this text.
- The framework of the *Canadian Standards of Psychiatric and Mental Health Nursing* is based on the seven domains of practice delineated in Patricia Benner's research on nursing practice. Expected competencies are associated with each domain.
- The PMH nurse interacts with other disciplines and many times acts as a coordinator in the delivery of care.
- PMH nurses need to be aware of team dynamics and their impact on care. When nurses practice in interdisciplinary settings, there may be an overlapping of professional roles. Nurses are accountable for both discrete and shared functions that they perform in their practice.
- New challenges for PMH nurses are emerging. Using technology well, including the protection of privacy and confidentiality; applying research findings to practice; and working to make the health care system more responsive to the mental health needs of Canadians are some of those challenges.
- Nurses and other health professionals practicing in psychiatric and mental health settings need to collaborate with consumers, families, and communities in all aspects of care.
- Several organizations provide leadership in shaping local, national, and international mental health care, providing an avenue for the PMH nurse to make a significant, positive difference.

CRITICAL THINKING CHALLENGES

1 Explain the biopsychosocial model and apply it to the following three clinical examples:
   a. A first-time father is extremely depressed after the birth of his child, who is perfectly healthy.
   b. A child is unable to sleep at night because of terrifying nightmares.
   c. A older woman is resentful of moving into a senior citizens' residence even though the decision was hers.

2 Identify some mental health needs of the Canadian population. Consider such needs across such factors as age, location, general health, and socioeconomic status.

3 Use the CD-ROM included with this book to access a complete version of the *Canadian Standards of Psychiatric and Mental Health Nursing*. Review the Beliefs/Values and the brief description of the history of PMH nursing included in the document.

4 Visit the website of the organizations listed in the Web Links section of this chapter and discover the role of each in promoting quality mental health care or supporting nursing practice.

5 Contrast *multidisciplinary* and *interdisciplinary* practice. Describe how and when nursing care plans and integrated care paths should be used.

MOVIES

Awakenings: 1990. Based on the book by Oliver Sacks, this film is the story of victims of an encephalitis epidemic who have remained in a catatonic state for years. A new physician arrives at the hospital where they "reside" and, desperate to help them, gets permission to try a potential chemical cure. His clients begin to awaken. We see the nurses engaging with the awakened individuals in a deeper way than they did when the clients were comatose. One client, played by Robert DeNiro, becomes paranoid and aggressive from too much of the dopamine treatment. This person, however, has much to teach the physician and nurses about living life fully.

VIEWING POINTS: Nurses practicing in psychiatric and mental health settings strive to engage therapeutically with those in their care. Consider the challenge of engaging with an unresponsive, catatonic person and with a person who is suspicious and aggressive. What ideas does this movie offer you in terms of meeting such challenges?

WEB LINKS

www.cna-nurses.ca Canadian Nurses Association website
www.cfmhn.org Canadian Federation of Mental Health Nurses website
www.miaw-ssmm.ca Canadian Alliance on Mental Illness and Mental Health website
www.cpa-apc.org Canadian Psychiatric Association website
www.ccmhi.ca Canadian Collaborative Mental Health Initiative website
www.nursingworld.org American Nurses Association website

www.apna.org   American Psychiatric Nurses Association website

www.ispn-psych.org   International Society of Psychiatric–Mental Health Nurses website

www.who.int   World Health Organization website

www.mdri.org   Mental Disability Rights International website

www.wfmh.org   World Federation for Mental Health website

REFERENCES

Abraham, I., Fox, J., & Cohen, B. (1992). Integrating the bio into the biopsychosocial: Understanding and treating biological phenomena in psychiatric–mental health nursing. *Archives of Psychiatric Nursing, 6*(5), 296–305.

American Nurses Association. (2001). *Code for nurses with interpretive statements.* Washington, DC: Author.

American Nurses Association, American Psychiatric Nurses Association, & International Society of Psychiatric–Mental Health Nurses. (2000). *Scope and standards of psychiatric–mental health nursing practice.* Washington, DC: American Nurses Publishing.

Austin, W., Gallop, R., Harris, D., & Spencer, E. (1996). A domain of practice approach to the standards of psychiatric and mental health nursing. *Journal of Psychiatric and Mental Health Nursing, 3,* 111–115.

Benner, P. (1984). *From novice to expert: Excellence and power in clinical nursing practice.* Menlo Park, CA: Addison-Wesley.

Burkhardt, M. A., & Nagai-Jackson, M. G. (1997). Spirituality and healing. In B. M. Dossey (Ed.), *Core curriculum for holistic nursing,* pp. 42–51. Gaithersburg, MD: Aspen.

Canadian Federation of Mental Health Nurses. (1998). *The Canadian standards of psychiatric and mental health nursing* (2nd ed.). Toronto: Author.

Canadian Federation of Mental Health Nurses. (2005). *The Canadian standards of psychiatric and mental health nursing* (3rd ed.). Toronto: Author.

Canadian Nurses Association (CNA). (2002). *Code of ethics for Registered Nurses.* Ottawa: Author.

Canadian Nurses Association. (1998, April). *A national framework for the development of standards for the practice of nursing: A discussion paper for Canadian Registered Nurses.* (ISBN 1-55119-033-8). Ottawa: Author.

Desjarlais, R., Eisenberg, L., Good, B., & Kleinman, A. (1995). *World mental health: Problems and priorities in low-income countries.* New York: Oxford University Press.

Health & Welfare Canada. (1988). Mental health for Canadians: Striking a balance (Cat. H39-128/1988E). Ottawa: Minister of Supply and Service Canada.

Mauk, K., & Schmidt, N. (2004). *Spiritual care in nursing practice.* New York: Lippincott Williams & Wilkins.

O'Reilly, M. (2004). Spirituality and mental health clients. *Journal of Psychosocial Nursing and Mental Health Service, 42*(7), 44–59.

U.S. Department of Health and Human Services. (1999). *Mental health: A report of the Surgeon General.* Rockville, MD: Author.

Varcoe, C., Rodney, P., & McCormick, J. (2003). Health care relationships in context: An analysis of three ethnographies. *Qualitative Health Research, 13*(7), 957–973.

World Health Organization (2001). *The World Health report 2001. Mental health: New understanding, new hope.* Geneva: Author.

For challenges, please refer to the **CD-ROM** in this book.

Theoretic Basis of Psychiatric and Mental Health Nursing

Mary Ann Boyd and Ginette Pagé

LEARNING OBJECTIVES

After studying this chapter, you will be able to:

- Discuss the need for theory-based psychiatric and mental health (PMH) practice.
- Compare key elements of theories that provide a basis for such practice.
- Describe common nursing models used in PMH nursing.
- Identify theories that contribute to our understanding of human beings and their behaviour.

KEY TERMS

behaviourism ▪ classical conditioning ▪ cognition ▪ collective unconscious ▪ connections ▪ conscious countertransference ▪ defence levels ▪ diathesis ▪ disconnections ▪ disinhibition ▪ ego ▪ empathy ▪ empathic linkages ▪ expressed emotion ▪ family dynamics ▪ formal support systems ▪ genetics ▪ genomics ▪ id ▪ informal support systems ▪ interpersonal relations ▪ modelling ▪ object relations ▪ operant behaviour ▪ preconscious ▪ role ▪ self-actualization ▪ self-efficacy ▪ self-system ▪ shaping ▪ social distance ▪ superego ▪ transaction ▪ transference ▪ unconscious

⬟ KEY CONCEPT

- theory

This chapter presents an overview of some of the nursing and other theories that serve as the knowledge base for PMH nursing practice. Many of the theories underlying this practice are evolving, and only some have research support to date. As acknowledged in the Canadian Standards of Psychiatric and Mental Health Nursing, PMH nurses use knowledge from nursing, the health sciences and related mental health disciplines in their practice. The chapter begins, then, with selected nursing theories and moves to some of the many theories that underlie our understanding of the biologic, psychological and social aspects of human thought and behaviour.

NURSING THEORIES

Nursing **theories** are essential in conceptualizing nursing practice. A nurse may choose to base his or her practice consistently on one nursing theory or may choose to use a specific theory depending on the care situation. For example, in nursing a person with schizophrenia who has problems related to maintaining self-care, Dorothea Orem's theory may be particularly useful. Hildegard Peplau's theory may be more helpful in addressing relationship issues.

> ⬢ **KEY CONCEPT** A **theory** is an account of a phenomenon that is composed of an interrelated set of definitions, concepts, and propositions.

Nightingale: The Visionary

Florence Nightingale (b. 1820), the founder of modern nursing, is recognized as the first nurse researcher and the pioneer of theory development in nursing. Many nurses believe that "if her model for nursing had been followed, the nursing profession would be in a much more advantageous position in society today" (MacPhail, 1988, p. 49). The respect for her legacy is apparent: International Nurses Day is celebrated on her birthday, May 12; Canada's National Nursing Week occurs the second week of May. Nightingale's model, developed in the mid-1800s, emerged from her work in hospitals and in the Crimean war, where unhealthy physical environments for the sick prevailed (Nightingale, 1859). This is the reason that the primary focus of her model, although not neglecting psychosocial needs, is on improving environmental conditions. Nightingale's intent was to create healthy surroundings that help alleviate suffering and promote well-being. Health, for her, included the ability to use "every power we have" (p. 334). For example, she considered that giving false reassurance to sick people was unacceptable behaviour. For Nightingale, the curative process was accomplished by nature alone: medicine and nursing do not cure. Nursing activities, therefore, were to "put the patient in the best condition for nature to act upon him [her]" (p. 133).

Interpersonal Relations Models

Hildegard Peplau: Interpersonal Relations

Hildegard Peplau's (b. 1909) theoretic perspectives continue to be an important base for the practice of PMH nursing. Influenced by Harry Stack Sullivan (discussed later in this chapter), Peplau introduced the first systematic theoretic framework for PMH nursing in her 1952 book *Interpersonal Relations in Nursing* (Peplau, 1952). One of her major contributions was the introduction of the nurse–patient relationship, including a conceptualization of its phases (see Chapter 8). Although her work continues to stimulate debate, she led PMH nursing out of the confinement of custodial care into theory-driven professional practice.

Peplau believed in the importance of the environment, defined as those external factors considered essential to human development (Peplau, 1992): cultural forces, presence of adults, secure economic status of the family, and a healthy prenatal environment. She believed in the importance of the "interpersonal environment," which included interactions between person and family, parent and child, or patient and nurse.

Peplau also emphasized the importance of empathic linkage, the ability to feel in oneself the feelings experienced by another person or people. The interpersonal transmission of anxiety or panic is the most common empathic linkage. According to Peplau, other feelings, such as anger, disgust, and envy, can also be communicated nonverbally by way of empathic transmission to others. She believed that if nurses pay attention to what they feel during a relationship with a patient, they can gain invaluable observations of feelings a patient is experiencing and has not yet noticed or talked about.

> ### CRNE Note
> In being empathic as a nurse, one should know that it is not enough to attempt to understand the patient's experience. Nurses need to communicate to their patients that they are attempting to understand.

The **self-system** is an important concept in Peplau's model. Drawing from Sullivan, Peplau defined the self as an "anti-anxiety system" and a product of socialization. The self proceeds through personal development that is always open to revision but tends toward a certain stability. For example, in parent–child relationships, patterns of approval, disapproval, and indifference are used by children to define themselves. If the verbal and nonverbal messages have been derogatory, children incorporate these messages and also view themselves negatively. The concept of need is important to

Peplau's model. Needs are primarily of biologic origin but need to be met within a sociocultural environment. When a biologic need is present, it gives rise to tension that is reduced and relieved by behaviours meeting that need. According to Peplau, nurses are not concerned about needs per se, but recognize the patients' patterns and style of meeting their needs in relation to their health status. Nurses interact with the patient to identify available resources, such as the quantity of food, availability of interpersonal support, and support for interaction patterns that help patients obtain what is needed.

Anxiety is a key concept for Peplau, who contends that professional practice is unsafe if this concept is not understood. If anxiety is not recognized, it continues to rise and escalates toward panic. There are various levels of anxiety (mild, moderate, severe, and panic levels), each having observable behavioural cues. These cues are sometimes called *defensive*, but Peplau argues that they are often "relief behaviours." For example, some people may relieve their anxiety by yelling and swearing, whereas others seek relief by withdrawing. In both instances, anxiety was generated by an unmet self-system security need.

Ida Jean Orlando: The Dynamic Nurse–Patient Relationship

In 1954, Ida Jean Orlando (b. 1926) studied the factors that enhanced or impeded the integration of mental health principles in the basic nursing curriculum. From this study, she published *The Dynamic Nurse–Patient Relationship*. Orlando identified three areas of nursing concern: the nurse–patient relationship, the nurse's professional role, and the identity and development of knowledge that is distinctly nursing (Orlando, 1961). A nursing situation involves the behaviour of the patient, the reaction of the nurse, and anything that does not relieve the distress of the patient. Patient distress is related to the inability of the individual to meet or communicate his or her own needs (Orlando, 1961; 1972).

Orlando's contribution to nursing practice focusses on the whole patient, rather than on the disease or institutional demands. Her ideas continue to be useful today, and current research supports her model (Olson & Hanchett, 1997). A small nursing study investigated whether Orlando's theory-based practice had a measurable impact on patients' immediate distress (n = 19) when compared with nonspecified nursing interventions (n = 11) (Potter & Bockenhauer, 2000). Orlando's approach consisted of the nurse validating the patient's distress before taking any action to reduce it. Patients being cared for by the Orlando group experienced significantly less stress than those being cared for with traditional nursing care.

Existential and Humanistic Theoretic Perspectives

Joyce Travelbee: Seeking Life Meaning

Influenced not only by Peplau and Orlando, Joyce Travelbee provided an existential perspective to nursing based on the works of Viktor Frankl, an existential philosopher who was a survivor of Nazi concentration camps. Existentialists believe that humans seek meaning in their life and experiences. "Suffering" is a feeling of displeasure ranging from simple and transitory mental, physical, or spiritual discomfort to extreme anguish, and to those phases beyond anguish, namely, the malignant phase of despair. Despair can be experienced as "not caring"; the terminal phase that follows is apathetic indifference (Travelbee, 1971). Travelbee also applied the concept of hope and defined it as a mental state characterized by the desire to gain an end or accomplish a goal combined with some degree of expectation that what is desired or sought is attainable.

Travelbee expanded the area of concern of PMH illness to include long-term physical illnesses. Focussing her attention on individuals who must learn to live with chronic illness, she believed that the nurse's spiritual values and philosophical beliefs about suffering would determine the extent to which the nurse could help ill people find meaning in these situations.

Travelbee's model was never subjected to empiric testing, and because of the philosophical underpinnings, it is unlikely that scientific research will be useful. However, her use of the interpersonal process as a nursing intervention and her focus on suffering and illness helped to define areas of concern and PMH nursing practice.

Jean Watson: Caring

The science of caring was initiated by Jean Watson (b. 1940). Watson believes that caring is the foundation of nursing and recommends that specific theories of caring be developed in relation to specific human conditions and health and illness experiences (Watson, 1990). She distinguishes between caring and curing, the work of medicine. The science of caring is based on 7 assumptions and 10 "carative" factors (Box 7-1).

Watson's theory is especially applicable to the care of those who seek help for mental illness. This model emphasizes the importance of sensitivity to self and others, the development of helping and trusting relations, the promotion of interpersonal teaching and learning, and provision for a supportive, protective, and corrective mental, physical, sociocultural, and spiritual environment. Research studies supporting the model use qualitative approaches (Baldursdottir & Jonsdottir, 2002).

Systems Models

Imogene M. King: Goal Attainment

The theory of goal attainment developed by Imogene M. King (b. 1923) is based on a systems model that includes three interacting systems: personal, interpersonal, and social (King, 1971). She believes that human beings interact with the environment and that the individual's perceptions influence reactions and interactions. For King, nursing involves caring for the human being, with the goal of health defined as adjusting to the stressors in both internal and external environments. She defines nursing as a "process of human interactions between nurse and patient whereby each perceives the other and the situation; and through communication, they set goals, explore means, and agree on means to achieve goals" (King, 1981, p. 144). The process is initiated to help the patient cope with a health problem that compromises his or her ability to maintain social roles, functions, and activities of daily living (King, 1992).

In this model, the person is goal oriented and purposeful, is reacting to stressors, and is viewed as an open system interacting with the environment. The variables in nursing situations are as follows:

- Geographic place of the transacting system, such as the hospital
- Perceptions of nurse and patient
- Communications of nurse and patient
- Expectations of nurse and patient
- Mutual goals of nurse and patient
- Nurse and patient as a system of interdependent roles in a nursing situation (King, 1981, p. 88)

The quality of nurse–patient interactions may have positive or negative influences on the promotion of health in any nursing situation. It is within this interpersonal system of nurse and patient that the healing process is performed. Interaction is depicted in which the outcome is a **transaction,** defined as the transfer of value between two or more people. This behaviour is unique, is based on experience, and is goal directed.

King's work reflects her understanding of the systematic process of theory development. She is a contemporary nursing theorist, and her model continues to be developed and applied in different settings, including psychiatric and mental health care. The King model was applied in group therapy for inpatient juvenile offenders, maximum security state offenders, and community parolees (Laben, Dodd, & Snead, 1991). This model has also been used as a nursing framework for individual psychotherapy (DeHowitt, 1992).

Betty Neuman: Systems and Stress

Betty Neuman (b. 1924) also used a systems approach as a model of nursing care. Neuman wanted to extend care beyond an illness model, incorporating concepts of problem finding and prevention and the newer behavioural science concepts and environmental approaches to wellness. Neuman developed her framework in the late 1960s as chairwoman of the University of California at Los Angeles graduate nursing program. The purpose of the model is to guide the actions of the professional caregiver through the assessment and intervention processes by focussing on two major components: the nature of the relationship between the nurse and patient, and the patient's response to stressors. The patient may be an individual, group (eg, a family), or community. The nurse is an "intervener" who attempts to reduce an individual's encounter with stress and to strengthen the person's ability to deal with stressors. The patient is viewed as a collaborator in setting health care goals and determining interventions. Neuman was one of the first PMH nurses to include the concept of stressors in understanding nursing care.

The model continues to be developed and applied. For example, the latest edition of the Neuman systems model is applied to a diversity of settings, including community health, family therapy, renal nursing, perinatal nursing, and mental health nursing of older adults (Neuman, Newman, & Holder, 2000). The model has also been applied to nursing care of patients with multiple sclerosis (Knight, 1990) and quality-of-life indicators defined as a perception of good physical health, being comfortable with socioeconomic status, and developing a psychospiritual self (Hinds, 1990). The Neuman Systems Model Trustee Group, Inc. was established in 1988 to preserve, protect, and perpetuate the integrity of the model for the future of nursing.

Dorothea Orem: Self-Care

Self-care is the focus of the general theory of nursing initiated by Dorothea Orem (b. 1914) in the early 1960s. The theory has three main focuses: self-care, self-care deficit, and a theory of nursing systems (Orem, 1991). Self-care is defined as those activities performed independently by an individual to promote and maintain personal well-being throughout life. Self-care deficits occur when an individual has a deficit in attitude (motivation), knowledge, or skill that impedes the meeting of self-care needs. Nurses can help individuals meet self-care requisites through five approaches: acting or doing for; guiding; teaching; supporting; and providing an environment to promote the patient's ability to meet current or future demands. The nursing systems theory refers to a series of actions a nurse takes to meet the patient's self-care requisites, varying from the individual being totally dependent on the nurse for care, to needing only some education and support. Orem's model is used extensively in psychiatric and mental health nursing because of its emphasis on promoting independence of the individual and on self-care activities (Campbell & Soeken, 1999).

Callistra Roy: Adaptation

Roy's nursing model is often selected by nurses working in inpatient psychiatric units because they find its concepts particularly relevant to their practice. This model, originating in 1964, describes humans as living adaptive systems with two coping mechanisms: the regulator and the cognator. The regulator copes with physiologic stimuli and the cognator with psychosociocultural stimuli. Manifestations of the coping mechanisms can be assessed by four adaptive modes: physiologic needs, self-concept, role function, and interdependence. In this model, the nursing process has four steps: nursing diagnosis, goal setting, intervention, and evaluation (Lutjens, 1991a) and involves the assessment of stimuli (focal, contextual, and residual).

Martha Rogers: Unitary Human Beings

The key concept of nursing for Martha Rogers (b. 1915) is **energy fields.** With its principles of homeodynamics—integrality, resonancy, and helicy—her abstract system offers a perspective of change as continuous and evolutionary (Rogers, 1994). Health and non-health are considered value laden, with the purpose of nursing being the promotion of human betterment. Important concepts are accelerating change, paranormal phenomena, and rhythmic manifestation of change. Rogers' science enables us to see human phenomena differently (Lutjens, 1991b). Roger's influence on other nursing theories such as Newman's (health as synthesis of disease and nondisease) and Parse's (health as human becoming) is evident.

BIOLOGIC THEORIES

Biologic theories are clearly important in understanding the manifestations of mental disorders and caring for people with these illnesses. Chapter 9 explains many of the important neurobiologic theories, and Chapter 13 focusses on psychopharmacology. Many of the biologically focussed interventions explained in Chapter 12 have their theoretic roots in basic nursing knowledge. This chapter describes two biologic approaches used to understand the expression of mental disorders.

Psychiatric Genetics

It has been noted for many decades that some families seem to have a susceptibility to a particular psychiatric illness. In fact, the 1823 archives of London's Bethlehem Royal Hospital ("Bedlam") indicate that the coversheet of case notes required the physician to answer "whether heredity?" (McGuffin & Southwick, 2003, p. 658). Paradoxically, recent discoveries in **genetics** (the study of specific DNA sequences or gene) and **genomics** (the study of the complete DNA structure or genome) make the answer to that question a more difficult and complex one, while at the same time providing evidence for the role of genes in psychopathology. The understanding of single gene disorders, such as Huntington's disease and early-onset familial Alzheimer disease, has advanced with research, but the pattern of inheritance of schizophrenia or bipolar disorders is more complex, involving multiple genes and environmental factors. For instance, there is some evidence of contributions to schizophrenia in linkage regions on chromosomes 8p, 13Q, and 22q and to bipolar disorder on chromosomes 13q and 22q regions, suggesting a genetic overlap (McGuffin & Southwick, 2003). The identifying role, if any, of genetics in some forms of addiction and in suicidal behaviour is also at an early stage (Courtet, 2005).

We do know, however, that genetics is not fate: nurture plays a role as well as nature. Environmental factors coact or interact with genes to increase (or to reduce) vulnerability to psychopathology (McGuffin & Southwick, 2003). The **diathesis-stress model** holds that certain genes or genetic combinations produce a diathesis, or constitutional predisposition or vulnerability to a disorder. When diathesis is combined with environmental stressors, abnormal behaviour results. According to this model, for a mental disorder to develop, there must be an interaction between diathesis and stress. Deciphering complicated gene–environment interaction in psychopathology is an exciting research area. Examples of relevant research include a study that shows how attribution of negative life events predicts alcohol use in undergraduate college students (Goldstein, Abela, Buchanan, & Buchanan, 2001) and one that reveals that maltreated children, with genotypes conferring low levels of monoamine oxidase A expression, developed conduct disorder, antisocial personality, and adult violent crime more often than children with high-activity genotypes (Moffitt, Caspi, & Rutter, 2005).

Studies in psychiatric genetics include twin and adoption studies (attempting to determine the role of heredity versus environment), linkage studies (finding the region of the genome that is inherited by affected people and not by unaffected people), and association studies (determining if an identified gene looks different in people with a disorder than in matched controls) (Conley, Steele, & Puskar, 2004). The ethical concerns related to psychiatric genetics must be addressed alongside the progress of this research. Atrocities have been committed in the name of "eugenics" (eg, the Nazi "extermination" of people with psychiatric illness), and information on an individual's genetic inheritance may lead to discrimination. Certainly, future findings in genetics will change the way mental disorders are understood and may affect the way individual responsibility is viewed (Corwin & Gill, 2003; Propping, 2005). Nurses need to keep abreast of the advances in genetic theory, testing, and intervention (Horner, 2004).

General Adaptation Syndrome

Hans Selye's landmark studies on stress described the interaction of environmental events and biologic responses (Selye, 1956). Selye looked for a link between illness and stressful events and identified the *general adaptation syndrome* (GAS), describing a three-stage process:

- alarm reaction
- resistance
- exhaustion

He hypothesized that during the alarm stage, patients exhibit an adrenocortical response associated with "fight-or-flight" behaviour. During the resistance phase, the body adapts to stress but functions at a lower than optimal level. If the adaptive mechanisms fail or wear out, the individual enters the third stage of exhaustion. At this point, the negative effects of the stressor spread to the entire organism, and Selye believed that ensuing illnesses could ultimately lead to death. Current research supports the relationship between illness and stressful events as argued by Selye, but new understandings about the specificity of responses, such as those within the neuroendocrine system, raise new questions about a general physical adaptation response.

Several nursing models refer to Selye's work. Roy's adaptation model, for instance, is linked to Selye's model by its physiologic mode of nursing assessment (Marriner-Tomey, 1994).

Applicability of Biologic Theories to Psychiatric and Mental Health Nursing

Both Selye's biophysical model and the diathesis-stress model are addressed by nurse theorists such as Neuman and Roy. Any holistic approach to care must acknowledge that humans are embodied beings with a genetic inheritance that shapes their responses to their environment and experiences.

PSYCHOLOGICAL THEORIES

Psychodynamic Theories

Psychodynamic theories explain human development processes, especially in early childhood, and their effects on thought and behaviour. The study of the unconscious is a key aspect of psychodynamic theory (Ellenberger, 1970). Many important concepts in PMH nursing began with the Austrian physician Sigmund Freud (1856–1939). Psychodynamic theories initially attempted to explain the cause of mental disorders, but etiologic explanations have not been consistently supported by empiric research. These theories, however, proved to be especially important in the development of therapeutic relationships, techniques, and interventions (Table 7-1).

Psychoanalytic Theory

Study of the Unconscious

In Freud's psychoanalytic model, the human mind was conceptualized in terms of **conscious** mental processes (an awareness of events, thoughts, and feelings with the ability to recall them) and **unconscious** mental processes (thoughts and feelings that are outside awareness and are not remembered). Freud believed that the unconscious part of the human mind is only rarely recognized by the conscious, as in remembered dreams. The term **preconscious** was used to describe unconscious material

Table 7.1	Psychodynamic Models		
Theorist	**Overview**	**Major Concepts**	**Applicability**
Psychoanalytic Models			
Sigmund Freud (1856–1939)	Founder of psychoanalysis. Believed that the unconscious could be accessed through dreams and free association. Developed a personality theory and theory of infantile sexuality.	Id, ego, superego Consciousness Unconscious mental processes Libido Object relations Anxiety and defence mechanisms Free associations, transference, and countertransference	Individual therapy approach used for enhancement of personal maturity and personal growth
Anna Freud (1895–1982)	Application of ego psychology to psychoanalytic treatment and child analysis with emphasis on the adaptive function of defence mechanisms.	Refinement of concepts of anxiety, defence mechanisms	Individual therapy, childhood psychoanalysis
Neo-Freudian Models			
Alfred Adler (1870–1937)	First defected from Freud. Founded the school of individual psychology.	Inferiority	Added to the understanding of human motivation
Carl Gustav Jung (1875–1961)	After separating from Freud, founded the school of psychoanalytic psychology. Developed new therapeutic approaches.	Redefined libido Introversion Extroversion Persona	Personalities are often assessed on the introversion and extroversion dimensions
Karen Horney (1885–1952)	Opposed Freud's theory of castration complex in women and his emphasis on the Oedipal complex. Argued that neurosis was influenced by the society in which one lived.	Situational neurosis Character	Beginning of feminist analysis of psychoanalytic thought
Interpersonal Relations			
Harry Stack Sullivan (1892–1949)	Impulses and striving need to be understood in terms of interpersonal situations.	Participant observer Parataxic distortion Consensual validation	Provided the framework for the introduction of the interpersonal theories in nursing
Humanist Theories			
Abraham Maslow (1921–1970)	Concerned himself with healthy rather than sick people. Approached individuals from a holistic-dynamic viewpoint.	Needs Motivation	Used as a model to understand how people are motivated and needs that should be met
Frederick S. Perls (1893–1970)	Awareness of emotion, physical state, and repressed needs would enhance the ability to deal with emotional problems.	Reality Here-and-now	Used as a therapeutic approach to resolve current life problems that are influenced by old, unresolved emotional problems
Carl Rogers (1902–1987)	Based theory on the view of human potential for goodness. Used the term *client* rather than *patient*. Stressed the relationship between therapist and client.	Empathy Positive regard	Individual therapy approach that involves never giving advice and always clarifying client's feelings

that is capable of entering consciousness. Uncovering unconscious material to help patients gain insight into unresolved issues was basic to the psychotherapy Freud developed.

Personality and Its Development
Freud's personality structure consisted of three parts: the id, ego, and superego (Freud, 1927). The id was formed by unconscious desires, primitive instincts, and unstructured drives, including sexual and aggressive tendencies that arose from the body. The **ego** consisted of the sum of certain mental mechanisms, such as perception, memory, and motor control, as well as specific defence mechanisms. The ego controlled movement, perception, and contact with reality. The capacity to form mutually satisfying relationships was a fundamental function of the

ego, which is not present at birth but is formed throughout the child's development. The **superego** was that part of the personality structure associated with ethics, standards, and self-criticism. A child's identification with important and esteemed people in early life, particularly parents, helped form the superego.

Object Relations and Identification

Freud introduced the concept of **object relations**, the psychological attachment to another person or object. He believed that the choice of a love object in adulthood and the nature of the relationship would depend on the nature and quality of the child's object relationships during the early formative years. The child's first love object was the mother, who is the source of nourishment and the provider of pleasure. Gradually, as the child separated from the mother, the nature of this initial attachment influenced any future relationships. The development of the child's capacity for relationships with others progressed from a state of narcissism to social relationships, first within the family and then within the larger community. Although the concept of object relations is fairly abstract, it can be understood in terms of a child who imitates her mother and then becomes like her mother in adulthood. This child has incorporated her mother as a love object, identifies with her, and becomes like her as an adult. This process becomes especially important in understanding an abused child who, under certain circumstances, becomes the adult abuser.

Anxiety and Defence Mechanisms

For Freud, anxiety was a specific state of unpleasantness accompanied by motor discharge along definite pathways, the reaction to danger of object loss. Defence mechanisms protected a person from unwanted anxiety. Although they are defined differently than in Freud's day, defence mechanisms still play an explanatory role in contemporary psychiatric and mental health practice. Defence mechanisms are discussed in Chapter 8; they are listed in Appendix H.

Sexuality

According to Freud, the energy or psychic drive associated with the sexual instinct, called the *libido*, literally translated from Latin to mean "pleasure" or "lust," resided in the id. When sexual desire was controlled and not expressed, tension resulted and was transformed into anxiety (Freud, 1905). Freud believed that adult sexuality was an end product of a complex process of development that began in early childhood and involved a variety of body functions or areas (oral, anal, and genital zones) that corresponded to stages of relationships, especially with parents.

Psychoanalysis

Freud (1949) developed *psychoanalysis*, a therapeutic process of accessing the unconscious and resolving the conflicts that originated in childhood with a mature adult mind. As a system of psychotherapy, psychoanalysis attempted to reconstruct the personality by examining free associations (spontaneous, uncensored verbalizations of whatever comes to mind) and the interpretation of dreams (Freud, 1955). Therapeutic relationships had their beginnings within the psychoanalytic framework.

Transference and Countertransference

Transference is the displacement of thoughts, feelings, and behaviours originally associated with significant others from childhood onto a person in a current therapeutic relationship (Moore & Fine, 1990). For example, a woman's feelings toward her parents as a child may be directed toward the therapist. If a woman were unconsciously angry with her parents, she may feel unexplainable anger and hostility toward her therapist. In psychoanalysis, the therapist uses transference as a therapeutic tool to help the patient understand emotional problems and their origin. It is considered an essential aspect to therapy. **Countertransference**, on the other hand, is defined as the direction of all the therapist's feelings and attitudes toward the patient. Feelings and perceptions caused by countertransference may interfere with the therapist's ability to understand the patient.

Neo-Freudian Models

Many of Freud's followers ultimately established their own forms of psychoanalysis. The various psychoanalytic schools have adopted other names because their doctrines deviated from Freudian theory.

Adler's Foundation for Individual Psychology

Alfred Adler (1870–1937), a Viennese psychiatrist and founder of the school of individual psychology, was an early colleague of Freud. He disagreed with Freud's focus on instinctual determination, and focussed instead on the social aspects of human existence. Adler believed mental health involves love, work, and community. For him, life goals are important. The motivating force in human life is a striving for superiority (Adler, 1963). Seeking perfection and security and trying to avoid feelings of inferiority can lead the individual to adopt a life goal that is unrealistic and frequently expressed as an unreasoning desire for power and dominance (ie, *inferiority complex*). Because inferiority is intolerable, the compensatory mechanisms set up by the mind may get out of hand, resulting in self-centred neurotic attitudes, overcompensation, and a retreat from the real world and its problems.

Adler focussed on growth, lifestyle, and becoming: humans are looking to realize their potential, to flourish within their community. Adlerian theory is based on principles of mutual respect, choice, responsibility, consequences, and belonging. Today, his theory and principles are applied to both psychotherapy (including family therapy) and education and exert a strong influence on the development of such psychotherapeutic approaches as Albert Ellis' Rational Emotive Therapy, in which people look to take risks and to become more responsible for their behaviour (Ellis, 1973).

Jung's Analytical Psychology

One of Freud's earliest colleagues, Carl Gustav Jung (1875–1961), a Swiss psychoanalyst, created a model called *analytical psychology*. For Jung, humans were influenced not only by their past, but also by what they were hoping for in the future. He supported the idea, not only of a personal unconscious, but of a second psychic system, the **collective unconscious**. The collective unconscious is universal, shared by all humans, and inherited, not individually developed. Within the collective unconscious are **archetypes**, forms or symbols common to all cultures. The image of Mother or Hero or Trickster, for instance, has a similar form in every society, important commonalities for humans (Jung, 1959). Jung described humans as having both feminine and masculine characteristics, and thought that therapy may be directed at helping an individual develop more fully as a person by embracing both aspects of himself or herself. His concept of **persona** (the mask one wears in society, one's public self) is similar to Freud's superego (Jung, 1966). The **shadow** is Jung's image for the dark side of every person, the side we do not like to recognize or show to others. For people to evolve as individuals, they need to become aware of and integrate their shadow into their personality, not attempt to extinguish it.

Jung believed in the existence of two psychological types: the **extrovert** (who finds meaning in the world) and the **introvert** (who finds meaning within). He also described four primary modes of orientation to the world: *thinking, feeling, intuition,* and *sensation*. Although he argued that each of these functions exists in an individual, certain preferences will dominate. Our unconscious is revealed often through our least developed mode. The Myers-Briggs Type Indicator tests are based on Jung's personality theory.

Horney's Feminine Psychology

Karen Horney (1885–1952), a German-American psychiatrist, challenged many of Freud's basic concepts and introduced principles of feminine psychology. Recognizing a male bias in psychoanalysis, Horney was the first to challenge the traditional psychoanalytic belief that women felt disadvantaged because of their genital organs. Freud believed that women felt inferior to men because their bodies were less completely equipped, a theory he described as "penis envy." Horney rejected this concept, as well as the Oedipal complex, arguing that there are significant cultural reasons why women may strive to obtain qualities or privileges that are defined by a society as being masculine. She argued that women truly were at a disadvantage because of the authoritarian culture in which they lived (Horney, 1939). Her primary concept

was that of basic anxiety: early (childhood) feelings of helplessness and isolation with which one strives to cope and resolve. This anxiety underlies all an individual's relationships. Behaviour can be understood as a reaction to basic anxiety. Horney named the unrealistic expectations that one puts on oneself "tyranny of the should" (Horney, 1950). Along with other Neo-Freudian, such as Eric Fromm, she introduced sociocultural dimensions of human behaviour into the psychoanalytical model.

Interpersonal Theories

Interpersonal theories were developed as an alternative explanation for human development and behaviour. Although there are similarities between psychoanalytic and interpersonal theories, the major difference is that interpersonal theories gave priority to relationships in personality development, with instincts and drives being less important. Childhood relationships with parenting figures are seen as especially significant and believed to influence important adult relationships, such as the choice of a mate.

Harry Stack Sullivan: Interpersonal Relations

Harry Stack Sullivan (1892–1949), an American psychiatrist, extended the concept of interpersonal relations to include characteristic interaction patterns. Sullivan studied personality characteristics that could be directly observed, heard, and felt. He believed that the health or sickness of one's personality was determined by the characteristic ways in which one dealt with other people. Health also depended on the constantly changing physical, social, and interpersonal environment as well as past and current life experiences (Sullivan, 1953).

Humanistic Theories

Humanistic theories were generated as a reaction against psychoanalytic premises of instinctual drives. Humanistic therapies are based on the views of human potential for goodness. Instead of focussing on instinctual drives, humanist therapists focus on one's ability to learn about oneself, acceptance of self, and exploration of personal capabilities. Within the therapeutic relationship, the patient begins to develop positive attitudes and view himself or herself as a person of worth. The focus is not on investigation of repressed memories, but on learning to experience the world in a different way.

Rogers' Client-Centred Therapy

Carl Rogers (1902–1987), an American psychologist, developed new methods of client-centred therapy. Rogers defined empathy as the capacity to assume the internal reference of the client in order to perceive the world in the same way as the client (Rogers, 1980). To use empathy in the therapeutic process, the counsellor must be non-directive, but not passive. Thus, the counsellor's attitude and nonverbal communication are crucial. He advocated that the therapist develop **unconditional positive regard**, a nonjudgmental caring for the client (Rogers, 1980) and believed that the therapist's emotional investment (ie, true caring) in the client is essential to the therapeutic process. Genuineness on the part of the therapist, in contrast with the passivity of the psychoanalyst, is seen as key.

Gestalt Therapy

Another humanistic approach created as a response to the psychoanalytic model was Gestalt therapy, developed by Frederick S. (Fritz) Perls (1893–1970), a German-born former psychoanalyst who immigrated to the United States. Perls believed that modern civilization inevitably produces neurotic anxiety because it forces people to repress natural desires and frustrates an inherent human tendency to adjust biologically and psychologically to the environment. For a person to be cured, unmet needs must be brought back to awareness. Perls did not believe that the intellectual insight gained through psychoanalysis enabled people to change. Instead, he devised individual and group exercises that enhanced the person's awareness of emotions, physical state, and repressed needs as well as physical and psychological stimuli in the here-and-now environment (Perls, 1969).

Abraham Maslow's Hierarchy of Needs

Abraham Maslow (1921–1970) developed a humanistic theory that is used in PMH nursing today (Maslow, 1998). His major contributions were to the understanding of needs and motivation (Maslow, 1970). He studied exemplary healthy persons (eg, Albert Einstein) whom he saw as self-actualizing and described their characteristics. For instance, he noted that they were creative and had a deep sense of kinship with others and a strong sense of ethics. People are self-actualized when they are making the most of their unique human potential. Maslow's view of human motivation was based on a hierarchy of needs, ranging from lower-level survival needs, such as air, water, basic food, and shelter, to higher-level needs, such as those for belonging and esteem and, finally, for **self-actualization** (Fig. 7-1). One must meet lower-level needs before moving to the higher-level ones. His theory offers a framework for assessment.

Frankl's Logotherapy

Viktor Frankl is considered a humanist and an existentialist. His perspective comes from his clinical back-

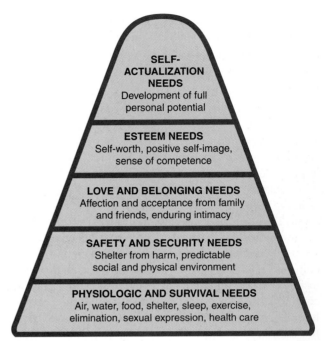

FIGURE 7.1 Maslow's hierarchy of needs.

ground and his personal experiences as a prisoner in Nazi concentration camps during World War II. Logotherapy is concerned with **meaning**. It is based on three assumptions: freedom of will, will to meaning, and meaning of life. Without meaning, life is empty. The goal of logotherapy is to help the person find meaning for herself or himself (Frankl, 1992).

Applicability of Psychodynamic Theories to Psychiatric and Mental Health Nursing

Several concepts in psychodynamic theories are core elements in PMH nursing practice, such as interpersonal relationships, needs, anxiety, defence mechanisms, transference, and countertransference. Many of these concepts are further developed within nursing theories. For instance, Freud's concept of anxiety contrasts with Peplau's (1952) levels of anxiety, and Frankl's logotherapy has commonalities with Travelbee's human-to-human relationship model. A key psychodynamic concept, the therapeutic relationship, is recognized as the core of PMH nursing intervention.

BEHAVIOURAL THEORIES

Behavioural theories, with roots in the discipline of psychology, offer important explanatory models for PMH nursing in terms of the way in which people act and learn (Table 7-2).

Table 7.2	**Behavioural Theorists**		
Theorist	**Overview**	**Major Concepts**	**Applicability**
Stimulus-Response Theories			
Edwin R. Guthrie (1886–1959)	Continued with understanding conditioning as being important in learning	Recurrence of responses tends to follow a specific stimulus	Important in analyzing habitual behaviour
Ivan P. Pavlov (1849–1936)	Classical conditioning	Unconditioned stimuli Unconditioned response Conditioned stimuli	Important in understanding learning of automatic responses such as habitual behaviours
John B. Watson (1878–1958)	Introduced behaviourism, believed that learning was classical conditioning called *reflexes;* rejected distinction between mind and body	Principle of frequency Principle of recency	Focusses on the relationship between the mind and body
Reinforcement Theories			
B. F. Skinner (1904–1990)	Developed an understanding of the importance of reinforcement and differentiated types and schedules	Operant behaviour Respondent behaviour Continuous reinforcement Intermittent reinforcement	Important in behaviour modification
Edward L. Thorndike (1874–1949)	Believed in the importance of effects that followed behaviour	Reinforcement	Important in behaviour modification programs
Cognitive Theories			
Albert Bandura (b. 1925)	Developed social cognitive theory, a model for understanding how behaviour is learned from others	Modelling Disinhibition Elicitation Self-efficacy	Important in helping patients learn appropriate behaviours
Aaron Beck (b. 1921)	Conceptualized distorted cognitions as a basis for depression	Cognitions Beliefs	Important in cognitive therapy
Kurt Lewin (1890–1947)	Developed field theory, a system for understanding learning, motivation, personality and social behaviour	Life space Positive valences Negative valences	Important in understanding motivation for changing behaviour
Edward Chace Tolman (1886–1959)	Introduced the concept of cognitions: believed that human beings act on beliefs and attitudes and strive toward goals	Cognition	Important in identifying person's beliefs

Early Stimulus-Response Theories

Pavlovian Theory

One of the earliest behavioural theorists was Ivan P. Pavlov (1849–1936), who was studying the gastric functioning of dogs when he noticed that stomach secretions of the dogs were stimulated by triggers other than food, such as the sight and smell of food. He became interested in this anticipatory secretion. Through his experiments, he was able to stimulate secretions with a variety of other laboratory nonphysiologic stimuli. Thus, a clear connection was made between thought processes and physiologic responses.

In Pavlov's model, there is an unconditioned stimulus (not dependent on previous training) that elicits an unconditioned (ie, specific) response. In his experiments, meat was the unconditioned stimulus, and salivation was the unconditioned response. Pavlov would then select other stimuli, such as a bell, a ticking metronome, and a triangle drawn on a large cue card, presenting this conditioned stimulus just before the meat, the unconditioned response. If the conditioned stimulus was repeatedly presented before the meat, eventually salivation was elicited by the conditioned stimulus. This phenomenon was called **classical** (Pavlovian) **conditioning** (Pavlov, 1927/1960).

John B. Watson and the Behaviourist Revolution

At about the same time Pavlov was working in Russia, John B. Watson (1878–1958) initiated the psychological revolution known as **behaviourism** in the United States. He developed two principles: frequency and recency. The principle of frequency states that the more often a given response is made to a given stimulus, the more likely the response to that stimulus will be repeated. The principle of recency states that the more recently a given response to a particular stimulus is made, the more likely it will be repeated. Watson's major contribution was the rejection of the distinction between body and mind and his emphasis on the study of objective behaviour (Watson & Rayner, 1917).

Reinforcement Theories

Edward L. Thorndike

A pioneer in experimental animal psychology, Edwin L. Thorndike (1874–1949) studied the problem-solving behaviour of cats to determine whether animals solved problems by reasoning or instinct. He found that neither choice was completely correct; animals gradually learn the correct response by "stamping in" the stimulus-response connection. The major difference between Thorndike and behaviourists such as Watson was that Thorndike believed in the importance of the effects that followed the response or the reinforcement of the behaviour. He was the first reinforcement theorist, and his view of learning became the dominant view in American learning theory (Thorndike, 1916).

B. F. Skinner

One of the most influential behaviourists, B. F. Skinner (1904–1990) recognized two different kinds of learning, each involving a separate kind of behaviour. *Respondent behaviour,* or the end result of classical conditioning, is elicited by specific stimuli. Given the stimulus, the response occurs automatically. The other kind of learning is referred to as *operant behaviour.* In this type of learning, the distinctive characteristic is the consequence of a particular behavioural response, not a specific stimulus. The learning of operant behaviour is also known as *conditioning,* but it is different from the conditioning of reflexes. If a behaviour occurs and is followed by reinforcement, it is probable that the behaviour will recur. For example, if a child climbs on a chair, reaches the faucet, and is able to get a drink of water successfully, it is more likely that the child will repeat the behaviour (Skinner, 1935). Skinner wrote a book about a utopian community based on the principles of behaviourism that he called *Walden II* (Skinner, 1976).

COGNITIVE THEORIES

The initial behavioural studies focussed attention on human actions without attention to the internal thinking process. As complex behaviour was examined and could not be accounted for by strictly behavioural explanations, thought processes became new subjects for study. Cognitive theories, an outgrowth of different theoretic perspectives, including the behavioural and the psychodynamic, attempted to link internal thought processes with human behaviour.

Albert Bandura's Social Cognitive Theory

Acquiring behaviours by learning from other people is the basis of social cognitive theory developed by the psychologist Albert Bandura, who was born in Mundare, Alberta (b. 1925). Bandura developed his ideas after being concerned about violence on television contributing to aggression in children. He believes that important behaviours are learned by internalizing behaviours of others. His initial contribution was identifying the process of **modelling:** pervasive imitation, or one person trying to be like another. According to Bandura, the model may not need to be a real person, but could be a character in history or generalized to an ideal person (Bandura, 1977).

The concept of **disinhibition** is important to Bandura's model and refers to the situation in which someone has learned not to make a response; then, in a given situation, when another is making the inhibited response, the individual becomes disinhibited and also makes the response. Thus, the response that was "inhibited" now becomes disinhibited through a process of imitation. For example, during severe dieting, an individual may have learned to resist eating large amounts of food. However, when at a party with a friend who eagerly fills a plate at a buffet, the person also eats large amounts of food.

In the instance of disinhibition, the desire to eat is already there, and the individual indulges that desire. However, in another instance, called **elicitation,** there is no desire present, but when one person starts an activity, others want to do the same. An example of this occurs when a child is playing with a toy, and the other children now want to play with the same toy even though they showed no interest in it before that time.

An important concept of Bandura's is **self-efficacy,** a person's sense of his or her ability to deal effectively with the environment (Bandura, 1993). Efficacy beliefs influence how people feel, think, motivate themselves, and behave. The stronger the self-efficacy, the higher the goals people set for themselves and the firmer their commitment to them.

Aaron T. Beck: Thinking and Feeling

American psychiatrist Aaron T. Beck (b. 1921) of the University of Pennsylvania devoted his career to understanding the relationship between cognition and mental health. For Beck, cognitions are verbal or pictorial events in the stream of consciousness. He realized the importance of cognitions when treating people with depression, finding that the depression improved when patients began thinking differently (Box 7-2).

BOX 7.2   RESEARCH FOR BEST PRACTICE

Aggression and Best Therapy

THE QUESTION: Of psychodynamic group psychotherapy and cognitive behaviour therapy, which has a better outcome for men with assaultive behaviour problems?

METHODS: To test the efficacy of a psychodynamic psychotherapy group (PPG) and a cognitive-behaviour group (CBG) for male veterans with a history of assault, a study was conducted in the Veterans Administration with 27 male subjects. The men were assigned randomly to a central group, PPG, or CBG. Data collected included the Addiction Severity Index, the Overt Aggression Scale, and the State-Trait Anger Expression Inventory. Analyses included an overall comparison of the groups as well as repeated-measures analyses and adjustments for covariates.

FINDINGS: The men in the PPG showed a trend toward improvement of overt aggression and significant improvement of trait aggression compared with the men in the CBG. There were no differences in stated aggression or efforts to control aggression. Both the PPG and CBG are effective treatments for aggression.

IMPLICATION FOR NURSING: This study provides hope to those who have difficulty controlling impulsive, aggressive behaviour. It is possible to decrease aggressive behaviour with more than one intervention.

Lanza, M. L., Anderson, J., Boisvert, C. M., LeBlanc, A., Fardy, M., & Steel, B. (2002). Assaultive behavior intervention in the Veterans Administration: Psychodynamic group psychotherapy compared to cognitive behavior therapy. *Perspective Psychiatric Care, 38*(3), 89–97.

He believed that people with depression had faulty information-processing systems that led to biased cognitions. These faulty beliefs cause errors in judgment that become habitual errors in thinking. These individuals incorrectly interpret life situations, judge themselves too harshly, and jump to inaccurate conclusions. A person may truly believe that he or she has no friends and therefore no one cares. On examination, the evidence for the beliefs is based on the fact that there has been no contact with anyone because of moving from one city to another. Thus, a distorted belief is the basis of the cognition. Beck and his colleagues developed cognitive therapy, a successful approach for the treatment of depression (see Chapter 18) (Beck, Thase, & Wright 2003). (See Chapter 14 for an overview of Cognitive Behavioural Therapy.) (See Box 7-2 for research comparing cognitive behavioural and psychodynamic group therapies.)

Applicability of Behavioural Theories to Psychiatric and Mental Health Nursing

Interventions based on behavioural theories are important in PMH nursing. For example, patient education interventions are usually based on learning principles derived from any number of the behavioural theories, and the teaching of new coping skills for patients regarding their symptoms of mental illnesses is usually based on behavioural theories. Changing an entrenched habit involves helping persons to identify what motivates them and how new lifestyle habits can become permanent. Examples of behavioural interventions used on in-patient hospital units include the privilege systems and token economies.

DEVELOPMENTAL THEORIES

The developmental theories explain normal human growth and development and focus on change over time. Many developmental theories are presented in terms of stages based on the assumption that normal development proceeds longitudinally from the beginning to the ending stage. Although this approach is useful, unless a stage model is truly supported by evidence, the model does not represent reality.

Erik Erikson: Psychosocial Development

Freud and Sullivan both published treatises on stages of human development, but Erik Erikson (1902–1994) outlined the psychosocial developmental model that is most often used in nursing. Erikson's model was an expansion of Freud's psychosexual development theory. Whereas Freud emphasized intrapsychic experiences, Erikson recognized the importance of culture. He believed that similar events may be experienced differently depending on a person's reaction, family background, and cultural situation.

Each of Erikson's eight stages is associated with a specific task that can be successfully or unsuccessfully resolved. The model is organized according to developmental conflicts by age: basic trust versus mistrust, autonomy versus shame and doubt, initiative versus guilt, industry versus inferiority, identity versus role diffusion, intimacy versus isolation, generativity versus stagnation, and ego integrity versus despair. Erikson's wife, Joan Serson Erickson, extended his theory to include old age as a ninth stage, gerotranscendence (Erikson & Erikson, 1997). Gerotranscendence theory focussed on the continued growth in dimensions such as spirituality and inner strength (see Chapter 29).

Within Erickson's theory, successful resolution of a crisis leads to essential strength and virtues. For example, a positive outcome of the trust versus mistrust crisis is the development of a basic sense of trust. If the crisis is unsuccessfully resolved, the infant moves into the next stage without a sense of trust. According to this model, a child who is mistrustful will have difficulty completing the next crisis successfully and, instead of developing a sense of autonomy, will more likely be full of shame and doubt (Erikson, 1963).

Identity and Adolescence

One of Erikson's major contributions was the recognition of the turbulence of adolescent development. Erikson wrote extensively about adolescence, youth, and identity formation. When adolescence begins, childhood ways must be given up, and body changes must be reconciled with the individual's social position, previous history, and identifications. An identity is formed. This task of reconciling how young people see themselves and how society perceives them can become overwhelming and lead to role confusion and alienation (Erikson, 1968).

Research Evidence for Erikson's Models

Two major areas of study support Erikson's models. One area of research focuses on the developmental stages and the second on gender differences. In one early study, male college students who measured low on identity also scored low on intimacy ratings (Orlofsky, Marcia, & Lesser, 1973). These results lend support to the idea that identity precedes intimacy. In still another study, intimacy was found to begin developing early in adolescence, before the development of identity (Ochse & Plug, 1986). Studying fathers with young children, Christiansen and Palkovitz (1998) found that generativity was associated with a paternal identity, psychosocial identity, and psychosocial intimacy. In addition, fathers who had a religious identification also had higher generativity scores than did others. These studies suggest that these well-known stages may be neither fixed nor sequential.

Evidence also suggests that girls' development is different than boys. One study shows that *generativity* (defined as the need or drive to produce, create, or effect a change) is associated with well-being in both males and females, but in males, generativity is related to the urge for self-protection, self-assertion, self-expansion, and mastery. In women, the antecedents may be the desire for contact, connection, and union (Ackerman, Zuroff, & Moskowitz, 2000).

Jean Piaget: Learning in Children

One of the most influential people in child psychology was Jean Piaget (1896–1980), who contributed more than 40 books and 100 articles on child psychology alone. Piaget viewed intelligence as an adaptation to the environment. He proposed that cognitive growth is like embryologic growth: an organized structure becomes more and more differentiated over time. Piaget developed a system that explains how knowledge develops and changes. Each stage of cognitive development represents a particular structure with major characteristics. Piaget's theory was developed through observation of his own children and therefore never received formal testing.

The major strength of his model was its recognition of the central role of cognition in development and the discovery of surprising features of young children's thinking. For PMH nursing, Piaget's model provides a framework on which to define different levels of thinking and use the data in the assessment and intervention processes. For example, the assessment of concrete thinking would be typical of people with schizophrenia who are unable to perform abstract thinking.

Carol Gilligan: Gender Differentiation

Carol Gilligan (b. 1936) argues that most development models are male centred and therefore inappropriate for girls and women. For Gilligan, attachment within relationships is the important factor for successful female development. After comparing male and female personality development, she highlighted the differences (Gilligan, 1982). Although the first primary relationship of both boys and girls is with the mother, in developing identity, boys separate from their mother and girls attach. Thus, girls probably learn to value relationships and become interdependent at an earlier age. They learn to value the ideal of care, begin to respond to human need, and want to take care of the world by sustaining attachments so that no one is left alone. According to Gilligan, female development does not follow a progression of stages but is based on experiences within relationships. However, some researchers suggest that relationships may also be equally important for boys in their development of a strong sense of self (Nelson, 1996).

Gilligan's conclusion that female development depends on relationships has implications for everyone who provides care to women. Traditional models that advocate separation as the primary goal of human development immediately place women at a disadvantage. By negating the value and importance of attachments within relationships, the natural development of women is impaired. If Erikson's model is applied to women, their failure to separate then becomes defined as a developmental failure (Gilligan, 1982). Currently, there is considerable debate about whether Erikson's developmental model is applicable to women.

Applicability of Developmental Theories to Psychiatric and Mental Health Nursing

Developmental theories are used in understanding childhood and adolescent experiences and their manifestations as adult problems. When working with children, nurses can use developmental models to help gauge development and mood. However, because most of the models are based on the assumptions of the linear progression of stages and have not been adequately tested, applicability has limitations. In addition, these models were based on a relatively small number of children who typically were raised in a Western middle-class environment. Most do not account for gender differences and diversity in lifestyles and cultures.

SOCIAL THEORIES

Numerous social theories underlie PMH nursing practice, and the nursing profession itself serves a specific societal function. This section represents a sampling of important social theories that nurses may use. This discussion is not exhaustive and should be viewed by the student as including only some of the theoretic perspectives that may be applicable.

Family Dynamics

Family dynamics are the patterned interpersonal and social interactions that occur within the family structure over the life of a family. Family dynamics models are based on systems theory describing a phenomenon in terms of a set of interrelated parts, in which the change of one part affects the total functioning of the system. A system can be "open" and interacting in the environment or "closed," completely self-contained and not influenced by the environment. The family is viewed organizationally as an open system in which one member's actions influence the functioning of the total system. Most of the theoretic explanations have emerged from treatment case studies, rather than from systematic development of theory based on generalizable research. Consequently, the limitation of available research should be considered when these models are used to understand family interactions and plan patient care (see Chapter 16).

Applicability of Family Theories to Psychiatric and Mental Health Nursing

Family theories are especially useful to nurses who are assessing family dynamics and planning interventions. Family systems models are used to help nurses form collaborative relationships with patients and families dealing with health problems. Generalist PMH nurses will not be engaged in family therapy. However, they will be caring for individuals and families. Understanding family dynamics is important in every nurse's practice. Many family interventions are consistent with these theories (see Chapter 16). Many of the symptoms of mental disorders, such as hallucinations or delusions, have implications for the total family and its interactions.

Balance Theory and Social Distance

A useful theory for understanding caregiving activities within a community is balance theory, proposed in 1966 by sociologist Eugene Litwak (b. 1925). This theory explains the importance of informal and formal support systems in the delivery of health care.

Formal support systems are large organizations, such as hospitals and nursing homes, that provide care to individuals. **Informal support systems** are family, friends, and neighbours. Litwak found that individuals with strong informal support networks actually live longer than those without this type of support. In addition, those without informal support have significantly higher mortality rates when the causes of death are accidents (eg, smoking in bed) or suicides (Litwak, 1985).

A key concept in balance theory is **social distance**, the degree to which the values of the formal organization and primary group members differ. The formal and informal groups are considered to be balanced when they are at a midpoint of social distance, that is, close enough to communicate, but not so close to destroy each other—neither enmeshment nor isolation (Litwak, Messeri, & Silverstein, 1990; Messeri, Silverstein, & Litwak, 1993). If the primary groups and the formal care system begin performing similar caregiving services, the formal system increases the social distance by developing linkages with the primary group. Thus, a balance is maintained between the two systems. For example, if a patient relies only on the health care provider for care and support (eg, calls the nurse every day, visits the physician weekly, refuses any help from family), the individual will be linked with an informal support system for help with some of the caregiving tasks. If the individual refuses any health promotion interventions from providers, the patient will be directly approached by the health care team.

Applicability of Balance Theory to Psychiatric and Mental Health Nursing

Balance theory is a practical model for conceptualizing delivery of mental health care in the community, particularly in rural areas where resources are limited. By using the framework of formal and informal support systems and social distance, mental health services can be developed and evaluated from this perspective. Nurse researchers at the Southeastern Rural Mental Health Research Center at the University of Virginia, Charlottesville developed a model for establishing linkages of formal and informal caregivers for mental health service for those with serious mental illnesses in rural areas (Fox, Blank, Kane, Hargrove, & David, 1994). In this model, case managers adjust the social distance between the formal and informal systems by identifying communication barriers and helping the two groups work together. For example, a patient misses an appointment because of a lack of transportation. The case manager helps the patient communicate the problem to the system to obtain another appointment. Informal caregivers are valued by the case manager, who recognizes the important services performed by family and friends. Thus, linkages between mental health providers (formal support) and the consumer network (informal support) are reinforced.

ROLE THEORIES

Perspectives

A role describes an individual's social position and function within an environment. Anthropologic theories explain members' roles that relate to a specific society. For example, the universal roles of healer may be assumed by a nurse in one culture and a spiritual leader in another. Societal expectations, social status, and rights are attached to these roles. Psychological theories, which are concerned about roles from a different perspective, focus on the relationship of an individual's role: the self. The responsibilities of a parent are often in conflict with the personal needs for time alone. All of the Neo-Freudian and humanist models that have been discussed focus on reciprocal social relationships or interactions that determine how the mind develops.

Applicability of Role Theories to Psychiatric and Mental Health Nursing

Role theories emphasize the importance of social interaction in either the individual's choice of a particular role or society's recognition of it. Several nursing models have role as a major concept: King (1971), Roy (1974), Peplau (1952). PMH nursing uses role concepts in understanding group interaction and the role of the patient in the family and community (see Chapters 15 and 16). In addition, milieu therapy approaches discussed in later chapters are based on the patient's assumption of a role within the psychiatric care environment.

SOCIOCULTURAL PERSPECTIVES

Margaret Mead: Culture and Gender

American anthropologist Margaret Mead (1901–1978) is widely known for her studies of small-scale non-Western societies and her contributions to social anthropology. She conducted studies in New Guinea, Samoa, and Bali and devoted much of her studies to the patterns of child rearing in various cultures. She was particularly interested in the cultural influences determining male and female behaviour (Mead, 1970). Although her research was often criticized as not having scientific rigor and

being filled with misinterpretations, it became accepted as a classic in the field of anthropology (Torrey, 1992). The importance of culture in determining human behaviour was acknowledged.

Madeleine Leininger: Transcultural Health Care

Concern about the impact of culture on the treatment of children with psychiatric and emotional problems led Madeleine Leininger (b. 1924), a nurse anthropologist, to develop a new field, transcultural nursing, directed toward holistic, congruent, and beneficent care. She used concepts from anthropology and nursing (from such theorists as Henderson [1966], Rogers [1994], and Watson [1990]) to depict universal and diverse dimensions of human caring. Because caring is an integral part of being human, as well as a learned behaviour, caring is culturally based (Leininger, 1991; 1999). Care is considered the essence of nursing, and caring manifestations include compassion, presence, and enabling (Leininger, 1993). Nursing care in one culture is different from that in another because definitions are different. Leininger developed a model to depict her theory symbolically. The model depicts the "world view, religion, kinship, cultural values, economics, technology, language, ethnohistory, and environmental factors that are predicted to explain and influence culture care" (1993, p. 27).

Applicability of Sociocultural Theories to Psychiatric and Mental Health Nursing

The use of sociocultural theories is especially important for PMH nurses. In any individual or family assessment, the sociocultural aspect is integral to mental health. It would be impossible to complete an adequate assessment without considering the role of the individual within the family and society. Interventions are based on the understanding and significance of family and cultural norms. It would be impossible to interact with the family in a meaningful way without an understanding of the family's cultural values. In the inpatient setting, the nurse is responsible for designing the social environment of the unit as well as ensuring that the patient is safe from harm. To accomplish this complex task, an understanding of the unit as a small social community helps the nurse use the environment in patient treatment (see Chapter 12). In addition, many group interventions are based on sociocultural theories (see Chapter 15).

SUMMARY OF KEY POINTS

◘ Nursing theories form the conceptual basis for nursing practice and are useful in a variety of psychiatric and mental health settings.

▢ The biologic framework forms a basis for nursing considerations based on such models as psychiatric genetics and the interaction of nature and nurture.

▢ The traditional psychodynamic framework helped form the basis of early nursing interpersonal interventions, including the development of therapeutic relationships and the use of such concepts as transference, countertransference, empathy, and object relations.

▢ The cognitive and behavioural theories are often used in strategies that help patients change behaviour and thinking.

▢ Sociocultural theories remain important in understanding and interacting with patients as members of families and cultures.

CRITICAL THINKING CHALLENGES

1 Compare and contrast the basic ideas of the nursing theorists.

2 Discuss the importance of the biologic theories in mental health practice. Compare Selye's model with the diathesis-stress model.

3 Discuss the similarities and differences between Freud's ideas and the Neo-Freudian, including Jung, Adler, Horney, and Sullivan.

4 Compare and contrast the basic ideas of psychodynamic and behavioural theories.

5 Compare and differentiate classical conditioning from operant conditioning.

6 Define the following terms and discuss their applicability to psychiatric and mental health nursing: classical conditioning, operant conditioning, positive reinforcement, and negative reinforcement.

7 List the major developmental theorists and their main ideas.

8 Discuss the way in which the cognitive therapy approaches can be used in psychiatric and mental health nursing practice.

WEB LINKS

www.sandiego.edu/nursing/theory The Hahn School of Nursing and Health Sciences offers this website on nursing theory.

www.florence-nightingale.co.uk This is the website of the Florence Nightingale Museum.

www.publish.uwo.ca/~cforchuk/peplau/hpcb.html This University of Western Ontario website has Hildegard Peplau's home page.

www.kumc.edu/gec/geneinfo.html Created for genetic professionals, this University of Kansas website has clinical information regarding genetic disorders, tests, and links to other sites.

www.freud.org.uk This is the website of the Freud Museum in London. It has pictures, publications, and links to other relevant sites.

www.jungianstudies.org This website of the International Association of Jungian Studies should be of interest to anyone interested in Jung's work.

M O V I E S

Florence Nightingale: 1985. This made-for-TV movie, starring Jaclyn Smith as Florence Nightingale, shows how the aristocratic Nightingale defied Victorian convention as a nurse in London and during the Crimean war. It is the fact-based story of "the Lady with the Lamp" and her efforts to reform health care (eg, hospital sanitation) that lead to the establishment of modern nursing.

VIEWING POINTS: Consider the opposition that Florence Nightingale faced in changing the thinking of her contemporaries. What qualities did she bring to this challenge and what strategies did she use that made her so successful?

Freud: 1962. This video depicts Sigmund Freud as a young physician, focussing on his early psychiatric theories and treatments. His struggles for acceptance of his ideas among the Viennese medical community are depicted. This fascinating film is well done and gives an interesting overview of the impact of psychoanalysis.

VIEWING POINTS: Watch for the impact of the political thinking on the gradual acceptance of Freud's ideas. Discuss the "dream sequence" and its impact on the development of psychoanalysis as a therapeutic technique.

REFERENCES

Ackerman, S., Zuroff, D. C., & Moskowitz, D. S. (2000). Generativity in midlife and young adults: Links to agency, communion, and subjective well-being. *International Journal of Aging and Human Development, 5*(1), 17–41.

Adler, A. (1963). The practice and theory of individual psychotherapy. Paterson, N.J.: Littlefield, Adams.

American Psychiatric Association. (2000). *Diagnostic and statistical manual of mental disorders* (4th ed., text revision). Washington, DC: Author.

Baldursdottir, G., & Jonsdottir, H. (2002). The importance of nurse caring behaviours as perceived by patients receiving care at an emergency department. *Heart & Lung, 31*(1), 67–75.

Bandura, A. (1977). *Social learning theory.* Englewood Cliffs, NJ: Prentice-Hall.

Bandura, A. (1993). Perceived self-efficacy in cognitive development and function. American Educational Research Association Annual Meeting. *Educational Psychologist, 28*(2), 117–148.

Beck, A. T., Thase, M. D., & Wright, J. H. (2003). Cognitive therapy. In R. E. Hales & S. C. Ydofsky (Eds.), *Textbook of clinical psychiatry* (4th ed., pp. 1245–1283), Washington, DC: American Psychiatric Publishers, Inc.

Campbell, J. C., & Soeken, K. L. (1999). Women's responses to battering: A test of the model. *Research in Nursing and Health, 22*(1), 49–58.

Christiansen, S. L., & Palkovitz, R. (1998). Exploring Erikson's psychosocial theory and development: Generativity and its relationship to paternal identity, intimacy, and involvement in childcare. *Journal of Men's Studies, 7*(1), 133–156.

Conley, Y. P., Steele, A. M., Puskar, K. R. (2004). Genetic susceptibility to psychiatric disorders. *MEDSURG Nursing, 13*(5), 319–325.

Corvin, A. & Gill, M. (2003). Psychiatric genetics in the post-genome age. *British Journal of Psychiatry, 182*, 95–96.

Courtet, P. (2005). The genetic basis of suicidal behavior. *Psychiatric Times, 22*(9).

DeHowitt, M. (1992). King's conceptual model and individual psychotherapy. *Perspectives in Psychiatric Care, 28*(4), 11–14.

Ellenberger, H. (1970). *The discovery of the unconscious: The history and evolution of dynamic psychiatry.* London: Allen Lane, Penguin Press.

Ellis, A. (1973). *Humanistic psychotherapy: The rational-emotive approach.* New York: McGraw-Hill.

Erickson, E., & Erikson, J., (1997). *The lifecycle completed, extended version.* New York: WW Norton.

Erikson, E. (1963). *Childhood and society* (2nd ed.). New York: Norton.

Erikson, E. (1968). *Identity: Youth and crisis.* New York: Norton.

Frankl, V. E. (1985). *Psychotherapy and existentialism.* New York: Washington Square Press.

Frankl, V. (1992). *Man's search for meaning: An introduction to logotherapy* (4th ed.). Boston: Beacon Press.

Freud, S. (1905). Three essays on the theory of sexuality. In J. Strachey, A. Freud, A. Strachey, & A. Tyson, (Eds.). (1953). *The standard edition of the complete psychological works of Sigmund Freud* (pp. 135–248). London: Hogarth Press.

Freud, S. (1927). The ego and the id. In E. Jones (Ed.). (1957). *The international psycho-analytical library* (No. 12). London: Hogarth Press.

Freud, S. (1949). *An outline of psychoanalysis.* New York: Norton.

Freud, S. (1955). *An interpretation of dreams.* London: Hogarth Press.

Fox, J., Blank, M., Kane, C., Hargrove, C. F., & David, S. (1994). Balance theory as a model for coordinating delivery of rural mental health services. *Applied and Preventive Psychology, 3*(2), 121–129.

Gilligan, C. (1982). *In a different voice.* Cambridge, MA: Harvard University Press.

Gilligan, C. (1994). Joining the resistance: Psychology, politics, girls and women. In M. Berger (Ed.), *Women beyond Freud: New concepts of feminine psychology* (pp. 99–145). New York: Brunner Mazel.

Goldstein, B., Abela, J. R., Buchanan, G. M., & Buchanan, M. E. (2001). Attributional styles and life events: A diathesis-stress theory of alcohol consumption. *Psychological Reports, 87*(3 Pt. 1), 949–955.

Henderson, V. (1966). *The nature of nursing: A definition and its implications for practice, research, and education.* New York: Macmillan.

Hinds, C. (1990). Personal and contextual factors predicting patients' reported quality of life: Exploring congruency with Betty Neuman's assumptions. *Journal of Advanced Nursing, 15*, 456–462.

Horner, K. (2004). Ethics and genetics: Implications for CNS practice. *Clinical Nurse Specialist, 18*(5), 228–231.

Horney, K. (1939). *New ways in psychoanalysis.* New York: Norton.

Horney, K. (1950). *Neurosis and human growth.* New York: Norton.

Jung, C. G. (1959). *The basic writings of C. G. Jung.* New York: Modern Library.

Jung, C. (1966). On the psychology of the unconscious. V. The personal and the collective unconscious. In C. Jung (Ed.), *Collected works of C. G. Jung* (2nd ed., Vol. 7, pp. 64–79). Princeton, NJ: Princeton University Press.

King, I., (1971). *Toward a theory for nursing: general concepts of human behavior.* New York: John Wiley and Sons.

King, I. (1981). *A theory for nursing: Systems, concepts, process.* New York: John Wiley and Sons.

King, I. (1992). King's theory of goal attainment. *Nursing Science Quarterly, 5*(1), 19–26.

Knight, J. (1990). The Betty Neuman systems model applied to practice: A client with multiple sclerosis. *Journal of Advanced Nursing, 15*, 447–455.

Laben, J., Dodd, D., & Snead, L. (1991). King's theory of goal attainment applied in group therapy for inpatient juvenile sexual offenders, maximum security state offenders, and community parolees, using visual aids. *Issues in Mental Health Nursing, 12*(1), 51–64.

Leininger, M. (1991). *Culture care diversity and universality: A theory of nursing.* New York: National League for Nursing.

Leininger, M. (1993). Assumptive premises of the theory. In C. Reynolds & M. Leininger (Eds.), *Madeleine Leininger: Cultural care diversity and universality theory. Notes on nursing theories* (Vol. 8, pp. 15–30). Newbury Park, CA: Sage.

Leininger, M. (1999). What is transcultural nursing and culturally competent care? *Journal of Transcultural Nursing, 10*(1), 9.

Litwak, E. (1985). Complementary roles for formal and informal support groups: A study of nursing homes and mortality rates. *Journal of Applied Behavioural Science, 21*(4), 407–425.

Litwak, E., Messeri, P., & Silverstein, M. (1990). The role of formal and informal groups in providing help to older people. *Marriage and Family Review, 15*(1–2), 171–193.

Lutjens, L. R., (1991a). *Callista Roy: an adaptation model.* CA: SAGE Publications, Inc.

Lutjens, L. R., (1991b). *Marta Rogers: The science of unatary human beings.* CA: SAGE Publications, Inc.

MacPhail, J., (1988). The professional image: Impact and strategies for change. In *Canadian nursing: Issues and perspectives* (pp. 47–58). Toronto, Canada: McGraw-Hill Ryerson.

Marriner-Tomey, A., (1994). *Nursing theorists and their work.* (3rd ed.), Missouri: Mosby.

Maslow, A. (1970). *Motivation and personality* (rev. ed.). New York: Harper & Brothers.

Maslow, A. (1998). *Toward a psychology of being* (3rd ed.). New York: John Wiley & Sons.

McGuffin, P., & Southwick, L., (2003). Fifty years of the double helix and its impact on psychiatry. *Australian and New Zealand Journal of Psychiatry 37*, 657–661.

Mead, M. (1970). *Culture and commitment: A study of the generation gap.* Garden City, NY: Natural History Press/Doubleday.

Messeri, P., Silverstein, M., & Litwak, E. (1993). Choosing optimal support groups: A review and reformulation. *Journal of Health and Social Behaviour, 34*(6), 122–137.

Moffitt, T., Caspi, A. & Rutter, M. (2005). Strategy for investigating interactions between measured genes and measured environments. *Archives of General Psychiatry, 62*, 473–481.

Moore, B., & Fine, B. (Eds.). (1990). *Psychoanalytic terms and concepts.* New Haven, CT: American Psychoanalytic Association and Yale University Press.

Nightingale, F. (1859). *Notes on nursing: What it is and what it is not.* London: Edward Stern and Company.

Nelson, M. (1996). Separation versus connection, the gender controversy: Implications for counseling women. *Journal of Counseling and Development, 74*(4), 339–344.

Neuman, B., Newman, D. M. L., & Holder, P. (2000). Leadership and scholarship integration: Using the Neuman system model for 21st century professional nursing practice. *Nursing Science Quarterly, 13*(1), 60–63.

Neuman, B. (1989). *The Neuman systems model* (2nd ed.). East Norwalk, CT: Appleton & Lange.

Ochse, R., & Plug, C. (1986). Cross-cultural investigation of the validity of Erikson's theory of personality development. *Journal of Personality and Social Psychology, 50*(6), 1240–1252.

Olson, J., & Hanchett, E. (1997). Nurse-expressed empathy, patient outcomes, and the development of a middle-range theory. *Image: The Journal of Nursing Scholarship, 29*(1), 71–76.

Orem, D. (1991). *Nursing concepts of practice.* St. Louis: Mosby–Year Book.

Orlando, I. J. (1961). *The dynamic nurse–patient relationship.* New York: G. P. Putnam's Sons.

Orlando, I. J. (1972). *The discipline and teaching of nursing process.* New York: G. P. Putnam's Sons.

Orlofsky, J., Marcia, J., & Lesser, I. (1973). Ego identity status and the intimacy versus isolation crisis of young adulthood. *Journal of Personality and Social Psychology, 27*(2), 211–219.

Pavlov, I. P. (1927/1960). *Conditioned reflexes.* New York: Dover Publications.

Peplau, H. (1952). *Interpersonal relations in nursing.* New York: G. P. Putnam & Sons.

Peplau, H. (1992). Interpersonal relations: A theoretical framework for application in nursing practice. *Nursing Science Quarterly, 5*(1), 13–18.

Perls, F. (1969). *In and out of the garbage pail.* Lafayette, CA: Real People Press.

Potter, M. L., & Bockenhauer, B. J. (2000). Implementing Orlando's nursing theory. *Journal of Psychosocial Nursing and Mental Health Services, 3813,* 14–21.

Propping, P. (2005). The biography of psychiatric genetics: From early achievements to historical burden, from an anxious society to critical geneticists. *American Journal of Medical Genetics: Neuropsychiatric Genetics 136*(1), 2–7.

Rogers, C. (1980). *A way of being.* Boston: Houghton Mifflin.

Rogers, M. E. (1994). The science of unitary human being: current perspectives. *Nursing Science Quarterly, 7*(1), 33–35.

Roy, C., (1974). The Roy adaptation model. In J. P. Riehl & C. Roy, (Eds.) *Conceptual models for nursing practice.* New York: Appleton-Century-Crofts.

Selye, H. (1956). *The stress of life.* New York: McGraw-Hill.

Skinner, B. F. (1935). The generic nature of the concepts of stimulus and response. *Journal of General Psychology, 12,* 40–65.

Skinner, B. F. (1976). *Walden II.* New York: Macmillan.

Sullivan, H. (1953). *The interpersonal theory of psychiatry.* New York: Norton.

Thorndike, E. L. (1916, c1906). *The principles of teaching, based on psychology.* New York: A. G. Seiler.

Torrey, E. (1992). *Freudian fraud.* New York: Harper Collins.

Travelbee, J. (1971). *Interpersonal aspects of nursing* (2nd ed.). Philadelphia: F. A. Davis.

Watson, J. (1990). Caring knowledge and informed moral passion. *Advances in Nursing Sciences, 13*(1), 15–24.

Watson, J. B., & Rayner, R. (1917). Emotional reactions and psychological experimentation. *American Journal of Psychology, 28,* 163–174

Wright, L., & Leahy, M. (2005). *Nurses and families: a guide to family assessment and intervention.* (3rd ed.). Philadelphia: FA Davis.

For challenges, please refer to the **CD-ROM** in this book.

CHAPTER 8

Communication and the Therapeutic Relationship

Cheryl Forchuk

LEARNING OBJECTIVES

After studying this chapter, you will be able to:

- Identify the importance of self-awareness in nursing practice.
- Develop a repertoire of verbal and nonverbal communication skills.
- Develop a process for selecting effective communication techniques.
- Explain how the nurse can establish a therapeutic relationship with clients by using rapport and empathy.
- Explain the physical, emotional, and social boundaries of the nurse–client relationship.
- Discuss the significance of defence mechanisms.
- Explain what occurs in each of the three phases of the nurse–client relationship: orientation, working, and resolution.

KEY TERMS

active listening ▪ boundaries ▪ communication blocks ▪ content themes ▪ defence mechanisms ▪ empathy ▪ empathic linkages ▪ nontherapeutic relationships ▪ nonverbal communication ▪ orientation phase ▪ passive listening ▪ process recording ▪ rapport ▪ resolution ▪ self-disclosure ▪ symbolism ▪ verbal communication ▪ working phase

⬠ KEY CONCEPTS

- nurse–client relationship ▪ self-awareness ▪ therapeutic communication

Clients with psychiatric disorders have special communication and relationship needs that require advanced therapeutic communication skills. In psychiatric and mental health (PMH) nursing, the nurse–client relationship is an important intervention tool that is used to reach treatment goals. The purposes of this chapter are (1) to help the nurse develop self-awareness and communication techniques needed for a therapeutic nurse–client relationship; (2) to examine the specific stages or steps involved in establishing the relationship; (3) to explore the specific factors that make a nurse–client relationship successful and therapeutic; and (4) to differentiate therapeutic from nontherapeutic relationships.

Self-Awareness

Self-awareness is the process of understanding one's own beliefs, thoughts, motivations, biases, and limitations and recognizing how they affect others. Without self-awareness, nurses will find it impossible to establish and maintain therapeutic relationships with clients. "Know thyself" is a basic tenet of PMH nursing (see Box 8-1).

To come to self-awareness, nurses can carry out self-examination, which can provoke anxiety and is rarely comfortable, either alone or with help from others. Self-examination without the benefit of another's perspective can lead to a biased view of self. Conducting self-examinations with a trusted individual who can give objective but realistic feedback is best. The development of self-awareness requires a willingness to be introspective and to examine personal beliefs, attitudes, and motivations.

> ⬢ **KEY CONCEPT Self-awareness** is the process of understanding one's own beliefs, thoughts, motivations, biases, and limitations and recognizing how they affect others.

BOX 8.1

"Know Thyself"

- Do you have any physical problems or illnesses?
- Have you had significant traumatic life events (e.g., divorce, death of significant person, abuse, disaster)?
- Did your family or significant others have prejudiced or embarrassing beliefs and attitudes about groups different than yours?
- Would sociocultural factors in your background contribute to being rejected by members of other cultures?
- If you answer "Yes" to any of these questions, how would these experiences affect your ability to care for clients with these characteristics?

THE BIOPSYCHOSOCIAL SELF

Each nurse brings a biopsychosocial self to nursing practice. The client perceives the biologic dimension of the nurse in terms of physical characteristics: age, gender, body weight, height, ethnic or racial background, and any other observed physical characteristics. The nurse, too, can have a certain genetic composition, chronic illness, or unobservable physical disability that may influence the quality or delivery of nursing care. The nurse's psychological state also influences how he or she analyzes client information and selects treatment interventions. An emotional state or behaviour can inadvertently influence the therapeutic relationship. For example, a nurse who has just learned that her child is using illegal drugs and who has a client with a history of drug use may inadvertently project a judgmental attitude toward her client, which would interfere with the formation of a therapeutic relationship. The nurse needs to examine underlying emotions, motivations, and beliefs and determine how these factors shape behaviour.

The nurse's social biases can be particularly problematic for the nurse–client relationship. Although the nurse may not verbalize these values to clients, some are readily evident in the nurse's behaviour and appearance, such as how the nurse acts or appears at work. Other sociocultural values may not be immediately obvious to the client; for example, the nurse's religious or spiritual beliefs or feelings about divorce, abortion, or homosexuality. These beliefs and thoughts can influence how the nurse interacts with a client who is dealing with such issues.

UNDERSTANDING PERSONAL FEELINGS AND BELIEFS AND CHANGING BEHAVIOUR

Nurses must understand their own personal feelings and beliefs and try to avoid projecting them onto clients. The development of self-awareness will enhance the nurse's objectivity and foster a nonjudgmental attitude, which is so important in building and maintaining trust throughout the nurse–client relationship. Soliciting feedback from colleagues and supervisors about how personal beliefs or thoughts are being projected onto others is a useful self-assessment technique. One of the reasons that ongoing clinical supervision is so important is that the supervisor really knows the nurse and can continually observe for inappropriate communication and question assumptions that the nurse may hold, as well as reinforce helpful behaviour.

Once a nurse has identified and analyzed personal beliefs and attitudes, behaviours that were driven by prejudicial ideas may change. The change process requires introspective analysis that may result in viewing the world differently. Through self-awareness and conscious effort, the nurse can change learned behaviours to engage effectively in therapeutic relationships with clients. Nevertheless, sometimes a nurse realizes that some attitudes are too ingrained to support a therapeutic relationship with a client with different beliefs. In such cases, the nurse should refer the client to someone who can be therapeutic.

Communication

Effective communication skills, including verbal and nonverbal techniques, are the building blocks for all successful relationships. The nurse–client relationship is built on therapeutic communication, the ongoing process of interaction through which meaning emerges (see Box 8-2). **Verbal communication**, which is principally achieved by spoken words, includes the underlying emotion, context, and connotation of what is actually said. **Nonverbal communication** includes gestures, expressions, and body language. Both the client and the nurse use verbal and nonverbal communication. **Empathic linkages** are the direct communication of feelings. To respond therapeutically in a nurse–client relationship, the nurse is responsible for assessing and interpreting all forms of client communication.

CRNE Note

In analyzing client–nurse communication, nonverbal behaviours and gestures are communicated first. If a client's verbal and nonverbal communication are contradictory, priority should be given to the nonverbal behaviour and gestures.

BOX 8.2

Principles of Therapeutic Communication

1. The client should be the primary focus of the interaction.
2. A professional attitude sets the tone of the therapeutic relationship.
3. Use self-disclosure cautiously and only when the disclosure has a therapeutic purpose.
4. Avoid social relationships with clients.
5. Maintain client confidentiality.
6. Assess the client's intellectual competence to determine the level of understanding.
7. Implement interventions from a theoretic base.
8. Maintain a nonjudgmental attitude. Avoid making judgments about the client's behaviour and giving advice. By the time the client sees the nurse, he or she has had plenty of advice.
9. Guide the client to reinterpret his or her experiences rationally.
10. Track the client's verbal interaction through the use of clarifying statements. Avoid changing the subject unless the content change is in the client's best interest.

> **KEY CONCEPT Therapeutic communication** is the ongoing process of interaction through which meaning emerges.

Therapeutic and social relationships are very different. In a therapeutic relationship, the nurse focuses on the client and client-related issues, even when engaging in social activities with that client. For example, a nurse may take a client shopping and out for lunch. Even though the nurse is engaged in a social activity, that trip should have a definite purpose, and conversation should focus only on the client. The nurse must not attempt to meet his or her own social or other needs during the activity.

USING VERBAL COMMUNICATION

The process of verbal communication involves a sender, a message, and a receiver. The client is often the sender, and the nurse is often the receiver (Fig. 8-1), but communication is always two-way. The client formulates an idea, encodes a message (puts ideas into words), and then transmits the message with emotion. The client's words and their underlying emotional tone and connotation communicate the individual's needs and emotional problems. The nurse receives the message, decodes it (interprets the message, including its feelings, connotation, and context), and then responds to the client. On the surface, this interaction is deceptively simple; unseen complexities lie beneath. Is the message the nurse receives consistent with the client's original idea? Did the nurse interpret the message as the client intended?

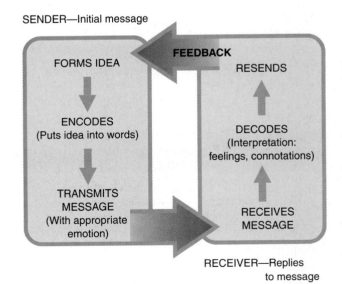

FIGURE 8.1 The communication process. (Adapted from Boyd, M. [1995]. Communication with clients, families, healthcare providers, and diverse cultures. In M. Strader & P. Decker [Eds.]. *Role transition to client care management* [p. 431]. Norwalk, CT: Appleton & Lange.)

Is the verbal message consistent with the nonverbal flourishes that accompany it? Validation is essential to ensure that the nurse has received the information accurately.

Self-Disclosure

One of the most important principles of therapeutic communication for the nurse to follow is to focus the interaction on the client's concerns. **Self-disclosure**, telling the client personal information, generally is not a good idea. The conversation should focus on the client, not the nurse. If a client asks the nurse personal questions, the nurse should elicit the underlying reason for the request. The nurse can then determine how much personal information to disclose, if any. In revealing personal information, the nurse should be purposeful and have identified therapeutic outcomes. For example, a male client who was struggling with the implications of marriage and fidelity asked a male nurse if he had ever had an extramarital affair. The nurse interpreted the client's statement as seeking role-modeling behaviour for an adult man and judged self-disclosure in this instance to be therapeutic. He honestly responded that he did not engage in affairs and redirected the discussion back to the client's concerns.

Nurses sometimes may feel uncomfortable avoiding clients' questions for fear of seeming rude. Sometimes they disclose too much personal information because they are trying to be "nice." However, being nice is not necessarily therapeutic. As appropriate, redirecting the client, giving a neutral or vague answer, or saying, "Let's talk about you" may be all that is necessary to limit self-disclosure. In some instances, nurses may need to tell the client directly that the nurse will not share personal information (Table 8-1).

Verbal Communication Techniques

Psychiatric and mental health nurses use many verbal techniques in establishing relationships and helping clients focus on their problems. Asking a question, restating, and reflecting are examples of such techniques. These techniques may at first seem artificial, but with practice, they can be useful.

Silence and Listening

One of the most difficult but often most effective techniques is the use of silence during verbal interactions. By maintaining silence, the nurse allows the client to gather thoughts and to proceed at his or her own pace.

Listening is another valuable tool. Silence and listening differ in that silence consists of deliberate pauses to encourage the client to reflect and eventually respond. Listening is an ongoing activity by which the nurse attends to the client's verbal and nonverbal communication. The art of listening is developed through careful attention to the content and meaning of the client's speech. There are two types of listening: passive and active. **Passive listening** involves sitting quietly and letting the client talk. A passive listener allows the client to ramble and does not focus or guide the thought process. Passive listening does not foster a therapeutic relationship.

Through **active listening**, the nurse focuses on what the client is saying to interpret and respond to the message objectively. While listening, the nurse concentrates only on what the client says and the underlying meaning. The nurse's verbal and nonverbal behaviour indicate active listening. The nurse usually responds indirectly, using techniques such as open-ended statements, reflection (Table 8-2), and questions that elicit additional responses from the client. In active listening, the nurse

Table 8.1	Self-Disclosure in Therapeutic vs. Social Relationships	
Situation	**Appropriate Therapeutic Response**	**Inappropriate Social Response With Rationale**
A client asks the nurse if she had fun over the weekend.	"The weekend was fine. How did you spend your weekend?"	"It was great. My boyfriend and I went to dinner and a movie." (*This self-disclosure has no therapeutic purpose. The response focuses the conversation on the nurse, not the client.*)
A client asks a student nurse if she has ever been to a particular bar.	"Many people go there. I'm wondering if you have ever been there?"	"Oh yes—all the time. It's a lot of fun." (*Sharing information about outside activities is inappropriate.*)
A client asks a nurse if mental illness is in his family.	"Mental illnesses do run in families. I've had a lot of experience caring for people with mental illnesses."	"My sister is being treated for depression." (*This self-disclosure has no purpose, and the nurse is missing the meaning of the question.*)
While shopping with a client, the nurse sees a friend, who approaches them.	To her friend: "I know it looks like I'm not working, but I really am. I'll see you later."	"Hi, Bob. This is Jane Doe, a client." (*Introducing the client to the friend is very inappropriate and violates client confidentiality.*)

Table 8.2	Verbal Communication Techniques		
Technique	**Definition**	**Example**	**Use**
Acceptance	Encouraging and receiving information in a nonjudgmental and interested manner	*Ct:* I have done something terrible. *Nurse:* I would like to hear about it. It's OK to discuss it with me.	Used in establishing trust and developing empathy
Confrontation	Presenting the client with a different reality of the situation	*Ct:* My best friend never calls me. She hates me. *Nurse:* I was in the room yesterday when she called.	Used cautiously to immediately redefine the client's reality. However, it can alienate the client if used inappropriately. A nonjudgmental attitude is critical for confrontation to be effective.
Doubt	Expressing or voicing doubt when a client relates a situation	*Ct:* My best friend hates me. She never calls me. *Nurse:* From what you have told me, that does not sound like her. When did she call you last?	Used carefully and only when the nurse feels confident about the details. It is used when the nurse wants to guide the client toward other explanations.
Interpretation	Putting into words what the client is implying or feeling	*Ct:* I could not sleep because someone would come in my room and rape me. *Nurse:* It sounds like you were scared last night.	Used in helping client identify underlying thoughts or feelings
Observation	Stating to the client what the nurse is observing	*Nurse:* You are trembling and perspiring. When did this start?	Used when a client's behaviours (verbal or nonverbal) are obvious and unusual for that client
Open-ended statements	Introducing an idea and letting the client respond	*Nurse:* Trust means. . . . *Ct:* That someone will keep you safe.	Used when helping client explore feelings or gain insight
Reflection	Redirecting the idea back to the client	*Ct:* Should I go home for the weekend? *Nurse:* Should you go home for the weekend?	Used when client is asking for the nurse's approval or judgment. Use of reflection helps nurse maintain a nonjudgmental approach.
Restatement	Repeating the main idea expressed; lets client know what was heard	*Ct:* I hate this place. I don't belong here. *Nurse:* You don't want to be here.	Used when trying to clarify what client has said
Silence	Remaining quiet, but nonverbally expressing interest during an interaction	*Ct:* I am angry!! *Nurse:* (Silence) *Ct:* My wife had an affair.	Used when client needs to express ideas but may not know quite how to do it. With silence, client can focus on putting thoughts together.
Validation	Clarifying the nurse's understanding of the situation	*Nurse:* Let me see if I understand.	Used when nurse is trying to understand a situation the client is trying to describe

should avoid changing the subject and instead follow the client's lead, although at times it is necessary to respond

CRNE Note

Self-disclosure can be used in very specific situations, but self-disclosure is not the first intervention to consider. In prioritizing interventions, active listening is one of the first to use.

directly to help a client focus on a specific topic or to clarify thoughts and beliefs.

Some verbal techniques block interactions and inhibit therapeutic communication (Table 8-3). One of the biggest blocks to communication is giving advice, particularly that which others have already given. Giving advice is different from supporting a client through decision making. The therapeutic dialogue presented in Box 8-3 differentiates between advice (telling the client what to do or how to act) and therapeutic communication, by

Table 8.3	Techniques That Inhibit Communication		
Technique	**Definition**	**Example**	**Problem**
Advice	Telling a client what to do	*Ct:* I can't sleep. It is too noisy. *Nurse:* Turn off the light and shut your door.	Nurse solves the client's problem, which may not be the appropriate solution, and encourages dependency on the nurse.
Agreement	Agreeing with a particular viewpoint of a client	*Ct:* Abortions are sinful. *Nurse:* I agree.	Client is denied opportunity to change view now that the nurse agrees.
Challenges	Disputing client's beliefs with arguments, logical thinking, or direct order	*Ct.* I'm a cowboy. *Nurse:* If you are a cowboy, what are you doing in the hospital?	Nurse belittles the client, and decreases self-esteem. Client will avoid relating to the nurse who challenges.
Reassurance	Telling a client that everything will be OK	*Ct:* Everyone thinks I'm bad. *Nurse:* You are a good person.	Nurse makes a statement that may not be true. Client is blocked from exploring feelings.
Disapproval	Judging client's situation and behaviour	*Ct:* I'm so sorry. I did not mean to kill my mother. *Nurse:* You should be. How could anyone kill their mother?	Nurse belittles the client. The client will avoid the nurse.

BOX 8.3

Therapeutic Dialogue: Giving Advice Versus Recommendations

Ms. J has just received a diagnosis of phobic disorder and been given a prescription for fluoxetine. She was referred to the home care agency because she does not want to take her medication. She is fearful of becoming suicidal. Two approaches are given below.

Ineffective Communication (Advice)

Nurse: Ms. J, the doctor has ordered the medication because it will help you.

Ms. J: I don't want to take the medication because I am afraid of becoming suicidal. I heard that some of this psychiatric medication does that. I haven't had any attacks for 2 weeks.

Nurse: This medication has rarely had that side effect. You should try it and see if you have any suicidal thoughts.

Ms. J: OK.

(The nurse leaves and Ms. J does not take the medication. Within a week, Ms. J is taken to the emergency room with a panic attack.)

Effective Communication

Nurse: Ms. J, how have you been doing?

Ms. J: So far, so good. I haven't had any attacks for 2 weeks.

Nurse: I understand that the doctor gave you a prescription for medication that may help with the panic attacks.

Ms. J: Yes, but I don't want to take it because I am afraid of becoming suicidal. I heard that some of this psychiatric medication does that.

Nurse: Have you ever had feelings of hurting yourself?

Ms. J: Not really.

Nurse: If you took the medication and had thoughts like that what would you do?

Ms. J: I don't know.

Nurse: I think I see your dilemma. This medication may help your panic attacks, but the suicidal thoughts are a real fear. Is that it?

Ms. J: Yeah, that's it.

Nurse: Are there any circumstances under which you would be able to try the medication?

Ms. J: If I knew that I would not have suicidal thoughts.

Nurse: I can't guarantee that, but I could call you every few days to see if you are having any of these thoughts and help you deal with them.

Ms. J: Oh, that will be OK.

(Ms. J successfully took the medication.)

Critical Thinking Challenge

- Contrast the communication in the first scenario with that in the second.
- What therapeutic communication techniques did the second nurse employ that may have contributed to a better outcome?
- Are there any cues in the first scenario that indicate that the client will not follow the nurse's advice? Explain.

BOX 8.4

RESEARCH FOR BEST PRACTICE

Boundaries Between Clients and Mental Health Nurses

THE QUESTION: What are the attitudes and behaviours of mental health nurses toward clients in the areas of attraction, dating, and sexual relationships?

METHODS: A self-administered survey with a majority of forced-choice, refined-response items was sent by mail to 2,009 nurses (896 Registered Nurses and 1,113 Registered Psychiatric Nurses) in Alberta. The response rate was 45.9%. The questionnaire was composed of 37 questions with 171 variables and took approximately 15 to 30 minutes to complete. Analysis involved examination of basic frequency distributions, percentage distributions, and cross-tabulations.

FINDINGS: Almost all respondents strongly agreed that it was inappropriate to go on a date with a current client (98.9%) or to have a sexual relationship with a current client (99.3%). Only one respondent reported having dated a current client (rarely), and nine respondents reported having dated a discharged client (rarely or sometimes). Six nurses reported that they had had a sexual relationship with a discharged client in the past.

IMPLICATIONS FOR NURSING: Nurses need to recognize that the potential for intimacy boundary violations with clients exists. Although most nurses in the study reported never dating or having sexual relationships with current or discharged clients, a few respondents reported having done so. Nurses who do engage in such inappropriate behaviours can face disciplinary action and lawsuits.

From Campbell, R. J., Yonge, O., & Austin, W. (2005). Intimacy boundaries between mental health nurses & psychiatric patients. *Journal of Psychosocial Nursing and Mental Health Services, 43*(5), 33–41.

which the nurse and client explore alternative ways of viewing the client's world. The client then can reach his or her own conclusions about the best approaches to use. Refer to Box 8-4 for a summary of a research study on boundaries between clients and psychiatric–mental health nurses.

USING NONVERBAL COMMUNICATION

Gestures, facial expressions, and body language actually communicate more than verbal messages. Under the best circumstances, body language mirrors or enhances what is verbally communicated. However, if verbal and nonverbal messages are conflicting, the listener will believe the nonverbal message. For example, if a client says that he feels fine but has a sad facial expression and is slumped in a chair away from others, the message of sadness and depression will be accepted, rather than the client's words. The same is true of a nurse's behaviour. If a nurse tells a client that she is happy to see him, but

her facial expression communicates indifference, the client will receive the message that the nurse is bored.

Because people with psychiatric problems often have difficulty verbally expressing themselves and interpreting the emotions of others, nurses need to assess continually the nonverbal communication needs of clients. Eye contact (or lack thereof), posture, movement (shifting in chair, pacing), facial expressions, and gestures are nonverbal behaviours that communicate thoughts and feelings. A client with low self-esteem may be unable to maintain eye contact and thus may spend a great deal of time looking toward the floor. A client who is pacing and restless may be upset or having a reaction to medication. A clenched fist usually indicates that a person feels angry or hostile.

Nonverbal behaviour is culturally specific. The nurse must therefore be careful to understand his or her own cultural context as well as that of the client. For example, in some cultures (such as Canadian Aboriginal nations), it is considered disrespectful to look a person straight in the eye. In other cultures, not looking a person in the eye may be interpreted as "hiding something" or low self-esteem. Whether one points with the finger, nose, or eyes and how much hand gesturing one uses are other examples of nonverbal communication that may vary considerably among cultures.

Nurses should use positive body language, such as sitting at the same eye level as the client with a relaxed posture that projects interest and attention. Leaning slightly forward helps engage the client. Generally, the nurse should not cross arms or legs during therapeutic communication because such postures erect barriers to interaction. Uncrossed arms and legs project openness and a willingness to engage in conversation (Fig. 8-2). Any verbal response should be consistent with nonverbal messages.

RECOGNIZING EMPATHIC LINKAGES

Empathic linkages are the communication of feelings (Peplau, 1952). This commonly occurs with anxiety.

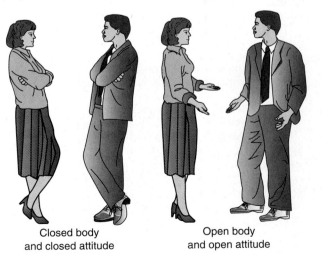

Closed body and closed attitude   Open body and open attitude

FIGURE 8.2   Open and closed body language.

For example, a nurse may be speaking with a client who is highly anxious, and the nurse may notice his or her own speech becoming more rapid in tandem with the client's. The nurse may also become aware of subjective feelings of anxiety. It may be difficult for the nurse to determine whether the anxiety was communicated interpersonally, or whether the nurse is personally reacting to some of the content of what the client is communicating. However, being aware of one's own feelings and analyzing them is crucial to determining the source of the feeling.

SELECTING COMMUNICATION TECHNIQUES

In therapeutic communication, the nurse chooses the best words to say and uses nonverbal behaviours that are consistent with these words. If a client is angry and upset, should the nurse invite the client to sit down and discuss the problem? walk quietly with the client? or simply observe the client from a distance and not initiate conversation? Choosing the best response begins with assessing and interpreting the meaning of the client's communication–both verbal and nonverbal.

CRNE Note

Applying communication techniques requires consideration of the ultimate goal and the ability of the client to benefit from the intervention. Giving advice rarely works.

Nurses should not necessarily take verbal messages literally, especially when a client is upset or angry. For example, one nurse walked into the room of a newly admitted client who accused, "You locked me up and threw away the key." The nurse could have responded defensively that she had nothing to do with the client being admitted; however, that response would have ended in an argument, and communication would have been blocked. Fortunately, the nurse recognized that the client was communicating frustration at being in a locked psychiatric unit and did not take the accusation personally.

The next step is identifying the desired client outcome. To do so, the nurse should engage the client with eye contact (if culturally appropriate) and quietly try to interpret the client's feelings. In this example, the desired outcome was for the client to clarify the hospitalization experience. The nurse responded that, "It must be frustrating to feel locked up." The nurse focused on the client's feelings, rather than the accusations, which reflected an understanding of the client's feelings. The client knew that the nurse accepted these feelings, which led to further discussion. It may seem impossible to plan reactions for each situation, but with

practice, the nurse will begin to respond consistently in a therapeutic way.

APPLYING COMMUNICATION CONCEPTS

When the nurse is interacting with clients, additional considerations can enhance the quality of communication. This section describes the importance of rapport, validation, empathy, and the role of boundaries and body space in nurse–client interactions.

Rapport

Rapport, interpersonal harmony characterized by understanding and respect, is important in developing a trusting, therapeutic relationship. Nurses establish rapport through interpersonal warmth, a nonjudgmental attitude, and a demonstration of understanding. A skilled nurse will establish rapport that will alleviate the client's anxiety in discussing personal problems.

People with psychiatric problems often feel alone and isolated. Establishing rapport helps lessen feelings of being alone. When rapport develops, a client feels comfortable with the nurse and finds self-disclosure easier. The nurse also feels comfortable and recognizes that an interpersonal bond or alliance is developing. All these factors—comfort, sense of sharing, and decreased anxiety—are important in establishing and building the nurse–client relationship.

Validation

Validation is explicitly checking out one's own thoughts or feelings with another person. To do so, the nurse must own his or her own thought or feeling by using "I" statements. The validation generally refers to observation, thoughts, or feelings and seeks explicit feedback. For example, a nurse who sees a client pacing the hallway before a planned family visit may conclude that the client is anxious. Validation may occur with a statement such as, "I notice you pacing the hallway. I wonder if you are feeling anxious about the family visit?" The client may agree, "Yes. I keep worrying about what is going to happen!" or disagree, "No. I have been trying to get into the bathroom for the last 30 minutes, but my roommate is still in there!"

Empathy

The use of empathy in a therapeutic relationship is central to PMH nursing. **Empathy** is the ability to experience, in the present, a situation as another did at some time in the past. It is the ability to put oneself in another person's circumstances and feelings. The nurse does not actually have to have had the experience but has to be able to imagine the feelings associated with it. For empathy to develop, there must be a giving of self to the other individual and a reciprocal desire to know each other personally. The process involves the nurse receiving information from the client with open, nonjudgmental acceptance and communicating this understanding of the experience and feelings so that the client feels understood.

Biopsychosocial Boundaries and Body Space Zones

Boundaries are the defining limits of individuals, objects, or relationships. Boundaries mark territory, or what is "mine" or "not mine." Human beings have many different types of boundaries. Material boundaries, such as fences around property, artificially imposed state lines, and bodies of water define territory as well as provide security and order. Personal boundaries can be conceptualized within the biopsychosocial model as including physical, psychological, and social dimensions. Physical boundaries are those established in terms of physical closeness to others—whom we allow to touch us or how close we want others to stand near us. Psychological boundaries are established in terms of emotional distance from others—how much of our innermost feelings and thoughts we want to share. Social boundaries, such as norms, customs, and roles, help us establish our closeness and place within the family, culture, and community. Boundaries are not fixed, but dynamic. When boundaries are involuntarily transgressed, the individual feels threatened and responds to the perceived threat. The nurse must elicit permission before implementing interventions that invade personal space and boundaries.

Personal Boundaries

Every individual is surrounded by four different body zones that provide varying degrees of protection against unwanted physical closeness during interactions. The actual sizes of the different zones vary according to culture. Some cultures define the intimate zone narrowly and the personal zones widely. Thus, friends in these cultures stand and sit close while interacting. People of other cultures define the intimate zone widely and are uncomfortable when others stand close to them. The variability of intimate and personal zones has implications for nursing. For a client to be comfortable with a nurse, the nurse needs to protect the intimate zone of that individual. The client usually will allow the nurse to enter the personal zone but will express discomfort if the nurse breaches the intimate zone. For the nurse, the difficulty lies in differentiating the personal zone from the intimate zone for each client.

The nurse's awareness of his or her own need for intimate and personal space is another prerequisite for therapeutic interaction with the client. It is important that a nurse feels comfortable while interacting with clients. Establishing a comfort zone may well entail fine-tuning the size of body zones. Recognizing this will help the nurse understand occasional inexplicable reactions to the proximity of clients.

Professional Boundaries

For nurses, professional boundaries are also essential to consider in the context of the nurse–client relationship. Clients often enter such relationships at a very vulnerable point, and nurses need to be aware of professional boundaries to avoid exploitation of the client. For example, in a friendship, there is two-way sharing of personal information and feelings, but as mentioned previously, the focus is on the client's needs, and the nurse generally does not share personal information or attempt to meet his or her own needs through the relationship. The client may seek a friendship or sexual relationship with the nurse (or vice versa), which would be inconsistent with the professional role.

Indicators that the relationship may be moving outside the professional boundaries are gift giving on either party's part, spending more time than usual with a particular client, strenuously defending or explaining the client's behaviour in team meetings, the nurse feeling that he or she is the only one who truly understands the client, keeping secrets, or frequently thinking about the client outside of the work situation (Gallop et al., 2002). Provincial regulatory bodies may have guidelines or firm rules, such as how long after a therapeutic relationship must be terminated before engaging in a romantic or sexual relationship. Guidelines are generally more vague about when a friendship would be appropriate, but such relationships are not appropriate when the nurse is actively providing care to the client. Exceptions may be when a relationship preceded the nursing context and another nurse is unavailable to provide care, such as in a nursing outpost (College of Nurses of Ontario, 1999). Similarly, relationships to meet the nurse's needs that are acquired through the nursing context, such as a relationship with a family member of the client, also breach professional boundaries. It is important to be familiar with the specific standards of practice related to boundaries and therapeutic relationships of your provincial regulatory and professional associations. Table 8-4 summarizes some of these. When concerns arise related to therapeutic boundaries, the nurse must seek clinical supervision or transfer the care of the client immediately.

Defence Mechanisms

Defence mechanisms (or coping styles) are the automatic psychological process protecting the individual

Table 8.4	Canadian Provincial Standards of Practice Regarding Therapeutic Nurse–Client Relationships	
Province Territory	**Standard of Practice/Best Practice Guidelines**	**Website**
Alberta	Registered Psychiatric Nurses Assoc. of Alberta: Standards of Practice 1998	http://www.rpnaa.ab.ca/Standardsof Practice.pdf
	College and Association of Registered Nurses of Alberta: Nursing Practice Standards	http://nurses.ab.ca/profconduct/npa. html
British Columbia	RN Assoc. of BC: Therapeutic Nurse–Client Relationship Professional Boundaries Practice Document	http://www.rnabc.bc.ca/pdf/406.pdf http://www.rnabc.bc.ca/pdf/389.pdf
Manitoba	RN Assoc. of Manitoba: Professional Boundaries for Therapeutic Relationship	http://www.crnm.mb.ca/downloads/ professionalboundaries_web.pdf
New Brunswick	Nurses Assoc. New Brunswick: Standards of Therapeutic Relationship	http://www.nanb.nb.ca/pdf_e/Publications/ General_Publications/Standards_for_the_ therapeutic_Nurse-Client_Relationship_ English.pdf
Newfoundland and Labrador	Assoc. of RNs of Newfoundland and Labrador: The Role of Psychiatric and Mental Health Nurses in the Community	http://www.arnn.nf.ca/links/position_ paper-the_role_of_psychiatric_and_mental_ health_nurses_in_the_community.htm
Northwest Territories	RN Assoc. of Northwest Territories and Nunavut: Standards of Practice	http://www.rnantnu.ca/standards.htm
Nova Scotia	College of Registered Nurses of Nova Scotia: Standard of Practice	http://www.crnns.ca/documents/stan- dardsfornurse practitioners.pdf
Ontario	College of Nurses of Ontario: Standards Therapeutic Relationship	http://www.cno.org/docs/prac/41033_ Therapeutic.pdf
	Registered Nurses Association of Ontario: Best Practice Guideline—Establishing Thera- peutic Relationships	http://rnao.org/bestpractices/com- pleted_guidelines/BPG_Guide_C2_TR.asp
Saskatchewan	Saskatchewan Registered Nurses Assoc.: Standards and Foundation Competencies Registered Psychiatric Nurses of Saskatchewan	http://www.srna.org/practice/standards_ foundation.pdf http://www.rpnas.com/public/jsp/con- tent/documentation/standards.jsp?print View=true
Yukon	RN Assoc. of Yukon: Standards of Practice	http://www.yrna.ca/pdf/standards.pdf
National	**Canadian Federation of Mental Health Nurses:** The Canadian Standards of Psychiatric and Mental Health Nursing Practice	http://www.cfmhn.org

against anxiety and from the awareness of internal or external dangers or stressors (Table 8-5; see Appendices for full list of defence mechanisms). Individuals often are unaware of these processes, although they mediate reactions to emotional conflicts and to internal and external stressors (American Psychiatric Association, 2000). Some defence mechanisms (eg, projection, split- ting, and acting out) are almost invariably maladaptive. Others, such as suppression and denial, may be either maladaptive or adaptive, depending on their severity and the context in which they occur.

As nurses develop therapeutic relationships, they will recognize their clients, and perhaps themselves, using defence mechanisms. With experience, the nurse will evaluate the purpose of a defence mechanism and then determine whether or not it should be discussed with the client. For example, if a client is using humor to alleviate an emotionally intense situation, that may be very appropriate. On the other hand, if someone con- tinually rationalizes antisocial behaviour, the use of the defence mechanism should be discussed. Defence mechanisms are grouped into seven related categories

Table 8.5	Specific Defence Mechanisms and Coping Styles*	
Defence Mechanism	**Definition**	**Example**
Denial	Refusing to acknowledge some painful aspect of external reality or subjective experience that would be apparent to others (*psychotic denial* used when there is gross impairment in reality testing)	A teenager's best friend moves away, but the adolescent says he does not feel sad.
Displacement	Transferring a feeling about, or a response to, one object onto another (usually less threatening), substitute object	A child is mad at her mother for leaving for the day, but says she is really mad at the sitter for serving her food she does not like.
Dissociation	Experiencing a breakdown in the usually integrated functions of consciousness, memory, perception of self or the environment, or sensory and motor behaviour	An adult relates severe sexual abuse experienced as a child, but does it without feeling. She says that the experience was as if she were outside her body watching the abuse.
Idealization	Attributing exaggerated positive qualities to others	An adult falls in love and fails to see the negative qualities in the other person.
Projection	Falsely attributing to another one's own unacceptable feelings, impulses, or thoughts	A child is very angry at a parent, but accuses the parent of being angry.
Rationalization	Concealing the true motivations for one's own thoughts, actions, or feelings through the elaboration of reassuring or self-serving but incorrect explanations	A man is rejected by his girlfriend, but explains to his friends that her leaving was best because she was beneath him socially and would not be liked by his family.
Reaction formation	Substituting behaviour, thoughts, or feelings that are diametrically opposed to one's own unacceptable thoughts or feelings (this usually occurs in conjunction with their repression)	A wife finds out about her husband's extramarital affairs and tells her friends that she thinks his affairs are perfectly appropriate. She truly does not feel, on a conscious level, any anger or hurt.
Repression	Expelling disturbing wishes, thoughts, or experiences from conscious awareness (the feeling component may remain conscious, detached from its associated ideas)	A woman does not remember the experience of being raped in the basement, but does feel anxious when going into that house.
Undoing	Words or behaviour designed to negate or to make amends symbolically for unacceptable thoughts, feelings, or actions	A man has sexual fantasies about his wife's sister. He takes his wife away for a romantic weekend.

* The following defence mechanisms and coping styles are identified in the *DSM-IV* as being used when the individual deals with emotional conflict or stressors (either internal or external).
Adapted from the American Psychiatric Association. (2000). *Diagnostic and statistical manual of mental disorders* (4th ed., Text revision, pp. 811–814). Washington, DC: Author.

called **defence levels.** These defence levels may be helpful in evaluating the meaning of the defence mechanism.

CRNE Note

When studying defence mechanisms, focus on those mechanisms and coping styles that are similar. For example, displacement, devoluation, and projection should be differentiated. Use these concepts in clinical assignments.

ANALYZING INTERACTIONS

Many people with psychiatric disorders have difficulty communicating. For example, perceptual, cognitive, and information-processing deficits, typical of people with schizophrenia, can interfere with the person's ability to express ideas, understand concepts, and accurately perceive the environment. Because of the complexity of communication, mental health professionals monitor their interactions with clients using various methods, including audio recording, video recording, and **process recording,** which entails writing a verbatim transcript of the interaction. A video or audio recording of an interaction provides the most accurate monitoring but is cumbersome to use. Process recording, one of the easiest methods to use, is adequate in most situations. Nurses should use it when first learning therapeutic communication and during times when communication becomes a problem.

In a process recording, the nurse records, from memory, the verbatim interaction immediately after the communication (Box 8-5).

The nurse then analyzes the content of the interaction in terms of the words and their meaning for both

BOX 8.5

Process Recording

Setting: The living room of Mr. S' home. His parents are in the room but cannot hear the conversation. Mr. S is sitting on the couch and the nurse is sitting on a chair. This is the nurse's first visit after Mr. S' discharge from the hospital.

Client	Nurse	Comments/Interpretation
	How are you doing, Mr. S?	*Plan:* Initially develop a sense of trust and initiate a therapeutic relationship.
I'm fine. It's good to be home. I really don't like the hospital.	You didn't like the hospital?	*Interpretation:* Mr. S does not want to return to hospital. Use reflection to begin to understand his experience.
NO. The nurses lock you up. Are you a nurse?	Yes. I'm a nurse. I'm wondering if you think that I will lock you up?	*Interpretation:* Mr. S is wondering what my role is and whether I will put him back in the hospital.
You could tell my mom to put me back in the hospital.	Any treatment that I recommend will be thoroughly discussed with you first. I am here to help you stay out of the hospital. I will not discuss anything with your mother unless you give me permission to do so.	Use interpretation to clarify Mr. S's thinking. Mr. S is wondering about my relationship with his mother. Explain my role.

the client and the nurse. The analysis is especially important because the ability to communicate verbally is often compromised in people with mental disorders. Words may not have the same meaning for the client as they do for the nurse. Clarification of meaning becomes especially important. The analysis can identify symbolic meanings, themes, and blocks in communication. **Symbolism,** the use of a word or phrase to represent an object, event, or feeling, is used universally. For example, automobiles are named for wild animals that represent speed, prowess, and beauty. In people with mental disorders, the use of words to symbolize events, objects, or feelings is often idiosyncratic, and they cannot explain their choices. For example, a person who is feeling scared and anxious may tell the nurse that bombs and guns are exploding. It is up to the nurse to make the connection between the bombs and guns and the client's feelings and then validate this with the client. Because of the client's cognitive limitations, the individual may express feelings only symbolically.

Some clients, for example some with developmental handicaps or organic brain difficulties, may have difficulty with abstract thinking and symbolism. Conversations may be interpreted literally. For example, in response to the question "What brings you to the hospital?" a client might reply, "the ambulance." In these situations, the nurse must be cautious to avoid using symbols or metaphors. Concrete language, that is, language reflecting what can be observed through the senses, will be more easily understood.

Verbal behaviour is also interpreted by analyzing **content themes**. Clients often express concerns or feelings repeatedly in several different ways. After a few sessions, a common theme emerges. Themes may emerge symbolically, as in the case with the client who constantly talks about the "guns and bombs." Alternatively, a theme may simply be identified as a recurrent thread of a story that a client retells at each session. For example, one client always explained his early abandonment by his family. This led the nurse to hypothesize that he had an underlying fear of rejection. The nurse was then able to test whether there was an underlying fear and to develop strategies to help the client explore the fear (Box 8-6). It is important to involve clients in analyzing themes so that they may learn this skill. Within the therapeutic relationship, the person who does the work is the one who develops the competencies, so the nurse must be careful to share this opportunity with the client (Peplau, 1952).

Communication blocks are identified by topic changes that either the nurse or the client makes. Topics are changed for various reasons. A client may change the topic from one that does not interest him or her to

BOX 8.6

Themes and Interactions

Session 1	Client discusses the death of his mother at a young age.
Session 2	Client explains that his sister is now married and never visits him.
Session 3	Client says that his best friend in the hospital was discharged and he really misses her.
Session 4	Client cries about a lost kitten.
Interpretation:	Theme of loss is pervasive in several sessions.

one that he or she finds more meaningful. However, an individual often changes the topic because he or she is uncomfortable with a particular subject. Once a topic change is identified, the nurse or client hypothesizes the reason for it. If the nurse changes the topic, he or she needs to determine why. The nurse may find that he or she is uncomfortable with the topic or may not be listening to the client. Beginning mental health nurses who are uncomfortable with silences or trying to elicit specific information from the client often change topics.

The nurse must also record and interpret the client's nonverbal behaviour in light of the verbal behaviour. Is the client saying one thing verbally and another nonverbally? The nurse must consider the client's cultural background. Is the behaviour consistent with cultural norms? For example, if a client denies any problems but is affectionate and physically demonstrative (which is antithetical to her naturally stoic cultural beliefs and behaviours), the nonverbal behaviour is inconsistent with what is normal behaviour for that person. Further exploration is needed to determine the meaning of the culturally atypical behaviour.

The Nurse–Client Relationship

The nurse-client relationship is a dynamic process that changes with time. It can be viewed in steps or phases with characteristic behaviours for both client and nurse. This text uses an adaptation of Hildegard Peplau's model that she introduced in her seminal work, *Interpersonal Relations in Nursing* (1952, 1992). The nurse–client relationship is conceptualized in three overlapping phases that evolve with time: orientation phase, working phase, and resolution phase.

The **orientation phase** is the phase during which the nurse and client get to know each other. During this phase, which can last from a few minutes to several months, the client develops a sense of trust in the nurse. The second is the **working phase,** in which the client uses the relationship to examine specific problems and learn new ways of approaching them. The final stage, **resolution,** is the termination stage of the relationship and lasts from the time the problems are actually resolved to the close of the relationship. The relationship does not evolve as a simple linear relationship. Instead, the relationship may be predominantly in one phase, but reflections of all phases can be seen in each interaction.

> **KEY CONCEPT** The **nurse–client relationship** is a dynamic process that changes with time. It can be viewed in steps or phases with characteristic behaviours for both the client and the nurse.

ORIENTATION PHASE

The orientation phase begins when the nurse and client meet and ends when the client begins to identify problems to examine. During the orientation phase, the nurse discusses the client's expectations, explains the purpose of the relationship and its boundaries, and facilitates the development of the relationship. It is natural for the nurse and client to be more nervous during the first few sessions. The goal of the orientation phase is to develop trust and security within the nurse–client relationship. During this initial phase, the nurse listens intently to the client's history and perception of problems and begins to understand the client and identify themes. The use of empathy facilitates the development of a positive therapeutic relationship.

First Meeting

During the first meeting, outlining both nursing and client responsibilities is important. The nurse is responsible for providing guidance throughout the therapeutic relationship, protecting confidential information, and maintaining professional boundaries. The client is responsible for attending agreed-upon sessions, interacting during the sessions, and participating in the nurse–client relationship. The nurse should also explain clearly to the client meeting times, handling of missed sessions, and the estimated length of the relationship. Issues related to recording information and how the nurse will work within the interdisciplinary team should also be made explicit.

Usually, both the nurse and the client feel anxious at the first meeting. The nurse should recognize the anxieties and attempt to alleviate them before the meeting. The client's behaviour during this first meeting may indicate to the nurse some of the client's problems in interpersonal relationships. For example, a client may talk nonstop for 15 minutes or may brag of sexual conquests. What the client chooses to tell or not to tell is significant. What a client first does or says may not accurately indicate his or her true feelings or the situation. In the beginning, clients may deny problems or choose not to discuss them as defence mechanisms or to prevent the nurse from getting to know them. The client is usually nervous and insecure during the first few sessions and may exhibit behaviour reflective of these emotions, such as rambling. Usually, by the third session, the client can focus on a topic.

Confidentiality in Treatment

Ideally, nurses include people who are important to the client in planning and implementing care. The nurse and client should discuss the issue of confidentiality in the first session. The nurse should be clear about any information that is to be shared with anyone else. Usually, the nurse shares significant assessment data and client progress with a supervisor and a physician. Most clients expect the nurse to communicate with other mental health professionals and are comfortable with this arrangement. Boundaries around what information can be shared with whom and under what circumstances are covered under provincial/territorial legislation such as Mental Health Acts and Health Information Acts.

Testing the Relationship

This first part of the orientation phase, called the "honeymoon phase," is usually pleasant. However, the therapeutic team typically hits rough spots before completing this phase. The client begins to test the relationship to become convinced that the nurse will really accept him or her. Typical "testing behaviours" include forgetting a scheduled session or being late. Clients may also express anger at something a nurse says or accuse the nurse of breaking confidentiality. Another common pattern is for the client to first introduce a relatively superficial issue as if it is the major problem. The nurse must recognize that these behaviours are designed to test the relationship and establish its parameters, not to express rejection or dissatisfaction with the nurse. The student nurse often feels personally rejected during the client's testing and may even become angry with the client. If the nurse simply accepts the behaviour as testing and continues to be available to the client and consistent in responses, these behaviours usually subside. Testing needs to be understood as a normal way that human beings develop trust.

WORKING PHASE

When the client begins identifying problems to work on, the working phase of the relationship has started. Problem identification can yield a wide range of issues, such as managing symptoms of a mental disorder, coping with chronic pain, examining issues related to sexual abuse, or dealing with problematic interpersonal relationships. Through the relationship, the client begins to explore the identified problems and develop strategies to resolve them. By the time the working phase is reached, the client has developed enough trust that he or she can examine the identified problems within the security of the therapeutic relationship. In the working phase, the nurse can use various verbal and nonverbal techniques to help the client examine problems.

Transference (unconscious assignment to others of the feelings and attitudes that the client originally associated with important figures) and countertransference (the provider's emotional reaction to the client based on personal unconscious needs and conflicts) become important issues in the working phase. For example, a client could be hostile to a nurse because of underlying resentment of authority figures; the nurse, in turn, could respond defensively because of earlier experiences of anger. The client uses transference to examine problems. During this phase, the client is psychologically vulnerable and emotionally dependent on the nurse. The nurse needs to recognize countertransference and prevent it from eroding professional boundaries.

Many times, nurses are eager to implement rehabilitation plans. However, this cannot be done until the client trusts the nurse and identifies what issues he or she wishes to work on in the context of the relationship.

RESOLUTION PHASE

The final stage of the nurse–client relationship is **resolution,** which begins when the actual problems are resolved and ends with the termination of the relationship. During this phase, the client is redirected toward a life without this specific therapeutic relationship. The client connects with community resources, solidifies a newly found understanding, and practices new behaviours. The client takes responsibility for follow-up appointments and interacts with significant others in new ways. New problems are not addressed during this phase, except in terms of what was learned during the working stage. The nurse assists the client in strengthening relationships, making referrals, and recognizing and understanding signs of future relapse.

Termination begins the first day of the relationship, when the nurse explains that this relationship is time limited and was established to resolve the client's problems and help him or her handle them. Because a therapeutic relationship is dependent, the nurse must constantly evaluate the client's level of dependence and continually support the client's move toward independence. Termination is usually stressful for the client, who must sever ties with the nurse who has shared thoughts and feelings and given guidance and support over many sessions. Depending on previous experiences with terminating relationships, some clients may not handle their emotions well during termination. Some may not show up for the last session at all to avoid their feelings of sadness and separation. Many clients display anger about the relationship ending. Clients may express anger toward the nurse or displace it onto others. For example, a client may shout obscenities at another client after being told that his therapeutic relationship with the nurse would end in a few weeks. One of the best ways to handle the anger is to help the client acknowledge it, to explain that anger is a normal emotion when a relationship is ending, and to reassure the

BOX 8.7

Therapeutic Dialogue: The Last Meeting

Ineffective Approach

Nurse: Today is my last day.
Client: I need to talk to you about something important.
Nurse: What is it?
Client: I have been hearing voices again.
Nurse: Oh, how often?
Client: Every night. You are the only one I'm going to tell.
Nurse: I think you should tell the new nurse.
Client: She is too new. She won't understand. I feel so bad about your leaving. Is there any way you can stay?
Nurse: Well, I could check on you tomorrow.
Client: Oh, would you? I would really appreciate it if you would give me your new telephone number.
Nurse: I don't know what the number will be, but it will be listed in the telephone book.

Effective Approach

Nurse: Today is my last day.
Client: I need to talk to you about something important.

Nurse: We talked about that. Anything "important" needs to be shared with the new nurse.
Client: But, I want to tell you.
Nurse: Saying good-bye can be very hard.
Client: I will miss you.
Nurse: Your feelings are very normal when relationships are ending. I will remember you in a very special way.
Client: Can I please have your telephone number?
Nurse: No, I can't give that to you. It is important that we say good-bye today.
Client: OK. Good-bye. Good luck.
Nurse: Good-bye.

Critical Thinking Challenge

- What were some of the mistakes the nurse in the first scenario made?
- In the second scenario, how does therapeutic communication in the termination phase differ from effective communication in the working phase?

client that it is acceptable to feel angry. The nurse should also reassure the client that anger subsides once the relationship is over.

Another typical termination behaviour is raising old problems that have already been resolved. The nurse may feel frustrated if clients in the termination phase present resolved problems as if they were new. The nurse may feel that the sessions were unsuccessful. In reality, clients are attempting to prolong the relationship and avoid its ending. Nurses should avoid addressing these problems. Instead, they should reassure clients that they already covered those issues and learned methods to control them. They should explain that the client may be feeling anxious about the relationship ending and redirect the client to newly found skills and abilities in forming new relationships, including support groups and social groups. The final meeting should focus on the future (see Box 8-7). The nurse can reassure the client that the nurse will remember him or her, but the nurse should not agree to see the client outside the relationship.

NONTHERAPEUTIC RELATIONSHIPS

Although it is hoped that all nurse–client relationships will go through the phases of the relationship described earlier, this is not always the case. Nontherapeutic relationships also go through predictable phases (Forchuk et al., 2000). These relationships also start in the orientation phase. However, trust is not established, and the relationship moves to a phase of grappling and struggling. The nurse and client both feel very frustrated and keep varying their approach with each other in an

attempt to establish a meaningful relationship. This is different from a prolonged orientation phase in that the efforts are not sustained; they vary constantly.

The nurse may try longer meetings, shorter meetings, being more or less directive, and varying the therapeutic stance from warm and friendly to aloof. Clients in this phase may try to talk about the past but then change to discussions of the "here and now." They may try talking about their family and in the next meeting talk about their work goals. Both grapple and struggle to come to a common ground, and both become increasingly frustrated with each other. Eventually the frustration becomes so great that the pair gives up on each other and moves to a phase of mutual withdrawal. The nurse may schedule seeing this client at the end of the shift and "run out of time" so that the meeting never happens. The client will leave the unit or otherwise be unavailable during scheduled meeting times. If a meeting does occur, the nurse will try to keep it short. "What's the point—we just cover the same old ground anyway." The client will attempt to keep it superficial and stay on safe topics. "You can always ask about your medications— nurses love to health teach, you know." Obviously no therapeutic progress can be made in such a relationship. The nurse may be hesitant to ask for a therapeutic transfer, assuming that a relationship would similarly fail with another nurse. However, each relationship is unique, and difficulties in one relationship do not predict difficulties in the next. Clinical supervision early on may assist the development of the relationship, but often a therapeutic transfer to another nurse is required.

BOX 8.8

RESEARCH FOR BEST PRACTICE

Therapeutic Relationships—From Psychiatric Hospital to Community

THE QUESTION: This study tested the effectiveness of a transitional discharge model (TDM) based on sustaining therapeutic relationships over the discharge process. The therapeutic relationships included staff and peer relationships.

METHODS: The authors provided a history and overview of TDM. The current study included 26 tertiary care psychiatric wards that were matched into 13 pairs of similar wards. Of these, one half implemented TDM (intervention group), and the other half continued with usual care (control group). There were 390 research subjects who were followed for 1 year after discharge. Comparisons of quality of life and use of services (costs) were made between the intervention and control groups.

FINDINGS: The quality of life and postdischarge costs were not significantly different between the intervention and control groups. However, the intervention group subjects were able to leave the hospital an average of 116 days sooner. This is equal to a savings of more than 12 million Canadian.

IMPLICATIONS FOR NURSING: Strategies focusing on developing and sustaining therapeutic relationships have the potential for significant health cost savings.

Forchuk, C., Martin, M. L., Chan, Y-C., & Jensen, E. (2005). Therapeutic relationships: From psychiatric hospital to community. *Journal of Psychiatric and Mental Health Nursing, 12*, 556–564

SUMMARY OF KEY POINTS

☑ To deal therapeutically with the emotions, feelings, and problems of clients, nurses must understand their own cultural values and beliefs and interpersonal strengths and limitations.

☑ The nurse–client relationship is built on therapeutic communication, including verbal and nonverbal interactions between the nurse and the client. Some communication skills include active listening, positive body language, appropriate verbal responses, and ability of the nurse to interpret appropriately and analyze the client's verbal and nonverbal behaviours.

☑ Two of the most important communication concepts are empathy and rapport.

☑ In the nurse–client relationship, as in all types of relationships, certain physical, emotional, and social boundaries and limitations need to be observed.

☑ The therapeutic nurse–client relationship consists of three major and overlapping stages or phases: the orientation phase, in which the client and nurse meet and establish the parameters of the relationship; the working phase, in which the client identifies and explores problems; and the resolution phase, in which the client learns to manage the problems and the relationship is terminated.

☑ The nontherapeutic relationship also consists of three major and overlapping phases: the orientation phase, the grappling and struggling phase, and the phase of mutual withdrawal.

CRITICAL THINKING CHALLENGES

1. Describe how you would communicate with a client who is concerned that a psychiatric diagnosis will negatively affect his or her social and work relationships.

2. Your client does not seem inclined to talk about his or her illness. Describe the measures you would take to initiate a therapeutic relationship with him or her. Who chooses the content to be discussed?

3. Your client does not appear for the last scheduled meeting. What will you do?

MOVIES

Good Will Hunting: 1997. Robin Williams plays a therapist to Will Hunting, a janitor identified as a mathematical genius, played by Matt Damon. Through a strong relationship, Will begins to realize his potential.

VIEWING POINTS: Watch closely how the relationship develops between the characters played by Williams and Damon. How does the relationship change as the characters move through different stages of their relationship?

Analyze This: 1999. In this comedy, Billy Crystal plays psychiatrist Dr. Ben Sobel. His client is Paul Vitti (Robert De Niro), a mobster who is having panic attacks. Dr. Sobel is intimidated into seeing his new client at all hours and places and into accepting expensive (stolen?) gifts from him. Power issues become very interesting in this unusual therapeutic relationship.

VIEWING POINTS: The issue of therapeutic boundaries is a source of comedy in this film. What normal therapeutic boundaries are being violated? Whose needs are being met throughout the film? What would be appropriate if a client evoked personal unresolved issues for the therapist?

REFERENCES

American Psychiatric Association. (2000). *Diagnostic and statistical manual of mental disorders* (4th ed., text revision). Washington, DC: Author.

Boyd, M. (1995). Communication with clients, families, healthcare providers, and diverse cultures. In M. Strader & P. Decker (Eds.), *Role transition to client care management* (p. 431). Norwalk, CT: Appleton & Lange.

Campbell, R. J., Yonge, O., & Austin, W. (2005). Intimacy boundaries between mental health nurses and psychiatric patients. *Journal of Psychosocial Nursing and Mental Health Services, 43*(5), 33–41.

College of Nurses of Ontario. (1999). *Standard for the therapeutic nurse–client relationship and registered nurses and registered practical nurses in Ontario*. Ontario, Canada: College of Nurses of Ontario.

Forchuk, C., Martin, M. L., Chan, Y-C., & Jensen, E. (2005). Therapeutic relationships: From psychiatric hospital to community. *Journal of Psychiatric and Mental Health Nursing, 12*, 556–564.

Forchuk, C., Westwell, J., Martin, M. L., Bamber-Azzapardi, W., Kosterewa-Tolman, D., & Hux, M. (2000). The developing nurse–client relationship: Nurses = perspectives. *Journal of the American Psychiatric Nurses Association, 6*(1), 3–10.

Gallop, R., Choiniere, J., Forchuk, C., Golea, G., Jonston, N., Levac, A. M., Martin, M. L., Robinson, T., Sogbein, S., Sutcliffe, H., & Wynn, F. (2002). *Nursing best practice guideline: Establishing therapeutic relationships*. Toronto, Canada: Registered Nurses Association of Ontario.

Peplau, H. E. (1952). The psychiatric nurse's family group. *The American Journal of Nursing, 52*(12), 1475–1477.

Peplau, H. E. (1972). The independence of nursing. *Imprint, 19*, 11.

Peplau, H. E. (1972). The nurse's role in health care delivery systems. *Pelican News, 28*, 12–14.

For more information, please access the Movie Viewing Guide on the **CD-ROM** in this book.

9

Biological Foundations of Psychiatric Nursing Practice

Anne Marie Creamer

LEARNING OBJECTIVES

After studying this chapter, you will be able to:

- Describe the association between biologic functioning and symptoms of psychiatric disorders.
- Describe approaches researchers have used to study the central nervous system and the significance of each approach.
- Locate brain structures primarily involved in psychiatric disorders; describe the primary functions of these structures.
- Assess symptoms of common psychiatric disorders in terms of central nervous system functioning.
- Describe the mechanisms of neuronal transmission.
- Identify the location and function of neurotransmitters significant to hypotheses regarding major mental disorders.
- Discuss the basic utilization of new knowledge gained from fields of study, including psychoendocrinology, psychoimmunology, and chronobiology.
- Discuss the role of genetics in the development of psychiatric disorders.

KEY TERMS

amino acids ▪ animal model ▪ autonomic nervous system ▪ basal ganglia ▪ biogenic amines ▪ biologic markers ▪ circadian cycle ▪ chronobiology ▪ cortex ▪ frontal, temporal, parietal, and occipital lobes ▪ genome ▪ hippocampus ▪ limbic system ▪ neurohormones ▪ neuropeptides ▪ psychoendocrinology ▪ psychoimmunology ▪ receptors ▪ risk factors ▪ symptom expression ▪ synapse ▪ zeitgebers

KEY CONCEPTS

- neurotransmitters ▪ plasticity

All behaviour recognized as human results from actions that originate in the brain and its amazing interconnection of neural networks. Modern research has increased understanding of how the complex circuitry of the brain interacts with external environment, memories, and experiences. Through the spinal column and peripheral nerves, along with other systems, such as the endocrine and immune systems, the brain constantly receives and processes information. As the brain shifts and sorts through the amazing amount of information it processes every hour, it decides on actions and initiates behaviours that allow each person to act in entirely unique and very human ways.

Foundational Concepts

This chapter reviews the basic information necessary for understanding neuroscience as it relates to the role of the psychiatric and mental health (PMH) nurse. It will review basic central nervous system (CNS) structures and functions; basic mechanisms of neurotransmission; general functions of the major neurotransmitters; basic structure and function of the endocrine system; genetic research; circadian rhythms; neuroimaging techniques; and biologic tests. The chapter assumes that the reader has a basic knowledge of human biology, anatomy, and pathophysiology. It is not intended as a full presentation of neuroanatomy and physiology, but rather as an overview of the structures and functions most critical to understanding the role of the PMH nurse.

THE BIOLOGIC BASIS OF BEHAVIOUR

As our understanding of the brain grows, evidence accumulates that most human behaviours have a biologic basis. Whether it is responding angrily, impulsively making a purchase, or struggling to make a decision, behaviours are in large part rooted in the neurocircuitry of the brain. So when common psychiatric symptoms manifest as abnormal behaviours (eg, seeing things that are not there, attempting suicide, talking in odd or unusual ways), we look to the brain. **Symptom expression** is a term referring to the behavioural symptoms seen in mental illness and the link to the neurobiologic basis of the symptom. Because symptoms of psychiatric illness are expressed mainly as behavioural disturbance, and because the behavioural symptoms are linked to anomalies in brain functioning, PMH nurses need to understand disease symptoms in relation to brain function.

Just as a breathing problem is often a symptom of respiratory disorders, psychiatric symptoms are often indicators of a CNS problem. Understanding this fundamental concept makes it much easier to understand

IN A LIFE

King George III (1739–1820)
Bipolar Illness Misdiagnosed

Public Personna
Crowned King of England at age 22, George III headed the most influential colonial power in the world at that time. England thrived in the peacetime after the Seven Year's War with France, but simultaneously taxed its American colonies so heavily and resolutely that the colonies rebelled. Could the American Revolution be blamed on King George III's (1739–1820) state of mind?

Personal Realities
At age 50, the king first experienced abdominal pain and constipation, followed by weak limbs, fever, tachycardia, hoarseness, and dark red urine. Later, he experienced confusion, racing thoughts, visual problems, restlessness, delirium, convulsions, and stupor. His strange behaviour included ripping off his wig and running about naked. Although he recovered and did not have a relapse for 13 years, he was considered to be mad. Relapses after the first relapse became more frequent, and the king was eventually dethroned by the Prince of Wales. It was believed that he suffered bipolar disorder.

However, was George's madness in reality a genetically transmitted blood disease that caused thought disturbances, delirium, and stupor? The genetic disease porphyria is caused by defects in the body's ability to make haem. The diseases are generally inherited in an autosomal dominant fashion. The retrospective diagnosis was not made until 1966 (Macalpine & Hunter, 1966).

Other members of the royal family who suffered from this hereditary disease were Queen Anne of Great Britain, Frederic the Great of Germany, George IV of Great Britain (son of George III), and George IV's daughter, Princess Charlotte, who died during childbirth from complications of the disease. After Charlotte's death, Victoria become Queen

From Macalpine, I., & Hunter, R. (1966). The insanity of King George 3d: A classic case of porphyria. *British Medical Journal, 5479*(1), 65–71.

the scientific rationale for many of the nursing care and treatment decisions presented in this book.

As you read this chapter, think about what you know about the symptoms of mental illness. PMH nurses must be able to make the connection among (1) patients' psychiatric symptoms, (2) the probable alterations in brain functioning linked to those symptoms, and the (3) rationale for treatment and care practices. Knowledge of the CNS is an inescapable aspect of modern PMH nursing.

Animal Modeling

How do scientists come to know about the workings of the brain? Animal modeling is the most common research method for studying the CNS. It involves using nonhuman organisms (animals such as rats and mice) to study biologic processes and how certain diseases affect those processes. Animal models resemble humans in anatomical structure, function, and genetics, allowing for research and learning that would not be possible to do with humans. Using animals, scientists can induce disease that occurs in humans and test treatments before attempting to treat humans who have that disease. Common examples of using animals to study human illness include studying cancer in mice, studying tissue reactions to transplanted cells in pigs, and analyzing DNA from a fly to study the genetic links of disease. Rats and mice are used in more than 90% of all medical research, and breeding mice for research is now a $200 million per year business in the United States (O'Rourke & Lee, 2003; Orth & Tabrizi, 2003). Animal models allow researchers to examine diseases such as high blood pressure, Parkinson's illness, depression, and Alzheimer's, as well as the neurobiology of normal behaviours, such as eating, mating, and learning. Researchers can then use the animal model to study what controls a behaviour or the way a disease progresses and how symptom expression occurs. Animal models are increasingly being used to explore psychiatric illnesses such as schizophrenia, bipolar disorder, and anxiety disorders, and to expand our knowledge of the illnesses, including the genetic basis for common psychiatric disorders. Every drug used to treat psychiatric disorders was first researched and tested in animal models.

Genetics

It has been known for some time that family members of individuals who have one of the major mental disorders, such as schizophrenia, bipolar, or panic disorder, have an increased risk for the same disorder. Animal models have greatly increased the ability of researchers to understand the influence of genetics on symptom expression in psychiatric disorders, and many of the common psychiatric disorders that nurses encounter have a known genetic component. As genetic knowledge increases, treatments that work at the genetic level are rapidly being developed (Johnson & Brensinger, 2000).

Genetic *processes* control how humans develop from a single-cell egg into an adult human. Genes control the regrowth of hair and skin cells, the growth and connection of nervous system cells, and our biologic reaction to stress. Genes make humans dynamic organisms, capable of growth, change, and development. The Human Genome Project, started in 1990, mapped the complete set of human genes, or genome, carried by all of us and transmitted to our offspring. The human genome is now completely identified, providing researchers with a road map of the exact sequence of the 3 billion nucleotide bases that make up human organisms. If printed out, the entire human genome sequence would fill a thousand 1,000-page telephone books. There are about 100,000 genes in the human genome, with the brain accounting for only about 1% of the body's DNA. Now that it is completed, the genome map can be used for studying the function of each gene and the disease-inducing capacity of those genes when they malfunction.

A gene comprises short segments of DNA and is packed with the instructions for making proteins that have a specific function. When genes are absent or malfunction, protein production is altered, and bodily functions are disrupted. In this fashion, genes play a role in cancer, heart disease, diabetes, and many psychiatric disorders.

Gene expression is the result of the genes' direction, or the production of these proteins. It is not a static condition fixed at some point in neuronal development. Individual nerve cells may respond to neurochemical changes outside the cell, producing different proteins for adaptation to the new environment. This dynamic nature of gene function highlights the manner in which the body and the environment interact and in how environmental factors influence gene expression.

Population Genetics

The study of molecular genetics in psychiatric disorders is in its infancy. Because the exact genetic basis of psychiatric disorder remains unclear, and animal models are hard to produce for some disorders, much of what we know about the genetics of psychiatric disorders comes from studies that trace given disorders within groups of people. This technique, called ***population genetics***, involves the analysis of genetic transmission of a trait within families and populations to determine risks and patterns of transmission. The risk for a given disorder occurring in the general population can then be compared with the risk within families and between groups of relatives. These studies rely on the initial identification of an individual who has the disorder and include the following principal methods:

- Family studies—analyze the occurrence of a disorder in first-degree relatives (biologic parents, siblings, and children), second-degree relatives (grandparents, uncles, aunts, nieces, nephews, and grandchildren), and so on.
- Twin studies—analyze the presence or absence of the disorder in pairs of twins. The *concordance rate* is the measure of similarity of occurrence in individuals with similar genetic makeup.
- Adoption studies—compare the risk for the illness developing in offspring raised in different environments. The strongest inferences may be drawn from studies that involve children separated from their parents at birth.

Few traits are completely heritable. Color blindness and blood type are examples of traits that exist because of heredity alone. Monozygotic twins have identical genetic contributions; therefore, both would have color blindness or the same blood type if they expressed that gene. This is 100% concordance. If a disorder were completely unrelated to genetics, then monozygotic twins would have the same concordance rates as dizygotic (fraternal) twins, who share roughly the same proportion of genes that ordinary siblings do—50%. If there is a genetic contribution with environmental influence, the concordance rates would be less than 100% for monozygotic twins but significantly greater than for dizygotic twins. Such is the case with several psychiatric disorders. Although no conclusive evidence exists for a complete genetic cause of most psychiatric disorders, significant evidence suggests strong genetic contributions exist for most (Harrison & Owen, 2003; Green et al., 2003; Lea, 2000; McGuffin et al., 2003; Merikanga & Avenevoli, 2000).

It is likely that psychiatric disorders are *polygenic*. This means that more than one gene is involved in producing a psychiatric disorder and that the disorder develops from genes interacting, which produces a risk factor, and environmental influences that lead to the expression of the illness. The environmental factors may include stress, infections, poor nutrition, catastrophic loss, complications during pregnancy, and exposure to toxins. Thus, genetic compositions convey vulnerability, or a risk for the illness, but the right set of environmental factors must be present for the disease to develop in the at-risk individual.

When considering information regarding risks for genetic transmission of psychiatric disorders, it is important to remember several key points:

- Psychiatric disorders have been described and labelled quite differently across generations, and errors in diagnosis may occur.
- Similar psychiatric symptoms may have considerably different causes, just as symptoms such as chest pain may occur in relation to many different causes.
- Genes that are present may not always cause the appearance of the trait.
- Several genes work together in an individual to produce a given trait or disorder.
- A biologic cause is not necessarily solely genetic in origin. Environmental influences alter the body's functioning and often mediate or worsen genetic risk factors.

As the public awareness of genetic evidence grows, it is likely that a PMH nurse will be faced with patients or family members requesting genetic testing or needing information regarding their likelihood of risk for a psychiatric disorder. As a result, psychiatric nurses increasingly will need greater understanding of the role genetics play in mental illness.

Risk Factors

The concept of genetic susceptibility suggests that an individual may be at increased risk for a psychiatric disorder. Research into *risk factors* is an important avenue of study. Just as knowledge of risk factors for diabetes and heart disease led to development of preventative interventions, learning more about risk factors for psychiatric disorders will lead to preventative care practices. Specific risk factors for psychiatric disorders are just beginning to be understood, and some of the environmental influences listed previously may be examples of risk factors. These events, circumstances, or demographic features are more likely to occur in individuals who experience a particular psychiatric disorder. In the absence of one specific gene for the major psychiatric disorders, risk factor assessment may be a logical alternative for predicting who is more likely to experience psychiatric disorders or certain conditions, such as aggression or suicidality. This is a growing area of psychiatric nursing.

Current Approaches and Technologic Advances

Neuroscience researchers have used several approaches to the study of the CNS structure and function. These approaches occur with both human research and animal models. The approaches, highlighted in Table 9-1, include the following:

- Comparative
- Developmental
- Chemoarchitectural
- Cytoarchitectural
- Functional

These different approaches to studying the CNS have significantly increased our understanding of normal CNS functioning and how disease affects behaviour and contributes to the development of psychiatric disorders. Research shows that areas of the brain, and the groups of nerve cells that constitute that area, often work together as functional units. A hierarchy of function exists in which primary sensory input is used in an increasingly more complex and integrated manner across areas of the brain. In addition, some areas of the brain, such as those that control basic levels of alertness and attention, must work correctly for information to be received, understood, and used by higher levels of the brain to organize a response. The brain's functional units work together to control or contribute to specific behaviours or emotions.

The *integrated approach* to brain development is the term used to describe the interactive working of brain areas and function. Understanding the work as an integration of parts allows us to understand that specific

Table 9.1	Approaches to the Study of Neuroanatomy		DSM IV

Approach	Purpose	Potential Limitations
Comparative	Explores and compares behaviour across animal nervous systems, from a simple primitive cordlike structure in some species to the large complex of the human brain	Difficult to correlate animal behaviour to human, especially emotional New brain structures do not necessarily correlate to new behaviour
Developmental	Studies nervous system structure within an individual or species of animal across different stages of development	Impossible to follow one human being's neuronal development Individual variation in development complicates comparisons of individuals across a specific point of time in development
Chemoarchitecture	Identifies differences in location of neurochemicals such as neurotransmitters throughout the brain	Boundaries between regional changes are subtle and may vary across individuals
Cytoarchitecture	Identifies differences or variations in cell type, structure, and density throughout the brain, mapping these variations by location	Boundaries between regional changes are subtle and may vary across individuals
Functional	Identifies location of predominant control over various behavioural functions within the brain Studies often conducted on the basis of dysfunction from a localized injury to the brain	Several regions or structures within the brain may contribute to one behaviour, making predominant control difficult to assign Controversy exists in correlating normal brain function to damaged brain tissue

areas of the brain control specific function. For example, there is a speech area in the brain, a mood area, an appetite area, and so on. Understanding the function of areas of the brain allows nurses to assess a patient's symptoms as, in large part, an expression of a problem with a specific brain area. Just as a person with an irregular heart beat is experiencing disruption in normal cardiac function, a person who fails to eat because of depression is experiencing a disruption in the brain's normal appetite and mood function.

> **KEY CONCEPT Plasticity** is the ability of the brain to change its structure and function in various ways to compensate for changes in the neuronal environment (Mohr & Mohr, 2001).

Neuroplasticity is an increasingly important concept when describing brain function. The changes in neural environment can come from internal sources, such as a change in electrolytes, or from external sources, such as a virus or toxin. With neuroplasticity, nerve signals may be rerouted, cells may learn new functions, sensitivity or number of cells may increase or decrease, or some nerve tissue may be regenerated in a limited way. Brains are most plastic during infancy and young childhood, when large adaptive learning tasks should normally occur. With age, brains become less plastic, which explains why it is easier to learn a second language at the age of 5 years than 55 years. Neuroplasticity contributes to understanding how function may be restored over time after brain damage occurs or how an individual may react over time to continuous pharmacotherapy regimens.

NEUROIMAGING

Since the 1980s, technologic advances in neuroimaging techniques have been a major aid to the current understanding of how the human brain functions. As knowledge grows, neuroimaging techniques are moving from research to routine clinical use, requiring PMH nurses to understand this technology. Two basic neuroimaging methods are structural and functional neuroimaging.

Structural Neuroimaging

Structural neuroimaging techniques were the first form of neuroimaging that allowed visualization of brain structures. Structural images show what normal structures of the brain look like and allow clinicians to identify tissue abnormalities, changes, or damage. Commonly used structural neuroimaging techniques include computed axial tomography (CT) scanning and magnetic resonance imaging (MRI). Although these techniques are useful in identifying what the brain looks like, they do not reveal anything about how the brain works.

Computed Axial Tomography

CT scanning first allowed scientists and clinicians to see structures inside the brain without more invasive and potentially dangerous methods. CT scans still use an x-ray beam passed through the head in serial slices. High-speed computers measure the decreased strength in the x-ray beam that results from absorption, and the computer assigns a shade of gray that reflects that change. The degree of energy absorbed by a tissue is proportionally related to its density. For example, cerebrospinal fluid (CSF) decreases the least, so it appears the darkest, whereas bone absorbs the most and appears light. White matter and gray matter are more difficult to discriminate with CT technology.

CT scans can be done with or without contrast material. Contrast materials are used to increase the visibility of certain tissues or blood vessels. If a contrast agent is used, an iodinated or other material is intravenously administered to enhance the CT image. Although CT scanning is a relatively safe, noninvasive procedure, the contrast material may have some adverse effects in some patients. Some patients receiving contrast materials report a metallic taste in the mouth, and some experience mild nausea, rashes, or joint pain. In rare instances, severe allergic responses, including anaphylaxis, may develop, so nurses must closely monitor patients who have received contrast media. In addition, because the equipment itself may frighten the patient, the nurse should educate the patient about the scan. Some patients may need to be accompanied during the procedure for ongoing reassurance.

Magnetic Resonance Imaging

MRI is performed by placing a patient into a long tube that contains powerful magnets. The magnetic field causes hydrogen-containing molecules (primarily water) to line up and move in symmetric ways around their axes. The magnetic field is then interrupted in pulses, causing the molecules to turn 90 or 180 degrees. Electromagnetic energy is released when the molecules return to their original position. The energy released is related to the density of the tissue and is detected by the MRI device, resulting in a scan measurement of the density of examined tissue. The CT scan is limited to one-dimensional images, but the MRI can produce three-dimensional images extremely clearly, allowing for discrimination of white and gray matter and other subtle changes in tissue.

MRI scans produce more information than CT images, but they also are more complicated and costly. In addition, MRI scans cannot be used for all patients. Because MRI uses magnet energy, individuals with pacemakers, metal plates, bone replacements, aneurysm clips, or other metal in their body cannot undergo the procedure; pregnant women also cannot have MRI scans. In addition, the loud noise of the equipment and the very narrow tube in which the patient must lie still trigger claustrophobic responses in some people. Adequate preparation of the patient by the nurse should eliminate any surprises. Assistance with shallow breathing techniques, mental distractions, or other anxiety-reducing strategies may help. Many MRI facilities are equipped with music to mask the whirring of the equipment and provide a distraction through the long testing period. Some tubes are now being made of clear plastic to decrease the claustrophobic sensation.

Functional Neuroimaging

Although structural imaging identifies what the brain looks like, the scans do not show how the brain is working. Functional neuroimaging techniques measure physiologic activities, providing insight into how the brain works. These methods let researchers study such activities as cerebral blood flow, neuroreceptor location and function, and distribution patterns of specific chemicals within the brain. Single photon emission computed tomography (SPECT) and positron emission tomography (PET) are the primary methods used to observe metabolic functioning. Both procedures require administering radioactive substances that emit charged particles, which are then measured by scanning equipment. Because these procedures measure function, the patient is usually asked to perform specific tasks during the test. The Wisconsin Card Sorting Test (WCST), which is commonly used, requires the individual to sort cards with different numbers, colors, and shapes into piles based on specified rules. This task requires use of the brain's frontal lobe, an important area for concept formation and decision making, and an area that often is disrupted in many psychiatric disorders. Figure 9-1 illustrates the differences between the frontal lobe activity of a pair of twins, one with schizophrenia and one without.

Positron Emission Tomography

PET measures glucose consumption in various brain regions. Because cells use glucose as fuel for cellular action, the higher the rate of glucose use detected by the PET scan, the higher the rate of metabolic activity in different areas of the brain. Abnormalities in glucose consumption, indicating more or less cellular activity, are found in Alzheimer's disease, seizures, stroke, tumor, and a number of psychiatric disorders. Scanning may be performed while the individual is at rest or performing a cognitive task. PET scans are often used to measure regional cerebral blood flow and neurotransmitter system functions.

Single Photon Emission Computed Tomography

SPECT is helpful in measuring regional cerebral blood flow. Evidence documents the use of SPECT scans in differentiating depression from dementia (Cho et al., 2002). Well documented in Alzheimer's disease (Vercelletto et al., 2002), decreased cerebral blood flow in specific areas of the brain is not found in depression. SPECT scans are also used to confirm changes in cerebral blood flow caused by certain drugs. For example, caffeine and nicotine cause a generalized decrease in cerebral blood flow.

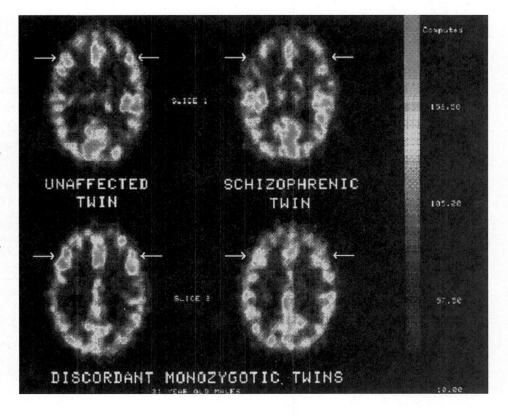

FIGURE 9.1 Differences in the frontal lobe activity of a pair of twins, one with the mental disorder of schizophrenia, and one who does not have the disorder. Figure courtesy of Drs. K. F. Berman and D. R. Weinberger, Clinical Brain Disorders Branch, National Institute of Mental Health.

New compounds have been developed recently to visualize the numbers or density of receptors in various areas of the brain, which may assist in understanding the effects of psychopharmacologic medications and neuroplastic changes in brain tissue over time.

Bridging the Structure–Function Gap

As structural and functional neuroimaging techniques advance, attempts are being made to develop imaging procedures that detail structure and function at the same time. Magnetic resonance spectroscopy (MRS) and functional magnetic resonance imaging (fMRI) are examples. The fMRI is useful for showing structure while localizing functioning and providing clear, high-resolution images. Like other forms of neuroimaging, the fMRI is noninvasive, but it requires no radioactive agent, making it economical and safer than PET and SPECT (Hennig, Speck, Koch, & Weiller, 2003).

MRS uses the same machinery as fMRI and provides precise and clear images of neuronal membranes as well as measures of metabolic cellular function (Heerschap, Kck, & Van De, 2003). In addition to these procedures, electromagnet encephalography (EEG/MEG) is being used. This procedure combines traditional EEG measurement (discussed later in this chapter) with imaging to visualize cellular electrical activity in the brain. Table 9-2 summarizes these neuroimaging methods. Although these neuroimaging procedures are used primarily as research tools, they also are becoming useful in clinical practice.

Neuroanatomy of the Central Nervous System

With advances in brain science comes greater understanding of the biologic basis of mental illnesses. Therefore, psychiatric–mental health nurses must increasingly be aware of the anatomic intricacy of the CNS as a foundation for modern psychiatric nursing assessments and interventions.

Although this section discusses each functioning area of the brain separately, each area is intricately connected with the others, and each functions interactively. The CNS contains the brain, brain stem, and spinal cord, whereas the total human nervous system includes the peripheral nervous system (PNS) as well. The PNS consists of the neurons that connect the CNS to the muscles, organs, and other systems in the periphery of the body. Whatever affects the CNS may also affect the PNS, and vice versa.

CEREBRUM

The largest part of the human brain, the cerebrum fills the entire upper portion of the cranium. The cortex, or outermost surface of the cerebrum, makes up about 80% of the human brain. The cortex is several millimeters thick and is composed of cell bodies mixed with capillary blood vessels. This mixture makes the cortex grey brown, thus the term *grey matter*. The cortex contains a number of bumps and grooves in a fully developed adult

Table 9.2   Methods of Neuroimaging

Method	Description	Considerations
Structural Imaging		

Computed tomography (CT), also called computerized axial tomography (CAT)	Uses X-ray technology to measure tissue density; is readily available; can be completed quickly, and less costly; may be used for screening, but many disease states are not clearly seen; use of contrast medium improves resolution	Contrast medium may produce allergic reactions; individuals with increased risk for contrast media complications include those with
		   History of previous reactions
		   Cardiac disease
		   Hypertension
		   Diabetes
		   Sickle cell disease
		Contraindications for use of contrast:
		   Iodine/shellfish allergies
		   Renal disease
		   Pregnancy

Magnetic resonance imaging (MRI)	Uses a magnetic field to magnetize hydrogen atoms in soft tissue, changing their alignment—this creates a tiny electric signal, which can be received to produce an image; produces greater resolution than a CT, diagnosing more subtle pathologic changes	Patients may experience headaches, dizziness, and nausea; symptoms of anxiety, claustrophobia, or psychosis can increase; contraindicated when patients have:
		   Aneurysm clips
		   Internal electrical, magnetic, or mechanical devices, such as pacemakers
		   Metallic surgical clips, sutures, and dental work distort the image
		   Claustrophobia

Functional Neuroimaging		
Positron emission tomography (PET)	Uses positron emitting isotopes (very short-lived radioactive entities such as oxygen-15) to image brain functioning; isotopes are incorporated into specific molecules to study cerebral metabolism, cerebral blood flow, and specific neurochemicals	Images appear blurry, lacking anatomic detail, but have been extremely useful in research to study distribution of neuroreceptors and the action of pharmacologic agents; invasive procedure, use of radioactivity limits the number of scans done with a single individual
Single photon emission computed tomography (SPECT)	Like PET, SPECT uses radioisotopes that produce only one photon; data are collected as a 3-dimensional volume and 2-dimensional images can be constructed on any plane	Less resolution and sensitivity than the PET, but inhalation methods may be used, allowing for some repeated studies
Functional magnetic resonance imaging (fMRI)	Combines spatial resolution of MRI with the ability to image neural activity; methods are still very early in development	Requires no radiation and can be completely noninvasive; individual can be imaged many times, in different clinical states, before or after treatments; removes many of the ethical constraints when studying children and adolescents with psychiatric disorders
Magnetic resonance spectroscopy (MRS)	Uses the same imaging equipment of the fMRI; by altering scanning parameters, signals represent specific chemicals in the brain	Noninvasive, repeatable, may be ideal for longitudinal studies, but has limited spatial resolution, especially with molecules that occur in low concentrations

brain, as shown in Figure 9-2. This "wrinkling" allows for a large amount of surface area to be confined in the limited space of the skull. The increased surface area allows for more potential connections between cells within the cortex. The grooves are called *fissures* if they extend deep into the brain and *sulci* if they are shallower. The bumps or convolutions are called *gyri*. Together, they provide many of the landmarks for the subdivisions of the cortex. The longest and deepest groove, the longitudinal fissure, separates the cerebrum into left and right hemispheres. Although these two divisions are nearly symmetric, there is some variation in the location and size of the sulci and gyri in each hemisphere. Substantial variation in these convolutions is found in the cortex of different individuals.

LEFT AND RIGHT HEMISPHERES

The cerebrum can be roughly divided into two halves, or hemispheres. For most people, one hemisphere is dominant, whereas about 5% of individuals have mixed dominance. Each hemisphere controls functioning

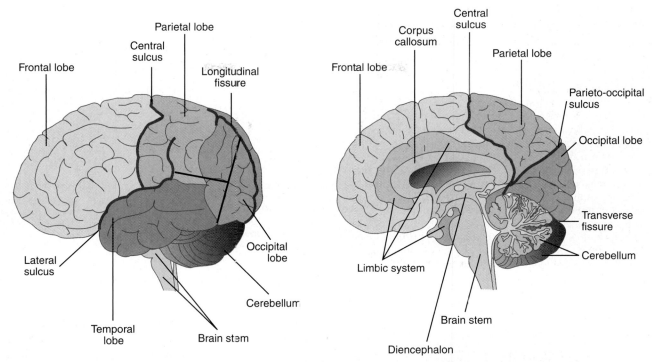

FIGURE 9.2   Lateral and medial surfaces of the brain. *Left*, the left lateral surface of the brain. *Right*, the medial surface of the right half of a sagittally hemisected brain.

mainly on the opposite side of the body. The left hemisphere, dominant in about 95% of people, controls functions mainly on the right side of the body. The right hemisphere provides input into receptive nonverbal communication, spatial orientation, and recognition; intonation of speech and aspects of music; facial recognition and facial expression of emotion; and nonverbal learning and memory. In general, the left hemisphere is more involved with verbal language function, including areas for both receptive and expressive speech control. In addition, the left hemisphere provides strong contributions to temporal order and sequencing, numeric symbols, and verbal learning and memory.

The two hemispheres are connected by the corpus callosum, a bundle of neuronal tissue that allows information to be exchanged quickly between the right and left hemispheres. An intact corpus callosum is required for the hemispheres to function in a smooth and coordinated manner.

Lobes of the Brain

The lateral surface of each hemisphere is further divided into four lobes: the **frontal, parietal, temporal, and occipital lobes** (Fig. 9-2). The lobes works in coordinated ways, but each is responsible for specific functions. Knowledge of these unique functions is helpful for understanding how damage to these areas produces the symptoms of mental illness and how medications that affect the functioning of these lobes can produce certain effects.

Frontal Lobes

The right and left frontal lobes make up about one fourth of the entire cerebral cortex and are proportionately larger in humans than in any other mammal. The precentral gyrus, the gyrus immediately anterior to the central sulcus, contains the primary motor area, or homunculi. Damage to this gyrus, or to the anterior neighbouring gyri, causes spastic paralysis in the opposite side of the body. The frontal lobe also contains Broca's area, which controls the motor function of speech. Damage to Broca's area produces expressive aphasia, or difficulty with the motor movements of speech. The frontal lobes are also thought to contain the highest or most complex aspects of cortical functioning, which collectively make up a large part of what we call personality. Working memory is an important aspect of frontal lobe function, including the ability to plan and initiate activity with future goals in mind. Insight, judgment, reasoning, concept formation, problem-solving skills, abstraction, and self-evaluation are all abilities that are modulated and affected by the action of the frontal lobes. These skills are often referred to as *executive functions* because they modulate more primitive impulses through numerous connections to other areas of the cerebrum.

When normal frontal lobe functioning is altered, executive functioning is decreased, and modulation of impulses can be lost, leading to changes in mood and personality. The importance of the frontal lobe and its

BOX 9.1

Frontal Lobe Syndrome

In the 1860s, Phineas Gage became a famous example of frontal lobe dysfunction. Mr. Gage was a New England railroad worker who had a thick iron-tamping rod propelled through his frontal lobes by an explosion. He survived, but suffered significant changes in his personality. Mr. Gage, who had previously been a capable and calm supervisor, began to show impatience, liable mood, disrespect for others, and frequent use of profanity after his injury (Harlow, 1868). Similar conditions are often called *frontal lobe syndrome.* Symptoms vary widely from individual to individual. In general, after damage to the dorsolateral (upper and outer) areas of the frontal lobes, the symptoms include a lack of drive and spontaneity. With damage to the most anterior aspects of the frontal lobes, the symptoms tend to involve more changes in mood and affect, such as impulsive and inappropriate behaviour.

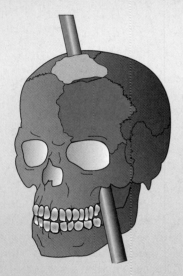

The skull of Phineas Gage, showing the route the tamping rod took through his skull. The angle of entry of the rod shot it behind the left eye and through the front part of the brain, sparing regions that are directly concerned with vital functions like breathing and heartbeat.

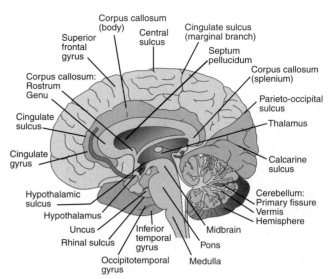

FIGURE 9.3   Gyri and sulci of the cortex.

sensory deficits, including neglect of contralateral sensory stimuli and spatial relationships. The parietal lobes contribute to the ability to recognize objects by touch, calculate, write, recognize fingers of the opposite hands, draw, and organize spatial directions, such as how to travel to familiar places.

Temporal Lobes

The temporal lobes contain the primary auditory and olfactory areas. Wernicke's area, located at the posterior aspect of the superior temporal gyrus, is primarily responsible for receptive speech. The temporal lobes also integrate sensory and visual information involved in control of written and verbal language skills as well as visual recognition. The hippocampus, an important structure discussed later, lies in the internal aspects of each temporal lobe and contributes to memory. Other internal structures of this lobe are involved in the modulation of mood and emotion.

Occipital Lobes

The primary visual area is located in the most posterior aspect of the occipital lobes. Damage to this area results in a condition called *cortical blindness.* In other words, the retina and optic nerve remain intact, but the individual cannot see. The occipital lobes are involved in many aspects of visual integration of information, including colour vision, object and facial recognition, and the ability to perceive objects in motion.

Association Cortex

Although not a lobe, the association cortex is an important area that allows the lobes to work in an integrated manner. Areas of one lobe of the cortex often share functions with an area of the adjacent lobe. When these neighbouring nerve fibers are related to the same sensory

role in the development of symptoms common to psychiatric disorders are emphasized in later chapters that discuss disorders such as schizophrenia, attention-deficit hyperactivity disorder, and dementia. Box 9-1 describes how altered frontal lobe function can affect mood and personality.

Parietal Lobes

The postcentral gyrus, immediately behind the central sulcus, contains the primary somatosensory area (Fig. 9-3). Damage to this area and neighbouring gyri results in deficits in discriminative sensory function, but not in the ability to perceive sensory input. The posterior areas of the parietal lobe appear to coordinate visual and somatosensory information. Damage to this area produces complex

modality, they are often referred to as *association* areas. For example, an area in the inferior parietal, posterior temporal, and anterior occipital lobes integrates visual, somatosensory, and auditory information to provide the abilities required for basic academic skills. These areas, along with numerous connections beneath the cortex, are part of the mechanisms that allow the human brain to work as an integrated whole.

Subcortical Structures

Beneath the cortex are layers of tissue composed of the axons of cell bodies. The axonal tissue forms pathways that are surrounded by glia, a fatty or lipid substance, which has a white appearance and give these layers of neuron axons their name—*white matter*. Structures inside the hemispheres, beneath the cortex, are considered subcortical. Many of these structures, essential in the regulation of emotions and behaviours, play important roles in our understanding of mental disorders. Figure 9-4 provides a coronal section view of the grey matter, white matter, and important subcortical structures.

Basal Ganglia

The **basal ganglia** are subcortical grey matter areas in both the right and left hemispheres that contain many cell bodies or nuclei. The basal ganglia are involved with motor functions and association in both the learning and the programming of behaviour or activities that are repetitive and, done over time, become automatic. The basal ganglia have many connections with the cere-bral cortex, thalamus, midbrain structures, and spinal cord. Damage to portions of these nuclei may produce changes in posture or muscle tone. In addition, damage may produce abnormal movements, such as twitches or tremors. The basil ganglia can be adversely affected by some of the medications used to treat psychiatric disorders, leading to side effects and other motor-related problems. The primary subdivisions of the basal ganglia are the putamen, globus pallidus, and caudate.

Limbic System

The **limbic system** is essential to understanding the many hypotheses related to psychiatric disorders and emotional behaviour in general. Basic emotions, needs, drives, and instinct begin and are modulated in the limbic system. Hate, love, anger, aggression, and caring are basic emotions that originate within the limbic system. Not only does the limbic system function as the seat of emotions, but also, because emotions are often generated based on our personal experiences, the limbic system is involved with aspects of memory. Hypothesized changes in the limbic system play a significant role in many theories of major mental disorders, including schizophrenia, depression, and anxiety disorders (discussed in later chapters). The limbic system is called a "system" because it comprises several small structures that work in a highly organized way. These structures include the hippocampus, thalamus, hypothalamus, amygdala, and limbic midbrain nuclei. See Figure 9-5 for identification and location of the structures within the limbic system and their relationship to other common CNS structures.

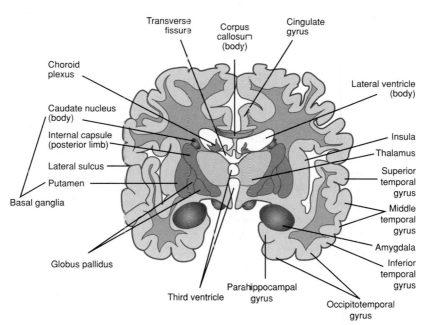

FIGURE 9.4   Coronal section of the brain, illustrating the corpus callosum, basal ganglia, and lateral ventricles.

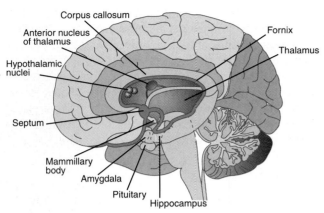

FIGURE 9.5 The structures of the limbic system are integrally involved in memory and emotional behaviour. Theories link changes in the limbic system to many major mental disorders, including schizophrenia, depression, and anxiety disorders.

Hippocampus

The **hippocampus** is involved in storing information, especially the emotions attached to a memory. Our emotional response to memories and our association with other related memories are functions of how information is stored within the hippocampus. Although memory storage is not limited to one area of the brain, destruction of the left hippocampus impairs verbal memory, and damage to the right hippocampus results in difficulty with recognition and recall of complex visual and auditory patterns. Deterioration of the nerves of the hippocampus and other related temporal lobe structures found in Alzheimer's disease produces the disorder's hallmark symptoms of memory dysfunction.

Thalamus

Sometimes called the "relay-switching center of the brain," the thalamus functions as a regulatory structure to relay all sensory information, except smell, sent to the CNS from the PNS. From the thalamus, the sensory information is relayed mostly to the cerebral cortex. The thalamus relays and regulates by filtering incoming information and determining what to pass on or not pass on to the cortex. In this fashion, the thalamus prevents the cortex from becoming overloaded with sensory stimulus. The thalamus is thought to play a part in controlling electrical activity in the cortex. Because of its primary relay function, damage to a very small area of the thalamus may produce deficits in many cortical functions, producing behavioural abnormalities.

Hypothalamus

Basic human activities, such as sleep–rest patterns, body temperature, and physical drives such as hunger and sex, are regulated by another part of the limbic system that rests deep within the brain and is called the hypothalamus. Dysfunction of this structure, whether from disorders or as a consequence of the adverse effect of drugs used to treat mental illness, produces common psychiatric symptoms, such as appetite and sleep problems.

Nerve cells within the hypothalamus secrete hormones: for example, antidiuretic hormone, which when sent to the kidneys, accelerates the reabsorption of water; and oxytocin, which acts on smooth muscles to promote contractions, particularly within the walls of the uterus. Because cells within the nervous system produce these hormones, they are often referred to as neurohormones and form a communication mechanism through the bloodstream to control organs that are not directly connected to nervous system structures.

Pituitary

The pituitary gland, often called the *master gland*, is directly connected by thousands of neurons that attach it to the ventral aspects of the hypothalamus. Together with the pituitary gland, the hypothalamus functions as one of the primary regulators of many aspects of the endocrine system. Its functions are involved in control of visceral activities, such as body temperature, arterial blood pressure, hunger, thirst, fluid balance, gastric motility, and gastric secretions. Deregulation of the hypothalamus can be manifested in symptoms of certain psychiatric disorders. For example, patients with schizophrenia often wear heavy coats during the hot summer months and do not appear hot. Before the role of the hypothalamus in schizophrenia was understood, psychological reasons were used to explain such symptoms. Now it is increasingly clear that such a symptom relates to deregulation of the hypothalamus's normal role in temperature regulation and is biologicly based (Shiloh et al., 2001).

Amygdala

The amygdala is directly connected to more primitive centers of the brain involving the sense of smell. It has numerous connections to the hypothalamus and lies adjacent to the hippocampus. The amygdala provides an emotional component to memory and is involved in modulating aggression and sexuality. Impulsive acts of aggression and violence have been linked to dysregulation of the amygdala, and erratic firing of the nerve cells in the amygdala is a focus of investigation in bipolar mood disorders (see Chapter 19).

Limbic Midbrain Nuclei

The limbic midbrain nuclei are a collection of neurons (including the ventral tegmental area and the locus ceruleus) that appear to play a role in the biologic basis of addiction. Sometimes referred to as the pleasure center or reward center of the brain, the limbic midbrain nuclei function to reinforce chemically certain behaviours, ensuring their repetition. Emotions such as feeling satisfied with good food, the pleasure of nurturing young, and the enjoyment of sexual activity originate in the limbic midbrain nuclei. The reinforcement of activities such as nutrition, procreation, and nurturing young are all primitive aspects of ensuring the survival of a species. When functioning in abnormal ways, the limbic midbrain nuclei can begin to reinforce unhealthy or risky behaviours, such as drug abuse. Exploration of this area of the brain is in its infancy but offers potential insight into addictions and their treatment.

OTHER CENTRAL NERVOUS SYSTEM STRUCTURES

The **extrapyramidal motor system** is a bundle of nerve fibers connecting the thalamus to the basal ganglia and cerebral cortex. Muscle tone, common reflexes, and automatic voluntary motor functioning, such as walking, are controlled by this nerve track. Dysfunction of this motor track can produce hypertonicity in muscle groups. In Parkinsons disease, the cells that compose the extrapyramidal motor system are severely affected, producing many involuntary motor movements. A number of medications, which are discussed in Chapter 13, also affect this system.

The **pineal body** is located above and medial to the thalamus. Because the pineal gland easily calcifies, it can be visualized by neuroimaging and often is a medial landmark. Its functions remain somewhat of a mystery, despite long knowledge of its existence. It contains secretory cells that emit the neurohormone melatonin and other substances. These hormones are thought to have a number of regulatory functions within the endocrine system. Information received from light–dark sources controls release of melatonin, which has been associated with sleep and emotional disorders. In addition, a modulation of immune function has been postulated for melatonin from the pineal gland.

The **locus ceruleus** is a tiny cluster of neurons that fan out and innervate almost every part of the brain, including most of the cortex, the thalamus and hypothalamus, the cerebellum, and the spinal cord. Just one neuron from the ceruleus can connect to more than 250,000 other neurons. Although it is very small, because of its wide-ranging neuronal connections, this tiny structure has influence in the regulation of attention, time perception, sleep–rest cycles, arousal, learning, pain, and mood and seems most involved with information processing of new, unexpected, and novel experiences. Some think its function/dysfunction may explain why individuals become addicted to substances and seek risky behaviours, despite awareness of negative consequences.

The **brain stem**, located beneath the thalamus and composed of the midbrain, pons, and medulla, has important life-sustaining functions. Nuclei of numerous neural pathways to the cerebrum are located in the brain stem. They are significantly involved in mediating symptoms of emotional dysfunction. These nuclei are also the primary source of several neurochemicals, such as serotonin, that are commonly associated with psychiatric disorders. Table 9-3 summarizes some of the key related nuclei.

The **cerebellum** is in the posterior aspect of the skull, beneath the cerebral hemispheres. This large structure controls movements and postural adjustments. To regulate postural balance and positioning, the cerebellum receives information from all parts of the body, including muscles, joints, skin, and visceral organs, as well as from many parts of the CNS.

Closely associated with the spinal cord, but not lying entirely within its column, is the **autonomic nervous system**, a subdivision of the PNS. It was originally given this name for being independent of conscious thought, that is, automatic. However, it does not necessarily function as autonomously as the name indicates. This system contains efferent (nerves moving away from the CNS) or motor system neurons, which affect target tissues such as cardiac muscle, smooth muscle, and the glands. It also contains afferent nerves, which are sensory and conduct information from these organs back to the CNS.

The autonomic nervous system is further divided into the sympathetic and parasympathetic nervous systems. These systems, although peripheral, are included here because they are involved in the emergency, or "fight-or-flight," response as well as the peripheral actions of many medications (see Chapter 13). Figure 9-6 illustrates the innervations of various target organs by the autonomic nervous system. Table 9-4 identifies the actions of the sympathetic and parasympathetic nervous systems on various target organs.

Neurophysiology of the Central Nervous System

At their most basic level, the human brain and connecting nervous system are composed of billions of cells (Fig. 9-7). Most are connective and supportive glial cells with ancillary functions in the nervous system.

NEURONS AND NERVE IMPULSES

About 10 billion cells are nerve cells, or neurons, responsible for receiving, organizing, and transmitting information. Each neuron has a cell body, or soma, which holds the nucleus containing most of the cell's genetic information. The soma also includes other

Table 9.3   Classic and Putative Neurotransmitters, Their Distribution and Proposed Functions

Neurotransmitter	Cell Bodies	Projections	Proposed Function
Acetylcholine			
Dietary precursor: choline	Basal forebrain Pons Other areas	Diffuse throughout the cortex, hippocampus Peripheral nervous system	Important role in learning and memory Some role in wakefulness, and basic attention Peripherally activates muscles and is the major neurochemical in the autonomic system
Monoamines			
Dopamine Dietary precursor: tyrosine	Substantia nigra Ventral tegmental area Arcuate nucleus Retina olfactory bulb	Striatum (basal ganglia) Limbic system and cerebral cortex Pituitary	Involved in involuntary motor movements Some role in mood states, pleasure components in reward systems, and complex behaviour such as judgment, reasoning, and insight
Norepinephrine Dietary precursor: tyrosine	Locus ceruleus Lateral tegmental area and others throughout the pons and medulla	Very widespread throughout the cortex, thalamus, cerebellum, brain stem, and spinal cord Basal forebrain, thalamus, hypothalamus, brain stem and spinal cord	Proposed role in learning and memory, attributing value in reward systems; fluctuates in sleep and wakefulness Major component of the sympathetic nervous system responses, including "fight or flight"
Serotonin Dietary precursor: tryptophan	Raphe nuclei Others in the pons and medulla	Very widespread throughout the cortex, thalamus, cerebellum, brain stem, and spinal cord	Proposed role in the control of appetite, sleep, mood states, hallucinations, pain perception, and vomiting
Histamine Precursor: histidine	Hypothalamus	Cerebral cortex Limbic system Hypothalamus Found in all mast cells	Control of gastric secretions, smooth muscle control, cardiac stimulation, stimulation of sensory nerve endings, and alertness
Amino Acids			
GABA	Derived from glutamate without localized cell bodies	Found in cells and projections throughout the CNS, especially in intrinsic feedback loops and interneurons of the cerebrum Also in the extrapyramidal motor system and cerebellum	Fast inhibitory response postsynaptically, inhibits the excitability of the neurons and therefore contributes to seizure, agitation, and anxiety control
Glycine	Primarily the spinal cord and brain stem	Limited projection, but especially in the auditory system and olfactory bulb Also found in the spinal cord, medulla, midbrain, cerebellum, and cortex	Inhibitory Decreases the excitability of spinal motor neurons but not cortical
Glutamate	Diffuse	Diffuse, but especially in the sensory organs	Excitatory Responsible for the bulk of information flow

Table 9.3   Classic and Putative Neurotransmitters, Their Distribution and Proposed Functions (*Continued*)

Neurotransmitter	Cell Bodies	Projections	Proposed Function
Neuropeptides			
Endogenous opioids, (ie, endorphins, enkephalins)	A large family of neuropeptides, which has three distinct subgroups, all of which are manufactured widely throughout the CNS	Widely distributed within and outside the CNS	Suppresses pain, modulates mood and stress Likely involvement in reward systems and addiction Also may regulate pituitary hormone release Implicated in the pathophysiology of diseases of the basal ganglia
Melatonin One of its precursors serotonin	Pineal body	Widely distributed within and outside the CNS	Secreted in dark and suppressed light, helps regulate the sleep–wake cycle as well as other biologic rhythms
Substance P	Widespread, significant in the raphe system and spinal cord	Spinal cord, cortex, brain stem and especially sensory neurons associated with pain perception	Involved in pain transmission, movement, and mood regulation
Cholecystokinin	Predominates in the ventral tegmental area of the midbrain	Frontal cortex where it is often colocalized with dopamine Widely distributed within and outside of the CNS	Primary intestinal hormone involved in satiety, also has some involvement in the control of anxiety and panic

organelles, such as ribosomes and endoplasmic reticulum, both of which carry out protein synthesis; the Golgi apparatus, which contains enzymes to modify the proteins for specific functions; vesicles, which transport and store proteins; and lysosomes, responsible for degradation of these proteins. Located throughout the neuron, mitochondria, containing enzymes and often called the "cell's engine," are the site of many energy-producing chemical reactions. These cell structures provide the basis for secreting numerous chemicals by which neurons communicate.

It is not just the vast number of neurons that accounts for the complexities of the brain but the enormous number of neurochemical interconnections and interactions between neurons. A single motor neuron in the spinal cord may receive signals from more than 10,000 sources of interconnections with other nerves. Although most neurons have only one axon, which varies in length and conducts impulses away from the soma, each has numerous dendrites, receiving signals from other neurons. Because axons may branch as they terminate, they also have multiple contacts with other neurons.

Nerve signals are prompted to fire by a variety of chemical or physical stimuli. This firing produces an electrical impulse. The cell's membrane is a double layer of phospholipid molecules with embedded proteins. Some of these proteins provide water-filled channels through which inorganic ions may pass (Fig. 9-8). Each of the common ions—sodium, potassium, calcium, and chloride—has its own specific molecular channel. These channels are voltage gated and thus open or close in response to changes in the electrical potential across the membrane. At rest, the cell membrane is polarized with a positive charge on the outside and about a 270-millivolt charge on the inside, owing to the resting distribution of sodium and potassium ions. As potassium passively diffuses across the membrane, the sodium pump uses energy to move sodium from the inside of the cell against a concentration gradient to maintain this distribution. An action potential, or nerve impulse, is generated as the membrane is depolarized and a threshold value is reached, which triggers the opening of the voltage-gated sodium channels, allowing sodium to surge into the cell. The inside of the cell briefly becomes positively charged and the outside negatively charged. Once initiated, the action potential becomes self-propagating, opening nearby sodium channels. This electrical communication moves into the soma from the dendrites or down the axon by this mechanism.

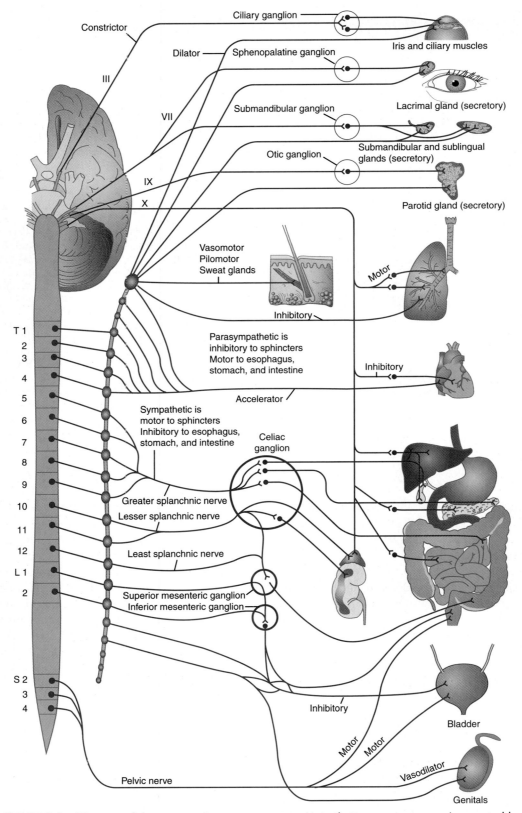

FIGURE 9.6   Diagram of the autonomic nervous system. Note that many organs are innervated by both sympathetic and parasympathetic nerves. (Adapted from Schaffe, E. E., & Lytle, I. M. [1980]. *Basic physiology and anatomy*. Philadelphia: J. B. Lippincott.)

Table 9.4	Peripheral Organ Response in the Autonomic Nervous System	
Effector Organ	**Sympathetic Response**	**Parasympathetic Response (Acetylcholine)**
Eye		
▪ Iris sphincter muscle	Preganglionic neurons— acetylcholine	Constriction
▪ Ciliary muscle	Postganglionic neurons— mostly norepinephrine Dilation Relaxation	Accommodation for near vision
Heart		
▪ Sinoatrial node	Increased rate	Decrease in rate
▪ Atria	Increased contractility	Decrease in contractility
▪ Atrioventricular node	Increased contractility	Decrease in conduction velocity
Blood vessels	Constriction	Dilation
Lungs		
▪ Bronchial muscles	Relaxation	Bronchoconstriction
▪ Bronchial glands		Secretion
Gastrointestinal Tract		
▪ Motility and tone	Relaxation	Increased
▪ Sphincters	Contraction	Relaxation
▪ Secretion		Stimulation
Urinary Bladder		
▪ Detrusor muscle	Relaxation	Contraction
▪ Trigone and sphincter	Contraction	Relaxation
Uterus	Contraction (pregnant) Relaxation (nonpregnant)	Variable
Skin		
▪ Pilomotor muscles	Contraction	No effect
▪ Sweat glands	Increased secretion	No effect
Glands		
▪ Salivary, lachrymal		Increased secretion
▪ Sweat		Increased secretion

SYNAPTIC TRANSMISSION

For one neuron to communicate with another, the electrical process described must change to a chemical communication. The synaptic cleft, a junction between one nerve and another, is the space where the electrical intracellular signal becomes a chemical extracellular signal. Various substances are recognized as the chemical messengers between neurons.

> ⬢ **KEY CONCEPT Neurotransmitters** are small molecules that directly and indirectly control the opening or closing of ion channels.

Neurotransmitters are small molecules that directly and indirectly control the opening or closing of ion channels. Neuromodulators are chemical messengers that make the target cell membrane or postsynaptic membrane more or less susceptible to the effects of the primary neurotransmitter. Some of these neurochemicals are synthesized quickly from dietary precursors, such as tyrosine or tryptophan, or enzymes inside the cytoplasm of the neuron, but most synthesis occurs in the terminals or the neuron itself. Some neurochemicals can reduce the membrane potential and enhance the transmission of the signal between neurons. These chemicals are called *excitatory neurotransmitters*. Other neurochemicals have the opposite effect, slowing down nerve impulses, and these substances are called *inhibitory neurotransmitters*.

As the electrical action potential reaches the ends of the axon, called *terminals*, calcium ion channels are opened, causing an influx of Ca^{++} ions into the **neuron**. This increase in calcium stimulates the release of neurotransmitters into the synapse. Rapid signaling between neurons requires a ready supply of neurotransmitter. These neurotransmitters are stored in small vesicles grouped near the cell membrane at the end of the axon. Because nerve terminals do not have the ability to manufacture proteins, the transmitters that fill these vesicles

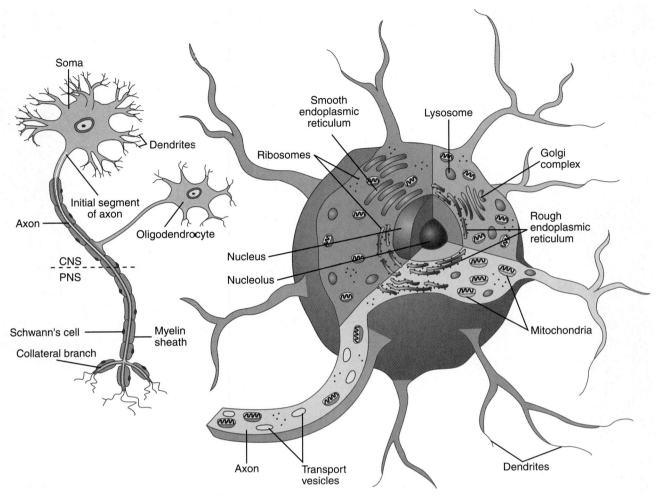

FIGURE 9.7   Cell body and organelles of an axon.

are small molecules, such as the bioamines (dopamine and norepinephrine) or the amino acids (glutamate or γ-aminobutyric acid [GABA]). The actions of these small molecules are discussed later in this chapter. When stimulated, the vesicles containing the neurotransmitter fuse with the cell membrane, and the neurotransmitter is released into the synapse (Fig. 9-9). The neurotransmitter then crosses the synaptic cleft to a receptor site on the postsynaptic neuron and stimulates adjacent neurons. This is the process of neuronal communication.

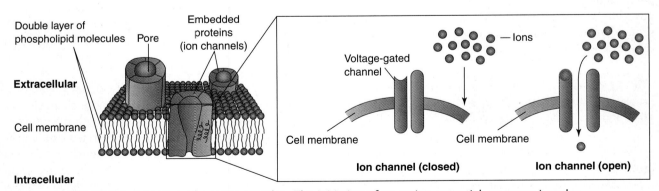

FIGURE 9.8   Initiation of a nerve impulse. The initiation of an action potential, or nerve impulse, involves the opening and closing of the voltage-gated channels on the cell membrane and the passage of ions into the cell. The resulting electrical activity sends communication impulses from the dendrites or axon into the body.

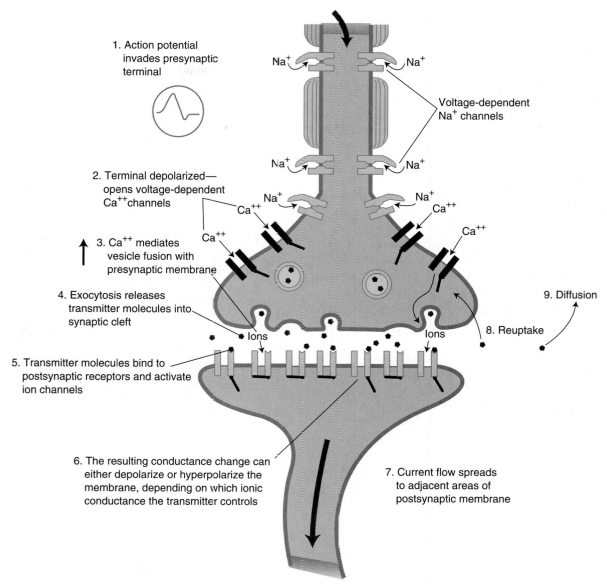

1. Action potential invades presynaptic terminal

Na^+

Na^+

Voltage-dependent Na^+ channels

Na^+

Na^+

2. Terminal depolarized—opens voltage-dependent Ca^{++} channels

Ca^{++}

Na^+

Na^+

Ca^{++}

Ca^{++}

Ca^{++}

3. Ca^{++} mediates vesicle fusion with presynaptic membrane

4. Exocytosis releases transmitter molecules into synaptic cleft

Ions

Ions

9. Diffusion

8. Reuptake

5. Transmitter molecules bind to postsynaptic receptors and activate ion channels

6. The resulting conductance change can either depolarize or hyperpolarize the membrane, depending on which ionic conductance the transmitter controls

7. Current flow spreads to adjacent areas of postsynaptic membrane

FIGURE 9.9   Synaptic transmission. The most significant events that occur during synaptic transmission: (1) the action potential reaches the presynaptic terminal; (2) membrane depolarization causes Ca^{++} terminals to open; (3) Ca^{++} mediates fusion of the vesicles with the presynaptic membrane; (4) transmitter molecules are released into the synaptic cleft, by exocytosis; (5) transmitter molecules bind to postsynaptic receptors and activate ion channels; (6) conductance changes cause an excitatory or inhibitory postsynaptic potential, depending on the specific transmitter; (7) current flow spreads along the postsynaptic membrane; and (8) transmitter remaining in the synaptic cleft returns to the presynaptic terminal by reuptake or (9) diffuses into the extracellular fluid. (Adapted and reproduced with permission from Schauf, C., Moffett, D., & Moffett, S. [1990]. *Human physiology.* St. Louis: Times Mirror/Mosby.)

Embedded in the postsynaptic membrane are a number of proteins that act as receptors for the released neurotransmitters. The "lock-and-key" analogy has often been used to describe the fit of a given neurotransmitter to its receptor site. Each neurotransmitter has a specific receptor, or protein, for which it and only it will fit. The target cell, when stimulated by the neurotransmitter, will then respond by evoking its own action potential and either producing some action common to that cell or acting as a relay to keep the messages moving throughout the CNS. This pattern of the electrical signal from one neuron, converted to chemical signal at the synaptic cleft, picked up by an adjacent neuron, again converted to an electrical action potential, and then to a chemical signal, occurs billions of times a day in billions of different brain cells. It is this electrical–chemical communication process that allows the structures of the brain to function together in a coordinated and organized manner.

When the neurotransmitter has completed its interaction with the postsynaptic receptor and stimulated that cell, its work is done, and it needs to be removed. It can be removed by natural diffusion away from the area of high neurotransmitter concentration at the receptors by being broken down by enzymes in the synaptic cleft, or through reuptake through highly specific mechanisms into the presynaptic terminal.

Many psychopharmacologic agents, particularly antidepressants, act by blocking the reuptake of the neurotransmitters, thereby increasing the available amount of chemical messenger. Presynaptic binding sites for neurotransmitters may serve not only as reuptake mechanisms but also as autoreceptors to perform various regulatory functions on the flow of neurotransmitter into the synapse. When these presynaptic autoreceptors are saturated, the neuron knows it is time to slow down or stop releasing neurotransmitter. The neurotransmitters taken back into the presynaptic neuron may be stored in vesicles for re-release, or they may be broken down by enzymes, such as monoamine oxidase, and removed entirely.

The primary steps in synaptic transmission are summarized in Figure 9-10. The preceding discussion contains only the basic mechanisms of neuronal communication. Many other factors that modulate or contribute to the communication between neurons are only beginning to be discovered. Examples include peptides that are released into the synapse and thought to behave like neurotransmitters or that also can appear in combination with another neurotransmitter. These peptides, known as *co-transmitters*, are believed to have a modulatory effect on the primary neurotransmitter.

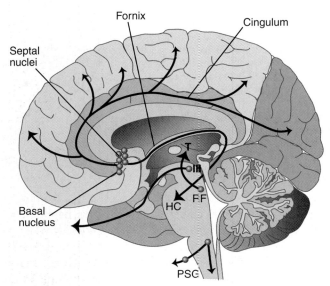

FIGURE 9.10 Cholinergic pathways. HC, hippocampal formation; PSG, parasympathetic ganglion cell; RF, reticular formation; T, thalamus. (Adapted from Nolte, J., & Angevine, J. [1995]. *The human brain: In photographs and diagrams.* St. Louis: Mosby.)

RECEPTOR ACTIVITY

Both presynaptic and postsynaptic receptors have the capacity to change, developing either a greater-than-usual response to the neurotransmitter, known as *supersensitivity*, or a less-than-usual response, called *subsensitivity*. These changes represent the concept of neuroplasticity of brain tissue discussed earlier in the chapter. The change in sensitivity of the receptor is most commonly caused by the effect of a drug on a receptor site or by disease that affects the normal functioning of a receptor site. Drugs can affect the sensitivity of the receptor by altering the strength of attraction or affinity of a receptor for the neurotransmitter, by changing the efficiency with which the receptor activity translates the message inside the receiving cell, or by decreasing over time the number of receptors.

These mechanisms may account for the long-term, sometimes severely adverse, effects of psychopharmacologic drugs, the loss of effectiveness of a given medication, or the loss of effectiveness of a medication after repeated use in treating recurring episodes of a psychiatric disorder. Disease may cause a change in the normal number or function of receptors, thereby altering their sensitivity (Garcia, Marin, & Perillo, 2002). It has been hypothesized that depression is caused by a reduction in the normal number of certain receptors, leading to an abnormality in their sensitivity to neurotransmitters such as serotonin and norepinephrine. A decreased response to continued stimulation of these receptors is usually referred to as *desensitization* or *refractoriness*. This suspected subsensitivity is referred to as *down-regulation* of the receptors.

RECEPTOR SUBTYPES

The nervous system uses many different neurochemicals for communication, and each specific chemical messenger requires a specific receptor on which the chemical can act. More than 100 different chemical messengers have been identified, with new ones being uncovered frequently as research on the functioning of the brain becomes more and more precise. In addition to the sheer number of receptors needed to accommodate these chemicals, the neurotransmitters may produce different effects at different synaptic sites. The ability of a neurotransmitter to produce different actions is, in part, because of the specialization of its receptors. The different receptors for each neurochemical messenger are referred to as *receptor subtypes* for the chemical. Each major neurotransmitter has several different subtypes of receptors, allowing the neurotransmitter to have different effects in different areas of the brain. For example, dopamine, a common neurotransmitter discussed in the next section, has five different subtypes of receptors that have been identified. Numbers usually name the receptor subtypes. In the example of dopamine, the various subtypes of receptors are called D1, D2, D3, and so on. Knowledge of the different subtypes helps in understanding both the effects and side effects of medications used to treat mental disorders.

NEUROTRANSMITTERS

Many substances have been identified as possible chemical messengers, but not all chemical messengers are neurotransmitters. Classic neurotransmitters are those that meet certain criteria agreed on by neuroscientists. The traditional criteria include the following:

- The chemical is synthesized inside the neuron.
- The chemical is present in the presynaptic terminals.
- The chemical is released into the synaptic cleft and causes a particular effect on the postsynaptic receptors.
- An exogenous form of the chemical administered as a drug causes identical action.
- The chemical is removed from the synaptic cleft by a specific mechanism.

Neurotransmitters can be grouped into categories that reflect chemical similarities of the neurotransmitter. Common practice classifies certain chemicals as neurotransmitters even though their ability to meet the strict traditional definition may be incomplete. For the purposes of this section, the classification of neurotransmitters will use this common system of classifying neurotransmitters. Common categories of neurotransmitters include:

- cholinergic neurotransmitters;
- biogenic amine neurotransmitters (sometimes called *monoamines* or *bioamines*);
- amino acid neurotransmitters;
- neuropeptide neurotransmitters.

Neurotransmitters are also classified by whether their action causes physiologic activity to occur or to stop occurring. All the neurotransmitters commonly involved in the development of mental illness or affected by the drugs used to treat these illnesses are excitatory except one, GABA, which is inhibitory. The significance of this concept is discussed later. Neurotransmitters are found wherever there are neurons. Neurons are contained in both the CNS and PNS, and psychiatric mental disorders occur in the CNS, so neurotransmitters are discussed from the perspective of the CNS.

Cholinergic

Acetylcholine (ACh) is the primary cholinergic neurotransmitter. Found in the greatest concentration in the PNS, ACh provides the basic synaptic communication for the parasympathetic neurons and part of the sympathetic neurons, which send information to the CNS. Understanding both the action of ACh and the receptor

subtypes for this neurotransmitter assists psychiatric mental health nurses in understanding the complex side effects of common medications used to treat mental disorders.

Cholinergic neurons, so named because they contain ACh, follow diffuse projections throughout the cerebral cortex and limbic system, arising primarily from cell bodies in the base of the frontal lobes. Pathways from this region also project throughout the hippocampus (Fig. 9-10). These connections suggest that ACh is involved in higher intellectual functioning and memory. Individuals who have Alzheimer's disease or Down syndrome often exhibit patterns of cholinergic neuron loss in regions innervated by these pathways (such as the hippocampus), which may contribute to their memory difficulties and other cognitive deficits. Some cholinergic neurons are afferent to these areas bringing information from the limbic system, highlighting the role that ACh plays in communicating emotional state to the cerebral cortex. ACh is an excitatory neurotransmitter, meaning that when released into a synapse, it causes the postsynaptic neuron to initiate some action.

The subtypes of ACh receptors are divided into two groups: the muscarinic receptors and the nicotinic receptors. Many psychiatric medications are anticholinergic agents, which block the effects of the muscarinic ACh receptors. This blocking effect of ACh causes common side effects, such as dry mouth, blurred vision, constipation, urinary retention, and tachycardia, which are seen in many psychotropic medications. Excessive blockade of ACh can cause confusion and delirium, especially in elderly patients, as discussed in Chapter 30. Table 9-4 lists the effects of ACh on various organs in the parasympathetic system.

Biogenic Amines

The **biogenic amines** (bioamines) consist of small molecules manufactured in the neuron that contain an amine group, thus the name. These include dopamine, norepinephrine, and epinephrine, which are all synthesized from the amino acid tyrosine; serotonin, which is synthesized from tryptophan; and histamine, manufactured from histidine. Of all the neurotransmitters, the biogenic amines are most central to current hypotheses of psychiatric disorders and thus are described individually in more detail.

Dopamine

Dopamine is an excitatory neurotransmitter found in distinct regions of the CNS, and it is involved in cognition, motor, and neuroendocrine functions. Dopamine levels are decreased in Parkinson's disease, and abnormally high production of dopamine has been associated with schizophrenia, discussed in more detail in Chapter 17.

Dopamine is also the neurotransmitter that stimulates the body's natural "feel good" reward pathways, producing pleasant euphoric sensation under certain conditions. Abnormalities of dopamine use within the reward system pathways are suspected to be a critical aspect of the development of drug and other addictions. The dopamine pathways are distinct neuronal areas within the CNS in which the neurotransmitter dopamine predominates. Three major dopaminergic pathways have been identified.

The mesocortical and mesolimbic pathways originate in the ventral tegmental area and project into the medial aspects of the cortex (mesocortical) and the medial aspects of the limbic system inside the temporal lobes, including the hippocampus and amygdala (mesolimbic). Sometimes they are considered to be one pathway and at other times two separate pathways. The mesocortical pathway has major effects on cognition, including such functions as judgment, reasoning, insight, social conscience, motivation, the ability to generalize learning, and reward systems in the human brain. It contributes to some of the highest seats of cortical functioning. The mesolimbic pathway also strongly influences emotions and has projections that affect memory and auditory reception. Abnormalities in these pathways have been associated with schizophrenia.

Another major dopaminergic pathway begins in the substantia nigra and projects into the basal ganglia, parts of which are known as the *striatum*. Therefore, this pathway is called the *nigrostriatal pathway*. This influences the extrapyramidal motor system, which serves the voluntary motor system and allows involuntary motor movements. Destruction of dopaminergic neurons in this pathway has been associated with Parkinson's disease.

The next or last dopamine pathway originates from projections of the mesolimbic pathway and continues into the hypothalamus, which then projects into the pituitary gland. Therefore, this pathway, called the *tuberoinfundibular pathway*, has an impact on endocrine function and other functions, such as metabolism, hunger, thirst, sexual function, circadian rhythms, digestion, and temperature control. Figure 9-11 illustrates the dopaminergic pathways.

Scientists have identified at least five subtypes of dopamine receptors in the CNS. These subtypes are distributed differently throughout the brain. For example, the D1 subtype receptor and its related receptor subtype, D5, predominate in areas that affect memory and emotions, such as the cortex, hippocampus, and amygdala. They have not been detected in the substantia nigra. D2 receptors are richly distributed throughout neurons in the extrapyramidal motor system, whereas D4 receptors are richly distributed in the frontal cortex, with few in the nigrostriatal system. Antipsychotic medications, discussed in Chapter 13, act

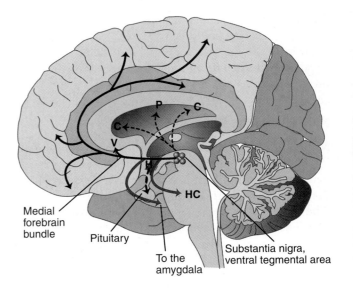

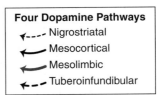

Four Dopamine Pathways
- Nigrostriatal
- Mesocortical
- Mesolimbic
- Tuberoinfundibular

FIGURE 9.11   Dopaminergic pathways. C, caudate nucleus; H, hypothalamus; HC, hippocampal formation; P, putamen; V, ventral striatum. (Adapted from Nolte, J., & Angevine, J. [1995]. *The human brain: In photographs and diagrams*. St. Louis: Mosby.)

by blocking the effects of dopamine at the receptor sites.

Many of the medications that are most effective on the acute symptoms of psychosis have a strong attraction or affinity for D2 receptors and a weaker but modest correlation with D1 receptors. Because D2 receptors predominate in the nigrostriatal pathway, medications that have a weaker blockade of D2 will have fewer extrapyramidal motor system effects. Side effects and adverse effects from the involuntary motor system are at times extremely debilitating to individuals. Based on the assumption that these dopamine receptor subtypes have different functions in the CNS, new medications are being designed to affect more predominantly one subtype than another, presumably avoiding effects on systems containing other subtypes and thus avoiding potential side effects of the medication. Researchers are attempting to develop new antipsychotic medications that avoid or minimize the effects on D2 and therefore diminish the occurrence of extrapyramidal effects.

Norepinephrine

Norepinephrine was first demonstrated to be the primary neurotransmitter of the PNS in 1946. Whereas it is commonly found in the PNS, norepinephrine is critical to CNS functioning as well. Norepinephrine is an excitatory neurochemical that plays a major role in generating and maintaining mood states. Decreased norepinephrine has been associated with depression, and excessive norepinephrine has been associated with manic symptoms (Montgomery, 2000). Because norepinephrine is so heavily concentrated in the terminal sites of sympathetic nerves, it can be released quickly to ready the individual for a fight-or-flight response to threats in the environment. For this reason, norepinephrine is thought to play a role in the physical symptoms of anxiety.

Nerve tracts and pathways containing predominantly norepinephrine are called *noradrenergic* and are less clearly delineated than the dopamine pathways. In the CNS, noradrenergic neurons originate in the locus ceruleus, where more than half of the noradrenergic cell bodies are located. Because the locus ceruleus is one of the major timekeepers of the human body, norepinephrine is involved in sleep and wakefulness. From the locus ceruleus, noradrenergic pathways ascend into the neocortex, spread diffusely (Fig. 9-12), and enhance the ability of neurons to respond to whatever input they may be receiving. In addition, norepinephrine appears to be involved in the process of reinforcement, which facilitates learning. Noradrenergic pathways innervate the hypothalamus and thus are involved to some degree in endocrine function. Anxiety disorders and depression are examples of psychiatric illnesses in which dysfunction of the noradrenergic neurons may be involved.

Serotonin

Serotonin (also called 5-hydroxytryptamine or 5-HT) is primarily an excitatory neurotransmitter that is diffusely distributed within the cerebral cortex, limbic system, and basal ganglia of the CNS. Serotonergic neurons also project into the hypothalamus and cerebellum. Figure 9-13 illustrates serotonergic pathways. Serotonin plays a role in emotions, cognition, sensory perceptions, and essential biologic functions, such as sleep and appetite. During the rapid-eye-movement (REM) phase of sleep, or the dream state, serotonin concentrations decrease, and muscles subsequently relax. Serotonin is also involved in the control of food intake, hormone secretion, sexual behaviour, thermoregulation, and cardiovascular regulation. Some serotonergic fibers reach the cranial blood vessels within the brain and the pia mater, where they have a vasoconstrictive effect. The potency of some new medications for migraine headaches is related to their ability to block serotonin transmission in the cranial blood vessels. Descending serotonergic pathways are important in central pain control. Depression and insomnia have been associated with decreased levels of 5-HT, whereas mania has been associated with increased 5-HT. Some of the most well-known antidepressant medications, such as Prozac and Zoloft, which are discussed in more depth in Chapter 13, function by raising serotonin levels within certain areas of the CNS (Harmer, Hill, Taylor, Cowen, & Goodwin, 2003). Obsessive-compulsive disorder,

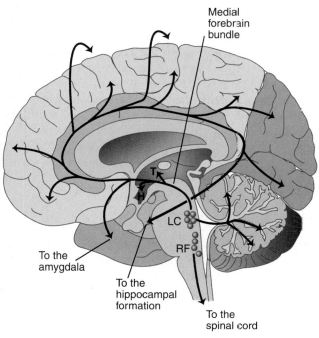

FIGURE 9.12   Noradrenergic pathways. H, hypothalamus; LC, locus ceruleus; RF, reticular formation; T, thalamus. (Adapted from Nolte, J., & Angevine, J. [1995]. *The human brain: In photographs and diagrams.* St. Louis: Mosby.)

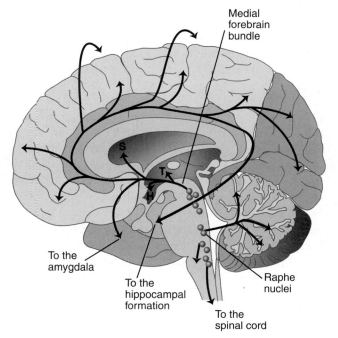

FIGURE 9.13   Serotonergic pathways. H, hypothalamus; S, septal nuclei; T, thalamus. (Adapted from Nolte, J., & Angevine, J. [1995]. *The human brain: In photographs and diagrams.* St. Louis: Mosby.)

panic disorder, and other anxiety disorders are believed to be associated with dysfunction of the serotonin pathways, explaining why these antidepressants have several uses in treating mental disorders (Kapczinski, Lima, Souza, & Schmitt, 2003).

Numerous subtypes of serotonin receptors also exist, and each of these appears to have a distinct function. 5-HT1a is involved in the control of anxiety, aggression, and depression. Drugs such as lysergic acid diethylamide (LSD) affect 5-HT2 and produce hallucinatory effects.

Histamine

Histamine has only recently been identified as a neurotransmitter. Its cell bodies originate predominantly in the hypothalamus and project to all major structures in the cerebrum, brain stem, and spinal cord. Its functions are not well known, but it appears to have a role in autonomic and neuroendocrine regulation. Many psychiatric medications can block the effects of histamine postsynaptically and produce side effects such as sedation, weight gain, and hypotension.

Amino Acids

Amino acids are the building blocks of proteins and have many roles in intraneuronal metabolism. In addition, amino acids can function as neurotransmitters in as many as 60% to 70% of the synaptic sites in the brain. Amino acids are the most prevalent neurotransmitters. Virtually all the neurons in the CNS are activated by excitatory amino acids, such as glutamate, and inhibited by inhibitory amino acids, such as GABA and glycine. Many of these amino acids coexist with other neurotransmitters.

γ-Aminobutyric Acid

GABA is the primary inhibitory neurotransmitter for the CNS. The pathways of GABA exist almost exclusively in the CNS, with the largest GABA concentrations in the hypothalamus, hippocampus, basal ganglia, spinal cord, and cerebellum. GABA functions in an inhibitory role in control of spinal reflexes and cerebellar reflexes. It has a major role in the control of neuronal excitability through the brain. In addition, GABA has an inhibitory influence on the activity of the dopaminergic nigrostriatal projections. GABA also has interconnections with other neurotransmitters. For example, dopamine inhibits cholinergic neurons, and GABA provides feedback and balance. Dysregulation of GABA and GABA receptors has been associated with anxiety disorders, and decreased GABA activity is involved in the development of seizure disorders.

Two specific subtype receptors have been identified for GABA: A and B. Two classes of medication, benzodiazepine antianxiety drugs and sedative-hypnotic barbiturate drugs, work because of their affinity for GABA receptor sites. Interest in the beneficial effects of these drugs has led to increased interest in GABA receptor sites. Researchers are finding endogenous chemicals that bind to the same receptor sites as benzodiazepines and serve as natural inhibitory regulators (Fritschy & Brunig, 2003).

Glutamate

Glutamate, the most widely distributed excitatory neurotransmitter, is the main transmitter in the associational areas of the cortex. Glutamate can be found in a number of pathways from the cortex to the thalamus, pons, striatum, and spinal cord. In addition, glutamate pathways have a number of connections with the hippocampus. Some glutamate receptors may play a role in the long-lasting enhancement of synaptic activity. In turn, in the hippocampus, this enhancement may have a role in learning and memory. Too much glutamate is harmful to neurons, and considerable interest has emerged regarding its neurotoxic effects.

Conditions that produce an excess of endogenous glutamate can cause neurotoxicity by overexcitation of neuronal tissue. This process, called excitotoxicity, increases the sensitivity of glutamate receptors, produces overactivation of the receptors, and is increasingly being understood as a critical piece of the cascade of events involved in physical symptoms of alcohol withdrawal in dependent individuals. Excitotoxicity is also believed to be part of the pathology of conditions such as ischemia, hypoxia, hypoglycemia, and hepatic failure. Damage to the CNS from chronic malfunctioning of the glutamate system may be involved in the psychiatric symptoms seen in neurodegenerative diseases such as Huntington's, Parkinson's, and Alzheimer's diseases; vascular dementia; amyotrophic lateral sclerosis; and acquired immune deficiency syndrome (AIDS)-related dementia (MacGregor, Avshalumov, & Rice, 2003). Degeneration of glutamate neurons has more recently been implicated in the development of schizophrenia (Kurup & Kurup, 2003).

Neuropeptides

Peptides are short chains of amino acids. Neuropeptides exist in the CNS and have a number of important roles as neurotransmitters, neuromodulators, or neurohormones. Neuropeptides were first thought to be pituitary hormones, such as adrenocorticotropin, oxytocin, and vasopressin, or hypothalamic-releasing hormones (eg, corticotropin-releasing hormone and thyrotropin-releasing hormone [TRH]). However, when an endogenous morphine-like substance was discovered in the 1970s, the term *endorphin*, or endogenous morphine, was introduced. Although the amino acids and monoamine neurotransmitters can be produced directly from dietary precursors in any part of the neuron, neuropeptides are, almost without exception, synthesized from messenger RNA in the cell body. Currently, two types of neuropeptides have been identified. Opioid neuropeptides, such as endorphins, enkephalins, and dynorphins, act in endocrine functioning and pain suppression. The nonopioid neuropeptides, such as substance P and somatostatin, play roles in pain transmission and endocrine functioning.

There are considerable variations in the distribution of individual neuropeptides, but some areas are especially rich in cell bodies containing neuropeptides. These areas include the amygdala, striatum, hypothalamus, raphe nuclei, brain stem, and spinal cord. Many of the interneurons of the cerebral cortex contain neuropeptides, but there are considerably fewer in the thalamus and almost none in the cerebellum.

By now, it should be obvious that the complexities of neuronal transmission are enormous. PMH nurses have a significant role in assessing symptoms and administering and monitoring medications for patients with psychiatric disorders. Knowledge of neurotransmitters is essential because even a single dose of a drug affecting this system may cause relief of symptoms or have adverse effects. The actions of psychopharmacologic agents and related nursing responsibilities are discussed more fully in Chapter 13. In addition, many nursing interventions designed to effect changes in such functions as sleep, diet, stress management, exercise, and mood modulation affect these neurotransmitters and neuropeptides, directly or indirectly. More research is clearly needed to understand the biopsychosocial aspects of nursing care.

New Fields of Study

As the complexity of the nervous system and its interrelationship with other body systems and the environment have become more fully understood, new fields of study have emerged. From the discussion of neuroanatomy and neurotransmitters, it is logical to deduce that understanding the endocrine system and its interrelationship with the nervous system is essential. Although it has long been observed that individuals under stress have compromised immune systems and are more likely to acquire common diseases, only recently have changes in the immune system been noted as widespread in some psychiatric illnesses. In addition, as biologic rhythms have become more fully understood and defined, new information suggests that dysfunction of these rhythms may not only result from a psychiatric illness but also contribute to its development. Therefore, the following sections provide a brief overview of psychoendocrinology, psychoimmunology, and chronobiology.

Psychoendocrinology

Psychoendocrinology examines the relationships among the nervous system, endocrine system, and behaviour. Messages are conveyed within the endocrine system mainly by hormones, and neurohormones are those substances excreted by special neurons within the nervous system. Neurohormones are cellular substances and are secreted into the bloodstream and transported to a site where they exert their effect. Of the several types of hormones, peptides are the most common hormones in the CNS.

The hypothalamus sends and receives information through the pituitary, which then communicates with structures in the peripheral aspects of the body. Figure 9-14 presents an example of the communication of the anterior pituitary with a number of organs and structures. Axes, the structures within which the neurohormones are providing messages, are the most often studied aspect of the neuroendocrine system. These axes always involve a feedback mechanism. For example, the hypothalamus–pituitary–thyroid axis regulates the

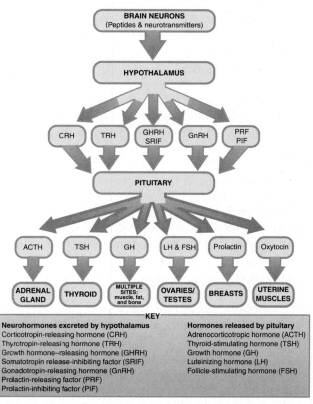

FIGURE 9.14 Hypothalamic and pituitary communication system. The neurohormonal communication system between the hypothalamus and the pituitary exerts effects on many organs and systems.

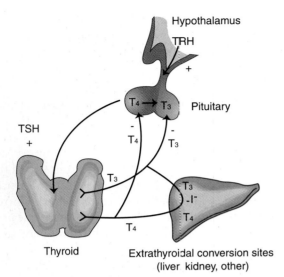

FIGURE 9.15   Hypothalamic–pituitary–thyroid axis. The regulation of thyroid-stimulating hormone (TSH or thyrotropin) secretion by the anterior pituitary. Positive effects of thyrotropin-releasing hormone (TRH) from the hypothalamus and negative effects of circulating triiodothyronine (T_3) and T_3 from intrapituitary conversion of thyroxine (T_4).

release of thyroid hormone by the thyroid gland using TRH hormone from the hypothalamus to the pituitary and thyroid-stimulating hormone (TSH) from the pituitary to the thyroid. Figure 9-15 illustrates the hypothalamic–pituitary–thyroid axis. The hypothalamic–pituitary–gonadal axis regulates estrogen and testosterone secretion through luteinizing hormone and follicle-stimulating hormone.

Interest in psychoendocrinology is heightened by various endocrine disorders that produce psychiatric symptoms. Addison's disease (hypoadrenalism) produces depression, apathy, fatigue, and occasionally psychosis. Hypothyroidism produces depression and some anxiety. Administration of steroids can cause depression, hypomania, irritability, and in some cases, psychosis. Some psychiatric disorders have been associated with endocrine system dysfunction. For example, some individuals with mood disorders show evidence of dysregulation in adrenal, thyroid, and growth hormone axes.

PSYCHOIMMUNOLOGY

Psychoimmunology is the study of immunology as it relates to emotions and behaviour. The immune system protects the body from foreign pathogens. Overactivity of the immune system can occur in autoimmune diseases such as systemic lupus erythematosus (SLE), allergies, or anaphylaxis. Too little activity may result from cancer and serious infections, as is the case with AIDS. Evidence suggests that the nervous system regulates many aspects of immune function. Specific immune system dysfunctions may result from damage to the hypothalamus, hippocampus, or pituitary and may produce symptoms of psychiatric disorders. Figure 9-16 illustrates the interaction between stress and the immune system. This figure also demonstrates the true biopsychosocial nature of the complex interrelationship of the nervous system, the endocrine system, the immune system, and environmental or emotional stress.

Immune dysregulation may also be involved in the development of psychiatric disorders. This can occur by allowing neurotoxins to affect the brain, damaging neuroendocrine tissue or damaging tissues in the brain at locations such as the receptor sites. Some antidepressants have been thought to have antiviral effects. Symptoms of diseases such as depression may follow an occurrence of serious infection, and prenatal exposure to infectious organisms may be associated with the development of schizophrenia. Stress and conditioning have specific effects on the suppression of immune function (Ekman, Persson, & Nilsson, 2002; Friedman, 2000; Ishihara, Makita, Imai, Hashimoto, & Nohara, 2003). In many cases, individuals with SLE experience symptoms of depression, insomnia, nervousness, and confusion. Although there is still much to learn about the relationship of psychiatric disorders and the immune system, it is clear that psychiatric–mental health nurses must develop and implement interventions designed to enhance immune function in psychiatric patients.

CHRONOBIOLOGY

Chronobiology involves the study and measure of time structures or biologic rhythms. Some rhythms have a circadian cycle, or 24-hour cycle, whereas others, such as the menstrual cycle, operate in different periods. Rhythms exist in the human body to control endocrine secretions, sleep–wake, body temperature, neurotransmitter synthesis, and more. These cycles may become deregulated and may begin earlier than usual, known as a phase advance, or later than usual, known as a phase delay.

Zeitgebers are specific events that function as time givers or synchronizers and that set biologic rhythms. Light is the most common example of an external zeitgeber. The suprachiasmatic nucleus of the hypothalamus is an example of an internal zeitgeber. Some theorists think that psychiatric disorders may result from one or more biologic rhythm dysfunctions. For example, depression may be, in part, a phase advance disorder, including early morning awakening and decreased time of onset of REM sleep. Seasonal affective disorder may be the result of shortened exposure to light during the winter months. Exposure to specific artificial light often relieves symptoms of fatigue, overeating, hypersomnia, and depression.

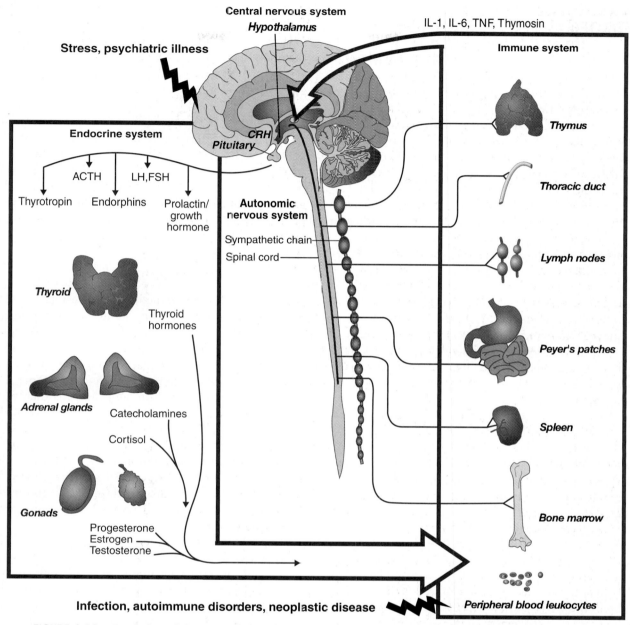

FIGURE 9.16 Examples of the interaction between stress or psychiatric illness and the immune system through the endocrine system. CRH, corticotropin-releasing hormone; IL, interleukin; TNF, tumor necrosis factor; ACTH, adrenocorticotropic hormone; LH, luteinizing hormone; FSH, follicle-stimulating hormone.

Diagnostic Approaches

Now that we understand more about neural transmission, brain functioning, and psychopharmacology, focus is shifting to applying the knowledge in order to find biologic markers for the psychiatric disorders previously thought to have only a psychological component. **Biologic markers** are diagnostic test findings that occur only in the presence of the psychiatric disorder and include such findings as laboratory and other diagnostic test results and neuropathologic changes noticeable in assessment. These markers increase diagnostic certainty and reliability, and may have predictive value, allowing for the possibility of preventive interventions to forestall or avoid the onset of illness.

In addition, biologic markers could assist in developing evidence-based care practices. If markers can be used reliably, it would be much easier to identify the most effective treatments and to determine the expected prognosis for given conditions. The PMH health nurse should be aware of the most current information on biologic markers so that information, limitations, and results can be discussed knowledgeably with the patient.

LABORATORY TESTS AND NEUROPHYSIOLOGIC PROCEDURES

For many years, laboratory tests have attempted to measure levels of neurotransmitters and other CNS substances in the bloodstream. Many of the metabolites of neurotransmitters can be found in the urine and CSF as well. However, these measures have had only limited utility in elucidating what is happening in the brain. Levels of neurotransmitters and metabolites in the bloodstream or urine do not necessarily equate with levels in the CNS. In addition, availability of the neurotransmitter or metabolite does not predict the availability of the neurotransmitter in the synapse, where it must act, or directly relate to the receptor sensitivity. Nonetheless, numerous research studies have focused on changes in neurotransmitters and metabolites in blood, urine, and CSF. These studies have provided clues but remain without conclusive predictive value and therefore are not routinely used.

Another laboratory approach to the study of some of the psychiatric disorders is the challenge test. A challenge test has been most often used in the study of panic disorders. These tests are usually conducted by intravenously administering a chemical known to produce a specific set of psychiatric symptoms. For example, lactate or caffeine may be used to induce the symptoms of panic in a person who has panic disorder. The biologic response of the individual is then monitored. These tests have been developed primarily for research purposes. However, endocrine stimulation tests, such as the TRH stimulation test and the dexamethasone suppression test, have some limited clinical utility.

In the TRH stimulation test, TRH is administered, and the TSH blood level is measured over time, usually at intervals during a period of 3 to 4 hours. The patient with hypothyroidism has an elevated TSH level. A blunted TRH stimulation test has been proposed as a biologic marker for major depression; however, only about 30% of individuals with major depression show the response. The dexamethasone suppression test involves administering 1 mg dexamethasone at 11 PM. Cortisol blood levels are then measured. In the healthy individual, dexamethasone suppresses cortisol levels, but results of numerous studies suggest that there is nonsuppression in certain types of depression. Typically, the cortisol levels are measured before administering the dexamethasone and then again at 8 AM, 4 PM, and 11 PM on the following day. Many medical conditions, such as diabetes mellitus, obesity, infection, pregnancy, recent surgery, and use of medications, such as carbamazepine or high doses of estrogen, may alter the test results, producing false-positive results. Overall, a positive result, or abnormal nonsuppression, appears to indicate major depression, but a negative result does not rule out depression. Considerable controversy exists regarding the clinical usefulness of this test.

Although no commonly used laboratory tests exist that directly confirm a mental disorder, laboratory tests are still an active part of care and assessment of psychiatric patients. Many physical conditions mimic the symptoms of mental illness, and many of the medications used to treat psychiatric illness can produce health problems. For these reasons, the routine care of patients with psychiatric disorders includes the use of laboratory tests such as complete blood counts, thyroid studies, electrolytes, hepatic enzymes, and other evaluative tests. PMH nurses need to be familiar with these procedures and assist patients in understanding the use and implications of such tests.

Electroencephalography

EEG is a tried and true method for investigating what is happening inside the living brain. Developed in the 1920s by Hans Berger, an EEG measures electrical activity in the uppermost nerve layers of the cortex. Usually, 16 electrodes are placed on the patient's scalp. The EEG machine, equipped with graph paper and recording pens, is turned on, and the pens then trace the electrical impulses generated over each electrode. Until the use of CT in the 1970s, the EEG was the only method for identifying brain abnormalities. It remains the simplest and most noninvasive method for identifying some disorders. It is increasingly being used to identify individual neuronal differences and most recently to predict a person's response to common antidepressant medication (Cook, et al., 2002).

An EEG may be used in psychiatry to differentiate possible causes of the patient's symptoms. For example, some types of seizure disorders, such as temporal lobe epilepsy, head injuries, or tumors, may present with predominantly psychiatric symptoms. In addition, metabolic dysfunction, delirium, dementia, altered levels of consciousness, hallucinations, and dissociative states may require EEG evaluation.

Spikes and wave-pattern changes are indications of brain abnormalities. Spikes may be the focal point from which a seizure occurs. However, abnormal activity often is not discovered on a routine EEG while the individual is awake. For this reason, additional methods are sometimes used. Nasopharyngeal leads may be used to get physically closer to the limbic regions. The patient may be exposed to a flashing strobe light while the examiner looks for activity that is not in phase with the flashing light or may be asked to hyperventilate for 3 minutes to induce abnormal activity if it exists. Sleep deprivation may also be used. This involves keeping the patient awake throughout the night before the EEG evaluation. The patient may then be drowsy and fall asleep during the procedure. Abnormalities are more likely to occur when the patient is asleep. Sleep may also be induced using medication; however, many medications change the wave patterns on an EEG. For example, the benzodiazepine class of drugs increases the rapid and fast beta activity. Many other prescribed and illicit drugs, such as lithium, which increases theta activity, can cause EEG alterations. In addition to reassuring, preparing, and educating the patient for the examination, the nurse should carefully assess the history of substance use and report this information to the examiner. If a sleep deprivation EEG is to be done, caffeine or other stimulants that might assist the patient in staying awake should be withheld because they may change the EEG patterns.

Polysomnography

Polysomnography is a special procedure that involves recording the EEG throughout a night of sleep. This test is usually conducted in a sleep laboratory. Other tests are usually performed at the same time, including electrocardiography and electromyography. Blood oxygenation, body movement, body temperature, and other data may be collected as well, especially in research settings. This procedure is usually conducted for evaluating sleep disorders, such as sleep apnea, enuresis, or somnambulism. However, sleep pattern changes are frequently researched in mental disorders as well.

Researchers have found that normal sleep divisions and stages are affected by many factors, including drugs, alcohol, general medical conditions, and psychiatric disorders. For example, REM latency, the length of time it takes an individual to enter the first REM episode, is shortened in depression. Reduced delta sleep is also observed. These findings have been replicated so frequently that some researchers consider them biologic markers for depression.

Other Neurophysiologic Methods

Evoked potentials (EPs), also called event-related potentials, use the same basic principles as an EEG. They measure changes in electrical activity of the brain in specific regions as a response to a given stimulus. Electrodes placed on the scalp measure a large waveform that stands out after the administration of repetitive stimuli, such as a click or flash of light. There are several different types of EPs to be measured, depending on the sensory area affected by the stimulus, the cognitive task required, or the region monitored, any of which can change the length of time until the wave occurrence. EPs are used extensively in psychiatric research. In clinical practice, EPs are used primarily in the assessment of demyelinating disorders, such as multiple sclerosis.

However, brain electrical activity mapping (BEAM) studies, which involve a 20-electrode EEG that generates computerized maps of the brain's electrical activity, have found a slowing of electrical activity in the frontal lobes of individuals who have schizophrenia. These findings are consistent with other findings that suggest a "hypofrontality" in schizophrenia (see Chapter 17). Nonetheless, neurophysiologic methods provide only rough approximations compared with current structural and functional neuroimaging techniques.

Integration of the Biologic, Psychological, and Social Domains

Basic knowledge in the neurosciences has become essential content for the practicing psychiatric nurse. In a truly holistic biopsychosocial model, all psychological and social influences are seen as interacting with the complex human biologic system. For example, treatment of generalized anxiety disorder would involve addressing etiologies in each of these areas (see Fig. 9-17). As research continues to increase our understanding of the biologic dimension of psychiatric disorders and mental health, nursing care will focus on human biology in increasingly sophisticated ways. Psychiatric nurses must integrate this information into all aspects of nursing management, including:

- *Assessment*—genetic, physical, and environmental factors that contribute to the symptoms of psychiatric disorders; biologic rhythm changes; cognitive abilities that may effect or complicate interventions;

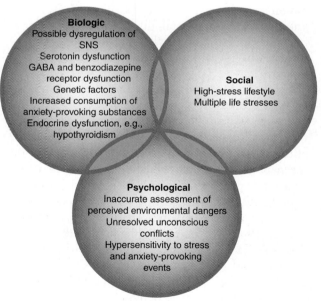

FIGURE 9.17 Biopsychosocial etiologies for patients with generalized anxiety disorders. GABA, γ-aminobutyric acid; SNS, sympathetic nervous system.

and risk factors that may predict development of psychiatric symptoms or disorders.

- *Diagnosis*—difficulties related to diet, exercise, or sleep that may change the individual's biology; quality-of-life difficulties based on biologic changes; knowledge deficits concerning the biologic basis of psychiatric disorders or treatment.
- *Interventions*—designed to modify biologic changes and physical functioning; designed to enhance biologic treatments; or modified to consider cognitive dysfunction related to psychiatric disorders.

SUMMARY OF KEY POINTS

◙ Neuroscientists now view behaviour and cognitive function as a result of complex interactions within the central nervous system and its plasticity, or its ability to adapt and change in both structure and function.

◙ Each hemisphere of the brain is divided into four lobes: the frontal lobe, which controls motor speech function, personality, and working memory—often called the *executive functions* that govern one's ability to plan and initiate action; the parietal lobe, which controls the sensory functions; the temporal lobe, which contains the primary auditory and olfactory areas; and the occipital lobe, which controls visual integration of information.

◙ The structures of the limbic system are integrally involved in memory and emotional behaviour. Dysfunction of the limbic system has been linked with major mental disorders, including schizophrenia, depression, and anxiety disorders.

◙ Neurons communicate with each other through synaptic transmission. Neurotransmitters excite or inhibit a response at the receptor sites and have been linked to certain mental disorders. These neurotransmitters include acetylcholine, dopamine, norepinephrine, serotonin, γ-aminobutyric acid, and glutamate.

◙ Psychoendocrinology examines the relationship between the nervous system and endocrine system and the effects of neurohormones excreted by special neurons to communicate with the endocrine system in effecting behaviour. Psychoimmunology focuses on the nervous system as regulating immune function, which may play a significant role in effecting psychological states and psychiatric disorders. Chronobiology focuses on the study and measure of time structures or biologic rhythms occurring in the body and associates dysregulation of these cycles as contributing factors to the development of psychiatric disorders.

◙ Biologic markers are physical indicators of disturbances within the central nervous system that differentiate one disease process from another, such as biochemical changes or neuropathologic changes.

These biologic markers can be measured by several methods of testing, including challenge tests, electroencephalography, polysomnography, evoked potentials, computed tomography scanning, magnetic resonance imaging, positron emission tomography, and single photon emission computed tomography, all of which the psychiatric–mental health nurse must be familiar with.

◙ Although no one gene has been found to produce any psychiatric disorder, significant evidence indicates there is for most psychiatric disorders a genetic predisposition or susceptibility. For individuals who have such genetic susceptibility, the identification of risk factors is crucial in helping to plan interventions to prevent development of that disorder or to prevent certain behaviour patterns, such as aggression or suicide.

CRITICAL THINKING CHALLENGES

1 Explain the significance of mental disorders being described as *polygenetic*.

2 A patient who is scheduled for magnetic resonance imaging asks how this test can possibly help explain why he is "all nerved up." He states that his friend had a "CT scan," and he wants that instead. What would the nurse say to assist this patient in understanding the difference between the two tests?

3 Five different approaches to the study of neuroanatomy are discussed in this chapter. Define each approach and discuss its utility in understanding mental disorders.

4 A woman who has experienced a "ministroke" continues to regain lost cognitive function months after the stroke. Her husband takes this as evidence that she never had a stroke. How would you approach patient teaching and counseling for this couple to help them understand this occurrence if the stroke did damage to her brain?

5 Choose a patient from whom you are caring. Review his or her psychotropic medications and discuss their impact on the patient's CNS. Discuss what side effects might be seen and why.

6 Mr. S. is unable to sleep after watching an upsetting documentary. Identify the neurotransmitter activity that may be interfering with sleep. (Hint: fight-or-flight.)

7 Describe what behavioural symptoms or problems may be present in a patient with dysfunction of the following brain area:
   a. Basal ganglia
   b. Hippocampus
   c. Limbic system
   d. Thalamus
   e. Hypothalamus
   f. Frontal lobe

8   Compare and contrast the functions of the sympathetic and parasympathetic nervous systems.

9   Discuss the steps in synaptic transmission, beginning with the action potential and ending with how the neurotransmitter no longer communicates its message to the receiving neuron.

10   Examine how a receptor's usual response to a neurotransmitter might change.

11   Compare the role of dopamine and acetylcholine in the CNS.

12   Explain how dopamine, norepinephrine, and serotonin all contribute to endocrine system regulation. Suggest some other transmitters that may affect endocrine function.

13   Discuss how the fields of psychoendocrinology, psychoimmunology, and chronobiology overlap.

14   Compare the methods used to find biologic markers of psychiatric disorders reviewed in this chapter. Consider the potential risks and benefits to the patient.

15   Determine the actions you would take in preparing a patient for an MRI scan.

REFERENCES

Cho, M. J., Lyoo, I. K., Lee, D. W., Kwon, J. S., Lee, J. S., Lee, D. S., Jung, J. K., & Lee, M. C. (2002). Brain single photon emission computed tomography findings in depressive pseudodementia patients. *Journal of Affective Disorders, 69*(1–3), 159–166.

Cook, I. A., Leuchter, A. F., & Morgan, M. (2002). *Neuropsychopharmacology, 27*(1), 120–131.

Duman, R. S. (2000). Neuronal plasticity and survival in mood disorder. *Biologic Psychiatry, 48,* 732–739.

Ekman, R., Persson, R., & Nilsson, C. L. (2002). Neurodevelopmental influences on the immune system reflecting brain pathology. *Neurotoxic Research, 4*(5–6), 565–572.

Friedman, M. J. (2000). What might the psychobiology of posttraumatic stress disorder teach us about the future approaches to pharmacotherapy? *Journal of Clinical Psychiatry, 61*(7), 44–51.

Fritschy, J. M., & Brunig, I. (2003). Formation and plasticity of GABAergic synapses: Physiological mechanisms and pathophysiological implications. *Pharmacologic Therapy, 98*(3) 299–323.

Garcia, D. A., Marin, R. H., & Perillo, M. A. (2002). Stress-induced decrement in the plasticity of the physical properties of chick brain membranes. *Molecular Membrane Biology, 19*(3), 221–230.

Green, R. C., Cupples, L. A., Kurz, A., Auerbach, S., Go, R., Sadovnick, D., Duara, R., Kukull, W. A., Chui, H., Edeki, T., Griffith, P. A., Friedland, R. P., Bachman, D., & Farrer, L. (2003). Depression as a risk factor for Alzheimer disease: The MIRAGE Study. *Archives of Neurology, 60*(5), 753–759.

Harlow, J. M. (1868). Recovery after severe injury to the head. *Publication of the Massachusetts Medical Society, 2,* 327.

Harmer, C. J., Hill, S. A., Taylor, M. J., Cowen, P. J., & Goodwin, G. M. (2003). Toward a neuropsychological theory of antidepressant drug action: Increase in positive emotional bias after potentiation of norepinephrine activity. *American Journal of Psychiatry, 160,* 990–992.

Harrison, P. J., & Owen, M. S. (2003). Genes for schizophrenia? Recent findings and their pathophysiological implications. *Lancet 361*(9355), 417–419.

Heerschap, A., Kok, R. D., & Van De, W. (2003). Antenatal proton MR spectroscopy of the human brain in vivo. *Childrens Nervous System, 17,* 44–46.

Hennig, J., Speck, O., Koch, M. A., & Weiller, C. (2003). Functional magnetic resonance imaging: A review of methodological aspects and clinical applications. *Journal of Magnetic Resonance Imaging, 18*(1), 1–15.

Ishihara, S., Makita, S., Imai, M., Hashimoto, T., & Nohara, R. (2003). Relationship between natural killer activity and anger expression in patients with coronary heart disease. *Heart Vessels, 18*(2), 85–92.

Johnson, K. A., & Brensinger, J. D. (2000). Genetic counseling and testing. *Clinics of North America, 35*(3), 615–621.

Kapczinski, F., Lima, M. S., Souza, J. S., Cunha, A., & Schmitt, R. (2003). Antidepressants for generalized anxiety disorder (Cochrane Review). *Cochrane Database System Review, 2,* CD003592.

Kurup, R. K., & Kurup, P. A. (2003). Hypothalamic digoxin: Central role in conscious perception, neuroimmunoendocrine integration and coordination of cellular function—relation to hemispheric dominance. *Medical Hypotheses, 60*(2), 243–257.

Lea, D. H. (2000). A clinician's primer in human genetics: What nurses need to know. *Nursing Clinics of North America, 35*(3), 583–614.

MacGregor, D. G., Avshalumov, M. V., & Rice, M. E. (2003). Brain edema induced by in vitro ischemia: Causal factors and neuroprotection. *Journal of Neurochemistry, 85*(6), 1402–1411.

McGuffin, P., Rijsdijk, F., Andrew, M., Sham, P., Katz, R., & Cardno, A. (2003). The heritability of bipolar affective disorder and the genetic relationship to unipolar depression. *Archives of General Psychiatry, 60,* 497–502.

Merikangas, K. R., & Avenevoli, S. (2000). Implications of genetic epidemiology for the prevention of substance use disorders. *Addictive Behaviors, 25,* 807–820.

Mohr, W., & Mohr, B. (2001). Brain, behavior, connections and implications: Psychodynamics no more. *Archives of Psychiatric Nursing, 15*(4), 171–181.

Montgomery, S. A. (2000). Understanding depression and its treatment: Restoration of chemical balance or creation of conditions promoting recovery. *Journal of Clinical Psychiatry, 61*(6), 3–6.

Nolte, J., & Angevine, J. (1995). *The human brain: In photographs and diagrams.* St. Louis: Mosby.

O'Rourke, J. L., & Lee, A. (2003). Animal models of *Helicobacter pylori* infection and disease. *Microbes Infection, 5*(8), 741–748.

Orth, M., & Tabrizi, S. J. (2003). Models of Parkinson's disease. *Movement Disorders, 7,* 729–737.

Sharma, J., Angelucci, A., & Sur, M. (2000). Induction of visual orientation modules in auditory cortex. *Nature, 404,* 841–847.

Shiloh, R., Weizman, A., Epstein, Y., Rosenberg, S. L., Valevski, A., Dorfman-Etrog, P., Wiezer, N., Katz, N., Munitz, H., & Hermesh, H. (2001). Abnormal thermoregulation in drug-free male schizophrenia patients. *European Neuropsychopharmacology, 11*(4), 285–288.

Vercelletto, M., Martinez, F., Lanier, S., Magne, C., Jaulin, P., & Bourin, M. (2002). Negative symptoms, depression and Alzheimer's disease. *International Journal of Geriatric Psychiatry, 17*(4), 383–387.

Interventions in Psychiatric and Mental Health Nursing Practice

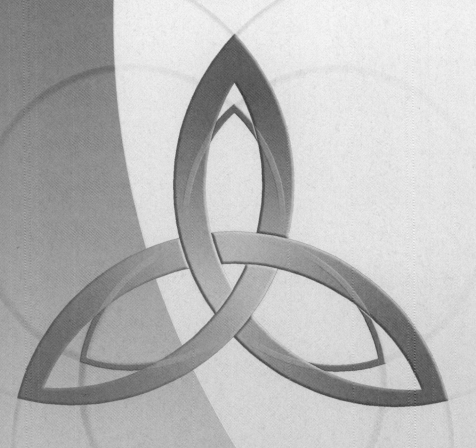

10

The Assessment Process

Gerri Lasiuk and Mary Ann Boyd

LEARNING OBJECTIVES

After studying this chapter, you will be able to:

- Identify assessment as part of the nursing process.
- Define assessment.
- Differentiate comprehensive and focussed assessments.
- Discuss the contributions of observation, interviewing, examination, and consultation to the psychiatric–mental health assessment.
- Discuss the synthesis of the biopsychosocial assessment data.
- Delineate important areas of assessment for the biologic, psychological, and social domains in completing the psychiatric nursing assessment.

KEY TERMS

affect ▪ assessment ▪ body image ▪ cognition ▪ comprehensive assessment ▪ delusion ▪ dysphoric ▪ euphoria ▪ euthymic ▪ focussed assessment ▪ hallucination ▪ illusion ▪ insight ▪ level of consciousness ▪ judgment ▪ mental status exam ▪ mood ▪ nursing process ▪ objective data ▪ orientation ▪ perception subjective data

▶ KEY CONCEPTS

assessment ▪ mental status examination

The *Code of Ethics for Registered Nurses* (Canadian Nurses Association, 2002) states that nurses value health, which includes

> health promotion and well-being and assisting persons to achieve their optimum level of health in situations of normal health, illness, injury, disability or at the end of life. (p. 8)

The **nursing process** is a problem-solving method by which nurses can translate that value into practice. The four essential components of the nursing process are assessment, planning, implementation, and evaluation. This chapter deals with **assessment**—activities involved with the collection, validation, analysis, synthesis, and documentation of information concerning clients' responses to health and illness.

ASSESSMENT AS A PROCESS

Standard II of the *Canadian Standards of Psychiatric and Mental Health Nursing* states:

> Effective assessment, diagnosis and monitoring is central to the nurse's role and is dependent upon theory, as well as upon understanding the meaning of the health or illness experience from the perspective of the client. This knowledge, integrated with the nurse's conceptual model of nursing practice, provides a framework for processing client data and for developing client-focussed plans of care. The nurse makes professional judgments regarding the relevance and importance of this data, and acknowledges the client as a valued and respected partner throughout the decision-making process. (Canadian Federation of Mental Health Nurses, 2005)

This underscores the importance of assessment as the basis for developing a plan of care.

Assessment is not a one-time activity. Rather, it is a purposeful, systematic, and dynamic process that is ongoing throughout the nurse's relationship with individuals in her or his care. Effective assessment involves:

1. A broad theoretical knowledge of human, social, and health sciences; the ability to think critically; and psychomotor and interpersonal skills
2. Collaboration with the client, family, and other members of the health care team to gather holistic information through observation, examination, interview, and consultation
3. Collection, validation, analysis, synthesis, organization, and documentation of client health–illness information
4. Refinement of client information through ongoing monitoring
5. Anticipation of potential problems in clients' health and functional status (eg, shifts in mood indicative of change in potential for self-harm) (Adapted from Canadian Federation of Mental Health Nurses, 2005)

> **KEY CONCEPT Assessment** is a purposeful, systematic, and dynamic process that is ongoing throughout the nurse's relationship with individuals in her or his care. It involves the collection, validation, analysis, synthesis, organization, and documentation of client health–illness information.

Types of Assessment

Depending on the client's needs and the context of care, an assessment may be comprehensive or focussed. A **comprehensive assessment** includes a health history and physical examination; considers the psychological, emotional, social, spiritual, ethnic, and cultural dimensions of health; attends to the meaning of the client's health–illness experience; and evaluates how all of this affects the individual's daily living (Fig. 10-1). It is typically done in collaboration with other members of the health care team. The purpose of a comprehensive assessment is to develop a holistic understanding of the individual's problems and needs as well as his or her strengths and resources. With this, the treatment team collaborates with the client to establish a diagnosis, identify treatment goals, and develop a plan of care.

Because of its broad scope and the time it takes to develop rapport, a comprehensive assessment may take days or even weeks to complete. Members of the health care team collect information from several sources, including the individual and his or her family, other health care providers, social service and justice personnel, educators, employers, and existing client records. All this is done while attending to issues of confidentiality and pertinent legal statutes.

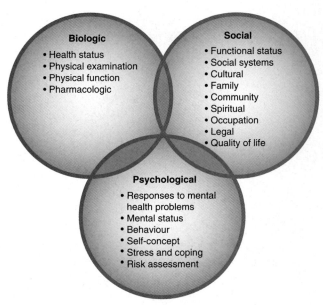

FIGURE 10.1 Biopsychosocial nursing assessment.

A **focussed assessment** is the collection of specific information about a particular need, problem, or situation. This may involve evaluation of such things as medications effects, risk for self-harm, knowledge deficits, or the adequacy of supports and resources. As the name suggests, focussed assessments are briefer, narrower in scope, and more present oriented than are comprehensive assessments. Focussed assessments are also used to screen individuals who are at high risk for particular problems or disorders. In these instances, nurses often employ standardized assessment tools (eg, Glasgow Coma Scale, Mini-Mental Status Exam, or Hamilton Depression Inventory).

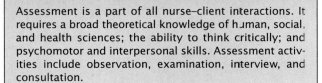

CRNE Note

Assessment is a part of all nurse–client interactions. It requires a broad theoretical knowledge of human, social, and health sciences; the ability to think critically; and psychomotor and interpersonal skills. Assessment activities include observation, examination, interview, and consultation.

The type of assessment most appropriate for a given situation rests on two key factors: the immediate needs of the client and the practice setting. Efforts to perform a comprehensive assessment during a psychiatric emergency (eg, when an individual is floridly psychotic or actively suicidal) can be both dangerous and futile. The quality and trustworthiness of information collected in these circumstances is biased by the client's symptoms and by the high emotionality of the situation. The priority in such situations is to perform a focussed assessment that provides the treatment team with sufficient information to treat the client's symptoms and to ensure the safety of all involved.

The type of assessment a nurse performs is also largely determined by the setting in which he or she works. The mandate of a psychiatric–mental health facility or program will determine the type of service it offers, which in turn dictates the nature of the assessment required. During the course of a first admission to a psychiatric unit, for example, an individual is likely to undergo a comprehensive assessment. In contrast, nurses working with a telehealth line or with a mobile mental health crisis team will collect only the information required to address the immediate problem or crisis.

Assessment Techniques

Psychiatric–mental health assessments involve observation of the individual at different times of the day and in different circumstances, interviews with the individual and family members, analyses and synthesis of findings from physical and mental examinations

into a care plan, and consultation with other health care providers.

Observation

Although verbal communication is vital to the assessment process, nonverbal cues also communicate important information about the client's health–illness experience (see Chapter 8). Nurses learn to engage all their senses and to seamlessly integrate assessment into all their encounters with clients. Close attention to nuances of dress, manner, facial expression, gestures, and interactions with others (particularly when the individual is not aware of being observed) provide important information that may not otherwise be revealed through conversation. For example, in addition to observing hygiene and personal grooming, the nurse considers whether the client's dress is appropriate to the season and situation. Other important observations include behavioural evidence of perceptual disturbances or disordered thought (eg, listening or talking to unseen others) and apparent inconsistencies between what an individual reports and what the nurse observes.

Examination

A comprehensive health assessment includes a health history, a physical examination, and diagnostic testing. This is particularly important in the provision of holistic psychiatric–mental health care because individuals with mental illness are at high risk for a range of physical problems and are less likely than those in the general population to seek regular medical care (Coghlan, Lawrence, Holman, & Jablensky, 2001; Hahm, & Segal, 2005; Phelan, Stradins, & Morrison, 2001). Common risk factors in this group include smoking, alcohol and drug use, obesity, poverty, and self-care deficits. It is also important to remain cognizant that medical conditions can mask, imitate, or exacerbate psychiatric symptoms and that psychiatric medications have significant short-term and long-term side effects. The situation is further complicated because some mental illnesses cause an individual to misattribute physical sensations, making it difficult to recognize and describe his or her symptoms.

The Mental Status Examination (MSE) is a structured approach to assessing an individual's psychological, emotional, social, and neurologic functioning. Although the components of the MSE are standard across clinical settings, the findings are highly subjective and rely heavily on the clinician's knowledge, communication skills, interpretation, and judgment. For this reason, it is important for clinicians to be self-reflective and to collaborate with colleagues to develop an unbiased understanding of the client's experience.

BOX 10.1

Factors that Facilitate Effective Interviewing

- As much as possible, **negotiate the terms of the interview with all the participants** (eg, choose a mutually agreeable time and place; clearly state your intent; and continually create opportunities for participants to express their thoughts, feelings, wants, and needs). This conveys respect, establishes a human connection, and fosters rapport.
- **The environment.** Choose a private and comfortable setting that is free from interruption.
- **Realistic time management.** Be clear at the outset how much time you have available for an interview and make a realistic plan about what you can achieve. Communicate that to participants.
- **Be attentive to your nonverbal communication.** Sit at the same level of other participants. Maintain an open body posture and actively attend to the encounter. If you intend to make notes, inform others

of this at the beginning of the interview. Keep your notes brief; most of your attentional resources should be focussed on the interaction.
- **Avoid jargon** and choose language that is clear, simple, and developmentally and culturally appropriate to all participants. Repeatedly check with participants to ensure that they understand what you are saying.
- **Begin with a less sensitive topic and move toward sensitive issues as rapport develops.**
- Leave some time at the end of the encounter for **closure and future planning.** The interviewer is responsible for time keeping. This involves monitoring the available time and notifying other participants when the interview is coming to an end. Closure activities help participants to disengage from the encounter and orient themselves to the future.

Interview

An assessment interview is a semistructured conversation aimed at building rapport, obtaining facts, clarifying perceptions and meanings, validating observations, and comparing understandings. Skillful interviewing is much more than peppering an individual with questions about signs and symptoms; it is both an art and a science and takes years of practice to develop (Box 10-1). Effective interviewers train themselves to be fully present to the individual before them, no matter how brief the encounter. They are genuinely warm and respectful and approach individuals in their care as collaborators working toward the same ends. Above all, competent interviewers engage in what Carl Rogers (1980) referred to as empathic listening, which he describes as

> entering the private perceptual world of the other and becoming thoroughly at home in it. [Empathic listening] involves being sensitive, moment by moment, to the changing felt meanings which flow in the other person, to the fear or rage or tenderness or confusion or whatever he or she is experiencing. It means temporarily living in the other's life, moving about in it delicately without making judgments.

Because many psychiatric symptoms are beyond an individual's awareness, sometimes only those around them are aware of them. For that reason, nurses may also interview family and friends to obtain client-related information. That being said, the Canadian *Privacy Act* imposes obligations on government departments and public agencies, including health-serving facilities, to respect privacy rights and to limit the collection, use, and disclosure of personal information. Today, every province and territory has privacy laws, and it is the

responsibility of every nurse to know the limits of information sharing under that legislation.

It is often the case that novice interviewers are so overwhelmed by their own anxieties about interviewing that they become unduly focussed on their own experience and on asking questions to elicit needed information. When this happens, the interpersonal nature of the interaction is forgotten. Box 10-2 identifies some interviewer behaviours that are barriers to effective interviewing.

Collaboration

Although nurses have long been vital contributors to interdisciplinary teams, recent health care reforms reiterate the importance of interdisciplinary collaboration. In large part, this is a response to concerns expressed both in the Romanow report (2002) and by the Health Council of Canada about the lack of continuity among health care providers and the institutions in which they work. The shift toward primary health care brings with it an emphasis on teams of health professionals who are accountable for providing comprehensive services to clients. There is a clear consensus that working partnerships among nurses, physicians, and other practitioners result in better health, improved access to services, more efficient use of resources, and higher levels of satisfaction for both consumers and health professionals.

Psychiatric–mental health teams typically include the client and his or her family, nurses, physicians, psychologists, social workers, pharmacists, occupational therapists, and recreational therapists. Depending on the treatment setting and the client's particular needs, however, other professionals (eg, teachers, clergy or spiritual leaders, other medical specialists) may be regular contributors to

---

BOX 10.2

Barriers to Effective Interviewing

- **Having a lack of clarity about the purpose and parameters of the interview** is like embarking on a journey without a clear idea of where you are going, your means of travel, and the time you have allotted for the trip. Although you may have some interesting experiences, you also risk missing some important things. A statement such as, "Mrs. Woods my name is Kate Donovan. I am a nurse on this Unit, and I would like to spend the next hour or so getting to know more about you and completing your admission assessment. Is that okay with you?" conveys respect, informs the client of your intent, and begins the process of negotiating a contract for the encounter.
- **Asking too many closed-ended questions.** Closed-ended questions invite brief responses and are most useful for eliciting specific facts, like those needed in a focussed assessment. Heavy reliance on them tends to orient the interview around the interviewer's desire for information and prevents the client from introducing or expanding on topics of importance to them.
- **Avoiding silence.** Often in response to their own discomfort or anxiety, interviewers rush to fill all silences with words. Pauses in the conversation allow both the client and interviewer time to reflect on their experience in the moment, to formulate or elaborate on their

responses, to switch speakers, or to turn the conversation to a new topic.
- **Asking complex questions.** A complex question is really several questions presented as one, as in, "Why did you come to the hospital today, who brought you, and how did you get here?" These types of questions are confusing to the respondent, who often does not know which to answer first. Successful interviewers ask one question at a time, listen carefully to the answer, and probe for more detail if it is not clear.
- **Making assumptions.** Effective interviewers are those who understand that each individual experiences and understands the world in their own unique way. The failure to clarify and validate what the client means results in misunderstanding and inaccuracies.
- **Avoiding or ignoring expressions of emotion.** Emotions are rich communications. They provide insight into the meaning an individual assigns to an experience or event. Minimizing or ignoring an expression of emotion sends a powerful message. For example, "There are parts of you that I do not acknowledge" or "Your emotions are frightening or unimportant." Competent practitioners need to maintain a high level of self-awareness in order to remain grounded in their own experience so that they can bear witness to others.

---

the team or participate on an *ad hoc* basis. One member of the team is usually assigned to be the client's primary therapist and takes on the role of coordinating team activities to address the client's needs. Teams meet together frequently to share information, to develop and evaluate treatment goals, and to provide ongoing support.

In most psychiatric–mental health treatment facilities, the interdisciplinary team works to develop a psychiatric diagnosis based on the *Diagnostic and Statistical Manual of Mental Health Disorders* (DSM-IV-TR; American Psychiatric Association, 2000). This diagnosis provides a framework for understanding clients' responses to mental illness.

BIOPSYCHOSOCIAL PSYCHIATRIC–MENTAL HEALTH NURSING ASSESSMENT

A biopsychosocial psychiatric–mental health nursing assessment rests on the assumption that humans are whole, integrated beings who live in constant and reciprocal relationship with their physical and social environments. One's state of health–illness reflects "the extent to which an individual or group is able to realize aspirations and satisfy needs and to change or cope with the environment" (Canadian Nurses Association, 2005). The biopsychosocial model presented in Chapter 6 provides a framework for assessing the physical, psychological, emotional, social, spiritual, ethnic, and cul-

tural dimensions of health. Whereas the goal of medical assessment is the diagnosis and treatment of disease and illness, nursing assessment aims to develop a holistic understanding of the individual's health–illness experience. As well as identifying health problems and deficits, it attends to strengths and resources and evaluates how these affect the individual's daily living.

Types and Sources of Information

Client information or data fall into two broad categories: *objective* and *subjective*. Objective data (also called *signs*) are directly observable and measurable. The physical examination, vital signs, and diagnostic tests all yield objective data. In contrast, subjective data (*symptoms*) are neither directly observable nor measurable. Subjective data are what the client and others report about their thoughts, attitudes, beliefs, emotions, perceptions, experiences, and motivations. A health history provides this type of data. Subjective information provides a window into an individual's inner experience. This experience is influenced by personal history, learning, ethnicity, culture, and spirituality and offers insight into the sense an individual makes of the world. It is critical for nurses to remember that individuals act and react to the *meanings they assign* to events and experiences, rather than to the events or experiences themselves.

Both objective and subjective data are generated from *primary* or *secondary* sources. The individual or client is the primary source of information about himself or herself. Secondary data, on the other hand, come from all others sources, including family, other health care providers, written reports, and client records.

Documentation

Health care records are important vehicles for communication as well as being legal documents. The type of information collected and how it is documented is regulated by the program or facility in which the nurse practices. In turn, programs and facilities develop documentation policies and procedures to comply with provincial and territorial legislation.

Generally speaking, there are two common approaches to documentation: *source-oriented* and *problem-oriented* documentation. In source-oriented documentation, each discipline is assigned a section of the client record (eg, nurse's notes or physician's notes). Although this approach clearly identifies the discipline of the person making the entry, it tends to fragment the data, which is antithetical to holistic care. In problem-oriented documentation, everyone involved with the care of an individual makes entries in the same section of the record. This not only facilitates interdisciplinary collaboration but also keeps team members oriented toward the client's identified goals, needs, and problems.

Information may be entered in the client record in several ways, including fill-in forms, flowsheets, checklists, and narrative notes. Computerized documentation is becoming more common because it is efficient, saves time, and facilitates electronic sharing of client information. In many settings, practitioners use the SOAP, DAR, or PIE methods to organize their notes (Box 10-3). Another approach to documentation is *charting by exception*, which involves documenting only those client health–illness responses that deviated from well-articulated standards.

BOX 10.3

Methods of Documentation

SOAP Method
S = Subjective data
O = Objective data
A = Assessment/clinical judgment
P = Plan/implementation/evaluation

DAR Method
D = Data
A = Action
P = Plan

PIE Method
P = Problem
I = Implementation
E = Evaluation

Biologic Domain

Health History

The health history (Table 10-1) establishes a subjective database about the client's current and past health–illness experience, identifies strengths and resources, identifies actual and potential health problems and deficits, and is an opportunity to build rapport. Depending on the practice setting, different members of the health care team may take responsibility for sections of the health history. For example, the social worker may perform the family and social assessments, the occupational therapist undertakes the occupational assessment, and the recreational therapist often assesses the individual's exercise and leisure activities. Box 10-4 outlines the components of a health history and relates the significance of important findings to mental health and illness.

Physical Examination

The physical examination is a process by which a clinician collects objective information about the client's health. Components include anthropomorphic measurements (eg, height and weight), vital signs, an examination of all body systems, and diagnostic testing appropriate to the individual's age, level of risk, and sex. The physical

---

BOX 10.4

PQRST Method of Symptom Analysis

Many practitioners use the PQRST acronym to guide their analysis of the nature and characteristics of reported symptoms.

P = Precipitating/ palliative factors	**Ask:** What were you doing when you first noticed it? What makes it better? Worse?
Q = Quality/ quantity	**Ask:** Describe the symptom in your own words. What does it feel/look/sound like? Has it changed during this episode? If yes, how? How often do you experience it? How does it affect your day-to-day life?
R = Region/radiation/ related symptoms	**Ask:** Point to where it is. Does it occur or spread anywhere else? What else have you noticed about it?
S = Severity	**Ask:** One a scale of 0 to 10, with 10 being the most severe that this symptom has ever been, where do you rate it at this moment? Using the same scale, what is the usual severity of this symptom?
T = Time	**Ask:** When was the first time you ever experienced it? How often does it occur? How long does it usually last? When did this episode begin?

Table 10.1	Health History and Significance to Psychiatric–Mental Health Problems
Data	**Considerations/Significance**
Source of Information	Ideally, the client is the primary source of information; consultation with secondary sources is necessary with minors or when the client is unable to do so. Note the apparent reliability and consistency of the information provided.
Identification/Biographic Information	Legal name/nicknames/aliases; date and place of birth; gender; address; telephone numbers; relationship status; next-of-kin; ethnicity; religious/spiritual affiliation; employer; education; provincial/territorial health insurance number. Because this information is relatively nonthreatening, it is a safe place to begin an assessment. It also provides important clues about an individual's current living situation.
Primary Reason for Seeking Care	Record this verbatim because it speaks to the client and family's perception of and insight into existing problems; their judgment; and goals for treatment.
Past Health Past illness, injury, and/or hospitalization	Note positive history of childhood diseases, especially viral infection, which have been linked to some psychiatric disorders (eg, schizophrenia). Inquire about surgeries and trauma, particularly those resulting in concussion or loss of consciousness. Ask about parental alcohol and drug use (especially during pregnancy); birth trauma; lengthy/repeated separation from parents/caregivers because of hospitalization; a pattern of injury suggestive of childhood abuse/neglect; and surgeries.
Chronic illnesses	Chronic illnesses (eg, diabetes and thyroid dysfunction), even when well-controlled, may affect mental status. Highlight known allergies, type of reaction, usual treatment, and effectiveness of treatment.
Family Health History	Record the name, age, and current health status of close relatives (spouse/partner, children, parents, siblings, grandparents, and aunts/uncles). If a family member is deceased, note the date and cause of death and indications of unresolved grief/loss. Inquire specifically about diseases/disorders that "run in the family," particularly psychiatric disorders and addictions. A genogram is a useful tool for recording this information. Many psychiatric disorders are genetically linked, so a family health history provides information about the client's risk factors. It also provides clues about social roles, the availability of social support, and family resources/stressors. Coping strategies, both effective and ineffective, are learned early in life from our family of origin. A family health history can help to identify these.
Developmental Considerations	Note social and educational difficulties, as well as failure to achieve expected developmental milestones. These may be indicative of attentional or interpersonal deficits; behavioural problems; a chaotic family environment; acquired brain injury; or childhood mental illness. Ask about early parental death or separation because these may be associated with alterations in attachment and later relationship difficulties. The Canadian Government's practice of removing aboriginal children to residential schools traumatized children, fragmented families, decimated cultures/languages, and contributed to serious social and psychological problems that still reverberate among First Nations people.
Immunization/HIV/ Hepatitis status	Individuals with severe and persistent mental illness often live in severe poverty and lack knowledge and resources for health promotion. In addition, many have lifestyles that put them at risk for serious communicable diseases.
Psychological Trauma	Ask: "Have you ever experienced or witnessed anything that threatened your life or safety or the life or safety of a loved one" If yes, probe for details.

(Continued)

Table 10.1	Health History and Significance to Psychiatric–Mental Health Problems (Continued)
Data	**Considerations/Significance**
	Psychological trauma associated with natural disasters, motor vehicle crashes, combat, abuse/assault (physical or sexual), and childhood neglect is associated with a number of psychiatric/mental health problems (eg, particularly Posttraumatic Stress Disorder, other anxiety disorders, and depression)
Current health status	Provides information about medical conditions that affect mental status, global functioning, and quality of life
	A systematic approach to performing a health history ensures thoroughness, helps the clinician to organize/cluster the data, and cues the informants memory
	Analyze significant symptoms (see Box 10.4)
Integumentary	Ask about problems/changes in the skin, hair, and nails. Note the presences of scars; piercings/body art; lesions/sores; rashes; discolouration; itching; or unusual sensations.
	Piercings and body art are expressions of one's personal aesthetic, which is part of self-concept. They may also indicate identification with particular social groups.
Sensory systems	Note sensory deficits and the use of eye glasses, contact lens, hearing aids, and dentures.
	Uncorrected sensory deficits can affect an individual's day-to-day function and ability to communicate.
	Record the report of unusual perceptions or sensations because these may be related to perceptual or thought disturbances.
Respiratory	Note problems/disease, recurrent infections, cough, sputum, shortness of breath, noisy respirations, and smoking history.
Cardiovascular/hematologic	Inquire about history of cardiac disease/problems; palpitations; arrhythmias; murmurs; dizzy spells; coldness/blueness/swelling of extremities; leg pain while walking.
	Individuals who experience panic episodes often present at emergency departments because their signs and symptoms mimic heart attack.
	Inquire about anemia, bleeding disorders, fatigue, blood transfusions, bruising, and cancers.
	Monitoring of some long-term neuroleptic medication use (eg, lithium and clozapine) requires regular blood tests.
Gastrointestinal	Ask about changes in appetite, weight, and bowel patterns; nausea, vomiting, indigestion, gastroesophageal reflux disease; antacid and laxative use; history of disease (eg, ulcers, irritable bowel syndrome, and cancer); and rectal discharge/bleeding.
	Alterations in gastrointestinal function are implicated in many psychiatric disorders. An individual may not notice hunger or have the energy to prepare food. Others may handle distressing emotions by eating more than usual.
	Anticholinergic effects of antipsychotic medication can cause constipation, whereas lithium carbonate can cause diarrhea.
Genitourinary	Note pain/burning on urination, frequency, urgency, dribbling/incontinence, hesitancy, colour of urine, history of urinary tract infection/kidney disease, and frequent night-time urination.
	Anticholinergic effects of antipsychotic medication can cause urinary hesitancy and/or retention.
Reproductive/breasts	Ask females about menarche; usual pattern of menses (frequency, duration, colour/amount of bleeding, and recent changes); obstetrical history (pregnancies, live births, miscarriages, abortions); infertility; dysmenorrhoea (pain, excessive bleeding); past or current infection/disease (eg, sexually transmitted infections, sores/lesions, unusual discharge or odour); date of last Pap smear; sexual orientation; sexual activity (including level of sexual desire, change in frequency of sexual activity, satisfaction with sexual relationships, painful intercourse); and contraceptive use.
	Ask males about number of children; infertility; past or current infection/disease (eg, sexually transmitted infections, sores/lesions, penile/rectal discharge); date of last testicular and prostate examinations; sexual orientation; sexual activity (including level of sexual desire, change in frequency of sexual activity, satisfaction with sexual relationships, painful intercourse, erectile/ejaculatory problems); and contraceptive use.

| Table 10.1 | Health History and Significance to Psychiatric–Mental Health Problems (Continued) |

Data	Considerations/Significance
	Ask both men and women about past disease; changes in breasts or nipples (eg, masses/lumps, pain, discharge); and breast self-examination. Note the date of female clients' last mammogram.
	Attitudes, beliefs, and expressions of sexuality provide important information about an individual's self-concept, gender identification, quality of relationships, and overall satisfaction with life.
	Changes in level of desire and frequency of sexual activity are common in many psychiatric disorders, including depression, anxiety, and mania.
	Side effects of selective serotonin reuptake inhibitors (SSRIs) are decreased sexual desire and erectile/ejaculatory dysfunction.
	Suicide rates among gay and lesbian youth are higher than the national average.
Musculoskeletal	Note problems with mobility; limited range of motion; pain or weakness; joint problems; disease/injury (eg, osteoporosis); use of prosthetics; and impairments to activities of daily living.
Endocrine	Ask about disease/illness (eg, diabetes, hypothyroidism/hyperthyroidism, and goitre); changes in height, weight, hair and skin, appetite, and energy level; excessive thirst; frequent urination; weakness; heat/cold intolerance; and current hormone therapy.
	Diseases of the endocrine system can imitate symptoms associated with psychiatric disorders (eg, depression, anxiety, mania, eating disorders, and dementia).
Neurologic	Ask about head trauma; alterations in consciousness; seizures; headaches; changes in cognition and memory; sensory and motor disturbances (numbness, tingling, and loss of sensation, tremors, lack of coordination, balance problems, and pain). As well, inquire about alterations in personality, speech, or ability to manage activities of daily living.
	Neurologic signs and symptoms are associated with many psychiatric disorders, as well as with side effects/toxicity of some neuroleptic medications (eg, neuroleptic malignant syndrome, serotonin syndrome, and lithium toxicity).
Current Medications	
(including over-the-counter preparations and herbal remedies)	Specify the name of the medication, purpose, usual dose, frequency, effectiveness, side-effects, prescriber, and length of time client has been taking it.
	This information helps to assess the client's health-promoting behaviours and potential knowledge deficits.
	Individuals with serious and persistent mental illness often take several different medications, which puts them at risk for drug–drug and drug–food interactions.
Health/Lifestyle	
Health promotion/maintenance	Ask individuals to describe what they do on a daily, weekly, and yearly basis to promote and maintain their health. Note the dates of their last physical examination, visit to a dentist, and eye examination.
Nutritional patterns	Ask about usual eating patterns and whether there have been any recent changes. Changes in eating patterns are associated with many affective states and psychiatric disorders.
	Particularly note dissatisfaction with weight and shape, as well as activities aimed at weight loss. Body dissatisfaction is a factor in eating disorders and contributes to self-concept. It is particularly common among girls/women, elite athletes, and those with occupations that emphasize physical appearance (eg, modelling, dancing).
	Psychiatric symptoms, neuroleptic medication, and poverty can all affect nutritional status.
	The weight gain associated with many neuroleptic medications increases individuals' risk for type II diabetes.

(Continued)

Table 10.1	Health History and Significance to Psychiatric–Mental Health Problems (Continued)
Data	**Considerations/Significance**
Sleep/rest patterns	Changes in sleep patterns can be a response to stress or symptoms of a psychiatric disorder.
	Probe a positive response about alterations in usual sleep patterns. Ask about *sleep onset* (latency between going to bed and falling asleep); *sleep maintenance* (frequency of wakening during the night and ease of falling back to sleep); *early morning wakening* (consistently waking up before one needs to be up). Also, ask about whether the individual generally feels rested/refreshed.
	Alterations in sleep patterns are common in many psychiatric disorders (eg, depression, mania, and schizophrenia). For many individuals with serious and persistent mental illness, sleep disturbances are early signs of relapse.
Activity/exercise	Ask about usual activity level and type and amount of exercise.
	Involvement in social activities and hobbies enhances health and reduces stress. Withdrawal from these things may be early signs of illness.
	Two of the negative symptoms of schizophrenia are anhedonia (decreased ability to experience pleasure) and avolition (lack of motivational drive and energy). This explains why many individuals with schizophrenia sleep excessively.
	Alterations in usual activities are associated with many mental disorders including depression, mania, schizophrenia, and some eating disorders.
Tobacco, alcohol and nonprescription drug use and problem gambling	*Tobacco.* Inquire about type (cigarettes, cigars, pipes, and chewing tobacco); age at first use; frequency; efforts to stop use.
	Alcohol. Ask about age at first use; preferred type (beer, wine, or spirits); usual pattern of drinking; and any recent changes to that pattern. It is also important to explore whether the individual or those close to the individual believe that alcohol is a problem in the individual's life. If yes, probe for details.
	Many people use alcohol to self-medicate—that is, to cope with stress, unpleasant emotions, sleep disturbances, and so forth.
	Nonprescription drugs. Ask about the age of first use, drug(s) of choice, dose, route, and frequency of nonprescription drug use. Probe for information about the effects of drug use (physical, psychological, emotional, social, legal, and economic).
	Problem gambling. Ask at what age it began, game(s) of choice, frequency, and average amount of money lost per month. Probe for information about the consequences (physical, psychological, emotional, social, legal, and economic).

examination aids in diagnosing disease or illness, establishes a baseline for evaluating change, and provides an opportunity to validate information provided in the health history. With respect to laboratory studies, particular attention is paid to any abnormalities of hepatic, renal, or urinary function because these systems metabolize or excrete many psychiatric medications. In addition, abnormal white blood cell and electrolyte levels are noted. See Table 10-2 for selected haematologic measures and their relevance to psychiatric disorders.

Psychological Domain

The psychological domain encompasses responses to mental health problems, mental status, stress and coping, and risk assessment.

Responses to Mental Health Problems

Psychiatric disorders are manifested as characteristic patterns of thought, behaviours, and affective states.

Like other illnesses, these disorders affect individuals and their families in many different ways. An important part of assessing the psychological domain is to explore the individual's experience of illness. Many have specific fears about losing their job, about their family, or about their personal safety. It is also important to identify the person's strategies for managing the illness and the effectiveness of those strategies. A simple question such as "How do you deal with your voices when you are with other people?" may initiate a discussion about a particular experience or symptom.

Mental Status Examination

The mental status examination (Box 10-5) is a systematic assessment of an individual's appearance, affect, behaviour, and cognitive processes. It reflects the examiner's observations and impressions at the time of the interview and is used in a variety of clinical settings to evaluate developmental, neurologic, and psychiatric disorders.

Table 10.2	Selected Hematologic Measures and Their Relevance to Psychiatric Disorders	

Test	Result	Implications
Complete Blood Count (CBC)		
Leukocyte count (WBC)	Leukopenia ($\downarrow$ WBC)	May be a side effect of phenothiazines, clozapine, carbamazepine
	Agranulocytosis ($\downarrow$ granulocytic WCB)	Lithium causes a benign mild to moderate increase (11,000–17,000/μL).
	Leukocytosis ($\uparrow$ WCB)	Neuroleptic malignant syndrome (NMS) can be associated with increases of 15,000 to 30,000/mm^3 in about 40% of cases.
WBC differential	"Shift to the left"—from segmented neutrophils to band forms	This shift suggests a bacterial infection but has been reported in about 40% of cases of NMS.
Red blood cell count (RBC)	Polycythemia ($\uparrow$ RBC)	Primary form (true polycythemia) is associated with several disease states; requires further evaluation.
		Secondary form is compensation for decreased oxygenation (eg, chronic obstructive pulmonary disease [COPD]).
		Blood is more viscous, which is exacerbated by being dehydrated.
	$\downarrow$ RBCs	Associated with some types of anemia; requires further evaluation
Hematocrit (Hct)	$\uparrow$ Hct	Associated with dehydration
	$\downarrow$ Hct	Associated with anemia; may be related to alterations in mental status, including asthenia, depression, and psychosis
		Twenty percent of women of childbearing age in North America have iron-deficiency anemia.
Hemoglobin (Hgb)	$\downarrow$ Hgb	Indicative of anemia; evaluation of cause requires review of erythrocyte indices.
Erythrocyte indices, such as red cell distribution width (RDW)	$\uparrow$ RDW	Finding suggests a combined anemia resulting from both vitamin B_{12} and folate acid deficiencies and iron deficiency, as in that found in chronic alcoholism
		Oral contraceptives also decrease vitamin B_{12}
Other Hematologic Measures		
Vitamin B_{12}	Deficiency	May be associated with neuropsychiatric symptoms such as psychosis, paranoia, fatigue, agitation, marked personality change, dementia, and delirium
Folate	Deficiency	Associated with alcohol use and with medications such as phenytoin, oral contraceptives, and estrogens
Platelet count	Thrombocytopenia ($\downarrow$ platelets)	Associated with use of some psychiatric medications, such as carbamazepine, phenothiazines, or clozapine and with other nonpsychiatric medications; may also cause thrombocytopenia
		Also associated with some disease states; requires further evaluation.
Serum Electrolytes		
Sodium	Hyponatremia (serum sodium)	Associated with significant alterations in mental status. May be related to Addison's disease; the syndrome of inappropriate secretion of antidiuretic hormone (SIADH); polydipsia; and carbamazepine use.

(Continued)

Table 10.2	Selected Hematologic Measures and Their Relevance to Psychiatric Disorders (Continued)	
Test	**Result**	**Implications**
Potassium	Hypokalemia (↓ serum potassium)	Associated with weakness, fatigue, electrocardiogram (ECG) changes, paralytic ileus, and muscle paresis
		Common in individuals exhibiting bulimic behaviour, psychogenic vomiting, misuse of diuretics, and/or excessive laxative use. Hypokalemia may be life threatening.
Chloride	Elevation	Chloride tends to increase to compensate for lower bicarbonate.
	Decrease	Associated with binging and purging behaviour.
Bicarbonate	Elevation	Associated with binging and purging, disordered eating, excessive laxative use, and/or psychogenic vomiting
	Decrease	May develop in individuals who hyperventilate (eg, panic disorder)
Renal Function Tests		
Blood urea nitrogen (BUN)	Elevation	Associated with alterations in mental status (eg, lethargy and delirium), dehydration, and medications excreted by the kidney, such as lithium and amantadine
Serum creatinine	Elevation	Indicative of decreased renal function; typically does elevate until 50% of nephrons in the kidney are damaged.
Serum Enzymes		
Amylase	Elevation	Associated with the binging and purging behaviour in eating disorders; tends to decline when these behaviours stop
	ALT > AST	This disparity is common in acute forms of viral and drug-induced hepatic dysfunction.
Alanine aminotransferase (ALT; formerly serum glutamic pyruvic transaminase, or SGPT)	Elevation	Mild elevations are common with use of sodium valproate.
Aspartate aminotransferase (AST; formerly serum glutamic oxaloacetic transaminase, or SGOT)	AST > ALT	Severe elevations are associated with chronic hepatic disease and myocardial infarction.
Creatine phosphokinase (CPK)	Elevations of the isoenzyme related to muscle tissue	Associated with muscle tissue injury Level is elevated in NMS and by repeated intramuscular injections (eg, depot antipsychotics).
Thyroid Function		
Serum triiodothyronine (T_3)	Decrease	Associated with hypothyroidism and other nonthyroid related disease
		Individuals with depression may convert less T_4 to T_3 peripherally, but not out of the normal range.
		Medications such as lithium and sodium valproate may suppress thyroid function, but clinical significance is unknown.
	Elevation	Indicative of hyperthyroidism; T_3 toxicosis is associated with alterations in mood, anxiety, and symptoms of mania.
Serum thyroxine (T_4)	Elevation	Indicative of hyperthyroidism

Table 10.2	Selected Hematologic Measures and Their Relevance to Psychiatric Disorders (Continued)	
Test	**Result**	**Implications**
Thyroid-stimulating hormone (TSH)	Elevation	Associated with hypothyroidism, which shares features of depression with the additional physical signs of cold intolerance, dry skin, hair loss, bradycardia, and so forth Lithium may also cause elevations.
	Decrease	Considered nondiagnostic; may be associated with hyperthyroidism, pituitary hypothyroidism, or even euthyroid status

⬟ **KEY CONCEPT** The **mental status examination** is a systematic assessment of an individual's appearance, affect, behaviour, and cognitive processes. It reflects the examiner's observations and impressions at the time of the interview and is used in a variety of clinical settings to evaluate developmental, neurologic, and psychiatric disorders.

General Observations

This section of the MSE provides a brief narrative summary of the examiner's observations and impressions of the individual at the time of the interview. Although an individual's health history remains relatively stable, his or her mental status is variable over time.

APPEARANCE. Describe the individual's general appearance and presentation. Note manner and appropriateness of dress, personal hygiene, odours, pupil size, and obvious identifying characteristics, such as tattoos and piercings. Physical signs such as skin tone (eg, duski-

---

BOX 10.5

Components of the Mental Status Exam

1. General observations
   a. Appearance
   b. Psychomotor behaviour
   c. Attitude toward interviewer
2. Mood
3. Affect
4. Speech characteristics
5. Perception
6. Thinking
   a. Content
   b. Process/form
7. Sensorium
   a. Level of consciousness
   b. Orientation (person, place, time)
   c. Memory (immediate retention and recall; recent, short-term, and long-term)
   d. Attention and concentration
   e. Comprehension and abstract reasoning
8. Insight
9. Judgment

---

ness, pallor, or flushing), nutritional status, and energy level (eg, catatonia, lethargy, or restlessness) provide clues to the person's general level of health–illness.

PSYCHOMOTOR ACTIVITY. Observe and note the individual's behaviour during the interview, including posture, gait, coordination, facial expression, mannerisms, gestures, and activity. Pay particular attention to cues to the person's emotional state (eg, perspiration, clamminess, muscle tension, repetitive movements, general activity level).

ATTITUDE TOWARD INTERVIEWER. The individual's attitude toward the interviewer and the interview process may be described as accommodating, cooperative, open, friendly, apathetic, bored, guarded, suspicious, hostile, or evasive. The following is an example of how the interviewer may describe the individual:

Mr. D. is a tall, thin, Caucasian man, who looks older than his stated age of 47 years. He is unshaven, his hair is uncombed, and he has a strong body odour. His clothing is stained and dishevelled but appropriate to the season. He reports feeling "jumpy," and he declined to sit during the interview, opting instead to pace around the interview room. His posture is erect and his movements are quick, purposeful, and well coordinated; he displays no unusual mannerisms. Mr. D. was cooperative to the interview process, although his verbal responses were brief, and he did not maintain eye contact.

Mood and Affect

In everyday usage, the terms *emotion, feelings,* and *mood* are used interchangeably. In the context of an MSE, however, these words refer to specific phenomena. **Emotion** is the individual's experience of a feeling state, whereas **mood** is "a pervasive and sustained emotion that colors the person's perception of the world" (Saddock & Saddock, 2003, p. 238). Mood is what the individual reports about his or her prevailing emotional state. Although mood does vary with internal and external changes, it tends to be stable over time and reflects the person's disposition or worldview. Mood can be assessed by asking a simple, open-ended question like, "How have you been feeling over the past while?" Whatever the person answers, the interviewer should probe to find whether this is typical or is a response to some recent life event. A person who is generally positive and content will remain so even when bad things happen. He or she will tend to view adversity as a temporary period of unpleasantness in a basically happy life. In contrast, an individual whose mood tends to be negative or depressed views life through dark-coloured glasses. He or she experiences life as difficult and sees happiness as fleeting.

Mood may be sustained for days or weeks, or it may fluctuate during the course of a day. For example, some depressed individuals have a diurnal variation in their mood; they experience their lowest mood in the morning, but as the day progresses, their mood lifts, and they feel somewhat better in the evening. Terms used to describe mood include **euthymic** (normal), **euphoric** (elated), and **dysphoric** (depressed, disquieted, restless).

Affect is the individual's emotional responsiveness during the interview and is inferred from facial expressions, vocalizations, and behaviour. During the assessment, an individual's affect may change as he or she talks about an immediate experience or recent life events. Affect is described in terms of its *range, intensity, appropriateness*, and *stability*. *Affective range* can be full or constricted. Individuals who express several emotions that are consistent with their stated feelings and the content of what they are saying are described as having a full range of affect that is congruent with the situation. On the other hand, a person who speaks of the recent, tragic death of a loved one in a monotone voice with little outward expression of his or her internal feeling state is described as having constricted affect. In evaluating the *appropriateness* of a particular response, the nurse must consider both the meaning of the event to the individual and cultural norms. Descriptions of *intensity* attempt to quantify an affective response. Intensity may be characterized as heightened, blunted, or flat. An example of heightened affect is the man who reacts to deaths of the victims of the September 11 attack as if they were all his personal friends. He states that his life stopped when the World Trade Center towers came down; he cried every day and could not eat or sleep for weeks afterward. The phrase *blunted affect* describes limited emotional expression, whereas *flat affect* is its near absence. The person whose affect is flat speaks in a monotone voice and has little or no facial expression. *Stability* of affect can be described as mobile (normal) or labile. If a person displays a wide range of strong emotions in a relatively short period of time, his or her affect is described as being labile.

Speech Characteristics

Patterns and characteristics of speech provide clues about the individual's thoughts, emotions, and cognitive organization. They also convey information about the person's understanding of the situation and ability to read and respond to social cues. Speech is described in terms of its *quantity*; *rate and fluency of production*; and *quality*. In assessing speech *quantity*, the individual may be described as talkative, verbose, garrulous, subdued, reticent, or taciturn. *Rate of speech production* may be slow, hesitant, fast, or pressured, whereas *fluency* refers to the apparent ease with which speech is produced. *Pressured speech* is speech that is rapid and increased in amount and difficult to understand; it is often associated with mania. Aphasic disturbances are problems of speech output and may be neurologic, cognitive, or emotional in origin. *Speech quality* refers to its characteristics, such as monotone, whispered, slurred, mumbled, staccato, or loud. During conversation, the interviewer also notes speech impediments (eg, stuttering), response latency (the length of time it takes for the individual to respond to a question or comment), and repetition, rhyming, or unusual use of words.

Perception

Perception is the complex series of mental events involved with taking in of sensory information from the environment and the processing of that information into mental representations. Two perceptual disturbances commonly associated with mental illness are hallucinations and illusions. **Hallucinations** are false sensory perceptions not associated with external stimuli and are not shared by others. Although auditory are the most common type of hallucination, they may occur in any of the five major sensory modalities: auditory, visual, tactile, olfactory, or gustatory. Most people are familiar with **hypnagogic hallucinations**—false sensory perceptions that occur while falling asleep; these are not associated with mental disorder. Of more concern are **command hallucinations**, the false perception of commands or orders that an individual feels obligated to obey. For example, a person may hear voices telling him or her to harm or kill oneself or someone else. **Illusions** are the misperception or misrepresentation of real sensory stimuli (eg, misidentifying the wind as a voice calling one's name or thinking that a label on a piece of clothing is an insect).

Thought

Because thought is not directly observable, it is assessed through language in terms of its content and process (form). **Thought content** is what the person is thinking about (eg, ideas, beliefs, preoccupations, and obsessions), and **thought process** is the manner in which thoughts are formed and expressed. Some individuals are very forthcoming about the content of their thoughts, whereas others are more reticent to talk about them. Assessing thought requires the clinician to carefully attend to and explore unusual or recurring themes in the individual's conversation. Box 10-6 lists some common disturbances of thought content.

BOX 10.6

Common Disturbances of Thought Content

Delusion—a false, fixed belief, based on an incorrect inference about reality. It is not shared by others and is inconsistent with the individual's intelligence or cultural background and cannot be corrected by reasoning.

Delusions of control—the belief that one's thoughts, feelings, or will are being controlled by outside forces. The following are some specific examples of delusions of control:

- **Thought insertion**—the belief that thoughts or ideas are being inserted into one's mind by someone or something external to one's self
- **Thought broadcasting**—the belief that one's thoughts are obvious to others or are being broadcast to the world
- **Ideas of reference**—the belief that other people, objects, and events are related to or have a special significance for one's self (eg, a person on television is talking to or about them)

Paranoid delusions—an irrational distrust of others and/or the belief that others are harassing, cheating, threatening, or intend one harm

Bizarre delusion—an absurd or totally implausible belief (eg, light waves from space communicate special messages to an individual)

Somatic delusion—a false belief involving the body or bodily functions

Delusion of grandeur—an exaggerated belief of one's importance or power

Religious delusion—the belief that one is an agent of or specially favoured by a greater being

Depersonalization—the belief that one's self or one's body is strange or unreal

Magical thinking—the belief that one's thought, words, or actions have the power to cause or prevent things to happen; similar to Jean Piaget's notion of preoperational thinking in young children

Erotomania—the belief that someone (often a public figure) unknown to the individual is in love with them or involved in a relationship with them

Nihilism—the belief that one is dead or nonexistent

Obsession—a repetitive thought, emotion, or impulse

Phobia—a persistent, exaggerated, and irrational fear

Saddock and Saddock (2003) define thinking as "the goal-directed flow of ideas, symbols, and associations initiated by a problem or task and leading toward a reality-oriented conclusion" (p. 282). A number of mental disorders are characterized by disturbances in the form or process of normal thinking. Box 10-7 lists some common disturbances of thought process.

Sensorium and Cognition

This portion of the MSE assesses brain function and cognitive abilities. The Mini-Mental Status Examination (MMSE; Folstein, Folstein, & McHugh, 1975) is a valid and reliable instrument, widely used to screen for gross impairments in these areas (Box 10-8). The MMSE evaluates orientation, memory, calculation, reading and writing, visuospatial ability, and language.

LEVEL OF CONSCIOUSNESS. Evaluating level of consciousness (LOC) assesses arousal or wakefulness. An altered LOC typically indicates organic brain impairment. If the individual is not conscious, the nurse applies increasing levels of stimulation (eg, verbal, tactile, and painful) to elicit a response. Terms used to describe LOC include alert, awake, lethargic, somnolent, stuporous, or comatose.

ORIENTATION. This reflects an individual's ability to perceive and grasp the significance of environmental information. The examiner determines orientation by asking questions about time, place, and person because

BOX 10.7

Common Disturbances of Thought Process

Loosening of association—the lack of a logical relationship between thoughts and ideas; conversation shifts from one topic to another in a completely unrelated manner, making it confusing and difficult to follow

Circumstantiality—the individual takes a long time to make a point because his or her conversation is indirect and contains excessive and unnecessary detail

Tangentiality—similar to circumstantiality, except that the speaker does not return to a central point or answer the question posed

Thought blocking—an abrupt pause or interruption in one's train of thought, after which the individual cannot recall what he or she was saying

Neologisms—the creation of new words

Flight of ideas—rapid, continuous verbalization, with frequent shifting from one topic to another

Word salad—an incoherent mixture of words and phrases

Perseveration—a persisting response to a stimulus even after a new stimulus has been presented

Clang Association—the use of words or phrases that have similar sounds but are not associated in meaning; may include rhyming or puns

Echolalia—the persistent echoing or repetition of words or phrases said by others

Verbigeration—the meaningless repetition of incoherent words or sentences; typically associated with psychotic states and cognitive impairment

Pressured speech—speech that is increased in rate and volume and is often emphatic and difficult to interrupt; typically associated with mania or hypomania

impairments tend to exist in this order (ie, a sense of time is impaired before a sense of place). The nurse begins with specific questions about the date, time of day, location of the interview, and name of the interviewer and moves to more general questions if necessary. For example, if the client knows the year, but not the exact date, the nurse can ask the season.

MEMORY. Memory function is traditionally divided into four spheres: *immediate retention and recall; recent memory; short-term memory;* and *remote or long-term memory.* To check immediate retention and recall, the nurse gives the person three unrelated words to remember and asks him or her to recite them immediately and at 5- and 15-minute intervals during the interview. To test recent memory, the nurse asks questions about events of the past few hours or days. Short-term memory involves things that occurred within the past few weeks or months. The nurse assesses remote or long-term memory by asking about events of years ago. If they are personal events and the answers seem incorrect, the nurse may check them with a family member.

ATTENTION AND CONCENTRATION. To test attention and concentration, the nurse asks the individual to count backward, aloud, from 100 by increments of 7 (eg, 93, 86, 79, and so on) or to start with 20 and subtract 3. The nurse must decide which is most appropriate for the patient considering education and understanding; subtracting 3s from 20 is the easier of the two tasks. Another way to test these areas is to ask the person to spell a simple word, such as house, backward.

COMPREHENSION AND ABSTRACT REASONING. To test abstract reasoning and comprehension, the nurse asks the person to interpret a simple proverb. Examples include "People in glass houses shouldn't throw stones," "A rolling stone gathers no moss," and "A penny saved is a penny earned." The examiner should keep in mind that proverbs are highly culturally bound and may not be appropriate for persons whose first language is not English. An alternative is to ask the individual to explain the similarities between everyday objects (eg, apple and orange) or concepts (eg, truth and beauty).

Insight and Judgment

Insight and judgment are related concepts that involve the ability to examine ideas, conceptualize facts, solve problems, and think abstractly. **Insight** is understanding the reality of a set of circumstances. It reflects the person's awareness of his or her own thoughts and feelings and an ability to compare them with the thoughts and feelings of others. For example, individuals with impaired insight may not believe that they have mental illness. They may have delusions and hallucinations or be hospitalized for bizarre and sometimes dangerous behaviour, but do not grasp that this is unusual or abnormal.

Judgment is the ability to reach a logical decision about a situation and to choose a course of action after examining and analyzing various possibilities. Throughout the interview, the nurse evaluates the person's problem-solving abilities and capacity to learn from past experience. For example, a nurse might conclude that an individual who repeatedly chooses partners who are abusive demonstrates poor judgment in selecting partners. Another way to assess judgment is to give a simple scenario and ask the person to identify the best response. An example of such a scenario is, "What would you do if you found a bag of money outside a bank on a busy street?" If the patient responds, "Run with it," his or her judgment is questionable.

Stress and Coping Patterns

Everyone lives with some degree of stress in their life (see Chapter 34 for a full discussion). For vulnerable individuals, however, stress may contribute to the development of mental disorders. Identification of major stressors in an individual's life helps the nurse to understand and support the use of successful coping behaviours in the future. The nurse should identify the individual's current stressors and coping strategies and evaluate the effectiveness of the latter. This information is vital to the overall plan of care because it highlights both problem areas and resources.

CRNE Note

A comprehensive assessment should always identify stressors and coping patterns. Identifying how an individual copes with stress can be used as a basis of care in all nursing situations. Review content from Chapter 34 when studying these concepts.

Risk Assessment

Risk factors are those characteristics, conditions, situations, and events that increase the individual's vulnerability to threats to safety or well-being. Throughout this text, assessment of risk factors focuses on risks to safety, risks for developing psychiatric–mental health disorders, and risks for increasing, or exacerbating, symptoms and impairment in individuals with an existing psychiatric disorder

The assessment of safety is a priority and a part of every encounter with clients. Examples include the risk for self-harm or suicide, risk for violence toward others, and risk for adverse events, such as falls, seizures, allergic reactions, or elopement. Nurses must assess these risk factors on a priority basis. For example, they must assess the risk for violence or suicide and take measures to prevent injury, such as implementing environmental constraints, before addressing other assessment factors.

Suicide

A suicide risk assessment involves garnering specific detail regarding:

Suicidal ideation—thoughts about self-harm or of self-inflicted death

Threats of suicide—a verbal or behavioural indication (direct or indirect) that an individual is planning to end his or her life

Suicide attempt—action taken to end one's life

To ascertain this information, the nurse asks specific questions about suicidal thoughts, previous suicide attempts (including dates and outcome), the existence and lethality of a suicide plan, access to means, and symptoms of hopelessness. See Chapter 37 for a full discussion.

- Do you have thoughts of suicide at this time? Have you thought about suicide in the past? If the answer to either of these questions is "yes," probe for details about when these thoughts occur and their frequency and intensity.
- Have you ever tried to harm or kill yourself? If the answer is "yes," probe for details about precipitating circumstances, means, and outcome. If the individual has thought about suicide but not acted on these thoughts, determine why not.
- Do you have a plan? If the answer is "yes," ask for details (eg, when, by what means).
- Do you have the means to carry out this plan?
- Have you made preparations for your death (eg, writing a good-bye note, putting finances in order, giving away possessions)?
- Has a significant episode in your life caused you to think this way? Probe for indications of hopelessness, a sense of helplessness, a loss of enjoyment in life, guilt or shame, anger, or impaired judgment.

From this assessment, the nurse and other members of the team determine the individual's level of risk for self-harm and intervene as necessary. Most psychiatric–mental health programs and facilities use rating scales to quantify an individual's risk for self-harm. Those deemed to be at high risk are usually hospitalized and constantly observed.

Assaultive or Homicidal Ideation

A safety assessment also includes an evaluation of the level of threat an individual poses to others. Of particular importance are delusions or hallucinations that involve harming or killing others. Questions to ask to ascertain assaultive or homicidal ideation are as follows:

- Do you intend to harm someone? If yes, who?
- Do you have a plan? If yes, what are the details of the plan?
- Do you have the means to carry out the plan? (If the plan requires a weapon, is it readily available?)

Social Domain

A comprehensive assessment also attends to social dimensions of an individual's life. Much of this information is elicited during the health history and the MSE and includes information about the individual's current living situation, the individual's family of origin, and the existence and quality of significant relationships (see Chapter 16). The treatment team also assesses work, education, and social and leisure activities. As well, the team observes the individual's interactions with those around them. This component of the assessment helps to identify important strengths and resources as well as problems and deficits.

Functional Status

Understanding how an individual functions in his or her day-to-day life is a vital part of assessment. Many mental health teams use the Global Assessment of Functioning (GAF) scale (discussed in Chapter 3) as a single measure of functioning.

Ethnic and Cultural Assessment

Ethnicity and culture profoundly affect an individual's worldview and frames the person's beliefs about life, death, health and illness, and roles and relationships. As part of a comprehensive assessment, the nurse must consider ethnic and cultural factors that influence health and illness. To understand these, the nurse should ask the following questions:

- Do you identify with a cultural group? If yes, which one?
- Do you identify with an ethnic group? If yes, which one?
- What does health mean to you?
- What does illness mean to you?
- How do you define good and evil?
- What do you do to enhance your physical and mental health?
- Whom do you see for help when you are physically or mentally ill?
- By what cultural rules or taboos do you live?
- Do you eat special foods?

Spiritual Assessment

Nurses must be clear about their own spirituality to ensure that it does not interfere with assessment of the patient's spirituality. See Chapter 6 for a definition of spirituality. Examples of questions that may foster an understanding of an individual's spirituality include:

- What gives your life meaning?
- What brings joy into your life?
- Do you believe in God or a higher power?
- Do you participate in any religious activities? If yes, which ones?
- Do you feel connected with the world?

CRNE Note

Data from spirituality assessment can serve as a basis for strengthening coping strategies.

SUMMARY OF KEY POINTS

◘ **Assessment** is a purposeful, systematic, and dynamic process that is ongoing throughout the nurse's relationship with individuals in her or his care. It involves the collection, validation, analysis, synthesis, organization, and documentation of client health–illness information.

◘ A **comprehensive assessment** includes a health history and physical examination; considers the psychological, emotional, social, spiritual, ethnic, and cultural dimensions of health; attends to the meaning of the client's health–illness experience; and evaluates how all this affects the individual's daily living. A **focussed assessment** is the collection of specific information about a particular need, problem, or situation. It is briefer, narrower in scope, and more present oriented than a comprehensive assessment.

◘ Techniques of data collection include observation, interview, physical and mental examinations, and collaboration.

◘ Biologic assessment includes health history, physical examination, and diagnostic testing.

◘ Assessment of the psychological domain includes understanding the individual's response to mental health problems, mental status examination, evaluation of stress and coping, and risk assessment.

◘ The mental status examination is a systematic assessment of an individual's appearance, affect, behaviour, and cognitive processes. It reflects the examiner's observations and impressions at the time of the interview and is used in a variety of clinical settings to evaluate developmental, neurologic, and psychiatric disorders.

◘ Risk factors are those characteristics, conditions, situations, or events that increase the individual's vulnerability to threats to safety or well-being. Examples include the risk for self-harm or suicide, violence toward others, and the risk for adverse events, such as falls, seizures, allergic reactions, or elopement.

◘ The social assessment involves a family and relationship assessment, evaluation of functional status, and information about the individual's ethnicity, culture, and spirituality.

CRITICAL THINKING CHALLENGES

1 A 23-year-old Caucasian woman is admitted to an acute psychiatric setting for depression and suicidal gestures. This admission is her first, but she has experienced bouts of depression since early adolescence. She and her fiancé have just ended their engagement and moved into separate apartments. She has not yet told anyone that she is pregnant. She reports that her mother believes that she was "living in sin" and that she would "pay for it." From this scenario, develop three assessment questions for each domain: biologic, psychological, and social.

2 Write a paragraph on your self-concept, including body image, self-esteem, and personal identity. Explore the type of clinical situations in which your self-concept can aid in your interactions with clients. Explore the types of clinical situations in which your self-concept can hinder your interactions with patients.

WEB LINKS

www.cfmhn.org/Home.htm Canadian Federation of Mental Health Nurses (CFMHN). This site provides the *Standards of Psychiatric and Mental Health Nursing* (2005), information about the CFMHN activities, and links to sites of interest to psychiatric–mental health nurses.

www.cna-nurses.ca Canadian Nurses Association. This website provides a copy of the *Code of Ethics for Registered Nurses* (2002), information about current issues of interest to nurses, position statements, and links to other Canadian nursing organizations.

www.hcc-ccs.com/index.aspx This site describes the mission, mandate, and activities of the Health Council of Canada.

www.laws.justice.gc.ca/en/P-21/95414.html This is the site of the Department of Justice Canada and contains the *Privacy Act*.

www.coping.org/adult_link/tests.htm This is a public service site that has several self-report mental health screening tests.

www.psychpage.com/learning/library/assess/index.html This site explains the process of a mental health status examination.

REFERENCES

American Psychiatric Association. (2000). *Diagnostic and statistical manual of mental disorders* (4th ed., Text revision). Washington, DC: Author.

Canadian Federation of Mental Health Nurses. (2005). *Canadian standards of psychiatric and mental health nursing* (3rd ed.). Retrieved June 15, 2005, from http://www.cfmhn.org/Documents/Standards%20%20english%20doc.htm.

Canadian Nurses Association. (2002). *Code of ethics for registered nurses.* Ottawa, ON: Author. Retrieved June 15, 2005, from http://www.cna-nurses.ca/CNA/documents/pdf/publications/CodeofEthics2002_e.pdf.

Canadian Nurses Association. (2005). *Canadian nurse practitioner core competency framework.* Ottawa, ON: Author.

Coghlan, R., Lawrence, D., Holman, D., & Jablensky, A. (2001). Duty to care: Preventable physical illness in people with mental illness. Crawley, WA: University of Western Australia. Retrieved June 15, 2005, from http://www.populationhealth.uwa.edu.au/welcome/research/chsr/chsr/consumer_info/duty_to_care/dtc_cons.pdf.

Folstein, M. F., Folstein, S. E., & McHugh, P. R. (1975). Mini-mental state: A practical method for grading the cognitive state of patients for the clinician. *Journal of Psychiatric Research, 12*, 189–198.

Hahm, H. C., & Segal, S. P. (2005). Failure to seek health care among the mentally ill. *American Journal of Orthopsychiatry, 75*(1), 54–62.

Phelan, M., Stradins, L., & Morrison, S. (2001). Physical health of people with severe mental illness. *British Medical Journal, 322*(7284), 443–444.

Rogers, C. R. (1980). *A way of being.* Boston: Houghton Mifflin.

Romanow, R. J. (2002). *Building on values: The future of health care in Canada. Final Report.* Ottawa, ON: National Library of Canada. Retrieved June 30, 2005, from http://www.hc-sc.gc.ca/english/pdf/romanow/pdfs/HCC_Final_Report.pdf.

Saddock. J., & Saddock, V. A. (2003). *Kaplan's & Saddock's synopsis of psychiatry: Behavioral sciences and clinical psychiatry* (9th ed.). Philadelphia: Lippincott Williams & Wilkins.

11

Diagnosis and Outcomes Development

Doris Bell, Lorraine D. Williams, and Christine Davis

LEARNING OBJECTIVES

After studying this chapter, you will be able to:

- Define components of nursing diagnoses.
- Discuss the use of nursing diagnoses in psychiatric and mental health care.
- Define and explore alternatives to nursing diagnosis, such as the Tidal Model.
- Discuss the relationship between client-centred care, patient outcomes, and quality care.
- Discuss the use of individual outcomes in psychiatric and mental health nursing.
- Describe the process of developing individual outcomes with clients.
- Write individual outcome statements for psychiatric and mental health nursing care.

KEY TERMS

- clinical domain outcome statements ▪ defining characteristics ▪ diagnosis-specific outcomes ▪ discharge outcomes ▪ humanitarian domain outcome statements ▪ indicators ▪ initial outcomes ▪ primary health care ▪ provider domain outcome statements ▪ public welfare domain outcome statements ▪ rehabilitative domain outcome statements ▪ revised outcomes

KEY CONCEPTS

- best practice guidelines ▪ client-centred care ▪ defining characteristics ▪ nursing diagnosis ▪ outcomes

After completing an assessment of the individual who is to receive care, the nurse generates appropriate nursing diagnoses based on the assessment data. With experience, the nurse can easily cluster the assessment data to support one nursing diagnosis over another. Mutually agreed-on goals flow from the nursing diagnoses and provide guidance in determining appropriate interventions. Initial outcomes are determined and then are monitored and evaluated throughout the care process. Measuring outcomes not only demonstrates clinical effectiveness but also helps to promote rational clinical decision making and is reflective of the nursing interventions. This chapter describes the development of nursing diagnosis, client-centred care, and individual outcomes in psychiatric and mental health (PMH) nursing within the context of the Canadian health care system.

EVOLUTION OF NURSING DIAGNOSIS AND INDIVIDUAL OUTCOMES

The concepts of nursing diagnosis and individual outcomes are not new ones. Florence Nightingale identified patient problems and analyzed patient outcomes during the Crimean War. As early as 1962, Mildred Aydelotte published one of the first nursing studies involving patient outcomes. In 1973, in the United States, Gebbie and Lavin (1975) called the first National Conference on Nursing Classification, which laid the groundwork for the development of nursing diagnosis and outcomes. Lang and Clinton (1984) proposed the following outcomes: physical health status, mental health status, social and physical functioning, health attitude, knowledge and behaviour, use of professional health resources, and patient perception of the quality of nursing care.

In 1989, Marek identified 15 outcome categories: physiologic measures, symptom control, frequency of service, home maintenance, psychosocial measures, well-being, functional status, goal attainment, patient behaviours, patient satisfaction, patient knowledge, rehospitalization, safety, cost, and resolution of nursing diagnoses. In the 1990s, efforts focussed on developing outcomes that could be used to evaluate nursing effectiveness.

In Canada, in the early 2000s, the Registered Nurses Association of Ontario (RNAO) was funded by the Ontario Ministry of Health and Long-Term Care to develop, implement, evaluate, and revise Best Practice Guidelines that would inform nursing practice in a number of areas. The Nursing Best Practice Guideline (BPG) Program connects research and practice to ensure that individuals and families participate in and receive the most up-to-date evidence-based care, ensuring better outcomes for individuals and thereby reducing costs (RNAO, 2005).

◆ **KEY CONCEPT** **Best practice guidelines (BPGs)**, also termed clinical practice guidelines (CPGs), are broad or specific recommendations for health care based on the best current evidence.

BOX 11.1

Examples of RNAO Practice Guidelines

Establishing therapeutic relationships
Client-centred care
Crisis intervention
Interventions for postpartum depression
Enhancing health adolescent development
Women abuse: screening, identification, and initial response

See Box 11-1 for examples of available RNAO guidelines. See Web Links for access information. BPGs support nurses in making make good clinical decisions. They are to be used flexibly and in conjunction with knowledge of the preferences of the people seeking care.

CURRENT TRENDS IN CANADA

The current trend in nursing in Canada is away from the nurse as expert about a patient's needs to a client-centred approach with the recognition that individuals, as whole and unique beings (RNAO, 2002), make meaning of their own lived experiences and participate in all aspects of their care (CCMHI, 2005).

◆ **KEY CONCEPT** **Client-centred care** is an approach to care in which the client is recognized as a whole person with the right to autonomy, self-determination, and participation in decision making (RNAO, 2002).

The Canadian Collaborative Mental Health Initiative (CCMHI), a consortium of 12 national organizations, representing community services, consumer, family and self-help groups, dietitians, family physicians, nurses, occupational therapists, pharmacists, psychologists, psychiatrists, and social workers was established in 2004 to enhance mental health services in primary health care. At the core of CCMHI's work are the needs of consumers or individuals (Gagne, 2005). Consumer "centredness," or client-centred care, involves individuals, families, and caregivers in all areas of care from treatment choices to evaluation (Gagne, 2005).

Although the importance of identifying outcomes of nursing interventions has been the subject of several nursing research studies since the 1960s, escalating health care costs have forced the demonstration of measurable outcomes. Concerns about quality, cost, and use of limited resources have contributed to the current emphasis on both evidence-based practice and individual outcomes. With the expansion of nursing knowledge gained through measuring intervention effectiveness, the nursing discipline itself will continue to evolve.

DERIVING A NURSING DIAGNOSIS

> **KEY CONCEPT** A **nursing diagnosis** is a clinical judgment about an identified problem or need that requires nursing interventions and nursing management. It is based on data generated from a nursing assessment. A formal nursing diagnosis statement includes defining characteristics and related factors (Carpenito-Moyet, 2004).

Because nursing diagnoses provide the basis for planning nursing interventions, they are used in diverse practice settings in multiple individual populations to assist individuals to achieve positive health outcomes (Delaney, Herr, Maas, & Specht, 2000). For nurses to improve their ability to make sound nursing diagnoses, they must actively apply nursing principles, concepts, and theories to the care of the individual (Kleinpell, 2003). A complete list of North American Nursing Diagnosis Association (NANDA) nursing diagnoses can be found on *the Point*.

> **KEY CONCEPT Defining characteristics** are key signs and symptoms (clues) that relate to each other and that validate a nursing diagnosis. The nurse analyzes these characteristic clues to formulate a cluster of data, which helps in selecting an appropriate diagnosis or diagnoses reflecting the actual or potential health status or problems of the individual.

Clusters of data lead the nurse to choose certain diagnoses over others. For example, when assessing an individual, the nurse observes that the individual's responses are often self-negating (eg, "I always mess things up," "I never get it right"). The nurse also observes that the individual shows indecisiveness and lacks problem-solving abilities (eg, "I can never decide what is the right thing to do, and when I do finally choose, it is always wrong"). Nonverbal and verbal information should be used to identify defining characteristics. Observations of the individual sitting with her head down, making no eye contact, and dressed in dirty clothes are important data that should be considered in support of a nursing diagnosis. Such observations support the hypothesis that the individual has a disturbance in self-esteem. Further assessment will help the nurse determine whether the self-esteem disturbance is chronic or situational.

Related factors are those that influence or change the individual's health status and are associated with the nursing diagnosis. Related factors are grouped into four categories: pathophysiologic (biologic or psychological or spiritual), treatment-related (medications, diagnostic studies, surgeries), situational (environmental, home, community, person), and maturational (age-related influences) (Carpenito-Moyet, 2004). To continue with the assessment example, the nurse learns that the individual has lost three jobs within the past year, resulting in financial problems. These situation-related factors further support the nursing diagnosis of Self-Esteem Disturbance.

In the real world, most PMH nurses practice in an interdisciplinary or multidisciplinary environment. Nursing diagnoses are dimensional, not categorical (as is the *Diagnostic and Statistical Manual of Mental Disorders*, 4th edition, text revision [DSM-IV-TR] psychiatric disorder diagnosis [American Psychiatric Association, 2000]), so they may be helpful to other members of the team because degrees of problems can be considered and outcomes that can be measured developed. Despite the use of nursing diagnosis by other disciplines, the nursing interventions need to be clearly specified.

DEVELOPING INDIVIDUAL OUTCOMES

> **KEY CONCEPT Outcomes** are the individual's response to nursing care at a given point in time. An outcome is concise, stated in few words and in neutral terms. Outcomes describe an individual's state, behaviour, or perception that is variable and can be measured (Table 11-1).

According to the *Canadian Standards of Psychiatric and Mental Health Nursing* and the *Scope and Standards of Psychiatric–Mental Health Nursing Practice*, outcomes are expected to be individualized to each individual (American Nurses Association, American Psychiatric Association, and International Society of Psychiatric–Mental Health Nurses, 2000; Canadian Federation of Mental Health Nurses, 2006) (Table 11-2). Individual outcomes are linked to nursing diagnoses through the nursing process. By linking outcomes to the nursing diagnosis, it is possible to monitor nursing practice and facilitate clinical decision making and knowledge development (Table 11-3).

Outcomes can be defined as an individual's response to care. Outcome identification has moved away from the clinical symptoms and laboratory signs that medicine has traditionally used to describe individual knowledge, behaviours, and quality of life. Outcomes are the end result of a process, a treatment, or a nursing intervention and should be monitored and documented over time and across clinical settings. **Diagnosis-specific outcomes** show that the intervention resolved the problem or nursing diagnosis (Table 11-4). At other times, the outcome is nonspecific (ie, not diagnosis-specific, meaning it does not show resolution of the diagnosis). In that case, the outcome is abstract or general (Table 11-5).

Indicators answer the question, "How close is the individual moving toward the outcome?" The indicator represents the dimensions of the outcome. Outcome indicators represent or describe individual status, behaviours, or perceptions evaluated during an individual's

Table 11.1   Example of Outcomes

Diagnosis	Outcome	Intervention
Spiritual distress Related to conflict between religious or spiritual beliefs and prescribed health regime	Will express religious or spiritual satisfaction **Indicators** a. Express decreased feelings of guilt and fear. b. State that conflict has been eliminated.	Provide accurate information about treatment plan. Encourage the client and the physician to consider alternative methods of therapy. Support client making informed decisions—even if decision conflicts with own values.

From Carpenito-Moyet, L. J. (2006). *Nursing Diagnosis: Application to clinical practice* (11th ed.). Philadelphia: Lippincott Williams & Wilkins.

Table 11.2   Clinical Path: Depression

Day	Assessment Parameters	Nursing Diagnosis	Nursing Interventions	Patient Outcomes
Day 1	Individual admits to having a suicide plan.	Risk for Self-Directed Violence	Institute suicide precautions.	Suicide: self-restraint
Day 2			Maintain suicide precautions.	Suicide: self-restraint
Day 3	Individual is apathetic, doesn't wash or dress self.	Ineffective Health Maintenance	Help individual with personal hygiene, exhibit patience.	Self-care: dressing and bathing

Table 11.3   Results of Nursing Interventions

Diagnosis	Patient Outcome	Nursing Intervention
Anticipatory Grieving	Grief resolution (adjusting to impending loss) **Indicators** a. Express feelings about loss. b. Express feelings about how life will change due to loss. c. Maintain relationships until death occurs. d. Maintain nutrition. e. Maintain social support. f. Practice skills and role function needed in the future.	Provide supportive feedback to verbal concerns and feelings.

Table 11.4   Example of Condition: Diagnosis-Specific Outcomes

Diagnosis	Outcome
Anxiety	a. Anxiety control b. Aggression control

Table 11.5   Example of System-Specific Outcome

Diagnosis	Outcome
Disturbed Sensory Perception (hallucination)	Movement disorder occurrence **Indicators** a. Initiation of antipsychotic drugs b. Demonstration of choreic movement c. Demonstration of pelvic gyrations d. Increase or decrease in dosage of antipsychotic drugs

Table 11.6	Example—Linkage of Nursing Diagnosis and Outcomes
Diagnosis	**Outcome**
1. Disturbed Body Image	Self-mutilation restraint
2. Chronic Confusion	Improved thought control
3. Ineffective Denial	Anxiety control

From Johnson, M., Maas, M., & Moorhead, S. (2000). *Iowa Outcomes Project, Nursing outcomes classification* (NOC) (2nd ed.). St. Louis: Mosby.

Table 11.8	Example of Discipline-Specific Outcome
Diagnosis	**Outcome**
Deficient Knowledge	Knowledge: medication
	Indicator
	Description of side effects of medications

assessment. Indicators are a measurement of individual progress in relation to the individual outcomes and can serve as intermediate outcomes in a clinical pathway or standardized care plan. See Table 11-6 for examples of outcomes linked to nursing diagnoses and Table 11-7 for examples of expected outcomes from nursing interventions.

Indicators are sensitive to nursing interventions; therefore, if other disciplines use the outcome, the indicators that are sensitive to nursing can be monitored to provide nursing accountability for care (Table 11-8). When two disciplines use the same outcomes, both of the indicators are related to the outcome but are discipline sensitive. For example, in Table 11-8, "description of side effects of medication" relates to a nursing intervention, whereas "description of potential of an adverse reaction when taking multiple drugs" is a pharmacy indicator.

In nursing care planning, outcomes can be **initial outcomes** (those written after the initial individual interview and assessment), **revised outcomes** (those written after each evaluation), or **discharge outcomes** (those outcomes to be met before discharge). Because of the decreased length of stay or days of service, discharge outcomes often are not met but are passed along to the community nurse. If these discharge outcomes continue to be relevant, they become initial outcomes in community or home care.

Documentation of Outcomes

Nurses are accountable for documentation of individual outcomes, nursing interventions, and any changes in diagnosis, care plan, or both. Individual responses to care are documented as changes in behaviour or knowledge and can include the degree of satisfaction with the health care provided (Kleinpell, 2003). Outcomes can be expressed in terms of the individual's actual responses (eg, no longer reports hearing voices) or the status of a nursing diagnosis at a point in time after implementation of nursing interventions, such as "Caregiver Role Strain resolved." This documentation is important for further research and quality of care studies.

Purposes of Individual Outcomes

The primary purposes of developing individual outcomes are to ensure the needs of the individual are being met and to ensure quality care. They provide guidelines for what is expected of the individual and direction for continuity of care that reflects current knowledge in the field of PMH nursing. The measurement of individual outcomes helps to meet the goal of continuous quality improvement (CQI). By identifying variations in individual outcomes and working to reduce or eliminate these variations, CQI occurs. Thus, outcomes drive the CQI process (Fig. 11-1).

In addition, outcomes motivate the individual by providing a sense of achievement when they are reached.

Table 11.7	Expected Outcomes From Nursing Interventions
Nursing Intervention	**Expected Outcome**
Provide educational information about mental illness	Knowledge: disease process
Educational group in caregiving	Caregiver: individual relationship
Group therapy	Improved thought control
Weight control counselling	Knowledge: diet
Health teaching	Knowledge: medication
Teaching limit setting	Coping
Reality orientation	Identity: self
Life review	Hope
Teaching anger management	Impulse control

Based on Johnson, M., Maas, M., & Mcorhead, S. (2000). *Iowa Outcomes Project, Nursing outcomes classification* (NOC) (2nd ed.). St. Louis: Mosby.

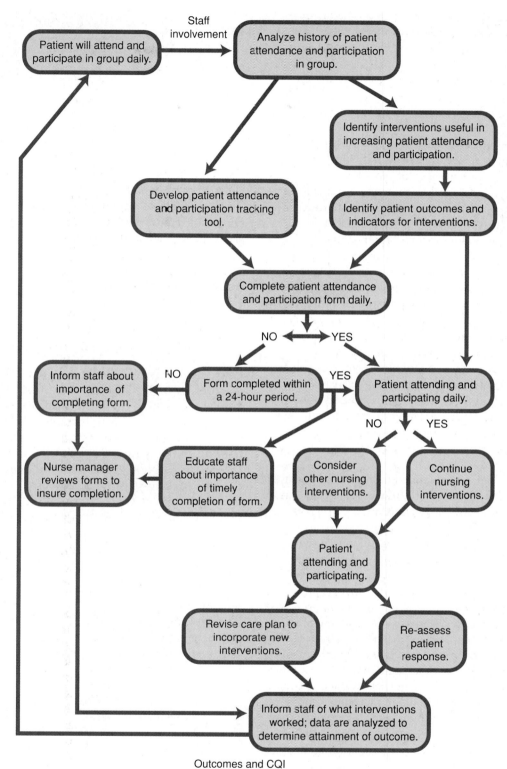

Staff involvement

Outcomes and CQI

FIGURE 11.1   Outcomes and continuous quality improvement (CQI).

Table 11.9	Example of Humanitarian Domain Outcome	
Diagnosis	**Outcome**	**Intervention**
Readiness for Enhanced Family Coping	Parents and adolescents talk to each other at breakfast about feelings and concerns.	Encourage family to spend time listening to each other's concerns and feelings.

Individuals feel empowered and successful when a particular outcome is realized. Positive individual outcomes have been linked to a number of biopsychosocial PMH nursing areas, including individual hygiene, nutrition and hydration, pressure sores/skin integrity, intravenous therapy, discharge planning, pain control, education/rehabilitation, and elimination. Other studies demonstrate effectiveness of nursing interventions in individual education, health promotion, cardiac rehabilitation, postoperative and preoperative care, anxiety prevention/reduction, and pain management. A review of the effectiveness of mental health nursing interventions shows significant improvements in depression, self-esteem, general health, and satisfaction (Doran, 2003).

PMH nurses work as members of interdisciplinary teams that usually develop one treatment plan. Nursing interventions should be clearly differentiated from outcomes associated with the other mental health disciplines. Outcomes and indicators also provide excellent nurse-to-nurse communication, which leads to good continuity of care.

Also, individual outcomes and indicators can be used to evaluate whether a specific nursing intervention is effective with a specific problem (Rantz, 2001), answering the question, "What are the expected results of the nurse's actions or interventions?" Outcomes can also be linked to measuring the performance effectiveness of the caregivers.

Accountability is an important concept in health care. Nursing and other disciplines are being pressured within health services systems to justify their practice, to demonstrate to consumers that they deliver quality care, and to control health care costs. Measurement of outcomes can be used to determine quality of care during a single episode of illness and across the continuum of care and can assist in discharge planning. Outcomes also can be used to determine quality of care in different systems and between systems.

From an economic viewpoint, identifying nursing interventions sensitive to individual outcomes can demonstrate the PMH nurse's contribution to multidisciplinary care. Increasingly, cost reduction is a guiding principle for health care. If the nursing contribution is not visible, it will not be recognized and therefore may become dispensable (Doran, 2003). Evaluation of individual outcomes can help validate nursing interventions by identifying which interventions are effective. Outcomes can also be a communication tool when working with other nurses, case managers, caregivers, and policy makers, and can be used to conduct program evaluations and develop research databases. Standardized labels (outcomes) provide effective and efficient ways to deliver the message that nursing is part of the health care system.

Outcomes Classification Systems

Outcomes can be classified in several ways. This section identifies two classification systems developed in the United States but relevant to Canadian health care as well. First, the National Institute of Mental Health (NIMH) framework provides a perspective that can be used by all disciplines. Second, the Nursing Outcome Classification (NOC) from the Iowa Outcome Projects provides nursing-sensitive outcomes.

NIMH Classification of Outcomes

In 1991, the NIMH defined four categories of outcome statements that are not necessarily nurse sensitive: humanitarian domain, public welfare domain, rehabilitative domain, and clinical domain. In their review of nursing outcome research, Merwin and Mauck (1995) added a fifth category—that of provider domain. Definitions and examples of each of the five categories of outcome statements are as follows:

- **Humanitarian domain outcome statements** spell out behaviours or responses that show a sense of well-being of individuals and personal fulfillment of individuals and family members (Table 11-9).
- **Public welfare domain outcome statements** show responses or behaviours that provide examples for preventing harm to self, family, and community (Table 11-10).

Table 11.10	Example of Public Welfare Domain Outcome	
Diagnosis	**Outcome**	**Intervention**
Risk for Other-Directed Violence (Hitting)	Individual verbalizes feelings (not act out).	Encourage individual to talk about feelings.

Table 11.11	Example of Rehabilitative Domain Outcome	
Diagnosis	**Outcome**	**Intervention**
Ineffective Coping (not attending school)	Individual demonstrates responsibility for behaviour (graduation from high school).	Assist individual in identifying stressors that hinder attendance in school.

- **Rehabilitative domain outcome statements** provide examples of improvement or restoration of social and vocational functioning and lead to independent living (Table 11-11).
- **Clinical domain outcome statements** indicate reduction in symptoms of illness or cure of a specific mental illness (Table 11-12).
- **Provider domain outcome statements** describe behaviours and attitudes of nursing staff and responses to nurse–individual relationships (Table 11-13).

Nursing Outcome Classification

These are the first nurse-sensitive outcomes that describe individual outcomes and indications for measurement and that are linked to nursing diagnoses. They were developed in the late 1990s by the Iowa Outcome Project. The Project's NOC is a three-level classification system currently composed of 7 domains, 29 outcome classes, and 330 outcomes (Moorhead, Johnson, & Maas, 2004). The outcomes are conceived as being on a continuum, rather than as discrete met or unmet goals. When nurses use NOC or the biopsychosocial model to develop outcome statements (Table 11-14), they can attend to all aspects of the individual and how he or she relates to the family and community (Fig. 11-2).

EVALUATION

Evaluation of individual outcomes involves answering the following questions:
- What were the benefits for the individual?
- What was the individual's level of satisfaction?

Table 11.12	Example of Clinical Domain Outcome	
Diagnosis	**Outcome**	**Intervention**
Disturbed Sensory Perception (auditory hallucinations)	Individual questions validity of voices.	Discuss possible explanations for the voices.

Table 11.13	Example of Provider Domain Outcome	
Diagnosis	**Outcome**	**Intervention**
Fear Related to Assault (Individual violence)	Nurses discuss fear of recurrence of event.	Supportive counselling (crisis intervention)

Table 11.14	Example of Diagnosis-Specific Outcome	
Diagnosis	**Outcome**	**Intervention**
Sleep Deprivation	a. Sleep b. Resting **Indicator** Determine number of hours of sleep. Describe factors that prevent sleep. Describe factors that promote sleep.	Teach individual relaxation techniques to use at bedtime.

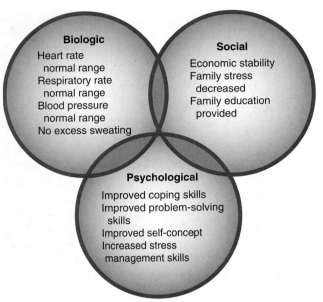

FIGURE 11.2 Biopsychosocial outcomes for an individual with anxiety.

- Was the outcome diagnosis specific or nonspecific?
- What is the cost-effectiveness of the intervention?

When measuring outcomes, nurses must consider the time frame. Identifying the intermediate outcome indicators that may be achieved in one setting versus the indicators that can be achieved in a second setting provides for a measurement of progression and enhances continuity of care. For example, in Table 11-15, the individual may be able to satisfy the first set of indicators—resolution of depression, demonstration of confidence, demonstration of self-esteem, and decreased suicide

attempts—during his or her stay in an institutional health care setting (hospital).

Nevertheless, not until the individual is discharged or moved to a community setting can he or she satisfy the second set of indicators: demonstration of confidence when alone at home, demonstration of positive interpersonal relationship with opposite sex, demonstration of confidence in role skills (worker/mother), and demonstration of self-advocacy behaviour. Together, the sets of indicators can measure the individual's progress.

Outcomes can be measured immediately after the nursing intervention or after time passes. Remember that outcomes based on health prevention and health promotion diagnoses can occur after considerable time has passed.

Future Practice Considerations

In some Canadian mental health settings, the NANDA nursing diagnosis taxonomy is seen to be less client centred and therefore less meaningful to the individual's lived experience. The antithesis of NANDA nursing diagnosis is the Tidal Model, a theory-based approach to mental health nursing emphasizing the "need for nurses to collaborate closely with the people by developing a therapeutic user-empowering relationship" (see Chapter 4). That change is life's only constant is a core element in this theory (hence the metaphor of the tide). Care is grounded on an understanding of the individual's present and future needs in the personal domains of world, self, and other (Barker, 2001). Box 11-2 outlines the "ten commitments" of care put forth in the Tidal Model.

Table 11.15	Progression in Care					
Diagnosis	**Outcome**					
Family Violence: Individual	Abuse recovery: emotional	None 1	Limited 2	Moderate 3	Substantial 4	Extensive 5
	Indicators a. Resolution of depression; demonstration of confidence; demonstration of self-esteem; decreased suicide attempts b. Demonstration of confidence when alone in home; demonstration of positive interpersonal relationship with opposite sex; demonstration of confidence in role skills (worker, mother); self-advocacy behaviour					

BOX 11.2

Ten Commitments of the Tidal Model

1. **Value the voice:** The person's story is the beginning and end point of the helping encounter. All nursing care plans and documents should be written in the person's own voice.
2. **Respect the language:** Each person has developed his or her own unique way of telling his or her story. It is not necessary to use the language of psychiatry and psychiatric nursing.
3. **Develop genuine curiosity:** Those who seek to be of assistance to the person need to develop ways of expressing genuine interest in the person's story so that they might better understand it and the storyteller.
4. **Become the apprentice:** The person is the expert/authority on his or her life story
5. **Reveal personal wisdom:** One of the key tasks for the helper is to assist in revealing the person's life wisdom that will sustain and guide recovery.
6. **Be transparent:** Both the person and the professional embody the opportunity to become a team. The pro-
fessional can support this by being transparent at all times, helping the person understand *what* is being done and *why*.
7. **Use the available tool kit:** The person's story contains numerous examples of "what has worked" or "what might work" for this person.
8. **Craft the step beyond:** The helper and the person work together to construct an appreciation of what needs to be done "now." The first step is the crucial step, revealing the power of change and pointing towards the ultimate goal of recovery.
9. **Give the gift of time:** There is no value in asking "how much time do we have?" The question is, "how do we use this time?"
10. **Know that change is constant:** The professional helper needs to become aware of how change is happening and discover the way that knowledge may steer the person out of danger and distress and remain on to the journey to recovery.

From Barker, P., & Buchanan-Barker, P. The 10 Commitments: Essential values of the Tidal Model. Available at: http://www.tidal-model.co.uk/ Ten%20Commitments.htm. Accessed on March 17, 2006.

SUMMARY OF KEY POINTS

☐ The Canadian Standards of Psychiatric and Mental Health Nursing (Canadian Federation of Mental Health Nurses, 2006) support the importance of outcome identification.

☐ Outcomes must be measurable and indicative of the individual's progress.

☐ More research is needed to identify individual outcomes as they relate to nursing interventions and nursing diagnosis.

☐ Nursing diagnoses, nursing interventions, and individual outcomes are initially derived from the assessment data.

☐ Initial, revised, and discharge outcomes can be included in a nursing care plan.

☐ Outcome statements can cover the biopsychosocial domains.

☐ Nursing care, from assessment to outcome measurement, needs to be client centred, with recognition of the client's right to participate in health care decisions.

CRITICAL THINKING CHALLENGES

1 Create a nursing care plan with outcomes for an individual who has a substance abuse problem.
2 Create a teaching plan that shows linkage of diagnoses and outcomes.
3 What are the potential barriers to implementing the Tidal Model within a psychiatric and mental health care setting?

WEB LINKS

www.rnao.org/bestpractices/index.asp This website offers RNAO Best Practice Guidelines.

www.tidal-model.co.uk This site has information regarding the Tidal Model.

REFERENCES

American Nurses Association, American Psychiatric Association, & International Society of Psychiatric–Mental Health Nurses. (2000). *Scope and standards of psychiatric–mental health nursing practice.* Washington, DC: American Nurses Publishing.

American Psychiatric Association. (2000). *Diagnostic and statistical manual of mental disorders* (4th ed., Text revision). Washington, DC: Author.

Aydelotte, M. K. (1962). The use of individual welfare as a criterion measure. *Nursing Research, 11,* 10–14.

Barker, P. (2001). The Tidal Model: Developing a person-centred approach to psychiatric and mental health nursing. *Perspectives in Psychiatric Care, 37,* 79–87.

Canadian Alliance on Mental Illness and Mental health (2005). Canadian Collaborative Mental Health Charter Discussion. Guelph, ON: Author.

Canadian Federation of Mental Health Nurses. (2006). Canadian Standards of Psychiatric and Mental Health Nursing. Available at: http://www.cfmhn.org.

Carpenito-Moyet, L. J. (2006). *Nursing diagnosis: Application to clinical practice* (11th ed.) Philadelphia: Lippincott Williams & Wilkins.

Carpenito-Moyet, L. J. (2004). *Nursing diagnosis: Application to clinical practice.* (10th ed.). Philadelphia: Lippincott Williams & Wilkins.

Delaney, C., Herr, K., Maas, M., & Specht, J. (2000). Reliability of nursing diagnoses documented in a computerized nursing information system. *Nursing Diagnosis, 11*(3), 121–135.

Doran, D. M. (2003). *Nursing sensitive outcomes: State of the science.* Sudbury, MA: Jones and Bartlett.

Gagne, M. A. (2005). What is collaborative mental health care? an introduction to the collaborative mental health care framework. Report prepared for the Canadian Mental Health Care Initiative. Mississauga, ON: Canadian Mental Health Care Initiative.

Gebbie, K. M., & Lavin, M. A. (Eds.). (1975). *Classification of nursing diagnoses: Proceedings of the First National Conference.* St. Louis: CV Mosby.

Green, P. M., & Slade, D. S. (2001). Environmental nursing diagnoses for aggregates and community. *Nursing Diagnosis, 12*(1), 5–11.

Kleinpell, R. M. (2003). Measuring advanced practice nursing outcome, strategies and resources. *Critical Care Nurse, February* (Suppl), 6–10.

Lang, N. M., & Clinton, J. F. (1984). Assessment of quality of nursing care. *Annual Review of Nursing Research, 2*, 135–163.

Marek, K. D. (1989). Outcome measurement in nursing. *Journal of Nursing Quality Assurance, 4*(1), 1–9.

Merwin, E., & Mauck, A. (1995). Psychiatric nursing outcome research: The state of the science. *Archives of Psychiatric Nursing, 9*(6), 311–331.

Moorhead, S., Johnson, M., & Maas, M. (2004). *Nursing outcomes classification* (NOC) (3rd ed.). St. Louis: Mosby.

Rantz, M. J. (2001). The value of a standardized language. *Nursing Diagnosis, 12*(3), 107–108.

Registered Nurses Association of Ontario (2002a). Client-centered care. Toronto, ON: Author.

Registered Nurses Association of Ontario (2002b). Establishing therapeutic relationships. Toronto, ON: Author.

Registered Nurses Association of Ontario Best Practice Guidelines. (2005). Available at: http://www.rnao.org/bestpractices/index.asp.

For challenges, please refer to the **CD-ROM** in this book.

Psychiatric and Mental Health Nursing Care

Mary Ann Boyd and Janet Landeen

LEARNING OBJECTIVES

After studying this chapter, you will be able to:

- Discuss the basis for selection of psychiatric and mental health nursing interventions.
- Discuss the application of nursing interventions for the biologic domain.
- Discuss the application of nursing interventions for the psychological domain.
- Discuss the application of nursing interventions for the social domain.

KEY TERMS

- automatic thinking ▪ behaviour modification ▪ behaviour therapy ▪ chemical restraint ▪ cognitive interventions ▪ conflict resolution ▪ containment ▪ counselling ▪ cultural brokering ▪ de-escalation ▪ distraction ▪ guided imagery ▪ home visits ▪ illogical thinking ▪ milieu therapy ▪ observation ▪ open communication ▪ physical restraint ▪ psychoeducation ▪ recovery ▪ reminiscence ▪ seclusion ▪ simple relaxation techniques ▪ spiritual support ▪ structured interaction ▪ token economy ▪ validation

⬟ KEY CONCEPT

- nursing interventions

Psychiatric and mental health (PMH) nursing interventions are nursing activities that promote mental health, prevent mental illness, assess dysfunction, assist clients to regain or improve their coping abilities and/or prevent further disabilities (American Nurses Association [ANA] et al., 2000; Canadian Federation of Mental Health Nurses, 2005). Based on clinical judgment and knowledge, nursing interventions include any treatment that a nurse performs to enhance client outcomes. These interventions are direct (performed through interaction with the client) or indirect (performed away from, but on behalf of, the client) (McCloskey & Bulechek, 2000). Interventions can be either nurse-initiated treatment, which is an autonomous action in response to a nursing diagnosis, or physician-initiated treatment, which is a response to a medical diagnosis as a result of a "physician's order. In PMH nursing, the *Canadian Standards of Psychiatric and Mental Health Nursing* describe the scope of practice, delineate nursing competencies, and guide the selection of interventions for implementation in the plan of care (CFMHN, 2005) (see Chapter 6).

> **KEY CONCEPT Nursing interventions** are nursing activities that promote and foster health, assess dysfunction, assist clients to regain or improve their coping abilities, or prevent additional disabilities (ANA et al., 2000).

After many different factors are considered, selection of nursing approaches involves integrating biologic, psychological, and social interventions into a comprehensive plan of care for the client with a psychiatric disorder (Fig. 12-1). PMH nurses deliver care in various roles. In some settings, such as an acute care hospital or the home, the nurse provides direct nursing care. In other settings, the nurse may assume the role of a case manager, who primarily coordinates care for all disciplines, including nursing. In this instance, the nurse may be responsible for all or part of direct nursing care as well as for ensuring that agreed-on care is appropriate for the client, even if other providers deliver it. The nurse may also be the leader or manager of a nursing unit and thus responsible for delegating the care to paraprofessional and nonprofessional providers; however, he or she remains accountable for the client's care. In all these instances, the nurse plans and initiates interventions that are safe and appropriate for the client.

Nursing Interventions and Psychiatric and Mental Health Nursing

The Nursing Interventions Classification (NIC) is an extensive system consisting of 486 specific interventions, with discrete activities for each (McCloskey & Bulechek, 2000). The NIC system is based on data collected from surveys of practicing nurses, who identified the interventions that were ultimately classified. The NIC taxonomy includes classes or groups of interventions categorized according to six domains: physiologic basic, physiologic complex, behavioural, safety, family, health system, and community. The intention of the NIC taxonomy is to represent both basic and specialty advanced nursing practice. For example, both basic and specialist nurses use interventions such as reinforcing positive behaviour; however, the advanced practice psychiatric nurse may actually develop the plan and also use it as part of psychotherapy with the client. This text uses many NIC interventions and those identified in the *Canadian Standards of Psychiatric and Mental Health Nursing* (CFMHN, 2005), as well as others reported in the PMH nursing literature (Box 12-1).

Interventions for the Biologic Domain

Biologic interventions focus on physical functioning and are directed toward the client's self-care, activities and exercise, sleep, nutrition, relaxation, hydration, and thermoregulation as well as pain management and medication management. In the NIC taxonomy, these interventions are found within the physiologic basic and physiologic complex domains.

PROMOTION OF SELF-CARE ACTIVITIES

Self-care is the ability to perform activities of daily living (ADLs) successfully. Many clients with psychiatric and

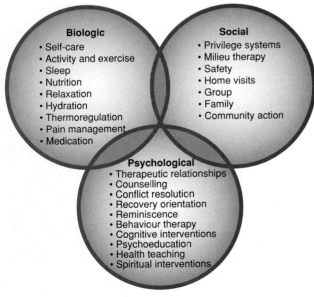

Biologic
- Self-care
- Activity and exercise
- Sleep
- Nutrition
- Relaxation
- Hydration
- Thermoregulation
- Pain management
- Medication

Social
- Privilege systems
- Milieu therapy
- Safety
- Home visits
- Group
- Family
- Community action

Psychological
- Therapeutic relationships
- Counselling
- Conflict resolution
- Recovery orientation
- Reminiscence
- Behaviour therapy
- Cognitive interventions
- Psychoeducation
- Health teaching
- Spiritual interventions

FIGURE 12.1   PMH nursing interventions.

BOX 12.1

Nursing Intervention Classification Taxonomy

I. Physiologic: Basic—Care That Supports Physical Functioning
  A. Activity and exercise management: Interventions to organize or assist with physical activity and energy conservation and expenditure
  B. Elimination management: Interventions to establish and maintain regular bowel and urinary elimination patterns and manage complications due to altered patterns
  C. Immobility management: Interventions to manage restricted body movement and the sequelae
  D. Nutrition support: Interventions to modify or maintain nutritional status
  E. Physical comfort promotion: Interventions to promote comfort using physical techniques
  F. Self-care facilitation: Interventions to provide or assist with routine activities of daily living
II. Physiologic: Complex—Care That Supports Homeostatic Regulation
  G. Electrolyte and acid–base management: Interventions to regulate electrolyte/acid–base balance and prevent complications
  H. Drug management: Interventions to facilitate desired effects of pharmacologic agents
  I. Neurologic management: Interventions to optimize neurologic function
  J. Perioperative care: Interventions to provide care before, during, and immediately after surgery (ECT)
  K. Respiratory management: Interventions to promote airway patency and gas exchange
  L. Skin/wound management: Interventions to maintain or restore tissue integrity
  M. Thermoregulation: Interventions to maintain body temperature within a normal range
  N. Tissue perfusion management: Interventions to optimize circulation of blood and fluids to the tissues
III. Behavioural—Care That Supports Psychosocial Functioning and Facilitates Lifestyle Changes
  O. Behavioural therapy: Interventions to reinforce or promote desirable behaviours or alter undesirable behaviours
  P. Cognitive therapy: Interventions to reinforce or promote desirable cognitive functioning or alter undesirable cognitive functioning

  Q. Communication enhancement: Interventions to facilitate delivering and receiving verbal and nonverbal messages
  R. Coping assistance: Interventions to assist another to build on own strengths, adapt to a change in function, or achieve a higher level of function
  S. Patient education: Interventions to facilitate learning
  T. Psychological comfort promotion: Interventions to promote comfort using psychological techniques
IV. Safety—Care That Supports Protection Against Harm
  U. Crisis management: Interventions to provide immediate, short-term help in both psychological and physiologic crises
  V. Risk management: Interventions to initiate risk reduction activities and continue monitoring risks over time
V. Family—Care That Supports the Family Unit
  W. Childbearing care: Interventions to assist in understanding and coping with the psychological and physiologic changes during the childbearing period
  X. Life span care: Interventions to facilitate family unit functioning and promote the health and welfare of family members throughout the life span
VI. Health System—Care That Supports Effective Use of the Health Care Delivery System
  Y. Health system mediation: Interventions to facilitate the interface between client/family and the health care system
  a. Health system management: Interventions to provide and enhance support services for the delivery of care
  b. Information management: Interventions to facilitate communication among health care providers
VII. Community—Care That Supports the Health of the Community
  a. Community Health Promotion: Interventions that promote health of community
  b. Community Risk Management: Interventions that assist in detecting or preventing health risk to the whole community

With permission from McCloskey, J., & Bulechek, G.(2000). *Nursing interventions classification* (NIC), 3rd ed., pp. 90–103. St. Louis: Mosby.

mental health problems can manage self-care activities such as bathing, dressing appropriately, selecting adequate nutrition, and sleeping regularly. (Although maintaining adequate nutrition and promoting normal sleep hygiene are considered self-care activities, they are discussed in separate sections because of their significance in mental health care.) Others cannot manage such self-care activities, either because of their symptoms or as a result of the side effects of medications. Because nursing is concerned with maintaining the client's health and well-being, a focus on ADLs can become a nursing priority.

Dorothea Orem's general nursing model is based on the concept of self-care deficit (see Chapter 7). This

model promotes the idea that self-care is learned and that these behaviours regulate human integrity, functioning, and development. This theory actually consists of three nursing theories: self-care deficit, self-care (the core theory), and nursing system. The emphasis on helping the individual develop independence is consistent with client outcomes in psychiatric nursing.

In the inpatient setting, the psychiatric nurse works with the client so that basic self-care activities are completed. During acute phases of psychiatric disorders, the inability to attend to basic self-care tasks, such as getting dressed, is very common. Thus, ability to complete personal hygiene activities (eg, dental care, grooming) is monitored, and clients are assisted in completing such activities. In a psychiatric facility, clients are encouraged and expected to develop independence in completing these basic self-care activities. In the community, monitoring these basic self-care activities is always a part of the nursing visit or clinic appointment.

ACTIVITY AND EXERCISE INTERVENTIONS

In some psychiatric disorders (eg, schizophrenia), people become sedentary and appear to lack the motivation to complete ADLs. This lack of motivation is part of the disorder and requires nursing intervention. In addition, side effects of medication include sedation and lethargy compounding the problem.

The nurse must attend to the client's level of activity. Encouraging regular activity and exercise can improve general well-being and physical health. In some instances, exercise behaviour becomes an abnormal focus of attention, such as in some clients with anorexia nervosa.

When assuming the responsibility of direct care provider, the nurse can help clients identify realistic activities and exercise goals. As leader or manager of a psychiatric unit, the nurse can influence ward routine. However, promoting a healthy lifestyle, including daily exercise, can help clients deal with the weight gain and type II diabetes associated with many psychotropic medications. Some institutions have other professionals (eg, recreational therapists) available for the implementation of exercise programs. As a case manager, the nurse should consider the activity needs of individuals when jointly setting goals.

SLEEP INTERVENTIONS

Many psychiatric disorders and medications are associated with sleep disturbances. Sleep is also disrupted in clients with dementia; such clients may have difficulty falling asleep or may frequently awaken during the night. In dementia of the Alzheimer type, individuals may reverse their sleeping patterns by napping during the day and staying awake at night.

Nonpharmacologic interventions are always used first because of the side-effect risks associated with the use of sedatives and hypnotics (see Chapter 13). Sleep interventions to communicate to clients include the following:
- Go to bed only when tired or sleepy.
- Establish a consistent bedtime routine.
- Avoid stimulating foods, beverages, or medications.
- Avoid naps in the late afternoon or evening.
- Eat lightly before retiring and limit fluid intake.
- Use bed only for sleep or intimacy.
- Avoid emotional stimulation before bedtime.
- Use behavioural and relaxation techniques.
- Limit distractions.

NUTRITION INTERVENTIONS

Psychiatric disorders and medication side effects can affect eating behaviours. For varying reasons, some clients eat too little, whereas others eat too much. For instance, homeless clients with mental illness have difficulty maintaining adequate nutrition because of their deprived lifestyle. Substance abuse also interferes with maintaining adequate nutrition, either through stimulation or suppression of appetite or neglecting nutrition because of drug-seeking behaviour. Thus, nutrition interventions should be specific and relevant to the individual's circumstances and mental health. In addition, recommended daily allowances are important in the promotion of physical and mental health, and nurses should consider them when planning care.

Some psychiatric symptoms involve changes in perceptions of food, appetite, and eating habits. If a client believes that food is poisonous, he or she may eat sparingly or not at all. Interventions are then necessary to address the suspiciousness as well as to encourage adequate intake of recommended daily allowances. Allowing clients to examine foods, participate in preparations, and test the safety of the meal by eating slowly or after everyone else may be necessary.

Obesity is common in people with mental disorders. Antipsychotics, antidepressants, and mood stabilizers are associated with weight gain, which is thought to be related to changes in metabolism and appetite that some of these types of medications cause. Many clients stop taking medications because of the weight gain. Excessive weight gain can be especially stressful to the individual's emotional well-being as well as detrimental to physical health. However, nurses should encourage clients to avoid quick-weight-loss programs because they are not effective. Furthermore, hypoglycemia can exacerbate a depressed mood and lead to suicidal thoughts. If weight gain is a problem, the best approach is to assist the client to monitor current intake and develop realistic strategies for changing eating patterns combined with a healthy lifestyle.

RELAXATION INTERVENTIONS

Relaxation promotes comfort, reduces anxiety, alleviates stress, eases pain, and prevents aggression. It can diminish the effects of hallucinations and delusions. The many different relaxation techniques used as mental health interventions range from simple deep breathing to biofeedback to hypnosis. Although some techniques such as biofeedback require additional training and, in some instances, certification, nurses can easily apply simple relaxation, distraction, and imagery techniques.

Simple relaxation techniques encourage and elicit relaxation to decrease undesirable signs and symptoms. **Distraction** is the purposeful focussing of attention away from undesirable sensations, and **guided imagery** is the purposeful use of imagination to achieve relaxation or direct attention away from undesirable sensations (Table 12-1). These interventions are helpful for people experiencing anxiety; guided imagery is especially useful in stress management.

As a direct care provider, the nurse may teach the client relaxation exercises. As a case manager, nurses can include relaxation exercises in the plan of care. The unit leader can be responsible for ensuring that appropriately prepared staff implement relaxation exercises.

Relaxation techniques that involve physical touch (eg, back rubs) usually are not used for people with mental disorders. Touching and massaging usually are not appropriate for clients with mental disorders, especially those who have a history of physical or sexual

---

Table 12.1   Relaxation Techniques: Descriptions and Implementation

Simple Relaxation Techniques	Distraction	Guided Imagery
<ul><li>Create a quiet, nondisrupting environment with dim lights and a comfortable temperature.</li><li>Instruct the client to assume a relaxed position, wearing loose and comfortable clothing.</li><li>Instruct the client to relax and to let the sensations happen.</li><li>Use a low tone of voice with a slow, rhythmic pace of words.</li><li>Instruct the client to take an initial slow, deep breath (abdominal breathing) while thinking about pleasant events.</li><li>Use soothing music (without words) to enhance relaxation.</li><li>Reinforce the use of relaxation by praising efforts and helping the client to schedule time regularly for it.</li><li>Evaluate and document the client's response to relaxation.</li></ul>	<ul><li>Distraction techniques include music, counting, television, reading, play, and exercise. Help the client choose a technique that will work for him or her.</li><li>Advise the client to practice the distraction technique before he or she will need to use it.</li><li>Have the client develop a specific plan for how and when he or she will use distraction.</li><li>Evaluate and document the client's response to distraction.</li></ul>	<ul><li>Help the client choose a particular guided imagery technique (alone or with others).</li><li>Discuss an image the client has experienced as pleasurable and relaxing, such as lying on a beach, watching snow fall, floating on a raft, or watching the sun set.</li><li>Individualize the images chosen, considering religious or spiritual beliefs, artistic interests, or other individual preferences.</li><li>Make suggestions to induce relaxation (eg, peaceful images, pleasant sensations, or rhythmic breathing).</li><li>Use modulated voice when guiding the imagery experience.</li><li>Have the client travel mentally to the scene, and assist in describing the setting in detail.</li><li>Use permissive directions and suggestions when leading the imagery, such as "perhaps," "if you wish," or "you might like."</li><li>Have the client slowly experience the scene. How does it look? smell? sound? feel? taste?</li><li>Use words or phrases that convey pleasurable images, such as floating, melting, and releasing.</li><li>Develop cleansing or clearing portion of imagery (eg, all pain appears as red dust and washes downstream in a creek as you enter).</li><li>Assist the client in developing a method of ending the imagery technique, such as counting slowly while breathing deeply.</li><li>Encourage expression of thoughts and feelings regarding the experience.</li><li>Prepare the client for unexpected (but often therapeutic) experiences, such as crying.</li><li>Evaluate and document the client's response.</li></ul>

Adapted from: McCloskey, J., & Bulechek, G. (2000). *Nursing interventions classification* (NIC) (3rd ed.). St. Louis: Mosby.

abuse. Such clients may find touching too stimulating or misinterpret it as being sexual or aggressive.

HYDRATION INTERVENTIONS

Assessing fluid status and monitoring fluid intake and output are often important interventions. Overhydration or underhydration can be a symptom of a disorder. For example, some clients with psychotic disorders experience chronic fluid imbalance. For these individuals, a treatment protocol that includes a target weight procedure can help prevent both overhydration and water intoxication and promote self-control (see Chapter 17). The nurse functions as the direct care provider (teaching client), unit leader (delegating weighing of the client to staff), or coordinator of the protocol.

Many psychiatric medications affect fluid and electrolyte balance (see Chapter 9). For example, when taking lithium carbonate, clients must have adequate fluid intake, with special attention paid to serum sodium levels. When sodium levels drop through perspiration, lithium is used in place of sodium, which in turn leads to lithium toxicity. Many psychiatric medications cause dry mouth, which in turn causes individuals to drink fluids excessively. Interventions that help clients understand the relationship of medications to fluid and electrolyte balance are important in their overall care.

THERMOREGULATION INTERVENTIONS

Many psychiatric disorders can disturb the body's normal temperature regulation. Thus, clients cannot sense temperature increases or decreases and consequently cannot protect themselves from extremes of hot or cold. This problem is especially difficult for people who are homeless or live in substandard housing such as some rooming houses. In addition, many psychiatric medications affect the ability to regulate body temperature.

Interventions include educating clients about the problem of thermoregulation, identifying potential extremes in temperatures, and developing strategies to protect the client from the adverse effects of temperature changes. For example, community nurses engage in active outreach to at-risk clients during extreme weather alerts.

PAIN MANAGEMENT

Emotional reactions are often manifested as pain. For instance, chronic, unexplained pain is one of the main symptoms of somatization disorder (see Chapter 21). Chronic pain is particularly problematic because often no cause for it is found.

PMH nurses are more likely to provide care to clients experiencing chronic pain than acute pain. However, a single intervention is seldom successful for relieving chronic pain. In some instances, pain is managed by medication; in other instances, nonpharmacologic techniques, such as simple relaxation techniques, distraction, or imagery, are used. Indeed, relaxation is one of the most widely used cognitive and behavioural approaches to pain. Psychoeducation, stress management techniques, and biofeedback are also used in pain management.

The key to managing pain is engaging the client in identifying how it is disrupting his/her personal, social, professional, and family life. Education focussing on the pain, use of medications for treatment, and development of cognitive skills are important pain management components. In some cases, redefining treatment success as improvement in functioning, rather than alleviation of pain, may be necessary. The interaction between stress and pain is important; that is, increased stress leads to increased pain. Clients can better manage their pain when stress is reduced.

MEDICATION MANAGEMENT

The PMH health nurse uses many medication management interventions to help clients maintain therapeutic regimens. Medication management involves more than the actual administration of medications. Nurses also assess medication effectiveness and side effects and consider drug–drug interactions. Treatment with psychopharmacologic agents can be lengthy because of the chronic nature of many disorders; many clients remain on medication regimens for years, never becoming medication free. Thus, medication education is an ongoing intervention that requires careful documentation. Medication follow-up may include home visits as well as telephone calls.

Interventions for the Psychological Domain

A major emphasis in PMH nursing is on the psychological domain: emotion, behaviour, and cognition. The nurse–client relationship serves as the basis for interventions directed toward the psychological domain. Because the therapeutic relationship was extensively discussed in Chapter 8, it is not covered in this chapter. This section does cover counselling, conflict resolution, recovery orientation, reminiscence, behaviour therapy, cognitive interventions, psychoeducation, health teaching, and spiritual interventions. Chapter 7 presents the theoretic basis for many of these interventions.

Nurses in the direct care role will use all of the psychological interventions to respond to the health care problems of their clients. Nurses in case manager roles will also frequently use interventions from the psychological domain to promote recovery and to empower the client to make changes. Case management relationships are based on trust. The nurse manager oversees the use of the psychological interventions and evaluates the staff's ability to use the interventions and assess outcomes.

COUNSELLING INTERVENTIONS

Counselling interventions are specific, time-limited interactions between a nurse and a client, family, or group experiencing immediate or ongoing difficulties related to their health or well-being. Counselling is usually short term and focusses on improving coping abilities, reinforcing healthy behaviours, fostering positive interactions, or preventing illness and disability. Counselling strategies are discussed throughout the text. Psychotherapy, which differs from counselling, is generally a long-term approach aimed at improving or helping clients regain previous health status and functional abilities. Mental health specialists, such as advanced practice nurses, use psychotherapy.

CONFLICT RESOLUTION

A conflict involves an individual's perception, emotions, and behaviour. In a conflict, a person believes that his or her own needs, interests, wants, or values are incompatible with someone else's. The individual experiences fear, sadness, bitterness, anger, hopelessness, or some combination of these emotions in response to the perceived threat. Consequently, the individual takes action to meet his or her own needs, a course of action that can potentially interfere with the other person's ability to do the same (Mayer, 2000).

Conflict resolution is a specific type of intervention through which the nurse helps clients resolve disagreements or disputes with family, friends, or other clients. Conflict can be positive if individuals see the problem as solvable and providing an opportunity for growth and interpersonal understanding. The nurse may be in the position of actually resolving a family conflict or teaching family members how to resolve their own conflicts positively. In addition, because nurses are in positions of leadership, they often need conflict resolution skills to settle employee conflicts.

Conflict Resolution Process

Calmness and objectivity are important in resolving any client or family conflict. The desired outcome of conflict resolution is a "win-win" situation—that is, each party feels good about the outcome. Conflict resolution includes the following steps:

1. helping those involved identify the problem;
2. developing expectations for a win-win situation;
3. identifying interests;
4. fostering creative brainstorming; and
5. combining options into a win-win situation (Littlefield, Love, Peck, & Wertheim, 1993).

The first step involves identifying the problem. Because the conflict exists, with each person thinking he or she has the solution, each must express a view of the problem and solution. During this phase, calming of emotions may be necessary. The next step involves developing expectations for a win-win situation by creating an atmosphere of mutual respect and trust. The nurse should avoid taking sides and reassure the involved parties that there may be a way to solve the problem and achieve an outcome about which everyone feels positive. Next, an exploration of underlying issues is important to elicit interest and response. Questions such as, "What do you really want?" or "What are you worried about?" often identify the real issues and target what could become acceptable outcomes. (Nurses need to determine whether they have any underlying issues by asking themselves the same questions.)

The next step, brainstorming creative options, can then occur. The nurse directs participants to create potential solutions. The nurse writes them down without allowing any criticism; deferring judgment of what has been said helps prevent premature rejection of good ideas. The final step involves combining the generated ideas into a win-win situation. The group develops solutions that meet many of the participants' key interests and usually represent new approaches that are acceptable to all (Littlefield et al., 1993).

Cultural Brokering in Client–System Conflicts

At times, clients who are politically and economically powerless find themselves in conflict with the health care system. Differences in cultural values and languages between clients and health care organizations contribute to feelings of powerlessness. For example, new immigrants, people who are homeless, and people who need to make informed decisions under stressful conditions may be unable to navigate the health care system. The nurse can help to resolve such conflicts through **cultural brokering**, the act of bridging, linking, or mediating messages, instructions, and belief systems between groups of people of differing cultural systems to reduce conflict or produce change (Tripp-Reimer, Brink, & Pinkham, 1999).

For the "nurse-as-broker" to be effective, he or she establishes and maintains a sense of connectedness or relationship with the client. In turn, the nurse also establishes and cultivates networks with other health care facilities and resources. Cultural sensitivity enables the nurse to be aware of and sensitive to the needs of clients from a variety of cultures. Cultural competence is necessary for the brokering process to be effective.

RECOVERY ORIENTATION

Interventions that have a recovery focus are becoming more prevalent in psychiatric and mental health nursing practice. Nurses apply this orientation to their everyday interactions with their clients. For individuals struggling with addictions, self-help, 12-step programs frequently refer to recovery as the abstinence from the addictive behaviour (see Chapter 6 for the 12 Steps of the Alcoholics Anonymous program).

For individuals with schizophrenia or bipolar disorder, a recovery orientation means helping the person regain functioning or "getting on with life," despite having ongoing symptoms of the psychiatric illness. Recovery may refer to what the client does, how the nurse functions, or how the mental health system is organized. One model of recovery suggests that there are **internal and external conditions that promote recovery.** The nurse facilitates the internal conditions on an individual level, which include a sense of **hope** (that recovery is possible), **healing** (having a sense of self outside the illness and some sense of control), **empowerment** (having some autonomy of action, having the courage to act, and taking responsibility for one's actions), and **connection** (having relationships and social roles). The nurse advocates for changes in external conditions, which include **human rights** (having access to basic human resources such as housing and safety and protection from stigma and discrimination), **a positive culture of healing** (having a health care environment that promotes respect and empathy), and **recovery-oriented services** (including a range of treatment and rehabilitation approaches) (Jacobson & Greenley, 2001).

REMINISCENCE

Reminiscence, the thinking about or relating of past experiences, is used as a nursing intervention to enhance life review in older clients. Reminiscence encourages clients, either in individual or group settings, to discuss their past and review their lives. Through reminiscence, individuals can identify past coping strategies that can support them in current stressful situations. Clients can also use reminiscence to maintain self-esteem, stimulate thinking, and support the natural healing process of life review. Activities that facilitate reminiscence include writing an account of past events, making a tape recording and playing it back, explaining pictures in old family albums, drawing a family tree, and writing to old friends.

BEHAVIOUR THERAPY

Behaviour therapy interventions focus on reinforcing or promoting desirable behaviours or altering undesirable ones. The basic premise is that, because most behaviours are learned, new functional behaviours can also be learned. Behaviours—not internal psychic processes—are the targets of the interventions. The models of behavioural theorists serve as a basis for these interventions (see Chapter 7).

Behaviour Modification

Behaviour modification is a specific, systematized behaviour therapy technique that can be applied to individuals, groups, or systems. The aim of behaviour modification is to reinforce desired behaviours and extinguish undesired ones. Desired behaviour is rewarded to increase the likelihood that clients will repeat it and, over time, replace the problematic behaviour with it. Behaviour modification is used for various problematic behaviours, such as dysfunctional eating and addictions, and often is used in the care of children and adolescents.

Token Economy

Used in inpatient settings, a **token economy** applies behaviour modification techniques to multiple behaviours. In a token economy, clients are rewarded with tokens for selected desired behaviours. They can use these tokens to purchase meals, leave the unit, watch television, or wear street clothes. In less restrictive environments, clients use tokens to purchase additional privileges, such as attending social events. Token economy systems have been especially effective in reinforcing positive behaviours in people who are developmentally disabled. The strategy also works with aggressive inpatient (Silverstein, Hatashita-Wong, & Bloch, 2002).

COGNITIVE INTERVENTIONS

Cognitive interventions are verbally structured interventions that reinforce and promote desirable, or alter undesirable, cognitive functioning. The belief underlying this approach is that thoughts guide emotional reactions, motivations, and behaviours. Cognitive interventions do not solve problems for clients but help clients develop new ways of viewing situations so that they can solve problems themselves. Nurses may use several models as the basis for cognitive interventions, but all models assume that, by changing the cognitive appraisal of a situation (view of the world) and by examining the meaning of events, clients can reinterpret situations. In turn, emotional changes will follow the cognitive changes, and, ultimately, behaviours will change.

CRNE Note

Use principles of teaching/learning in health promotion. This applies across all areas of nursing.

Because people develop their thinking patterns throughout their lifetime, many thoughts become so automatic that they are outside individuals' awareness. Thus, a person may be unaware of the automatic thoughts that influence his or her actions or other thoughts. **Automatic thinking** is often subject to errors or tangible distortions of reality that contradict objective appraisals. For example, a client with depression may be convinced that no one cares about him when, in fact, his family and friends are deeply concerned. **Illogical thinking,** another thinking error, occurs when a person draws a faulty conclusion. For example, a college student is so devastated by failing an examination that she perceives her college career to be over.

To engage in cognitive treatment, the client must be capable of introspection and reflection about thoughts and fantasies. Cognitive interventions are used in a wide range of clinical situations, from short-term crises to persistent mental disorders. Cognitive interventions also include thought stopping, contracting, and cognitive restructuring. These specific interventions are discussed in Chapter 14.

PSYCHOEDUCATION

Psychoeducation uses educational strategies to teach clients the skills they lack because of a psychiatric disorder. The goal of psychoeducation is a change in knowledge and behaviour. Nurses use psychoeducation to meet the educational needs of clients by adapting teaching strategies to their disorder-related deficits. As clients gain skills, functioning improves. Some clients may need to learn how to maintain their morning hygiene. Others may need to understand their illness and cope with hearing voices that others do not hear.

Specific psychoeducation techniques are based on adult learning principles, such as beginning at the point the learner is currently at and building on his or her current experiences. Thus, the nurse assesses the client's current skills and readiness to learn. From there, the nurse individualizes a teaching plan for each client. He or she can conduct such teaching in a one-to-one situation or a group format.

Psychoeducation is a continuous process of assessing, setting goals, developing learning activities, and evaluating for changes in knowledge and behaviour. Nurses use it with individuals, groups, families, and communities. Psychoeducation serves as a basis for psychosocial

rehabilitation, a service-delivery approach for those with severe and persistent mental illness (see Chapter 17).

HEALTH TEACHING

Teaching-coaching is one of the standards of care for the psychiatric nurse (CFMHN, 2005). According to this standard, the PMH nurse "attempts to understand the life experience of the client and uses this understanding to support and promote learning related to health and personal development" (CFMHN, 2005, p. 10). Based on principles of teaching, health teaching involves collaborating with the client to determine learning needs and transmitting new information, "while considering the context of the client's life experiences. [The nurse] considers readiness, culture, literacy, language, preferred learning style, and resources available" (CFMHN, 2005, p. 10). According to the *Canadian Standards of Psychiatric and Mental Health Nursing,* "all interactions between the nurse and patient are potentially teaching/learning situations" (CFMHN, 2005, p. 10). Thus, in health teaching, the PMH nurse attends to potential health care problems in addition to mental disorders and emotional problems. For example, if a person has diabetes mellitus and is taking insulin, the nurse provides health care teaching related to diabetes and the interaction of this problem with the mental disorder (Fig 12.2).

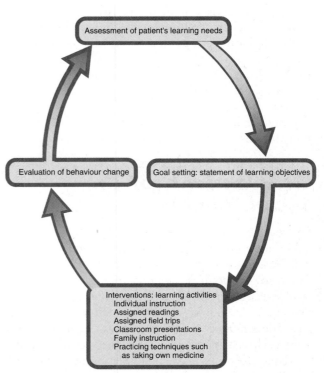

FIGURE 12.2 Teaching evaluation model. (Adapted from Rankin, S., & Stallings, K. [1990]. *Patient education* [p. 252]. Philadelphia: J. B. Lippincott.)

CRNE Note

Nursing competencies include intervening in mental health crises and facilitating the client's reintegration with family and community.

BOX 12.2

Hold the Hope

One concept that cuts across all nursing interventions is hope. Promoting hope in the client has long been identified as one of the key ingredients of psychotherapy. Without being unrealistically hopeful, the nurse conveys that some positive outcome is possible. Given that many psychiatric illnesses are characterized by a lack of hope, and that suicide rates can be distressingly high, it is important for the nurse to combat hopelessness.

Strategies to promote hope begin with deep listening to the client's story. Showing respect for the client's perspective while believing that recovery is possible helps the client and nurse to connect at a deeper level. By careful listening to the story, the nurse can begin to understand what is important to this unique human being. Talking openly about the future with a view to assisting the client to set and meet small goals can promote hope, as can promoting supportive connections with others.

One participant in a qualitative research study on hope and schizophrenia described the role of nurses in helping her to be hopeful.

I'd say the most important thing is to listen to the person and try to understand why they don't feel hopeful, which is probably because they have an illness over which they have very little control. To try and understand, it's something that until you've experienced it, you can't understand. But it's important for others to try and see themselves in that person's shoes and have empathy for them. It is important to realize that hope is something that is difficult for them to achieve, but it's not impossible. If you can hold the hope for someone who has no hope, at that moment when they start to feel better, you can pass the hope back over to them. It's nice to have someone who holds the hope for you, especially when you feel like you have no hope.

From Kirkpatrick, H., Landeen, J., Woodside, H., & Byrne, C. (2001). How people with schizophrenia build their hope. *Journal of Psychosocial Nursing, 39*(1), 46–53.

SPIRITUAL INTERVENTIONS

Spiritual care is based on an assessment of the client's spiritual needs. A nonjudgmental relationship and just "being with" (not doing for) the client are keys to providing spiritual intervention. In some instances, clients ask to see a religious leader. Nurses should always respect and never deny these requests. To assist people in spiritual distress, the nurse should know and understand the beliefs and practices of various spiritual groups. **Spiritual support,** assisting clients to feel balance and connection within their relationships, involves listening to expressions of loneliness, using empathy, and providing clients with desired spiritual articles.

Fostering hope is an important aspect of all nursing interventions, including spiritual ones. See Box 12-2.

Interventions for the Social Domain

The social domain includes the individual's environment and its affect on his or her responses to mental disorders and distress. Interventions within the social domain are geared toward couples, families, friends, and large and small social groups, with special attention given to ethnicity and community interactions. In some instances, nurses design interventions that affect a client's environment, such as helping a family member decide to place a loved one in long-term care. In other instances, the nurse actually modifies the environment to promote positive behaviours. Group and family interventions are discussed in Chapters 15 and 16, respectively.

SOCIAL BEHAVIOUR AND PRIVILEGE SYSTEMS INPATIENT UNITS

In psychiatric units, unrelated strangers who have problems interacting live together in close quarters. For this reason, most psychiatric units develop a list of behavioural expectations, called *unit rules*, that staff members post and explain to clients upon admittance. Their purpose is to facilitate a comfortable and safe environment and have little to do with the clients' reasons for admission. Getting up at certain times, showering before breakfast, making the bed, and not visiting in others' rooms are typical expectations. It is usually the nurse manager who oversees the operation of the unit and implementation of privilege systems.

Most psychiatric facilities use a privilege system to protect clients and to reinforce unit rules and other appropriate behaviour (also see the previous section discussing a token economy). The more appropriate the behaviour, the more privileges of freedom the person has. Privileges are based on the assessment of a client's risk to harm himself or herself or others and ability to follow treatment regimens. For example, a client with few privileges may be required to stay on the unit and eat only with other clients. A client with full privileges may have freedom to leave the unit and go outside the hospital and into the community for short periods.

MILIEU THERAPY

Milieu therapy provides a stable and coherent social organization to facilitate an individual's treatment. (The terms *milieu therapy* and *therapeutic environment* are often used interchangeably.) In milieu therapy, the design of the physical surroundings, structure of client activities, and promotion of a stable social structure and cultural setting enhance the setting's therapeutic potential. A therapeutic milieu facilitates client interactions and promotes personal growth. Milieu therapy is the responsibility of the nurse in collaboration with the client and other health care providers. The key concepts of milieu therapy include containment, validation, structured interaction, and open communication.

Containment

Containment is the process of providing safety and security and involves the client's access to food and shelter. In a well-contained milieu, clients feel safe from their illnesses and protected against social stigma. The physical surroundings are also important in this process and should be clean and comfortable, with special attention paid to promoting a noninstitutionalized environment. Pictures on walls, comfortable furniture, and soothing colours help clients relax. Most facilities encourage clients and nursing staff to wear street clothes, which helps decrease the formalized nature of hospital settings and promotes nurse–client relationships.

Therapeutic milieus emphasize client involvement in treatment decisions and operation of the unit; nurses should encourage freedom of movement within the contained environment. Clients participate in maintaining the quality of the physical surroundings, assuming responsibility for making their own beds, attending to their own belongings, and keeping an acceptable living area. Families are viewed as a part of the client's life, and ties are maintained. In most inpatient settings, specific times are set for family interaction, education, and treatment. Family involvement is often a criterion for admission for treatment, and the involvement may include regular family attendance at therapy sessions.

Validation

In a therapeutic environment, **validation** is another process that affirms client individuality. Staff–client interactions should constantly reaffirm the client's humanity and human rights. Any interaction a staff member initiates with a client should reflect his or her respect for that client. Clients must believe that staff members truly like and respect them.

As stated, clients should participate in treatment decisions. When possible, the roles between clients and nurses are blurred, and nurses view clients as responsible human beings in charge of their own treatment decisions. Such expectations validate the humanity of clients.

Structured Interaction

One of the most interesting milieu concepts is **structured interaction**, purposeful interaction that allows clients to interact with others in a useful way. For instance, the daily community meeting provides structure to explain unit rules and consequences of violations. Ideally, clients who are either elected or volunteer for the responsibility assume leadership for these meetings. In the meeting, the group discusses behavioural expectations, such as making beds daily, appropriate dress, and rules for leaving the unit. Usually, there are other rules, such as no fighting or name calling (Table 12-2).

Table 12.2	Client–Staff Community Meeting
Goal	**Implementation**
Plan ahead.	• Designate leader and several deputy leaders. • Hold brief meeting with staff.
Operate the meeting.	• Establish rules and norms. • Announce the purpose, format, and rules (include clients who know the routine). • Keep meeting brief. • Refer treatment questions to outside of meeting.
Get everyone involved.	• Ask everyone to introduce themselves. • Address individuals by name. • Use structured exercises to engage all clients. • Delegate tasks of meeting to individuals.
Infuse energy.	• Use exercises to mobilize energy. • Use humour and empathy. • Maintain a lively and interesting approach.
Choose relevant topics.	• Focus on discussion of issues that affect all. • Deal with difficult issues calmly and frankly. • Affirm rules and norms.
Address unit process.	• Discuss needs of unit at each meeting: containment, structure, support, involvement, validation. • Discuss strategies.

From Kahn, F. (1994). The patient–staff community meeting: Old tools, new rules. *Journal of Psychosocial Nursing, 32*(8), 23–26.

In some instances, the treatment team assigns structured interactions to specific clients as part of their treatment. Specific attitudes or approaches are directed toward individual clients who benefit from a particular type of interaction. Nurses consistently assume indulgence, flexibility, passive or active friendliness, matter-of-fact attitude, casualness, watchfulness, or kind firmness when interacting with specific clients. For example, if a client is known to overreact and dramatize events, the staff may provide a matter-of-fact attitude when the client engages in dramatic behaviour.

Open Communication

In **open communication,** staff and client willingly share information. Staff members invite client self-disclosure within the support of a nurse–client relationship. In addition, they provide a model of effective communication when interacting with one another as well as with clients. They arrange an environment to facilitate optimal interaction and resocialization. Support, attention, praise, and reassurance given to clients improves self-esteem and increases confidence. Client education is also a part of this support, as are directions to foster coping skills.

Milieu Therapy in Different Settings

Milieu therapy is applied in various settings. In long-term care settings, the therapeutic milieu becomes essential because clients may reside there for months or years. These clients typically have schizophrenia or developmental disabilities. Structure in daily living is important to the successful functioning of the individuals and the overall group but must be applied within the context of individual needs. For example, if a client cannot get up one morning in time to complete assigned tasks (eg, showering or making a bed) because of a personal crisis the night before, the nurse should consider the situation compassionately and flexibly, not applying the "consequences" rule or taking away the client's privileges. In turn, the nurse must weigh individual needs against the collective needs of all the clients. For the client who is consistently late for treatment activities, the nurse should apply the rules of the unit, even if it means taking away privileges.

Recently, concepts of milieu therapy have been applied to short-term inpatient and community settings. In acute-care inclient settings, nursing actions provide limits to and controls on client behaviour and provide structure and safety for the clients. Milieu treatments are based on the individual needs of the clients and include relaxation groups, discussion groups, and medication groups. Spontaneous and planned activities are possible on a short-term unit as well as in a long-term setting. In the community, it is possible to apply milieu

therapy approaches in day treatment centers, group homes, and single dwellings.

PROMOTION OF CLIENT SAFETY ON PSYCHIATRIC UNITS

Although the use of social rules of conduct and privilege systems can enhance smooth operation of a unit, some potentially serious problems can be associated with these practices. A most critical aspect of PMH nursing is the promotion of client safety, especially in inpatient units.

Observation

Observation is the ongoing assessment of the client's mental status to identify and subvert any potential problem. An important process in all nursing practice, observation is particularly important in psychiatric nursing. In psychiatric settings, clients are ambulatory and thus more susceptible to environmental hazards. In addition, judgment and cognition impairment are symptoms of many psychiatric disorders. Often, clients are admitted because they pose a danger to themselves or others. In PMH nursing, observation is more than just "seeing" clients. It means continually monitoring them for any indication of harm to themselves or others.

All clients who are hospitalized for psychiatric reasons are continually monitored. The intensity of the observation depends on their risk to themselves and others. Some clients are merely asked to "check in" at different times of the day, whereas others have a staff member assigned to only them, such as in instances of potential suicide. Mental health facilities and units all have policies that specify levels of observation for clients at varying degrees of risk.

De-escalation

De-escalation is an interactive process of calming and redirecting a client who has an immediate potential for violence directed toward self or others. This intervention involves assessing the situation and preventing it from escalating to one in which injury occurs to the client, staff, or other clients. Once the nurse has assessed the situation, he or she calmly calls to the client and asks the individual to leave the situation. The nurse must avoid rushing toward the client or giving orders (see Chapter 35). Nurses can use various interventions in this situation, including distraction, conflict resolution, and cognitive interventions.

Seclusion

Seclusion is the involuntary confinement of a person in a room or an area where the person is physically prevented

BOX 12.3 RESEARCH FOR BEST PRACTICE

Seclusion Perceived as Punishment

THE QUESTION: What are patients' perceptions of seclusion?

METHODS: Twelve patients receiving acute inpatient psychiatric care participated in semistructured interviews to elicit their perceptions of seclusion. Assessed areas of interest included perceptions of the reasons for seclusion, feelings while in seclusion, perceptions of staff about the seclusion experience, and attitudes about the seclusion environment.

FINDINGS: Five themes recurred. Most patients felt that they were secluded inappropriately and experienced seclusion as punishment. The experience generated negative emotions. Patients reported feeling angry before, during, and after the seclusion episode and directed their anger primarily toward the staff involved. Anger usually gave way to a sense of powerlessness. The social isolation and physical characteristics of the seclusion room combined to distort reality, making some patients feel as if they were "going mad" or "losing control." Patients did develop several strategies to assist them in coping with their restricted environment, including talking to themselves, singing, and pacing. Finally, the level of interaction with staff during and after seclusion was a source of dissatisfaction. Patients believed that if communication had been more effective, they would not have ended up in seclusion.

IMPLICATIONS FOR NURSING: This study supports avoiding the use of seclusion as a control measure. The experience is negative and does not foster positive mental health. Patients view seclusion as punishment, blocking effective nurse–patient communication.

Meehan, T., Vermeer, C., & Windsor, C. (2000). Patients' perceptions of seclusion: A qualitative investigation. *Journal of Advanced Nursing*, 31(2), 370–377.

from leaving (Centers for Medicare & Medicaid Services [CMS], 2002). A client is placed in seclusion for purposes of safety or behavioural management. The seclusion room has no furniture except a mattress and a blanket. The walls usually are padded. The room is environmentally safe, with no hanging devices, electrical outlets, or windows from which the client could jump. Once a client is placed in seclusion, he or she is observed at all times.

There are several types of seclusion arrangements. Some facilities have seclusion rooms next to the nurses' stations that have an observation window. Other facilities use a modified client room and assign a staff member to view the client at all times.

Seclusion is an extremely negative client experience; consequently, its use is seriously questioned (Meehan, Vermeer, & Windsor, 2000), and many facilities have completely abandoned its practice (Box 12-3). Client outcomes may actually be worse if seclusion is used. In one study, secluded subjects exhibited poorer attitudes toward the hospital and had longer lengths of stay than did their nonsecluded cohorts (Legris, Walters, & Browne, 1999). If units are adequately staffed and personnel are trained in dealing with assaultive clients, seclusion is rarely needed. If seclusion is used, it must follow the same guidelines as the use of restraints (discussed next).

Restraints

In Canada, the laws for restricting the freedom of clients against their will are specific to each province. Restraint is the most restrictive safety intervention and is only used in the most extreme circumstances and as a measure of last resort. Provincial laws, such as the Mental Health Act of Ontario, govern the situations under which restraint may be used.

Chemical restraint is the use of medication to control clients or manage their behaviour. This is distinct from medication used to treat their psychiatric illness. In several provinces, it is possible for a client to be competent to refuse medical treatment but be required to stay in the hospital for psychiatric assessment.

A **physical restraint** is any manual method or physical or mechanical device attached or adjacent to the client's body that restricts freedom of movement or normal access to one's body, material, or equipment and cannot be easily removed. Holding a patient in a manner that restricts movement constitutes restraint for that client (CMS, 2002). Different types of physical restraints are available. Wrist restraints restrict arm movement. Four-point restraints are applied to the wrists and ankles in bed. When five-point restraints are used, all extremities are secured, and another restraint is placed across the chest.

In addition to following provincial law, the nurse must also adhere to hospital policies regarding restraint. A physician's order is necessary for restraint, and nurses should document all of the previously tried de-escalation interventions before the application of restraint. Nurses should limit use of restraints to times when an individual is judged to be a danger to self or others; they should apply restraints only until the client has gained control over behaviour. When a client is in physical restraints, the nurse should closely observe the client and protect him or her from self-injury.

Given the negative consequences to the client, and the impact on the nurse–client relationship, it is essential that nurses treat the client with respect and dignity at all times during a psychiatric emergency that necessitates seclusion or restraint. Every incident should be followed by a thorough debriefing to identify how the situation might have been avoided (See Chapter 5).

HOME VISITS

Clients usually have been hospitalized or have received treatment for acute psychiatric symptoms before being referred to psychiatric home service. The goal of **home visits**, the delivery of nursing care in the client's living environment, is to maximize the client's functional ability within the nurse–client relationship and with the family or partner as appropriate. The PMH nurse who makes home visits needs to be able to work independently, is skilled in teaching clients and families, can administer and monitor medications, and uses community resources for the client's needs.

Traditional home visits are regaining popularity, particularly when the client has concomitant psychiatric and physical illnesses.

Home visits are especially useful in several different situations, including helping reluctant clients enter therapy, conducting a comprehensive assessment, strengthening a support network, and maintaining clients in the community when their condition deteriorates. Home visits are also useful in helping individuals become compliant in taking medication. One major advantage of home visits is the opportunity to provide family members with information and education and to engage them in planning and interventions.

Home visits also help providers develop cultural sensitivity to families from a variety of backgrounds. Home-based interventions allow the nurse to assess the family structure and interactions, including the roles various members play, how the family functions in terms of responsibilities, and the family life cycle. See Chapter 15. A family's cultural background influences all these factors, and culture is important to consider when planning interventions.

The home visit process consists of three steps: the previsit phase, the home visit, and the postvisit phase. During previsit planning, the nurse sets goals for the home visit based on data received from other health care providers or the client. In addition, the nurse and client agree on the time of the visit. As the nurse travels to the home, he or she should assess the neighbourhood for access to services, socioeconomic factors, and safety.

The actual visit can be divided into four parts. The first is the greeting phase, in which the nurse establishes rapport with family members. Greetings, which are usually brief, establish the communication process and the atmosphere for the visit. Greetings should be friendly but professional. In cultures that consider greetings important, this phase may involve more formal interactions, such as taking food or tea with family members. The next phase establishes the focus of the visit. Sometimes the purpose of the visit is medication administration, health teaching, or counselling. The client and family must be clear regarding the purpose. The implementation of the service is the next phase and

should use most of the visit time. If the purpose of the visit is problem solving or decision making, the family's cultural values may determine the types of interaction and decision-making approaches. Closure is the last phase, the end of the home visit. It is a time to summarize and clarify important points. The nurse should also schedule any additional visits and reiterate client expectations between visits. Usually, the nurse is the only provider to see the client regularly. The nurse should acknowledge family members on leaving if they were not a part of the visit.

The post-visit phase includes documentation, reporting, and follow-up planning. This time is also when the nurse meets with the supervisor and presents data from the home visit at the team meeting.

COMMUNITY ACTION

Nurses have a unique opportunity to promote mental health awareness and support humane treatment for people with mental disorders. Activities range from being an advisor to support groups to participating in the political process through lobbying efforts and serving on community mental health boards. These unpaid activities are usually outside the realm of a particular job. However, an important role of professionals is to provide community service in addition to service through income-generating positions.

SUMMARY OF KEY POINTS

- Nurses develop nursing interventions from assessment data and organize them around nursing diagnoses. The client outcomes and the *Canadian Standards of Psychiatric and Mental Health Nursing* (2005) guide their selection.
- The ability of clients with psychiatric disorders to manage self-care activities varies. The Orem self-care model is often used in conceptualizing client needs and implementing interventions.
- Interventions focussing on the biologic areas include activity and exercise; sleep, nutrition, relaxation, hydration, and thermoregulation interventions; pain management; and medication management. Nutritional interventions are used with most clients with psychiatric disorders. Medication management is a priority because of the long-term nature of the disorders and the importance of medication compliance.
- Interventions focussing on the psychological dimensions include counselling, behaviour therapy, cognitive interventions, psychoeducation, health teaching, and others. Implementation of these interventions requires a broad theoretic knowledge base.
- Interventions focussing on the social dimensions include group and family approaches, milieu therapy,

safety interventions, home visits, and community action. On an inpatient psychiatric unit, the nurse uses milieu therapy to maximize the treatment effects of the client's environment.

CRITICAL THINKING CHALLENGES

1 Tom, a 25-year-old man with schizophrenia, lives with his parents, who want to retire to Vancouver Island. Tom goes to work each day but relies on his mother for meals, laundry, and reminders to take his medication. Tom believes that he can manage the home, but his mother is concerned. She asks the nurse for advice about leaving her son to manage on his own. Identify a nursing diagnosis and interventions that would meet some of Tom's potential responses to his changing lifestyle.

2 Joan, a 35-year-old married woman, is admitted to an acute psychiatric unit for stabilization of her mood disorder. She is extremely depressed but refuses to consider a recommended medication change. She asks the nurse what to do. Using a nursing intervention, explain how you would approach Joan's problem.

3 A nurse reports to work for the evening shift. The unit is chaotic. The television in the day room is loud; two clients are arguing about the program. Visitors are mingling in clients' rooms. The temperature of the unit is hot. One client is running up and down the hall yelling, "Help me, help me." Using a milieu therapy approach, what would you do to calm the unit?

WEB LINKS

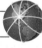

www.cfmhn.org   The Canadian Federation for Mental Health Nurses is an Associate member of the Canadian Nurses Association. The website contains conference information and standards related to psychiatric nursing practice in Canada.

www.rnao.org/bestpractices   The Registered Nurses Association of Ontario publishes best practice guidelines related to all aspects of nursing.

www.cmha.ca   The Canadian Mental Health Association website contains information for health professionals and the general public about a broad range of mental health issues.

REFERENCES

American Nurses Association (ANA), American Psychiatric Nurses Association, & International Society of Psychiatric–Mental Health Nurses. (2000). *Scope and standards of psychiatric and mental health nursing practice.* Washington, DC: American Nurses Publishing.

Burks, K. J. (1999). A nursing model for chronic illness. *Rehabilitation Nursing, 24*(5), 197–200.

Bustillo, J. R., Lauriello, J., Horan, W. P., et al. (2001). The psychosocial treatment of schizophrenia: An update. *American Journal of Psychiatry, 158,* 163–175.

Campbell, J. C., & Soeken, K. L. (1999). Women's responses to battering: A test of the model. *Research in Nursing & Health, 22*(1), 49–58.

Canadian Federation of Mental Health Nurses. (2005). *Canadian standards of psychiatric and mental health nursing practice* (2nd ed.). Retrieved September 15, 2005, from http://www.cfmhn.org/documents/standards.

Centers for Medicare & Medicaid Services. (2002). *Interpretive guidelines for hospital CoP for patients rights. Quality of care information, quality standards.* Available at: www.cms.hhs.gov/manuals.

Jacobson, N., & Greenley, D. (2001). What is recovery? A conceptual model and explication. *Psychiatric Services, 52*(4), 482–485.

Kahn, E. (1994). The patients–staff community meeting: Old tools, new rules. *Journal of Psychosocial Nursing, 32*(8), 23–26.

Legris, J., Walters, M., & Browne, G. (1999). The impact of seclusion on the treatment outcomes of psychotic inpatients. *Journal of Advanced Nursing, 30*(2), 448–459.

Littlefield, L., Love, A., Peck, C., & Wertheim, E. (1993). A model for resolving conflict: Some theoretical, empirical and practical implications. Special issue: The psychology of peace and conflict. *Australian Psychologist, 28*(2), 80–85.

Mayer, B. (2000). *The dynamics of conflict resolution.* San Francisco: Jossey-Bass.

McCloskey, J., & Bulechek, G. (2000). *Nursing interventions classification* (NIC) (3rd ed.) St. Louis: Mosby Year Book

Meehan, T., Vermeer, C., & Windsor, C. (2000). Patients' perceptions of seclusion: A qualitative investigation. *Journal of Advanced Nursing, 3*(2), 370–377.

Rankin, S., & Stallings, K. (1990). *Patient education.* Philadelphia: J.B. Lippincott.

Silverstein, S. M., Hatashita-Wong, M., & Bloch, A. (2002). A second chance for people with 'treatment-refractory' psychosis. *Psychiatric Services, 53*(4), 480.

Tripp-Reimer, T., Brink, P., & Pinkham, C. (1999). Cultural brokerage. In J. McCloskey, & G. Bulechek (Eds.), *Nursing interventions: Effective nursing treatments* (pp. 637–649). Philadelphia: W. B. Saunders.

13

Psychopharmacology

Kathleen Hegadoren and Susan McCabe

LEARNING OBJECTIVES

After studying this chapter, you will be able to:

- Explain the key role of neurotransmitter chemicals and their receptor sites in the action of psychopharmacologic medications.
- Explain the role of receptors in the brain and other organ systems in the actions of psychotropic medications.
- Define the three properties that determine the strength and effectiveness of a medication.
- Describe hypothesized mechanisms of action for major classes of psychopharmacologic medication.
- Describe the major therapeutic effects as well as prevalent side effects of various classes of psychotropic medications.
- Suggest appropriate nursing methods to administer medications that facilitate efficacy.
- Implement interventions to minimize side effects of psychopharmacologic medications.
- Differentiate acute and chronic medication-induced movement disorders.
- Identify aspects of patient teaching that nurses must implement for successful maintenance of patients using psychotropic medications.
- Analyze the potential benefits and risks associated with other forms of somatic treatments, including electroconvulsive therapy, light therapy, and nutrition therapy.
- Evaluate potential causes of nonadherence and implement interventions to improve adherence with treatment regimens.

KEY TERMS

absorption ▪ adherence ▪ adverse reactions ▪ affinity ▪ agonists ▪ akathisia ▪ antagonists ▪ bioavailability ▪ biotransformation ▪ desensitization ▪ distribution ▪ dystonia ▪ efficacy ▪ excretion ▪ first-pass effect ▪ half-life ▪ intrinsic activity ▪ kindling ▪ metabolism ▪ pharmacogenomics ▪ phototherapy ▪ protein binding ▪ pseudoparkinsonism ▪ selectivity ▪ side effects ▪ solubility ▪ tardive dyskinesia ▪ target symptoms ▪ therapeutic index ▪ tolerance ▪ toxicity

KEY CONCEPTS

- psychopharmacology ▪ receptors

Throughout history, treatment choices for mental disorders have been linked to the prevailing assumptions about the aetiology of these illnesses. In the early 1900s, Emil Kraeplin classified mental disorders based on clusters of observed symptoms, providing the basic tenets of the contemporary biologic approach to understanding and treating psychiatric disorders. However, this approach fell out of favour as psychoanalytic, psychodynamic, interpersonal, and other therapies flourished and mental disorders were increasingly assumed to have primarily a psychological aetiology. In the 1950s, when it was discovered that the phenothiazine medications, such as chlorpromazine (Thorazine), relieved many of the symptoms of psychosis, and iproniazid, a medication for treating tuberculosis, elevated mood, there was renewed interest in neurophysiology and biologic treatments.

Recent scientific and technologic developments have renewed awareness of the biologic basis of mental disorders, leading to a proliferation of new medications that act at the cellular level, producing major behavioural and psychological change. These medications provide relief from debilitating symptoms in millions of individuals with psychiatric disorders. They have become the dominant form of treatment and are the cornerstones of all psychiatric treatment.

Most psychiatric–mental health nurses work with individuals who are receiving psychopharmacologic agents as part of their treatment. As awareness of the prevalence of mental disorders increases, these medications are increasingly prescribed in primary care settings, and even nurses working in nonpsychiatric settings now need an in-depth knowledge of these medications to care for their patients in any setting (Hegadoren, 2004).

> ⬢ **KEY CONCEPT Psychopharmacology** is a subspecialty of pharmacology that studies medications that affect the brain and behaviours and that are used to treat psychiatric disorders. It is important to remember, however, that many drugs used to treat other conditions, such as pain syndromes and heart disease, have powerful effects in the brain.

This chapter reviews the major classes of psychopharmacologic drugs used in treating mental disorders, including antipsychotics, mood stabilizers, antidepressants, antianxiety medications, and stimulants, and provides a basis for understanding the specific biologic treatments of psychiatric disorders that are described more fully in later chapters.

The target for psychiatric medications is predominantly the central nervous system (CNS) at the cellular and synaptic level, although the autonomic nervous system often contributes to the pharmacologic profile of psychiatric drugs. For this reason, this chapter focuses on understanding the impact of psychotropic medications on the basic unit of CNS functioning, the synapse, and on receptors embedded in neuronal cell membranes. This basic understanding allows the psychiatric–mental health nurse to accept the role and responsibilities of administering medications, monitoring and treating side effects, and educating the patient and family, which is crucial to successful psychopharmacologic therapy. In addition to psychopharmacologic therapy, other biologic treatments (sometimes referred to as *somatic treatments*) are used. These therapies include electroconvulsive therapy, light therapy, and nutritional therapy and are discussed later.

PHARMACODYNAMICS

A comparatively small amount of medication can have a significant and large impact on cell function and resulting behaviour. When tiny molecules of medication are compared with the vast amount of cell surface in the human body, the fraction seems disproportionate. Yet the drugs used to treat mental disorders often have profound effects on behaviour. To understand how this occurs, one needs to understand both where and how drugs work.

Targets of Drug Action: Where Drugs Act

Drug molecules do not act on the entire cell surface, but rather at receptor sites. Many psychopharmacologic drugs, especially older classes, act at multiple receptors. Newer agents are more specific to one type of receptor, but none is exclusive to one type of receptor. Another key to understanding drug effects is the distribution of receptors within the body. Differing types of receptors and subtypes of receptors can be concentrated in specific brain regions. Thus, there is a close relationship between drug effects and the functions associated with a brain region.

> ⬢ **KEY CONCEPT** Receptors are associated with the work of German chemist Paul Erhlich, who in 1900 suggested that a receptive substance exists within the cell membrane. The biologic action of a drug depends on how its structure interacts with a specific receptor. The importance of receptor sites is now firmly established and is a key to understanding how drugs work in the body.

Receptors are proteins that exist within the cell membrane and have binding sites for both naturally occurring chemicals (called endogenous substances) and administered drugs. Endogenous brain chemicals involved in neurotransmission, such as dopamine and serotonin, adhere to specific groups of receptors. Administered drugs may compete with neurotransmitters for these receptors by

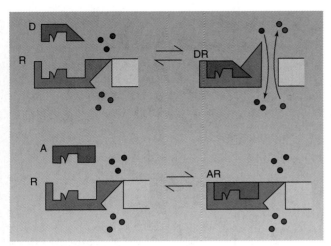

FIGURE 13.1   Agonist and antagonist drug actions at a receptor site. This schematic drawing represents drug–receptor interactions. At *top,* drug D has the correct shape to fit receptor R, forming a drug–receptor complex, which results in a conformational change in the receptor and the opening of a pore in the adjacent membrane. Drug D is an agonist. At *bottom,* drug A also has the correct shape to fit the receptor, forming a drug–receptor complex, but in this case, there is no conformational change and, therefore, no response. Drug A is, therefore, an antagonist.

mimicking or blocking the action of the neurotransmitter. In this chapter, **receptor** refers only to those membrane proteins to which a neurotransmitter can specifically adhere to produce a change in the cell membrane, serving a physiologic regulatory function (such as those discussed in Chapter 9). These include ligand-gated ion channels or the G-protein–coupled receptors.

Receptors

Many drugs have been developed to act specifically at the receptor sites. Their chemical structure is similar to the neurotransmitter substance for that receptor. When attached, these drugs act as **agonists**—chemicals producing the same biologic action as the neurotransmitter itself—or as **antagonists**—chemicals blocking the biologic action of an agonist at a given receptor. Figure 13-1 illustrates the action of an agonist and an antagonist drug at a receptor site.

Selectivity

A drug's ability to interact with a given receptor type may be judged by three properties. The first property, called **selectivity,** is the ability of the drug to be specific for a particular receptor. If a drug is highly selective, it will interact only with its specific receptors in the areas of the body where these receptors occur and, therefore, not affect tissues and organs where its receptors do not occur. Using a "lock-and-key" analogy, only a specific, highly selective key will fit a given lock. The more selective or structurally specific a drug is, the more

likely it will affect only the specific receptors for which it is meant. The more receptors for other neurochemicals are affected, the more unintended effects, or **side effects,** are produced. Selectivity is important to understand because it helps explain the concept of side effects caused by medications, a major cause of concern in medication treatment. The distribution of receptors in specific brain regions also plays a role in the side-effect profile. For example, dopamine antagonists can produce dystonic movements because high concentrations of dopamine receptors are found in the region of the brain that controls fine motor movement.

Affinity

The second property is that of **affinity,** which is the degree of attraction or strength of the bond between the drug and its receptor. Normally, these bonds are produced by relatively weak electrochemical attractions. Basic to the action of most drugs within the body is their ability to bind to a receptor, produce a response, and then easily move off the receptor. Although most drugs used in psychiatry have this on–off property in relation to their target receptors, some drugs, specifically the monoamine oxidase inhibitors (discussed later), have a different type of bond, called a *covalent bond.* This type of bond is stronger and irreversible at normal temperatures. The effects of the drugs that form covalent bonds are often called "irreversible" because new receptors must be produced, a process taking several weeks.

Intrinsic Activity

The final property of a drug's ability to interact with a given receptor is that of **intrinsic activity** or the ability of the drug to produce a biologic response once it becomes attached to the receptor. Some drugs have selectivity and affinity but produce no biologic response; therefore, an important measure of a drug is whether it produces a change in the cell containing the receptor. Drugs that act as agonists have all three properties: selectivity, affinity, and intrinsic activity. However, antagonists have only selectivity and affinity because they produce no biologic response by attaching to that receptor. However, in complex biologic systems such as the brain, preventing an agonist from binding can yield multiple cellular and ultimately behavioural responses. An example of this is the antipsychotic class, all members of which are antagonists.

Some drugs act as *partial agonists.* When a stronger agonist with high intrinsic activity is combined with a weaker agonist (low intrinsic activity) that has high affinity for a given receptor, the net effect is that the weaker agonist will act as an antagonist to the stronger agonist. Because it has some intrinsic activity (although weak), it is referred to as a *partial agonist.* A drug may act as an agonist at one receptor and an antagonist for another. For some drugs, their activity is dose dependent: at low doses they act as agonists, but at higher doses they act more as antagonists. Medications that have both agonist and antagonist effects are called *mixed agonist–antagonists*.

Ion Channels

Some drugs act directly on ion channels imbedded in the nerve cell membrane. Examples include local anaesthetics that block the entry of sodium into the cell, preventing a nerve impulse, and nicotine that acts as an agonist at nicotinic acetylcholine receptors. In psychiatry, the utility of calcium-channel blockers has been investigated for use with the symptoms of mania, a state of increased activity, euphoria, difficulty sleeping, racing thoughts, and rapid and forced speech (see Chapter 19). Operating on the hypothesis that mania is related to too much neurotransmitter released into the synapse, researchers suggested that modulating the influx of calcium (which stimulates the vesicles to release neurotransmitter) might decrease the symptoms of mania. Although this theory is overly simplistic, it is an example of how neurotransmission may be changed by different drug actions.

The benzodiazepine drugs, frequently used in psychiatry, decrease the symptoms of anxiety and are an example of drugs that affect the ion channels of the nerve cell membrane. The benzodiazepine molecule, in such drugs as diazepam (Valium), works by binding to a region of the gamma-aminobutyric acid (GABA)-receptor chloride channel complex. They facilitate GABA in opening the chloride ion channel, rather than replacing GABA, and have a modulatory effect in opening the ion channel.

Enzymes

Enzymes are complex proteins that catalyze specific biochemical reactions within cells and are the targets for some drugs used to treat mental disorders. For example, monoamine oxidase is the enzyme required to break down most bioamine neurotransmitters, such as norepinephrine, serotonin, and dopamine, and can be inhibited by medications from a group of antidepressants called monoamine oxidase inhibitors (MAOIs). Strong covalent bonds are formed between the medication and the enzyme, which inhibit the ability of the enzyme to inactivate the bioamine neurotransmitters after they have been used, resulting in increased amounts of these neurotransmitters ready for release in the nerve terminals. The inhibitory effect is greater for norepinephrine and serotonin than it is for dopamine. This increase in available norepinephrine and serotonin is thought to initiate the cascade of cellular changes that ultimately relieve the symptoms of depression.

Carrier Proteins: Uptake Receptors

Neurotransmitters are small organic molecules that are released in response to a change in the polarity of the cell membrane (called an action potential), interact with receptors, and then are transported back into the neuronal cell by carrier proteins. In much the same way as receptors, these transporters (also referred to as *uptake receptors*) have recognition sites specific for the type of molecule to be transported. After a neurotransmitter, such as serotonin, has activated receptors in the synapse, its actions are terminated by these transporters that take serotonin back up into the presynaptic cell. Medications specific for this site may block or inhibit this transport and, therefore, increase the amount of the neurotransmitter in the synaptic space available for action on the receptors.

A primary action of most of the antidepressants is to increase the amount of neurotransmitters in the synapse by blocking their reuptake. Older antidepressants block the reuptake of more than one neurotransmitter. The newer antidepressants, such as fluoxetine (Prozac) and sertraline (Zoloft), are more selective for serotonin, whereas reboxetine is more selective for norepinephrine. These newer medications are called selective serotonin reuptake inhibitors (SSRIs) and selective norepinephrine reuptake inhibitors, respectively. These medications have reduced the number of side effects experienced by the patients by acting more selectively. Figure 13-2 illustrates the reuptake blockade of serotonin by an SSRI.

Efficacy and Potency: How Drugs Act

Efficacy is another characteristic of medications to be considered when selecting a drug for treatment of a particular set of symptoms. **Efficacy** is the ability of a drug to produce a desired response. It is important to remember that the degree of receptor occupancy contributes to efficacy, yet it is not the only variable. A drug may occupy a large number of receptors but not produce a response. In contrast, **potency** considers the amount of drug required to produce the desired biologic response. One drug may be able to achieve the

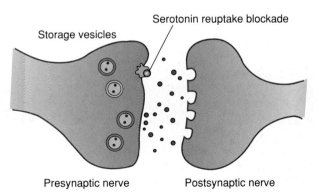

FIGURE 13.2 Reuptake blockade of a carrier molecule for serotonin by a selective serotonin reuptake inhibitor.

same clinical effect as another drug but at a lower dose, making it more potent. Although the drug given at the lower dose is more potent, because both drugs achieve similar effects, they may be considered to have equal efficacy. However, side effects are often related to dose, so a potent drug that can produce a therapeutic response at a lower dose may be preferable.

Loss of Effect: Biologic Adaptation

In some instances, the effects of medications diminish with time, especially when they are given repeatedly, as in the treatment of chronic psychiatric disorders. This loss of effect can be a form of physiologic adaptation that may develop as the cell attempts to regain homeostatic control to counteract the effects of the drug. **Desensitization** is a rapid decrease in drug effects that may develop in a few minutes of exposure to a drug. This process is rare with most psychiatric medications but can occur with some medications used to treat serious side effects (e.g., physostigmine, sometimes used to relieve severe anticholinergic side effects). **Tolerance** is a gradual decrease in the action of a drug at a given dose or concentration in the blood. This decrease may take days or weeks to develop and results in loss of therapeutic effect of a drug. This loss of effect is often called *treatment refractoriness*. There are many reasons for decreased drug effectiveness (Box 13-1). A rapid decrease can occur with some drugs because of immediate transformation of the receptor when the drug molecule binds to the receptor. Other drugs cause a decrease in the number of receptors. Some drugs may deplete cellular stores of neurotransmitter. Examples include d-amphetamine, which depletes dopamine stores, whereas the recreational drug "Ecstasy" depletes serotonin stores. Drug tolerance is also caused by an increase in the **metabolism** (breakdown) of the medication, such as with barbiturates, which trigger an increase in the amount of hepatic enzymes responsible for their metabolism and result in a precipitous drop in the blood level of the anticonvulsant carbamazepine (Tegretol) if used in combination with phenobarbital, for example. Cycling female hormones can also affect response to drugs. Progesterone and its metabolites

---

BOX 13.1

Mechanisms Causing Decrease in Medication Effects

- Change in receptor affinity
- Loss of receptors
- Depletion of neurotransmitter supply
- Increased metabolism of the drug
- Physiologic adaptation
- Interaction with female hormones

---

bind to the same GABA receptor as do the benzodiazepines and can affect the efficacy and potency of benzodiazepines at certain stages of the menstrual cycle.

Other forms of physiologic adaptation result in a gradual tolerance that may be helpful in the case of unpleasant side effects, such as drowsiness or nausea. This information is important for the nurse to communicate to patients experiencing such side effects so that they can be reassured that the effects will subside. The psychiatric nurse must also know when tolerance will not occur and when a lack of tolerance to a significant side effect warrants discontinuation of the medication.

Target Symptoms and Side Effects

Psychiatric medications are indicated for specific symptoms, referred to as **target symptoms**. Target symptoms are those measurable specific symptoms expected to improve with medication use. The target symptoms for each class of medication are discussed more fully in later sections of this chapter. Because receptors for neurotransmitters such as serotonin are found in all regions of the brain and in the periphery, serotonin-related drugs produce widespread effects in many body systems. For example, these drugs interact with receptors in the gastrointestinal tract and in facial motor nerves, causing gastrointestinal upset and bruxism (clenching and grinding of teeth) These unwanted effects of medications are called **side effects** or **untoward effects**. Some unwanted effects may have serious physiologic consequences, referred to as **adverse reactions**. Although technically different, these three terms are often used interchangeably in the literature.

Knowledge of a medication's affinity for receptors and subtypes of receptors may give some indication of the likelihood that specific target symptoms might improve and what side effects might be predicted. Table 13-1 provides a brief summation of possible physiologic effects from drug actions on specific neurotransmitters. For example, antagonists with high affinity for acetylcholine receptors of the muscarinic subtype will be more likely to cause such side effects as dry mouth, blurred vision, constipation, urinary hesitancy or retention, and nasal congestion. This information should serve only as a guide in predicting side effects because of considerable interindividual variability in drug responses and not all underlying mechanisms have been elucidated. A psychiatric–mental health nurse should use this information to focus assessment on these areas. If the symptoms are mild, simple nursing interventions suggested in Table 13-2 should be implemented. If symptoms persist or are severe, the prescriber should be notified immediately.

Drug Toxicity

All drugs have the capacity to be harmful as well as helpful. **Toxicity** generally refers to the point at which

Table 13.1 Drug Affinity for Specific Neurotransmitters and Receptors and Subsequent Effects

Neurotransmitter/ Receptor Action	Physiologic Effects	Example of Drugs That Exhibit High Affinity
Receptor Blockade		
Norepinephrine reuptake inhibition	Antidepressant action	desipramine
	Potentiation of pressor effects of norepinephrine	reboxetine
	Interaction with guanethidine	
	Side effects: tachycardia, tremors, insomnia, erectile and ejaculation dysfunction	
Serotonin reuptake inhibition	Antidepressant action	fluoxetine
	Antiobsessional effect	paroxetine
	Increase or decrease in anxiety, dose dependent	
	Side effects: gastrointestinal distress, nausea, headache, nervousness, motor restlessness and sexual side effects, including anorgasmia	
Dopamine reuptake inhibition	Antidepressant action	buproprion
	Antiparkinsonian effect	
	Side effects: increase in psychomotor activity, aggravation of psychosis	
Reuptake Inhibition		
Histamine receptor blockade (H$_1$)	Side effects: sedation, drowsiness, hypotension, and weight gain	quetiapine imipramine clozapine olanzapine
Acetylcholine receptor blockade (muscarinic)	Side effects: anticholinergic (dry mouth, blurred vision, constipation, urinary hesitancy and retention, memory dysfunction) and sinus tachycardia	imipramine amitriptyline thioridazine clozapine
Norepinephrine receptor blockade (α_1 receptor)	Potentiation of antihypertensive effect of prazosin and terazosin	amitriptyline
	Side effects: postural hypotension, dizziness, reflex tachycardia, sedation	clomipramine clozapine
Norepinephrine receptor blockade (α_2 receptor)	Increased sexual desire (yohimbine)	amitriptyline
	Interactions with antihypertensive medications, blockade of the antihypertensive effects of clonidine	clomipramine clozapine trazodone
	Side effect: priapism	yohimbine
Norepinephrine receptor blockade (β_1 receptor)	Antihypertensive action (propranolol)	propranolol
	Side effects: orthostatic hypotension, sedation, depression, sexual dysfunction (including impotence and decreased ejaculation)	
Serotonin receptor blockade (5-HT$_{1a}$)	Antidepressant action	trazodone
	Antianxiety effect	risperidone
	Possible control of aggression	ziprasidone
Serotonin receptor blockade (5-HT$_2$)	Antipsychotic action	risperidone
	Some antimigraine effect	clozapine
	Decreased rhinitis	olanzapine
	Side effects: hypotension, ejaculatory problems, weight gain, metabolic disorders	ziprasidone haloperidol
Dopamine receptor blockade (D$_2$)	Antipsychotic action	ziprasidone
	Side effects: extrapyramidal symptoms, such as tremor, rigidity (especially acute dystonia and parkinsonism); endocrine changes, including elevated prolactin levels	

concentrations of the drug in the bloodstream are high enough to become harmful or poisonous to the body. However, what is considered harmful? Side effects can be harmful but not toxic, and individuals vary widely in their responses to medications. Some patients experi- ence adverse reactions more easily than others. **Therapeutic index,** a concept often used to discuss the toxicity of a drug, is a ratio of the maximum nontoxic dose to the minimum effective dose. A high therapeutic index means that there is a large range between the dose at

Table 13.2 Managing Common Side Effects of Psychiatric Medications

Side Effect or Discomfort	Intervention
Blurred vision	Reassurance (generally subsides in 2 to 6 wk)
Dry eyes	Warn ophthalmologist; no eye exam for new glasses for at least 3 wk after a stable dose
	Artificial tears may be required; increased use of wetting solutions for those wearing contact lens
Dry mouth and lips	Frequent rinsing of mouth, good oral hygiene, sucking sugarless candies, lozenges, lip balm, lemon juice, and glycerin mouth swabs
Constipation	High-fiber diet, encourage bran, fresh fruits and vegetables
	Metamucil (must consume at least 16 oz of fluid with dose)
	Increase hydration
	Exercise, increase fluids
	Mild laxative
Urinary hesitancy or retention	Monitor frequently for difficulty with urination, changes in starting or stopping stream
	Notify prescriber if difficulty develops
	A cholinergic agonist, such as bethanechol, may be required
Nasal congestion	Nose drops, moisturizer, *not* nasal spray
Sinus tachycardia	Assess for infections
	Monitor pulse for rate and irregularities
	Withhold medication and notify prescriber if resting rate exceeds 120 bpm
Decreased libido and ejaculatory inhibition	Reassurance (reversible)
	Consider change to another drug in same class or change class of drug
Postural hypotension	Frequent monitoring of lying-to-standing blood pressure during dosage adjustment period, immediate changes and accommodation, measure pulse in both positions
	Advise patient to get up slowly, sit for at least 1 min before standing (dangling legs over side of bed), and stand for 1 min before walking or until light-headedness subsides
	Increase hydration, avoid caffeine
	Elastic stockings if necessary
	Notify prescriber if symptoms persist or significant blood pressure changes are present; medication may have to be changed if patient does not have impulse control to get up slowly
Photosensitivity	Protective clothing
	Dark glasses
	Use of sun block, remember to cover *all* exposed areas
Dermatitis	Stop medication usage
	Consider medication change, may require a systemic antihistamine
	Initiate comfort measures to decrease itching
Impaired psychomotor functions	Advise patient to avoid dangerous tasks, such as driving
	Avoid alcohol, which increases this impairment
Drowsiness or sedation	Encourage activity during the day to increase accommodation
	Avoid tasks that require mental alertness, such as driving
	May need to adjust dosing schedule or, if possible, give single daily dose at bedtime
	May need a cholinergic medication if sedation is the problem
	Avoid driving or operating potentially dangerous equipment
	May need change to less-sedating medication
	Provide quiet and decreased stimulation when sedation is the desired effect
Weight gain	Exercise and diet teaching
	Caloric control and regular monitoring of blood glucose levels
Edema	Check fluid retention
	Reassurance
	May need a diuretic
Irregular menstruation	Reassurance (reversible)
Amenorrhea	May need to change class of drug
	Reassurance and counselling (does not indicate lack of ovulation)
	Instruct patient to continue birth control measures
Vaginal dryness	Instruct in use of lubricants

which the drug begins to take effect and a dose that would be toxic to the body. Drugs with a low therapeutic index have a narrow range and are often carefully monitored through routine assessment of blood levels. This concept has some limitations. The concept of toxicity is only vaguely defined. The range can also be affected by drug tolerance. For example, individuals increasing their dosages of barbiturates as they became increasingly more tolerant to the effects and requiring larger doses to make them sleep have caused accidental suicides. The therapeutic index of a medication also may be greatly changed by the coadministration of other medications or drugs. For example, alcohol consumed with most CNS depressant drugs will have added depressant effects, greatly increasing the likelihood of toxicity or death.

Despite the limitations of the therapeutic index, it is a helpful guide for nurses, particularly when working with potentially suicidal individuals. Psychiatric–mental health nurses must be aware of the potential for overdose and closely monitor the availability of drugs for these patients. In some cases, prescriptions may have to be dispensed every few days or each week until a suicidal crisis has passed to ensure that patients do not have a lethal dose available to them.

PHARMACOKINETICS: HOW DRUGS MOVE THROUGH THE BODY

The field of pharmacokinetics describes, often in mathematical models, how a drug moves throughout the body to get to its target receptors and then is eliminated. The processes of absorption, distribution, metabolism, and excretion are of central importance. Overall, the goal in pharmacokinetics is to describe and predict the time course of drug concentrations throughout the body and factors that may interfere with these processes. Together with the principles of pharmacodynamics, this information can be helpful to the psychiatric nurse in such ways as facilitating or inhibiting drug effects and predicting behavioural response.

Absorption and Routes of Administration

The first phase of drug disposition in the human body is **absorption,** defined as the movement of the drug from the site of administration into the plasma. It is important to consider the impact of routes by which a drug is administered on the process of absorption. Not all potential routes of administration are available for medications used to treat psychiatric disorders. The primary routes available include oral (both tablet and liquid), sublingual, intramuscular (short- and long-acting agents), and intravenous (rarely used for treatment of the primary psychiatric disorder, but instead for rapid

treatment of adverse reactions). The psychiatric–mental health nurse needs to know about the advantages and disadvantages of each route and the subsequent effects on absorption (Table 13-3).

Drugs taken orally are usually the most convenient for the patient; however, this route is also the most variable because absorption can be slowed or enhanced by a number of factors. Taking certain drugs orally with food or antacids may slow the rate of absorption or change the amount of the drug absorbed. For example, the β-receptor antagonist propranolol exhibits increased blood levels when taken with food. Antacids containing aluminium salts decrease the absorption of most antipsychotic drugs; thus, antacids must be given at least 1 hour before administration or 2 hours after.

Oral preparations absorbed from the gastrointestinal tract into the bloodstream first go to the liver through the portal vein. There, they may be metabolized in such a way that most of the drug is inactivated before it reaches the rest of the body. Some drugs are also subjected to metabolism in the gastrointestinal wall. These losses of orally administered drugs before entering the systemic circulation are termed the *first-pass effect.* The consequence of first-pass effect is that the fraction of the drug reaching systemic circulation is reduced, sometimes substantially. Drugs that commonly undergo first-pass include nortriptyline, meperidine, and propranolol.

First-pass explains why the dose of propranolol given intravenously is so much less than the oral dose. However, even drugs with first-pass effect reach the rest of the body, but other factors affecting absorption should be considered when administering drugs with known first-pass effect. Liver disease and dysfunction can alter the first-pass effect and result in increased drug levels and thus an increased risk for side effects. Gastric motility also affects how the drug is absorbed. Increasing age, many disease states, and concurrent medications can reduce motility and slow absorption. Other factors, such as blood flow in the gastrointestinal system, drug formulation, and chemical factors, may also interfere with absorption. Nurses must be aware of a patient's physical condition and use of medications or other substances that can interfere with drug absorption.

In full strength, many liquid preparations, especially antipsychotics, irritate the mucosal lining of the mouth, oesophagus, and stomach and must be adequately diluted. Nurses must be careful when diluting liquid medications because some liquid concentrate preparations are incompatible with certain juices or other liquids. If a drug is mixed with an incompatible liquid, a white or grainy precipitant usually forms, indicating that some of the drug has bound to the liquid and inactivated. Thus, the patient actually receives a lower dose of the medication than intended. Precipitants can also form from combining two liquid medications in one diluent, such

Table 13.3   Selected Forms and Routes of Psychiatric Medications

Preparation and Route	Examples	Advantages	Disadvantages
Oral tablet	Basic preparation for most psychopharmacologic agents, including antidepressants, antipsychotics, mood stabilizers, anxiolytics, etc.	Convenience	Variable rate and extent of absorption, depending on the drug May be affected by the contents of the intestines May show first-pass metabolism effects May not be easily swallowed by some individuals
Oral liquid	Also known as concentrates Many antipsychotics, such as haloperidol, chlorpromazine, thioridazine, risperidone The antidepressant fluoxetine Antihistamines, such as diphenhydramine Mood stabilizers, such as lithium citrate	Ease of incremental dosing Easily swallowed In some cases, more quickly absorbed	More difficult to measure accurately Depending on drug: ▪ Possible interactions with other liquids such as juice, forming precipitants ▪ Possible irritation to mucosal lining of mouth if not properly diluted
Rapid-dissolving tablet	Atypical antipsychotics, such as olanzapine	Dissolves almost instantaneously in mouth Handy for people who have trouble swallowing or for patients who let medication linger in the cheek for later expectoration Can be taken when water or other liquid is unavailable	Patient needs to remember to have completely dry hands and to place tablet in mouth immediately Tablet should not linger in the hand
Sublingual	Lorazepam	Rapid action, no first-pass metabolism	Increased risk for tolerance and psychological dependance
Intramuscular	Some antipsychotics, such as haloperidol, chlorpromazine, and risperidone Anxiolytics, such as lorazepam Anticholinergics, such as diphenhydramine and benztropine mesylate No antidepressants No mood stabilizers	More rapid acting than oral preparations No first-pass metabolism	Injection-site pain and irritation Some medications may have erratic absorption if heavy muscle tissue at the site of injection is not in use High-potency antipsychotics in this form may be more prone to adverse reactions, such as neuroleptic malignant syndrome
Intramuscular depot (or long-acting)	Haloperidol decanoate, fluphenazine decanoate, risperidone	May be more convenient for some individuals who have difficulty following medication regimens	Significant pain at injection site
Intravenous	Anticholinergics, such as diphenhydramine, benztropine mesylate Anxiolytics, such as diazepam, lorazepam, and chlordiazepoxide The antipsychotic haloperidol (unlabeled use)	Rapid and complete availability to systemic circulation	Inflammation of tissue surrounding site Often inconvenient for patient and uncomfortable Continuous dosage requires use of a constant-rate IV infusion

as juice. Sometimes, precipitants may be difficult to see, such as in orange juice, so nurses must be aware of the compatibilities of liquid preparations. If a precipitant forms in a medication cup, it will also form in the stomach, causing additional inactivation of the drugs. Therefore, some medications should be given at least an hour apart. With new technologies come novel administration routes and drug forms, one of which is the rapid-dissolving oral pill. Different manufacturers have different procedures for developing rapid-dissolving drugs, and the different methods are patented and named differently. Common forms include the DuraSolv and QuickTab technologies. Many drugs are currently available in rapid-dissolving form, including the atypical antipsychotic olanzapine (Zyprexa, Zydis), risperidone (Risperdal M-Tab), and mirtazapine (Remeron SolTab). Nurses need to be aware of the special administration and patient-teaching requirements of the rapid-dissolving drug forms.

To take an orally disintegrating tablet, the nurse or patient should use dry hands to peel back the foil packaging, immediately take out the tablet, and place it into the mouth. The tablet will quickly dissolve and can be swallowed with saliva. No water is needed to swallow disintegrating tablets. This is advantageous when a patient cannot swallow well or is unwilling to swallow pills, or when water is not readily available.

Bioavailability

Bioavailability describes the amount of the drug that actually reaches systemic circulation. The route by which a drug is administered significantly affects bioavailability. With some oral drugs, the amount of drug entering the bloodstream is decreased by first-pass metabolism and bioavailability is lower (Pandolfi et al., 2003). On the other hand, some rapid-dissolving oral medications have increased bioavailability.

Bioavailability is a concept often used to compare one drug with another, obviously implying that increased bioavailability makes one drug "better" than another. The U.S. Food and Drug Administration (FDA) uses bioavailability as one measure for comparing the equivalency of the drugs when generic forms of a drug are developed. Although increased bioavailability of a drug may sound impressive, it is important to remember that this is not a characteristic solely of the drug preparation. It may be low if absorption is incomplete. Wide individual variations in the enzyme activity of the intestine or liver, gastric pH, and intestinal motility will all affect it. In practice, bioavailability is difficult to quantify.

Psychiatric–mental health nurses must remember that many factors on any particular occasion may affect the absorption and bioavailability of the drug for an individual patient.

Distribution

Even after a drug enters the bloodstream, several factors affect how it is distributed in the body. **Distribution** of a drug reflects how easy it is for a drug to pass out of the systemic circulation and move into other types of tissues, such as brain, abdominal organs, skin, or bone, where target receptors are found. Factors that affect medication distribution to specific tissues in the body include the amount of blood flow or perfusion within the tissue, how lipophilic ("fat-loving") the drug is, plasma **protein binding,** and anatomic barriers, such as the blood–brain barrier, that the drug must cross. A drug may have rapid absorption and high bioavailability, but if it cannot cross the blood–brain barrier to reach the CNS, it is of little use in psychiatry. Table 13-4 provides a summary of how some significant factors affect distribution. Two of these factors, ionic characteristics and protein binding, warrant additional discussion with regard to how they relate to psychiatric medications.

Ionic Characteristics of Drugs

Drugs in the bloodstream can be charged molecules (in the form of positive or negative ions) or can be

Table 13.4	Factors Affecting Distribution of a Drug
Factor	**Effect on Drug Distribution**
Size of the organ	Larger organs require more drug to reach a concentration level equivalent to other organs and tissues.
Blood flow to the organ	The more blood flow to and within an organ (perfusion), the greater the drug concentration. The brain has high perfusion.
Ionic characteristics	Drugs with no electrical charge move easily across cell membranes and thus will be widely distributed
Plasma protein binding	If a drug binds well to plasma proteins, particularly to albumin, it will stay in the body longer but have a slower distribution.
Anatomic barriers	Both the gastrointestinal tract and the brain are surrounded by layers of cells that control the passage or uptake of substances. Lipid-soluble substances are usually readily absorbed and pass the blood–brain barrier.

uncharged. Within cell membranes there are many charged components. Thus, drugs that have an electrical charge cannot passively cross through a cell membrane; instead, they must be transported by carrier proteins. Uncharged drugs (also called lipophilic or "fat-loving" drugs) can move easily across cell membranes. Most psychiatric drugs are very lipophilic and can move into major organ systems, as well as cross the blood–brain barrier. However, this characteristic means that psychopharmacologic agents can also cross the placenta. It also means that these agents can be taken into fat stores. Drugs stored in fatty tissue are only slowly released back into the systemic circulation for eventual elimination. This is why a lipophilic drug can be detected long after discontinuation in older women and overweight individuals. It may account for unexpected drug–drug interactions when substitute drugs regimes are initiated quickly.

Protein Binding

Many drugs bind to large carrier proteins in the bloodstream. The degree to which a drug is bound to these plasma proteins affects the drug's ability to interact with receptors. Only unbound or "free" drugs can move across membranes to their target receptors. High protein binding can prolong the duration of action of the drug. Many of the psychiatric drugs are more than 90% protein bound. Chronic disease and normal aging can decrease the amounts of plasma protein and thus can shift the ratio of bound to free drug. For highly bound drugs like the classic antipsychotics, a decrease of only 10% of bound drug (eg, from 90% to 80%) would translate into a doubling of free drug and significantly increase the risk for side effects.

Metabolism

The duration of drug action depends to a large degree on the body's ability to change or alter a drug chemically. **Metabolism,** also called **biotransformation,** is the process by which the drug is altered, often broken down into smaller substances known as *metabolites.* Through the processes of metabolism, lipid-soluble drugs become more water soluble so that they may be excreted more readily.

Most metabolism occurs in the liver, but it can also occur in the kidneys, lungs, and intestines. The outcome of this process is usually an inactive metabolite. However, metabolism can also change a drug to an active metabolite with either similar or very different actions as the parent compound. For instance, the antidepressant imipramine is metabolized to a pharmacologically active substance, desipramine, which also has antidepressant effects. This becomes important when measuring the therapeutic blood level of imipramine. It is more clinically relevant and accurate to obtain both imipramine and desipramine levels, even though the patient may be taking only the drug imipramine. Prozac (fluoxetine), an SSRI antidepressant, is metabolized in the liver and forms an active metabolite, norfluoxetine, which has a very long half-life. Metabolism may also change an inactive drug (called a prodrug) to an active one or an active drug to a toxic metabolite. Codeine is an example of a prodrug that must be metabolized before having analgesic properties. *N*-hydroxyacetaminophen is formed with an acetaminophen overdose and is further oxidized to a toxic chemical that can destroy liver cells.

The cytochrome P-450 superfamily of metabolic enzymes (or CYP450s) is responsible for most drug metabolism. The classification of the CYP450 superfamily uses a combination of numbers and letters to denote families, subfamilies, and individual enzymes. Specific genes encode each enzyme, but polymorphisms are common. Most psychiatric drugs are metabolized by members of the 1A, 2D, and 3A subfamilies of CYP450 enzymes. The 3A family is the most abundant, constituting more than 60% of the liver enzyme weight. The metabolizing activity of some of the CYP450 enzymes can be altered by drugs and environmental chemicals. Some drugs like phenobarbital induce CYP450 activity. This increases enzymatic action and thus decreases drug levels of any drug taken concomitantly with phenobarbital. Subthreshold drug levels may affect efficacy. Other common substances, such as cigarette smoke, chronic alcohol consumption, and coal tar in charcoal-broiled foods, can induce the CYP450 enzyme system. Alternately, drugs can inhibit CYP450 activity and thus increase drug levels, potentially into toxic ranges. A CYP enzyme that is responsible for a wide variety of therapeutic agents and is often inhibited is CYP2D6. Acute alcohol ingestion and the antiulcer medication cimetidine (Tagamet), available over the counter, can inhibit CYP2D6. Some of the SSRIs are also potent inhibitors of CYP2D6. Grapefruit juice is an inhibitor of CYP3A enzymes. Not all SSRIs are equal in their potency to inhibit CYP2D6. Paroxetine (Paxil) is the most potent, producing more than 90% inhibition of this enzyme subfamily, whereas sertraline exhibits mild effects, with only 20% to 50% inhibition (Dalfen & Stewart, 2001). The newer SSRI citalopram has minimal inhibiting properties.

The metabolism of many of the older drugs has not been thoroughly investigated. Indeed, information about the specific CYP450 enzyme responsible for metabolism is available for only about 20% of commonly prescribed medications. In addition, a drug can be metabolized by more than one CYP450. A minor route of metabolism can become the major route under conditions of liver disease or dysfunction or if the individual has a genetic mutation of that enzyme, rendering it with only low intrinsic activity.

CYP450 enzymes contribute to the enormous differences in the reaction of individuals to medications. More than 100,000 people die each year of adverse reactions to medications that are safe and beneficial to others. Another 2.2 million experience serious side effects, whereas others experience no response to the same medications. Differences and changes in CYP450 enzymatic activity among people alter how individuals experience response to medications. These differences in the enzymes often are caused by genetic variations (Bachmann, 2002). DNA variants in the CYP450 system and the enzymes encoded by these genes have been investigated for several CYP enzymes in relation to specific ethnic and racial groups. For example, about 3% of Caucasians and more than 20% of Japanese are poor metabolizers of CYP2C19. About 2% of Chinese, but up to 10% of Caucasians, are poor metabolizers of CYP2D6 (Baker et al., 1998).

The emerging science of **pharmacogenomics** blends pharmacology with genetic knowledge and is concerned with understanding and determining an individual's specific CYP450 makeup, then individualizing medications to match the person's CYP450 profile. Increasingly, psychiatric medications are prescribed after testing to determine the patient's CYP450 genotype to guide treatment with the most effective drugs for the person, and to drastically reduce potential drug–drug interactions. For example, dextromethorphan is used to assess intrinsic activity of CYP2D6 and classify the individual into low, normal, or extensive metabolizers. Within the next decade, it is expected that scientists will begin to connect DNA variants with individual responses to medical treatments, identify particular subgroups of patients, and develop drugs customized for those populations.

Nurses should remain alert to the possibilities of drug–drug interactions when patients are receiving more than one medication. Pharmacology texts and dedicated websites are helpful reference sources. In addition, if an individual receiving a medication experiences an unusual reaction or suddenly loses effect from a medication that had previously been working, the nurse should carefully assess other substances that the person has recently consumed, including prescription medications, nonprescription remedies, dietary supplements or changes, and substances of abuse. The widespread use of herbal products has introduced another potential source of drug–drug interaction. A good example of this is St. John's wort, a botanical product used extensively for mild depression. Drug–drug interactions have been reported for St. John's Wort and alprazolam, amitriptyline, and cyclosporine (Izzo, 2004).

Excretion

Excretion refers to the elimination of drugs from the body either unchanged or as metabolites. Clearance refers to the total volume of blood, serum, or plasma from which a drug is completely removed from the bloodstream per unit of time. The driving force that determines the time required to eliminate a drug is the concentration of drug and the clearance rate. The elimination **half-life** ($t_{1/2}$) refers to the time required for plasma concentrations of the drug to be reduced by 50%. For example, 50% of a drug is cleared in one $t_{1/2}$. In the next $t_{1/2}$, 50% of the remaining concentration would be eliminated (leaving 25% of the original concentration), then after the third $t_{1/2}$, there would be 12.5% remaining. Thus, it usually takes four to seven half-lives for a drug to be completely eliminated from the body. Notable exceptions to this decrease by percent concentration include alcohol and acetylsalicylic acid, in which the specific enzymes responsible for metabolism limit the speed at which elimination can occur. For this reason, elimination is at a set rate irrespective of concentration, which is why in the case of alcohol, it can be calculated how many drinks it takes per hour to reach a blood alcohol level of 0.8 (a common legal level indicative of impairment) and the time required to eliminate all alcohol from the system. In the case of acetylsalicylic acid overdose, increasing the renal clearance through changes in pH or increasing fluid volume will not affect the time required for elimination because it is determined by enzyme activity, not blood flow.

As indicated previously, the goal of most metabolic processes is to decrease the lipophilic nature of drugs by increasing their ionic characteristics. Drugs that are in a more ionic form in the bloodstream can be easily removed by the kidney and excreted through urine. However, many psychiatric medications are large molecules and thus can also be removed through bile and eliminated in feces. Lithium, a mood stabilizer, is a notable exception. It is a very small cation and is dependent on renal excretion. Any impairment in renal function or renal disease, or even temporary dehydration (eg, from flu symptoms or even strenuous exercise) may lead to severe toxic symptoms. Biliary elimination can lead to "enteroportal recirculation," a process by which active drug or metabolites that were excreted in bile into the small intestine are reabsorbed into the portal circulation, go through the liver again, and end up back into the systemic circulation. A well-known example of this is oral contraceptives. Oral antibiotics change the intestinal environment, can decrease recirculation, and thus affect the contraceptive efficacy. This same process of reabsorption may also contribute to the plasma concentration of psychiatric drugs over time.

Dosing refers to the administration of medication over time, so that therapeutic levels may be achieved or maintained without reaching toxic levels. In general, it is necessary to give a drug at intervals no greater than the half-life of the medication to avoid excessive fluctuation of concentration in the plasma between doses. With repeated dosing, a certain amount of the drug is accumulated in the body. This accumulation slows as dosing continues and plateaus when absorption equals excretion. This is called *steady-state plasma concentration* or simply *steady state*. The rate of accumulation is determined by the half-life of the drug. Drugs generally reach steady state in four to five times the elimination half-life. However, because elimination or excretion rates may vary significantly, fluctuations may still occur, and dose schedules may need to be individualized.

The nurse should remember that although these principles can support best practice, they are not substitutes for ongoing individual assessment of indicators of treatment response or unwanted effects and recording individual perceptions about drug effects.

Individual Variations in Drug Effects

Many factors affect drug absorption, distribution, metabolism, and excretion. These factors may vary among individuals, depending on their age, genetics, and ethnicity. Nurses must be aware of and consider these individual variations in the effects of medications.

Age

Pharmacokinetics is influenced by life cycle stages. Gastric absorption changes with age. Gastric pH in the newborn is 6 to 8 and decreases to 1 to 3 over the first 24 hours (in the premature infant, the pH stays up). This significantly affects drug absorption. Changes in drug absorption is also seen in elderly people because of increased gastric pH, decreased gastric emptying, slowed gastric motility, and reduced splanchnic circulation. Normally, these changes do not significantly impair oral absorption of a medication, but addition of common conditions, such as diarrhoea, may significantly alter and reduce absorption. The use of multiple drug therapies (termed polypharmacy) in the elderly can also significantly alter pharmacokinetic properties of each individual drug (Hogan et al.,1995; Jacelon, 1999).

Renal function is also altered in both very young and elderly patients. Infants who are exposed in utero to medications that are excreted through the kidneys may experience toxic reactions to these medications because renal function in the newborn is only about 20% that of an adult. In less than a week, renal function develops to adult levels, but in premature infants, the process may take longer. Renal function also declines with age. Creatinine clearance in a young adult is normally 100 to 120 mL/min, but after age 40 years, this rate declines by about 10% per decade. Medical illnesses, such as diabetes and hypertension, may further the loss of renal function. When creatinine clearance falls below 30 mL/min, the excretion of drugs by the kidneys is significantly impaired, and potentially toxic levels may accumulate.

Metabolism changes across the life span, especially in infancy and childhood. At birth, many of the liver enzymes are not fully functional, whereas in early childhood, there is evidence of increased activity compared with adulthood. For example, CYP1A2 activity is reduced in the first 4 months, but increased between ages 1 and 2 years; CYP2D6 activity is reduced until ages 3 to 5 years, and CYP3A4 is reduced in the first month of life, but increased between ages 1 and 4 (Kearns et al., 2003; Leader & Kearns, 1997). Thus, paediatric pharmacotherapeutics cannot be simply based on relative dosing by weight. With age, blood flow to the liver and the mass of liver tissue both decrease. The activity of hepatic enzymes also slows with age. As a result, the ability of the liver to metabolize medications may show as much as a fourfold decrease between the ages of 20 and 70 years. Again, the use of multiple drugs in elderly people adds to metabolic burden, potentially increasing drug levels of each individual drug.

Most psychiatric medications are bound to proteins. Albumin is one of the primary circulating proteins to which drugs bind. Production of albumin by the liver is lower in neonates and generally declines with age. In addition, a number of medical conditions change the ability of medications to bind to albumin. Malnutrition, cancer, and liver disease decrease the production of albumin, which translates to more free drug available to interact with target receptors and an increased risk for adverse or toxic effects.

Less information is known about age-related changes in pharmacodynamics. There is evidence of pharmacodynamic differences in cyclosporine effects in infants (Marshall & Kearns, 1999). Higher digoxin doses are required in infants because of lower affinity in target myocardial receptors (Soldin & Soldin, 2002). Changes in the parasympathetic nervous system produce a greater sensitivity in elderly patients to the anticholinergic side effects of specific psychiatric drugs.

Ethnicity and Genetic Makeup

Although only a small amount of information is available at this time, it is clear that genetics plays a significant role in the metabolism of medications. Studies of identical and nonidentical twins show that much of the individual variability in elimination half-life of a given drug is genetically determined. Individuals of Asian descent have decreased activity of enzymes involved in the metabolism of ethanol compared with Caucasians and thus produce higher concentrations of acetaldehyde, resulting in such adverse symptoms as flushing, palpitations, and headache. Asian research subjects have been found to be more susceptible to the effects of drugs such as propranolol than are Caucasian individuals, whereas individuals of African descent were less sensitive (Bachmann, 2002). Several case reports indicate that Asians require one half to one third the dose of antipsychotic medications required by Caucasians and that they may be more sensitive to side effects because of higher blood levels (Zhou, 2003). Lower doses of antidepressant medications are also often required for individuals of Asian descent. Although many of these variations appear to be related to the cytochrome P-450 genetic differences discussed earlier, more research is needed to understand fully the underlying mechanisms and to identify groups that may require different approaches to medication treatment.

PHASES OF DRUG TREATMENT

The psychiatric–mental health nurse is involved in all the phases of medication treatment. Considerations in terms of assessment, treatment issues such as **adherence** (keeping with the therapeutic regimen), prevalence and severity of side effects, and expected time lines for symptom relief vary across the phases of treatment, but all involve potential nursing actions. These phases include initiation, stabilization, maintenance, and discontinuation of the medication. Psychiatric–mental health nurses must be concerned with treatment phases as a guide for what may be expected as they administer medications and monitor individuals receiving medications across each of these phases. The following subsections discuss some of the knowledge required and the assessments and interventions to be performed by the psychiatric–mental health nurse within each phase.

Initiation Phase

Before beginning to take medications, patients must undergo several assessments.

- A psychiatric evaluation, including past history and previous medication treatment response, will clarify diagnosis and determine target symptoms for medication use.
- An open discussion regarding adherence issues: attitudes toward drug treatments, patient-specific goals for the drug therapy, any lifestyle issues that affect the structuring of a drug regimen (shift work, cigarette smoker, type of occupation and current job responsibilities, reproductive issues), and any health insurance issues related to prescription benefits will help to identify barriers to the patient's willingness and ability to comply with the medication regimen.
- Physical examination and indicated laboratory tests, often including baseline determinations such as a complete blood count (CBC), liver and kidney function tests, electrolyte levels, and urinalysis, and possibly thyroid function tests and electrocardiogram (ECG), will help determine whether a physical condition may be causing the symptoms and establish that it is safe to initiate use of a particular medication.
- Any other current medications, including over-the-counter medications, herbal remedies and mixtures from health food stores or naturopathic or homeopathic visitations, and recreational drug use (including regular amount of alcohol) should be identified to prevent harmful drug interactions.

Nurses should perform their own premedication evaluations, including physical assessments that focus on preexisting symptoms, such as gastrointestinal distress, or restrictions in range of motion that may later be confused with side effects. Side effects are difficult to assess if baseline status has not been evaluated. An assessment of cognitive functioning will assist the nurse in assessing whether memory aids or other supports are necessary to assist the individual in accurately completing the medication regimen. Information from the psychosocial and lifestyle assessment should be reviewed in consultation with the prescriber and other members of the multidisciplinary team to develop a plan that is acceptable to the patient and that will improve functioning, minimize side effects, and improve quality of life.

In all situations, recommendations and treatment alternatives should be developed and reviewed with input from the individual seeking treatment. Doing so will allow the patient to ask questions and receive complete information about target effects and the most common adverse effects, thus allowing for fully informed consent to the selected approach. Patients are often overwhelmed during the initial phases of treatment and may have symptoms that make it difficult for them to participate fully in treatment planning. Information is often forgotten or may need to be repeated and provided in written form for ongoing reference. Nurses must keep their detailed drug knowledge current to be able to answer questions and provide ongoing education.

When use of the medication is initiated, psychiatric–mental health nurses should treat the first dose as if it were a "test" dose. They should observe the patient closely for sensitivity to the medication, such as changes in blood pressure, pulse, or temperature; changes in mental status; allergic reactions; dizziness; ataxia; or gastric distress. Other common side effects that may occur with even one dose of medication should also be closely monitored. A protocol to reporting side effects and which ones should trigger immediate contact should be in place.

Stabilization Phase

During stabilization, the medication dosage is often being adjusted and increased to achieve the maximum amount of improvement with a minimum of side effects. This process is sometimes referred to as *titration*. Psychiatric–mental health nurses must continue to assess target symptoms, looking for change or improvement and side effects. If medications are being increased rapidly, such as in a hospital setting, nurses must closely monitor temperature, blood pressure, pulse, mental status, common side effects, and unusual adverse reactions.

On an outpatient basis, nurses must provide both verbal and written materials to individuals who are receiving the medication as to the expected outcome and potential side effects. This educational support should include factors that may influence the effectiveness of the medication, such as whether to take the medication with food, common interventions that may minimize side effects if they develop, and what side effects require immediate attention. Again, a plan is needed to clearly identify what to do if adverse reactions develop. The plan should include emergency telephone numbers or available emergency treatment and be reviewed frequently.

Therapeutic drug monitoring is important in this phase of treatment for drugs with narrow therapeutic windows, such as lithium, valproate, and carbamazepine. Nurses must be aware of when and how these levels are to be determined and assist patients in learning these procedures. Plasma levels of other psychiatric medications can be evaluated, for example, to rule them out as a potential source of treatment nonresponse related to increased metabolism. Unfortunately, the first medication chosen often does not adequately improve the patient's target symptoms. In treatment of depression, for example, studies have shown that up to 60% of individuals fail to respond to any given antidepressant (Thase, 2002). This can be very discouraging, particularly in a population in which powerlessness and hopelessness are inherent in the disorder. This possibility must be discussed before initiating antidepressant drug therapy. Most of the time, a substitute drug from the same class or a drug from a new class will be given. Medications may also be changed when adverse reactions or seriously uncomfortable side effects occur or these effects substantially interfere with the individual's quality of life. Nurses should be familiar with the pharmacokinetics of both drugs to be able to monitor side effects and possible drug–drug interactions during this transition period.

At times, an individual may show only partial improvement from a medication, and the prescriber may try an augmentation strategy. *Augmentation* refers to the addition of another medication to enhance or potentiate the effects of the first medication. For example, a prescriber may add a mood stabilizer, such as lithium, to an antidepressant to improve the overall efficacy of the antidepressant. These strategies are often used with so-called treatment-resistant situations. Treatment resistance has various definitions, but most often it means that after several medication trials, the individual has gained, at best, only partial improvement. Treatment-resistant symptoms often require multiple medications. Multiple medications may affect different physiologic processes and, in combination, provide overall synergistic or additive pharmacologic effects. Nurses must be familiar with the potential effects, side effects, drug interactions, and rationale for this type of complex treatment regimen.

Maintenance Phase

Once the individual's target symptoms have improved, medications may be continued to prevent relapse or reoccurrence. Relapse usually refers to re-emerging symptoms in response to premature discontinuation of treatment, whereas **reoccurrence** refers to an entirely new episode that occurs over time after full remission was achieved. Higher risk for relapse in depression is associated with those who are older, have chronic episodes, have severe symptoms or psychotic symptoms, or have three or more previous or more frequent episodes (Viguera et al., 1998). Other reasons for re-emerging symptoms, despite continued use of the medication, include loss of efficacy, metabolic induction, comorbid medical illness, psychosocial stressors, and concurrent use of prescription or nonprescription medications. Whatever the reason, patients must be educated about their target symptoms and have a plan of action if the symptoms return. The psychiatric–mental health nurse has a central role in assisting individuals to monitor their own symptoms, manage psychosocial stressors, and avoid other factors that may cause exacerbation of symptoms that were previously under control.

Some side effects or adverse reactions emerge only after the individual has been receiving the medication for an extended period. Specific examples are discussed in later sections of this chapter.

Discontinuation Phase

Many psychiatric medications require a tapered discontinuation. Tapering involves slowly reducing dosage while monitoring closely for re-emergence of key symptoms, such as a drop in mood, increased anxiety, sleep disturbance, thought disorder, or decreased level of self-care. Some psychiatric disorders, such as mild depression or adjustment disorder, may respond to several months of treatment and not recur. Other disorders, such as bipolar disorder, chronic major depressive disorder, and schizophrenia, usually require continued medication treatment for extended periods of time. A withdrawal syndrome, affecting up to 25% of individuals after abrupt cessation of the SSRIs, has been described and includes such symptoms as dizziness, restlessness, increased anxiety and mood lability, GI upset, and fatigue (Ditto, 2003). Restoration of the drug therapy relieves the symptoms within 24 hours. Untreated, the symptoms can last 1 to 3 weeks. Withdrawal effects have also been described for abrupt discontinuation of benzodiazepines.

Nurses must be aware of the potential for these symptoms, monitor them closely, and implement measures to minimize their effects. They should support individuals throughout this process, whether they can successfully stop taking the medication or must continue the treatment. Even if patients can successfully discontinue use of the medication without a return of symptoms, nurses may help implement preventive measures to avoid recurrence of the psychiatric disorder. In the roles of advocate, patient educator, and provider of interpersonal support, psychiatric–mental health nurses often have a central role in helping patients incorporate preventative mental health strategies into their daily routine.

ANTIPSYCHOTIC MEDICATIONS

It is hard to image how psychiatric illnesses were treated before the development of psychopharmacologic medications. Antipsychotic medications were among the very first drugs ever used to treat psychiatric disorders. First synthesized by Paul Charpentier in 1950, chlorpromazine became the interest of Henri Lorit, a French surgeon, who was attempting to develop medications that controlled preoperative anxiety. Administered in intravenous doses of 50 to 100 mg, chlorpromazine produced drowsiness and indifference to surgical procedures. At Lorit's suggestion, a number of psychiatrists began to administer chlorpromazine to agitated psychotic patients. In 1952, Jean Delay and Pierre Deniker, two French psychiatrists, published the first report of chlorpromazine's calming effects with psychiatric patients. They soon discovered it was especially effective in relieving hallucinations and delusions associated with schizophrenia. As more psychiatrists began to prescribe the medication, the use of restraints and seclusion in psychiatric hospitals dropped sharply, ushering in a revolution in psychiatric treatment.

Since that time, numerous antipsychotic medications have been developed. Older, typical antipsychotic medications, available since 1954, are equally effective, inexpensive drugs that vary in the degree to which they cause certain groups of side effects. Table 13-5 provides a list of selected antipsychotics grouped by the nature of their chemical structure and indicating the likelihood of certain side effects. These medications treat the symptoms of psychosis, such as hallucinations, delusions, bizarre behaviour, disorganized thinking, and agitation.

Typical and Atypical Antipsychotics

Initially, the term *major tranquilizer* was applied to this group of medications. Later, major tranquilizers were known as *neuroleptics*, which more accurately describes the action of drugs such as chlorpromazine and haloperidol. Neuroleptic means "to clasp the neuron." The term reflects the common and often significant neurologic side effects produced by these types of drugs. The development of newer antipsychotic drugs that have less significant neurologic side effects has led to these older agents being used as secondary, not first-line, drugs. The term *typical antipsychotic* now identifies the older antipsychotic drugs with greater risk for neurologic side effects, and *atypical antipsychotic* identifies the newer generation of antipsychotic drugs with fewer adverse neurologic effects.

Indications and Mechanism of Action

Antipsychotic medications generally are indicated for treating acute psychosis or severe agitation. Possible target symptoms for the antipsychotics include hallucinations, delusions, paranoia, agitation, assaultive behaviour, bizarre ideation, disorientation, social withdrawal, catatonia, blunted affect, thought blocking, insomnia, and anorexia, when these symptoms are the result of a psychotic process. (These symptoms are described more fully in later chapters.)

In general, the older, typical antipsychotics, such as haloperidol (Haldol), chlorpromazine, and thioridazine (Mellaril), are equally effective in relieving hallucinations, delusions, and bizarre ideation, termed "positive" symptoms of schizophrenia. The "negative" symptoms—blunted affect, social withdrawal, lack of interest in usual activities, lack of motivation, poverty of speech, thought blocking, and inattention—respond less well to the typical antipsychotics and in some cases may even be worsened by such agents. Newer atypical antipsychotics, such as clozapine, risperidone (Risperdal), olanzapine (Zyprexa), quetiapine (Seroquel), and ziprasidone (Geodon), are more effective at improving negative symptoms. Although antipsychotic medications are the primary treatment for schizophrenia and related illnesses, such as schizoaffective disorder, schizophreniform disorder, and brief psychotic disorder, they are increasingly being used to treat other psychiatric and medical illnesses. Psychotic symptoms that occur during a major depressive episode, anxiety, or bipolar affective disorder can be treated with antipsychotics, primarily on a short-term basis. Olanzapine (Zyprexa) is now approved by the FDA for the short-term treatment of acute mania, and some manufacturers of atypical antipsychotics are seeking FDA approval for their use in depression without psychosis. These medications reduce agitation, aggressiveness, and inappropriate

Table 13.5   Side-Effect Comparison of Selected Antipsychotic Medications

Drug Category Drug Name	Sedation	Extrapyramidal	Anticholinergic	Orthostatic Hypotension
Standard (Typical) Antipsychotics				
PHENOTHIAZINES				
ALIPHATICS				
chlorpromazine (Thorazine)	+4	+2	+3	+4
PIPERIDINES				
thioridazine (Mellaril)	+3	+1	+4	+4
mesoridazine (Serentil)	+3	+1	+4	+3
PIPERAZINES				
fluphenazine (Prolixin)	+1	+4	+1	+1
perphenazine (Trilafon)	+2	+3	+2	+2
trifluoperazine (Stelazine)	+1	+3	+1	+1
THIOXANTHENES				
thiothixene (Navane)	+1	+4	+1	+1
DIBENZOXAZEPINES				
loxapine (Loxitane)	+2	+3	+2	+3
BUTYROPHENONES				
haloperidol (Haldol)	+1	+4	+1	+1
DIHYDROINDOLONES				
molindone (Moban)	+2	+3	+2	+1
Atypical Antipsychotics				
DIBENZODIAZEPINES				
clozapine (Clozaril)	+4	+/0	+4	+4
BENZISOXAZOLE				
risperidone (Risperdal)	+1	+/0	+/0	+2
THIENOBENZODIAZEPINE				
olanzapine (Zyprexa)	+4	+/0	+2	+1
DIBENZOTHIAZEPINE				
quetiapine fumarate (Seroquel)	+4	+/0	+/0	+3
MONOHYDROCHLORIDE				
ziprasidone HCl (Geodon)	+1	+/0	+1	+2
DIHYDROCARBOSTYRILS				
aripiprazole (Abilify)	+1	+/0	+/0	+1

behaviour in pervasive developmental disorders, such as autism or severe mental retardation. Within the typical antipsychotics, haloperidol and pimozide are approved for treating Tourette's syndrome, reducing the frequency and severity of vocal tics. Some of the typical antipsychotics, particularly chlorpromazine, are used as antiemetics or for postoperative intractable hiccoughs.

Off-label uses of the drug have also been effective. Chlorpromazine and haloperidol are both effective in treating drug-related psychosis, such as that caused by phencyclidine. Atypical antipsychotics have been effective and safe in controlling behavioural disturbances in elderly patients who have dementia by reducing symptoms of agitation, hyperactivity, hallucinations, suspiciousness, and hostility. Some evidence exists for their efficacy in treating psychiatric sequelae of trauma, especially in the case of significant dissociation and mood reactivity arising from childhood interpersonal abuse (Grootens & Verkes, 2005). Antipsychotic medications may also be useful in treating migraine

headaches, Huntington's chorea, and some other neurologic disorders.

The typical antipsychotic drugs generally are effective in decreasing the so-called positive target symptoms because they are potent postsynaptic dopamine antagonists. Chapter 17 discusses the link between dopamine and disorders such as schizophrenia and provides additional detail about how lowering dopamine levels helps reduce target symptoms. The atypical antipsychotic medications differ from the typical antipsychotics in that they block serotonin receptors as well as dopamine receptors. The differences between the mechanism of action of the typical and atypical antipsychotics helps to explain their differences in efficacy in relation to both positive and negative symptoms and side-effect profiles.

Pharmacokinetics

Antipsychotic medications administered orally have a variable rate of absorption complicated by the presence of food, antacids, smoking, and even the coadministration of anticholinergics, which slow gastric motility. Clinical effects begin to appear in about 30 to 60 minutes. Absorption after intramuscular (IM) administration is less variable because this method avoids the first-pass effects. Therefore, IM administration produces greater bioavailability, but increases risk for side effects. It is important to remember that IM medications are absorbed more slowly when patients are immobile, such as when restrained for long periods of time, because erratic absorption may occur when muscles are not in use. For example, the patient's arm may be more mobile than the buttocks. The deltoid has better blood perfusion, and thus medications are more readily absorbed. The nurse must also remember that plastic syringes may absorb some medications. This is true of the antipsychotics, and injectable medications should never be allowed to remain in the syringe longer than 15 minutes.

Metabolism of these drugs occurs almost entirely in the liver, where hepatic microsomal enzymes convert these highly lipid-soluble substances into water-soluble metabolites that can be excreted through the kidneys. Therefore, these medications are subjected to the effects of other drugs that induce or inhibit the cytochrome P-450 system described earlier. Table 13-6 summarizes many of the possible medication interactions with antipsychotics, including those resulting from changes in hepatic enzymes. Careful observance of concurrent medication use, including prescribed, over-the-counter, and substances of abuse, is required to avoid drug–drug interactions.

Excretion of these substances tends to be slow because the drugs can easily accumulate in fat stores. Most antipsychotics have a half-life of 24 hours or longer, but many also have active metabolites with longer half-lives. These two effects make it difficult to

Table 13.6 Chemical Interactions With Antipsychotic Medications

Agent	Effect
Alcohol	Phenothiazines potentiate CNS depressant effects. Extrapyramidal reactions may occur
Barbiturates	Speed action of liver microsomal enzymes so antipsychotic is metabolized more quickly, reducing phenothiazine and haloperidol plasma levels; barbiturate levels may also be reduced by phenothiazines; potentiate CNS depressant effect
Tricyclic antidepressants	Can lead to severe anticholinergic side effects; some antipsychotics (especially phenothiazines or haloperidol) can raise the plasma level of the antidepressant, probably by inhibiting metabolism of the antidepressant
hydrochlorothiazide and hydralazine	Can produce severe hypotension
Guanethidine	Antihypertensive effect is blocked by phenothiazines, haloperidol, and possibly thiothixene
Aluminum salts (antacids)	Impair gastrointestinal absorption of the phenothiazines, possibly reducing therapeutic effect. Administer antacid at least 1 h before or 2 h after the phenothiazine
Nicotine	Heavy consumption requires larger doses of antipsychotic because of hepatic microsomal enzyme induction
Charcoal (and charbroiled food)	Decreases absorption of phenothiazines
Anticholinergics	May reduce the therapeutic actions of the phenothiazines, increase anticholinergic side effects, lower serum haloperidol levels, worsen symptoms of schizophrenia, increase symptoms of tardive dyskinesia
meperidine	May result in excessive sedation and hypotension when coadministered with phenothiazines
fluoxetine	Case report of serious extrapyramidal symptoms when used in combination with haloperidol
lithium	May induce disorientation, unconsciousness, extrapyramidal symptoms, or possibly the risk for neuroleptic malignant syndrome when combined with phenothiazines or haloperidol
carbamazepine	Decreases haloperidol serum levels, decreasing its therapeutic effects
phenytoin	Increase or decrease in phenytoin serum levels; thioridazine and haloperidol serum levels may be decreased
methyldopa	May potentiate the antipsychotic effects of haloperidol or may produce psychosis. Serious elevations in blood pressure may occur with methyldopa and trifluoperazine
General anesthesia (barbiturates)	Antipsychotic may potentiate effect of anesthetic; may increase the neuromuscular excitation or hypotension

predict elimination time, and metabolites of some of these agents may be found in the urine months later. If a patient experiences side effects from a medication severe enough to discontinue use of the drug and begin use of a new one, the adverse effects of the first drug may not necessarily immediately subside. The patient may continue to experience and sometimes need treatment for the adverse effects for several days. Similarly, patients who have discontinued use of antipsychotic drugs may still derive therapeutic benefit for several days to weeks after drug discontinuation.

Typical antipsychotics are best administered in divided doses to minimize side effects, but the long elimination time does allow the medication to be given in once-daily dosing. This schedule increases adherence and reduces the impact of the peak occurrence of some side effects, such as sedation during the day.

High lipid solubility, accumulation in the body, and other factors have also made it difficult to correlate blood levels with therapeutic effects. Dose–response curves have not been established, and the dose required for an individual to experience treatment effects varies widely. Plasma levels of these medications are only partially helpful. Although these can be measured for a number of antipsychotics, their correlation with therapeutic response has been inconsistent. Haloperidol and clozapine correlate well and may be helpful in determining whether an adequate blood level has been reached and maintained during a trial of medication. Table 13-7 shows the therapeutic ranges available for some of the antipsychotic medications. Plasma levels may also be helpful in identifying absorption problems or metabolic differences (high or low metabolizer), determining adherence, and identifying adverse reactions from drug–drug interactions.

Potency of the antipsychotics also varies widely and is of specific concern when considering typical antipsychotic drugs. As Table 13-7 indicates, 100 mg chlorpromazine is roughly equivalent to 2 mg haloperidol and 5 mg trifluoperazine. Although drugs that are more potent are not inherently better than less potent drugs, differentiating low-potency versus high-potency

Table 13.7   Antipsychotic Medications

Generic (Trade) Drug Name	Usual Dosage Range (mg/d)	Half-Life (h)	Therapeutic Blood Level	Approximate Equivalent Dosage (mg)
Standard (Typical) Antipsychotics				
PHENOTHIAZINES				
ALIPHATICS				
chlorpromazine (Thorazine)	50–1200	2–30	30–100 mg/mL	100
PIPERIDINES				
thioridazine (Mellaril)	50–600	10–20	1–1.5 ng/mL	100
mesoridazine (Serentil)	50–400	24–48	Not available	50
PIPERAZINES				
fluphenazine (Prolixin)	2–20	4.5–15.3	0.2–0.3 ng/mL	2
perphenazine (Trilafon)	12–64	Unknown	0.8–12.0 ng/mL	10
trifluoperazine (Stelazine)	5–40	47–100	1–2.3 ng/mL	5
THIOXANTHENES				
thiothixene (Navane)	5–60	34	2–20 ng/mL	4
DIBENZOXAZEPINES				
loxapine (Loxitane)	20–250	19	Not available	15
BUTYROPHENONES				
haloperidol (Haldol)	2–60	21–24	5–15 ng/mL	2
DIHYDROINDOLONES				
molindone (Moban)	50–400	1.5	Not available	10
Atypical Antipsychotics				
DIBENZODIAZEPINES				
clozapine (Clozaril)	300–900	4–12	141–204 ng/mL	50
BENZISOXAZOLE				
risperidone (Risperdal)	2–8	20	Not available	1
THIENOBENZODIAZEPINE				
olanzapine (Zyprexa)	5–10	21–54	Not available	Not available
DIBENZOTHIAZEPINE				
quetiapine fumarate (Seroquel)	150–750	7	Not available	Not available
MONOHYDROCHLORIDE				
ziprasidone HCl (Geodon)	40–160	7	Not available	Not available
DIHYDROCARBOSTYRILS				
aripiprazole (Abilify)	10–30	75–94	Not available	Not available

antipsychotics may be somewhat helpful in predicting side effects. Roughly speaking, high-potency medications, such as haloperidol and fluphenazine, produce a greater frequency of extrapyramidal symptoms, and low-potency antipsychotics, such as chlorpromazine and thioridazine, produce more sedation and hypotension.

Ultimately, selection of medication from the group of typical antipsychotics depends predominately on predicted side effects, prior history of treatment response, whether or not a depot preparation will be needed during maintenance, concurrent medications, and other medical conditions.

Drug Formulations: Long-Acting Preparations

Currently, in Canada, two typical antipsychotic drugs, haloperidol and fluphenazine, are available in long-acting, depot forms. These two antipsychotics may be administered by injection once every 2 to 4 weeks. After administration, the drug is slowly released from the injection site; therefore, these forms of the drugs are referred to as *depot preparations*. Long-acting injectable medications maintain a fairly constant blood level between injections. Because they bypass problems with gastrointestinal absorption and first-pass metabolism, this method may enhance therapeutic outcomes for the patient. Lower rates of relapse have been reported for patients receiving long-acting injectable medication compared with those taking oral medications. Depot preparations are used when individuals have difficulty remembering to take their oral medications and are able to keep appointments reliably or attend a program regularly where the injection may be administered. Fluphenazine decanoate and haloperidol decanoate are equally effective in treating the symptoms of psychosis. Long-acting forms of fluphenazine are available as fluphenazine decanoate and fluphenazine enanthate. The latter has a markedly increased risk for extrapyramidal side effects and is rarely used. Nurses should be aware that the injection site may become sore and inflamed if certain precautions are not taken. The liquids are viscous, and a large-gauge needle (at least 21-gauge) should be used to withdraw the drug from the ampoule. However, there is emerging evidence that glass particles can be drawn up with the liquid, especially if using an 18-gauge needle, and thus a filtered needle is preferred for long-term use of depot medications (Preston & Hegadoren, 2004). Because the medication is meant to remain in the injection site, the needle should be dry, and a deep IM injection should be given by the Z-track method. (Note: Do not massage the injection site. Rotate sites and document in the patient's record.) A change to depot preparation from oral antipsychotic is done on a gradual basis after the patient is fully informed and consents and has taken several oral doses to ensure no significant immediate adverse reactions are likely to occur.

Recently, an atypical antipsychotic, risperidone, has become available in a long-acting formulation. It differs from the conventional depot form in that it is aqueous based and thereby better tolerated. Long-acting risperidone is unique in that microspheres (encapsulated polymers containing the medication) gradually break down, releasing the active form of the medication. This medication is administered intramuscularly every 2 weeks. Initiation of this medication regimen requires that an oral antipsychotic be given during the first 3 weeks to reach a therapeutic blood level.

Side Effects, Adverse Reactions, and Toxicity

Various side effects and interactions can occur with antipsychotics (see Tables 13-6 and 13-7), with the typical drugs producing more significant side effects than the atypical antipsychotics. The side effects vary largely based on their degree of attraction to different neurotransmitter receptors and their subtypes.

Cardiovascular Side Effects

Cardiovascular side effects, such as orthostatic hypotension, depend on the degree of blockade of α-adrenergic receptors. Low-potency typical antipsychotics, such as chlorpromazine and thioridazine, and the atypical antipsychotic clozapine have a high degree of affinity for α-adrenergic receptors and therefore produce considerable orthostatic hypotension. Other cardiovascular side effects from typical antipsychotics have been rare, but occasionally they cause ECG changes that have a benign or undetermined clinical effect. Thioridazine (Mellaril) and ziprasidone (Geodon) have both been associated with prolonged QT intervals and should be used cautiously in patients who have increased Q-T intervals or are taking other medications that may prolong the Q-T interval (Taylor, 2003).

Anticholinergic Side Effects

Anticholinergic side effects resulting from blockade of acetylcholine are another common concern with the typical and some of the atypical antipsychotic drugs. Dry mouth, slowed gastric motility, constipation, urinary hesitancy or retention, vaginal dryness, blurred vision, dry eyes, nasal congestion, and confusion or decreased memory are examples of these side effects. Interventions for decreasing the impact of these side effects are outlined in Table 13-2. This group of side effects occurs with many of the medications used for psychiatric treatment. Sometimes, a cholinergic medication, such as bethanechol, may reduce the peripheral effects but not the CNS effects. Using more than one medication with anticholinergic effects often increases the symptoms. Elderly patients are often most susceptible to a potential toxicity that results from high blockade of acetylcholine. This toxicity is called an *anticholinergic* crisis and is described, along with its treatment, in Chapter 17. The likelihood of anticholinergic side effects, along with sedation and extrapyramidal side effects, from antipsychotics, is explored in Table 13-5.

Weight Gain

Other clinically important effects also occur with the antipsychotic medications. Weight gain from increased appetite is common with the low-potency antipsychotics but occurs in highest proportion with clozapine and olanzapine. Weight gain has been associated with antipsychotic drugs since chlorpromazine was developed and is of increasing concern with the increased use of atypical drugs such as clozapine and olanzapine. The weight gain related to antipsychotic medications is linked to an increased risk for diabetes, heart disease, and hyperlipidemia. A Quebec study (N = 19,582) showed that the risk for initiation of a pharmacologic treatment for diabetes or dyslipidemia is significantly higher with olanzapine than risperidone (Moisan et al., 2005). Awareness of these risks emphasizes the need for early, preventive intervention with diet and exercise, as well as careful consideration in the choice of the specific atypical agent for at-risk populations. The chronic health problems of diabetes and cardiovascular illness occur much more often in individuals with mental illness than in the general population, making it essential for nurses to assist patients in dealing effectively with issues of weight gain. Ziprasidone (Geodon) and quetiapine (Seroquel) are two atypical antipsychotics associated with little to no weight gain during clinical trials.

Endocrine and Sexual Side Effects

Endocrine and sexual side effects result primarily from the blockade of dopamine in the tuberoinfundibular pathways of the hypothalamus. As a result, blood levels of prolactin may increase with almost all the typical antipsychotics but less commonly with the atypical antipsychotics. Increased prolactin causes breast enlargement and rare but potential galactorrhoea (milk production and flow), decreased sexual drive, amenorrhea, menstrual irregularities, and increased risk for growth in preexisting breast cancers. Bromocriptine, a dopamine agonist, may be helpful, but more likely these symptoms necessitate a change in medication. The prescriber should be notified immediately. Endocrine side effects can occur in males as well. Retrograde ejaculation (backward flow of semen) is rare, but it may be painful and can occur with all the antipsychotics. A more common side effect is erectile dysfunction, including difficulty achieving and maintaining an erection. Anorgasmia, or the inability to achieve orgasm, may develop in women.

Blood Disorders

Blood dyscrasias are rare but have received renewed attention since the introduction of clozapine. Agranulocytosis is an acute reaction that causes the individual's white blood cell count to drop to very low levels, and concurrent neutropenia, a drop in neutrophils in the blood, develops. In the case of the antipsychotics, the medication suppresses the bone marrow precursors to blood factors. The exact mechanism by which the drugs produce this effect is unknown. The most notable symptoms of this disorder include high fever, sore throat, and mouth sores. Although benign elevations in temperature have been reported in individuals taking clozapine, no fever should go uninvestigated. Untreated agranulocytosis can be life threatening. Although agranulocytosis can occur with any of the antipsychotics, the risk with clozapine is 10 to 20 times greater than with the other antipsychotics (Bilici, Tekelioglu, Efendioglu, Ovali, & Ulgen, 2003). Therefore, prescription of clozapine requires weekly blood samples for the first 6 months of treatment, and then every 2 weeks after that for as long as the drug is taken. Drawing of these samples must continue for 4 weeks after clozapine use has been discontinued. If sore throat or fever develops, medications should be withheld until a leukocyte count can be obtained. Hospitalization, including reverse isolation to prevent infections, is usually required. Agranulocytosis is more likely to develop during the first 18 weeks of treatment. Some research indicates that it is more common in women. The requirement for regular blood monitoring and added cost of laboratory services with clozapine has limited its use in community psychiatry with chronically mentally ill populations.

Miscellaneous

Photosensitivity reactions to antipsychotics, including severe sunburns or rash, most commonly develop with the use of low-potency typical medications. Sun block must be worn on all areas of exposed skin when taking these drugs. In addition, sun exposure may cause pigmentary deposits to develop, resulting in discoloration of exposed areas, especially the neck and face. This discoloration may progress from a deep orange color to a blue grey. Skin exposure should be limited and skin tone changes reported to the prescriber. Pigmentary deposits may also develop on the retina of the eye, especially with high doses of thioridazine, even for a few days. This condition is called *retinitis pigmentosa* and can lead to significant visual impairment. Therefore, thioridazine should never be administered in doses greater than 800 mg/d.

Antipsychotics may also lower the seizure threshold. Patients with an undetected seizure disorder may experience seizures early in treatment. Those who have a preexisting condition should be monitored closely.

Neuroleptic malignant syndrome (NMS) and water intoxication are two serious complications that may result from antipsychotic medications. Characterized by rigidity and high fever, NMS is a rare condition that may occur abruptly with even one dose of medication. Temperature must always be monitored when administering antipsychotics, especially high-potency medications. Water intoxication may develop gradually with long-term use. This condition is characterized by the patient's consumption of large quantities of fluid (polydipsia) and the resulting effects of sodium depletion (hyponatremia). Both of these conditions are discussed more fully in Chapter 17.

Medication-Related Movement Disorders

Medication-related movement disorders are a group of side effects or adverse reactions that are commonly caused by typical antipsychotic medications but less commonly with atypical antipsychotic drugs. These disorders of abnormal motor movements can be divided into two groups: acute extrapyramidal syndromes (EPS), which are acute abnormal movements developing early in the course of treatment (sometimes after just one dose); and chronic syndromes, which develop from longer exposure to antipsychotic drugs. The atypical antipsychotic drugs are most likely to cause movement disorders.

Acute Extrapyramidal Syndromes

Acute EPS occur in as many as 90% (Glazer, 2000) of all patients receiving typical antipsychotic medications. These syndromes include dystonia, parkinsonism, and **akathisia** (an involuntary movement disorder). They develop early in treatment, sometimes from as little as one dose. Although the abnormal movements are treatable, they are at times dramatic and frightening, causing physical and emotional impairments that often prompt patients to stop taking their medication. Some milder forms of EPS may occur with classes of medication other than antipsychotics, including the SSRIs. The acute EPS often are mistaken for aspects of anxiety, rather than medication side effects. Nurses play a vital role in the early recognition and treatment of these syndromes. Early recognition can save the patient considerable discomfort, fear, and impairment. All nurses must be aware of these symptoms, notifying the prescriber as soon as possible and implementing selected medication changes and other interventions. Several medications can control these acute extrapyramidal symptoms (Table 13-8).

Dystonia, sometimes referred to as an *acute dystonic reaction,* is impaired muscle tone that generally is the first extrapyramidal symptom to occur, usually within a few days of initiating use of an antipsychotic. Dystonia is characterized by involuntary muscle spasms, especially of the head and neck muscles. Patients usually first complain of a thick tongue, tight jaw, or stiff neck.

The syndrome can progress to a protruding tongue, oculogyric crisis (eyes rolled up in the head), torticollis (muscle stiffness in the neck, which draws the head to one side with chin pointing to the other), and laryngopharyngeal constriction. Abnormal postures of the upper limbs and torso may be held briefly or sustained. In severe cases, the spasms may progress to the intercostal muscles, producing more significant breathing difficulty for patients who already have respiratory impairment from asthma or emphysema.

Drug-induced parkinsonism is sometimes referred to as **pseudoparkinsonism** because its presentation is identical to Parkinson's disease without the same destruction of dopaminergic cells. These symptoms include the classic triad of rigidity, slowed movements (akinesia), and tremor. The rigid muscle stiffness is usually seen in the arms. Akinesia can be observed by the loss of spontaneous movements, such as the absence of the usual relaxed swing of the arms while walking. In addition, masklike facies or loss of facial expression and a decrease in the ability to initiate movements also are present. Usually, tremor is more pronounced at rest, but it can also be observed with intentional movements, such as eating. If the tremor becomes severe, it may interfere with the patient's ability to eat or maintain adequate fluid intake. Hypersalivation is possible as well. Pseudoparkinsonism symptoms may occur on one or both sides of the body and develop abruptly or subtly but usually within the first 30 days of treatment.

Akathisia is characterized by the inability to sit still. The person will pace, rock while sitting or standing, march in place, or cross and uncross the legs. All these repetitive motions have an intensity that is frequently beyond the explanation of the individual. In addition, akathisia may be present as a primarily subjective experience without obvious motor behaviour. This subjective experience includes feelings of anxiety, jitteriness, or the inability to relax, which the individual may or may not be able to communicate. It is extremely uncomfortable for a person experiencing akathisia to be forced to sit still or be confined. These symptoms are sometimes misdiagnosed as agitation or an increase in psychotic symptoms, but if the nurse administers an antipsychotic medication PRN (as needed), the symptoms will not abate and will often worsen. Differentiating akathisia from agitation may be aided by knowing the person's symptoms before the introduction of medication. Psychotic agitation does not usually begin abruptly after antipsychotic medication use has been started, whereas akathisia may occur after administration. In addition, the nurse may ask the patient if the experience is felt primarily in the muscles (akathisia) or in the mind or emotions (agitation).

Akathisia is the most difficult acute medication-related movement disorder to relieve. It does not usually respond well to anticholinergic medications and is

Table 13.8   Drug Therapies for Acute Medication-Related Movement Disorders

Agents	Typical Dosage Ranges	Routes Available	Common Side Effects
Anticholinergics			
benztropine (Cogentin)	2–6 mg/d	PO, IM, IV	Dry mouth, blurred vision, slowed gastric motility causing constipation, urinary retention, increased intraocular pressure; overdose produces toxic psychosis
trihexyphenidyl (Artane)	4–15 mg/d	PO	Same as benztropine, plus gastrointestinal distress Elderly people are most prone to mental confusion and delirium
biperiden (Akineton)	2–8 mg/d	PO	Fewer peripheral anticholinergic effects Euphoria and increased tremor may occur
Antihistamines			
diphenhydramine (Benadryl)	25–50 mg qid to 400 mg daily	PO, IM, IV	Sedation and confusion, especially in elderly people
Dopamine Agonists			
amantadine (Symmetrel)	100–400 mg daily	PO	Indigestion, decreased concentration, dizziness, anxiety, ataxia, insomnia, lethargy, tremors, and slurred speech may occur on higher doses Tolerance may develop on fixed dose
β-Blockers			
propranolol (Inderal)	10 mg tid to 120 mg daily	PO	Hypotension and bradycardia Must monitor pulse and blood pressure Do not stop abruptly as may cause rebound tachycardia
Benzodiazepines			
lorazepam (Ativan)	1–2 mg IM 0.5–2 mg PO	PO, IM	All may cause drowsiness, lethargy, and general sedation or paradoxical agitation Confusion and disorientation in elderly people
diazepam (Valium)	2–5 mg tid	PO, IV	Most side effects are rare and will disappear if dose is decreased
clonazepam (Klonopin)	1–4 mg/d	PO	Tolerance and withdrawal are potential problems

uncommon in patients receiving atypical antipsychotics. It is thought that the pathology of akathisia may involve more than just the extrapyramidal motor system. It may include serotonin changes that also affect the dopamine system (Kulkarni & Naidu, 2003). A number of medications have been used to reduce symptoms, including β-adrenergic blockers, anticholinergics, antihistamines, and low-dose antianxiety agents (Sajatovic, 2000). The usual approach to treatment is to change to an atypical antipsychotic if possible. If not, reducing the dose of typical antipsychotic medication can be tried. During this time, psychiatric–mental health nurses must closely assess for worsening of symptoms. Then, β-adrenergic blockers, such as propranolol (Inderal), given in doses of 30 to 120 mg/d, have been most successful. Nurses must monitor the patient's pulse and blood pressure because propranolol can cause hypotension and bradycardia. If the patient's pulse falls below 60 bpm, propranolol should be withheld and the prescriber notified. Normal signs of hypoglycaemia may be blocked by propranolol; therefore, patients with diabetes must monitor their blood or urine glucose levels carefully, especially because they are under physical stress from the disorder.

A number of nursing interventions may reduce the impact of these syndromes. Individuals with acute extrapyramidal symptoms need frequent reassurance that this is not a worsening of their psychiatric condition but instead is a treatable side effect of the medication. They also need validation that what they are experiencing is real and that the nurse is concerned and will be responsive to changes in these symptoms. Physical and psychological stress appears to increase the symptoms and further frighten the patient; therefore, decreasing stressful situations becomes important. These symptoms are often physically exhausting for the patient, and nurses should ensure that the patient receives adequate rest and hydration. Because tremors, muscle rigidity, and motor restlessness may interfere with the individual's ability to eat, the nurse may need to assist the patient with eating and drinking fluids to maintain nutrition and hydration.

Risk factors for acute EPS syndromes include previous episodes of extrapyramidal symptoms. Listen closely when patients say they are "allergic" or have had "bad reactions" to antipsychotic medications. Often, they are describing one of the medication-related movement disorders, particularly dystonia, rather than a rash or other allergic symptoms. About 90% of the individuals who have experienced extrapyramidal symptoms in the past will again have these symptoms if use of an antipsychotic medication is restarted (Arana, 2000; Nasrallah, 2002). High-potency medications, such as haloperidol and fluphenazine, are more likely to cause extrapyramidal symptoms. Age and gender appear to be risk factors for specific syndromes. Acute dystonia occurs most often in young men, adolescents, and children; akathisia is more common in middle-aged women. Elderly patients are at the greatest risk for experiencing pseudoparkinsonism (O'Hara et al., 2002). Although the occurrence of EPS is decreasing as atypical medications are more commonly used, acute EPS remains a serious clinical concern.

Chronic Syndromes

Chronic syndromes develop from long-term use of antipsychotics. They are serious and afflict about 20% of the patients who receive typical antipsychotics for an extended period. These conditions are typically irreversible and cause significant impairment in self-image, social interactions, and occupational functioning. Early symptoms and mild forms may go unnoticed by the person experiencing them because they frequently remain beyond the individual's awareness. Therefore, psychiatric–mental health nurses in contact with individuals who are taking antipsychotic medications for months or years must be vigilant for symptoms of these typical chronic conditions.

First identified in 1957, tardive dyskinesia is the most well-known of the chronic syndromes. It involves irregular, repetitive involuntary movements of the mouth, face, and tongue, including chewing, tongue protrusion, lip smacking, puckering of the lips, and rapid eye blinking. Abnormal finger movements are common as well. In some individuals, the trunk and extremities are also involved, and in rare cases, irregular breathing and swallowing lead to belching and grunting noises. These

symptoms usually begin no earlier than after 6 months of treatment or when the medication is reduced or withdrawn. Once thought to be irreversible, considerable controversy now exists as to whether or not this is true.

Part of the difficulty in determining the irreversibility of tardive dyskinesia is that any movement disorder that persists after discontinuation of antipsychotic medication has been described as tardive dyskinesia. Atypical forms are now receiving more attention because some researchers believe they may have different underlying mechanisms of causation. Some of these forms of the disorder appear to remit spontaneously. Symptoms of what is now called *withdrawal tardive dyskinesia* appear when use of an antipsychotic medication is reduced or discontinued and remit spontaneously in 1 to 3 months. Tardive dystonia and tardive akathisia have also been described. Both appear in a manner similar to the acute syndromes but continue after the antipsychotic medication has been withdrawn. More research is needed to determine whether these syndromes are distinctly different in origin and outcome.

The risk for experiencing tardive dyskinesia increases with age. Although the prevalence of tardive dyskinesia averages 15% to 20%, the rate rises to 50% to 70% in elderly patients receiving antipsychotic medications (O'Hara et al., 2002; Yeung et al., 2000). Cumulative incidence of tardive dyskinesia appears to increase 5% per year of continued exposure to antipsychotic medications (Levy et al., 2002). Women are at higher risk than men. Individuals with affective disorders, particularly depression, are at higher risk than are those who have schizophrenia. Any individual receiving antipsychotic medication may experience tardive dyskinesia; therefore, nurses must be particularly alert to individuals at higher risk. Risk factors are summarized in Box 13-2. The causes of tardive dyskinesia remain unclear. Lack of a consistent theory of aetiology for the chronic medication-related movement disorder syndromes has led to inconsistent and disappointing treatment approaches. No one medication relieves the symptoms. Dopamine agonists, such as bromocriptine, and many other drugs have been tried. Even dietary precursors of acetylcholine, such as lethicin, and nutritional therapies, such as vitamin E supplements, may prove to be beneficial.

BOX 13.2

Risk Factors for Tardive Dyskinesia

- Age more than 50 years
- Female
- Affective disorders, particularly depression
- Brain damage or dysfunction
- Increased duration of treatment
- Standard antipsychotic medication
- Possible—higher doses of antipsychotic medication

The best approach to treatment remains avoiding the development of the chronic syndromes. Preventive measures include use of atypical antipsychotics, using the lowest possible dose of typical medication, minimizing use of PRN medication, and closely monitoring individuals in high-risk groups for development of the symptoms of tardive dyskinesia. All members of the mental health treatment team who have contact with individuals taking antipsychotics for longer than 3 months must be alert to the risk factors and earliest possible signs of chronic medication-related movement disorders.

Monitoring tools, such as the Abnormal Involuntary Movement Scale (AIMS), should be used routinely to standardize assessment and provide the earliest possible recognition of the symptoms. Standardized assessments should be performed at a minimum of 3- to 6-month intervals. The earlier the symptoms are recognized, the more likely they will resolve if the medication can be changed or its use discontinued. Newer, atypical antipsychotic medications have a much lower risk for causing tardive dyskinesia and are increasingly being considered first-line medications for treating schizophrenia. Other medications are under development to provide alternatives that limit the risk for tardive dyskinesia.

MOOD STABILIZERS (ANTIMANIA MEDICATIONS)

Mood stabilizers, or antimania medications, are psychopharmacologic agents used primarily for stabilizing mood swings, particularly those of mania in bipolar affective disorders. For a number of years, lithium was the only drug known to stabilize the symptoms of mania. Although it remains the gold standard of treatment for acute mania and maintenance of bipolar affective disorders, not all individuals experience response to lithium, and increasingly other drugs are being used as first-line agents. In the 1970s, carbamazepine (Tegretol) and later valproate, both anticonvulsants approved for treating epilepsy, were found to have mood-stabilizing effects. Other medications, such as calcium-channel blockers, have been used as adjunctive treatment for the symptoms of mania. At present, three drugs have FDA approval for the short-term treatment of acute mania. They include lithium, olanzapine (Zyprexa), and valproic acid (Depakote). Lithium is the only drug with approved FDA indication for the prevention and treatment of both manic and depressive episodes. Many other drugs, including other anticonvulsants, atypical antipsychotics, adrenergic blocking agents, and calcium-channel blockers, are frequently used to treat bipolar disorder.

Lithium

Lithium, a naturally occurring element, was first discovered in the early 1800s. It has been in medical use in a variety of forms, including tonics and elixirs, since that time. As an element that acts as a salt substitute, the unregulated use of lithium produced a number of cases of toxicity and, as a result, lost favour in the 1940s. Rediscovered in 1949 by the Australian John Cade, lithium was found to reduce agitation in some patients experiencing psychosis, and in the 1950s, Mogens Schou published reports that lithium controlled and prevented the symptoms of mania. In 1970, the FDA approved lithium for use in treating manic episodes in bipolar affective disorder. Since then, it has become a mainstay in psychopharmacology. Lithium is effective in only about 40% of patients with bipolar disorder, and patients who do experience response often have limited clinical improvement. Although lithium is not a perfect drug, a great deal is known regarding its use—it is inexpensive, it has restored stability to the lives of thousands of people, and it remains the gold standard of bipolar pharmacologic treatment.

Indications and Mechanisms of Action

The target symptoms for lithium are the symptoms of mania, such as rapid speech, jumping from topic to topic (flight of ideas), irritability, grandiose thinking, impulsiveness, and agitation. Other psychiatric indications include using lithium for its mild antidepressant effects in treating depressive episodes of bipolar illness and in patients experiencing major depression that has only partially responded to antidepressants alone. Used in patients who have experienced only partial response, lithium has been used in augmentation as a potentiator (enhancing the effects) of antidepressant medications. It also has been shown to be helpful in reducing impulsivity and aggression in certain psychiatric patients.

Lithium has been effective in treating several nonpsychiatric disorders, such as cluster headaches. Because lithium stimulates leukocytosis, it often improves the neutrophil counts of patients who are undergoing chemotherapy or who have other conditions that cause neutropenia. In addition, lithium has been investigated as an antiviral agent because it appears to inhibit the replication of several DNA viruses, including herpes virus. Additional research is needed to fully understand the mechanisms of these effects.

Lithium is actively transported across cell membranes, altering sodium transport in both nerve and muscle cells. It replaces sodium in the sodium–potassium pump and is retained more readily than sodium inside the cell. Conditions that alter sodium content in the body, such as vomiting, diuresis, and diaphoresis, also alter lithium retention. The results of lithium influx into the nerve cell lead to increased storage of catecholamines within the cell, reduced dopamine neurotransmission, increased norepinephrine reuptake, increased GABA activity, and increased serotonin receptor sensitivity (Bschor et al., 2003; Solomon et al., 2000). Lithium also alters the distribution of calcium and magnesium ions and inhibits second messenger systems within the neuron. The specific mechanisms by which lithium improves the symptoms of mania are complex, most likely involving the sum of all or part of these actions and more. Genetic research in bipolar disorder considers lithium response as an important criterion for subgrouping the bipolar population (Alda, 2004).

Pharmacokinetics

Lithium carbonate is available orally in capsule, tablet, and liquid forms. Slow-release preparations are also available. Lithium is readily absorbed in the gastric system and may be taken with food, which does not impair absorption. Peak blood levels are reached in 1 to 4 hours, and the medication is usually completely absorbed in 8 hours. Slow-release preparations are absorbed at a slower, more variable rate.

Lithium is not protein bound, and its distribution into the CNS across the blood–brain barrier is slow. The onset of action is usually 5 to 7 days and may take as long as 2 weeks. The elimination half-life is 8 to 12 hours, and 18 to 36 hours in individuals whose blood levels have reached steady state and whose symptoms are stable. Lithium is almost entirely excreted by the kidneys but is present in all body fluids. Conditions of renal impairment or decreased renal function in elderly patients decrease lithium clearance and may lead to toxicity. Several medications affect renal function and therefore change lithium clearance. See Chapter 19 for a list of these and other medication interactions with lithium. About 80% of lithium is reabsorbed in the proximal tubule of the kidney along with water and sodium. In conditions that cause sodium depletion, such as dehydration caused by fever, strenuous exercise, hot weather, increased perspiration, and vomiting, the kidney attempts to conserve sodium. Because lithium is a salt, the kidney retains lithium as well, leading to increased blood levels and potential toxicity. Significantly increasing sodium intake causes lithium levels to fall.

Lithium is usually administered in doses of 300 mg two to three times daily. During the acute phases of mania, blood levels of 0.8 to 1.4 mEq/L are usually attained and maintained until symptoms are under control. During maintenance, the dosage is reduced, and dosages are adjusted to maintain blood levels of 0.4 to 1 mEq/L. As a drug with a narrow therapeutic range or index, blood levels are monitored frequently during acute mania, while the dosage is increased every 3 to 5 days. These increases may be slower in elderly patients or patients who experience uncomfortable side effects. Blood levels should be monitored 12 hours after the last dose of medication. In the hospital setting, nurses should withhold the morning dose of lithium until the serum sample is drawn to avoid falsely elevated levels. Individuals who are at home should be instructed to have their blood drawn in the morning about 12 hours after their last dose and before they take their first dose of medication.

Lithium clears the body relatively quickly after discontinuation of its use. Withdrawal symptoms are rare, but occasional anxiety and emotional lability have been reported. It is important to remember that almost half of the individuals who discontinue lithium treatment abruptly experience a relapse of symptoms within a few weeks (Goodwin & Ghaemi, 2000; Kennedy et al., 2003). Some research suggests that discontinuation of the use of lithium for individuals whose symptoms have been stable may lead to lithium losing its effectiveness when use of the medication is restarted. Patients should be warned of the risks in abruptly discontinuing their medication and should be advised to consider the options carefully in consultation with their prescriber.

Side Effects, Adverse Reactions, and Toxicity

At lower therapeutic blood levels, side effects from lithium are relatively mild. These reactions correspond with peaks in plasma concentrations of the medication after administration, and most subside during the first few weeks of therapy. Frequently, individuals taking lithium complain of excessive thirst and an unpleasant metallic-like taste. Sugarless throat lozenges may be useful in minimizing this side effect. Other common side effects include increased frequency of urination, fine head tremor, drowsiness, and mild diarrhoea. Weight gain occurs in about 20% of the individuals taking lithium. Nausea may be minimized by taking the medication with food or by use of a slow-release preparation. However, slow-release forms of lithium increase diarrhoea. Muscle weakness, restlessness, headache, acne, rashes, and exacerbation of psoriasis have also been reported. See Chapter 19 for a summary of selected nursing interventions to minimize the impact of common side effects associated with lithium treatment. Patients most frequently discontinued their own medication use because of concerns with mental slowness, poor concentration, and memory problems.

As blood levels of lithium increase, the side effects of lithium become more numerous and severe. Early signs of lithium toxicity include severe diarrhoea, vomiting, drowsiness, muscular weakness, and lack of coordination. Lithium should be withheld and the prescriber consulted if these symptoms develop. Lithium toxicity can easily be resolved in 24 to 48 hours by discontinuing the medication, but haemodialysis may be required in severe situations. See Chapter 19 for a summary of the side effects and symptoms of toxicity associated with various blood levels of lithium.

Monitoring of creatinine concentration, thyroid hormones, and CBC every 6 months during maintenance therapy helps to assess the occurrence of other potential adverse reactions. Kidney damage is considered an uncommon but potentially serious risk for long-term lithium treatment. This damage is usually reversible after discontinuation of the lithium use. A gradual rise in serum creatinine and decline in creatinine clearance indicate the development of renal dysfunction. Individuals with preexisting kidney dysfunction are susceptible to lithium toxicity.

Lithium may alter thyroid function, usually after 6 to 18 months of treatment. About 30% of the individuals taking lithium exhibit elevations in thyroid-stimulating hormone, but most do not show suppression of circulating thyroid hormone. Thyroid dysfunction from lithium treatment is more common in women, and some individuals require the addition of thyroxine to their care. During maintenance, thyroid-stimulating hormone levels may be monitored. Nurses should observe for dry skin, constipation, bradycardia, hair loss, cold intolerance, and other symptoms of hypothyroidism. Other endocrine system effects result from hypoparathyroidism, which increases parathyroid hormone levels and calcium. Clinically, this change is not significant, but elevated calcium levels may cause mood changes, anxiety, lethargy, and sleep disturbances. These symptoms may erroneously be attributed to depression if hypocalcaemia is not investigated.

Lithium use must be avoided during pregnancy because it has been associated with birth defects, especially when administered during the first trimester. If lithium is given during the third trimester, toxicity may develop in a newborn, producing signs of hypotonia, cyanosis, bradykinesia, cardiac changes, gastrointestinal bleeding, and shock. Diabetes insipidus may persist for months. Lithium is also present in breast milk, and women should not breast-feed while taking lithium. Women expecting to become pregnant should be advised to consult with their physician before discontinuing use of birth control methods.

Anticonvulsants

Six anticonvulsants are commonly used to treat bipolar disorder: valproic acid, carbamazepine, gabapentin (Neurontin), topiramate (Topamax), lamotrigine (Lamictal), and oxcarbazepine (Trileptal). Although lithium alone has provided tremendous relief to thousands of individuals experiencing bipolar affective disorder, 20% to 40% of those affected by the disorder do not respond, most often those with rapid cycling episodes. The psychopharmacologic properties of some anticonvulsant medications have been reported since the 1960s,

but it was not until the 1970s in Japan that carbamazepine was demonstrated to have mood-stabilizing effects in patients with bipolar affective disorders. Concern about blood dyscrasias delayed its release in the United States, and the increased risks for aplastic anaemia and agranulocytosis with carbamazepine use still require close monitoring of CBCs during treatment. Valproate and its derivatives have had a similar course of development. With the exception of gabapentin (Neurontin), for which little evidence exists, the benefit of anticonvulsant use in bipolar disorder has been well established.

Indications and Mechanisms of Action

Anticonvulsant medications in general are primarily indicated for treating seizure disorders. Target symptoms for the use of anticonvulsants with bipolar affective disorder include all the symptoms of mania discussed earlier. However, anticonvulsants are often used for individuals who have not experienced response to lithium or who are identified as having rapid cycling. Studies have shown some common traits in these individuals. Those who do not experience response to lithium most often are those who have a dysphoric or mixed mania. These individuals experience the increase in physical activity during manic episodes without any elevation in mood. They often are referred to as *mixed states* because they have elements of both depression and mania. These individuals exhibit symptoms of high anxiety, agitation, and irritability, which are then target symptoms for the use of anticonvulsants. Empirical data show carbamazepine and valproic acid to be effective in mood stabilization. The data are less clear for gabapentin, which for that reason is often an adjunctive, not primary, medication for treating patients with bipolar disorder (Grunze & Walden, 2002).

The term *rapid cycling* is applied when individuals experience four or more episodes of either depression or mania during a 12-month period. This occurs more often in women than in men. These patients make up a group of individuals who experience poor response to lithium treatment. Mood instability is also a target symptom of anticonvulsant medications. The theory of the mechanism of action of the anticonvulsants involves the concept of kindling as it applies to mood disorders.

Kindling refers to the emergence of spontaneous firing of nerve cells in response to repeated subthreshold electrical stimulation. Once brain regions such as the amygdala have been "kindled," it takes considerably less stimulation to initiate a seizure. In the case of mood disorders, it is hypothesized that "kindled" brain regions include the areas associated with emotional regulation. Stimulation of these regions by increasingly minor stressors or other environmental factors produces mood swings, instead of a seizure.

Anticonvulsants have "antikindling" properties and decrease the sensitization of affected cells, making them less easy to stimulate. In general, the anticonvulsant mood stabilizers have many actions, but it is their effects on ion channels, reducing repetitive firing of action potentials in the nerves, that most directly decreases manic symptoms. In addition, drugs such as carbamazepine affect the release and reuptake of several neurotransmitters, including norepinephrine, GABA, dopamine, and glutamate. They also change several second messenger systems. No single mechanism has yet accounted for the anticonvulsants' ability to stabilize mood. Divalproex sodium also has been shown to have numerous neurotransmission effects. The most widely held theory of how it stabilizes mood swings relates to its effects on GABA. As the major inhibitory neurotransmitter in the CNS, increased levels of GABA and improved responsiveness of the neurons to GABA lead to control of epileptic activity. Divalproex sodium increases levels of GABA in the CNS by activating its synthesis, inhibiting the catabolism (destructive metabolism) of GABA, increasing its release, and increasing receptor density (Loscher, 2002; Solomon et al., 2000). Although the exact mechanisms of action for the anticonvulsants remain unknown, these theories related to kindling and the enhanced functioning of GABA hold promise for the future of new developments in treatment.

Pharmacokinetics

Carbamazepine is an unusual drug and is absorbed in a somewhat variable manner. The liquid suspension is absorbed more quickly than the tablet form, but food does not appear to interfere with absorption. Peak plasma levels occur in 2 to 6 hours. Because high doses influence peak plasma levels and increase the risk for side effects, carbamazepine should be given in divided doses two or three times a day. The suspension, which has higher peak plasma levels and lower trough levels, must be given more frequently than the tablet form.

Valproic acid is more rapidly absorbed, but the enteric coating of divalproex sodium adds a delay of as long as 1 hour. Peak serum levels occur in about 1 to 4 hours. The liquid form (sodium valproate) is absorbed more rapidly and peaks in 15 minutes to 2 hours (Loscher, 2002). Food appears to slow absorption, but does not lower bioavailability of the drug. Valproate is a good example of the importance of considering **bioequivalence**, a term referring to the abilities of two formulations of the same drug to induce a therapeutic response of similar magnitude and duration (Zintzaras, 2005). For example, divalproex, an enteric coated formulation, has a half-life of 12 to 16 hours; is not affected by food intake and achieves more consistent plasma levels than valproic acid, which has a shorter half-life (8 hours), should not be taken with food, and produces gastrointestinal irritation in about 40% of patients.

Carbamazepine and valproic acid are highly protein bound; therefore, patients who are older, medically ill, or malnourished may experience the effects of increased unbound levels of both drugs. When given with other drugs that are competing for the same protein-binding sites, higher levels of unbound drug may occur. In both cases, these individuals risk more side effects and fluctuations in medication plasma levels. Newer agents for treatment of bipolar affective disorder, such as gabapentin, have little protein binding and therefore are not subject to some of these effects. Carbamazepine and valproic acid also cross easily into the CNS and move into the placenta as well. Both are associated with an increased risk for birth defects, including spina bifida, and carbamazepine accumulates in foetal tissue. Carbamazepine and valproic acid are metabolized by the cytochrome P-450 system of microsomal hepatic enzymes. However, one of the metabolites of carbamazepine is potentially toxic. When other, concurrent medications inhibit the enzymes that break down this toxic metabolite, severe adverse reactions are often the result. Medications that inhibit this breakdown include erythromycin, verapamil, and cimetidine (now available in nonprescription form).

Carbamazepine activates its own metabolism through induction of the P-450 microsomal hepatic enzymes. As long as 2 to 3 months after steady state has been achieved, patients receiving carbamazepine may experience a precipitant drop in therapeutic blood levels and a relapse in symptoms if the dosage is not increased. Although valproic acid is also affected by other medications that stimulate the P-450 system, it does not enhance its own metabolism. Both carbamazepine and valproic acid are available in slow-release, extended-action forms, allowing for decreased daily dosing and improved **adherence.**

Teaching Points

Nurses need to educate patients about potential drug interactions, especially with nonprescription medications. Nurses can also inform other health care practitioners who may be prescribing medication that these patients are taking carbamazepine. It is important to note that oral contraceptives may become ineffective, and female patients should be advised to use other methods of birth control.

Side Effects, Adverse Reactions, and Toxicity of Anticonvulsants

The most common side effects of carbamazepine are dizziness, drowsiness, tremor, visual disturbance, nausea, and vomiting. These side effects may be minimized by initiating treatment in low doses. Patients should be advised that these symptoms will diminish, but care should be taken when changing positions or performing tasks that require visual alertness. Giving the drug with food may diminish nausea. Valproic acid also causes gastrointestinal disturbances, tremor, and lethargy. In addition, it can produce weight gain and alopecia (hair loss). These symptoms are transient and should diminish with the course of treatment. Dietary supplements of zinc and selenium may be helpful to patients experiencing hair loss. Constipation and urinary retention occur in some individuals. Nurses should monitor urinary output and assist patients to increase fluid consumption to decrease constipation.

Transient elevations in liver enzymes occur with both carbamazepine and valproic acid, but rarely do symptoms of hepatic injury occur. If the patient reports abnormal pain or shows signs of jaundice, the prescriber should be notified immediately. Several blood dyscrasias are associated with carbamazepine, including aplastic anaemia, agranulocytosis, and leucopenia. Patients should be advised to report fever, sore throat, rash, petechiae, or bruising immediately. In addition, advise patients of the importance of completing routine blood tests throughout treatment.

Both valproic acid and carbamazepine may be lethal if high doses are ingested. Toxic symptoms appear in 1 to 3 hours and include neuromuscular disturbances, dizziness, stupor, agitation, disorientation, nystagmus, urinary retention, nausea and vomiting, tachycardia, hypotension or hypertension, cardiovascular shock, coma, and respiratory depression. Carbamazepine appears to be more lethal at lower doses, but valproic acid is absorbed rapidly, and gastric lavage may be ineffective, depending on time from ingestion.

Of the newer anticonvulsant drugs, gabapentin (Neurontin) has relatively few side effects. Lamotrigine (Lamictal) in rare cases produces severe, life-threatening rashes that usually occur within 2 to 8 weeks of treatment. This risk is highest in children. Use of lamotrigine should be immediately discontinued if a rash is noted. Topamax (Topiramate) carries an increased risk for kidney stone formation. It can also cause a decrease in serum digoxin levels and may decrease effectiveness of oral birth control agents. In addition, ongoing ophthalmologic monitoring is required because of reports of acute myopia with secondary glaucoma. Trileptal (oxcarbazepine) has the potential for causing hyponatremia and may also decrease the effectiveness of oral birth control agents. Because of the potentially significant adverse reactions that the anticonvulsants can produce, careful patient teaching and monitoring are required.

ANTIDEPRESSANT MEDICATIONS

Researchers in the 1950s who were investigating other drugs related to the phenothiazines for treatment of psychosis discovered that imipramine, a related compound, relieved the symptoms of depression. Imipramine was the first of a number of medications that contained a three-ring structure in their chemical makeup and produced improvement in depression. These medications became known as tricyclic antidepressants (TCAs). Table 13-9 lists other related TCAs still in use today.

Concurrent with the discovery of TCAs, an antibiotic, iproniazid, used in treating tuberculosis, alleviated the symptoms of depression. Iproniazid increased the bioamine neurotransmitters by inhibiting monoamine oxidase, the enzyme that breaks down these neurotransmitters inside the nerve cell. Iproniazid is no longer used, but related, more effective drugs, phenelzine and tranylcypromine, make up a subgroup of antidepressants called the monoamine oxidase inhibitors (MAOIs).

TCAs, MAOIs, and More

Throughout the 1960s and 1970s, the TCAs and MAOIs were the primary medications for treating depression. Research continued to develop new agents with increased effectiveness, while decreasing the side effects and potential lethal effects. In the 1980s, several medications that were significantly different in chemical structure were introduced. Bupropion (Wellbutrin), introduced in 1987, had actions that were significantly different from those of previous antidepressants, but concern about the risk for seizures and other side effects limited initial excitement about its use. In 1988, the release of fluoxetine (Prozac) received much public attention and resulted in increased awareness of depression and its treatment. Fluoxetine was the first of a class of drugs that acted "selectively" on one group of neurotransmitters, in this case serotonin. Other similarly selective medications, sertraline (Zoloft), paroxetine (Paxil), and fluvoxamine (Luvox), soon followed and together make up the SSRIs. The newest SSRIs include citalopram (Celexa) and escitalopram oxalate (Lexapro). Reboxetine is the only norepinephrine selective reuptake inhibitor available in Canada.

Citalopram is a racemate, which means it contains equal proportions of two isomers. Isomers are molecules with the same chemical formula but with a different spatial arrangement of the atoms, which may cause different effects in the human body or have different side-effect profiles. The two isomers of citalopram were separated, and escitalopram, one of the isomers, is marketed as an antidepressant in its own right.

Since the initial introduction of the SSRIs, several new chemical compounds have been introduced that have unique structure or actions, making them difficult to categorize. These medications differ in which neurotransmitters they affect and in what side effects are common. This subgroup of antidepressants includes such drugs as mirtazapine (Remeron) and venlafaxine (Effexor). In the Canadian clinical guidelines for the

Table 13.9 Antidepressant Medications

Generic (Trade) Drug Name	Usual Dosage Range (mg/d)	Half-Life (h)	Therapeutic Blood Level (ng/mL)
Tricyclic—Tertiary Amines			
amitriptyline (Elavil)	50–300	31–46	110–250
clomipramine (Anafranil)	25–250	19–37	80–100
doxepin (Sinequan)	25–300	8–24	100–200
imipramine (Tofranil)	30–300	11–25	200–350
Tricyclics—Secondary Amines			
amoxapine (Asendin)	50–600	8	200–500
desipramine (Norpramin)	25–300	12–24	125–300
nortriptyline (Aventyl)	30–100	18–44	50–150
protriptyline (Vivactil)	15–60	67–89	100–200
Selective Serotonin Reuptake Inhibitors			
fluoxetine (Prozac)	20–80	2–9 days	72–300
sertraline (Zoloft)	50–200	24	Not available
paroxetine (Paxil)	10–50	10–24	Not available
fluvoxamine (Luvox)	50–300	17–22	Not available
citalopram (Celexa)	20–50	35	Not available
escitalopram (Lexapro)	10–20	27–32	Not available
Other Antidepressant Medications			
PHENETHYLAMINE			
venlafaxine (Effexor)	75–375	5–11	100–500
TETRACYCLIC			
maprotiline (Ludiomil)	50–225	21–25	200–300
TRIAZOLOPYRIDINE			
trazodone (Desyrel)	150–600	4–9	650–1,600
PHENYLPIPERAZINE			
nefazodone (Serzone)	100–600	2–4	Not available
AMINOKETONE			
bupropion (Wellbutrin)	200–450	8–24	10–29
PIPERAZINOAZEPINES			
mirtazapine (Remeron)	15–45	20–40	Not available
Monoamine Oxidase Inhibitors			
moclobemide (Manerix)	300–600	6–10	Not available
phenelzine (Nardil)	15–90	24 (effect lasts 3–10 d)	Not available
tranylcypromine (Parnate)	10–60	24 (effect lasts 3–10 d)	Not available

treatment of depressive disorders developed by the CANMAT Depression Working Group (Kennedy et al., 2001), first-line treatment for a major depressive episode is either an SSRI or venlafaxine.

Indications and Mechanisms of Action

The TCAs have multiple effects on a variety of receptors in the CNS, including reuptake inhibition at serotonin and norepinephrine transporters, down-regulation of specific serotonin and noradrenergic receptors, and blockade of cholinergic, adrenergic and histamine receptors. On the other hand, the MAOIs are more specific in their actions. They inhibit MAO, an enzyme that breaks down biogenic amines, such as serotonin, thereby increasing synaptic neurotransmission, resulting in clinical improvement.

The primary indication for antidepressant medications is depression, thus the name "antidepressant." Symptoms such as loss of interest in the person's usual activities (anhedonia), depressed mood, lethargy or decreased energy, insomnia, decreased concentration, loss of appetite, and suicidal ideation usually respond (see Chapter 19 for a more complete discussion of the symptoms of depression). Antidepressants are also used to treat other symptoms and disorders, and increasingly the name antidepressant might be somewhat misleading.

Antidepressants are prescribed to treat the whole range of anxiety disorders (see Chapter 20). Antidepressants are also used to treat eating disorders (see Chapter 22), depression in bipolar affective disorders, dysthymia, chronic pain disorders, and premenstrual syndrome. More sedating antidepressants are sometimes used in small doses to improve sleep disturbance.

Trazodone, amitriptyline, mirtazapine, and other agents have been used alone or as adjunctive interventions for sleep disturbance. Antidepressants are also used for other sleep disorders, such as sleep apnoea. Symptoms of some psychiatric disorders of childhood (see Chapter 27), such as attention deficit hyperactivity disorder (ADHD), enuresis (bed wetting), and school phobia, often respond to antidepressant medication.

At times, the symptoms of depression present in an "atypical" manner, which is called *atypical depression*. Individuals with atypical depression have a mixture of anxiety and depression, hypersomnia, mood swings, worsening of the symptoms in the evening, and oversensitivity to such interpersonal feelings as rejection. These target symptoms of atypical depression often respond better to the MAOIs, such as phenelzine (Nardil), or to the mixed action antidepressants (those that have both direct neurotransmitter receptor action and reuptake properties) like trazodone or nefazedone.

Pharmacokinetics

All of the antidepressant medications are well absorbed from the gastrointestinal system; however, some individual variations exist. For example, food slightly increases the amount of trazodone absorbed but decreases its maximum blood concentrations and lengthens the time to peak effects from 1 hour on an empty stomach to 2 hours with food. Food also increases the maximum concentrations of sertraline in the bloodstream and decreases the time to peak plasma levels, whereas fluoxetine and fluvoxamine are unaffected, although food may delay the absorption of fluoxetine. Food has little effect on the TCAs.

Psychiatric–mental health nurses should review pharmacokinetic information as it applies to each individual medication. They must consider how this information will affect the patient's use of the medication given the target symptoms for which the drug is intended. For example, if trazodone is being used on a continuous dose schedule for its antidepressant effect, the effects of food probably matter very little. However, if trazodone is being used in a small dose at bedtime to assist a patient to sleep, an empty stomach becomes important because food would lengthen the time of onset of clinical effects, in this case, sleep.

The TCAs undergo considerable first-pass metabolism but reach peak plasma concentrations in 2 to 4 hours. The TCAs are highly bound to plasma proteins, which make the association between blood levels and therapeutic clinical effects difficult. However, some plasma ranges have been established. Table 13-9 includes the available ranges for therapeutic blood levels of the TCAs. In addition, times to steady-state plasma levels have wide variations, and the effective dose of medication must be individualized. Other antidepressants are also highly protein bound, which means that drugs that compete for these binding sites may cause fluctuations in blood levels of the antidepressants. Venlafaxine has the lowest protein binding; therefore, drug interactions of this type are not expected with this medication. Blood level changes caused by the presence of other drugs competing with binding sites are not expected.

Onset of action also varies considerably, depending on specific symptom. For example, improvement in sleep often occurs earlier than effects on overall mood or anhedonia. Complete relief of symptoms may take several weeks. Full enzyme inhibition with the MAOIs may take as long as 2 weeks, but the energizing effects may be seen within a few days. Overcoming issues such as social stigma, viewing depression as a personal failing, fear about taking a medication, and the decreased energy and motivation associated with depression have made deciding to seek treatment a major hurdle. Indeed, in both U.S. and Canadian community surveys, only about one third of individuals with depression had sought treatment for their symptoms (Regier et al., 1993; Satcher, 1999). The variable onset of action may add to their sense of discouragement and powerlessness. Psychiatric–mental health nurses and families are often involved in providing encouragement and other supportive interventions to assist the patient in "getting through" this period of time.

Although antidepressants are primarily excreted by the kidneys, their routes of metabolism vary. Most of the TCAs have active metabolites that act in much the same manner as the parent drug. Therefore, in determining the rate of elimination, one must consider the half-lives of these metabolites. Most of these antidepressants may be given in a once-daily single dose. If the medication causes sedation, this dose should be given at bedtime. The SSRIs frequently cause more activation of energy and are often given in the morning. Venlafaxine, nefazodone, and bupropion are examples of antidepressants whose shorter half-life periods and other factors require administration two or three times per day. Fluoxetine and its active metabolite have particularly long half-lives, remaining present for as long as 5 to 6 weeks. This may affect a number of decisions. For example, women who wish to have children and are taking fluoxetine ideally should discontinue use of the agent at least 6 weeks before attempting to conceive. They should be advised to consult their prescriber before making this decision. Fluoxetine would also not be a good choice for intermittent use for premenstrual dysphoric disorder. Table 13-9 provides information about the average elimination half-lives of most of the antidepressants.

Most of the antidepressants are metabolized by the P-450 enzyme system, so that drugs that induce this system tend to decrease blood levels of the antidepressants, and inhibitors of this system increase antidepressant blood levels. This effect varies according to the subfamily that is induced. For example, fluvoxamine (Luvox) substantially inhibits CYP1A2. Thus, other drugs that are metabolized by the system experience slower metabolism. These include such medications as amitriptyline, clomipramine, imipramine, clozapine, propranolol, theophylline, and caffeine (Cozza, Armstrong, & Oesterheld, 2003). Paroxetine and fluoxetine are very potent inhibitors of CYP2D6, as well as mild inhibitors of CYP2C19 and CYP2C9.

Side Effects, Adverse Reactions, and Toxicity

Side effects of the antidepressant medications vary considerably. Because the TCAs act at several types of receptors, in addition to serotonin and norepinephrine receptor, these drugs have many unwanted effects. Conversely, the SSRIs are more selective for serotonin and have comparatively fewer and better tolerated side effects. Attention to a patient's ability to tolerate side effects is critical because uncomfortable side effects are the primary reason patients discontinue medication treatment. With the TCAs, sedation, orthostatic hypotension, and anticholinergic side effects are the most common sources of discomfort for patients receiving these medications. See Chapter 19 for a comparison of side effects of antidepressant medications.

Receptor affinities may be helpful in predicting which side effects are most likely to occur with a given medication. Table 13-1 provides a summary of major receptor targets for common antidepressants. Using this table in conjunction with Chapter 19, nurses may be able to predict which side effects will be most common with each medication. Interventions to assist in minimizing these side effects are listed in Table 13-2.

Tolerance develops gradually to the sedation and anticholinergic side effects caused by TCAs, but these may be minimized when the prescriber begins with a low dose and increases gradually. Other side effects of the TCAs include tremors, restlessness, insomnia, nausea and vomiting, confusion, pedal edema, headache, and seizures. Blood dyscrasias may also occur, and any fever, sore throat, malaise, or rash should be reported to the prescriber.

Sexual dysfunction is a relatively common side effect with most antidepressants. Erectile and ejaculation disturbances occur in men and anorgasmia in women. This side effect is often difficult to assess if the nurse has not obtained a sexual history before initiation of use of the medication. Anorgasmia is particularly common with the SSRIs and often goes unreported, frequently because nurses and other health care providers do not ask. Bupropion and nefazodone (Serzone) appear to be least likely to cause sexual disturbance. In addition, when sexual dysfunction is related to the medication, several treatment options are available. These include a change in dose or type of antidepressant or, less frequently, using other medications to treat this side effect. Nurses must take responsibility for discussing the potential for sexual side effects before initiation of drug treatment and for continuing to reassess during follow up visits. The TCAs have the potential for cardiotoxicity, which limits their use in the elderly. Symptoms include prolongation of cardiac conduction that may worsen preexisting cardiac conduction problems. TCAs are contraindicated with second-degree atrioventricular block and should be used cautiously in patients who have other cardiac problems. Occasionally, they may precipitate heart failure, myocardial infarction, arrhythmias, and stroke. The newer antidepressants, such as the SSRIs and bupropion, are less cardiotoxic, and nefazodone currently exhibits no evidence of cardiotoxicity.

Antidepressants that block the dopamine (D_2) receptor, such as amoxapine, have produced symptoms of neuroleptic malignant syndrome. Mild forms of extrapyramidal symptoms and endocrine changes, including galactorrhea and amenorrhea, may develop. Amoxapine should be avoided in elderly patients because it may be associated with the development of tardive dyskinesia with this age group. Rare occurrences and only mild forms of extrapyramidal symptoms, such as tightness in the jaw and muscle spasms, may occur with any of the TCAs or SSRIs (Zullino, Delacrausaz, & Baumann, 2002).

The most common side effects of the SSRIs include headache, anxiety, insomnia, transient nausea, vomiting, and diarrhea. Sedation may also occur, especially with fluvoxamine. Most often, these medications are given in the morning, but if daytime sedation occurs, they may be given in the evening. Higher doses, especially of fluoxetine, are more likely to produce sedation.

Venlafaxine (Effexor) has little effect on acetylcholine and histamine; thus, the risks for sedation and anticholinergic symptoms are low. However, higher doses are associated with sexual dysfunction, sedation, diastolic hypertension, increased perspiration, constipation, dry mouth, tremors, blurred vision, and asthenia or muscle weakness. Elevations in blood pressure have been described, and nurses should monitor blood pressure, especially in patients who have a preexisting history of hypertension. Nurses need to be very familiar with nefazodone (Serzone) and the clinical issues related to its side effects. Nefazodone is a phenylpiperazine antidepressant that is structurally related to trazodone. Its most common side effects include sedation, dizziness, orthostatic hypotension; less common is increased risk for seizures. Drug–drug interactions between nefazodone and triazolam and alprazolam have been reported, with increased plasma levels of these benzodiazepines, resulting in an enhancement of the psychomotor impairment caused by these agents. Bupropion (Wellbutrin) has a chemical structure unlike any of the other antidepressants. Some of its pharmacologic profile is due to effects on dopamine systems, in addition to effects on serotonin and norepinephrine. Bupropion's activating effects may be experienced as agitation or anxiety by some patients. Others also experience insomnia and appetite suppression. Rarely, bupropion has produced psychosis, including hallucinations and delusions. Most likely, this is secondary to stimulation of dopamine systems. Dopamine is also associated with reward and motivated behaviour, which accounts for the increasingly common use of bupropion, under the trade name of Zyban, as a smoking cessation agent. The slightly increased risk for experiencing seizures with bupropion use has received the most attention. It has been found that if the total daily dose of bupropion is no more than 450 mg and no individual dose is greater than 150 mg, the risk for seizures with bupropion is no greater than the risk with the other TCAs (Ferry & Johnston, 2003). Most important, bupropion has not caused sexual dysfunction and often is used in individuals who are experiencing these side effects.

The MAOIs can produce anticholinergic side effects (dizziness, dry mouth, blurred vision, constipation, nausea, peripheral edema, urinary hesitancy), but at a much reduced rate compared with the TCAs. Orthostatic hypotension is common; thus, frequent assessment of lying and standing blood pressures is required, especially in elderly patients, who may be at risk for falls and subsequent bone fractures and require assistance in changing position. Sexual dysfunction, including decreased libido, impotence, and anorgasmia, can occur with MAOIs.

The most serious side effect of the MAOIs is their interaction with food and certain medications. The food interaction occurs because MAOIs block the breakdown of tyramine, a trace amine with vasoconstrictor properties. Increased levels of tyramine can cause severe headaches and hypertension, stroke, and in rare instances, death. Patients who are taking MAOIs are placed on a low-tyramine diet. This diet has been difficult for some individuals to follow, and concerns about the risk for severe hypertension have led many clinicians to rarely use the MAOIs (see Table 13-10).

MAOIs in current use in Canada include phenelzine (Nardil) and tranylcypromine (Parnate). These are considered irreversible MAOIs because they form unbreakable covalent bonds with monoamine oxidase. It takes at least 2 weeks to produce replacement enzyme molecules after discontinuation of use of the medication. Moclobemide is an example of a reversible MAOI that is available in Europe and Canada. Although it acts in

Table 13.10 Example of a Tyramine-Restricted Diet

Category of Food	Food to Avoid	Food Allowed
Cheese	All matured or aged cheeses. All casseroles made with these cheeses, pizza, lasagna, etc. *Note:* All cheeses are considered matured or aged except those listed under "foods allowed"	Fresh cottage cheese, cream cheese, ricotta cheese, and processed cheese slices. All fresh milk products that have been stored properly (e.g., sour cream, yogurt, ice cream)
Meat, fish, and poultry	Fermented/dry sausage: pepperoni, salami, mortadella, summer sausage, etc. Improperly stored meat, fish, or poultry. Improperly stored pickled herring	All fresh packaged or processed meat; (e.g., chicken loaf, hot dogs), fish, or poultry. Refrigerate immediately and eat as soon as possible
Fruits and vegetables	Fava or broad bean pods (not beans). Banana peel	Banana pulp. All others except those listed in "food to avoid"
Alcoholic beverages	All tap beers	Alcohol: No more than two domestic bottled or canned beers or 4-fluid-oz glasses of red or white wine per day; this applies to non-alcoholic beer also; please note that red wine may produce a headache unrelated to a rise in blood pressure
Miscellaneous foods	Marmite concentrated yeast extract. Sauerkraut. Soy sauce and other soybean condiments	Other yeast extracts (e.g., brewer's yeast). Soy milk

Adapted from Gardener, D. M., Shulman, K. I., Walker, S. E., & Tailor, S. A. N. (1996). The making of a user friendly MAOI diet. *Journal of Clinical Psychiatry, 57,* 99–104.

the same way as the irreversible MAOIs, moclobemide forms weaker bonds that are short lasting. Therefore, a less restrictive diet may be used with moclobemide. In addition to food restrictions, many prescription and nonprescription medications that stimulate the sympathetic nervous system (sympathomimetics) produce the same risk for hypertensive crisis as do foods containing tyramine. The nonprescription medication interactions involve primarily diet pills and cold remedies. Patients should be advised to check the labels of any nonprescription drugs carefully for a warning against use with antidepressants, especially the MAOIs, and then consult their prescriber or pharmacist before consuming these medications. In addition, symptoms of other serious drug–drug interactions may develop, such as coma, hypertension, and fever, which may occur when patients receive meperidine (Demerol) while taking an MAOI. Patients should notify other health care providers, including dentists, that they are taking an MAOI before being prescribed or given any other medication.

Suicide is a major concern when working with individuals who are depressed. Systematic suicide risk assessment should be done routinely before initiating antidepressant therapy, in the first 2 to 4 weeks of treatment and for longer if indicated. Some of these medications are more lethal than others. For example, the TCAs pose a significant risk for overdose and are more lethal in children. Symptoms of overdose and treatment are discussed more fully in Chapter 19, but for now, it is important to remember that this potential exists. Sometimes, the prescriber will provide the patient with only small amounts of the medication, requiring more frequent visits, and will closely monitor use. In general, newer antidepressant medications, such as the SSRIs, are associated with less risk for toxicity and lethality in overdose. Box 13-3 highlights some of the newest antidepressants being tested in clinical trials.

ANTIANXIETY AND SEDATIVE-HYPNOTIC MEDICATIONS

Sometimes called *anxiolytics*, antianxiety medications and sedative-hypnotic medications come from various pharmacologic classifications, including benzodiazepines, nonbenzodiazepines, and nonbarbiturate sedative-hypnotics, such as chloral hydrate. These drugs represent some of the most widely prescribed medications today for the short-term relief of anxiety or anxiety associated with depression.

Benzodiazepines

Commonly prescribed benzodiazepines include chlordiazepoxide (Librium), diazepam (Valium), lorazepam (Ativan), flurazepam (Dalmane), oxazepam (Serax), clonazapam (Rivotril), and triazolam (Halcion).

BOX 13.3

Novel Antidepressant Drug Development

Research into the neurobiology of depression has implicated other neurotransmitter and neuroendocrine systems in the etiology of depression. This has led to the development of new antidepressants, many of which are currently in clinical trials.

For example, the hypothalamic-pituitary-adrenal (HPA) axis, a major stress hormone system, shows evidence of overactivity and blunted feedback control in depression. The principal activator of the HPA axis is a hormone called *corticotropin-releasing hormone* (CRH). This hormone is produced in the hypothalamus and stimulates the pituitary to release adrenocorticotrophic hormone (ACTH), which stimulated release of cortisol from the adrenal gland. In depression, excessive CRH leads to increased levels of cortisol. Increased levels of cortisol are associated with some of the symptoms in depression, like difficulties concentrating, sleep disturbance, and lowered energy. This led to the CRH theory of depression (Nemeroff, 2002) and prompted the development of CRH antagonists and glucocorticoid receptor antagonists as potential antidepressants.

Glutamate is the major excitatory neurotransmitter and has been implicated in many psychiatric and neuropsychiatric disorders, including depression. Some evidence exists for increased glutamate in depression (Krystal et al., 2002). Thus, glutamate antagonists are also being tested for any antidepressant properties.

Indications and Mechanisms of Action

Benzodiazepines act as positive modulators at GABA ion channels, increasing the ease of GABA binding to its binding site. This enhancement of GABA binding increases both the duration and frequency of channel opening and decreases the firing rate of the nerve cell. This inhibition of nerve cell firing allows this class of drugs to act as anticonvulsants, antianxiety medications, or hypnotics, depending on dose and pharmacokinetic properties. Other neurotransmitter systems are also involved in the effects of benzodiazepines. Of the various benzodiazepines in use to relieve anxiety (and treat insomnia), oxazepam (Serax) and lorazepam (Ativan) are often preferred for patients with liver disease and for elderly patients because of their short half-lives.

Pharmacokinetics

The variable rate of absorption of the benzodiazepines determines the speed of onset. Table 13-11 provides relative indications of the speed of onset, from very fast to slow, for some of the commonly prescribed benzodiazepines.

Chlordiazepoxide (Librium) and diazepam (Valium) are slow, erratic, and sometimes incompletely absorbed when given intramuscularly, whereas lorazepam (Ativan) is rapidly and completely absorbed when given IM.

Table 13.11   Antianxiety and Sedative-Hypnotic Medications

Generic (Trade) Drug Name	Usual Dosage Range (mg/d)	Half-Life (h)	Speed of Onset After Single Dose
Benzodiazepines			
diazepam (Valium)	4–40	30–100	Very fast
chlordiazepoxide (Librium)	15–100	50–100	Intermediate
clorazepate (Tranxene)	15–60	30–200	Fast
prazepam (Centrax)	20–60	30–200	Very slow
flurazepam (Dalmane)	15–30	47–100	Fast
lorazepam (Ativan)	2–8	10–20	Slow-intermediate
oxazepam (Serax)	30–120	3–21	Slow-intermediate
temazepam (Restoril)	15–30	9.5–20	Moderately fast
triazolam (Halcion)	0.25–0.5	2–4	Fast
alprazolam (Xanax)	0.5–10	12–15	Intermediate
clonazepam (Livotril)	1.5–20	18–50	Intermediate
Nonbenzodiazepines			
buspirone (BuSpar)	15–30	3–11	Very slow
zolpidem (Ambien)	5–10	2.6	Fast

Lorazepam is also well absorbed by the sublingual route.

All the benzodiazepines are highly lipid soluble and highly protein bound. They are distributed throughout the body and enter the CNS quickly. Other drugs that compete for protein-binding sites may produce drug–drug interactions. The degree to which each of these drugs is lipid soluble affects its duration of action. Most of these drugs have active metabolites, but the degree of activity of each metabolite affects duration of action and elimination half-life. Most of these drugs vary markedly in length of half-life. Oxazepam, which is itself an active metabolite of diazepam, and lorazepam have no active metabolites and thus have shorter half-lives. Sustained presence of these drugs after discontinuation may be observed in elderly or obese patients.

Side Effects, Adverse Reactions, and Toxicity

The most commonly reported side effects result from the sedative and CNS depression effects of these medications. Drowsiness, intellectual impairment, anterograde memory impairment, ataxia, and reduced motor coordination are common adverse effects. If used for sleep, many of these medications, especially long-acting benzodiazepines, produce significant "hangover" effects experienced on awakening. Flunitrazepam (Rohypnol), otherwise known as the "date rape" drug, because of its ability to impair anterograde memory, is illegal in Canada. Elderly patients receiving repeated doses of medications such as flurazepam (Dalmane) at bedtime may experience paradoxical confusion, agitation, and delirium, sometimes after the first dose. In addition, daytime fatigue, drowsiness, and cognitive impairments may continue while the person is awake. For most patients, the effects subside as tolerance develops; however, alcohol increases all these symptoms and potentiates the CNS depression. Individuals using these medications should be warned to be cautious when driving or performing other tasks that require mental alertness. If these tasks are part of the person's work requirements, another medication may be chosen. Administered intravenously, benzodiazepines often cause phlebitis and thrombosis at the intravenous sites, which should be monitored closely and changed if redness or swelling develops.

Because tolerance develops to most of the CNS depressant effects, individuals who wish to experience the feeling of "intoxication" from these medications may be tempted to increase their own dosage. Psychological dependence is more likely to occur when using these medications for a longer period, as well as for the short-acting forms. Abrupt discontinuation of the use of benzodiazepines may result in a recurrence of the target symptoms, such as rebound insomnia or anxiety. Other withdrawal symptoms appear rapidly, including tremors, increased perspiration, palpitations, increased sensitivity to light, abdominal discomfort or pain, and elevations in systolic blood pressure. These symptoms may be more pronounced with the short-acting benzodiazepines, such as lorazepam. Gradual tapering is recommended for discontinuing use of benzodiazepines after long-term treatment. When tapering short-acting medications, the prescriber may switch the patient to a long-acting benzodiazepine before discontinuing use of the short-acting drug.

Individual reactions to the benzodiazepines appear to be associated with sensitivity to their effects. Some patients feel apathy, fatigue, tearfulness, emotional lability, irritability, and nervousness. Benzodiazepines do little for depression symptoms, except for sleep disturbance, and may even exacerbate anhedonia and difficulties concentrating. As such, their use in depression, even with significant comorbid anxiety, should be closely monitored. Gastrointestinal disturbances, including nausea, vomiting, anorexia, dry mouth, and constipation, may develop. These medications may be taken with food to ease the gastrointestinal distress.

Elderly patients are particularly susceptible to incontinence, memory disturbances, dizziness, and increased risk for falls when using benzodiazepines. Pregnant patients should be aware that these medications cross the placenta and are associated with increased risk for birth defects, such as cleft palate, mental retardation, and pyloric stenosis. Infants born addicted to benzodiazepines often exhibit flaccid muscle tone, lethargy, and difficulties sucking. All the benzodiazepines are excreted in breast milk, and breast-feeding women should avoid using these medications. Infants and children metabolize these medications more slowly; therefore, more drug accumulates in their bodies.

Toxicity can develop with liver dysfunction or disease. Symptoms include worsening of the CNS depression, ataxia, confusion, delirium, agitation, hypotension, diminished reflexes, and lethargy. Rarely do the benzodiazepines cause respiratory depression or death. In overdose, these medications have a high therapeutic index and rarely result in death unless combined with another CNS depressant drug, such as alcohol.

Nonbenzodiazepines: Buspirone and Zolpidem

One of the nonbenzodiazepines, buspirone (BuSpar), was first synthesized in 1968 by Michael Eison, who was searching for an improved antipsychotic medication. Later, it was found that buspirone was effective in controlling the symptoms of anxiety but had no effect on panic disorders and little effect on obsessive-compulsive disorder. Another nonbenzodiazepine, zolpidem (Ambien), is a medication for sleep that acts on the benzodiazepine–GABA receptor complex.

Indications and Mechanisms of Actions

These drugs are effective for treating anxiety disorders without the CNS depressant effects or the potential for abuse and withdrawal syndromes. Buspirone is indicated for treating generalized anxiety disorder; therefore, its target symptoms include anxiety and related symptoms, such as difficulty concentrating, tension, insomnia, restlessness, irritability, and fatigue. Because buspirone does not add to depression symptoms, it has been tried for treating anxiety that coexists with depression. In some instances, it is thought to potentiate the antidepressant actions of other medications.

Buspirone has no effect on the benzodiazepine–GABA complex but instead appears to control anxiety by blocking the serotonin subtype of receptor, 5-HT1a, at both presynaptic reuptake and postsynaptic receptor sites. It has no sedative, muscle relaxant, or anticonvulsant effects. It also lacks potential for abuse.

Zolpidem (Ambien), which is indicated for short-term insomnia treatment, appears to increase slow-wave (deep) sleep and to modulate GABA receptors in a similar fashion to benzodiazepines, but with less risk for tolerance or withdrawal issues.

Pharmacokinetics

Buspirone is rapidly absorbed but undergoes extensive first-pass metabolism. Food slows absorption but appears to reduce first-pass effects, increasing the bioavailability of the medication. Buspirone is given on a continual dosing schedule of three times a day because of its short half-life of 2 to 3 hours. Clinical action depends on reaching steady-state concentrations; taking this medication with food may facilitate this process.

Buspirone is highly protein bound but does not displace most other medications. However, it does displace digoxin and may increase digoxin levels to the point of toxicity. It is metabolized in the liver and excreted predominantly by the kidneys but also through the gastrointestinal tract. Patients with liver or kidney impairment should be given this medication with caution.

Buspirone cannot be used on a PRN basis; rather, it takes 2 to 4 weeks of continual use for symptom relief to occur. It is more effective in reducing anxiety in patients who have never taken a benzodiazepine.

Buspirone does not block the withdrawal of other benzodiazepines. Therefore, a switch to buspirone must be initiated gradually to avoid withdrawal symptoms. Nurses should closely monitor patients who are undergoing this change of medication for emergence of withdrawal symptoms from the benzodiazepines and report such symptoms to the prescriber.

Zolpidem is metabolized by the liver; it crosses the placenta, and enters breast milk. It has a short half-life of 3 hours, which makes it an ideal hypnotic and is excreted in the urine.

Side Effects, Adverse Reactions, and Toxicity

Common side effects from higher-dose buspirone include dizziness, drowsiness, nausea, excitement, and headache. Most other side effects occur at an incidence of less than 1%. There have been no reports of death from an overdose of buspirone alone. Elderly patients, pregnant women, and children have not been adequately studied. For now, buspirone can be assumed to cross the placenta and is present in breast milk; therefore, its use should be avoided in pregnant women, and women who are taking this medication should not breast-feed.

Rebound effects, such as insomnia and anxiety, from zolpidem are minimal. There are minimal effects on respiratory function and little potential for abuse.

STIMULANTS

Amphetamines were first synthesized in the late 1800s but were not used for psychiatric disorders until the 1930s. Initially, amphetamines were prescribed for a variety of symptoms and disorders, but their high abuse potential soon became obvious.

Methylphenidate, Pemoline, and Modafinil

Among the medications known as stimulants are methylphenidate (Ritalin), used for attention deficit disorders; pemoline (Cylert), a CNS stimulant also used for hyperactivity and attention deficit disorders; and modafinil (Provigil), used for narcolepsy, a sleep disorder.

Indications and Mechanisms of Action

Medical use of these drugs is now restricted to a few disorders, including narcolepsy, ADHD—particularly in children—and obesity unresponsive to other treatments. However, stimulants are increasingly being used as an adjunctive treatment in depression and other mood disorders to address the anhedonia and low energy common to these conditions.

Dextroamphetamine (or d-amphetamine, indicating the d-isomer; Dexadrine) indirectly stimulate the sympathetic nervous system, producing alertness, wakefulness, vasoconstriction, suppressed appetite, and hypothermia. Tolerance develops to some of these effects, such as suppression of appetite, but the CNS stimulation continues. Although the exact mechanism of action is not completely understood, stimulants cause a release of catecholamines, particularly norepinephrine and dopamine, into the synapse from the presynaptic nerve cell. They also block reuptake of these catecholamines. Methylphenidate is structurally similar to the amphetamines but produces a milder CNS stimulation. Pemoline is structurally dissimilar from the amphetamines but produces the same pharmacologic actions. Pemoline predominantly affects the dopamine system and therefore has less effect on the sympathetic nervous system.

Although the stimulant effects of these medications may seem logically indicated for narcolepsy, a disorder in which the individual frequently and abruptly falls asleep, the indications for childhood ADHD seem less obvious. The aetiology and neurobiology of ADHD remain unclear, but psychostimulants produce a paradoxic calming of the increased motor activity characteristic of ADHD. Studies show that medication decreases disruptive activity during school hours, reduces noise and verbal activity, improves attention span and short-term memory, improves ability to follow directions, and decreases distractibility and impulsivity. Although these improvements have been well documented in the literature, the diagnosis of ADHD and subsequent use of psychostimulants with children remains a matter of controversy (see Chapter 27).

Off-Label Use

Psychostimulants have also been used for other psychiatric disorders, and nurses must be aware that these medications are outside of Health Canada–approved indications for the medications. Used alone, stimulants are not indicated for treating depression. However, research has found that these medications may be beneficial as adjunctive medications, especially in those with severe psychomotor retardation. All appetite depressants are stimulants, but most are not related to the amphetamines and have a low potential for abuse. However, psychostimulants have been used for treating obesity when other treatments have failed. In addition, these medications have relieved lethargy, boosted mood, and reduced cognitive deficits associated with chronic medically debilitating conditions, such as chronic fatigue syndrome, acquired immunodeficiency syndrome, and some types of cancer, but more research is needed. Increasingly, psychostimulants are being used to improve the residual symptoms of attention deficit disorder in adults, such as inattention, impulsivity, decreased concentration, anxiety, and irritability. This use remains a matter of controversy, and psychostimulants should be used very cautiously in individuals who have a history of substance abuse.

Modafinil (Alertec) is a new wake-promoting agent used for treating excessive daytime sleepiness (EDS) associated with narcolepsy and other health states. Patients with EDS cannot stay awake in the daytime, even after getting enough night-time sleep. They fall asleep when they want to stay awake. Although modafinil is approved by Health Canada only for treating narcolepsy, it is being used for people with EDS and general fatigue found in many diverse disorders, including fibromyalgia and major depression. Its use by long distance truckers and shift workers has created controversy, and more research is needed.

Pharmacokinetics

Psychostimulants are rapidly absorbed from the gastrointestinal tract and reach peak plasma levels in 1 to 3 hours. Considerable individual variations occur between the drugs in terms of bioavailability, plasma levels, and half-life. Table 13-12 compares the primary psychostimulants

Table 13.12 Psychostimulant Medications

Generic (Trade) Drug Name and Half-Life	Usual Dosage Range (mg/d)	Side Effects
dextroamphetamine (Dexedrine); 6–7 h	5–40	• Overstimulation • Restlessness • Dry mouth • Palpitations • Cardiomyopathy (with prolonged use or high dosage) • Possible growth retardation (greatest risk); risk reduced with drug holidays
methylphenidate (Ritalin); 2–4 h	10–60	• Nervousness • Insomnia • Anorexia • Tachycardia • Impaired cognition (with high doses) • Moderate risk for growth suppression
pemoline (Cylert); 12 h (mean)	37.5–112.5	• Insomnia • Anorexia with weight loss • Elevated liver function tests (ALT, AST, LDH) • Jaundice • Least risk for growth suppression

ALT, alanine aminotransferase; AST, aspartate aminotransferase; LDH, lactic dehydrogenase.

used in psychiatry. Some of these differences are age dependent because children metabolize these medications more rapidly, producing shorter elimination half-lives. Methylphenidate (Ritalin) is available in a sustained-release form and should not be chewed or crushed.

The psychostimulants appear to be unaffected by food in the stomach and should be given after meals to reduce the appetite-suppressant effects when indicated. However, changes in urine pH may affect the rates of excretion. Excessive sodium bicarbonate alkalizes the urine and reduces amphetamine secretion. Increased vitamin C or citric acid intake may acidify the urine and increase its excretion. Starvation from appetite suppression may have a similar effect. All these drugs are highly lipid soluble, crossing easily into the CNS and the placenta. Psychostimulants undergo metabolic changes in the liver, where they may affect, or be affected by, other drugs. They are primarily excreted through the kidneys; therefore, renal dysfunction may interfere with excretion.

The precise action of modafinil (Alertec) in promoting wakefulness is unknown. It does appear to have wake-promoting actions similar to sympathomimetic agents such as amphetamine and methylphenidate, although the pharmacologic profile is not identical. It is absorbed rapidly and reaches peak plasma concentration in 2 to 4 hours. Absorption of modafinil may be delayed by 1 to 2 hours if taken with food. Modafinil is eliminated through liver metabolism, with subsequent excretion of metabolites through renal excretion. Modafinil may interact with drugs that inhibit, induce, or are metabolized by CYP2C19 isoenzymes, including phenytoin, diazepam, and propranolol. Concurrent use of modafinil and other

drugs metabolized by CYP2C19 may lead to increased circulating blood levels of the other drugs.

Psychostimulants are usually begun at a low dose and increased weekly, depending on improvement of symptoms and occurrence of side effects. Initially, children with ADHD are given a morning dose so that their school performance may be compared from morning to afternoon. Rebound symptoms of excitability and talkativeness may occur when use of the medication is withdrawn or after dose reduction. These symptoms also begin about 5 hours after the last dose of medication, which may affect the dosing regimen for some individuals. The return of symptoms in the afternoon for children with ADHD may require that a second dose be given at school. Prescribers should work with parents to implement other interventions after school and on weekends when the psychostimulants are not used. Severity of symptoms may require that the medications be continued during these times, but this dosing schedule should be determined after careful evaluation on an individual basis. Use of these medications should not be stopped abruptly, especially with higher doses, because the rebound effects may last for several days.

Side Effects, Adverse Reactions, and Toxicity

Side effects associated with psychostimulants typically arise within 2 to 3 weeks after use of the medication begins. From most to least common, these side effects include appetite suppression, insomnia, irritability, weight loss, nausea, headache, palpitations, blurred vision, dry mouth, constipation, and dizziness. Because of the effects on the sympathetic nervous system, some individuals experience blood pressure changes (both hypertension and hypotension), tachycardia, tremors, and irregular heart rates. Blood pressure and pulse should be monitored initially and after each dosage change. Pemoline is associated with elevated liver enzymes and produces hepatotoxicity in 1% to 3% of children taking the medication; therefore, liver function tests should be obtained at least every 6 months. Liver function returns to normal when use of the medication is discontinued.

Rarely, psychostimulants suppress growth and development in children. These effects are a matter of controversy, and research has produced conflicting results. Although suppression of height seems unlikely to some researchers, others have indicated that psychostimulants may have an effect on cartilage. More reports of suppressed growth have occurred with d-amphetamine (Dexedrine) than methylphenidate (Ritalin), and both of these drugs are associated with greater growth suppression than is pemoline. Height and weight should be monitored several times annually for children taking these medications and compared with prior history of growth. Weight should be monitored especially closely during the initial phases of treatment. These effects also may be minimized by drug "holidays," such as during school vacations.

Rarely, individuals may experience mild dysphoria, social withdrawal, or mild to moderate depression. These symptoms are more common at higher doses and may require discontinuation of use of medication. Abnormal movements and motor tics may also increase in individuals who have a history of Tourette's syndrome. Psychostimulants should be avoided by patients with Tourette's symptoms or a positive family history of the disorder. In addition, dextroamphetamine has been associated with an increased risk for congenital abnormalities. Because there is no compelling reason for a pregnant woman to continue to take these medications, patients should be informed and should advise their prescriber immediately if they plan to become pregnant or if pregnancy is a possibility.

Death is rare from overdose or toxicity of the psychostimulants, but a 10-day supply may be lethal, especially in children. Symptoms of overdose include agitation, chest pain, hallucinations, paranoia, confusion, and dysphoria. Seizures may develop, along with fever, tremor, hypertension or hypotension, aggression, headache, palpitations, rashes, difficulty breathing, leg pain, and abdominal pain. Maximum dosage for children is 40 mg/day, with potential death resulting from a 400-mg dose. Parents should be warned regarding the potential lethality of these medications and take preventive measures by keeping the medication in a safe place.

Side effects associated with modafinil include nausea, nervousness, headache, dizziness, and trouble sleeping. If the effects continue or are bothersome, patients should consult the prescriber. Modafinil is generally well tolerated, with few clinically significant side effects. It is potentially habit forming and must be used with great caution in individuals with a history of substance abuse or dependence.

NEW MEDICATIONS

Each country has its own approval process for new medications. In Canada, this process is controlled by Health Canada. Through various phases of drug testing, a new drug must be determined to have therapeutic benefit based on known physiologic processes, animal testing, and laboratory models of human disease and its potential toxicity predicted at doses likely to produce clinical improvement in humans (see Box 13-4

BOX 13.4

Phases of New Drug Testing

- *Phase I:* Testing defines the range of dosages tolerated in healthy individuals
- *Phase II:* Effects of the drug are studied in a limited number of individuals with the target disorder.
- *Phase III:* Extensive clinical trials are conducted at multiple sites throughout the country with larger numbers of patients. Efforts focus on corroborating the efficacy identified in phase II. Phase III concludes with a new drug application (NDA) being submitted to Health Canada.
- *Phase IV:* Postmarketing surveillance continues to detect new or rare adverse reactions and potentially new indications. During this period, adverse reactions from the new medication are required to be reported to Health Canada

Implications for Mental Health Nurses

Throughout the phases, side effects and adverse reactions are monitored closely. The studies are tightly controlled, and strict regulations are enforced at each step.

Clinical trials for new drugs usually involve patient populations that have no other health problems but the one under study. This is important to test the drug's effectiveness, but in clinical practice, many patients have other health problems, and postmarketing surveillance helps identify unforeseen benefits or adverse effects in most heterogeneous patient populations.

A newly approved drug is approved only for the indications for which it has been tested. However, there is often a widening of application for other health problems over time (called *off-label* uses).

In Canada, the pharmaceutical companies must follow strict guidelines in terms of product advertising and interaction with health professionals. For example, the companies are not permitted to advertise directly to the public, and there are stringent guidelines regarding any potential sales incentives offered to health professionals. This is to address potential ethical issues around influencing prescriber preferences.

for more information). Then, the pharmaceutical company can begin research with human volunteers after filing an *investigational new drug* (IND) application. Many new psychiatric medications, particularly the atypical antipsychotics and novel antidepressants, are in various phases of clinical testing and are expected to be released in the coming years. Keeping the phases of new drug development in mind will assist the psychiatric-mental health nurse in understanding what to expect from drugs newly released to the market.

OTHER BIOLOGIC TREATMENTS

Biological treatment is the term applied to treatments that work at a somatic, physical level but are nonpharmacologic in nature. There is a long history of using somatic therapies to treat neuropsychiatric illnesses. Throughout history, numerous treatments have been developed and used to change the biologic basis of what was thought, at the time, to cause psychiatric disorders. Insulin coma, atropine coma, hemodialysis, hyperbaric oxygen therapy, continuous sleep therapy, and ether and carbon dioxide inhalation therapies are examples of some of the treatments that seemed to relieve some symptoms, but results could not be replicated, or potential adverse effects proved too great a risk. Although the primary biologic interventions remain pharmacologic, some somatic treatments continue to show efficacy, whereas others have gained acceptance, remain under investigation, or show promise for the future. These include neurosurgery, electroconvulsive therapy (ECT), and most recently, transcranial magnetic stimulation (TMS) and vagus nerve stimulation (VNS).

Electroconvulsive Therapy

For hundreds of years, seizures have been known to produce improvement in some psychiatric symptoms. Camphor-induced seizures were used in the 16th century to reduce psychosis and mania. With time, other substances, such as inhalants, were tried, but most were difficult to control or produced adverse reactions, sometimes even fatalities. ECT was formally introduced in Italy in 1938. It is one of the oldest medical treatments available and remains safely in use today. It is one of the most effective treatments for severe depression but has been used for other disorders, including mania and schizophrenia, when other treatments have failed.

With ECT, a brief electrical current is passed through the brain to produce generalized seizures lasting 25 to 150 seconds. The patient does not feel the stimulus or recall the procedure. A short-acting anaesthetic and a muscle relaxant are given before induction of the current. A brief pulse stimulus, administered unilaterally on the nondominant side of the head, is associated with less confusion after ECT. However, some individuals require bilateral treatment for effective resolution of depressive symptoms. Induction of a seizure is necessary to produce positive treatment outcomes. Because individual seizure thresholds vary and increase with age, the electrical impulse and treatment method also may vary. In general, the lowest possible electrical stimulus necessary to produce seizure activity is used. Blood pressure and the ECG are monitored during the procedure. This procedure is repeated two or three times a week, usually for a total of 6 to 12 treatments. Because there is no particular difference in treatment efficacy and a twice-weekly regimen produces less accumulative memory loss, this treatment course is often chosen. After symptoms have improved, antidepressant medications are used to prevent relapse. Some patients who cannot take or do not experience response to antidepressant treatment may go on maintenance ECT treatments. Usually, once-weekly treatments are gradually decreased in frequency to once monthly. The number and frequency vary depending on the individual's response.

Although ECT produces rapid improvement in depressive symptoms, its exact mechanism of antidepressant action remains unclear. It is known to down-regulate β-adrenergic receptors in much the same way as antidepressant medications. However, unlike antidepressant therapy, ECT produces an up-regulation in serotonin, especially 5-HT2. ECT also has several other actions on neurochemistry, including increased influx of calcium and effects on second messenger systems.

Brief episodes of hypotension or hypertension, bradycardia or tachycardia, and minor arrhythmias are among the adverse effects that may occur during and immediately after the procedure but usually resolve quickly. Common after-effects from ECT include headache, nausea, and muscle pain. Memory loss is the most troublesome long-term effect of ECT. Many patients do not experience amnesia, whereas others report some memory loss for months or even years (Abrams, 2002). Evidence is conflicting on the effects of ECT on the formation of memories after the treatments and on learning, but most patients experience no noticeable change. Memory loss occurring as part of the symptoms of untreated depression presents a confounding factor in determining the exact nature of the memory deficits from ECT. It is important to remember that patient surveys are positive, with most individuals reporting that they were helped by ECT and would have it again (Hirose, 2002).

ECT is contraindicated in patients with increased intracranial pressure. Risk also increases in patients with recent myocardial infarction, recent cerebrovascular accident, retinal detachment, or pheochromocytoma (a tumor on the adrenal cortex) and in patients at high risk for complications from anaesthesia.

BOX 13.5

Interventions for the Patient Receiving Electroconvulsive Therapy

- Discuss treatment alternatives, procedures, risks, and benefits with patient and family. Make sure that informed consent for electroconvulsive therapy (ECT) has been given in writing.
- Provide initial and ongoing patient and family education.
- Assist and monitor the patient who must take nothing by mouth (NPO) after midnight the evening before the procedure.
- Make sure that the patient wears loose, comfortable, nonrestrictive clothing to the procedure.
- If the procedure is performed on an outpatient basis, ensure that the patient has somone to accompany him or her home and stay with him or her after the procedure.
- Ensure that pretreatment laboratory tests are complete, including complete blood count, serum electrolytes,

urinalysis, electrocardiogram, chest radiograph, and physical examination.
- Teach the patient to create memory helps, such as lists and notepads, before the ECT.
- Explain that no foreign or loose objects can be in the patient's mouth during the procedure. Dentures will be removed, and a bite block may be inserted.
- When the patient is fully conscious and vital signs are stable, assist him or her to get up slowly, sitting for some time before standing.
- Monitor confusion closely; patient may need reorientation to the bathroom and other areas.
- For outpatients, advise family members to observe how patient manages at home, provide assistance as needed, and report any problems.
- Assist the patient to keep or schedule follow-up appointments.

Although ECT is a safe and effective treatment, its use carries substantial social stigma, and nurses need to allow patients and their families to share their concerns and beliefs. Although the actual procedure is usually completed by a physician and anaesthetist, nurses are involved in many aspects of care. These various roles are listed in Box 13-5.

Light Therapy (Phototherapy)

Human circadian rhythms are set by time clues (zeitgebers) inside and outside the body. One of the most powerful regulators of these body patterns is the cycle of daylight and darkness.

Research findings indicate that some individuals with depressive symptoms that worsen at specific times of the year (have a seasonal pattern) may experience disturbance in these normal body patterns or of circadian rhythms. For example, some individuals are more depressed during the winter months, when there is less light, and they improve spontaneously in the spring. (Refer to Chapter 19 for a complete description of depression and mood disorders.) These individuals usually have symptoms that are somewhat different from classic depression, including fatigue, increased need to sleep, increased appetite and weight gain, irritability, and carbohydrate craving. Administering artificial light to these patients during winter months has reduced these depressive symptoms.

Light therapy, sometimes called **phototherapy**, involves exposing the patient to an artificial light source to relieve seasonal depression. Artificial light is believed to trigger a shift in the patient's circadian rhythm to an earlier time. Research remains ongoing. The light source must be very bright, full-spectrum light, usually 2500 lux, which is about 200 times brighter than normal indoor lighting. Harmful ultraviolet light is filtered out.

Exposure to this light source has produced improvement and relief of depressive symptoms for significant numbers of seasonally depressed individuals. It produces no change for individuals who are not seasonally depressed.

Studies have shown that morning phototherapy produces a better response than either evening or morning and evening timing of the phototherapy session. Light banks with full-spectrum light may be put together by the individual or obtained from various companies now producing these light sources. Light visors, visors containing small, full-spectrum light bulbs that shine on the eyelids, have also been developed. The patient is instructed to sit in front of the lights at a distance of about 3 feet, engaging in a variety of other activities, but glancing directly into the light every few minutes. This should be done immediately on arising and is most effective before 8 AM. The duration of administration may begin with as little as 30 minutes and increase to 2 to 5 hours. One to 2 hours is usually sufficient, and the antidepressant response begins in 1 to 4 days, with the full effect usually complete after 2 weeks. Full antidepressant effect is usually maintained with daily sessions of 30 minutes.

Side effects of phototherapy are rare, but eye strain, headache, and insomnia are possible. An ophthalmologist should be consulted if the patient has a preexisting eye disorder. In rare instances, phototherapy has been reported to produce mania. Irritability is a more common complaint. Follow-up visits with the prescriber or therapist are needed to help manage side effects and assess positive results. Phototherapy should be implemented only by a provider knowledgeable in its use.

Nutritional Therapies

The neurotransmitters necessary for normal healthy functioning are produced from amino acids taken in with the foods we eat. Many nutritional deficiencies may produce symptoms of psychiatric disorders. Fatigue, apathy, and depression are caused by deficiencies in iron, folic acid, pantothenic acid, magnesium, vitamin C, or biotin. Logically, treating these deficiencies with nutritional supplements should improve the psychiatric symptoms. The question becomes: Can nutritional supplements actually treat psychiatric disorders?

In 1967, Linus Pauling espoused the theory that ascorbic acid deficiency produced many psychiatric disorders. He implemented a treatment for schizophrenia that included large doses of ascorbic acid and other vitamins. This treatment was referred to as *megavitamin therapy* or *orthomolecular therapy*. Many psychiatrists showed interest in Pauling's proposal, but his research and claims could never be substantiated, and most researchers and clinicians became highly sceptical of this hypothesis. Nonetheless, a small group remains committed to orthomolecular approaches.

Older theories and related diets are based on the belief that food controls behaviour. High sugar intake was once thought to produce hyperactivity in children, and Benjamin Feingold developed a diet to eliminate food additives that he believed increased hyperactivity. More recently, advances in technology have led research to new investigations regarding dietary precursors for the bioamines. For example, tryptophan, the dietary precursor of serotonin, has been most extensively investigated as it relates to low serotonin levels and increased aggression. Individuals who have low tryptophan levels are prone to have lower levels of serotonin in the brain, resulting in depressed mood and aggressive behaviour (Young & Leyton, 2002). Some individuals with mild depression do respond to large amounts of tryptophan, and tryptophan has been used as an adjunct to antidepressant drugs. Many individuals are turning to dietary herbal preparations to address psychiatric symptoms. More than 17% of the adult population has used herbal preparations to address their mood or emotions. From St. John's wort for depression, to ginkgo for cognitive impairment, to kava for anxiety, herbal preparations are increasingly being used (McCabe, 2002). Nurses need to include an assessment of these agents into their overall patient assessment to understand the needs of the patient.

Medications may also influence the development of nutritional deficiencies that may worsen psychiatric symptoms. For example, drugs with strong anticholinergic activity often produce impaired or enhanced gastric motility, which may lead to generalized malabsorption of vitamins and minerals. In addition, many nutritional supplements have toxicities of their own when given in excess. For example, daily ingestion of more than 100 mg pyridoxine (vitamin B_6) can produce neurotoxic symptoms, photosensitivity, and ataxia.

More research is needed to identify the underlying mechanisms and relationships of dietary supplements and dietary precursors of the bioamines to mood and behaviour and psychopharmacologic medications. For now, it is important for the psychiatric–mental health nurse to recognize that diet can have a significant impact on behaviour in sensitive individuals and that supplements can be a potential source of drug–drug interaction.

New Somatic Therapies

Repetitive transcranial magnetic stimulation (rTMS) and vagus nerve stimulation (VNS) are two emerging somatic treatments for psychiatric disorders. Both are ways to directly affect brain activity by stimulating nerve cell firing rates. Transcranial magnetic stimulation was introduced in 1985 as a noninvasive, painless method to stimulate the cerebral cortex. Undergirding this procedure is the hypothesis that a time-varying magnetic field will induce an electrical field, which, in brain tissue, activates inhibitory and excitatory neurons (Kanno, Matsumoto, Togashi, Yoshioka, & Mano, 2003), thereby modulating neuroplasticity in the brain. The low-frequency electrical stimulation from rTMS triggers lasting anticonvulsant effects in rats, and the therapeutic benefits of rTMS in humans are thought to be related to action similar to that produced by anticonvulsant medication. The rTMS has been used for both clinical and research purposes. The rTMS stimulation of the brain's prefrontal cortex may help some depressed patients in much the same way as ECT but without its side effects (Martis et al., 2003). Thus, it has been proposed as an alternative to ECT in managing symptoms of depression. The rTMS treatment is administered daily for at least a week, much like ECT, except that subjects remain awake. Although proven effective for depression, rTMS does have some side effects, including mild headaches.

Vagus nerve stimulation (VNS) is the newest of the currently available somatic treatments. For years, scientists have been interested in identifying how autonomic functions modulate activity in the limbic system and higher cortex. The vagus nerve has traditionally been considered a parasympathetic efferent nerve that was responsible only for regulating autonomic functions, such as heart rate and gastric tone. However, the vagus nerve (cranial X) also carries sensory information to the brain from the head, neck, thorax, and abdomen, and research has identified that the vagus nerve has extensive projections of its sensory afferent connections to many brain areas (Armitage, Husain, Hoffmann, & Rush, 2003). Although the basic mechanism of action of VNS is unknown, incoming sensory, or afferent, connections of the left vagus nerve directly project into many of the very same brain regions implicated in neuropsychiatric disorders. These connections help us to understand how VNS is helpful in treating psychiatric disorders. Vagus nerve stimulation changes levels of several neurotransmitters implicated in the development of major depression, including serotonin, norepinephrine, GABA, and glutamate (Forbes, Macdonald, Eljamel, & Roberts, 2003).

PSYCHOSOCIAL ISSUES IN BIOLOGIC TREATMENTS

Many factors influence successful medication and other biologic therapies. Of particular importance are issues related to adherence. Adherence refers to following the therapeutic regimen, self-administering medications as prescribed, keeping appointments, and following other treatment suggestions. Adherence exists on a continuum and can be conceived of as full, partial, or nil. Partial adherence, whereby a patient either attempts to take medications but misses doses or takes more than prescribed, is by far the most common. Recent estimates indicate that on the average, 50% or more of the individuals with schizophrenia taking antipsychotic medications stop taking the medications or do not take them as prescribed. It should be remembered that problems with adherence are an issue with many chronic health states, including diabetes and arthritis, not just psychiatric disorders. Box 13-6 lists some of the common reasons for nonadherence.

The most often sited reasons for nonadherence are related to side effects of the medication. Improved functioning may be observed by health care professionals but not felt by the patient. Side effects may interfere with work performance or other important aspects of the individual's life. For example, a construction worker cannot afford to be drowsy and sedated while operating a crane at a construction site, or a woman in an intimate relationship may find anorgasmia intolerable. Nurses need to be sensitive to the patient's ability to tolerate side effects and to the impact that side effects have on the patient's life. Medication choice, dosing schedules,

and prompt treatment of side effects may be crucial factors in helping patients to continue their treatment, even if the symptoms for which they initially sought help have improved.

Cognitive deficits associated with some psychiatric disorders may make it difficult for the individual to self-monitor, develop insight, make choices, remember to fill prescriptions, or keep appointments. Family members may have beliefs and attitudes that influence the individual not to take the medication. They may misunderstand or deny the illness; for example, "My wife's better, so she doesn't need that medicine anymore." Family members may be distressed when observable side effects occur. Akinesia, which has been linked to suicidal thoughts as a way to relieve the subjective discomfort, may be the most distressing side effect for family members of individuals who have schizophrenia (Fischer, Ferger, & Kuschinsky, 2002; Meltzer, 2000). Patients may also be reluctant to disclose financial constraints, especially in relation to the cost of newer agents, and may try to stretch out the prescription or just not fill their prescription. Adherence concerns must not be dismissed as the patient's or family's problem. Psychiatric nurses should actively address this issue. A positive therapeutic relationship between the nurse and patient and family must provide a strong sense of trust that side effects and other difficulties in treatment will be addressed and minimized. When individuals report distressing side effects, the nurse should immediately respond with assessment and interventions to reduce these effects. It is important to assess adherence often, asking questions in a nonthreatening, nonjudgmental manner. It also may be helpful to seek information from others who are involved with the patient.

Adherence can be improved by psychoeducation. This approach is most helpful if it addresses the individual's specific symptoms and concerns. For example, if the patient is having difficulty with understanding the purpose of the medication, it may be helpful to link taking it to reduction of specific unwanted symptoms or improved functioning, such as continuing to work. Family members should also be included in these discussions.

Other factors that interfere with adherence should also be assessed and plans developed to minimize their effect. For example, an individual who is being considered for clozapine therapy may have missed a number of appointments in the past. On assessment, the nurse may discover that it takes the individual 2 hours on three different busses each way to reach the clinic. The nurse can then assist with arranging for a home health nurse to visit the patient's apartment, draw blood samples for analysis, and assess side effects, thus decreasing the number of trips the patient must make to the clinic.

BOX 13.6

Common Reasons for Nonadherence with Medication Regimens

- Uncomfortable side effects and those that interfere with quality of life, such as work performance or intimate relationships
- Lack of awareness of or denial of illness
- Stigma
- Feeling better
- Confusion about dosage or timing
- Difficulties in access to treatment
- Substance abuse

SUMMARY OF KEY POINTS

◙ Psychopharmacology is the study of medications used to treat psychiatric disorders, including the drug categories of antipsychotics, mood stabilizers, antidepressants, antianxiety medications, and psychostimulants.

◙ Pharmacodynamics refers to the actions of drugs on living tissue and the human body, with the focus primarily on drug actions at receptor sites and transporters and on ion channel sites and enzyme activity.

◙ The importance of receptors is recognized in current psychopharmacology. Biologic action of many drugs depends on how their structure interacts with a specific receptor, functioning either as an agonist, reproducing the same biologic action as a neurotransmitter, or as an antagonist, blocking the response.

◙ A drug's ability to interact with a given receptor type may be judged on three qualities: selectivity—the ability to interact with specific types of receptors; affinity—the attraction the drug has for the binding site; and intrinsic activity—the ability to produce a certain biologic response.

◙ Many characteristics of specific drugs affect how well they act and how they affect patients. Psychiatric–mental health nurses must be familiar with characteristics, adverse reactions, and toxicity of certain drugs to administer psychotropic medications safely, educate patients regarding their safe use, and encourage therapeutic adherence.

◙ Pharmacokinetics refers to how drugs move within the human body to get to their target tissues and how drugs are removed from the body. Bioavailability describes the amount of the drug that actually reaches the systemic circulation. The wide variations in pharmacokinetic properties across individuals are related to physiologic differences caused by age, genetic makeup, other disease processes, and chemical interactions.

◙ Antipsychotic medications are drugs used in treating psychotic disorders, such as schizophrenia. They act primarily by blocking dopamine or serotonin postsynaptically. In addition, they have a number of actions on other neurotransmitters. Older typical antipsychotic drugs work on positive symptoms, are inexpensive, but produce many side effects. Newer atypical antipsychotic drugs work on positive and negative symptoms; are much more expensive, but have far fewer anticholinergic side effects; are better tolerated by patients, but increase risk for metabolic disorders.

◙ Medication-related movement disorders are a particularly serious group of side effects that principally occur with the typical antipsychotic medications and that may be acute syndromes, such as dystonia, pseudoparkinsonism, and akathisia, or chronic syndromes, such as tardive dyskinesia.

◙ The mood stabilizers, or antimania medications, are drugs used to control wide variations in mood related to mania, but these agents may also be used to treat other disorders. Lithium and the anticonvulsants are chemically unrelated and act in different ways to stabilize mood.

◙ Antidepressant medications are drugs used primarily for treating symptoms of depression, but are also used extensively for anxiety disorders and eating disorders. They act by blocking reuptake of one or more of the bioamines, especially serotonin and norepinephrine. These medications vary considerably in their structure and action. Newer antidepressants, such as the selective serotonin reuptake inhibitors, have fewer side effects and are less lethal in overdose than the older tricyclic antidepressants.

◙ Antianxiety medications also include several subgroups of medications, but benzodiazepines and non-benzodiazepines are those principally used in psychiatry. Benzodiazepines act by enhancing the actions of GABA, whereas the nonbenzodiazepine buspirone acts on serotonin. Benzodiazepines can be used on a PRN basis, whereas buspirone must be taken regularly.

◙ Psychostimulants enhance neurotransmitter activity, acting at a number of different receptors sites. These medications are most often used for treating symptoms related to attention deficit hyperactivity disorder and narcolepsy.

◙ Electroconvulsive therapy uses the application of an electrical pulsation to induce seizures in the brain. These seizures produce a number of effects on neurotransmission that result in the fairly rapid relief of depressive symptoms.

◙ Repetitive transcranial magnetic stimulation and vagus nerve stimulation are two emerging somatic treatments for psychiatric disorders. They are both means to directly affect brain function through stimulation of the nerves that are direct extensions of the brain.

◙ Phototherapy involves the application of full-spectrum light in the morning hours, which appears to reset circadian rhythm delays related to seasonal affective disorder and other forms of depression. Nutritional therapies are in various stages of investigation.

◙ Adherence refers to the ability of an individual to self-administer medications as prescribed and to follow other instructions related to medication treatment. It can be either full, partial, or nil. Nonadherence is related to factors such as medication side effects, cost, stigma, and family influences. Nurses play a key role in educating patients and helping them to improve adherence.

CRITICAL THINKING CHALLENGES

1 Discuss why it is essential that nurses have knowledge of the following concepts: neurotransmitter, receptor, agonist, and antagonist.

2 Discuss how the concepts of affinity with selectivity and intrinsic activity have meaning for nurses.

3 Discuss the usefulness of the concept of bioavailability for nurses. What does it mean to nurses, and how would nursing actions change if it were considered?

4 Delineate the ethical issues of nursing management activities associated with each phase of drug treatment: initiation, stabilization, maintenance, and discontinuation.

5 Discuss how you would go about identifying the target symptoms for a specific patient for the following medications: antipsychotic, antidepressant, and antianxiety drugs.

6 Discuss the ways in which you might explain to a patient the differences between typical and atypical antipsychotic medications.

7 Explain the health problems associated with anticholinergic side effects of the antipsychotic medications.

8 Compare the type of movements that characterize tardive dyskinesia with those that characterize akathisia and dystonia and explore which one is easier for a patient to experience.

9 Explain how your nursing care would be different for a male patient taking lithium carbonate than for a female patient.

10 Discuss contrasting views why the antidepressant class of medications has become so commonly prescribed.

11 Discuss the efficacy of anticonvulsive therapy and its mechanism of action.

12 Compare different approaches that you might use with a patient with schizophrenia who has decided to stop taking his or her typical antipsychotic medication because of intolerance to side effects.

REFERENCES

Abrams, H. (2002). Does brief-pulse ECT cause persistent or permanent memory impairment? *Journal of ECT, 18*(2), 71–73.

Alda, M. (2004). The phenotype spectra of bipolar disorder. *European Neuropsycopharmacology, 14*(Suppl 1), S94–99.

Allison, D. B., Mentore, J. L., & Heo, M. (1999). Antipsychotic-induced weight gain: A comprehensive research synthesis. *American Journal of Psychiatry, 156*, 1686–1696.

American Nurses Association (ANA). (1994). Psychopharmacology guidelines for psychiatric mental health nurses. In ANA (Ed.), *Psychiatric mental health nursing psychopharmacology project* (pp. 41–45). Washington, DC: Author.

Arana, G. W. (2000). An overview of side effects caused by typical antipsychotics. *Journal of Clinical Psychiatry, 61*(Suppl. 8), 5–13.

Armitage, R., Husain, M., Hoffmann, R., & Rush, A. J. (2003). The effects of vagus nerve stimulation on sleep EEG in depression: A preliminary report. *Journal of Psychosomatic Research, 54*(5), 475–482.

Bachmann, J. (2002). Genotyping and phenotyping the cytochrome p-450 enzymes. *American Journal of Therapeutics, 9*(4), 309–316.

Baker, G. B., Urichuk, L. J., & Coutts, R. T. (1998). Drug metabolism and metabolic drug-drug interactions in psychiatry. *Child and Adolescent Pharmacology News Suppl, 1*, 1–8.

Bilici, M., Tekelioglu, Y., Efendioglu, S., Ovali, E., & Ulgen, M. (2003). The influence of olanzapine on immune cells in patients with schizophrenia. *Progress in Neuropsychopharmacology and Biological Psychiatry, 27*(3), 483–485.

Bschor, T., Baethge, C., Adli, M., Lewitzka, U., Eichmann, U., & Bauer, M. (2003). Hypothalamic-pituitary-thyroid system activity during lithium augmentation therapy in patients with unipolar major depression. *Journal of Psychiatry Neuroscience, 28*(3), 210–216.

Ditto, K. E. (2003). SSRI discontinuation syndrome. Awareness as an approach to prevention. *Postgraduate Medicine, 114*, 79–84.

Dalfen, A. K., & Stewart, D. E. (2001). Who develops severe or fatal adverse drug reactions to selective serotonin reuptake inhibitors? *Canadian Journal of Psychiatry, 46*(3), 258–263.

Ferry, L., & Johnston, J. A. (2003). Efficacy and safety of bupropion SR for smoking cessation: Data from clinical trials and five years of postmarketing experience. *International Journal of Clinical Practice, 57*(3), 224–230.

Fischer, D. A., Ferger, B., & Kuschinsky, K. (2002). Discrimination of morphine- and haloperidol-induced muscular rigidity and akinesia/catalepsy in simple tests in rats. *Behavioural Brain Research, 21*; 134(1–2), 317–321.

Forbes, R. B., Macdonald, S., Eljamel, S., & Roberts, R. C. (2003). Cost-utility analysis of vagus nerve stimulators for adults with medically refractory epilepsy. *Seizure, 12*(5), 249–256.

Gardener, D. M., Shulman, K. I., Walker, S. E., & Tailor, S. A. N. (1996). The making of a user-friendly MAOI diet. *Journal of Clinical Psychiatry, 57*, 99–104.

Glazer, W. M. (2000). Extrapyramidal side effects, tardive dyskinesia, and the concept of atypicality. *Journal of Clinical Psychiatry, 61*, 16–21.

Goodwin, F. K., & Ghaemi, S. N. (2000). The impact of mood stabilizers on suicide in bipolar disorder: A comparative analysis. *CNS Spectrums, 5*(2), 12–19.

Grootens, K. P., & Verkes, R. J. (2005). Emerging evidence for the use of atypical antipsychotics in borderline personality disorder. *Pharmacopsychiatry, 38*(1), 20–23.

Grunze, H., & Walden, J. (2003). Relevance of new and newly rediscovered anticonvulsants for atypical forms of bipolar disorder. *Journal of Affective Disorders, 72*(Suppl. 1), S15–21.

Haddad, P. (1998). The SSRI discontinuation syndrome. *Journal of Psychopharmacology 12*(3), 305–313.

Hegadoren, K. M. (2004). Assessment and treatment of depression: A review in high risk populations. *Journal of Wound, Ostomy and Continence Nursing, 31*, 100–112.

Hirose, S. (2002). ECT for depression with amnesia. *Journal of ECT, 18*(1), 60.

Hirschfeld, R. M., Calabrese, J. R., & Weissman, N. M. (2002). Prevalence of bipolar disorders in US adults. Program and abstracts of the American Psychiatric Association 155th Annual Meeting, May 18–23. Philadelphia Industry-Supported Symposium No. NR247.

Hogan, D., Ebly, E., & Fung, T. (1995). Regional variations in use of potentially inappropriate medications by Canadian seniors participating in the Canadian Study of Health and Aging. *Canadian Journal of Clinical Pharmacology, 2*(4), 167–174.

Izzo, A. A. (2004). Drug interactions with St. John's Wort (Hypericum perforatum): A review of the clinical evidence. *International Journal of Pharmacology and Therapeutics. 42*(3), 139–148.

Jacelon, C. S. (1999). Preventing cascade iatrogenesis in hospitalized elders. *Journal of Gerontological Nursing, 25*(1), 27–33.

Kanno, M., Matsumoto, M., Togashi, H., Yoshioka, M., & Mano, Y. (2003). Effects of repetitive transcranial magnetic stimulation on behavioural and neurochemical changes in rats during an elevated plus-maze test. *Journal of the Neurological Sciences, 211*(1–2), 5–14.

Kaplan, G. B., & Hammer, R. P. (2002). *Brain circuitry and signaling in psychiatry: Basic science and clinical implications.* Washington, DC: APA.

Kearns, G. L. (2000). Impact of developmental pharmacology on pediatric study design: Overcoming the challenges. *Journal of Allergy and Clinical Immunology, 106*(3), 128–138.

Kearns, G. L., & Winter, H. S. (2004). Proton pump inhibitors in pediatrics: Relevant pharmacokinetics and pharmacodynamics. *Journal of Pediatric Gastroenterology and Nutrition, 37*(Suppl. 1), S52–59.

Keck, P. E. (2002). Clinical management of bipolar disorder. Clinical update. Retrieved September 20, 2005, from www.medscape.com/viewprogram/135_pnt.

Kennedy, S. H., Lam, R. W., Cohen, N. L., Ravindran, A. V., & the CANMAT Depression Work Group. (2001). Clinical guidelines for the treatment of depressive disorders. IV. Medications and other biological treatments. *Canadian Journal of Psychiatry, 46*(S1), 38S–58S.

Kennedy, S. H., Segal, Z. V., Cohen, N. L., Levitan, R. D., Gemar, M., & Bagby, R. M. (2003). Lithium carbonate versus cognitive therapy as sequential combination treatment strategies in partial responders to antidepressant medication: An exploratory trial. *Journal of Clinical Psychiatry, 64*(4), 439–444.

Krystal, J. H., Sancora, G., Blumberg, H., Anand, A., Charney, D. S., Marek, G., Epperson, C. N., Goddard, A., & Mason, G. F. (2002). Glutamate and GABA systems as targets for novel antidepressant and mood-stabilizing treatments. *Molecular Psychiatry, 7*(Suppl 1), S71–80.

Kulkarni, S. K., & Naidu, P. S. (2003). Pathophysiology and drug therapy of tardive dyskinesia: Current concepts and future perspectives. *Drugs Today (Barc), 39*(1), 19–49.

Leeder, J. S., & Kearns, G. L. (1997). Pharmacogenetics in pediatrics. *Pediatric Clinics of North America, 44*(1), 55–77.

Levy, G., Schupf, N., Tang, M. X., Cote, L. J., Louis, E. D., Mejia, H., Stern, Y., & Marder, K. (2002). Combined effect of age and severity on the risk of dementia in Parkinson's disease. *Annals of Neurology, 51*(6), 722–729.

Loscher, W. (2002). Basic pharmacology of valproate: A review after 35 years of clinical use for the treatment of epilepsy. *CNS Drugs, 16*(10), 669–694.

Madhusoodanan, S., Brenner, R., & Cohen, C. I. (2000). Risperidone for elderly patients with schizophrenia or schizoaffective disorder. *Psychiatric Annals, 30*(3), 175–180.

Marshall, J. D., & Kearns, G. L. (1999). Developmental pharmacodynamics of cyclosporine. *Clinical Pharmacology and Therapeutics, 66*, 66–75.

Martin, J. L., Barbanoj, M. J., Schlaepfer, T. E., Thompson, E., Perez, V., & Kulisevsky, J. (2003). Repetitive transcranial magnetic stimulation for the treatment of depression. Systematic review and meta-analysis. *British Journal of Psychiatry, 182*, 480–491.

Martis, B., Alam, D., Dowd, S. M., Hill, S. K., Sharma, R. P., Rosen, C., Pliskin, N., Martin, E., Carson, V., & Janicak, P. G. (2003). Neurocognitive effects of repetitive transcranial magnetic stimulation in severe major depression. *Clinical Neurophysiology, 114*(6), 1125–1132.

McCabe, S. (2002). Complementary herbal and alternative drugs in clinical practice. *Perspectives in Psychiatric Care, 38*(3), 98–107.

Meltzer, H. Y. (2000). Introduction. Side effects of antipsychotic medications: Physician's choice of medication and patient compliance. *Journal of Clinical Psychiatry, 61*(Suppl. 8), 3–4.

Moisan, J., Gregoire, J., Gaudet, M., Cooper, D. (2005) Exploring the risk of diabetes mellitus and dyslipidemia among ambulatory users of atypical antipsychotics: A population-based comparison of risperidone and olanzapine. *Pharmacoepidemiology and Drug Safety 14*, 427–436.

Nasrallah, H. A. (2002). Pharmacoeconomic implications of adverse effects during antipsychotic drug therapy. *American Journal of Health-System Pharmacy, 59*(22 Suppl 8), S16–S21.

Nemeroff, C. B. (2002). New directions in the development of antidepressants: The interface of neurobiology and psychiatry. *Human Psychopharmacology, 17*(Suppl 1), S13–16.

Nihart, M. A. (1995). *Managing the symptoms of schizophrenia: A nursing perspective.* American Psychiatric Nursing Association, Slide Kit, p. 29. Belle Mead, NJ: Excerpta Medica.

O'Hara, R., Thompson, J. M., Kraemer, H. C., Fenn, C., Taylor, J. L., Ross, L., Yesavage, J. A., Bailey, A. M., & Tinklenberg, J. R. (2002). Which Alzheimer patients are at risk for rapid cognitive decline? *Journal of Geriatric Psychiatry Neurology, 15*(4), 233–238.

Pandolfi, A., Grilli, A., Cilli, C., Patruno, A., Giaccari, A., DiSilvestre, S., De Lutiis, M. A., Pellegrini, G., Capani, F., Consoli, A., & Felaco, M. (2003). Phenotype modulation in cultures of vascular and smooth muscle cells from diabetic rats: Association with increased nitric oxide synthase expression and superoxide anion generation. *Journal of Cellular Physiology, 196*(2), 378–385.

Regier, D. A., Narrow, W. E., Rae, D. S., Manderscheid, R.W., Locke, B. Z., Goodwin, F. K. (1993). The de facto US mental and addictive disorders service spectrum. Epidemiological catchment area prospective 1-year prevalence rates of disorders and services. *Archives of General Psychiatry, 50*(2), 85–94.

Riederer, P., Lachenmayer, L., Laux, G. (2004). Clinical applications of MAO-inhibitors. *Current Medicinal Chemistry, 11*, 2033–2043

Sajatovic, M. (2000). Clozapine for elderly patients. *Psychiatric Annuals, 30*(3), 170–174.

Soldin, O. P., & Soldin, S. J. (2002). Review: Therapeutic drug monitoring in pediatrics. *Therapeutic Drug Monitoring, 24*, 1–8.

Solomon, D. A., Keitner, G. I., Ryan, C. E., et al. (2000). Lithium plus valproate as maintenance polypharmacy for patients with bipolar I disorder: A review. *CNS Spectrums, 5*(2), 19–28.

Satcher, D. (1999). Mental health: A report of the surgeon general. Available at: http://www.surgeongeneral.gov.

Taylor, D. (2003). Ziprasidone in the management of schizophrenia: The QT interval issue in context. *CNS Drugs, 17*(6), 423–430.

Thase, M. (2002). Studying new antidepressants: If there were a light at the end of the tunnel, could we see it? *Journal of Clinical Psychiatry, 63*(Suppl. 2), 24–28.

Viguera, A. C., Baldessarini, R. J., & Friedberg, J. (1988). Discontinuing antidepressant treatment in major depression. *Harvard Reviews in Psychiatry, 5*, 293–306.

Yeung, P. P., Tariot, P. N., & Schneider, L. S., et al. (2000). Quetiapine for elderly patients with psychotic disorders. *Psychiatric Annuals, 30*(3), 197–201.

Young, S. N., & Leyton, M. (2002). The role of serotonin in human mood and social interaction. Insight from altered tryptophan levels. *Pharmacology, Biochemistry and Behavior, 71*, 857–865.

Zhou, H. (2003). Pharmacokinetic strategies in deciphering atypical drug absorption profiles. *Journal of Clinical Pharmacology, 43*(3), 211–227.

Zintzaras, E. (2005). Statistical aspects of bioequivalence testing between two medicinal products. *European Journal of Drug Metabolism and Pharmacokinetics, 30*(1–2), 41–46.

Zullino, D., Delacrausaz, P., & Baumann, P. (2002). The place of SSRIs in the treatment of schizophrenia. *Encephale, 28*(5 Pt 1), 433–438.

For challenges, please refer to the **CD-ROM** in this book.

14

Cognitive-Behavioural Therapy

Tracey Tully and Ruth Gallop

LEARNING OBJECTIVES

After studying this chapter, you will be able to:

- Describe the cognitive model.
- Discuss the levels of cognition, including core beliefs, intermediate beliefs, automatic thoughts, and their interrelationship.
- Identify and describe the ten principles of cognitive-behavioural therapy.
- Discuss cognitive treatment techniques.
- Discuss behavioural treatment techniques.

KEY TERMS

- automatic thoughts ▪ cognitive schema ▪ core beliefs ▪ intermediate beliefs

⬠ KEY CONCEPTS

- Cognitive-behavioural therapy ▪ cognitive restructuring

One of the more exciting and significant achievements in modern psychotherapy is the advancement of cognitive-behavioural therapy (CBT). CBT is a form of psychotherapy that emphasizes the centrality of thought or cognition in the development of core beliefs about self and the world. The aim of CBT is to identify, analyze, and ultimately change the habitually inflexible and negative cognitions about oneself, others, and the world at large that contribute to distressing emotional states and problematic behaviours (Ingram, Miranda, & Segal, 1998). Through modifying thinking, emotion and behaviour also change. CBT is the most widely researched form of psychotherapy and, given the robust findings from numerous controlled clinical trials, is recognized by many as the treatment of choice for many mental disorders, including posttraumatic stress disorder, bulimia nervosa, panic disorder, and depression.

> 🔷 **KEY CONCEPT Cognitive-behavioural therapy** is psychotherapy focussed on identifying, analyzing, and ultimately changing the habitually inflexible and negative cognitions about oneself, others, and the world that contribute to distress and problematic behaviours.

Although the assumptions underlying CBT can be traced back to ancient times and the Stoic philosopher, Epictetus, Aaron Beck, a psychiatrist, and Albert Ellis, a psychologist, are acknowledged with founding CBT as we know it today. In the mid-1950s to early 1960s, when experimental and clinical psychology and psychiatry were ruled by behaviourism and psychoanalytic theory, Ellis and Beck, independently of each other, became increasingly dissatisfied with both the ability of psychoanalysis to explain the struggles of their patients and its lack of scientific rigor. In treating their patients, they noted certain biases toward irrational and inflexible thought patterns that negatively influenced mood and behaviour. They proposed that if these rigid and negative thought patterns could be changed, mood would improve, and behaviour would become more functional. Although this theory is now widely accepted, at the time, a cognitively focussed psychotherapy was viewed as radical. Beck and Ellis remain international leaders in clinical practice, teaching and training, and empirical study of CBT. Although CBT is a mental health treatment, it is based on a cognitive model that is applicable to the experience of all humans in all situations. Beck and Ellis envision that future generations will be educated in the foundations of CBT so as to provide important life skills for coping with distress and problem solving.

THE COGNITIVE MODEL

The cognitive model forms the foundation of CBT, the essence of which is that humans respond primarily to

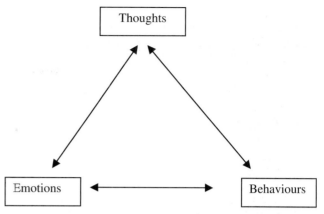

FIGURE 14.1   Interconnection between thoughts, emotions, and behaviours

cognitive representations of the environment, and that cognition mediates affect and behaviour (Ingram, Miranda, & Segal, 1998). In simpler terms, the way we *think* about situations influences our *emotions* and our *behaviour*. Our emotions, behaviours, and thoughts all interact in complex and interconnected ways; however, the cognitive model places particular importance on thoughts as the "director" of our experience (Fig. 14-1).

Cognitive theory suggests that one's perception of situations and events is particularly salient in guiding emotional and behavioural responses (Beck, 1995). Events in and of themselves do not cause us to feel and act in particular ways; rather, it is how we *understand* or think about what happens to us that affects how we feel about it and what we do about it. For example, think about what would go through your mind if you entered a party where the only other guest you knew had not yet arrived. Would you think, "This is a great opportunity to introduce myself to others. Maybe I'll meet some interesting people," or would you think, "Everyone is staring at me because I'm alone. If my friend does not show up in the next 15 minutes, I'm leaving"? The party itself is a relatively neutral event, but how you interpret the event will affect how you feel at the party and what you do or how you act. If your thought process tends toward the former, your emotions of excitement and enjoyment will propel you to stay and mingle with the other partygoers (your behaviour). If your thought process is more consistent with the latter, your anxiety and uncertainty will compel you to flee (your behaviour).

The different ways that individuals evaluate and respond to a particular situation or event are as varied as the individuals themselves. The particular reasons why individuals are so varied in their perceptions of situations, and thereby their emotional and behavioural responses, are in part accounted for by their core beliefs. See Box 14-1 for an example of students responding differently to the same situation. In summary, the cognitive model posits that: when an emotion is felt, a thought is

Affect of Cognition on Feelings and Behaviour

In this example, four student nurses in the same clinical group respond to the same situation in four different ways, owing to different patterns of thinking, feeling, and acting.
The situation: A nursing instructor informs the clinical group that by the end of their shift today, each student is expected to seek out an opportunity to insert their first intravenous line. All students received the appropriate classroom teaching and lab practice with this skill.

SUSAN thinks, "I have been waiting so long to perform advanced clinical skills. I can hardly wait to give it a try." She feels excited and responds behaviourally by informing all staff in morning report of her learning opportunity. She requests that any new intravenous starts be directed to her.

DAVID thinks, "I understand the theory behind intravenous insertion, but I did not have much success in the lab. I know I need to fulfill this requirement, but I am not sure how I am going to do it without hurting someone and embarrassing myself." He feels anxious and uncertain and responds behaviourally by reluctantly informing his buddy nurse, midway through the shift, that he is required to meet this expectation.

JENNIFER thinks, "There is absolutely no way I am ready for this. I do not have the confidence or skill set to perform this task." She feels terrified and responds behaviourally by speaking to the clinical instructor privately informing her that she is feeling nauseous and must return home for the day.

PAULINE thinks, "Once again I'm being told what to do without any regard for my own learning needs. No one can force me to comply." She feels outraged and angry and responds behaviourally by refusing to complete the skill as required.

All the students were presented with the identical situation, and all received similar training to perform the required skill. The way in which each student *thought about* the situation, however, was very different and consequently led to emotions as varied as excitement and terror and behaviours as varied as approach and avoidance. It is not the situation itself that influenced how each of the students responded, but rather each individual's unique interpretation of the situation.

behind it; and when behaviour is enacted, a thought is behind it.

LEVELS OF COGNITION

At this point, it has been established that cognition is given primary importance in CBT. Now the three levels of cognition that are considered in CBT are explored, beginning with the deepest level and moving toward the most superficial.

Core Beliefs

Cognitive theory posits the existence of core knowledge structures that hold, organize, and interpret all information about one's view of self, others, and the world (Hollon & Kriss, 1984; Needleman, 1999; Sperry, 1999). These structures, referred to as **core beliefs** or **cognitive schema**, comprise basic beliefs so fundamental that they are often not articulated in explicit words but rather are accepted as absolute truths (Beck, 1995). Core beliefs assist in evaluating and assigning meaning to events and influencing the subsequent range of affective and behavioural responses (Beck & Emery, 1985). The deeply rooted nature of core beliefs and their difficulty in being accessed, or explicitly identified, means that they are difficult to change. Examples of core beliefs are: I am inadequate; I am unlovable; Others are not trustworthy; and The world is an unsafe place.

Core beliefs hold both general and specific information about the self, others, and the world and influence the manner in which one negotiates one's way through life. If, for example, an individual holds the belief that she is a person worthy of love, she will likely engage in mutually respectful and fulfilling relationships. Conversely, if the world is believed to be a hostile place in which people are not to be trusted, she may have an approach of hypervigilance and suspiciousness and may experience relationships as potentially dangerous. As one moves through life gathering and considering information, beliefs are processed in a way that is consistent with the view of self, others, and the world and become solidified (Hollon & Kriss, 1984). As such, core beliefs are self-confirming and self-perpetuating in nature which contributes to their rigidity and global application (Beck, 1995).

Intermediate Beliefs

Existing at a more accessible level than core beliefs are cognitive products, which are often separated into two categories: **intermediate beliefs** and **automatic thoughts** (Beck, 1995; Hollon & Kriss, 1984). Intermediate beliefs consist of attitudes, rules or expectations, and assumptions that influence one's perceptions, affect, and behaviours. They often take the form of "if... then," "should," or "must" statements that are rigid and unrealistic. Assumptions, rules, and expectations may have arisen from the direct teaching or observation of important others early in life. One's cultural background also plays a role in one's understanding and tolerance for what is acceptable. Examples of intermediate beliefs include:

- If I'm not liked by everyone, it means I've failed.
- Assume the worst will happen because it usually does.
- If I show my vulnerability, I make myself open to attack.
- I must be the best in everything that I endeavour.
- Relationships make you open to rejection.

Automatic Thoughts

At an even more superficial level than intermediate beliefs are automatic thoughts. Automatic thoughts are the "knee-jerk" in-the-moment words and images generated in a particular situation (Beck, 1995). They may not be logical and are often difficult to "shut off." Automatic thoughts are the most superficial and accessible of the levels of cognition and thus are generally the first to be targeted in treatment. Although automatic thoughts are accessible, we are not always immediately conscious of their presence. Instead, we may be more aware of the accompanying emotion rather than the preceding spontaneous thought. In fact, the presence of a strong emotion is often a signal that an important thought is present. For example, when a car cuts you off on the freeway, you might be more likely to respond with anger than to be aware of the thought behind the emotion of anger ("Who do you think you are? You put the safety of my family at risk."). Part of the early therapeutic work of CBT is to bring automatic thoughts into our awareness.

Relationship Between Levels of Cognition

The relationship between automatic thoughts, intermediate beliefs, and core beliefs is demonstrated in the following two examples. There is a situation in which an individual is standing in a line and someone steps into the position in front of her. In the moment, the individual tells herself, "This person must not have realized I was already in line. I will tell him that I was first in line so that he can take his place behind me." These automatic thoughts occur spontaneously and reside at the most superficial level of cognition. The deeper intermediate beliefs, rules, and expectations that support these automatic thoughts may be, "People do not intend to be malicious, but can cause inconvenience," "It is necessary to follow social norms," and "The ability to assert oneself is important." Underlying these automatic thoughts and intermediate rules and expectations is a core belief, the deepest level of cognition, of "I am a valuable person who is worthy of respect." This example of the relationship between the three levels of cognition is illustrated in Figure 14-2. Another individual may process this same situation very differently. The same three levels of cognition still exist, although the content of each level is different. She may tell herself, "This person saw me standing here, and he intentionally stepped in front of me. He must think I am someone that can be easily exploited." The intermediate beliefs and rules that gave rise to these automatic thoughts are, "I am not capable of speaking up for myself," "I expect that people will treat me with a lack of respect," and "I can't speak up for myself, therefore I'll never get anywhere in life." In this example, the automatic thoughts and expectations are driven by core beliefs rooted in a sense of unworthiness, such as, "I'm not deserving of respect."

Early experiences, past events, messages from others, and direct observations contribute to the formation of

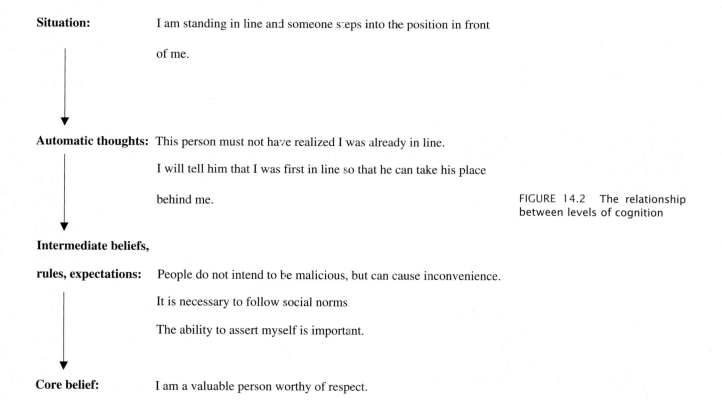

Situation: I am standing in line and someone steps into the position in front of me.

Automatic thoughts: This person must not have realized I was already in line.

I will tell him that I was first in line so that he can take his place behind me.

Intermediate beliefs,

rules, expectations: People do not intend to be malicious, but can cause inconvenience.

It is necessary to follow social norms.

The ability to assert myself is important.

Core belief: I am a valuable person worthy of respect.

FIGURE 14.2 The relationship between levels of cognition

core beliefs and subsequent intermediate beliefs and automatic thoughts. In the individual whose early experiences were primarily nurturing, reliable, and positive, core beliefs are generally an accurate, realistic, and functional reflection of reality. However, the individual who experienced inconsistency, emotional unavailability, and cruelty may develop hypercritical beliefs about the self, others, and the world that are rigid, overgeneralized, and an inaccurate reflection of current reality. These core beliefs contribute to emotions and behaviours that are intensely negative and harmful.

CRNE Note

Understanding the way thinking affects emotions and behaviour can be helpful in working with clients who are having difficulty adhering to treatment regimens.

PRINCIPLES OF COGNITIVE-BEHAVIOURAL THERAPY

CBT is grounded in a set of specific principles. The particular treatment strategies employed in CBT are specific to the disorder being treated; however, the basic principles remain common across all disorders. The ten principles that appear in Box 14.2 and discussed below are based on the work of Beck (1995), Beck and Emery (1985), and Fennell (1989).

Cognitive-Behavioural Formulation

A cognitive-behavioural formulation begins during the initial assessment of the client and is reviewed and revised over the course of therapy. It outlines the typical thoughts and problematic behaviours that contribute to current distress. The client who presents with

BOX 14.2

Ten Principles of Cognitive-Behavioural Therapy

1. CBT is based on a cognitive-behavioural formulation of the client.
2. CBT requires a strong therapeutic alliance.
3. CBT is time limited and brief.
4. CBT is goal oriented, problem focussed, and change oriented.
5. CBT is structured and directive.
6. CBT is educative.
7. CBT requires therapeutic collaboration.
8. CBT employs inductive reasoning.
9. CBT uses Socratic questioning.
10. CBT uses self-reflective exercises to apply and hone skills learned from therapy in day-to-day situations.

From Beck (1995), Beck and Emery (1985), and Fennell (1989).

social anxiety may have the thoughts, "Showing my nervousness is a sign of weakness" and "I appear incompetent when I make presentations." Problematic behaviours that flow from these negative thoughts may include avoidance of any situation in which he might be the centre of attention (eg, speaking up in meetings), over-preparing (eg, memorizing a brief statement to be made during a meeting), and use of alcohol (eg, reliance on several glasses of beer before attending a party where socializing is an expectation). The next component of the formulation involves collecting information on the factors that precipitated the onset of the current problem. The precipitating factor for the socially anxious client may be starting a new job where there is an expectation to chair meetings, conduct staff training, and give presentations to outside agencies. A cognitive-behavioural formulation also outlines the developmental issues that contributed to and continue to reinforce the current problem. For example, harsh criticism by parents for being less than perfect, being ridiculed and mocked by students while speaking in front of the class, and receiving below-average grades on oral presentations may all be predisposing factors for the socially anxious client. Over his life, he may have systematically ignored his multiple successes and amplified his perceived social failures, which served to strengthen his beliefs about weakness and inadequacy.

The cognitive-behavioural formulation is shared with the client as part of the collaborative relationship (see Box 14-2, principle 7). It is presented as a working framework that can be added to and changed by both the therapist and client as new information becomes available. In addition to providing both a framework for guiding treatment and a means to enhancing therapeutic collaboration, it also demonstrates to the client how part of one's experience can be broken down in order to gain a better understanding of the whole; that one's seemingly overwhelming problems are composed of smaller and more manageable parts.

Strong Therapeutic Alliance

Much of the emphasis of CBT is on therapy technique and strategies; however, therapeutic change would not be achievable without a strong therapeutic relationship consisting of trust, mutual respect, safety, empathy, warmth, and acceptance. Most clients enter therapy afraid, uncertain, and perhaps unsure if it will be helpful. Many have struggled for years on their own, too ashamed to seek help. Further, the personal histories of some clients render them highly mistrustful of those in positions of perceived power. It is the primary task of the therapist to create an environment in which clients feel free to disclose their anxieties and take risks, in which they feel attended to, listened to, and understood. The therapeutic relationship is discussed further in Chapter 8.

Time Limited and Brief

Some forms of psychotherapy, in particular the insight-oriented psychotherapies, are open ended with respect to length of treatment (see Chapter 7). Given the nature and goals of psychodynamic therapy, treatment may not be completed for a number of years. In contrast, CBT is a short-term form of treatment. For example, a maximum of 25 sessions of CBT are recommended for depression (Fennell, 1989; Kaplan, Sadock, & Greeb, 1994), whereas 5 to 20 sessions are recommended for anxiety disorders (Clark, 1998). The treatment guidelines for panic disorder recommend 12 sessions of CBT (American Psychiatric Association, 1998). The standard number of sessions for social phobia when it is delivered in group CBT, as determined by Heimberg's extensive study in the field, is 12 (Heimberg & Becker, 2002). Individuals who present with simple phobias generally require even fewer sessions, as few as 1 or 2 sessions in certain cases. When determining the number of sessions required, the therapist considers the severity and duration of the presenting problem, client motivation, and the client's ability to form and maintain a therapeutic relationship.

Goal Oriented, Problem Focussed, and Change Oriented

Clients enter CBT with a clear idea of that with which they are struggling. The therapist and client collaboratively set realistic and measurable goals to be attained within the treatment period. Using cognitive and behavioural strategies (to be discussed), the client works toward analyzing the current accuracy and logic of negative thinking patterns. Distortions in thinking are tested and are replaced with more accurate and flexible ways of evaluating self, others, and the world. Potential barriers to goal attainment are considered, and methods to overcome these obstacles are planned.

Structured and Directive

Although the content of each therapy session changes from week to week, sessions follow a similar structure throughout the course of treatment. The structure of CBT provides clarity, reassurance, and a sense of control to the client as well as maintains focus and maximizes the ability to use the session effectively. An additional benefit of the structured nature of CBT is that it supports the client to be his or her own therapist upon therapy termination.

The therapist begins the session with a mood check, asks for a brief summary of the client's week, collaboratively decides which problem areas will be discussed in the session (often referred to as agenda setting), requests feedback about the previous session, reviews and discusses the self-reflective exercise (see Box 14-2,

principle 10), addresses the agenda items, provides new self-reflective exercises, and elicits feedback about the session. Throughout the session, the therapist offers summaries of key areas. As the therapy progresses, the client takes on the responsibility of providing these summaries and managing the structure in general.

Educative

The initial sessions of CBT are more therapist directed than later sessions and include education about the client's presenting problem and the cognitive model of their particular disorder in addition to socializing the client to CBT. For example, the first four sessions of a group CBT intervention for self-injuring women who have a history of sexual abuse included therapist-led content on the cognitive model of childhood sexual abuse and self-injury; the cognitive, affective, and behavioural patterns that emerge from early experiences of abuse; and the functions and purposes of self-injury (Tully, 2005). Further on in CBT, therapists teach clients how to engage in cognitive restructuring, the process whereby habitually negative thought patterns are identified, evaluated, and modified. Providing clients information on the nature and course of their disorder not only helps them to understand their current struggles, but also empowers clients to engage in a collaborative approach to their care. An additional benefit of the educative nature of CBT is that it assists in preparing clients for the process of self-therapy; that is, it helps ensure that clients adopt the skills necessary to continue change and prevent relapse after the specific therapy has ended.

Therapeutic Collaboration

Cognitive-behavioural therapists practice from the stance that therapy is a collaborative effort. The client and therapist each bring essential and different ingredients to the relationship, and both are vital in achieving therapeutic change. The client assumes the role of equal partner in agenda setting, problem solving, and generating self-reflective exercises (see Box 14-2, principle 10). Because the content and process of CBT are demystified and made transparent, it is possible for clients to truly take on a collaborative role. The therapist remains an active participant in the treatment; neither a neutral nor authoritative stance would be appropriate in CBT.

Inductive Reasoning

Clients entering therapy often view their thoughts and feelings as facts and unshakeable truths; for example, "I know I am a stupid person. When I'm depressed, it means I'm weak." Clients of CBT are encouraged to view their thoughts and feelings as hypotheses; they are not rigid facts, but are plausible explanations that will be put to test and revised as needed. The goal is to assist the client in attending to all the available facts and information in their hypothesis testing, not merely the "old ruts" of thinking in which they generally find themselves stuck. Clients are encouraged to "think like a scientist and search for objective facts" or "play detective to find all the evidence" when examining the validity and accuracy of their thoughts.

Socratic Questioning

Cognitive-behavioural therapists adopt a questioning stance, referred to as Socratic questioning, as a method to reveal information about negative thought patterns and to aid in developing balanced thoughts. When a question is posed by the therapist, possible answers are generated. The client is encouraged to view these answers as hypotheses capable of being examined and tested in the therapy. The intention of Socratic questioning is not for the client to feel interrogated; rather, it is for the client to come to his or her own broader perspective about the validity, accuracy, and functionality of his or her thought process.

Self-Reflective Exercises

One of the most effective ways of helping clients reflect on and practice newly developed skills and monitor progress is through the use of self-reflective exercises, sometimes referred to as homework exercises. Extensive empirical study indicates that homework compliance is a significant predictor of positive treatment outcome (Kazantzis, Deane, & Ronan, 2000). Self-reflective exercises are provided at the end of each session with the expectation that the client will work on them throughout the week and be prepared to discuss them at the beginning of the following session. It is essential that therapists review the assigned exercise with the client at the following session because this reinforces the therapist's commitment and investment in the process. Clients will be less likely to complete the exercises if they have little accountability and if they do not observe the therapist valuing the assignments. Review of the exercises also provides the therapist with clinically useful information. If clients state that they do not feel like completing the exercise, are too busy, or do not see the point, this provides the therapist with clinically relevant material that should be explored further in the therapy. For example, a client may avoid attempting the exercises because he does not feel as though it will be done "right" or "good enough," or that he will appear "stupid, just like I always do," which would lead to humiliation. The therapist would then take the opportunity to explore these thoughts, thoughts that may represent negative patterns of thinking that are generalized to situations beyond the completion of the exercises and warrant ana-

lyzing and modification. If a client insists that she does not have adequate time to complete the exercises, further exploration may reveal that either the exercises as assigned were in fact too detailed and labour intensive, or that the client has difficulty committing the personal time necessary to effect therapeutic change. It is also equally important for the therapist to know whether the client is experiencing new insights and a sense of accomplishment through completing the exercises because this assists in gauging where next to direct the therapy.

TREATMENT STRATEGIES

CBT uses both cognitive and behavioural techniques to effect change. The strategies outlined here represent those basic to CBT. Additional strategies are used, but because of their advanced application, are beyond the scope of this text. Training in CBT is generally obtained at the graduate level, and although treatment strategies are described here, advanced training through course work, clinical practicum, and clinical supervision is essential before delivery of the treatment.

Cognitive Techniques

Cognitive techniques revolve primarily around cognitive restructuring, which is a process that follows a particular path of identifying, analyzing, and modifying the three levels of cognition, beginning with automatic thoughts and working through to core beliefs.

> ◆ **KEY CONCEPT** Cognitive restructuring is a process in which cognitions (automatic thoughts, intermediate and core beliefs) are identified, analyzed, and modified to effect positive change in mood and behaviour.

Identifying Automatic Thoughts

Awareness of one's thinking is the first step toward change. Early in treatment, clients are often unaware of their running internal negative dialogue about themselves, others, and the world. As previously discussed, the accompanying emotion may be much more apparent to the client than the underlying negative and inflexible thought process. When introducing clients to the skill of identifying automatic thoughts, a useful place to begin is to have them attend to shifts in or intensification of their emotions. When a strong emotion is felt or a new emotion is experienced, the question is asked, "What was going through your mind just then?" (Beck, 1995). This question often helps clients to attend to their thinking that drives their emotional experience. Another technique to elicit automatic thoughts is to ask the client to recount a very recent problematic situation. The client is encouraged to play back the situation in his or her mind using all the senses. As the client visualizes the details of what happened, he or she is asked, "What does this situation say about you?" "What does it mean for how others will view you?" "What is the most distressing aspect of this situation?" "If the worst case scenario came from this situation, what do you think would happen?" (Greenberger & Padesky, 1995). Once automatic thoughts are identified, the next step of evaluating their accuracy and usefulness is undertaken.

Evaluating Automatic Thoughts

The goal of evaluating automatic thoughts is to examine thoughts in detail to determine their accuracy. Clients consider both the evidence that supports and the evidence that does not support their automatic thoughts. It is important that clients focus on objective facts rather than interpretations, assumptions, or opinions when generating evidence that supports their automatic thoughts, although this may be difficult initially (Greenberger & Padesky, 1995). The task of finding evidence that does not support automatic thoughts can be aided by key questions such as, "What experiences have I had that show this thought is not always completely true?" "If someone I cared deeply about had this thought, what would I tell them?" "If someone who cared deeply about me knew I was thinking this, what would they say to me?" "What evidence is there that this thought is not 100% true?" (Greenberger & Padesky, 1995). When evaluating automatic thoughts, often clients conclude that the evidence for the automatic thought is weaker than the evidence against and therefore that the thought is no longer as accurate and valid as it was once believed to be.

The following case example illustrates the process of evaluating automatic thoughts. A situation occurred in which the client, Elizabeth, was reprimanded by her employer for not completing her monthly report, an essential part of her job. After exploring the emotions she experienced in this situation (fear and shame), she identified several negative automatic thoughts, including, "My boss hates me," "I might lose my job," "He thinks I'm incompetent," "I'm not a responsible or trustworthy employee," and "I'm nothing but a screw up." The therapist helped Elizabeth determine which automatic thought was most distressing to her ("I'm nothing but a screw up"), and it was this thought that became the one to be evaluated. Elizabeth was asked to find evidence to support the thought, "I'm nothing but a screw up." Given that she was instructed to consider only objective information, and not her opinion, the following evidence was generated: "I failed two courses in one semester during my first year of university because I partied more than I studied," "I am sometimes late paying my credit card bill," and "I once had a boyfriend who told me I wouldn't get anywhere in life." Elizabeth's next task was to find evidence that does not support her thought, "I'm nothing but a screw up." In reviewing the key questions with her therapist, she was able to find the following nonsupporting evidence: "I generally receive above average yearly performance appraisals from my boss," "In addition to working this job, I volunteer in my son's classroom two times a month where I have been called invaluable," "My best friend tells me that I'm a very organized mother."

Another aspect of the process of evaluating one's automatic thoughts involves identifying cognitive distortions. Cognitive distortions, also referred to as thinking errors or problematic thinking styles, are the characteristic and habitual ways in which people make errors in thinking about themselves or others (Burns, 1989). Thinking errors are problematic because they keep people locked into patterns of negative thinking and behaviour. Burns (1989) initially identified 10 types of thinking errors, a list that has been adapted and added to by others over time (Box 14-3). People have a tendency to engage in patterns of thinking errors that are similar across a variety of situations. All people engage in distorted thinking; it is not a phenomenon limited to people with mental disorders. In CBT, the therapist works with the client to first identify which thinking errors are being used. Clients are commonly given a handout listing all the cognitive errors with relevant examples of each. This handout guides clients through the process of identifying and labelling thinking errors. The next step is to examine the usefulness and validity of this style of thinking so that clients can respond to their thoughts in a more realistic and balanced manner, thus achieving a more accurate view of themselves and others. Through the process of correcting thinking errors, clients see that the negative automatic thoughts and beliefs they held about themselves, others, and the world at large are no longer valid. It is important to catch oneself when making the errors and inject a clearer way of looking at the situation. When we give ourselves more options for how to think, we give ourselves more options for how to feel and how to respond.

Returning to the previous case of Elizabeth, she identified that she routinely engages in distorted thinking by jumping to conclusions ("I might lose my job," "He thinks I'm incompetent") and overgeneralization ("I'm not a responsible or trustworthy employee," "I'm nothing but a screw up"). Elizabeth worked with her therapist to increase her awareness of how frequently she engages in this style of thinking. Further, her therapist helped Elizabeth to realize the inaccuracy and destructiveness of this style of thinking.

Modifying Automatic Thoughts

Identifying and evaluating automatic thoughts are two important aspects of CBT; however, given the focus on

BOX 14.3

Ten Thinking Errors

1. **All-or-nothing thinking:** The tendency to see things in black-and-white categories, with no shades of grey. Things are seen in extremes, either very good or very bad. "If I don't get a perfect evaluation, I'm a failure."

2. **Overgeneralization:** The assumption that one error/problem means a lifetime of this error/problem. "If I lose this job, I will never succeed in making a living."

3. **Mental filter:** Filtering out the good things that happen and retaining only the negative. "When I received that award, I could see that Jane didn't think I deserved it."

4. **Magnification/minimization:** Overexaggeration of fears, imperfections, or errors. "There is absolutely no way I could have passed that exam. I've totally blown the course."

5. **Jumping to conclusions:** Concluding things that are not justified based on available evidence. "I saw Peter yawn during my presentation. Everyone was bored." Includes **mind reading:** "My co-worker didn't say hello to me today because she's starting to dislike me" and **fortune telling:** "He didn't call me tonight. That's it. He'll never call again."

6. **Labelling:** Putting a negative label on yourself or others, a way to believe that no one can change. "My roommate is a slob. I have to keep everything tidy."

7. **Personalization and blame:** Making yourself feel responsible for things out of your control. "It is my fault our team lost the game. If only I hadn't dropped the ball in the first half."

8. **Should/must statements:** Thinking in terms of "should" and "must." "I must make no mistakes during the skill laboratory, no matter what."

9. **Discounting the positives:** Refusing to credit the positive aspects of situations. "John said that I looked great today. He must think that I look terrible most days."

10. **Emotional reasoning:** Believing something must be true because one "feels" it so strongly, ignoring any evidence to the contrary. "I know I've had people in my life who say I'm a good person, but it's hard to believe because I feel like I'm so bad."

From Burns, D. D. (1989). *The feeling good handbook: Using the new mood therapy in everyday life.* New York: Morrow.

change in CBT, modification of automatic thoughts is an essential component of the treatment. The client makes use of everything he has learned and acquired in identifying and evaluating automatic thoughts to move toward modification. Modifying thoughts involves weighing both the evidence for and the evidence against an automatic thought in an effort to generate a new and more balanced way of thinking. It must be emphasized that this new way of thinking does not simply involve replacing negative thoughts with positive ones. Unquestioning acceptance of a positive stance can be as destructive as negative thinking because it does not take into account all available evidence (Greenberger & Padesky, 1995). The new way of thinking considers all aspects of one's experience so that one can arrive at a more broadened way of viewing oneself, others, or the world. In Elizabeth's case, she examined all her available evidence and recognized an alternative way of understanding her situation: "I have exceedingly high expectations of myself and find it very hard to give myself a break when I've done something I perceive as less than acceptable. I have screwed up in the past, but it's been relatively infrequently, and I do learn from my mistakes." It can also be useful for clients to make a summary statement of all the evidence that supports and does not support their automatic thought to help develop balanced thinking. For example, Elizabeth summarized her evidence by saying, "I've done things that are not responsible and have received negative messages from others of the same kind, but I also am currently successful in juggling many demanding roles and receive praise for my efforts." With this expanded view, clients generally report that they experience a positive shift in mood.

One very useful and commonly used tool to achieve the goals of identifying, evaluating, and modifying automatic thoughts is the Thought Record (Greenberger & Padesky, 1995). A Thought Record is a structured worksheet that records all the pertinent information about problematic and distressing situations and helps clients to make sense of why they feel and react in particular ways. Thought Records take all aspects of one's experience and organize it into information presented in seven columns: the situation, moods, automatic thoughts, evidence that supports the thoughts, evidence that does not support the thoughts, formation of balanced or alternative thoughts, and re-rating of moods. At various points throughout the Thought Record, thoughts and emotions are rated and re-rated on their degree of strength and believability (0% to 100%). Once the Thought Record is completed, the goal is for the client to experience a balanced or alternative thought that is rated as more believable than their original negative automatic thought accompanied by a decrease in the intensity of their originally identified emotions. Thought Records are often completed during therapy sessions, as well as between sessions when problematic or distressing situations arise.

Students undergoing cognitive-behavioural training are generally required to routinely complete their own Thought Records to gain an increased awareness of their own thinking patterns and resulting emotions and behaviours and to encourage self-reflection and self-monitoring. Thought Records are often shared with supervisors and discussed in supervision sessions. Completing Thought Records is also very important for helping students in training become intimately acquainted with the process of completing the record. Although deceptively simple, Thought Records require much practice to achieve mastery.

Identifying and Modifying Intermediate Beliefs

Many of the same techniques used for identifying and modifying automatic thoughts are also used with intermediate beliefs or assumptions. There are some additional techniques that are employed, given that assumptions exist at a deeper level than automatic thoughts. Identifying assumptions can be aided by attending to the patterns of negative thoughts that emerge over the course of therapy. These themes suggest an underlying assumption or perhaps even a core belief. It can also be useful to help clients identify the rules that they live by and expect of others. A commonly used method to uncover assumptions behind an automatic thought is the downward arrow technique (Burns, 1980), in which the therapist questions the meaning of the client's thought until an assumption, or a core belief, about self, others, or the world is revealed. See Box 14-4 for an example. This technique can also be used to reveal assumptions about others (What does x mean about other people?) or the world in general (What does x say about how the world works?). Once the assumption is revealed, the process of restructuring the assumption is initiated wherein the evidence for and against the assumption and alternative responses are considered. Behavioural experiments (to be discussed) are also an effective means to modify assumptions because they allow clients to use real-life situations to test the accuracy of beliefs.

Identifying and Modifying Core Beliefs

All the techniques discussed thus far, especially the downward arrow technique, are useful for identifying core beliefs. Additional strategies may be required

because of the deeply rooted nature of core beliefs. Discussing the early life experiences of the client can often facilitate the identification of core beliefs. Through this process, the client and therapist examine the influence of early experiences in developing and maintaining core beliefs. Often, core beliefs are better understood when the context in which they developed is considered. However, this is an advanced technique beyond the scope of this chapter. The exploration must be approached with care and conducted in a manner that is containing for the client; in-depth exploration wherein clients relive painful early experiences is not appropriate in CBT.

Beck (1995) encourages the use of Core Belief Worksheets to identify core beliefs, to strengthen the believability of new core beliefs, and to weaken the influence of old core beliefs. The client first identifies his old core belief and rates it out of 100 (eg, "I'm undesirable," 70%), followed by his new core belief ("Once people get to know me, they can see that I'm a likeable person," 40%). Similar to the process of evaluating automatic thoughts, the client gathers evidence that contradicts his old belief and supports his new belief ("Last week someone in my running group gave me her number so we can arrange to go for a run together," "I have one friend who has stayed by my side despite all the things I've been through"). The final step is to gather evidence that supports the old belief with the addition of a cognitive reframe ("When my last girlfriend broke up with me, she said she could never love a person like me, but I was struggling with depression during our relationship, therefore I couldn't bring much to the relationship," "People don't readily seek out my friendship, but I'm now realizing that I have given off signals to people to stay away. This was my way of protecting myself from the rejection I believed was inevitable"). A broader perspective is achieved through this process, one that takes into account both past and current experiences.

Behavioural Techniques

Increasingly, practitioners of CBT recognize the importance of behavioural experiments if core beliefs are to be modified. The validity and accuracy of old core beliefs are tested in real life situations, thus strengthening new ones.

Behavioural strategies are primarily utilized in CBT as a way to test and challenge both old maladaptive thinking patterns and newly acquired rational thoughts. They may also be used to modify symptoms when conducted in a manner that supports a change in cognition (Wells, 1997). Behavioural techniques must be considered and implemented within the larger scope of CBT. They are not employed in isolation, nor are they

---

BOX 14.4

A Dialogue Using the Downward Arrow Technique

Client: I didn't do the self-reflective exercise this week because it was too hard.
Therapist: What does that say about you that you found it too hard?
Client: It says that I didn't pay enough attention in the session last week.
Therapist: And if that were true, that you didn't pay enough attention last week, what would that say about you?
Client: It would say that I'm lazy.
Therapist: If it was true that you were lazy, what would that say about you?
Client: It would say that I'm useless.

implemented without being linked back to the cognitive model of the particular disorder being treated.

Behavioural Strategies to Test Beliefs

Behavioural experiments to test and challenge core beliefs have always been considered an essential treatment strategy in CBT; however, recent evidence suggests that they are more important for promoting and solidifying change than Thought Records (Bennett-Levy, 2003; Bennett-Levy, Westbrook, Fennell, Cooper, Rouf, & Hackmann, 2004). Behavioural experiments offer clients the opportunity to put their newly modified cognitions to test in real-life situations, thereby increasing the believability of alternative thoughts (Bennett-Levy, 2003). Without this behavioural component, the process of challenging the accuracy and validity of old thoughts and generating new thoughts may be little more than an intellectual exercise and may not lead to meaningful cognitive, emotional, or behavioural change. Behavioural experiments can be challenging for clients because the prospect of putting new thoughts into action and testing old destructive ways of thinking can be anxiety producing.

Behavioural experiments can be presented to clients as an opportunity to "test drive" their new thoughts to see what will really happen as a result. A typical behavioural experiment consists of the therapist and client collaboratively constructing an experiment to test a new belief. For example, the new belief, "I'm a likeable person" could be tested by constructing an experiment in which the client plans to call an acquaintance from his running group and invite her to go for a run. The client makes a prediction about what might happen in the course of the experiment ("She'll agree to go with me, but she'll find me a bit uninteresting"). Potential obstacles are considered ("I will become very nervous and talk very little, therefore she'll think I'm boring"), as well as action that can be taken to manage the obstacles ("Remind myself that being nervous is okay when you are getting to know people for the first time. Remind myself that even if I don't talk much, I can't jump to the conclusion that she will think I'm boring"). The actual result of the experiment is reported ("We ran together for one hour and talked about our interests. I found out that we have many things in common, including that we both like classic films and we're both shy people. She told me that *Citizen Kane* is playing in 2 weeks and suggested that we see it together"). The client then rates how much the result of the experiment supports his new belief (90%) and finally reflects on what was learned in the process of the experiment ("If I take more risks and show people who I really am, they can see that I'm a nice person and worth getting to know better"). Behavioural experiments are a powerful means of altering beliefs because they compel clients to take action on a

thought. When clients are able to directly see the outcome of testing their beliefs, they are more likely to actually modify their beliefs.

Behavioural Strategies to Modify Symptoms

Numerous types of behavioural strategies for symptom reduction are available, including exposure techniques, relaxation training, and activity monitoring. Exposure therapies, including in vivo exposure, interoceptive exposure, graded exposure, and imaginal flooding, are utilized in panic disorder, panic disorder with agoraphobia, posttraumatic stress disorder, social phobia, and obsessive-compulsive disorder. The common thread among all types of exposure is that they put the client in contact with feared or avoided thoughts, emotions, behaviours, or situations (Needleman, 1999). Through this process, three possible outcomes may occur: the client's anticipated catastrophic outcome may be disconfirmed; the client may become desensitized to the feared response; and the client's ability to cope with the feared situation may be improved (Needleman, 1999). Exposure-based techniques are very specific to the disorder being treated, and the protocols are extensive and comprehensive. Several treatment manuals for specific disorders are available and clearly outline the rationale and steps for conducting exposure therapy. The following authors may be referred to for further reading on exposure techniques: Antony and Swinson (2000), Taylor (2000), Foa and Rothbaum (1998), Swinson, Antony, Rachman, and Richter (1998).

Relaxation strategies, such as breathing retraining and progressive muscle relaxation, may be employed with clients who have generalized anxiety disorder, panic disorder, and posttraumatic stress disorder. Breathing retraining is the practice of learning how to breath at an appropriate pace and depth so that this skill can be called on when faced with feared stimuli. Clients are also educated about how the physiologic effects of hyperventilation or breath holding, such as increased blood pressure and disturbance of the oxygen–carbon dioxide balance, may worsen anxiety symptoms (Needleman, 1999). Progressive muscle relaxation, or Jacobsonian relaxation (Jacobson, 1938) involves the practice of deliberately tensing and relaxing 12 groups of muscles, beginning with the feet and moving upward to the face. The technique teaches clients how to relax muscles and induce a sense of physical and mental calmness. Other relaxation techniques may be employed, although they are not discussed here, such as mindfulness-based meditation and guided imagery.

Depressed individuals often benefit from activity scheduling, wherein daily activities and accompanying moods are recorded in a diary format (Beck, 1995). Many depressed clients become immobilized and

Ross, C. J. M., Davis, T. M. A., & MacDonald, G. F. (2005). Cognitive-behavioural treatment combined with asthma education for adults with asthma and coexisting panic disorder. *Clinical Nursing Research, 14*, 131–157.

BOX 14.5 RESEARCH FOR BEST PRACTICE

Cognitive-Behavioural Therapy for Asthma and Coexisting Panic Disorder

THE QUESTION: Does group-administered CBT, combined with asthma education for adults with coexisting asthma and panic disorder, lead to statistically significant changes in panic and asthma outcome measures?

METHODS: Forty-eight participants diagnosed with both panic disorder and asthma were randomly assigned to a treatment group or a wait-list control group. The CBT treatment occurred in 12 sessions over 8 weeks and was focussed on four areas: anxiety and panic education; CBT techniques to identify, analyze, and modify cognitions related to anxiety and panic; breathing retraining; and interoceptive exposure. The asthma education focussed on six components: airway inflammation and bronchospasm, medication inhaler techniques, self-monitoring symptoms and peak flow, asthma triggers and strategies for control, and action plans. Outcomes were measured by standardized panic disorder measures, a panic diary, asthma symptoms diaries, and an asthma quality-of-life measure.

FINDINGS: Statistically significant posttreatment improvements were demonstrated by CBT participants as compared with the control group, on measures of panic frequency (88% were panic free at posttreatment), general anxiety, and anxiety sensitivity, as well as on measures of asthma-related quality of life and morning peak expiratory flow.

IMPLICATIONS: CBT combined with asthma education has potential as treatment for individuals with panic disorder with comorbid asthma. Nurses can assist patients in differentiating between panic episodes, asthma episodes, and combined panic–asthma episodes, as well as preventing and/or controlling these episodes. The treatment is cost effective and can be delivered by nurses with the appropriate level of training.

believe that they must wait to feel better before engaging in activities. Activity monitoring encourages depressed individuals to instead engage in activity as a way to improve mood. Activity scheduling is useful for scheduling both pleasurable and avoided tasks and monitoring moods (Beck, 1995). It is also beneficial for challenging beliefs ("There isn't anything that I enjoy doing," "I'm not good at doing anything") (Beck, Rush, Shaw, & Emery, 1979). See Box 14-5 for an example of CBT research.

CONCLUSION

The simple idea that emotion and behaviour are influenced by cognition has generated decades of empirical study, which indicates that CBT is a highly effective and cost-efficient treatment for individuals struggling with certain mental disorders. The active and collaborative nature of CBT, combined with its orientation toward change, makes it an easy fit with nursing, as is evidenced by the interest and broad appeal of CBT among nurses. Psychiatric and mental health nurses are strong advocates of self-reflection and awareness of how one's own experiences influence the therapeutic relationship. With appropriate training, nurses will find CBT to be useful to their therapeutic repertoire. CBT offers an empirically and theoretically sound means to improve the mental health of their clients.

SUMMARY OF KEY POINTS

- The cognitive model is based on the idea that the way we think about situations influences our emotion and behaviour.
- Cognitive-behavioural therapy (CBT) is based on changing negative thought patterns as a means to improve mood and behaviour.
- CBT is the most widely researched form of psychotherapy used to treat many mental disorders, including posttraumatic stress disorder, bulimia nervosa, panic disorder, and depression.
- There are 10 principles of cognitive-behavioural therapy: cognitive-behavioural formulation; strong therapeutic alliance; time limited and brief; goal oriented, problem focussed, and change oriented; structured and directive; educative; therapeutic collaboration; inductive reasoning; Socratic questioning; and self-reflective exercises.
- Cognitive techniques involve cognitive restructuring, a process that follows the steps of identifying, analyzing, and modifying automatic thoughts through to core beliefs.
- Behavioural techniques are used within the cognitive model and are seen as opportunities to test new beliefs.

CRITICAL THINKING CHALLENGES

1 How would you explain the cognitive model to a fellow student with no previous knowledge of CBT? What aspects of the model do you think are most important to emphasize?
2 Think about an incident that you experienced in the past week that caused you mild upset. Using the cognitive model, how would you differentiate between various aspects of your experience?
3 Describe the differences and interplay between core beliefs and automatic thoughts. Are there automatic thoughts that you routinely experience?
4 How do thinking errors contribute to emotional distress?
5 Why are behavioural experiments an essential aspect of CBT?
6 How are the principles of CBT different from and similar to other forms of psychotherapy you have studied?

WEB LINKS

www.cbt.ca   This website, with self-help tools and a referral directory for the public and clinical tools and a directory of education opportunities for mental health practitioners, is supervised by Dr. Greg Dubord of the International Academy of Cognitive Therapy (IACT), based in Toronto.

www.cognitivetherapynyc.com   This is the website of the American Institute for Cognitive Therapy, a group of clinical psychologists and psychotherapists that provide CBT which was founded in 1985.

www.cognitivetherapy.com/basics.html   This website is supervised by John Winston Bush, PhD of the New York Institute for Cognitive and Behavioral Therapies and contains basic information about cognitive therapy.

www.cognitivetherapy.com/outlinks.html   This website is a link to www.resources on cognitive-behavioural therapy.

MOVIES

The Matrix: 1999. This science fiction story stars Keanu Reeves as Thomas Anderson, a computer hacker who learns that human life on Earth is not what is seems. Humans like Thomas think that they are living at the end of the 20th century. The truth is that it is actually two centuries later, and the world has been taken over by forms of cyber intelligence. These machines exist by "farming" the energy of captured humans, placating them by manipulating their minds into believing they are leading ordinary lives. A few humans, led by Morpheus, know the truth, and they lead Thomas to reality and to a new identity as Neo, The One.

VIEWING POINTS: Consider the way in which this movie illustrates the power of the mind to create and shape our reality and thus our actions. How difficult is it for Thomas to change his ideas about his life? Relate the premise of this movie to the assumptions underlying cognitive behavioural theory.

REFERENCES

American Psychiatric Association. (1998). *Practice guidelines for the treatment of panic disorder.* Arlington, VA: American Psychiatric Publishing.

Antony, M. M., & Swinson, R. P (2000). *Phobic disorders and panic in adults: A guide to assessment and treatment.* Washington, DC: American Psychological Association.

Beck, A. T., & Emery, G. (1985). *Anxiety disorders and phobias: A cognitive perspective.* New York: Basic Books.

Beck, A. T., Rush, A. J., Shaw, B. F., & Emery, G. (1979). *Cognitive therapy of depression.* New York: Guilford Press.

Beck, J. (1995). *Cognitive therapy: Basics and beyond.* New York: Guilford.

Bennett-Levy, J. (2003). Mechanisms of change in cognitive therapy: The case of automatic thought records and behavioural experiments. *Behavioural and Cognitive Psychotherapy, 31,* 261–277.

Bennett-Levy, J., Westbrook D., Fennell, M, Cooper, M., Rouf, K., & Hackmann, A. (2004). Behavioural experiments: Historical and conceptual underpinnings. In J. Bennett-Levy, G. Butler, M. Fennell, A. Hackmann, M. Mueller, & D. Westbrook (Eds.), *Oxford guide to behavioural experiments in cognitive therapy* (pp. 1–20). Oxford, UK: Oxford University Press.

Burns, D. D. (1980). *Feeling good: The new mood therapy.* New York: Morrow.

Burns, D. D. (1989). *The feeling good handbook: Using the new mood therapy in everyday life.* New York: Morrow.

Clark, D. M. (1998). Anxiety states: Panic and generalized anxiety. In K. Hawton, P. M. Salkovskis, J. Kirk, & D. M. Clark (Eds.), *Cognitive behaviour therapy for psychiatric problems* (pp. 52–96). Oxford, UK: Oxford University Press.

Fennell, M. J. V. (1989). Depression. In K. Hawton, P. M. Salkovskis, J. Kirk, & D. M. Clark (Eds.), *Cognitive behaviour therapy for psychiatric problems* (pp. 169–234). Oxford, UK: Oxford University Press.

Foa, E. B., & Rothbaum, B. O. (1998). *Treating the trauma of rape: Cognitive behavioral therapy for PTSD.* New York: Guilford Press.

Greenberger, D., & Padesky, C. A. (1995). *Mind over mood.* New York: Guilford Press.

Heimberg, R. G., & Becker, R. E. (2002). *Cognitive-behavioral group therapy for social phobia.* New York: Guilford Press.

Hollon, S., & Kriss, M. (1984). Cognitive factors in clinical research and practice. *Clinical Psychology Review, 4,* 35–76.

Ingram, R. E., Miranda, J., & Segal, Z. V. (1998). *Cognitive vulnerability to depression.* New York: Guilford Press.

Jacobson, E. (1938). *Progressive relaxation.* Chicago: University of Chicago Press.

Kaplan, H. I., Sadock, B. J., & Grebb, J. A. (1994). *Kaplan and Sadock's synopsis of psychiatry: Behavioral sciences, clinical psychiatry.* Baltimore: Williams & Wilkins.

Kazantzis, N., Deane, F. P., & Ronan, K. R. (2000). Homework assignments in cognitive and behavioral therapy: A meta-analysis. *Clinical Psychology: Science & Practice, 7,* 189–202.

Needleman, L. D. (1999). *Cognitive case conceptualization.* Mahwah, NJ: Lawrence Erlbaum.

Sperry, L. (1999). *Cognitive behavior therapy of DSM-IV personality disorders.* Philadelphia: Brunner/Mazel.

Swinson, R. P., Antony, M. M., Rachman, S., & Richter, M. A. (Eds.). (1998). *Obsessive compulsive disorder: Theory, research, and treatment.* New York: Guilford Press.

Taylor, S. (2000). *Understanding and treating panic disorder: Cognitive and behavioral approaches.* New York: Wiley.

Tully, T. L. (2005). The development and pilot testing of a cognitive-behavioural group psychotherapy intervention for women with a history of childhood sexual abuse who engage in self-injury. Doctoral dissertation, University of Toronto, 2003. Dissertation Abstracts International, 66/06, 3064.

Wells, A. (1997). *Cognitive therapy of anxiety disorders.* Chichester, UK: John Wiley & Sons.

Interventions With Groups

Mary Ann Boyd and Carol Ewashen

LEARNING OBJECTIVES

After studying this chapter, you will be able to:

- Discuss group concepts useful in understanding and leading groups.
- Compare the different roles of group members.
- Identify important aspects of leading a group, such as member selection, leadership skills, seating arrangements, and ways of dealing with challenging group members.
- Differentiate types of groups: psychoeducational, cognitive-behavioural, supportive therapy, psychotherapy, and self-help.
- Compare different nursing intervention groups.

KEY TERMS

closed group ▪ leadership styles ▪ formal group roles ▪ group ▪ group dynamics ▪ groupthink ▪ structured groups ▪ interactive groups ▪ informal group roles ▪ maintenance functions ▪ open group ▪ task functions ▪ self-help groups ▪ group cohesion ▪ group leadership ▪ therapeutic factors

KEY CONCEPTS

group ▪ group process

Participation in therapeutic groups has powerful treatment effects. Group treatment is an effective and efficient modality for patients to develop understanding of self through interaction with others, gain new knowledge and social skills, conquer unwanted thoughts and feelings, and change behaviour. For effective interventions, the nurse must possess leadership skills that can shape, enhance, and monitor group interactions. Competent group skill development for the psychiatric–mental health nurse requires the ability to critically select and modify techniques to best accommodate the particular practice conditions. This applies across diverse situations from providing patient education or conducting support groups to direct care provision, case management, and unit leadership. A challenge in group intervention is the shift from a primarily individual focus to consideration of interpersonal and whole group interactions. This chapter presents relevant group concepts for psychiatric nurses. Group leadership is explored, with special emphasis on the groups relevant to psychiatric–mental health nursing practice.

GROUP: DEFINITIONS AND CONCEPTS

There are many different definitions of a group. Psychoanalytic tradition draws from the work of Sigmund Freud and considers group interaction as a recapitulation of the family of origin, interpreting unconscious conflicts and reexamining them. Contemporary psychodynamic theories consider groups a combination of group dynamics and interpersonal and intrapsychic transactions (Rutan & Stone, 2001). Irving Yalom (1983, 1998, 2005) suggests that group is a social microcosm of interpersonal dynamics and advocates a "here and now," self-reflective approach. The cognitive-behavioural approach considers group a social arena for corrective change in maladaptive thinking and behaviour patterns; whereas according to systems theory, a group consists of parts or components that exist to perform some activity or purpose. As group members interact, subsystems form, challenging leaders to understand boundary realignments and the effects of subcomponents on the system and to improve interpersonal communication. A global, but rather simple, definition of a group is two or more people who are in an interdependent relationship with one another. The simplicity of the definition is misleading because interactions within groups, or **group dynamics,** are anything but simple. Group dynamics influence the group's development and process. In fact, it takes an astute observer to determine the real dynamics of a group and the effects. No matter the type of group, its theoretic orientation, or its purpose, group dynamics influence the effectiveness of a group intervention.

In this text, a group is defined as "a social system with structure, norms and usual ways of doing things" (Dimock & Devine, 1994, p. 54). Groups can be further defined according to the number of people or the relationship of members. A **dyad** is a group of two people such as a married couple, siblings, or parent and child. A **triad** is a group of three people. A family is a special type of group and is discussed in Chapter 16.

> **KEY CONCEPT** A **group** is "a social system with structure, norms and usual ways of doing things" (Dimock & Devine, 1994, p. 54).

Open Versus Closed Groups

A group can be viewed as either an open or a closed system. In an **open group**, new members are welcomed and provided time to learn group norms and expectations. For example, a newly admitted patient may join an anger management group that is part of an ongoing program in an inpatient unit. With new members, it is important to help them engage with the group by inviting member-to-member interaction. The advantage of an open group is that participants can join at any time. In addition, these groups can function on an ongoing basis and thus can be available to more people.

In a **closed group**, members begin the group at one time, and no new members are admitted. If a member of a closed group leaves, no replacement joins. Advantages of a closed group are that the participants get to know one another at the same time, the group is more cohesive, and members move through the group process concurrently. However, implementing closed-group interventions is often difficult, especially in tertiary settings, because patients are not always available at the same time.

Group Size

Group size is an important consideration in forming group programs. Many mental health professionals favour small groups, but large groups can also be effective. Whether to form a large or small group depends on the purpose, abilities, and availability of the participants and the skills of the leader. Small groups (usually no more than 8 to 10 members) become more cohesive, are less likely to form subgroups, and can provide a richer interpersonal experience than large groups. Small groups may function with one group leader, although many small groups are led by two people. An ideal small group is about seven to eight people in addition to the leader or leaders (Yalom, 2005).

CRNE Note

Size of group will depend on the overall patient goals and abilities. Patients with challenging behaviours should be carefully screened and assigned to smaller groups.

Small groups often are used for patients who are trying to deal with complex emotional issues, such as depression, anxiety, sexual abuse, eating disorders, or trauma. They are also ideal for individuals who require more individualized intervention. These groups work best if they are closed to new members or if new members are gradually introduced. One disadvantage of small groups relates to the loss of members. If places are unfilled, the group's dynamics change, which may interfere with the therapeutic process.

A large group (more than 10 members) can also be therapeutic, as well as cost-effective in clinical settings. Some research suggests that large treatment groups are effective for specific problems, such as smoking, or settings, such as the workplace (Moher, Hey, & Lancaster, 2003). A large group can be ongoing and open-ended. In large group intervention, a challenge for the nurse leader is to include all members in discussion, preventing a sense of alienation with the potential for member dropout.

Leading a group, whether large or small, is complex because of the number of potential interactions, relationships, and conflicts that can form. The leader needs both presentation and group leadership skills. Barbara Posthuma (2001) suggests that it is insufficient to be purely a leader—a leader must practice in a therapeutic or facilitative manner. Practitioners who take on leadership of groups require education and training for competent, accountable group practices. In large groups, the leader is often both a presenter of educative information and a facilitator of experiential learning among participants. In-depth reflection on participants' feelings and thoughts may not be the focus of group work. Depending on the theoretic orientation and the purpose of the group, leadership style and interventions must change to be effective in meeting goals of small or large groups.

Group Development

In the same way that the development of the therapeutic relationship is a process, so is the development of a group (see Chapter 8). Many researchers view group development as a sequence of phases, particularly in small groups (Table 15-1). Although models of group development differ, most follow a pattern of a begin-ning, middle, and ending phase (Alvarez, 2002). These stages should be thought of not as a straight line with one preceding another, but as a dynamic process that is constantly revisiting and reexamining group interactions and behaviours, as well as progressing forward.

> **KEY CONCEPT Group process** is the "what is happening" in the group, how members are interacting and relating as individuals and as a whole group, including nonverbal communications.

Beginning Stage

When a group begins, group members get to know one another and the group leader. The length of the beginning stage depends on, among other variables, the purpose of the group, the number of members, and the skill of the leader. It may last for only a few sessions or several. "Honeymoon" behaviour characterizes this stage in the beginning, but "conflict" dominates at the end. During the initial sessions, members usually display polite, congenial behaviour typical of those in new social situations. They are "good patients" and often intellectualize their problems; that is, these patients deal with emotional conflict or stress by excessively using abstract thinking or generalizations to minimize disturbing feelings. Members are usually anxious and sometimes display behaviour that does not truly represent their feelings. In the first few sessions, members test whether they can trust one another. Sometime after the initial sessions, group members usually experience a period of conflict, either among themselves or with the leader. This conflict is a normal part of group development, and many believe that conflict is necessary to move into any working phase. Sometimes, one or more group members become the scapegoat. Such situations challenge the leader to guide the group during this period by avoiding taking sides and treating all members respectfully.

Working Stage

The working stage of groups involves a real sharing of ideas and the development of closeness. A group per-

Table 15.1	**Comparison of Models of Group Development**	
Robert Bales (1955)	**William Schutz (1960)**	**Bruce Tuckman (1965)**
■ *Orientation:* What is the problem? ■ *Evaluation:* How do we feel about it? ■ *Control:* What should we do about it?	■ *Inclusion:* Deal with issues of belonging and being in and out of the group. ■ *Control:* Deal with issues of authority (who is in charge?), dependence, and autonomy. ■ *Affection:* Deal with issues of intimacy, closeness, and caring, versus dislike and distancing.	■ *Forming:* Get to know one another and form a group. ■ *Storming:* Tension and conflict occur; subgroups form and clash with one another. ■ *Norming:* Develop norms of how to work together. ■ *Performing:* Reach consensus and develop cooperative relationships.

sonality may emerge that is distinct from the individual personalities of its members. The group develops its own rules and rituals and has its own behavioural norms; for example, groups develop regular patterns of seating and interaction. During this stage, the group realizes its purpose. If the purpose is education, the participants engage in learning new content or skills. If the aim of the group is to share feelings and experiences, these activities consume group meetings. During this phase, the group starts on time, and the leader often needs to remind members when it is time to stop.

Termination Stage

Termination can be difficult for a group, especially a successful one. During the final stages, members begin to grieve for the loss of the group's closeness and begin to reestablish themselves as individuals. Individuals terminate from groups as they do from any relationship. One person may not show up at the last session, another person may bring up issues that the group has already addressed, and others may demonstrate anger or hostility. Most members of successful groups are sad as the group terminates. During the last meetings, members may make arrangements for meeting after group. These plans rarely materialize or continue. Leaders should recognize these plans as part of the farewell process—saying good-bye to the group.

Roles of Group Members

There are two official or **formal group roles,** the leader and the members; however, in small groups, members often assume **informal group roles** or positions in the group with rights and duties that are directed toward one or more group members. These roles can either help or hinder the group's process. One of the first and oldest models is Benne and Sheats' (1948) list of task, maintenance, and individual roles. **Task functions** involve the business of the group or "keeping things focussed." Individuals who provide this function keep the group focussed on a main purpose. For any group to be successful, it must have members who assume some of these task roles, such as *information seeker* (asks for clarification), *coordinator* (spells out relationships between ideas), and *recorder* (keeper of the minutes). **Maintenance functions** help the group stay together by ensuring it starts on time, assisting individuals to compromise, and determining membership. These individuals are more interested in maintaining the group's cohesiveness than focusing on the group's tasks. The *harmonizer, compromiser*, and *standard setter* are examples of maintenance roles. In a successful group, members assume both group task and maintenance functions (Table 15-2).

Individual roles are those member roles that either enhance or detract from the group's functioning. These roles have nothing to do with the group's purpose or cohesion; for example, someone who monopolizes the group inhibits the group's work. People who are participating in the group may be meeting personal needs, such as feeling important or being an expert on a subject. However, when individual roles predominate, the risk is that dominant individuals may contribute to neither the task nor the maintenance of the group.

In selecting members and analyzing the progress of the group, the leader must pay attention to the balance between the task and maintenance functions. If too many group members assume task functions and too few assume maintenance functions, the group may have difficulty developing cohesion. If too many members assume maintenance functions, the group may never finish its work. Although it is usually impossible to select individuals only because of their group role, tracking the group in terms of how well it functions and how much it actually gets done is important.

Group Communication

One of the responsibilities of the group leader is to facilitate both verbal and nonverbal communication to meet the treatment goals of the individual members and the entire group. Because of the number of people involved, developing trusting relationships within groups is more complicated than is developing a single relationship with a patient. The communication techniques used in establishing and maintaining individual relationships are similar for groups, but the leader also attends to the communication patterns among the members.

Verbal Communication

Group interaction can be viewed as a communication network that becomes patterned and predictable. In a group, verbal comments are linked in a chain formation.

Communication Network
Asking a colleague to observe and record the content and interaction is a useful technique in determining the interaction pattern within a group; the leader may also use an audio or video recorder. In some groups, one person may always change the subject when another raises a sensitive topic. One person may always speak after another. People who sit next to each other tend to communicate among themselves. By analyzing the content and patterns, the leader can determine the existence of communications pathways—who is most liked in the group, who occupies a position of power, what subgroups have formed, and who is isolated from the group. Moreno's (1953) sociometric diagrams of interpersonal choice provide a way to identify stars, isolates, and overchosen and underchosen group members. Usually, those

Table 15.2 Roles and Functions of Group Members

Task Roles	Maintenance Roles	Individual Roles
Initiator-contributor suggests or proposes new ideas or a new view of the problem or goal.	*Encourager* praises, agrees with, and accepts contributions of others.	*Aggressor* deflates the status of others; expresses disapproval of the values, acts, or feelings of others; attacks the group or problem; jokes aggressively; tries to take credit for the work.
Information seeker asks for clarification of the values pertinent to the group activity.	*Harmonizer* mediates differences among members and relieves tension in conflict situations.	
Information giver offers "authoritative" facts or generalizations or gives own experiences.	*Compromiser* operates from within a conflict and may yield status or admit error to maintain group harmony.	*Blocker* tends to be negative and resistant, disagrees and opposes without or beyond "reason," and attempts to bring back an issue after group has rejected it.
Opinion giver states belief or opinions with emphasis on what should be the group's values.	*Gate-keeper* attempts to keep communication channels open by encouraging or facilitating the participation of others or proposes regulation of the flow of communication through limiting time.	*Recognition-seeker* calls attention to self through such activities as boasting, reporting on personal achievements, acting in unusual ways.
Elaborator spells out suggestions in terms of examples, develops meanings of ideas and rationales, tries to deduce how an idea would work.	*Standard setter* expresses standards for the group to achieve.	*Self-confessor* uses group setting to express personal, non–group-oriented feelings or insights.
Coordinator shows or clarifies the relationships among various ideas and suggestions.	*Group observer* keeps records of various aspects of group processes and interprets data to group.	*Playboy* makes a display of lack of involvement in group's processes.
Orienter defines the position of the group with respect to its goals.	*Follower* goes along with the movement of the group.	*Dominator* tries to assert authority or superiority in manipulating the group or certain members of the group through flattery, being directive, interrupting others.
Evaluator-critic measures the outcome of the group against some standard.		*Help-seeker* attempts to call forth sympathy from other group members through expressing insecurity, personal confusion, or depreciation of self beyond reason.
Energizer attempts to stimulate the group to action or decision.		
Procedural technician expedites group movement by doing things for the group such as distributing copies, arranging seating.		*Special interest* pleader speaks for a special group, such as "grass roots," usually representing personal prejudices or biases.
Recorder writes suggestions, keeps minutes, serves as group memory.		

who are well liked or display leadership abilities tend to be chosen for interactions more often than do those who are less well liked (Fig. 15-1). In one study of communication networks, members who exhibited more dominant behaviours or who the group perceived as being dominant emerged as more central to the group's communication networks and both sent and received more messages. The study also found that the task at hand affects the communication network. Groups that worked on low-complexity tasks had more centralized communication than when they worked on high-complexity tasks (Brown & Miller, 2000).

Group Themes

Group themes are the collective conceptual underpinnings of a group and express the members' underlying concerns or feelings, regardless of the group's purpose. Themes that emerge in groups help members to understand group dynamics. Different groups have different themes. For example, three themes emerged for a support group for grieving children, including their vulnerability, the importance of maintaining memories, and the contribution of the group to the process of grieving (Graham & Sontag, 2001). Although some predictable themes occur in groups, the obvious or assumed themes at the beginning may actually wind up differing from reality as the process continues. In one hospice support group, the members seemed to be focussing on the memories of their loved ones. However, upon examination of the content of their interactions, discussions were revolving around financial planning for the future

Nonverbal Communication

Nonverbal communication is important to understanding group behaviour. All members, not just the group leader, observe the eye contact, posture, and body gestures of the participants. What is expressed is the result

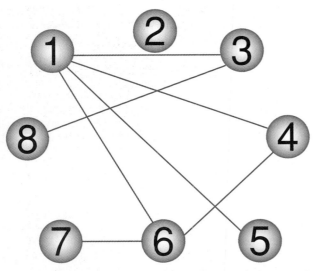

FIGURE 15.1 Sociometric analysis of group behaviour. In this sociometric structure, response pattern was recorded during member interaction. Group members interacted with number 1 the most. Therefore, number 1 is the overchosen person. Numbers 5 and 7 are underchosen. Number 2 is never chosen and is determined to be the isolate.

of individual and group, as well as internal and external processes. For example, if one member is explaining a painful experience and another member looks away and tries to engage still another, the self-disclosing member may feel devalued and rejected because he or she interprets the disruptive behaviour as disinterest. However, if the leader interprets the disruptive behaviour as anxiety over the topic, he or she may try to engage the other member in discussing the source of the anxiety.

The leaders should monitor the nonverbal behaviour of group members during each session. Often, one or two people can set the overall mood of the group. Someone who comes to a session very sad or angry can set a tone of sadness or anger for the whole group. An astute group leader recognizes the effects of an individual's mood on the total group. If the purpose of the group is to deal with emotions, the group leader may invite the member to discuss emotional issues at the beginning of the session. The leader thus acknowledges the mood of the one person experiencing it and encourages discussion regarding the effect on other group members. If the group's purpose is inconsistent with self-disclosure of personal problems, the nurse should acknowledge the individual members' distress yet maintain the group focus. In this instance, the nurse would limit repeated episodes of self-disclosure from that member or others.

Group Norms and Standards

Groups develop norms or rules and standards that establish acceptable group behaviours. Some norms are for-

malized, such as beginning group on time, but others are never really formalized. These standards encourage conformity of behaviour among group members. The group discourages deviations from these established norms. A group member has four options in relation to norms: conform, change the norm, be deviant, or leave the group (Posthuma, 2001). Open discussion that encourages healthy interacting while addressing unhelpful or problematic behaviours is one of the most successful ways of renegotiating group norms. Leadership is critical in establishing group norms consistent with the group goals to effect desired changes.

Group Cohesion

One of the goals of most group leaders is to foster **group cohesion,** a sense of "we-ness" as a group, with high levels of participation and involvement among members. Group cohesion is analogous to the therapeutic alliance in one-to-one relationships (MacKenzie, 1997). One of the first tasks of a good leader is to develop group cohesion through engaging all members in the group process. This involves close monitoring of the group climate or atmosphere to develop a sense of belonging and commitment to the group goals. A particularly effective intervention for enhancing group cohesion is encouraging member-to-member interaction. In supportive and educational groups, leaders can promote social interaction with minimal supervision, through organizing refreshment periods and team-building exercises. Cohesiveness is especially important in health education groups that focus on health maintenance behaviours such as exercise and weight control. These groups typically have high dropout rates, but members are more likely to attend when a group is cohesive (Annesi, 1999).

Dimock and Devine (1994) state that cohesion is like the glue that holds the group together and that if cohesion decreases, the group may begin to fall apart. Cohesion is a powerful force that motivates members and correlates with outcomes. In cohesive groups, members are committed to the existence of the group. In large heterogeneous groups, cohesiveness tends to be decreased, with subsequent decreased performance among group members in completing tasks. When members are strongly committed to completing a task and the leader encourages equal participation, cohesiveness promotes job satisfaction and higher performance (Steinhardt, Dolbier, Gottlieb, & McCalister, 2003). However, cohesiveness can be a double-edged sword. In very cohesive groups, members are more likely to transgress personal boundaries. Too much cohesiveness can exert powerful social pressure to conform to group standards with low tolerance for difference, while too little cohesiveness can result in mistrust, lack of engagement, and eventual disbanding of the group.

Groupthink and Decision Making

Groups that are strong and healthy encourage creativity, risk taking, and change while remaining respectful of all members. Healthy groups encourage conformity to group norms and standards while remaining respectful of each member's unique contributions. In a healthy group, conformity to group norms does not mean uniformity of member behaviour because a cohesive group is both productive and constructive (Dimock & Devine, 1994). However, if feelings of unity become too intense, and members are overly invested in maintaining the status quo, a phenomenon of **groupthink** can occur (Kurtz, 1992). **Groupthink** is the tendency of many groups to avoid conflict and adopt a normative pattern of thinking that is often consistent with the ideas of the group leader (Janis, 1972, 1982). In groupthink, striving for unanimity overrides the motivation of members to appraise realistically alternative courses of action. Members may not give honest feedback to each other for fear of censure. Many catastrophes, such as the *Challenger* explosion and Bay of Pigs invasion, have been attributed to groupthink, but the empiric evidence of groupthink's negative implications in organizations is small. Studies have shown that closed leadership style and external threat, particularly time pressure, appear to promote symptoms of groupthink and defective decision making (Neck & Moorhead, 1995). The relationship between cohesiveness and groupthink is still inconclusive.

Current research suggests that groupthink can have positive effects on the group. In one study, groupthink was positively associated with group activities and team performance and negatively associated with concurrence (pressure for everyone to agree) and defective decision making (Choi & Kim, 1999).

Nurse leaders are responsible for mobilizing therapeutic factors to support healthy group development and prevent a stagnating groupthink. Which factors to mobilize and when depend on the type, purpose, and developmental stage of the group. Supportive factors often emerge spontaneously and include universality, altruism, hope, and acceptance (MacKenzie, 1997). Other therapeutic factors proposed by Yalom (1983, 2005) are imparting information, corrective recapitulation of the primary family group, development of socializing techniques, imitative behaviours, catharsis, existential factors, cohesiveness, and interpersonal learning (Box 15-1).

GROUP LEADERSHIP

In the beginning, the group leader establishes the presence of each member, constructs a working environment, builds a working relationship with the group and among participants, and clarifies outcomes, processes, and skills related to the group's purpose (Alf & Wilson, 2001). While attempting to understand the group process, the

---

BOX 15.1 RESEARCH FOR BEST PRACTICE

Using the CORE-R Battery to Improve Group Practices

THE PROJECT: Collaborative project sponsored by the Humboldt Foundation and the American Group Psychotherapy Association Research Special Interest Group, with the aim to revise and update the AGPA CORE battery (Clinical Outcomes Results Standardized measures) to develop clinically useful measures sensitive to patient change with ability to graph patient change and provide immediate feedback on patient status.

QUESTIONS: *Empirical:* Does this treatment work for this diagnostic indication? *Practice guideline:* What treatment components are most important? *Patient-focussed:* Is this treatment working for this patient?

METHODS: Extensive review and metasynthesis of group literature from an empirical and clinical perspective. Review of the original CORE battery as well as AGPA Roy MacKenzie and Gary Burlingame course on process and outcome instruments.

FINDINGS: Revision and update to offer CORE-R battery, a tool developed internationally to measure group processes and outcomes. Meta-analysis indicates that empirically supported treatment techniques explain only

10% of patient improvement. The claim of superior outcomes on one treatment over another has little empirical support. Recommend evidence-based models coupled with patient-focussed treatment that consider patient response and therapist variability. Specific areas addressed by the CORE-R battery include: selection of patients for group, pre-group preparation, and an extensive, empirically validated selection of process and outcome measures.

IMPLICATIONS FOR INTERDISCIPLINARY PRACTICES: Clinical uses of the CORE-R process measures: gauging the quality of the group therapeutic environment, frequent process assessments to clarify the nature of group development over time, clarifying process dimensions that may be absent or negatively affect individual participants or the group as a whole, and increase awareness of group dynamics. Clinical use of CORE-R outcome measures: supplements clinical judgment, expands patient communication through written and verbal involvement, and provides ongoing feedback to the group leader regarding how much change as well as clinically significant changes.

From Burlingame, G., Strauss, B., Joyce, A. S., MacNair-Semands, R., MacKenzie, K. R., Ogrodniczuk, J. S., & Taylor, S. (2004). The American Group Psychotherapy Association's CORE Battery—Revised (CORE-R). Draft report submitted at the 62nd Annual Meeting of the AGPA, New York City, March 7–12, 2005.

leader must also consider when and how to participate. Depending on the purpose of the group and the stage of development, the leader position shifts, for example, from a primarily supportive role, to educative with provision of information, to interpretive of group dynamics. The leader reflects on, evaluates, and responds to promote effective group work. Leader intervention skills include attention to process while considering timing of interventions, when to clarify and when to interpret, when to intervene at the individual level, and when to intervene at the whole group level. The use of various techniques enhances the leader's ability to lead the group effectively and to help the group meet its goals (Table 15-3).

One of the most important leadership skills is listening. A leader who practices active listening provides group members with someone who is responsive to what they say. A group leader who listens also models listening behaviour for others, helping them improve their skills. Listening enables the leader to process events and track interactions. The leader should be able to listen to the group members and formulate responses based on an understanding of the discussion. Members may need to learn to listen to one another, track discussions without changing the subject, and not speak while others are talking.

The leader tracks the verbal and nonverbal interactions throughout the group. Depending on the group's purpose, the leader may keep this information to himself or herself to understand the group process or may share the observations with the group. For example, if the purpose of the group is psychoeducational, the leader may use the information to facilitate the best learning environment. If the purpose of the group is to improve the self-awareness and interaction skills of members, the leader may point out the observations. The leader needs to be clear about the purpose of the group and tailor leadership strategies accordingly.

Understanding different leadership styles can be useful in deciding which style fits which group situation. Often leaders have a dominant style that fits more comfortably with who they are; however, developing a repertoire of different styles offers a wider range of interventions. Regardless of style, a leader remains fair and respectful, avoiding favouritism and encouraging participation and involvement of all members with each other. Other important skills include providing everyone with an opportunity to contribute and respecting everyone's ideas. A leader must also consider the degree of neutrality warranted in each situation. In supportive and educative groups, leaders tend to be more expressive and interactive. A good rule of thumb in relation to leader self-disclosure is to consider whether the disclosure furthers the purposes of the group. A leader is responsible for understanding the intent and impact of leader self-disclosure on both individual members and the group as a whole.

Some generally accepted guidelines in leading groups include setting start and stop times, arranging for the introduction of new members, and listening while other people talk. Leaders should explain these rules at the first group meeting and re-emphasize them at different points. A group should always begin at its scheduled time; otherwise, members who tend to be late will not change their behaviour, and those who are on time will resent waiting for the others. A group should also end on time. Members should understand from the beginning that either new people can attend without the group knowing about it or that the group will discuss the introduction of new members before their attendance. Whatever the group decides, the leader must also follow the rules.

Choosing Leadership Styles

A group is led within the context of the group leader's theoretic background and the group's purpose. For example, a leader with training in cognitive-behavioural therapy may focus on treating depression by asking members to think differently about situations, which in turn leads to feeling better. A leader with a psychodynamic orientation may focus on the feelings of depression by examining situations that generate the same feelings. Whatever the leader's theoretic background, his or her leadership behaviour can be viewed on a continuum of direct to indirect. In **direct leadership behaviour,** the leader controls the interaction by giving directions and information and allowing little discussion. The leader literally tells the members what to do. On the other end of the continuum is the **indirect leader,** who primarily reflects the group members' discussion and offers little guidance or information to the group. Sometimes the group needs more direct leadership; other times it needs a leader who is indirect. The challenge of providing leadership is to give sufficient direction that the group can meet its goals and develop its own group process but enough freedom that members can make mistakes and recover from their thinking errors in a supportive, caring, learning environment.

Selecting the Members

Individuals can self-refer or be referred to groups by treatment teams or clinicians. The leader is responsible for assessing the individual's suitability to the group. In instances when a new group is forming, the leader selects and invites members so that the group can be well functioning and successful. The leader should consider the following criteria when selecting members:

- Does the purpose of the group match the treatment goals of the potential member?
- Does the potential member have the social skills to function comfortably in the group?

Table 15.3	Techniques in Leading Groups	
Technique	**Purpose**	**Example**
Support: giving feedback that provides a climate of emotional support	Helps a person or group continue with ongoing activities Informs group about what the leader thinks is important Creates a climate for expressing unpopular ideas Helps the more quiet and fearful members speak up	"We really appreciate your sharing that experience with us. It looked like it was quite painful."
Confrontation: challenging a participant (needs to be done in a supportive environment)	Helps individuals learn something about themselves Helps reduce some forms of disruptive behaviour Helps members deal more openly and directly with one another	"Tom, this is the third time that you have changed the subject when we have talked about spouse abuse. Is something going on?"
Advice and suggestions: sharing expertise and knowledge that the members do not have	Provides information that members can use once they have examined and evaluated it Helps focus group's task and goals	"The medication that you are taking may be causing you to be sleepy."
Summarizing: statements at the end of sessions that highlight the session's discussion, any problem resolution, and unresolved problems	Provides continuity from one session to the next Brings to focus still-unresolved issues Organizes past in ways that clarify; brings into focus themes and patterns of interaction	"This session we discussed Sharon's medication problems, and she will be following up with her physicians."
Clarification: restatement of an interaction	Checks on the meanings of the interaction and communication Avoids faulty communication Facilitates focus on substantive issues rather than allowing members to be side tracked into misunderstandings	"What I heard you say was that you are feeling very sad right now. Is that correct?"
Probing and questioning: a technique for the experienced group leader that asks for more information	Helps members expand on what they were saying (when they are ready to) Gets at more extensive and wider range of information Invites members to explore their ideas in greater detail	"Could you tell us more about your relationship with your parents?"
Repeating, paraphrasing, highlighting: a simple act of repeating what was just said	Facilitates communication among group members Corrects inaccurate communication or emphasizes accurate communication	*Member:* "I forgot about my wife's birthday." *Leader:* "You forgot your wife's birthday."
Reflecting feelings: identifying feelings that are being expressed	Orients members to the feelings that may lie behind what is being said or done Helps members deal with issues they might otherwise avoid or miss	"You sound upset."
Reflecting behaviour: identifying behaviours that are occurring	Gives members an opportunity to see how their behaviour appears to others and to evaluate its consequences Helps members to understand others' perceptions and responses to them	"I notice that when the topic of sex is brought up, you look down and shift in your chair."

Adapted from Sampson, E., & Marthas, M. (1990). *Group process for the health professions* (pp. 222–224). Albany, NY: Delmar.

- Can the potential member make a commitment to attending group meetings?

Arranging Seating

Spatial and seating arrangements contribute to group communication. Group members tend to sit in the same places. Those who sit close to the group leader are more likely to have more power in the group than those who sit far away. Communication flows better when no physical barriers, such as tables, are between members. Arranging a group in a circle with chairs comfortably close to one another without a table enhances group work. No one should sit outside the group. If a table is necessary, a round table is better than a rectangular one, which implicitly increases the power of those who sit at the ends.

The session should be held in a quiet, pleasant room with adequate space and privacy. Holding a session in too large or too small a room inhibits communication. Group sessions should not be held in rooms to which nonparticipants have access because of compromised confidentiality and potential distractions.

Dealing With Challenging Group Behaviours

Problematic behaviours occur in all groups. They can be challenging to the most experienced group leaders and frustrating to new leaders. In dealing with any problematic behaviour or situation, the leader must remember to support the integrity of the individual members and the group as a whole.

Monopolizer

Some people tend to monopolize a group by constantly talking or interrupting others. This behaviour is common in the beginning stages of group formation and usually represents anxiety that the member displaying such behaviour is experiencing. Within a few sessions, this person usually relaxes and no longer attempts to monopolize the group. However, for some people, monopolizing discussions is part of their normal personality and will continue. Other group members usually find the behaviour mildly irritating in the beginning and extremely annoying as time passes. Members may drop out of the group to avoid that person. The leader needs to decide if, how, and when to intervene. The best case scenario is when savvy group members remind the monopolizer to let others speak. The leader can then support the group in establishing rules that allow everyone the opportunity to participate. However, the group often waits for the leader to manage the situation. There are a couple of ways to deal with the situation. The leader can interrupt the monopolizer by acknowledging the member's contribution but redirecting the discussion to others, or the leader can become more directive and limit the discussion time per member.

"Yes, But. . ."

Some people have a patterned response to any suggestions from others. Initially, they agree with suggestions others offer them, but then they add "yes, but" and give several reasons why the suggestions will not work for them. Leaders and members can easily identify this patterned response. In such situations, it is best to avoid problem solving for the member and encourage the person to develop his or her own solutions. The leader can serve as a role model of the problem-solving behaviour for the other members and encourage them to let the member develop a solution that would work specifically for him or her.

Disliked Member

In some groups, members clearly dislike one particular member. This situation can be challenging for the leader because it can result in considerable tension and conflict. This person could become the group's scapegoat. The group leader may have made a mistake by placing the person in this particular group, and another group may be a better match. One solution may be to move the person to a better-matched group. Whether the person stays or leaves, the group leader must stay neutral and avoid displaying negative verbal and nonverbal behaviours that indicate that he or she too dislikes the group member or that he or she is displeased with the other members for their behaviour. Often, the group leader can manage the situation by showing respect for the disliked member and acknowledging his or her contribution. In some instances, getting supervision from a more experienced group leader is useful. Defusing the situation may be possible by using conflict resolution strategies and discussing the underlying issues.

Group Conflict

Most groups experience periods of conflict. The leader first needs to decide whether the conflict is a natural part of the group process or whether the group needs to address some issues. Member-to-member conflict can be handled through the previously discussed conflict resolution process (see Chapter 12). Leader-to-member conflict is more complicated because the leader has the formal position of power. In this instance, the leader can use conflict resolution strategies but should be sensitive to the power differential between the leader's role and the member's role.

TYPES OF GROUPS

Structured Groups

Psychoeducational Groups

Psychoeducational groups are directed to specific concepts and teaching-learning aims. The process is primarily didactic with opportunity for questions, discussion, and activities related to the topic. The group leader primarily imparts information, promotes discussion, and facilitates experiential learning through structured activities. Psychoeducational groups include task groups that focus on completion of specific activities (such as planning a week's menu), and teaching groups that are used to enhance knowledge, improve skills, or solve problems. Other examples include medication groups, anger management groups, and stress management groups. Psychoeducational groups are formally planned, and members are purposefully selected. Members are asked to join specific groups because of the focus of the group. These groups are time limited and last for only a few sessions (Box 15-2).

Cognitive Behavioural Groups

The leader in cognitive groups identifies specific distorted thought patterns as the focus of change, whereas in behavioural groups, the leader targets specific behaviours to be modified. Cognitive interventions and behavioural interventions may be combined to offer cognitive-behavioural group interventions. Cognitive interventions aim to modify distortions in attitudes and beliefs about self, the situation, and the future. Behavioural interventions modify behavioural excess such as overly aggressive or sexual behaviour, behavioural deficits such as social isolation or extreme passivity, and behaviours interfering with living such as phobias and panic attacks (see Chapter 14). Groups are often very structured with homework expectations for members.

Interactive Groups

Supportive Therapy Groups

Supportive therapy groups are usually less intense than psychotherapy groups and focus on helping individuals cope with their illnesses and problems as well as build interpersonal connection. Implementing supportive therapy groups is one of the basic functions of the psychiatric nurse. In conducting this type of group, the nurse focuses on helping members cope with situations that are common for other group members. Counselling strategies are used. For example, a group of patients with bipolar illness whose illness is stable may discuss at a monthly meeting how to tell other people about the illness or how to cope with a family member who seems insensitive to the illness. Family caregivers of people with mental illnesses benefit from the support of the group, as well as additional information about providing care for an ill family member.

Psychotherapy Groups

Groups that rely primarily on interpretive interventions are known as group psychotherapies. Psychotherapy

---

BOX 15.2   RESEARCH FOR BEST PRACTICE

Psychoeducational Codependency Support Groups for Older Adults

THE QUESTION: What are the benefits of a psychoeducational support group for older adults with codependency issues?

METHODS: Older adults who have loved ones dependent on alcohol or drugs often experience the adverse effects of a codependent relationship. Many experience anxiety, low self-esteem, depression, and even suicidal thoughts. To promote well-being and reduce adverse effects of codependency among older adults, a pilot psycheducational codependency support group curriculum was developed by the authors. A convenience sample of 22 older adults (age 65 years and older) who resided in an eastern Canada community participated in six 90-minute psychoeducational group sessions held over a 2-month period. A pretest and posttest were administered. Irvin Yalom's (1998) Therapeutic Factors were used to evaluate the group process.

FINDINGS: Results indicated that older adults do benefit from a psychoeducational support group format. A majority (82%) were dealing with an adult child. Most of the seniors were female and older than the age of 75. All openly participated in the group; common themes were present and all participants acknowledged positive change in their knowledge about addictions and codependency. An increase in healthy behaviours and attitudes was seen and a reduction in codependency issues, for example, increased self-esteem and a reduced sense of personal isolation.

IMPLICATIONS FOR NURSING: The projects provided both insight and direction for health care providers in using the group model to serve older adults who live in a codependent relationship. Providing a supportive environment in which life experiences and various coping strategies could be shared allowed these seniors to work through sensitive and painful issues. Future studies should be conducted using a larger sample size, a more diverse group of seniors, and standardized pretest and posttest instruments.

From McInnis-Perry, G. J., Good, J. M. (in press). A psychosocial codependency support group for older adults who reside in the community: Friends supporting friends. *Journal of Gerontological Nursing.*

groups differ depending on the theoretic perspective, including psychodynamic, interpersonal, and existential. These groups focus primarily on increasing cognitive and emotional insight as well as improving interpersonal relations to help members face their life situations. In group psychotherapy, "therapeutic change is an enormously complex process" (Yalom, 1998, p. 7). At times, these groups can be extremely intense. Psychotherapy groups provide an opportunity for members to examine and resolve psychological and interpersonal issues within a safe environment. Mental health specialists who have a minimum of a master's degree and are trained in group psychotherapy lead such groups. When providing nursing care, communication with the group therapist is important for continuity and collaboration of care.

Self-Help Groups

Self-help groups are led by lay people, often a mental health consumer who has experienced a specific problem or life crisis. These groups are generally structured, with supportive interaction among members. These groups do not explore psychodynamic issues in depth. Professionals usually do not attend these groups or serve as consultants. Alcoholics Anonymous, Overeaters Anonymous, and One Day at a Time (a grief group) are examples of self-help groups.

COMMON NURSING INTERVENTION GROUPS

Common intervention groups led by nurses include medication, symptom management, anger management, and self-care groups. In addition, nurses lead many other groups, including stress management, relaxation groups, and women's groups. The key, as a nurse, to being a good group leader is to critically select and modify group interventions to best accommodate the primary focus of therapeutic change in relation to the unique conditions of the clinical setting and the group membership (Garrick & Ewashen, 2001).

Medication Groups

Nurse-led medication groups are common in psychiatric nursing. Not all medication groups are alike, so the nurse must be clear regarding the purpose of each specific medication group (Box 15-3). A medication group can be used primarily to transmit information about medications, such as action, dosage, and side effects, or it can focus on issues related to medications, such as compliance, management of side effects, and lifestyle adjustments. Many nurses incorporate both perspectives.

Assessing a member's medication knowledge is important before he or she joins the group to determine what the individual would like to learn. People with mental illness may have difficulty remembering new information, so assessment of cognitive abilities is important. Assessing attention span, memory, and problem-solving skills gives valuable information that nurses can use in designing the group. The nurse should determine the members' reading and writing skills to select effective patient education materials.

An ideal group is one in which all members use the same medication. In reality, this situation is rare. Usually, the group members are using various medications. The nurse should know which medications each member is taking, but to avoid violating patient confidentiality, the nurse needs to be careful not to divulge that information to other patients. If group members choose, they can share the names of their medications with one another. A small group format works best, and the more interaction, the better. Using a lecture method of teaching is less effective than involving the members in the

---

BOX 15.3

Medication Group Protocol

PURPOSE: Develop strategies that reinforce a self-medication routine.

DESCRIPTION: The medication group is an open, ongoing group that meets once a week to discuss topics germane to self-administration of medication. Members will not be asked to disclose the names of their medications.

MEMBER SELECTION: The group is open to any person taking medication for a mental illness or emotional problem who would like more information about medication, side effects, and staying on a regimen. Referrals from mental health providers are encouraged. Each person will meet with the group leader before attending the group to determine if the group will meet the individual's learning needs.

STRUCTURE: Format is a small group, with no more than eight members and one psychiatric nurse group leader

facilitating a discussion about the issues. Topics are rotated.

TIME AND LOCATION: 2:00–3:00 PM, every Wednesday at the Mental Health Center

Cost: No Charge for attending

TOPICS:
- How Do I Know If My Medications Are Working?
- Side Effect Management: Is It Worth It?
- Hints for Taking Medications Without Missing Doses!
- Health Problems that Medication Affects
- (Other topics will be developed to meet the needs of group members.)

EVALUATION: Short pretest and posttest for instructor's use only

learning process. The nurse should expose the members to various audio and visual educational materials, including workbooks, videotapes, and handouts. The nurse should ask members to write down information to help them remember and learn through various modes. Evaluation of the learning outcomes begins with the first class. Nurses can develop and give pretests and posttests, which in combination can measure learning outcomes.

Symptom Management Groups

Nurses often lead groups that focus on helping patients deal with a severe and persistent mental illness. Handling hallucinations, being socially appropriate, and staying motivated to complete activities of daily living are a few common topics. In symptom management groups, members also learn when a symptom indicates that relapse is imminent and what to do about it. Within the context of a symptom management group, patients can learn how to avoid relapse.

Anger Management Groups

Anger management is another common topic for a nurse-led group, often in the inpatient setting. The purposes of an anger management group are to discuss the concept of anger, identify antecedents to aggressive behaviour, and develop new strategies to deal with anger other than verbal and physical aggression (see Chapter 35). The treatment team refers individuals with a history of being verbally and physically abusive, usually to family members, to these groups to help them better understand their emotions and behavioural responses. Impulsiveness and emotional lability are problems for many of the group members. Anger management usually includes a discussion of associated stressful situations, events that trigger anger, feelings about the situation, and unmet personal needs.

Self-Care Groups

Another common nurse-led psychiatric group is a self-care group. People with psychiatric illnesses often have self-care deficits and benefit from the structure that a group provides. These groups are challenging because members usually know how to perform these daily tasks (eg, bathing, grooming, performing personal hygiene), but their illnesses cause them to lose the motivation to complete them. The leader not only reinforces the basic self-care skills but also, more importantly, helps identify strategies that can motivate the patients and provide structure to their daily lives.

Reminiscence Groups

Reminiscence therapy has been shown to be a valuable intervention for elderly clients. In this type of group,

members are encouraged to remember events from past years. Such a group is easily implemented. Usually, a simple question about an important family event will spark memories. Reminiscence groups are usually associated with people who have dementia and are having difficulty with recent memory. Recalling distant memories is comforting to elderly people and improves well-being. Reminiscence groups can also be used in caring for people with depression (Jones & Beck-Little, 2002) and in conjunction with cognitive therapy for affective symptoms in older adults (Puentes, 2004).

SUMMARY OF KEY POINTS

- The definition of group can vary according to theoretic orientation. A general definition of group is "a social system with structure, norms and usual ways of doing things" (Dimock & Devine, 1994, p. 54). Group dynamics are the interactions within a group that constitute group development and process.

- Groups can be *open*, with every session available to new membership, or *closed*, with membership determined at the first session. Leading a group, whether small or large, is complex because dynamics change depending on different sizes of groups and clinical conditions.

- The group development process occurs in phases: beginning, middle, and termination. These stages are not fixed but dynamic. Each phase challenges the leader to intervene in different ways. Success at the beginning phase prepares the group to take responsibility for addressing its purpose during the working stage.

- Although there are only two formal group roles, leader and member, there are many informal group roles. These roles are usually categorized according to purpose—task functions, maintenance functions, and individual roles. Members who assume task functions encourage the group members to stay focused on the group's task. Those who assume maintenance functions worry more about the group working together than the actual task itself. Individual roles can either enhance or detract from the work of the group.

- Verbal communication includes the communication network and group themes. Nonverbal communication is more complex and involves eye contact, body posture, and mood of the group.

- Nurse leaders are responsible for mobilizing therapeutic factors to support healthy group development and prevent a stagnating groupthink. Which factors to mobilize and when depend on the type, purpose, and developmental stage of the group.

- Seating arrangements affect group interaction. The fewer physical barriers there are, such as tables, the better the potential for interactive communication. Everyone should be engaged as a member of the group and be invited to join in. In most interactive groups, members face one another in a circle.

☐ Leadership skills involve listening, tracking verbal and nonverbal behaviours, remaining fair and respectful, avoiding favouritism, and encouraging participation and involvement of all members with each other.

☐ The leader should address challenges to the leadership, group process, or other members to determine whether to intervene, and how. In some instances, the leader redirects a monopolizing member; at other times the leader supports the group to deal with the behaviour. Periods of group conflict occur in most groups during the transition from beginning to working phase.

☐ There are many different types of groups. Psychiatric nurses lead psychoeducational and supportive therapy groups. Mental health specialists who are trained to provide intensive therapy lead psychotherapy groups and cognitive-behavioural groups. Consumers lead self-help groups, and professionals assist only as requested.

☐ Medication, symptom management, anger management, and self-care groups are common nurse-led groups.

CRITICAL THINKING CHALLENGES

1 Group members are very polite to one another and are superficially discussing topics. You would assess the group as being in which phase? Explain your answer.

2 After three sessions of a supportive therapy group, two members begin to share their frustration with having a mental illness. The group is moving into which phase of group development? Explain your answer.

3 Define the roles of the task and maintenance functions in groups. Observe your clinical group and identify classmates who are assuming task functions and maintenance functions.

4 Observe a patient group for at least five sessions. Discuss the seating pattern that emerges. Identify the communication network and the group themes. Then identify the group's norms and standards.

5 Discuss the conditions that lead to groupthink. When is groupthink positive? When is groupthink negative? Explain.

6 List at least six characteristics that are important for effective group leadership. Justify your answers.

7 During the first meeting, one member seems very anxious and tends to monopolize the conversation. Discuss how you would assess the situation and whether you would intervene.

8 At the end of the fourth meeting, one group member angrily accuses another of asking too many questions. The other members look on quietly. How would you assess the situation? Would you intervene? Explain.

WEB LINKS

www.cdngrppsych.ca The Canadian Group Psychotherapy Association (CGPA) is a national organization dedicated to the promotion of group therapy practice and the enhancement of clinical knowledge and skills through training, continuing education, and research. CGPA is multidisciplinary, resulting in a rich and diverse membership. The association is responsible for setting national training standards and for accrediting regional training programs. CGPA has three levels of membership, reflecting a broad range of expertise and experience, from internationally acclaimed members to students of the mental health professions.

www.mentalhelp.net/selfhelp This website serves as an online self-help resource containing information on many different self-help groups.

www.princeton.edu This website includes an Outdoor Action Guide to Group Dynamics and Leadership, which reviews how to teach a skill, leadership concepts, and group dynamics.

MOVIES

12 Angry Men: 1998. In this excellent film, a young man stands accused of fatally stabbing his father. A jury of his "peers" is deciding his fate. This jury is portrayed by an excellent cast, including Jack Lemmon, George C. Scott, Tony Danza, and Ossie Davis. At first, the case appears to be "open and shut." This film depicts an intense struggle to reach a verdict and is an excellent study of group process and group dynamics.

VIEWING POINTS: Identify the leaders in the group. How does leadership change throughout the film? Do you find any evidence of groupthink? How does the group handle conflict?

REFERENCES

Alf, L., & Wilson, K. (2001). Facilitating group beginnings. 1. A practice model. *Groupwork, 13*(1), 6–30.

Alvarez, A. (2002). Pitfalls, pratfalls, shortfalls and windfalls: Reflection on forming and being formed by groups. *Social Work With Groups, 25*(1), 93–105.

Annesi, J. (1999). Effects of minimal group promotion on cohesion and exercise adherence. *Small Group Research, 30*(5), 542–557.

Benne, K., & Sheats, P. (1948). Functional roles of group members. *Journal of Social Issues, 4*(2), 41–49.

Brown, T., & Miller, C. (2000). Communication networks in task-performing groups: Effects of task complexity, time, pressure, and interpersonal dominance. *Small Group Research, 31*(2), 131–157.

Choi, J., & Kim, M. (1999). The organizational application of group-think and its limitations in organizations. *Journal of Applied Psychology, 84*(2), 297–306.

Dimock, H. G., & Devine, I. (1994). *Making workgroups effective* (3rd ed.). North York, Ontario: Captus Press.

Garrick, D., & Ewashen, C. (2001). An integrated model for adolescent inpatient group therapy. *Journal of Psychiatric and Mental Health Nursing, 8*, 165–171.

Graham, M., & Sontag, M. (2001). Art as an evaluative tool: A pilot study. *Art Therapy, 18*(1), 37–43.

Janis, I. (1972). *Victims of groupthink.* Boston: Houghton-Mifflin.

Janis, I. (1982). *Groupthink* (2nd ed.). Boston: Houghton-Mifflin.

Jones, E. D., & Beck-Little, R. (2002). The use of reminiscence therapy for the treatment of depression in rural-dwelling older adults. *Issues in Mental Health Nursing, 23*, 279–280.

Kurtz, L. F. (1992). Group environment in self-help groups for families. *Small Group Research, 23*, 199–215.

MacKenzie, R. K. (1997). Time-managed group psychotherapy: *Effective clinical applications.* Washington, DC: American Psychiatric Press.

Moreno, J. (1953). *Who shall survive?* Beacon, NY: Beacon House.

Neck, C. P., & Moorhead, G. (1995). Groupthink remodeled: The importance of leadership, time pressure, and methodical decision-making procedures. *Human Relations, 48*(5), 537–557.

Posthuma, B. (2001). *Small groups in counseling and therapy: Process and leadership* (4th ed.). Boston: Pearson Education Canada.

Puentos, W. J. (2004). Cognitive therapy integrated with life review techniques: An eclectic treatment approach for affective symptoms in older adults. *Journal of Clinical Nursing, 13*, 84–89.

Rutan, J. S., & Stone, W. N. (2001). *Psychodynamic group psychotherapy* (3rd ed.). New York: Guilford Press.

Sampson, E., & Marthas, M. (1990). Group process for the health professions. Albany, NY: Delmar.

Steinhardt, M. A., Dolbier, C. L., Gottlieb, N. H., & McCalister, K. T. (2003). The relationship between hardiness, supervisor support, group cohesion, and job stress as predictors of job satisfaction. *American Journal of Health Promotion, 17*(6), 382–389.

Yalom, I. D. (1983). *Inpatient group psychotherapy.* New York: Basic Books.

Yalom, I. D. (1998). *The Yalom Reader: Selections from the work of a master therapist and storyteller.* New York: Basic Books.

Yalom, I. D. (2005) *The theory and practice of group psychotherapy* (5th ed.). New York: Basic Books.

For challenges, please refer to the **CD-ROM** in this book.

16

Family Assessment and Interventions

Mary Ann Boyd and Lori Houger Limacher

LEARNING OBJECTIVES

After studying this chapter, you will be able to:

- Discuss the balance of family mental health with family functioning.
- Develop a genogram that depicts the family history, relationships, and mental disorders across at least three generations.
- Develop a plan for a comprehensive family assessment.
- Apply family nursing diagnoses to families who need nursing care.
- Discuss nursing interventions that are useful in caring for families.

KEY TERMS

boundaries ▪ differentiation of self ▪ emotional cutoff ▪ extended family ▪ family development ▪ family life cycle ▪ family projection process ▪ family structure ▪ genogram ▪ multigenerational transmission process ▪ nuclear family ▪ nuclear family emotional process ▪ sibling position ▪ subsystems ▪ transition times ▪ triangles

⬟ KEY CONCEPTS

- comprehensive family assessment ▪ family

A family is a group of people connected emotionally, by blood, or in both ways, and a group who have well developed patterns of interaction and relationships. Family members have a shared history and a shared future (Carter & McGoldrick, 1999b). A **nuclear family** is two or more people living together and related by blood, marriage, or adoption. An **extended family** is several nuclear families whose members may or may not live together and function as one group. Traditional definitions of family suggest that they are unique in that, unlike other organizations, they generally incorporate new members by birth, adoption, or marriage, and members leave only by divorce or death.

A more inclusive definition, beyond these traditional conceptions, focuses on belonging, affection, and durability of the relationships in a person's life; family is then defined as "who they say they are" (Wright & Leahey, 2005).

> **KEY CONCEPT Family** is a group of people connected emotionally, or by blood, or in both ways, and a group who have well developed patterns of interaction and relationships. Family members have a shared history and a shared future (Carter & McGoldrick, 1999b).

The psychiatric and mental health (PMH) nurse interacts with families in various ways. Because of the interpersonal and chronic nature of many mental illnesses, psychiatric nurses often have frequent and long-term contact with families. Involvement may range from meeting family members only once or twice to treating the whole family as a patient. Unlike a therapeutic group (see Chapter 15), the family system has a history and continues to function when the nurse is not there. The family reacts to past, present, and anticipated future relationships within at least a three-generation family system. This chapter explains how to integrate important family concepts into the nursing process when providing PMH nursing care to families experiencing mental health problems.

Family Mental Health

In a mentally healthy family, members live in harmony among themselves and within society. These families support and nurture their members throughout their lives. However, mental illness can affect a family's overall mental health and daily functioning.

The word *dysfunctional* has been used to describe a family whose interactions, decisions, or behaviours appear to interfere with the positive development of the family and its individual members. Sometimes a mentally healthy family appears dysfunctional after a crisis or stressful situation that the family lacks the coping skills to handle. A family can be mentally healthy and at the same time have a member who has a mental illness. Conversely, a family can appear dysfunctional and have no member with a diagnosable mental illness.

Psychiatric and mental health nurses must be cautious when using the language of "dysfunction" to describe clients or their families. This word falls short of capturing the whole of families' experiences, strengths, resources, and capabilities. Exclusively focusing on dysfunction when talking to a family risks shaping the conversation toward noticing and drawing forth only problems and deficits, obscuring the equally powerful strengths and resources. Nurses must challenge themselves to recognize both sides of what they observe with families, that is, the strengths, resources, and capabilities, alongside the challenges and difficulties.

EFFECTS OF MENTAL ILLNESS ON FAMILY FUNCTIONING

Families of people with persistent mental disorders have special needs. Many of these adults live with their parents well into their 30s and beyond. For adults with persistent mental illness, the family serves several functions that those without mental illness do not need. Such functions include the following:

Providing support. People with mental illness often have difficulty maintaining nonfamilial support networks and may rely exclusively on their families.

Providing information. Families often have complete and continuous information about care and treatment over the years.

Monitoring services. Families observe the progress of their relative and report concerns to those in charge of care.

Advocating for services. Family groups advocate for money for residential care services.

Conflicts can occur between parents and mental health workers who place a high value on independence. Members of the mental health care system may criticize families for being overly protective when, in reality, the patient with mental illness may face real barriers to independent living. Housing may be unavailable; when available, quality may be poor. The patient may fear leaving home, may be at risk for relapse if he or she does leave, or may be too comfortable at home to want to leave (Hatfield, 1992). When long-term caregivers die, patients with mental illness experience housing disruptions and potentially traumatic transitions. Few families actually plan for this difficult eventuality (Smith, Hatfield, & Miller, 2000).

Nurses must remain sensitive when discussing independence and dependence with the family. Family emotions often obscure the underlying issues, but nurses can diffuse such emotions so that everyone can explore the alternatives comfortably. Although separation must eventually occur, the timing and process vary according to each family's particular situation. Parents may be highly anxious when their adult children first leave home and need reassurance and support.

INFLUENCE OF CULTURAL BELIEFS AND VALUES ON FAMILY FUNCTIONING

Conceptualizations of normal family functioning vary among different cultural groups. For example, some Asian cultures expect a mother-in-law to move in with her married child and his or her spouse to help care for the couple's children. In some families of European descent, a mother-in-law's presence is construed as unusual or an interference with family functioning. One challenge of PMH nursing is to avoid classifying certain family patterns as pathologic just because they deviate from either dominant cultural norms or the nurse's theoretically based or theoretically driven values. On the other hand, the nurse must be careful not to over attribute symptoms and dysfunctional patterns to culture when such difficulties reflect actual problems. For instance, the nurse might overlook a patient's withdrawal as a symptom of depression if he or she attributes such behaviour to a "cultural" tendency.

Beliefs about seeking help for mental health problems are also culturally based and vary among groups. Although most families experience some discomfort in sharing family problems with outsiders, uneasiness with disclosure is particularly prominent in families from ethnic minority groups (Celano & Kaslow, 2000).

Comprehensive Family Assessment

A comprehensive family assessment is the collection of all relevant data related to family health, psychological well-being, and social functioning to identify problems for which the nurse can help generate nursing interventions. The assessment consists of a face-to-face interview with family members and can be conducted during several sessions. Nurses should conduct a comprehensive family assessment whenever they care for patients and their families, especially when a patient's mental health problems are so complex that family support is important for optimal care (Box 16-1).

> ⬟ **KEY CONCEPT** A **comprehensive family assessment** is the collection of all relevant data related to family health, psychological well-being, and social functioning to identify problems for which the nurse can generate nursing interventions.

RELATIONSHIP BUILDING

In preparing for a family assessment, nurses must concentrate on developing a relationship with the family. Although necessary when working with any family, relationship development is particularly important for families from ethnic minority cultures. Developing a relationship takes time, so the nurse may need to complete the assessment during several meetings, rather than just one.

To develop a positive relationship with a family, nurses must establish credibility with the family and address its immediate intervention needs. To establish credibility, the family must see the nurse as willing to listen to their concerns, and as knowledgeable and skillful. Possessing culturally competent nursing skills and projecting a professional image are crucial to establishing credibility. With regard to immediate intervention needs, a family who needs shelter or food is not ready to discuss a member's medication regimen until the first needs are met. The nurse will make considerable progress in establishing a relationship with a family when he or she helps members meet their immediate needs.

GENOGRAMS

Families possess various structural configurations (eg, single-parent, multigenerational, same-gender relationships). The nurse can facilitate taking the family history by completing a **genogram**, which is a multigenerational schematic diagram that lists family members and their relationships. The genogram is a skeleton of the family that the nurse can use as a framework for exploring relationships and patterns of health and illness.

A genogram includes the age, dates of marriage and death, and geographic location of each member. Squares represent men and circles represent women; ages are listed inside the squares and circles. Horizontal lines represent marriages with dates; vertical lines connect parents and children. Genograms can be particularly useful in understanding family history, composition, relationships, and illnesses (Fig. 16-1).

Genograms vary from simple to elaborate. The patient's and family's assessment needs guide the level of detail. In a small family with limited problems, the genogram can be rather general. In a large family with multiple problems, the genogram should reflect these complexities. Thus, depending on the level of detail required, nurses collect various data. They can study important events such as marriages, divorces, deaths, and geographic movements. They can include cultural or religious affiliations, education and economic levels, and the nature of the work of each family member. Psychiatric nurses should always include mental disorders and other significant health problems in the genogram.

Analyzing and Using Genograms

For a genogram to be useful in assessment, the nurse needs to analyze the data for family composition, relationship problems, and mental health patterns. Nurses can begin with composition. How large is the family?

BOX 16.1

Family Mental Health Assessment

Family Name: _____

Family Members Present at Interview: _____

_____

_____

_____

Nurse Interviewer: _____

1. Referral route and presenting problem (include psychiatric diagnosis, and current treatment): _____

_____

_____

2. Family composition (complete and attach a family genogram)
3. Family life cycle stage (include stage and any pertinent transitional issues): _____

_____

_____

4. Pertinent history of the problem:
   a. Explore why the family is presenting for assistance at this point in time.
   b. Explore the effects of the mental health concern on all family members.
   c. Developmental history (including family of origin, health or medical events)
   d. Communication patterns (for solving day to day issues or problems)
   e. Previous solutions
   f. Ethnicity/culture
   g. Social supports (informal and formal programs)
   h. Financial and legal status
5. Strengths and problems (identify the family strengths, resources and capabilities): _____

_____

_____

6. Summary (include a hypothesis about the presenting problem, any pertinent history, patterns of communicating, subsystems, or boundary issues): _____

_____

_____

7. Goals/plans (list interventions and family responses): _____

_____

8. Nursing diagnosis: _____

_____

_____

Adapted from Wright, L. M., & Leahey, M. (2005). *Nurses and families: A guide to family assessment and intervention.* Philadelphia: F. A. Davis.

Where do family members live? A large family whose members live in the same city is more likely to have support than a family in which distance separates members. Of course, this is not always the case. Sometimes even when family members live geographically close, they are emotionally distant from one another.

The nurse should also study the genogram for relationship and illness patterns. For instance, in terms of relationship patterns, the nurse may find a history of divorces or family members who do not keep in touch with the rest of the family. The nurse can then explore the significance of these and other relationships. In terms of illness patterns, alcoholism, often seen across several generations, may be prevalent in men on one side of a family. The nurse can then hypothesize that alcoholism is one of the mental health risks for the family and design interventions to reduce the risk. The nurse can also explore how some family members managed to "escape" alcoholism, as a means of exploring potential solutions with a family.

FAMILY BIOLOGIC DOMAIN

In the family biologic domain, the family assessment includes a thorough picture of physical and mental health status and how the status affects family functioning. The family with multiple health problems, both physical and mental, will be trying to manage these problems as well as obtain the many financial and health care resources it needs.

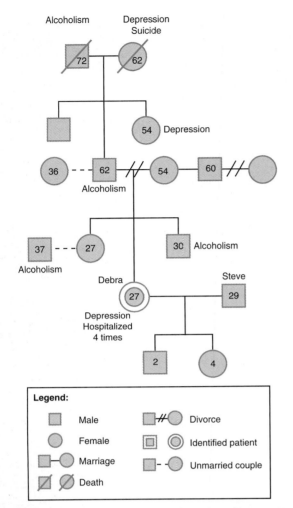

Legend:

▢	Male	▢–//–◯	Divorce
◯	Female	▣ ◎	Identified patient
▢—◯	Marriage	▢- -◯	Unmarried couple
▨ ⌀	Death		

FIGURE 16.1   Analysis of genogram for Debra. Illness patterns are depression (maternal aunt, grandmother [suicide]) and alcoholism (brother, father, grandfather). Relationship patterns show that parents are divorced and neither sibling is married.

Physical Health Status

The family health status includes the physical illnesses and disabilities of all members; the nurse can record such information on the genogram and also include the physical illnesses and disabilities of other generations. However, the illnesses of family members are an indication not only of their physical status but also of the stress currently being placed on the family and its resources. Thus, the nurse should pay particular attention to any physical problems that affect family functioning. For example, if a member requires frequent visits to a provider or hospitalizations, the whole family will feel the effects of focusing excessive time and financial resources on that member. The nurse should explore how such situations specifically affect other members.

Mental Health Status

Exploring a family's history and experience with a mental disorder may be a sensitive topic for discussion. In

our Western culture, families often experience an element of shame or stigma associated with mental health concerns. This cultural discourse, or pressure, may invite a family into silencing or burying their concerns, especially with people outside the family. This sometimes leads to families maintaining a shroud of secrecy around their difficulties or challenges, a process referred to as a "family secret."

Directly and calmly, the nurse should ask family members to identify anyone who has had or has a mental illness. He or she should record the information on the genogram as well as in the narrative. If family members do not know whether anyone in the family had or has a mental illness, the nurse should ask if anyone was treated for "nerves" or had a "nervous breakdown." Overall, a good family history of mental illness across multiple generations helps the nurse understand the significance of mental illness in the current generation. If one family member has a serious mental illness, the whole family will be affected. Usually, siblings of the mentally ill member receive less parental attention than the affected member.

FAMILY PSYCHOLOGICAL DOMAIN

Assessment of the family's psychological domain focuses on the family's development and life cycle, communication patterns, stress and coping abilities, and problem-solving skills. One aim of the assessment is to understand the relationships within the family. Although family roles and structures are important, the true value of the family is in its relationships, which are irreplaceable. For example, if a parent leaves or dies, another person (eg, stepparent, grandparent) can assume some parental functions but can never really replace the emotional relationship with the missing parent.

Family Development

Family development is a broad term that refers to all the processes connected with the growth of a family, including changes associated with work, geographic location, migration, acculturation, and serious illness. In optimal family development, family members are relatively differentiated (capable of autonomous functioning) from one another, anxiety is low, and the parents have good emotional relationships with their own families of origin.

Family Life Cycles

Family development differs from the concept of the family life cycle, which refers to family stages based on significant events related to the arrival and departure of family members, such as birth or adoption, child rearing, departure of children from home, occupational retirement, and death. However, as second marriages, career changes in midlife, and other phenomena occur with increasing frequency, this traditional model is being challenged, modified, and redesigned to address such contemporary structural and role changes. This model also may not fit many cultural groups.

CRNE Note

Apply family life cycle stages to a specific family with a member who has a psychiatric disorder. Identify the emotional transitions and the required family changes.

Thus, the **family life cycle** is a process of expansion, contraction, and realignment of relationship systems to support the entry, exit, and development of family mem-

bers in a functional way (Carter & McGoldrick, 1999b) (Table 16-1). A family's life cycle is conceptualized in terms of stages throughout the years. To move from one stage to the next, the family system undergoes changes. Structural and potential structural changes within stages can usually be handled by rearranging the family system (first-order changes), whereas transition from one stage to the next requires changes in the system itself (second-order changes). In first-order changes, the family system is rearranged, such as when all the children are finally in school and the stay-at-home parent returns to work. The system is rearranged, but the structure remains the same. In second-order changes, the family structure does change, such as when a member moves away from the family home to live independently.

As suggested, the nurse should not view this model as the "normal" life cycle for every family and should limit

---

Table 16.1 Stages of the Family Life Cycle

Family Life Cycle Stage	Emotional Transition	Required Family Changes
1. Leaving home: single young adults	Accepting emotional and financial responsibility for self	Differentiation of self in relation to family of origin Development of intimate peer relationships Establishment of self regarding work and financial independence
2. The joining of families through marriage: the new couple	Commitment to new system	Formation of marital system Realignment of relationships with extended families and friends to include spouse
3. Families with young children	Accepting new members into the system	Adjusting marital system to make space for children Joining in childrearing, financial, and household tasks Realignment of relationships with extended family to include parenting and grandparenting roles
4. Families with adolescents	Increasing flexibility of family boundaries to include children's independence and grandparents frailties	Shifting of parent–child relationships to permit adolescent to move in and out of system Refocus on midlife marital and career issues Beginning shift toward joint caring for older generation
5. Launching children and moving on	Accepting multitude of exits from and entries into the family system	Renegotiation of marital system as a dyad Development of adult–adult relationships between grown children and their parents Realignment of relationships to include in-laws and grandchildren Dealing with disabilities and death of parents (grandparents)
6. Families in later life	Accepting the shifting of generational roles	Maintaining own and couple functioning interests in face of physiologic decline, exploration of new familial and social role options Support for a more central role of middle generation Making room in the system for the wisdom and experience of the elderly, supporting the older generation without overfunctioning for them Dealing with loss of spouse, siblings, and other peers and preparation for own death

From Carter B., & McGoldrick, M. (1999b). Overview: The expanded family life cycle. In B. Carter & M. McGoldrick (Eds.). *The expanded family life cycle* (p. 2). New York: Allyn & Bacon.

Table 16.2   The Divorcing Family

Family Life Cycle Stage	Prerequisite Attitude	Developmental Issues
Divorce		
1. Decision to divorce	Acceptance of inability to resolve marital tensions sufficiently to continue relationship	Acceptance of one's own part in the failure of the marriage
2. Planning the breakup of the system	Supporting viable arrangements for all parts of the system	Working cooperatively on problems of custody, visitation, and finances Dealing with extended family about the divorce
3. Separation	Willingness to continue cooperative co-parental relationship and joint financial support of children Work on resolution of attachment to spouse	Mourning loss of intact family Restructuring marital and parent–child relationships and finances; adaptation to living apart Realignment of relationships with extended family; staying connected with spouse's extended family
4. The divorce	More work on emotional divorce: overcoming hurt, anger, guilt, etc.	Mourning loss of intact family: giving up fantasies of reunion Retrieval of hopes, dreams, expectations from the marriage Staying connected with extended families
Postdivorce Family		
1. Single-parent (custodial household or primary residence)	Willingness to maintain financial responsibilities, continue parental contact with ex-spouse, and support contact of children with ex-spouse and his or her family	Making flexible visitation arrangements with ex-spouse and family Rebuilding own financial resources Rebuilding own social network
2. Single-parent (noncustodial)	Willingness to maintain parental contact with ex-spouse and support custodial parent's relationship with children	Finding ways to continue effective parenting relationship with children Maintaining financial responsibilities to ex-spouse and children Rebuilding own social network

From Carter, B., & McGoldrick, M. (1999a). The divorce cycle: A major variation in the American family life cycle. In B. Carter & M. McGoldrick (Eds.), *The expanded family life cycle* (p. 375). New York: Allyn & Bacon.

its use to those families it clearly fits. Variations of the family life cycle are presented for the divorced family (Table 16-2) and the remarried family (Table 16-3).

Transition times are any times of addition, subtraction, or change in status of family members. During transitions, family stresses are more likely to cause symptoms or difficulties. Significant family events, such as the death of a member or the introduction of a new member, also affect the family's ability to function. During these times, families may seek help from the mental health system.

Culture, Ethnicity, and Race

The terms *culture*, *ethnicity*, and *race* are often used interchangeably in discussions about diversity in psychiatric settings. This mingling of terms can create confusion, given that these words can mean very different things (Fine, Wieling, & Allen, 2004; Hartrick Doanne & Varcoe, 2005). Culture generally refers to the beliefs, values, and norms that guide and shape the way a family lives, whereas ethnicity is associated with more distinctive traits, like national heritage, social class, race, and religion. Race is generally considered a biologic dimension.

Given Canada's multicultural climate, it is important for nurses in psychiatric settings to consciously attend to diversity. One method for increasing sensitivity to culture has been by trying to identify distinctive characteristics, or responses to life cycle transitions, or disruptions like mental illness, within specific ethnic communities. Becoming conscious of the characteristics of particular ethnic groups is an important step toward developing an appreciation for diversity, as long as these norms are remembered to be gross generalizations. Labeling and categorizing ethnic groups' behaviours according to general rules can help raise our awareness of difference, but it can equally obscure the uniqueness of each family that we encounter. For the nurse, appreciating and validating ethnic differences, while at the same time acknowledging similarities, can feel like a delicate balancing act (McGoldrick, 2003).

For example, if a nurse anticipates that an Indo-Canadian, Italian-Canadian, or Aboriginal-Canadian's extended family (aunts, uncles, and cousins) will be

Table 16.3   Remarried Family Formulations

Family Life Cycle Stage	Prerequisite Attitude	Developmental Issues
1. Entering the new relationship	Recovery from loss of first marriage (adequate 'emotional divorce")	Recommitment to marriage and to forming a family with readiness to deal with the complexity and ambiguity
2. Conceptualizing and planning new marriage and family	Accepting one's own fears and those of new spouse and children about remarriage and forming a stepfamily. Accepting need for time and patience for adjustment to complexity and ambiguity of multiple new roles Boundaries: space, time, membership, and authority Affective issues: guilt, loyalty conflicts, desire for mutuality, unresolvable past hurts	Work on openness in the new relationships to avoid pseudomutuality Plan for maintenance of cooperative financial and co-parental relationships with ex-spouses Plan to help children deal with fears, loyalty conflicts, and membership in two systems Realignment of relationships with extended family to include new spouse and children Plan for maintenance of connections for children with extended family of ex-spouses
3. Remarriage and reconstitution of family	Final resolution of attachment to previous spouse and ideal of "intact" family Acceptance of a different model of family with permeable boundaries	Restructuring family boundaries to allow for inclusion of new spouse-stepparent Realignment of relationships and financial arrangement throughout subsystems to permit interweaving of several systems Making room for relationships of all children with biologic (noncustodial) parents, grandparents, and other extended family Sharing memories and histories to enhance stepfamily integration

From Carter, B., & McGoldrick, M. (1999a). The divorce cycle: A major variation in the American family life cycle. In B. Carter & M. McGoldrick (Eds.), *The expanded family life cycle* (p. 377). New York: Allyn & Bacon.

more involved in mental health treatment decisions and hospital visitation (Hartrick Doanne & Varcoe, 2005; McGoldrick & Giordano, 1996), or assumes that Chinese-Canadian families will be less likely to seek mental health treatment because they will not recognize or attend to mental illness in the same way (Casado & Leung, 2001), a generalization based on ethnicity is likely occurring. In the clinical example provided in Box 16-2, a particular generalization is at play in the description of Judy's rich familial connections and her location in a particular geographic region of Canada. This is another example of a cultural assumption.

Developing sensitivity to one's own beliefs about what constitutes normalcy and functionality in a family is a challenging and important endeavour. It is only in this process of self-reflection that the nurse will develop an awareness of the cultural norms and values that are guiding and creating the template against which the nurse is judging and assessing even the family life cycle (Hartrick Doanne & Varcoe, 2005). It is the dominant, white, middle-class, cultural rules that generally become the gold standard, the norm against which all other ethnic groups are measured and assessed. This can be problematic if the nurse is not aware of the power, and hence oppression, that might accompany these norms. Developing and maintaining sensitivity to ethnicity,

culture, and power is important in helping the nurse to recognize issue of diversity (see Chapter 3).

Families in Poverty

The family life cycle of those living in poverty may vary from those with adequate financial means. People living in poverty struggle to make ends meet, and members may face difficulties in meeting their own or other members' basic developmental needs. To be poor does not mean that a family is dysfunctional. But poverty is an important factor that can force even the healthiest families to crumble. In studying African American families living in poverty, Hines (1999) observed four distinguishing characteristics: condensed life cycle, female-headed households of the extended-family type, chronic stress and untimely losses, and reliance on institutional supports.

When the life cycle is condensed, family members leave home, mate, have children, and become grandparents at much earlier ages than their working-class and middle-class counterparts. Consequently, many individuals in such families assume new roles and responsibilities before they are developmentally capable.

The condensed life cycle creates adolescents whose educational opportunities are compromised (no time to

BOX 16.2

John and Judy Jones

John and Judy Jones were married 3 years ago, after their graduation from a small University in Eastern Canada. Judy's career choice required that she live on the East Coast, where she should be near her large family. John willingly moved with her and quickly found a satisfying position. After about 6 months of marriage, John became extremely irritable and depressed. He kept saying that his life was not his own. Judy was very concerned but could not understand his feelings of being overwhelmed. His job was going well, and they had a very busy social life, mostly revolving around her family, whom John loved. They decided to seek counselling and completed the following genogram:

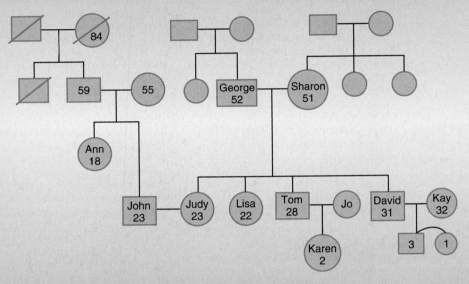

After looking at the genogram, both John and Judy began to realize that part of John's discomfort had to do with the number of family members who were involved in their lives. Judy and John began to redefine their social life, allowing more time with friends and each other.

complete school given family demands), limiting their employment skills. Therefore, the cycle of poverty is reinforced.

The second characteristic that Hines observed is female-headed households of the extended-family type, in which a woman, her children, and her daughter's children often live together without clear delineation of their respective roles. This scenario can create economic and emotional burdens for the older woman who is the principal breadwinner, and difficulty for the younger women in assuming parental responsibilities.

Despite possible poor health, elderly family members continue to work to support their children and grandchildren into later life (Hines, 1999).

The third characteristic is chronic stress and untimely losses. Families living in poverty are subject to disruption via abrupt loss of members, loss of unemployment compensation, illness, death, imprisonment, or alcohol or drug addiction. Men may die relatively young compared with their middle-class counterparts. Ordinary problems, such as transportation or a sick child, can become major crises because of a lack of resources.

Reliance on institutional supports is the final distinguishing characteristic. Poor families are often forced to seek public assistance, which ultimately can result in additional stress in having to deal with a governmental agency.

Communication Patterns

Family communication patterns develop over a lifetime. Some family members communicate more openly and honestly than others. In addition, family subgroups may have unique communication patterns with one another. Just as in any assessment interview, the nurse should observe the verbal and nonverbal communication of the family members. Who sits next to each other? Who talks to whom? Who answers most questions? Who volunteers information? Who changes the subject? Which subjects seem acceptable to discuss? Which topics are not discussed? How are partners intimate with each other? How are the family secrets or sensitive topics revealed? Does the nonverbal communication match the verbal communication? Nurses can use this information to help identify family problems, strengths, and communication issues.

Nurses should also assess the family for its daily communication patterns. Identifying which family members confide in one another is a place to start examining ongoing communication. Other areas include how often children talk with parents, which child talks to the parents most, and who is most likely to discipline the children. Another question considers how family members express positive and negative feelings. In determining how open or closed the family is, the nurse explores the type of information the family shares with nonfamily members. For example, one family may tell others about a member's mental illness, whereas another family may not discuss any illnesses with those outside the family.

Stress and Coping Abilities

One of the most important assessment tasks is to determine how family members deal with major and minor stressful events and their available coping skills. Some families seem able to cope with overwhelming stresses, such as the death of a member, major illness, or severe conflict, whereas other families seem to fall apart over relatively minor events. It is important for the nurse to listen to which situations a family appraises as stressful and help the family identify usual coping responses. The nurse can then evaluate these responses. If the family's responses are maladaptive (eg, substance abuse, physical abuse), the nurse will discuss the need to develop coping skills that lead to family well-being (see Chapter 34).

CRNE Note

Identifying stressful events and coping mechanisms should be a priority in a family assessment.

Problem-Solving Skills

Nurses assess family problem-solving skills by focusing on the more recent problems the family has experienced and determining the process that members used to solve them. For example, a child is sick at school and needs to go home. Does the mother, father, grandparent, or baby-sitter receive the call from the school? Who then cares for the child? Underlying the ability to solve problems is the decision-making process. Who makes and implements decisions? How does the family handle conflict? All these data provide information regarding the family's problem-solving abilities. Once these abilities are identified, the nurse can build on these strengths in helping families deal with additional problems.

FAMILY SOCIAL DOMAIN

An assessment of the family's social domain provides important data about the operation of the family as a system and its interaction within its environment. Areas of concern include the system itself, social and financial status, and formal and informal support networks.

Family Systems

Just as any group can be viewed as a system, a family can be understood as a system with interdependent members. Family system theories view the family as an open system whose members interact with their environment as well as among themselves. One family member's change in thoughts or behaviour can cause a ripple effect and change everyone else's. For example, a mother who decides not to pick up her children's clothing from their bedroom floors anymore invites the children to deal with cluttered rooms and dirty clothes in a different way than before.

One common scenario in the mental health field is the effect of a patient's improvement on the family. With new medications and treatment, patients are more likely to be able to live independently, which subsequently changes the responsibilities and activities of family caregivers. Although on the surface members may seem relieved that their caregiving burden is lifted, in reality, they must adjust their time and energies to fill the remaining void. This transition may not be easy because it is often less stressful to maintain familiar activities than to venture into uncharted territory. Families may seem as though they want to keep an ill member dependent, but in reality they are struggling with the change in their family system.

Several system models are used in caring for families: the Wright-Leahey Calgary model, Bowen's family system, and Minuchin's structural family system.

The language used in these three models to describe families and family interactions have permeated many psychiatric settings. Tracing the history of these words and terms is important in understanding the cultural norms that dominate and shape our current understanding of family nursing.

Calgary Family Model

Lorraine M. Wright and Maureen Leahey developed the Calgary Family Assessment Model (CFAM) and the Calgary Family Intervention Model (CFIM). These nursing models are based on systems, cybernetics, and communication and change theories (Wright and Leahey, 2005). Families seek help when they have family health and illness problems, difficulties, and suffering. These two models are multidimensional frameworks that conceptualize the family into structural, developmental, and functional categories. Each assessment category contains several subcategories. Structure is further categorized into internal (family, gender, sexual orientation, etc.), external (extended family and larger systems), and context (ethnicity, race, social class, religion, spirituality, environment).

Family developmental assessment is organized according to stages, tasks, and attachments. Functional assessment areas include instrumental (activities of daily living) and expressive (communication, problem-solving roles, beliefs, etc.).

The CFAM and CFIM are built around four stages: engagement, assessment, intervention and termination. The *engagement* stage is the initial stage in which the family is greeted and made comfortable. In the *assessment* stage, problems are identified, and relationships between family and health providers develop. During this stage, the nurse opens space for the family to tell its story. The *intervention* stage is the core of the clinical work and involves providing a context in which the family can make changes (see the Family Interventions section in this chapter). The *termination* phase refers to the process of ending the therapeutic relationship (Wright and Leahey, 2005).

Family Systems Therapy Model

Murray Bowen recognized the power of a system and believed that there is a balance between the family system and the individual. Bowen developed several concepts that professionals often use today when working with families (Bowen, 1975, 1976):

Differentiation of self involves two processes: intrapsychic and interpersonal. Intrapsychic differentiation means separating thinking from feeling: a differentiated individual can distinguish between thoughts and feelings and can consequently think through behaviour. For example, a person who has experienced intrapsychic differentiation, even though angry, will think through the underlying issue before acting; however, the feeling of the moment will drive the behaviour of an undifferentiated individual. Interpersonal differentiation is the process of freeing oneself from the family's emotional chaos. That is, the individual can recognize the family turmoil but avoid re-entering arguments and issues. For Bowen, the individual must resolve attachment to this chaos before he or she can differentiate into a mature, healthy personality.

Triangles: According to Bowen, the triangle is a three-person system and the smallest stable unit in human relations. Cycles of closeness and distance characterize a two-person relationship. When anxiety is high during periods of distance, one party "triangulates" a third person or thing into the relationship. For example, two partners may have a stable relationship when anxiety is low. When anxiety and tension rise, one partner may be so uncomfortable that he or she confides in a friend instead of the other partner. In these cases, triangulating reduces the tension but freezes the conflict in place. In families, triangulating occurs when a husband and wife diffuse tension by focusing on the children. To maintain the status quo and avoid the conflict, one of the parents develops an overly intense relationship with one of the children, which tends to produce symptoms in the child (eg, bed wetting, fear of school).

Family projection process: Through this process, the triangulated member becomes the centre of the family conflicts; that is, the family projects its conflicts onto the child or other triangulated person. Projection is anxious, enmeshed concern. For example, a husband and wife are having difficulty deciding how to spend money. One of their children is having difficulty with interpersonal relationships in school. Instead of the parents resolving their differences over money, one parent focuses on the child's needs and becomes intensely involved in the child's issues. The other parent then relates coolly and distantly to the involved parent.

Nuclear family emotional process: This concept describes patterns of emotional functioning in a family in a single generation. This emotional distance is a patterned reaction in daily interactions with the spouse.

Multigenerational transmission process: Bowen believed that one generation transfers its emotional processes to the next generation. Certain basic patterns between parents and children are replicas of those of past generations, and generations to follow will repeat them as well. The child who is the most involved with the family is least able to differentiate from his or her family of origin and passes on conflicts from one generation to another. For example, a spouse may stay emotionally distant from his partner, just as his father was with his mother.

Sibling position: Children develop fixed personality characteristics based on their **sibling position** in their families. For example, a first-born child may have more confidence and be more outgoing than the second-born child, who has grown up in the older child's shadow. Conversely, the second-born child may be more inclined to identify with the oppressed and be more open to other experiences than the first-born child. These attitudinal and behavioural patterns become fixed parts of both children's personalities. Knowledge of these general personality characteristics may be helpful in predicting the family's emotional processes and patterns.

Emotional cutoff: If a member cannot differentiate from his or her family, that member may just flee from the family, either by moving away or avoiding personal subjects of conversation. Yet a brief visit from parents can render these individuals helpless.

In using this model, the nurse can observe family interactions to determine how differentiated family members are from one another. Are members autonomous in thinking and feeling? Do triangulated relationships develop during periods of stress and tension? Are family members interacting in the same manner as their parents or grandparents? How do the personalities of older siblings compare with those of younger siblings? Who lives close to one another? Does any family member live in another city? The Bowen model can provide a way of assessing the system of family relationships.

Family Structure Model

Salvador Minuchin emphasizes the importance of family structure. In his model, the family consists of three essential components: structure, subsystems, and boundaries (Minuchin, Lee, & Simon, 1996).

Family structure is the organized pattern in which family members interact. As two adult partners come together to form a family, they develop the quantity of their interactions, or how much time they spend interacting. For example, a newly married couple may establish their evening interaction pattern by talking to each other during dinner but not while watching television. The quality of the interactions also becomes patterned. Some topics are appropriate for conversation during their evening walk (eg, reciting daily events), whereas controversial or emotionally provocative topics are relegated to other times and places.

Family rules are important influences on interaction patterns. For example, "family problems stay in the family" is a common rule. Both the number of people in the family and its development also influence the interaction pattern. For instance, the interaction between a single mother and her children changes when she remarries and introduces a stepfather. Over time, families repeat interactions, which develop into enduring patterns. For example, if a mother tells her son to straighten his room and the son refuses until his father yells at him, the family has initiated an interactional pattern. If this pattern continues, the child will come to see the father as the disciplinarian and the mother as incompetent. However, the mother will be more affectionate to her son, and the father will remain the disciplinarian on the "outside."

Subsystems develop when family members join together for various activities or functions. Minuchin views each member, as well as dyads and other larger groups that form, as a subsystem. Obvious groups are parents and children. Sometimes, there are "boy" and "girl" systems. Such systems become obvious in an assessment when family members talk about "the boys going fishing with dad" and "the girls going shopping with mother." Family members belong to several different subgroups. A mother may also be a wife, sister, and

daughter. Sometimes, these roles can conflict. It may be acceptable for a woman to be very firm as a disciplinarian in her role as mother. However, in her sister, wife, or daughter role, similar behaviour would provoke anger and resentment.

Boundaries are invisible barriers with varying permeabilities that surround each subsystem. They regulate the amount of contact a person has with others and protect the autonomy of the family and its subsystems. If family members do not take telephone calls at dinner, they are protecting themselves from outside intrusion. When parents do not allow children to interrupt them, they are establishing a boundary between themselves and their children. According to Minuchin, the spouse subsystem must have a boundary that separates it from parents, children, and the outside world. A clear boundary between parent and child enables children to interact with their parents but excludes them from the spouse subsystem.

Boundaries vary from rigid to diffuse. If boundaries are too rigid and permit little contact from outside subsystems, disengagement results, and disengaged individuals are relatively isolated. On the other hand, rigid boundaries permit independence, growth, and mastery within the subsystem, particularly if parents do not hover over their children, telling them what to do or fighting their battles for them. Enmeshed subsystems result when boundaries are diffuse. That is, when boundaries are too relaxed, parents may become too involved with their children, and the children learn to rely on the parents to make decisions, resulting in decreased independence. According to Minuchin, if children see their parents as friends and treat them as they would peers, enmeshment exists.

Indeed, autonomy and interdependence are key concepts, important both to individual growth and family system maintenance. Relationship patterns are maintained by universal rules governing family organization (especially power hierarchy) and mutual behavioural expectations. In the well-functioning family, boundaries are clear, and a hierarchy exists with a strong parental subsystem. Problems result when there is a malfunctioning of the hierarchical arrangement or boundaries or a maladaptive reaction to changing developmental or environmental requirements. Minuchin believes in clear, flexible boundaries by which all family members can live comfortably.

In the family structural theory, what distinguishes normal families is not the absence of problems but a functional family structure to handle them. Normal husbands and wives must learn to adjust to each other, rear their children, deal with their parents, cope with their jobs, and fit into their communities. The types of struggles change with developmental stages and situational crises. The PMH nurse assesses the family structure and the presence of subsystems or boundaries. He or she uses these data to determine how the subsystems and boundaries affect the family's functioning. Helping family members change a subsystem, such as including girls in the boys' activities, may improve family functioning.

Social and Financial Status

Social status is often linked directly to financial status. The nurse should assess the occupations of the family members. Who works outside the home and inside the home? Who is primarily responsible for the family's financial support? Families of low social status are more likely to have limited financial resources, which can place additional stresses on the family. Nurses can use information regarding the family's financial status to determine whether to refer the family to social services.

Cultural expectations and beliefs about acceptable behaviours may cause additional stress. For example, in one qualitative study of 12 black West Indian depressed women who emigrated to Canada or were first-born Canadians, the women rarely sought professional help because of the strong culturally defined stigma against mental disorders. Instead, they managed depression by "being strong," which meant that they tried not to dwell on their feelings, focussed on diversions, tried to regain composure, or used other approaches. The researchers concluded that "being strong" may be a factor in inducing depression or slowing or preventing recovery for some women (Schreiber, Noerager Stern, & Wilson, 2000).

Formal and Informal Support Networks

According to balance theory (see Chapter 7), both formal and informal networks are important in providing support to individuals and families. These networks are the link among the individual, families, and the community. Assessing the extent of formal support (eg, hospitals, agencies) and informal support (eg, extended family, friends, neighbours) gives a clearer picture of the availability of support. In assessing formal support, the nurse should ask about the family's involvement with government institutions and self-help groups such as Alcoholics Anonymous. Assessing the informal network is particularly important in cultural groups with extended family networks or close friends because these individuals can be major sources of support to patients. If the nurse does not ask about the informal network, these important people may be missed. Nurses can inquire whether family members volunteer at schools, local hospitals, or nursing homes. They can also ask whether the family attends religious services or activities.

Family Nursing Diagnoses

From the assessment data, nurses can choose several possible nursing diagnoses. Interrupted Family Processes; Ineffective Therapeutic Regimen Management; or Compromised, Disabling, or Ineffective Family Coping are all possibilities. Nurses choose Interrupted Family Processes if a usually supportive family is experiencing stressful events that challenge its previously effective functioning. They choose Ineffective Family Therapeutic Regimen Management if the family is experiencing difficulty integrating into daily living a program for the treatment of illness and the sequela of illness that meets specific health goals. They select Ineffective Family Coping when the primary supportive person is providing insufficient, ineffective, or compromised support, comfort, or assistance to the patient in managing or mastering adaptive tasks related to the individual's health challenge (Carpenito, 2003).

Family Interventions

Family interventions focus on supporting the biopsychosocial integrity and functioning of the family as defined by its members. Although family therapy is reserved for mental health specialists, the generalist PMH nurse can implement several biopsychosocial interventions, such as counselling promotion of self-care activities, supportive therapy, education and health teaching, and the use of genograms.

In implementing any family intervention, flexibility is essential, particularly when working with culturally diverse groups. To implement successful, culturally competent family interventions, nurses need to be open to modifying the structure and format of the sessions. Longer sessions are often useful, especially when a translator or interpreter is used. Nurses also need to respect and work with the changing composition of family and nonfamily participants (eg, extended family members, intimate partners, friends and neighbours, community helpers) in sessions. Because of the stigma that some cultural groups associate with seeking help, nurses may need to hold intervention sessions in community settings (eg, churches and schools) or at the family's home. Finally, termination may need to be gradual or delayed (Celano & Kaslow, 2000).

COUNSELLING

Nurses often use counselling when working with families because it is a short-term problem-solving approach that addresses current issues. If the assessment reveals complex, longstanding relationship problems, the nurse needs to refer the family to a family therapist. If the family is struggling with psychiatric problems of one or more family members or the family system is in a life cycle transition, the nurse should use short-term counselling. The counselling sessions should focus on specific issues, problems, and strengths using sound group process theory. Usually, a problem-solving approach works well once an issue has been identified (see Chapter 14).

PROMOTING SELF-CARE ACTIVITIES

Families often need support in changing behaviours that promote self-care activities. For example, families may inadvertently reinforce a family member's dependency out of fear of the patient being taken advantage of in work or social situations. A nurse can help the family explore how to meet the patient's need for work and social activity and at the same time help alleviate family fears.

Caregiver distress or role strain can occur in families responsible for the care of members with long-term illness. Family interventions can help families deal with the burden of caring for members with psychiatric disorders. An analysis of 16 studies indicated that family interventions can affect relatives' burden, psychological distress, and the relationship between patient and relative and family functioning. These interventions varied from education sessions to intensive family treatment. In most interventions, information on mental illness was presented, as well as discussion. Interventions with more than 12 sessions had more profound effects than did shorter interventions (Cuijpers, 1999). Identifying community resources, groups, and volunteers that can help care for the caregiver will assist in alleviating distress (Cuellar & Butts, 1999).

SUPPORTING FAMILY FUNCTIONING AND COHESIVENESS

Supporting family functioning involves various nursing approaches. In meeting with the family, the nurse should identify and acknowledge its values. In developing a trusting relationship with the family, the nurse should confirm that all members have a sense of self and self-worth. One way this can be accomplished is for the nurse to actively notice and distinguish the family's strengths, resources, and capabilities in the form of a verbal **commendation** (Houger Limacher & Wright, 2003; Wright, Watson, & Bell, 1996). For a family who has been challenged, often for many years, with a serious mental health issue, experiencing a direct, specific comment about their positive actions and solutions can be a powerful intervention. It can be as simple as a nurse stating to a family, "I am impressed with your strength, your detailed knowledge about the medication regime, and the way that you have stuck together to support one another by visiting the hospital and attending this family meeting." Supporting family subsystems, such as encouraging the children to play while

BOX 16.3

RESEARCH FOR BEST PRACTICE

The Therapeutic Relationship Holds Great Power

QUESTION: What makes a difference to clients and families in therapeutic conversations, and what contributes to change?

METHOD: Reviewed and analyzed more than 40 years of existing outcome research

FINDINGS: Consistent with Lambert's (1992) findings, these authors concluded that change was mostly dependent on four common factors. The first factor, predicted to account for 40% of change, included client variables that fell outside the therapy encounter. The second most powerful variable was the therapeutic relationship, accounting for 30% of change, followed by the placebo effect (or hope) and therapy techniques, each at 15%.

IMPLICATIONS FOR PRACTICE: The development of a meaningful therapeutic relationship with a family does matter and is important to change. Be empathic, listen, and build on the client's and family's strengths and competencies. The power of change begins within this special relationship.

From Hubble, M. A., Duncan, B. L., & Miller, S. D. (1999). *The heart and soul of change: What works in therapy.* Washington, DC: American Psychological Association.

meeting with the spouses, reinforces family boundaries. Based on assessment of the family system's operation and communication patterns, the nurse can reinforce open, honest communication.

In communicating with the family, the nurse needs to observe boundaries and avoid becoming triangulated into family issues. A warm, empathic, and open leadership style can set the tone for the family sessions.

See Box 16-3 for a summary of a research study on the therapeutic relationship.

PROVIDING EDUCATION AND HEALTH TEACHING

One of the most important family interventions is education and health teaching, particularly in families with mental illness. Families have a central role in the treatment of mental illnesses. Members need to learn about mental disorders, medications, actions, side effects, and overall treatment approaches and outcomes. For example, families are often reluctant to have members take psychiatric medications because they believe the medications will "drug" the patient or become addictive. The family's beliefs about mental illnesses and treatment will affect how patients manage their illness.

USING GENOGRAMS

Genograms not only are useful in assessment, but also can be used as intervention strategies. Nurses can use genograms to help family members understand current feelings and emotions as well as the family's evolution over several generations. Genograms allow the family to examine relationships from a factual, objective perspective. Often, family members gain new insights and can begin to understand their problems within the context of their family system. For example, families may begin to view depression in an adolescent daughter with new seriousness when they see it as part of a pattern of several generations of women who have struggled with depression. A husband, raised as an only child in a small town, may better understand his feelings of being overwhelmed after comparing his family structure with that of his wife, who comes from a large family of several generations living together in an urban centre (Box 16-2).

USING FAMILY THERAPY

Family therapy is useful for families who are having difficulty maintaining family integrity. Various theoretic perspectives are used in family therapy; the Minuchin and Bowen models discussed in the assessment section offer two examples. Family therapy can be short term or long term and is conducted by mental health specialists, including advanced practice PMH nurses.

SUMMARY OF KEY POINTS

- A family is a group of people who are connected emotionally, by blood, or in both ways and who have developed patterns of interactions and relationships. Families come in various compositions, including nuclear, extended, multigenerational, single-parent, and same-gender families. Cultural values and beliefs define family composition and roles.
- Nurses complete a comprehensive family assessment when they care for families for extended periods or if a patient has complex mental health problems.
- In building relationships with families, nurses must establish credibility and competence with the family. Unless the nurse listens and addresses the family's immediate needs first, the family will have difficulty engaging in the challenges of caring for someone with a mental disorder.
- The genogram is an assessment and intervention tool that is useful in understanding health problems, relationship issues, and social functioning across several generations.
- In assessing the family biologic domain, the nurse determines physical and mental health status and its effects on family functioning.
- Family members are often reluctant to discuss the mental disorders of family members because of the stigma associated with mental illness. In many instances, family members do not know whether mental illnesses were present in other generations.
- The family psychological assessment focuses on family development, the family life cycle, communication patterns, stress and coping abilities, and problem-solving skills. One assessment aim is to begin to understand family interpersonal relationships.
- The family life cycle is a process of expansion, contraction, and realignment of the relationship systems to support the entry, exit, and development of family members in a functional way. The nurse should determine whether a family fits any of the life cycle models. Families living in poverty may have a condensed life cycle.
- In assessing the family social domain, the nurse compiles data about the system itself, social and financial status, and formal and informal support networks.
- The family system model proposes that a balance should exist between the family system and the individual. A person needs family connection but also needs to be differentiated as an individual. Important concepts include triangles, family projection process, nuclear family emotional process, multigenerational transmission, sibling position, and emotional cutoff.
- The family structure model explains patterns of family interaction. Subsystems develop that also influence interaction patterns. Boundaries can vary from rigid to relaxed. The rigidity of the boundaries affects family functioning.
- Family interventions focus on supporting the family's biopsychosocial integrity and functioning as defined by its members. Family psychiatric nursing interventions include counselling, promotion of self-care activities, noticing strengths and resources, purposefully commending the family, supportive therapy, education and health teaching, and the use of genograms. Mental health specialists, including advanced practice nurses, conduct family therapy.
- Education of the family is one of the most useful interventions. Teaching the family about mental disorders, life cycles, family systems, and family interactions can help the family develop a new understanding of family functioning and the effects of mental disorders on the family.

CRITICAL THINKING CHALLENGES

1 Differentiate between a nuclear and extended family. How can a group of people who are unrelated by blood consider themselves a family?
2 Interview a family with a member who has a mental illness and identify who provides support to the individual and family during acute episodes of illness.
3 Interview someone from a different ethnic background regarding family beliefs about mental illness. Compare them to your own.

4 Develop a genogram for your family. Analyze the genogram in terms of its pattern of health problems, relationship issues, and social functioning.

5 A female patient, divorced with two small children, reports that she is considering getting married again to a man whom she met 6 months ago. She asks for help in considering the advantages and disadvantages of remarriage. Using the remarried family formulations life cycle model, develop a plan for structuring the counselling session.

6 Define Minuchin's term *family structure* and use that definition in observing your own family and its interaction.

7 Discuss what happens to a family that has rigid boundaries.

8 A family is finding it difficult to provide transportation to a support group for an adult member with mental illness. The family is committed to his treatment but is also experiencing severe financial stress because of another family illness. Using a problem-solving approach, outline a plan for helping the family explore solutions to the transportation problem.

WEB LINKS

www.aamft.org The American Association for Marriage and Family Therapy website offers help in finding a therapist and information on families and health. It also provides resources for practitioners.

www.bcfamily.com B-C Family Productions provides training products for advocates and providers in developing comprehensive systems of care for children and families.

www.fame.volnetmmp.net The Family Association for Mental Health Everywhere (FAME) "is an organization for family support when mental illness of any form is an issue." FAME is "run for and by families to reduce the stress of coping with mental illness by strengthening and supporting family members in their role as caregivers."

http://www.vifamily.ca The Vanier Institute of the Family was established in 1965 to promote the well-being of Canadian families. This national charitable organization offers support for students, educators, policy makers, and families. This site offers a newsroom and a virtual library.

http://mentalhelp.net Mental Help Net is one of the oldest mental health Internet guides for education and resources.

MOVIES

New Waterford Girl: 1999. Mooney Pottie, 15 years of age, lives in the coal-mining town of New Waterford on Cape Breton with her parents and four siblings. She feels confined within the bounds of her small-town life and yearns to leave. Her new friend, Lou, has moved with her mother from the Bronx to Cape Breton in an effort to get away from her boxer father. Though she sees the town and Mooney's warm family through different eyes, Lou helps Moonie with her plan to escape to the big city.

VIEWING POINTS: Consider the differences between Moonie's and Lou's families. How does the location and context of one's home and family influence family relationships? This story is set in the 1970s. Do you think things are different now in New Waterford?

Flower and Garnet: 2002. This very engaging story of a family living in British Columbia reveals the confusion of a young boy, Garnet, as he tries to understand his family and his world. Garnet's mother died giving birth to him, and Flower, Garnet's sister, has taken over the mothering role. His father's grief at the death of his wife remains unresolved. This award-winning film is both funny and moving in its portrayal of family dynamics.

VIEWING POINTS: What are the issues facing this family? What kind of support from the health care system would be helpful? What kind of efforts at support might not be suitable for this family?

REFERENCES

Bowen, M. (1975). Family therapy after twenty years. In S. Arieti, D. Freedman, & J. Dyrud (Eds.), *American handbook of psychiatry* (2nd ed., vol. 5, pp. 379–391). New York: Basic Books.

Bowen, M. (1976). Theory in the practice of psychotherapy. In P. Guerin (Ed.), *Family therapy: Theory and practice* (pp. 42–90). New York: Gardner Press.

Carpenito, L. (2003). *Nursing diagnosis: Application to clinical practice* (10th ed.). Philadelphia: Lippincott Williams & Wilkins.

Carter, B., & McGoldrick, M. (1999a). The divorce cycle: A major variation in the American family life cycle. In B. Carter & M. McGoldrick (Eds.), *The expanded family life cycle* (pp. 373–398). New York: Allyn & Bacon.

Carter, B., & McGoldrick, M. (1999b). Overview: The expanded family life cycle. Individual, family, and social perspectives. In B. Carter & M. McGoldrick (Eds.), *The expanded family life cycle* (pp. 1–26). New York: Allyn & Bacon.

Celano, M., & Kaslow, N. (2000). Culturally competent family interventions: Review and case illustrations. *American Journal of Family Therapy, 28,* 217–228.

Cuellar, N., & Butts, J. (1999). Caregiver distress: What nurses in rural settings can do to help. *Nursing Forum, 34*(3), 24–30.

Cuijpers, P. (1999). The effects of family interventions of relatives' burden: A meta-analysis. *Journal of Mental Health, 8*(3), 275–285.

Hartrick Doane, G., & Varcoe, C. (2005). *Family nursing as relational inquiry: Developing health-promoting practice.* Philadelphia: Lippincott Williams & Wilkins.

Hatfield, A. (1992). Leaving home: Separation issues in psychiatric illness. *Psychosocial Rehabilitation Journal, 15*(4), 37–47.

Hines, P. M. (1999). The family life cycle of African American families living in poverty. In B. Carter & M. McGoldrick (Eds.), *The expanded family life cycle* (pp. 327–345). New York: Allyn & Bacon.

Houger Limacher, L., & Wright, L. M. (2003). Commendations: Listening to the silent side of a family intervention. *Journal of Family Nursing, 9*(2), 130–150.

Hubble, M. A., Duncan, B. L., & Miller, S. D. (1999). *The heart and soul of change: What works in therapy*. Washington, DC: American Psychological Association.

Lambert, M. J. (1992). Implications of outcome research for psychotherapy integration. In J. C. Norcross & M. R. Goldfried (Eds.), *Handbook of psychotherapy integration* (pp. 94–129). New York: Basic Books.

McGoldrick, M., & Giordano, F. (1996). Overview: Ethnicity and family therapy. In M. McGoldrick, J. Giordano, & J. K. Pearce (Eds.), *Ethnicity and family therapy* (pp. 1–27). New York: The Guilford Press.

McGoldrick, M. (2003). Culture: A challenge to concepts of normality. In F. Walsh (Ed.), *Normal family processes: Growing diversity and complexity* (3rd ed., pp. 235–239). New York: Guilford Press.

Minuchin, S., Lee, W., & Simon, G. (1996). *Mastering family therapy: Journey of growth and transformation*. New York: John Wiley & Sons.

Schreiber, R., Noerager Stern, P., & Wilson, C. (2000). Being strong: How Black West-Indian Canadian women manage depression and its stigma. *Journal of Nursing Scholarship, 32*(1), 39–45.

Smith, G. C., Hatfield, A. B., & Miller, D. C. (2000). Planning by older mothers for the future care of offspring with serious mental illness. *Psychiatric Services, 51*(9), 1162–1166.

Turner, W. L., Wieling, E., & Allen, W. D. (2004). Becoming culturally effective family-based research programs: Implications for family therapists. *Journal of Mental and Family Therapy, 30*(3), 257–270.

Wright, L. M., & Leahey, M. (2005). *Nurses and families: A guide to family assessment and intervention*. Philadelphia: F. A. Davis.

Wright, L. M., Watson, W. L., & Bell, J. M. (1996). *Beliefs: The heart of healing in families and illness*. New York: The Guilford Press.

For challenges, please the **CD-ROM** in this book.

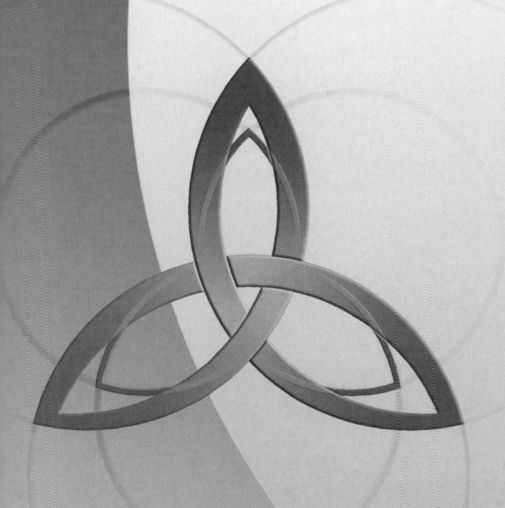

UNIT IV

Care of Persons with Psychiatric Disorders

CHAPTER 17

Schizophrenia

Andrea C. Bostrom, Mary Ann Boyd, and Hélène Provencher

LEARNING OBJECTIVES

After studying this chapter, you will be able to:

- Distinguish key symptoms of schizophrenia.
- Analyze the prevailing biologic, psychological, and social theories that are the basis for understanding schizophrenia.
- Analyze human response to schizophrenia with emphasis on hallucinations, delusions, and social isolation.
- Formulate nursing diagnoses based on a biopsychosocial assessment of people with schizophrenia.
- Formulate nursing interventions that address specific diagnoses based on a continuum of care.
- Analyze special concerns within the nurse–patient relationship common to treating those with schizophrenia.
- Identify expected outcomes and their evaluation.

KEY TERMS

affective flattening or blunting ▪ affective lability ▪ aggression ▪ agitation ▪ agranulocytosis ▪ akathisia ▪ alogia ▪ ambivalence ▪ anhedonia ▪ apathy ▪ autistic thinking ▪ avolition ▪ catatonic excitement ▪ circumstantiality ▪ clang association ▪ concrete thinking ▪ confused speech and thinking ▪ delusions ▪ echolalia ▪ echopraxia ▪ expressed emotion ▪ extrapyramidal side effects ▪ flight of ideas ▪ hallucinations ▪ hypervigilance ▪ hypofrontality ▪ illusions ▪ loose associations ▪ metonymic speech ▪ neologisms ▪ neuroleptic malignant syndrome ▪ oculogyric crisis ▪ paranoia ▪ paranoid schizophrenia ▪ polyuria ▪ pressured speech ▪ prodromal ▪ referential thinking ▪ regressed behaviour ▪ retrocollis ▪ stereotypy ▪ stilted language ▪ tangentiality ▪ tardive dyskinesia ▪ torticollis ▪ verbigeration ▪ waxy flexibility ▪ word salad

⬟ KEY CONCEPTS

disorganized symptoms ▪ negative symptoms ▪ neurocognitive impairment ▪ positive symptoms

Schizophrenia has fascinated and confounded healers, scientists, and philosophers for centuries. It is one of the most severe mental illnesses and is present in all cultures, races, and socioeconomic groups. Its symptoms have been attributed to possession by demons, considered punishment by gods for evils done, or accepted as evidence of the inhumanity of its sufferers. These explanations have resulted in enduring stigma for people with diagnoses of the disorder. Today the stigma persists, although it has less to do with demonic possession than with society's unwillingness to shoulder the tremendous costs associated with housing, treating, and rehabilitating patients with schizophrenia. All nurses need to understand this disorder.

Clinical Course

In the late 1800s, Emil Kraepelin first described the course of the disorder he called *dementia praecox*. In the early 1900s, Eugen Bleuler renamed the disorder *schizophrenia*, meaning *split minds*, and began to determine that there was not just one type of schizophrenia, but rather a group of schizophrenias. More recently, Kurt Schneider differentiated behaviours associated with schizophrenia as "first rank" symptoms (psychotic delusions, hallucinations) and "second rank" symptoms (all other experiences and behaviours associated with the disorder). These pioneering physicians had a great influence on the current diagnostic conceptualizations of schizophrenia that emphasize the heterogeneity of the disorder in terms of symptoms, course of illness, and positive and negative symptoms.

OVERVIEW OF SCHIZOPHRENIA

The clinical picture of schizophrenia is complex; individuals differ from one another; and the experience for a single individual may be different from episode to episode. The unique and deteriorating course of schizophrenia has been challenged by a number of longitudinal studies (Marengo, 1994). Ciompi (1989) identified eight possible long-term trajectories of schizophrenia. About 25% of people with schizophrenia experience a complete remission after one or several psychotic episodes (Westermeyer & Harrow, 1988; Wing, 1988). Early intervention, including pharmacologic and psychosocial interventions, is also promising for increasing the rate of recovery in people with first-onset schizophrenia (Liberman & Kopelowicz, 2005).

Acute Illness Period

Initially, the illness behaviours may be both confusing and frightening to the patient and the family. The changes may be subtle; however, at some point, the changes in thought and behaviour become so disruptive or bizarre that they can no longer be overlooked. These might include episodes of staying up all night for several nights, incoherent conversations, or aggressive acts against self or others. For example, one patient's parents reported their son walking around the apartment for several days holding his arms and hands as if they were a machine gun, pointing them at his parents and siblings, and saying "rat-a-tat-tat, you're dead." Another father described his son's first delusional–hallucination episode as so convincing that it was frightening. His son began visiting cemeteries and making "mind contact" with the deceased. He saw his deceased grandmother walking around in the home and was certain that there were pipe bombs in objects in his home. Another patient believed he had been visited by space aliens who wanted to unite their world with earth and assured him that he would become the leader of his country.

As symptoms progress, patients are less and less able to care for basic needs, such as eating, sleeping, and bathing. Substance use is common. Functioning at school or work deteriorates. Dependence on family and friends increases, and those individuals recognize the need for treatment. In the acute phase, these individuals with schizophrenia are at high risk for suicide. Patients usually are hospitalized to protect themselves or others.

The initial treatment focuses on alleviation of symptoms through initiation of medications, decreasing the risk for suicide through safety measures, normalizing sleep, and reducing substance use. Functional deficits persist during this period, and the patient and family must begin to learn to cope with these. Emotional blunting diminishes the ability and desire to engage in hobbies, vocational activities, and relationships. Limited participation in social activities spirals into numerous skill deficits, such as difficulty engaging others interpersonally. Cognitive deficits lead to problems recognizing patterns in situations and transferring learning and behaviours from one circumstance to another similar one.

Stabilization Period

After the initial diagnosis of schizophrenia and initiation of treatment, stabilization of symptoms becomes the focus. Symptoms become less acute but may be present. Treatment is intense during this period as medication regimens are established and patients and their families begin to adjust to the idea of a family member having a long-term severe mental illness. Ideally, the use of substances is eliminated. Socialization with others begins to increase, and rehabilitation begins.

Maintenance and Recovery Period

After the patient's condition is stabilized, the patient focuses on regaining the previous level of functioning and quality of life. Medication treatment of schizophrenia has generally contributed to an improvement in the lifestyle of people with this disorder; however, no medication has cured it. Faithful medication management tends to make the impairments in functioning less severe when they occur and to diminish the extremes an individual might experience. As with any chronic illness, stresses of life and major crises can contribute to exacerbations of symptoms.

Clearly family support and involvement are extremely important at this time. Once the initial diagnosis is made, patients and families must be educated to anticipate and expect relapse and know how to cope with it. This is one of the important themes throughout the nursing process for people with schizophrenia.

Relapses

Relapses can occur at any time during treatment and recovery. Relapse is not inevitable; however, it occurs with sufficient regularity to be a major concern in the treatment of schizophrenia. Relapses can occur and are very detrimental to the successful management of this disorder. With each relapse, there is a longer period of time to recover. Combining medications and psychosocial treatment greatly diminishes the severity and frequency of recurrent relapses (van Meijel, van der Gaag, Kahn, & Grypdonck, 2003).

One of the major reasons for relapse is noncompliance with medication regimen. Even with newer medication, compliance leading to relapse continues to be a problem (Leucht et al., 2003). Stopping use of medications almost certainly leads to a relapse and may actually be a stressor that causes a severe and rapid relapse (Baldessarini, 2002). Lower relapse rates are, for the most part, among groups who were following a treatment regimen.

Many other factors trigger relapse: the degree of impairment in cognition and coping that leaves patients vulnerable to stressors; the accessibility of community resources, such as public transportation, housing, entry-level and low-stress employment, and social services; income supports that buffer the day-to-day stressors of living; the degree of stigmatization that the community holds for mental illness that attacks the self-concept of patients; and the responsiveness of family members, friends, and supportive others (such as peers and professionals) when patients need help.

DIAGNOSTIC CRITERIA

The current definition outlined in the American Psychiatric Association's *Diagnostic and Statistical Manual of Mental Disorders*, 4th edition, text revision (*DSM-IV-TR*) (APA, 2000) states that schizophrenia is a mixture of positive and negative symptoms that present for a significant portion of a 1-month period but with continuous signs of disturbance persisting for at least 6 months.

Positive symptoms can be thought of as symptoms that exist but should not and negative symptoms as ones that should be there but are not.

> **KEY CONCEPT Positive symptoms** reflect an excess or distortion of normal functions, including delusions and hallucinations.

> **KEY CONCEPT Negative symptoms** reflect a lessening or loss of normal functions, such as restriction or flattening in the range and intensity of emotion (**affective flattening** or **blunting**); reduced fluency and productivity of thought and speech (**alogia**); withdrawal and inability to initiate and persist in goal-directed activity (**avolition**); and inability to experience pleasure (**anhedonia**).

The *DSM-IV-TR* criteria for diagnosing schizophrenia include necessary symptomatology, duration of symptoms, evaluation of functional impairment, and elimination of alternate hypotheses that might account for the symptoms (APA, 2000). Several schizophrenia subtypes are currently recognized: paranoid, disorganized, catatonic, undifferentiated, and residual. There is a growing belief that this subtyping is not useful for predicting the course and response to treatment. The diagnostic criteria and current subtypes are listed in Table 17-1 and Box 17-1, respectively.

Positive Symptoms of Schizophrenia

Delusions are erroneous fixed beliefs that usually involve a misinterpretation of experience. For example, the patient believes someone is reading his or her thoughts or plotting against him or her. Various types of delusions include the following:

- *Grandiose:* the belief that one has exceptional powers, wealth, skill, influence, or destiny
- *Nihilistic:* the belief that one is dead or a calamity is impending
- *Persecutory:* the belief that one is being watched, ridiculed, harmed, or plotted against
- *Somatic:* beliefs about abnormalities in bodily functions or structures

Hallucinations are perceptual experiences that occur without actual external sensory stimuli. They can involve any of the five senses, but they are usually *visual* or *auditory*. Auditory hallucinations are more common than visual ones. For example, the patient hears voices carrying on a discussion about his or her own thoughts or behaviours.

Table 17.1   Key Diagnostic Characteristics of Schizophrenia

Diagnostic Criteria and Target Symptoms

Diagnostic Criteria

- Two or more of the following characteristic symptoms present for a significant portion of time during a 1-month period: delusions; hallucinations; disorganized speech; grossly disorganized or catatonic behaviour; negative symptoms
- One or more major areas of social or occupational functioning (such as work, interpersonal relations, self-care) markedly below previously achieved level
- Continuous signs persisting for at least 6 months
- Absence or insignificant duration of major depressive, manic, or mixed episodes occurring concurrently with active symptoms
- Not a direct physiologic effect of a substance or medical condition
- Prominent delusions or hallucinations present when a prior history of autistic disorder or another pervasive developmental disorder exists

Target Symptoms and Associated Findings

- Inappropriate affect
- Loss of interest or pleasure
- Dysphoric mood (anger, anxiety, or depression)
- Disturbed sleep patterns

Associated Findings

- Lack of interest in eating or refusal of food
- Difficulty concentrating
- Some cognitive dysfunction, such as confusion, disorientation, memory impairment
- Lack of insight
- Depersonalization, derealization, and somatic concerns
- Motor abnormalities

Associated Physical Examination Findings

- Physically awkward
- Poor coordination or mirroring
- Motor abnormalities
- Cigarette-related pathologies, such as emphysema and other pulmonary and cardiac problems

Associated Laboratory Findings

- Enlarged ventricular system and prominent sulci in the brain cortex
- Decreased temporal and hippocampal size
- Increased size of basal ganglia
- Decreased cerebral size
- Slowed reaction times
- Abnormalities in eye tracking

Negative Symptoms of Schizophrenia

Negative symptoms are not as dramatic as positive symptoms, but they can interfere greatly with the patient's ability to function day to day. Because expressing emotion is

IN A LIFE

Émile Nelligan (1879–1941)
Canadian Poet

Public Persona
Considered one of the most important poets of Québec, Émile Nelligan had his first poem, *Rêve fantasque,* published (under a pseudonym) when he was only 17. *Romance du vin,* the poem that he dramatically presented at his only public reading, and *Vaisseau d'or* are two poems for which he is particularly famous. His work, however, includes 170 poems, sonnets, rondels, songs, and prose poems. Lyrical in nature with strong symbolic imagery, these works were collected and published in 1904.

Personal Realities
Émile Nelligan was born in Montréal to an Anglophone father who came to Canada from Ireland and a Francophone mother, known as a gifted musician. He was a handsome, sensitive young man who was torn between the two cultures of his parents. At the age of 20 years, just as he was gaining fame as a literary genius, he became ill with what was most likely schizophrenia. He spent the rest of his life in a psychiatric hospital, dying in the Hôpital Saint-Jean-de-Dieu on November 18, 1941.

difficult for them, people with schizophrenia laugh, cry, and get angry less often. Their affect is flat, and they show little or no emotion when personal loss occurs. They also suffer from **ambivalence**, which is the concurrent experience of equally strong opposing feelings so that it is impossible to make a decision. The avolition may be so profound that simple activities of daily living, such as dressing or combing hair, may not get done. Anhedonia prevents the person with schizophrenia from enjoying activities. People with schizophrenia have limited speech and difficulty saying anything new or carrying on a conversation. These negative symptoms cause the person with schizophrenia to withdraw and suffer feelings of severe isolation.

Neurocognitive Impairment

Neurocognitive impairment exists in schizophrenia and may be independent of positive and negative symptoms. Neurocognition includes memory (short- and long-term), vigilance or sustained attention, verbal fluency or the ability to generate new words, and executive functioning, which includes volition, planning, purposive action, and self-monitoring behaviour. Working memory is a concept that includes short-term memory and the ability to store and process information.

◆ KEY CONCEPT Neurocognitive impairment in memory, vigilance, and executive functioning is related to poor functional outcome in schizophrenia (Green, Kern, Braff, & Mintz, 2000).

BOX 17.1

Key Diagnostic Characteristics of Schizophrenia Subtypes

Paranoid Type: DSM-IV-TR 295.30
- Preoccupation with delusions or auditory hallucinations
- Lacks disorganized speech, disorganized or catatoric behaviour, or flat or inappropriate affect

Disorganized Type: DSM-IV-TR 295.10
- Disorganized speech, disorganized behaviour, and flat or inappropriate affect

Catatonic Type: DSM-IV-TR 295.20
At least two of the following characteristics present:
- Motor immobility or stupor
- Excessive purposeless motor activity
- Extreme negativism
- Posturing, stereotyped movements, prominent mannerisms, or prominent grimacing
- Echolalia or echopraxia

Undifferentiated Type: DSM-IV-TR 295.90
- Only characteristic symptoms present, but does not meet criteria for other subtypes

Residual Type: DSM-IV-TR 295.60
- Absence of prominent delusions, hallucinations, disorganized speech, and grossly disorganized or catatonic behaviour
- Negative symptoms persist, or two or more positive symptoms are present in attenuated form, such as odd beliefs or unusual perceptual experiences.

This impairment is independent of the positive symptoms. That is, cognitive dysfunction can exist even if the positive symptoms are in remission. Not all areas of cognitive functioning are impaired. Long-term memory and intellectual functioning are not necessarily affected. However, many people with the disorder appear to have low intellectual functioning, which may be related to lack of educational opportunities, which is common for people with mental illnesses. Neurocognitive dysfunction often is manifested in disorganized symptoms.

> ⬟ **KEY CONCEPT Disorganized symptoms** of schizophrenia are those things that make it difficult for the person to understand and respond to the ordinary sights and sounds of daily living. These include **confused speech and thinking** and **disorganized behaviour.**

Disorganized Thinking

Examples of disturbed speech and thinking patterns are to be found in Chapter 10, specifically in Boxes 10-6 and 10-7.

Disorganized perceptions often create an oversensitivity to colors, shapes, and background activities. **Illusions** occur when the person misperceives or exaggerates stimuli that actually exist in the external environment. This is in contrast to hallucinations, which are perceptions in the absence of environmental stimuli. Ancillary symptoms that may accompany schizophrenia include anxiety, depression, and hostility.

Disorganized Behaviour

Disorganized behaviour (which may manifest as very slow, rhythmic, or ritualistic movement), coupled with disorganized speech, makes it difficult for the person to partake in daily activities. Examples of disorganized behaviour include the following:

- **Aggression**—behaviours or attitudes that reflect rage, hostility, and the potential for physical or verbal destructiveness (usually comes about if the person believes someone is going to do him or her harm)
- **Agitation**—inability to sit still or attend to others, accompanied by heightened emotions and tension
- **Catatonic excitement**—a hyperactivity characterized by purposeless activity and abnormal movements such as grimacing and posturing
- **Echopraxia**—involuntary imitation of another person's movements and gestures
- **Regressed behaviour**—behaving in a manner of a less mature life stage; childlike and immature
- **Stereotypy**—repetitive, purposeless movements that are idiosyncratic to the individual and to some degree outside of the individual's control
- **Hypervigilance**—sustained attention to external stimuli as if expecting something important or frightening to happen
- **Waxy flexibility**—posture held in odd or unusual fixed position for extended periods of time

SCHIZOPHRENIA IN SPECIAL POPULATIONS

Children

The diagnosis of schizophrenia is rare in children before adolescence. When it does occur in children aged 5 or 6 years, the symptoms are essentially the same as in adults. In this age group, hallucinations tend to be visual and delusions less developed. Because disorganized speech and behaviour may be explained better by other disorders that are more common in childhood, those disorders should be considered before applying the diagnosis of schizophrenia to a child (APA, 2000).

However, new studies suggest that the likelihood of children later experiencing schizophrenia can be predicted. Developmental abnormalities in childhood, including delays in attainment of speech and motor development, problems in social adjustment, and poorer academic and cognitive performance have been found to be present in individuals who experience schizophrenia in adulthood. Specific factors that appear to predict schizophrenia in adulthood include problems in motor and neurologic development, deficits in attention and verbal short-term memory, poor social competence, positive formal thought disorder–like symptoms, and severe instability of early rearing environment (Niemi, Suvisaari, Tuulio-Henriksson, & Lonnqvist, 2003).

Older Adults

People with schizophrenia do grow old. For older persons who have had schizophrenia since young adulthood, this may be a time in which they experience some improvement in symptoms or relapse fluctuations. For instance, admission to general hospitals for older persons (age 65 years of older) with schizophrenia is more likely to be for an associated condition (Health Canada, 2002). Their lifestyle probably is dependent on the effectiveness of earlier treatment, the support systems that are in place (including relationships with family members and professionals), and the interaction between environmental stressors and the patient's functional impairments.

In late-onset schizophrenia, the diagnostic criteria are met after age 45 years. Women are affected more than men. The presentation of late-onset schizophrenia is most likely to include positive symptoms, particularly paranoid or persecutory delusions. Cognitive deterioration and affective blunting occur less frequently. Social functioning is more intact. Many individuals with diagnoses of late-onset schizophrenia have disturbances in sensory functions, primarily hearing and vision losses (APA, 2000). The cost of caring for older persons with schizophrenia remains high because many are no longer cared for in an institution, and community-based treatment has developed more slowly for this age group than for younger adults. We have little information regarding the effects of gender and ethnicity (Reeves, Stewart, & Howard, 2002).

Epidemiology

Schizophrenia occurs in all cultures and countries. The incidence and prevalence rates are similar across studies, with variations explained by the definition of schizophrenia and the sampling method used. It occurs in about 1.3% of the population, or more than 400,000 people in Canada (Goldner, Hsu, Waraich, & Somers, 2002). Its economic costs are enormous. Direct costs include treatment expenses, and indirect costs include lost wages, premature death, and incarceration. In addition, employment among people with schizophrenia is one of the lowest of any group with disabilities (New Freedom Commission on Mental Health, 2003).

The costs of schizophrenia in terms of individual and family suffering probably are inestimable.

People with schizophrenia tend to cluster in the lowest social classes in industrialized countries and urban communities. The symptoms of the illness are so pervasive that it is difficult for these individuals to maintain any type of gainful employment. Homelessness is a problem for the severely mentally ill (eg, people with schizophrenia or bipolar illness). People with schizophrenia may make up 11% to 14% of the homeless population, compared with 1% to 1.3% of the general population (U.S. DHHS, 2001).

RISK FACTORS

Risk factors for schizophrenia include stresses in the perinatal period (starvation, poor nutrition, infections), obstetrical complications, and genetic and family susceptibility. There has been recent evidence that parental age may also be a risk factor (Byrne, Agerbo, Ewald, Eaton, & Mortensen, 2003). Birth cohort studies suggest that the incidence may be higher among individuals born in urban settings than those born in rural ones and may be somewhat lower in later-born birth cohorts (Harrison et al., 2003). Infants affected by these maternal stressors may have conditions that create their own risk, such as low birth weight, short gestation, and early developmental difficulties. In childhood, stressors may include central nervous system infections.

AGE OF ONSET

Most people who experience schizophrenia have the disorder diagnosed in late adolescence and early adulthood. When schizophrenia begins earlier than age 25 years, symptoms seem to develop more gradually, and negative symptoms predominate throughout the course of the disease. People with early-onset schizophrenia experienced a greater number of neuropsychological problems. Finally, disruptions occur in milestone events of early adulthood, such as achieving in education, work, and long-term relationships (Csernansky, 2003).

GENDER DIFFERENCES

A gender difference for age of onset exists, with men having the disorder diagnosed earlier than women. The median age of onset for men is in the middle 20s, whereas the median age of onset for women is in the late 20s (APA, 2000). These gender differences have received attention because of hypotheses about sex-linked genetic etiologies. For instance, estrogen may play a protective role against the development of schizophrenia that disappears as estrogen levels drop during menopause (Hafner, 2003). This would account for the higher median age of onset and a more favorable treatment outcome in women.

ETHNIC AND CULTURAL DIFFERENCES

Increasingly, efforts are being made to consider culture and ethnic origin when diagnosing the disorder and treating individuals with symptoms of schizophrenia (APA, 2000; U.S. DHHS, 1999). Although symptoms of schizophrenia appear to be clearly defined, it is possible to find cultures in which what appears to be a hallucination may be considered a vision or a religious experience. In addition, behaviours such as averting eyes during a conversation or minimizing emotional expression may be culturally bound yet easily misinterpreted by clinicians of a different cultural or ethnic background.

Individuals of various racial groups may have varying diagnosis rates of schizophrenia. These findings may represent correct diagnosis or may reflect a misdiagnosis of the disorder based on a cultural bias of the clinician. Prevalence studies indicate a lower prevalence of schizophrenia in Asian versus non-Asian countries. It is not known if this difference is due to methodologic, genetic, environmental, or sociologic variables, such as stigma and underreporting (Goldner, Hsu, Waraich, & Somers, 2002).

FAMILIAL DIFFERENCES

First-degree biologic relatives (children, siblings, parents) of an individual with schizophrenia have a 10 times greater risk for schizophrenia than the general population (APA, 2000). Other relatives may have an increased risk for disorders within the "schizophrenia spectrum" (a group of disorders with some similarities of behaviour, such as schizoaffective disorder and schizotypal personality disorder) (APA, 2000).

COMORBIDITY

Several somatic and psychological disorders coexist with schizophrenia. It is estimated that nearly 50% of patients with schizophrenia have a comorbid medical condition (Box 17-2), but many of these illnesses are misdiagnosed or undiagnosed (Goldman, 1999). Recently, more attention has been paid to the causes of mortality among people with schizophrenia. Several physical disorders have been identified, including vision and dental problems, hypertension, diabetes, and sexually transmitted diseases (U.S. DHHS, 1999).

Substance Abuse and Depression

Among the behavioural comorbidities, substance abuse is common. Depression may also be observed in patients with schizophrenia. This is an important symptom for several reasons. First, depression may be evidence that the diagnosis of a mood disorder is more appropriate (see Chapters 19 and 23). Second, depression is not unusual in chronic stages of schizophrenia and deserves attention. Third, the suicide rate (10%) among individuals with schizophrenia is higher than that of the general population. Risk factors for suicide are male gender, chronic illness with frequent relapses, frequent short hospitalizations, a negative attitude

---

BOX 17.2 RESEARCH FOR BEST PRACTICE

Disordered Water Balance

THE QUESTION: The St. Louis Target Weight Procedure (STWP) was developed to help patients with disordered water balance control their fluid intake. It required establishing baseline and target weights and monitoring weight throughout the day. The baseline weight was determined as an early morning weight before dressing, after voiding, and before any oral intake. The target weight was calculated to be 105% of the baseline weight. The purpose of this study was to determine whether the STWP was useful in controlling hyponatremia. Patients with disordered water balance were weighed throughout the day; when their target weight was elevated, fluids were restricted.

METHODS: Thirty subjects hospitalized in a long-term care facility who met the criteria for disordered water balance volunteered for the 6-week study. The subjects were randomly assigned to one of two groups. Urine specific gravities served as the dependent variable and were collected daily at 4:00 PM. It was reasoned that urine specific gravities would approach normal if fluid balance was normalized. Baseline data on both groups were collected for the first 3 weeks. During weeks 4 through 6, the STWP was used for the treatment group. This group was weighed throughout the day and was restricted from drinking when their target weight was reached. The other group served as a control.

FINDINGS: Study results showed that the STWP group significantly increased its urine specific gravities, thus improving fluid balance. These findings demonstrated the clinical utility of the STWP.

IMPLICATIONS FOR NURSING: A nurse working in a long-term psychiatric setting used the results of this study to introduce a target weight procedure as a new nursing intervention for patients with water intoxication or fluid imbalance. The procedure was modified for use in this particular institution and was piloted on one unit before being introduced to the whole hospital.

From Boyd, M., Williams, L., Evenson, R., Eckert, A., Beaman, M., & Carr, T. R. (1992). A target weight procedure for disordered water balance in long-term care facilities. *Journal of Psychosocial Nursing and Mental Health Services, 30*(12), 22–27.

toward treatment, impulsive behaviour, parasuicide (nonfatal self-harm or gesture), psychosis, and depression (De Hert, McKenzie, & Peuskens, 2001). More recently, periods of untreated psychosis exceeding 1 year and treatment with older typical antipsychotic drugs also have been associated with a higher risk for suicide attempts (Altamura, Bassetti, Bignotti, Pioli, & Mundo, 2003).

Diabetes Mellitus

There is a renewed interest in the relationship of diabetes mellitus and schizophrenia. Years ago, an association was established between glucose regulation and psychiatric disorders (Franzen, 1970; Schimmelbusch, Mueller, & Sheps, 1971). In fact, insulin shock therapy was used in treating severe disorders. Also of growing concern is the possibility that people with schizophrenia may be more prone to type II diabetes than is the general public. Some suggest (Ryan, Collins, & Thakore, 2003) that this may be attributable to inherent characteristics. Evidence that supports this view includes a higher rate of type II diabetes in first-degree relatives of people with schizophrenia and higher rates of impaired glucose tolerance and insulin resistance among people with schizophrenia. However, obesity, which is associated with type II diabetes, is a growing problem in North America in general and is complicated in schizophrenia treatment by the tendency of individuals to gain weight once their disease is managed with medications. Weight gain in some individuals may be attributed to a return to a healthier living situation in which regular meals are available and symptoms that interfere with obtaining food regularly (eg, delusions) are decreased. For other individuals, weight gain may result from the antipsychotic drug (either typical or atypical) selected for treatment.

Disordered Water Balance

Patients with schizophrenia, particularly of early onset, may experience disordered water balance. Often this takes the form of water intoxication characterized by abnormally high water intake, followed by a rapid drop in serum sodium levels. The alteration in sodium level leads to diverse neurologic signs, ranging from ataxia to coma and possibly death. The prevalence rates of disordered water balance reportedly range from 6% (Mercier-Guidez & Loas, 2000) to 17.5% (Blum et al., 1983). The apparent decrease in prevalence may represent a real change or a difference in definition of water imbalance.

The cause of water intoxication is unknown. Research studies, conducted primarily in the 1990s, suggest multiple causes, including impaired renal excretion because of increased production of the antidiuretic hormone (ADH) arginine vasopressin; an abnormality in the hippocampal area of the brain causing stereotypical repetitive drinking behaviour; faulty osmoregulation of fluid intake; and a neurobiologic dysfunction that affects the ADH thirst and salt-appetite mechanisms (Boyd & Lapierre, 1996).

Disordered water balance generally precedes water intoxication. Patients characteristically begin compulsively drinking excessive amounts of water (polydipsia) in the morning, followed by diurnal (daytime) weight gain in the afternoon. The fluid weight gain produces generalized edema, cellular dysfunction, diminished serum osmolality, and dilution of serum sodium. By midday as fluid volumes increase and serum sodium levels decrease, symptoms of chronic hyponatremia appear (Box 17-3). These symptoms generally resolve overnight as excess fluid is excreted and sodium levels gradually rise. Often a benign condition, disordered water balance may go undetected for months to years; however, ingesting large amounts of water over a prolonged period may lead to complications, such as renal dysfunction, urinary incontinence, flaccid bladder, hydronephrosis, cardiac failure, malnutrition, hernia, dilation of the gastrointestinal tract, or permanent brain damage (Boyd & Lapierre, 1996).

Water intoxication, a complication that is life threatening, occurs when unusually large volumes of ingested water overwhelm the kidneys' capacity to excrete water. As a result, serum sodium levels rapidly fall below the normal range of 135 to 145 mEq/L to a level of 120 mEq/L or less (acute hyponatremia; see Box 17-3). This rapid decrease in sodium produces muscle twitching and irritability and puts the patient at risk for seizures or coma. The physiologic signs and symptoms of disordered water balance and its progression are presented in Box 17-4.

Behaviourally, these patients seem to be "driven to drink" (polydipsia) and may consume between 4 and 10 liters of fluid a day. They carry soda cans and water bottles with them, hoard cups or other water containers, and drink frequently from fountains and showers and sometimes from toilets. They make frequent trips to the bathroom because of the excessive need to urinate (**polyuria**). Generally the amount of urine excreted reflects the amount of fluid ingested. The patient's urine becomes very dilute with a very low specific gravity, which may

---

BOX 17.3

Signs and Symptoms of Hyponatremia

Chronic Hyponatremia
Generalized weakness, giddiness, headache, irritability, loss of appetite, muscle cramps, nausea, restlessness, slight confusion, and vomiting.

Acute Hyponatremia
Coma, confusion, decreased serum osmolality, decreased urine osmolality, increased urinary volume, lethargy, muscle twitching, seizures, specific urine gravity < 1.010, and weakness.

BOX 17.4

Physiologic Signs and Symptoms of Disordered Water Balance

Mild Disordered Water Balance

- Increased diurnal weight gain
- Urine specific gravity (1.011–1.025)
- Normal serum sodium (135–145 mEq/L)

Moderate Disordered Water Balance

- Increased diurnal weight gain
- Urine specific gravity (1.010–1.003)
- Possible facial puffiness
- Periodic nocturia

Severe Disordered Water Balance

- Possible evidence of stomach or bladder dilation
- Urine specific gravity (1.003–1.000)
- Frequent signs of nausea, vomiting
- Possible history of major motor seizure
- Possible change in blood pressure or pu se
- Polyuria
- Polydipsia
- Urinary incontinence during the night

From Snider, K., & Boyd, M. (1991). When they drink too much: Nursing interventions for patients with disordered water balance. *Journal of Psychosocial Nursing, 29*(7), 13.

BOX 17.5

Deficits That Cause Vulnerability In Schizophrenia

Cognitive Deficits

- Deficits in processing complex information
- Deficits in maintaining a steady focus of attention
- Inability to distinguish between relevant and irrelevant stimuli
- Difficulty forming consistent abstractions
- Impaired memory

Psychophysiologic Deficits

- Deficits in sensory inhibition
- Poor control of autonomic responsiveness

Social Skills Deficits

- Impairments in processing interpersonal stimuli, such as eye contact or assertiveness
- Deficits in conversational capacity
- Deficits in initiating activities
- Deficits in experiencing pleasure

Coping Skills Deficits

- Overassessment of threat
- Underassessment of personal resources
- Overuse of denial

Adapted from McGlashan, T. H. (1994). Psychosocial treatments of schizophrenia: The potential relationships. In N. C. Andreasen (Ed.), *Schizophrenia: From mind to molecule* (pp. 189–215). Washington, DC: American Psychiatric Press.

---

reflect a condition called hyposthenuria, in which the specific gravity falls below 1.008. Because of increased urgency and incontinence, especially at nighttime, the patient's clothing and room may smell like urine. Some patients may become highly agitated when efforts are made to limit access to water and other fluids. Other emotional/behavioural responses, such as increased psychotic symptoms, irritability, and lability, are caused by changes in sodium levels and the rapidity with which they occur.

Etiology

Since the 1970s, hypothetical causes of schizophrenia have changed dramatically, (Gur & Gur, 2005; Murray & Bramon, 2005; Walker et al., 2004). Purely psychological theories have been replaced by a neurobiologic model that says that patients with schizophrenia have a biologic predisposition or vulnerability that is exacerbated by environmental stressors. Those with schizophrenia are thought to have a genetically or biologically determined sensitivity that leaves them vulnerable to an overwhelming onslaught of stimuli from without and within (U.S. DHHS, 1999). These inherent vulnerabilities include cognitive, psychophysiologic, social competence, and coping deficits that alter the individual's ability, both cognitively and emotionally, to manage life events and interpersonal situations (Box 17-5 and Fig. 17-1).

Biologic Theories

Theories and research about the biologic vulnerability for schizophrenia focus on incorporating multiple observations into a coherent explanation. These observations include the course of the illness already

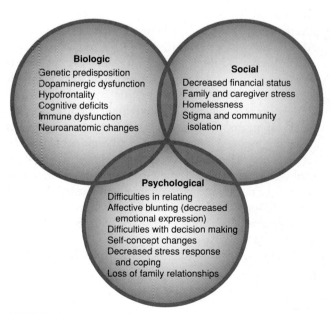

FIGURE 17.1 Biopsychosocial etiologies for patients with schizophrenia.

described, possible brain structure changes identified by postmortem and neuroimaging techniques, familial patterns, and pharmacologic effects on behaviour and neurotransmitter functions in the brain. One of the more recent theories about the cause of schizophrenic vulnerability focuses on neurodevelopment of the brain from the prenatal period through adolescence. This section describes the various observations and current theories about the cause of schizophrenia. However, the exact cause of schizophrenia remains elusive.

Neuroanatomic Findings

Postmortem and neuroimaging brain studies of patients with schizophrenia show four consistent changes in brain anatomy:

- decreased blood flow to the left globus pallidus early in the disease
- absence of normal blood flow increase in frontal lobes during tests of frontal lobe functioning, such as working memory tasks
- thinner cortex of the medial temporal lobe and a smaller anterior portion of the hippocampus
- decreases in gray matter and enlarged lateral and third ventricles and widened sulci (Chance, Esiri, & Crow, 2003)

These findings are being used as a basis for exploring the influence of genetic loading, obstetric complications, and differences in familial and nonfamilial patients with schizophrenia (Falkai et al., 2003; McDonald et al., 2002).

Familial Patterns

Evidence supports a familial or genetic base for schizophrenia. First-degree relatives (including siblings and children) are 10 times more likely to experience schizophrenia than are individuals in the general population (APA, 2000; U.S. DHHS, 1999). Concordance for schizophrenia is higher among monozygotic (identical) twins than among dizygotic (fraternal) twins, although the rate is not perfectly concordant.

Genetic researchers have sought to identify specific genes responsible for schizophrenia, but replicated results are emerging very slowly (Tsuang, Stone, & Faraone, 2001). The infrequency of reproducible results is likely attributable to the heterogeneity of the disorder, which may not be consistent with a single gene theory. A model that includes several genes is more likely to explain the development of schizophrenia (U.S. DHHS, 1999). Two possible locations are on the long arm of chromosome 22 and on chromosome 6 (Kandel, Schwartz, & Jessell, 2000).

Neurodevelopment

Current theory and research attempt to explain how genes or events early in life (especially perinatal events

such as infections or obstetric irregularities) would cause schizophrenia yet manifest symptoms only after years—in adolescence or young adulthood. The neurodevelopmental theory explains and reconciles the inconsistent neuroanatomic brain changes that have been found and links them to early development.

Brain development from prenatal periods through adolescence requires several coordinated molecular activities, including cell proliferation, cell migration, axonal outgrowth, pruning of neuronal connections, programmed cell death, and myelination. All these activities require coordinated development, usually through activation and inactivation of proteins by genes. Any of these processes could be disrupted by (1) inherited genes that place the individual at risk for schizophrenia, (2) a wild-type allele of this gene that is activated in adolescence or early adulthood; or (3) genetic sensitizing that leaves the individual susceptible to environmental causes or lesioning during some adverse perinatal event. In addition, several maturational events normally occur during puberty that may affect brain development: (1) changes in dopaminergic, serotonergic, adrenergic, glutamatergic, gamma-aminobutyric acid (GABA)-ergic, and cholinergic neurotransmitter systems and substrates; (2) a complex combination of synaptic pruning along with substantial brain growth in some areas of the cortex; and (3) changes in the steroid-hormonal environment (Chou, Halldin, & Farde, 2003).

Neurotransmitters, Pathways, and Receptors

Theories about the cause and pathophysiology of schizophrenia have been generated from decades of pharmacologic research and management of the disorder. For years, the leading hypothesis about the neurobiology of schizophrenia has been based on observations of drug actions. The *dopamine hypothesis* of schizophrenia arose from observations that antipsychotic drugs (Table 17-2), which so successfully ameliorate or reduce the positive symptoms of schizophrenia, act primarily by blocking postsynaptic dopamine receptors in the brain. In addition, other drugs that enhance dopamine function, such as amphetamines or cocaine, cause behavioural symptoms similar to those of **paranoid schizophrenia** in humans and bizarre stereotyped behaviour in monkeys. Antipsychotic drugs stop these drug-induced behaviours. Based on these observations, researchers concluded that schizophrenia was a syndrome of hyperdopaminergic action in the brain.

This old, straightforward hypothesis of dopamine hyperactivity is clearly complicated by recent findings. Positron emission tomography (PET) scan findings suggest that in schizophrenia, there is a general reduction in brain metabolism, with a relative hypermetabolism in the left side of the brain and in the left temporal lobe. Abnormalities exist in specific areas of the brain, such as in the

Table 17.2	Selected Antipsychotic Drugs	
Generic Name	**Trade Name**	**Dosage Range for Adults (mg/d)**
Selected Conventional Antipsychotic Drugs *Used to Treat Psychosis in the United States*		
First-Generation		
chlorpromazine	Thorazine	30–800
fluphenazine	Prolixin; Permitil	0.5–20
haloperidol	Haldol	1–15
loxapine	Loxitane	20–250
mesoridazine	Serentil	100–300
molindone	Moban	15–225
perphenazine	Trilafon	4–32
pimozide	Orap*	1–10
prochlorperazine	Compazine[†]	15–25
thiothixene	Navane	5–25
trifluoperazine	Stelazine	5–25
triflupromazine	Vesprin	60–150
Second-Generation		
aripiprazole	Abilify	10–15
clozapine	Clozaril	200–600
risperidone	Risperdal	4–16
olanzapine	Zyprexa	10–20
quetiapine	Seroquel	300–400
ziprasidone	Geodon	40–160

*Approved in the United States for Tourette's syndrome.
[†]Adapted from Stahl, S. (2000). *Essential psychopharmacology: Neuroscientific basis and practical application* (2nd ed., p. 404). Cambridge, UK: Cambridge University Press.

left globus pallidus (Sedvall, 1994). These findings support further exploration of differential brain hemisphere function in schizophrenia (Fig. 17-2). Other PET studies show **hypofrontality**, or a reduced cerebral blood flow and glucose metabolism in the prefrontal cortex of people with schizophrenia and hyperactivity in the limbic area (Buchsbaum, 1990) (Figs. 17-3 and 17-4). In addition, several types of dopamine receptors (labeled D_1, D_2, D_3, D_4, and D_5) and dopamine are found in four pathways (mesolimbic, mesocortical, nigrostriatal, and tuberoinfundibular) that innervate different parts of the brain (Kandel et al., 2000) (see Chapter 8). Based on the current understanding of schizophrenia, the following discussion relates the neurobiologic changes to the clinical symptoms.

Positive Symptoms: Hyperactivity of Mesolimbic Tract

Positive symptoms of schizophrenia (hallucinations and delusions) are thought to be caused by dopamine *hyperactivity* in the mesolimbic tract, which regulates memory and emotion. It is hypothesized that this hyperactivity could result from overactive modulation of neurotransmission from the nucleus accumbens (Kandel et al., 2000). Another explanation for dopaminergic hyperactivity in

the mesolimbic tract is hypoactivity of the mesocortical tract, which normally inhibits dopamine activity in the mesolimbic tract by some type of feedback mechanism. In schizophrenia, the primary defect may be in the mesocortical tract, where dopaminergic function is diminished, thereby decreasing the inhibitory effects on the mesolimbic tract. This disinhibition may be responsible for the overactivity of dopamine in the mesolimbic tract, resulting in the positive symptom cluster (Kandel et al., 2000).

Support for this interconnection between mesocortical and mesolimbic tracts has been found in laboratory animals. Destruction of the mesocortical tract of animals resulted in increased activity in the mesolimbic tract, especially in the nucleus accumbens. A compensatory increase in mesolimbic neurons is a suggested mechanism by which this overactivity occurs.

Negative Symptoms and Cognitive Impairment: Hypoactivity of the Mesocortical Tract

Negative symptoms and cognitive impairment are thought to be related to hypoactivity of the mesocortical dopaminergic tract, which by its association with the

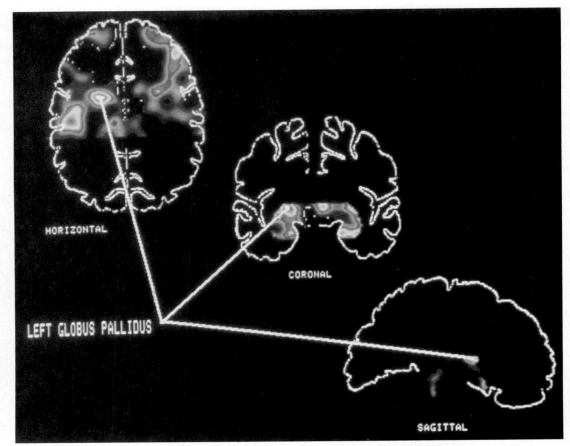

FIGURE 17.2   Area of abnormal functioning in a person with schizophrenia. These three views show the excessive neuronal activity in the left globus pallidus (portion of the basal ganglia next to the putamen). (Courtesy of John W. Haller, PhD, Departments of Psychiatry and Radiology, Washington University, St. Louis, MO.)

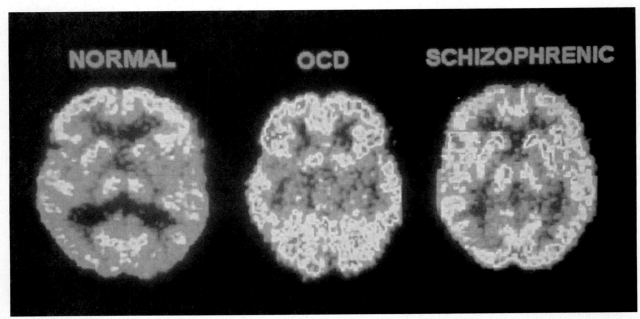

FIGURE 17.3   Metabolic activity in a control subject (*left*), a subject with obsessive-compulsive disorder (center), and a subject with schizophrenia (*right*). (Courtesy of Monte S. Buchsbaum, MD, The Mount Sinai Medical Center and School of Medicine, New York, NY.)

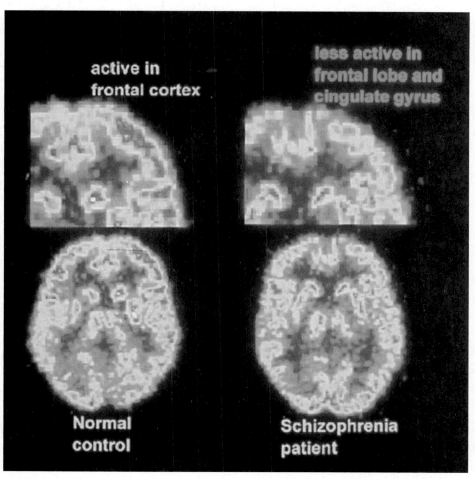

FIGURE 17.4 Positron emission tomography (PET) scan with ^{18}F-deoxyglucose shows metabolic activity in a horizontal section of the brain in a control subject (*left*) and in an unmedicated patient with schizophrenia (*right*). Red and yellow indicate areas of high metabolic activity in the cortex; green and blue indicate lower activity in the white-matter areas of the brain. The frontal lobe is magnified to show reduced frontal activity in the prefrontal cortex of the patient with schizophrenia. (Courtesy of Monte S. Buchsbaum, MD, The Mount Sinai Medical Center and School of Medicine, New York, NY.)

prefrontal and neocortex contributes to motivation, planning, sequencing of behaviours in time, attention, and social behaviour (Jibson & Tandon, 2000; Kandel et al., 2000). Negative symptoms, such as poor motivation and planning and flat affect, are remarkably similar to symptoms of patients who underwent lobotomy procedures in the late 1940s and early 1950s to disconnect the frontal cortex from the rest of the brain. Monkeys who have had dopamine in the prefrontal cortex depleted have difficulty with cognitive tasks. Finally, PET scans of energy metabolism suggest a reduced metabolism in frontal and prefrontal areas (Davidson & Heinrichs, 2003).

Role of Other Dopamine Pathways

The tuberoinfundibular dopaminergic tract is active in prolactin regulation and may be the source of neuroendocrine changes observed in schizophrenia. The nigrostriatal dopaminergic tract modulates motor activity and is believed to be the site of the **extrapyramidal side effects** of antipsychotic drugs, such as pseudoparkinsonism and tardive dyskinesia. This may also be the site of some motor symptoms of schizophrenia, such as stereotypic behaviour.

Role of Other Receptors

Other receptors are also involved in dopamine neurotransmission, especially serotonergic receptors. It is becoming clear that schizophrenia does not result from dysregulation of a single neurotransmitter or biogenic amine (eg, norepinephrine, dopamine, or serotonin). Investigators are also hypothesizing a role for glutamate and GABA (Ghose et al., 2003) because of the complex interconnections of neuronal transmission and the complexity and heterogeneity of schizophrenia symptoms. The N-methyl-D-aspartate (NMDA) class of glutamate receptor is being studied because of the actions of phencyclidine (PCP) at these sites and the similarity of the psychotic behaviours that are produced when someone takes PCP (see Figs. 17-2, 17-3, and 17-4).

Neural Connectivity

Manifestations of poor mental coordination include difficulty in a variety of functions, such as measuring time or space, making inferences about relationships, and coordinating the processing, priority setting, retrieval, and expression of information. It is now being hypothesized that there may be a basic developmental disorder of the neural connectivity involving multiple molecular mechanisms (Benes, 2000; Penn, 2001; Sallet et al., 2003).

PSYCHOLOGICAL THEORIES

Several psychological frameworks have been used to explain the etiology of schizophrenia. Before new biologic and neurochemical discoveries, these psychological theories, held by the mental health community, viewed the primary cause of schizophrenia to be dysfunctional parenting in early childhood development. Families often were blamed and alienated by mental health professionals. These theories are no longer held valid, and neurochemical-biologic theories have replaced them.

SOCIAL THEORIES

There are no social theories believed to explain schizophrenia, but some theories focus on patterns of family interaction that seem to affect the eventual outcome and social adjustment of individuals with schizophrenia. The theory of **expressed emotion** (EE) correlates certain family communication patterns with an increase in symptoms and relapse in patients with schizophrenia. Families are classified as high-EE families when they make comments about family members; when there are aspects of speech that connote criticism, hostility, and negativity about the patient; and when they are emotionally overly involved with the patient, such as overprotective or self-sacrificing. Low-EE families make fewer negative comments and show less overinvolvement with the patient. Families that rate high in the areas of criticism, hostility, and battles for control are hypothesized to be associated with increases in the patient's positive symptoms and relapse.

Research related to emotional expressiveness is contradictory. Although families categorized as low in EE have been shown to accept the patient as having a legitimate illness and have an understanding that interpersonal problems can exacerbate the illness (Weisman, Gomes, & Lopez, 2003), families high in EE have not been associated with either a greater family history of schizophrenia or the chronicity of the illness (Subotnik, Goldstein, Nuechterlein, Woo, & Mintz, 2002; Wuerker, Long, Haas, & Bellack, 2002).

Although this research might contribute to the understanding of how negative family interaction affects the patient, there are drawbacks to categorizing families in this manner. Professionals may tend to blame families for causing schizophrenia or limit the patient's contact with family, thus further alienating families who are so vital to the care and support of the patient.

There are numerous social barriers that prevent people with mental illness from getting the care they need. One of the major ones is the social stigma that surrounds mental illnesses (see Chapter 3). Box 17-6 describes the impact of living with a stigmatized illness. Another obstacle, unfair treatment limitation and financial requirements placed on mental health benefits and private health insurance, inhibits quality and continuity of care. Finally, the mental health service delivery system is fragmented, and the quality and types of services vary from community to community (New Freedom Commission on Mental Health, 2003).

Interdisciplinary Treatment

The most effective treatment approach for individuals with schizophrenia involves a variety of disciplines, including nursing (both generalist and advanced practice psychiatric nurses), psychiatry, psychology, social work, occupational and recreational therapy, and pastoral counselling. Pharmacologic management is the responsibility of the physicians and nurses; various psychosocial interventions can be implemented by all the members of the mental health team. Individuals with

---

BOX 17.6

Clinical Vignette: Graduate Student in Peril

BGW, born in 1973, spent most of his teenage years using drugs and alcohol, behaviour that started when he was 11. He and his small group of friends spent their teenage years outside of school running around on bicycles. He failed 8th grade, repeated it, and made it to 10th grade. He was removed permanently from school at the age of 16 years. His dress included a dirty denim jacket or Army fatigues, torn tee shirts with rock band logos, and tight-fitting jeans. At age 16, he was hospitalized for a psychotic episode initiated by LSD; it was the scariest moment of his life. His mind had been getting fuzzier every day; he had dabbled with black magic and Satanism. Later, he admitted that for years he had been trapped in a fantasy land, only partially explained by his drug use.

Years of treatment followed, and even with abstinence from drugs, his mental status fluctuated. Once antipsychotic agents were prescribed, he began to feel like himself. He was motivated to complete his high school diploma and entered college. He kept his mental illness a secret. While in graduate school, his thoughts, feelings, and behaviours began to change. His thinking became delusional, his moods unpredictable, and his behaviours illogical. Finally, he was hospitalized once again, and his condition was stabilized with medication. Currently, he is reapplying to graduate school and this time vowing to keep people close to him aware of his mental status.

Adapted from First Person Account: Graduate Student in Peril. (2002). *Schizophrenia Bulletin, 28*(4), 745–755.

general education in psychology, sociology, and social work often serve as case managers, nursing aids or technicians, and other support personnel in hospitals and community treatment agencies. These varied professionals and paraprofessionals are necessary because of the complex nature of the symptoms and chronic course of schizophrenia.

A considerable amount of overlap exists among these professionals and the therapeutic interventions and services they perform. Advanced practice nurses, along with psychiatrists, may monitor or prescribe psychoactive medications, depending on state nurse practice acts. Individual, group, and family counselling may be performed by advanced practice nurses, psychiatrists, psychologists, certified social workers, and pastoral counsellors. Nurses, along with occupational and recreational therapists, can help patients with schizophrenia cope with the disruptions in their day-to-day functioning caused by cognitive and social deficits associated with negative symptoms. Teams of professionals working from all these perspectives create the best environment for stabilizing and enhancing the lives of people who have schizophrenia. However, barriers to this type of treatment abound and include inadequate funding and reimbursements, staff shortages, huge caseloads, and insufficient community facilities to serve patients whose time in inpatient care facilities is all too brief.

Despite the barriers, nurses can play a central role in multidisciplinary teams because of nursing's emphasis on patients' responses to their illness, patients' functional adaptation, and patients' holistic needs, including their physical and psychosocial requirements.

Priority Care Issues

Several special concerns exist when working with people with schizophrenia. About 20% to 50% of people with the diagnosis of schizophrenia attempt suicide, and 10% commit suicide either as a result of psychosis in acute stages or in response to depression in the chronic phase (De Hert et al., 2001). Suicide assessment always should be done with a person who is experiencing his or her first psychotic episode. In an inpatient unit, patient safety concerns extend to potential aggressive actions toward staff and other patients during episodes of psychoses. A priority of care during times of acute illness is treatment with antipsychotic medications. During the chronic phase of schizophrenia, patients need help in accepting their illness and developing expectations for their future that are realistic. They also need help to avoid social isolation through improved social and vocational skills and living arrangements that ensure contact with others (De Hert et al., 2001). Interventions that focus on these goals may address the hopelessness that leads to suicide.

Family Response To Disorder

Few families have had experience with mental illness to help them deal with the manifestations of schizophrenia. The initial episodes are often accompanied by mixed emotions of disbelief, shock, fear, and care and concern for the family member. Hope that this is an isolated or transient episode may also be present. Families initially may seek reasons, attributing the episode to taking illicit drugs or to extraordinary stress or fatigue. They do not know how to comfort their disturbed family member and may find themselves fearful of his or her behaviours. If the patient is hostile and aggressive toward family members, the family may respond with anger and hostility along with fear, confusion, and anxiety. During these episodes, some families seek help from police to control the situation.

The initial period of illness for a patient and family who receive a diagnosis of schizophrenia is extraordinarily difficult. Families may deny the severity and chronicity of the illness, engage in the activities of their previous lifestyle, and only partially engage in treatment within the mental health system. Often, during the initial phase of treatment, explanation and education about the illness may be minimal. As families acknowledge the severity of the diagnosis and the long-term care and extensive rehabilitation required, they may feel overwhelmed, angry, and depressed.

NURSING MANAGEMENT: HUMAN RESPONSE TO DISORDER

The nursing management of the patient with schizophrenia lasts many years. Different phases of the illness require various nursing interventions. During exacerbation of symptoms, many patients are hospitalized for stabilization. During periods of relative stability, the nurse helps the patient maintain a therapeutic regimen, develop positive mental health strategies, and cope with the stress of having a severe, chronic illness.

Because of the complexity of this major psychiatric disorder, the nursing management for each domain is discussed separately. In reality, the nursing process steps overlap in all domains. For example, medication management is a direct biologic intervention; however, the effects of medications also are seen in psychological functioning. In the clinical area, effective nursing management requires an integration of the assessment data from all domains into meaningful interventions. Nursing interventions should cover all aspects of functioning, including biologic, psychological, social, and family functioning. See Nursing Care Plan 17-1 and the Interdisciplinary Treatment Plan that follows.

Many nursing diagnoses apply to a person with schizophrenia. This is particularly true given that schizophrenia affects so many aspects of an individual's functioning and

NURSING CARE PLAN 17.1

Patient With Schizophrenia

JT is a 19-year-old man who was brought to the hospital following his return from college, where he had locked himself in his room for 3 days. He was talking to nonexistent people in a strange language. His room was covered with small pieces of taped paper with single words on them. His parents immediately made arrangements for him to be hospitalized.

SETTING: PSYCHIATRIC INTENSIVE CARE UNIT

Baseline Assessment: JT is a 6'1", 145-lb young man whose appearance is disheveled. He has not slept for 4 days and appears frightened. He is hypervigilant, pacing, and mumbling to himself. He is vague about past drug use, but his parents do not believe that he has used drugs. He appears to be hallucinating, conversing as if someone is in the room. He is confused and unable to write, speak, or think coherently. He is disoriented to time and place. Lab values are within normal limits except Hgb, 10.2 and Hct, 32. He has not eaten for several days.

Associated Psychiatric Diagnosis	Medications
Axis I: Schizophrenia, paranoid Axis II: None Axis III: None Axis IV: Educational problems (failing) Social problems (withdrawn from peers) GAF = Current 25 Potential?	Risperidone (Risperdal), 2 mg bid, then titrate to 3 mg if needed Lorazepam (Ativan) 2 mg PO or IM for agitation PRN

NURSING DIAGNOSIS 1: DISTURBED THOUGHT PROCESSES

Defining Characteristics	Related Factors
Inaccurate interpretation of stimuli (people thinking his thoughts) Cognitive impairment—attention, memory, and executive function impairment Suspiciousness Hallucinations	Uncompensated alterations in brain activity

Outcomes

Initial	Long-Term
Decrease or eliminate hallucinations Accurate interpretation of environment (stop thinking people are thinking his thoughts) Improvement in cognitive functioning (improved attention, memory, executive functioning)	Use coping strategies to deal with hallucinations or delusions if they reappear Communicate clearly with others Maintain cognitive functioning

Interventions

Interventions	Rationale	Ongoing Assessment
Initiate a nurse–patient relationship by using an accepting, nonjudgmental approach. Be patient.	A therapeutic relationship will provide patient support as he begins to deal with a devastating disorder. Be patient because his brain is not processing information normally.	Determine the extent to which JT is willing to trust and engage in a relationship.
Administer risperidone as prescribed. Observe for effect, side effects, and adverse effects. Begin teaching about the medication and its importance, once symptoms subside.	Risperidone is a D_2 and $5\text{-}HT_{2A}$ antagonist and is indicated for the management of psychotic disorders.	Make sure JT swallows pills. Monitor for relief of positive symptoms and assess side effects, especially extrapyramidal. Monitor BP for orthostatic hypotension and body temperature increase (NMS).

NURSING CARE PLAN 17.1 (Continued)

Interventions

Interventions	Rationale	Ongoing Assessment
During hallucinations and delusional thinking, assess significance (is it frightening, voices telling him to hurt himself or others?). Reassure JT that you will keep him safe. (Do not try to convince JT that his hallucinations are not real.) Redirect to the here-and-now. Assess ability for self-care activities.	It is important to understand the context of the hallucinations and delusions to be able to provide the appropriate interventions. By avoiding arguments about the content, the nurse will enhance communication. Disturbed thinking may interfere with JT's ability to carry out ADLs.	Assess the meaning of the hallucination or delusion to the patient. Determine whether he is a danger to himself or others. Determine whether patient can be redirected. Continue to assess: Determine whether patient can manage own self-care.

Evaluation

Outcomes	Revised Outcomes	Interventions
Hallucinations and delusions began to decrease within 3 days. Is oriented to time, place, and person. Attention and memory improving.	Participate in unit activities according to ITP. Agree to continue to take antipsychotic medication as prescribed.	Encourage attendance at treatment activities. Teach JT about medications. Teach JT about schizophrenia.

NURSING DIAGNOSIS 2: RISK FOR VIOLENCE

Defining Characteristics	Related Factors
Assaultive toward others, self, and environment Presence of pathophysiologic risk factors: delusional thinking	Frightened, secondary to auditory hallucinations and delusional thinking Poor impulse control Dysfunctional communication patterns

Outcomes

Initial	Long-Term
Avoid hurting self or assaulting other patients or staff. Decrease agitation and aggression.	Control behaviour with assistance from staff and parents.

Interventions

Interventions	Rationale	Ongoing Assessment
Acknowledge patient's fear, hallucinations, and delusions. Be genuine and empathetic. Offer patient choices of maintaining safety: keeping distance from others, medication for relaxation. Administer lorazepam 2 mg for agitation. Oral route is preferable over injection.	Hallucinations and delusions change an individual's perception of environmental stimuli. Patient who is frightened will respond because of his need to stay safe. By having choices, he will begin to develop a sense of control over his behaviour. Exact mechanisms of action are not understood, but medication is believed to potentiate the inhibitory neurotransmitter GABA, relieving anxiety and producing sedation.	Determine whether patient is able to hear you. Assess his response to your comments and his ability to concentrate on what is being said. Observe patient's nonverbal communication for evidence of increased agitation. Observe for decrease in agitated behaviour.

Evaluation

Outcomes	Revised Outcomes	Interventions
JT gradually decreased agitated behaviour. Lorazepam was given regularly for first 2 days.	Demonstrate control of behaviour by resisting hallucinations and delusions.	Teach JT about the effects of hallucinations and delusions. Problem-solve ways of controlling hallucinations if they occur. Emphasize the importance of taking medications.

INTERDISCIPLINARY TREATMENT PLAN 17.1

Patient With Schizophrenia

Admission Date	Date of This Plan	Type of Plan: Check Appropriate Box					
		☐ Initial	☐ Master	☐ 30	☐ 60	☐ 90	☐ Other

Treatment Team Present:
A. Barton, MD; J. Jones, RNC; C. Anderson, CNS; B. Thomas, PhD; T. Toon, Mental Health Technician (MHT);
J. Barker, MHT.

DIAGNOSIS (*DSM-IV-TR*):

AXIS I: Schizophrenia, paranoid
AXIS II: None
AXIS III: None
AXIS IV: Educational problems (failing)
            Social problems (withdrawn from peers)
AXIS V: Current GAF: 25
            Highest-Level GAF This Past Year: 90

ASSETS (MEDICAL, PSYCHOLOGICAL, SOCIAL, EDUCATIONAL, VOCATIONAL, RECREATIONAL):

1. First episode of psychosis. No evidence of drug use.
2. Premorbid functional level appears to be normal.
3. Maintained good grades in high school.
4. Has supportive family members.

Prob. No.	Date	Problem/Need	Code	Change Code	Change Date
1	3/5/06	Is hallucinating and had delusional thoughts. Unable to communicate with parents or staff.	T		
2	3/5/06	Is aggressive and is striking out at staff and unfamiliar people.	T		
3	3/5/06	Dropped out of college because of thoughts and behaviours.	X		
4	3/5/06	Family members are very upset about their son's psychiatric symptoms.	T		

CODE   T = Problem must be addressed in treatment.
        N = Problem noted and will be monitored.
        X = Problem noted, but deferred/inactive/no action necessary.
        O = Problem to be addressed in aftercare/continuing care.
        I = Problem incorporated into another problem.
        R = Resolved.

INDIVIDUAL TREATMENT PLAN PROBLEM SHEET

#1 Problem/Need	Date Identified	Problem Resolved Discontinuation Date
	3/5/06	

Is hallucinating and has delusional thoughts. Unable
to communicate with parents or staff.

Objective(s)/Short-Term Goals	Target Date	Achievement Date
1. Reduce report and observations of hallucinations and delusions.	3/15/06	

INTERDISCIPLINARY TREATMENT PLAN 17.1 (Continued)

Treatment Interventions	Frequency	Person Responsible
1. Antipsychotic therapy for hallucinations and delusions. Administer and monitor for adherence, effect, and side effects.	As prescribed	MD/RN
2. Monitor frequency of hallucinations and delusions.	Close obsevation for 24–48 hours, then according to RN judgment	RN/MHT
3. Attend Symptom Management group as symptoms subside.	Daily	PhD, RN

#2 Problem/Need	Date Identified	Problem Resolved/Discontinuation Date
	3/5/06	

Is aggressive and is hitting out at staff and unfamiliar people.

Objective(s)/Short-Term Goals	Target Date	Achievement Date
1. De-escalate aggressive behaviour.	3/15/06	

Treatment interventions	Frequency	Person Responsible
1. Keep patient in a quiet, nonstimulating environment. Assign private room.	Ongioing	RN
2. Administer antianxiety medication as needed.	PRN	MD/RN
3. Use de-escalation techniques when approaching patient.	Ongoing	Everyone
4. Assign to anger management group if needed when psychotic symptoms decrease.	In 1 week	CNS

#3 Problem/Need	Date Identified	Problem Resolved/Discontinuation Date
	3/5/06	

Family members are very upset about their son's psychiatric symptoms.

Objective(s)/Short-Term Goals	Target Date	Achievement Date
Increase family's comfort levels with mental illness.	3/15/06	

Treatment Interventions	Frequency	Person Responsible
1. Meet with family each time they visit. Provide counselling and education to family.	Ongoing	CNS/RN/MD/PhD
2. Encourage family to attend family support group.	Weekly	PhD
3. Provide community resources for the treatment of mental illness.	When visiting	CNS

Responsible QMHP   **Client or Guardian**   **Staff Physician**

_____ _____   _____ _____   _____ _____
Signature   Date   Signature   Date   Signature   Date

that symptoms can be observed in cognitive, emotional, family, social, and physical functioning. The applicable diagnoses can be categorized into the phases in which they are most likely to appear. However, it is important to note that even though they have been sorted into these categories, they may still represent problems in other phases. It is also important to note that the quieter periods between exacerbations of symptoms are actually very active and important phases for intervention.

Biologic Domain

Biologic Assessment

The following discussion highlights the important assessment areas for people with schizophrenia.

Current and Past Health Status and Physical Examination

It is important to conduct a thorough history and physical examination to rule out medical illness or substance abuse that could cause the psychiatric symptoms. It is also important to screen for comorbid medical illnesses that need to be treated, such as diabetes mellitus, hypertension, and cardiac disease or a family history of such disorders. People with schizophrenia have a higher mortality rate from physical illness and often have smoking-related illnesses, such as emphysema, and other pulmonary and cardiac problems. The nurse should determine whether the patient smokes or chews tobacco, which not only affects the patient's health but also can affect the clearance of medications.

Physical Functioning

The negative symptoms of schizophrenia are often manifested in terms of impairment in physical functioning. Self-care often deteriorates, and sleep may be nonexistent during acute phases. Information regarding physical functioning may best be collected from family members.

CRNE Note

When assessing a patient with schizophrenia, the nurse should prioritize the severity of the current responses to the disorder. If hallucinations are impairing function, then managing hallucinations is a priority, and medications are needed immediately. If hallucinations are not a problem, coping with the negative symptoms becomes a priority.

Nutritional Assessment

A nutritional history should be completed to determine baseline eating habits and preferences. Medications can alter normal nutrition, and the patient may need to limit calories or fat consumption.

Fluid Imbalance Assessment

The nurse should remain alert for signs of polydipsia and polyuria to identify disordered water balance. Patients with these symptoms make frequent trips to the water fountain or display other excessive water-drinking behaviours; their excessive water intake may cause them to become disoriented, confused, or agitated. Polydipsia is difficult to detect in patients who do not drink fluid more often than normal but simply consume large volumes (Boyd & Lapierre, 1996). Patients suspected of having disordered water balance should be assessed for signs and symptoms of hyponatremia, water intoxication, excessive urination, incontinence, or periodically elevated blood pressure. Signs and symptoms of hypervolemia that may be evident include puffiness of the face or eyes, abdominal distention, and hypothermia. These patients should be weighed daily, and their urine specific gravity and serum sodium levels should be monitored.

Pharmacologic Assessment

Baseline information about initial psychological and physical functioning should be obtained before initiation of medication (or as early as possible). Side effects of medications should be assessed. Patients are often physically awkward and have poor coordination, motor abnormalities, and abnormal eye tracking. Before medication begins, standardized assessment of abnormal motor movements should be conducted using one of several assessment tools designed for that purpose, such as the Abnormal Involuntary Movement Scale (AIMS) (see Appendix D); the Dyskinesia Identification System (DISCUS) (Sprague & Kalachnik, 1991) (Table 17-3), or the Simpson-Angus Rating Scale (see Appendix C) (Simpson & Angus, 1970), which is designed for Parkinson's symptoms.

Nursing Diagnoses for Biologic Domain

Typical nursing diagnoses focusing on the biologic domain for the person during all phases of schizophrenia include Self-Care Deficit and Disturbed Sleep Pattern. During a relapse, Ineffective Therapeutic Regimen Management, Imbalanced Nutrition, Excess Fluid Volume, and Sexual Dysfunction are possible diagnoses. Constipation may occur if the patient takes anticholinergic medications.

CRNE Note

Monitoring actions and side effects of medications is a priority nursing intervention. Atypical antipsychotics are drugs of choice and should be easily recognized. The older medications will be used occasionally.

Table 17.3   The Dyskinesia Identification System (DISCUS)

_____ (facility)

Dyskinesia Identification System:
Condensed User Scale (DISCUS)

_____

CURRENT PSYCHOTROPICS/ANTI-
CHOLINERGIC AND TOTAL MG/DAY

_____ _____ mg

_____ _____ mg

_____ _____ mg

_____ _____ mg

See Instructions on Other Side

NAME _____   I.D. _____

EXAM TYPE (check one)
- ☐ 1. Baseline
- ☐ 2. Annual
- ☐ 3. Semi annual
- ☐ 4. D/C—1 mo
- ☐ 5. D/C—2 mo
- ☐ 6. D/C—3 mo
- ☐ 7. Admission
- ☐ 8. Other

COOPERATION (check one)
- ☐ 1. None
- ☐ 2. Partial
- ☐ 3. Full

SCORING

0—**Not present** (movements not observed or some movements observed but not considered abnormal)

1—**Minimal** (abnormal movements are difficult to detect or movements are easy to detect but occur only once or twice in a short nonrepetitive manner)

2—**Mild** (abnormal movements occur infrequently and are easy to detect)

3—**Moderate** (abnormal movements occur frequently and are easy to detect)

4—**Severe** (abnormal movements occur almost continuously **and** are easy to detect)

NA—**Not assessed** (an assessment for an item is not able to be made)

ASSESSMENT
DISCUS Item and Score (circle one score for each item)

FACE
1. Tics.. 0 1 2 3 4 NA
2. Grimaces............................... 0 1 2 3 4 NA

EYES
3. Blinking................................. 0 1 2 3 4 NA

ORAL
4. Chewing/Lip Smacking......... 0 1 2 3 4 NA
5. Puckering/Sucking/
   Thrusting Lower Lip.............. 0 1 2 3 4 NA

LINGUAL
6. Tongue Thrusting/
   Tongue in Cheek.................. 0 1 2 3 4 NA
7. Tonic Tongue....................... 0 1 2 3 4 NA
8. Tongue Tremor..................... 0 1 2 3 4 NA
9. Athetoid/Myokymic/
   Lateral Tongue..................... 0 1 2 3 4 NA

HEAD NECK/ TRUNK
10. Retrocollis/Torticollis........... 0 1 2 3 4 NA
11. Shoulder/Hip Torsion........... 0 1 2 3 4 NA

UPPER LIMB
12. Athetoid/Myokymic
    Finger–Wrist–Arm................ 0 1 2 3 4 NA
13. Pill Rolling........................... 0 1 2 3 4 NA

LOWER LIMB
14. Ankle Flexion/
    Foot Tapping...................... 0 1 2 3 4 NA
15. Toe Movement.................... 0 1 2 3 4 NA

COMMENTS/OTHER

_____

_____

_____

_____

TOTAL SCORE (items 1–15 only) _____

EXAM DATE _____

RATER SIGNATURE AND TITLE

NET EXAM DATE

EVALUATION

1. Greater than 90 days
   neuroleptic exposure?   :   YES   NO
2. Scoring/intensity level met?   :   YES   NO
3. Other diagnostic conditions?   :   YES   NO
   (if yes, specify)

_____

_____

4. Last exam date: _____
   Last total score: _____
   Last conclusion: _____

Preparer signature and title for items 1–4 (if different from physician):

5. Conclusion (circle one):
   A. No TD (if scoring prerequisite met, list other diagnostic condition or explain in comments)
   B. Probable TD
   C. Masked TD
   D. Withdrawal TD
   E. Persistent TD
   F. Remitted TD
   G. Other (specify in comments)

6. Comments:

_____

_____

_____

_____

_____

_____

_____

CLINICIAN SIGNATURE   DATE

From Sprague, R. L., & Kalachnik, J. E. (1991). Reliability, validity, and a total score cutoff for the Dyskinesia Identification System, Condensed User Scale (DISCUS) with mentally ill and mentally retarded populations. *Psychopharmacology Bulletin, 27*(1), 51–58.

Interventions for Biologic Domain

Nursing interventions during the initial acute phase of schizophrenia include prompt, safe, and informed administration of antipsychotic medications. During any stage, attention to self-care needs and the patient's ability to maintain hygiene and adequate nutrition are important.

Promotion of Self-Care Activities

For many with schizophrenia, the plan of care will include specific interventions to enhance self-care, nutrition, and overall health knowledge. Negative symptoms commonly leave patients unable to initiate these seemingly simple activities. Developing a daily schedule of routine activities (such as showering and shaving) can help the patient structure the day. Most patients actually know how to perform self-care activities (eg, hygiene, grooming) but are not motivated (avolition) to carry them out consistently. Interventions include developing a schedule with the patient for various hygiene activities and emphasizing the importance of maintaining appropriate self-care activities. Given the problems related to attention and memory in people with schizophrenia, education about these areas requires careful planning.

Activity, Exercise, and Nutritional Interventions

Encouraging activity and exercise is necessary, not only to maintain a healthy lifestyle, but also to counteract the side effects of psychiatric medications that cause weight gain. Because the diagnosis is usually made in late adolescence or early adulthood, it is possible to establish solid exercise patterns early.

During episodes of acute psychosis, patients are unable to focus on eating. Often when patients begin antipsychotic medication, normal satiety and hunger responses change, and overeating or weight gain can become a problem. Promoting healthy nutrition is a key intervention. Maintaining healthy nutrition and monitoring calorie intake also become important because of the effect many medications have on eating habits. Patients report that appetite increases and cravings for food develop when some medications are initiated.

Weight gain is one of the reasons some patients become resistant to taking medication. It also may be a contributing factor to the development of type II diabetes mellitus. As such, this places patients at greater risk for several health complications and early death. Monitoring for diabetes and managing weight are important activities for all care providers (Stahl, 2002). Patients should be screened for risk factors of diabetes, such as family history, obesity as indicated by a body mass index (BMI) exceeding or equal to 27, and age older than 45 years. Patients' weight should be measured at regular intervals and the BMI calculated. Blood pressure readings should be taken regularly. Laboratory findings for triglycerides, HDL cholesterol, and glucose level should be monitored and reviewed regularly. All providers should be alert to the development of diabetic ketoacidosis, particularly in patients known to have diabetes who begin taking new antipsychotic agents. A program to address weight gain should be initiated at the earliest sign of weight gain (probably between 5 and 10 pounds over desired body weight). Reduced caloric intake may be accomplished by increasing the patient's access to affordable, healthful, and easy-to-prepare foods. Behavioural management of weight gain includes keeping a food diary, diet teaching, and support groups.

Thermoregulation Interventions

Patients with schizophrenia may have disturbed body temperature regulation. In winter, they may seem to be oblivious to cold weather. In the heat of summer, they may dress for winter. Observing patients' responses to temperatures helps in identifying problems in this area. In patients who are taking psychiatric medications, body temperature needs to be monitored, and the patient needs to be protected from extremes in temperature.

Promotion of Normal Fluid Balance and Prevention of Water Intoxication

Nursing interventions for disordered water balance include teaching and assisting the patient to develop self-monitoring skills. Fluid intake and weight gain should be monitored to control fluid intake and reduce the likelihood of developing water intoxication.

Patients can be classified as having mild, moderate, or severe disordered water balance based on the signs and symptoms outlined in Box 17-2 (Snider & Boyd, 1991). Patients with mild disordered water balance are easily treated in outpatient settings and benefit from educational programs that teach them to monitor their own urine specific gravity and daily weight gains. Patients classified with moderate disordered water balance may respond well to education but have a more difficult time controlling their own fluid intake. Using a targeted weight procedure, a baseline weight is established, a targeted weight is calculated, and the patient is regularly weighed throughout the day (Box 17-7). Patients are taught that a 5- to 7-pound weight gain in 1 to 3 hours indicates too much fluid. Exceeding the targeted weight places the patient at risk for water intoxication. Patients with severe disordered water balance require considerable assistance to restrict their continual water-seeking behaviour. These patients may create considerable disruption in an inpatient setting but often are best managed by one-on-one observation to redirect their behaviour. For more information see Box 17-2.

BOX 17.7

Water Intoxication Protocol

I. Observation: evidence of polydipsia and polyuria
II. Assessment of fluid balance
  A. History of polydipsia and polyuria
  B. Hyponatremia: serum Na$^+$ <135 mEq/L
  C. Hyposthenuria: urine specific gravity <1.005
III. Interventions:
  A. If the above symptoms are present institute the following interventions
    1. Target weight procedure
    2. Assess behavioural changes daily
    3. Monitor urine specific gravity daily
    4. Identify specific interventions for helping patient develop control over fluid intake and learn self-monitoring skills
      a. Cognitive therapy approaches
      b. Individual or group therapy approaches
      c. Arrange access to sugarless candies, gum, and fruit to reduce feelings of thirst
      d. Limit access to fluids during the day
  B. If weight reaches or exceeds target weight, initiate the following:
    1. Prohibit fluid intake
    2. Restrict to program and residential area
    3. Assess vital signs q1h × 2
    4. Provide low-fluid diet after symptoms subside
  C. If more severe symptoms develop, notify physician and transfer patient to a medical unit.
IV. Evaluation
  A. Patient gains control over fluid balance as evidenced by developing strategies to stay under target weight.
  B. If there is no evidence of water intoxication and there is evidence that patient is gaining control over fluid balance, the target weight procedure and daily assessments of behaviour and urine specific gravity can be discontinued.

Pharmacologic Interventions

Early in the 20th century, somatic treatment of schizophrenia included hydrotherapy (baths), wet-pack sheets, insulin shock therapy, electroconvulsive therapy, psychosurgery, and occupational and physical therapy. But in the early 1950s, treatment of schizophrenia drastically changed with the accidental discovery that a drug, chlorpromazine, used to induce anesthesia also calmed patients with schizophrenia. Optimism persists as older medications continue to be used effectively while offering clues into the workings of the brain and as new discoveries about the brain lead to more precise medications for treating schizophrenia.

Antipsychotic drugs have the general effect of blocking dopamine transmission in the brain by blocking D$_2$ receptors to some degree (see Chapter 13). Some also block other dopamine receptors and receptors of other neurotransmitters to varying degrees. For the most part, the antidopamine effects are not specific to the mesolimbic and mesocortical tracts associated with schizophrenia, but instead travel to all the dopamine receptor sites throughout the brain. This results in desirable antipsychotic effects but also creates some unpleasant and undesirable side effects. The effects of these drugs on other neurotransmitter systems account for additional side effects.

The newer antipsychotic drugs risperidone (Risperdal) (Box 17-8), olanzapine (Zyprexa), quetiapine (Seroquel), ziprasidone (Geodon), and aripiprazole (Abilify) appear to be more efficacious and safer than conventional antipsychotics. They are available in a variety of formulations. Risperidone is also available in a long-acting injectable form (Consta). They are effective in treating negative and positive symptoms. These newer drugs (see Box 17-8) also affect several other neurotransmitter systems, including serotonin. This is believed to contribute to their antipsychotic effectiveness (see Chapter 9).

Monitoring and Administering Medications

Antipsychotic medications are the treatment of choice for patients with psychosis. The use of conventional antipsychotics (eg, haloperidol, Thorazine) decreased dramatically with the introduction of the second generation of antipsychotics. Generally, it takes about 1 to 2 weeks for antipsychotic drugs to effect a change in symptoms. During the stabilization period, the type of drug selected should be given an adequate trial, generally 6 to 12 weeks, before considering a change in the drug prescription. If treatment effects are not seen, another antipsychotic agent may be tried. Clozapine (Clozaril) use may be initiated when no other atypical antipsychotic is effective (see Box 17-9 for more information about clozaril).

Adherence to a prescribed medication regimen is the best approach to preventing relapse. Unfortunately, patient compliance with medication with atypical antipsychotic agents is not much different from that with conventional antipsychotic agents (Dolder, Lacro, Dunn, & Jeste, 2002). The use of long-acting injectables is expected to improve compliance outcomes. In these days of managed care, even state and veterans' facilities are discharging patients before a judgment can be made about the efficacy of a given drug treatment. Nurses and other mental health professionals are charged to ensure continuation of these stabilization protocols and to ensure that outpatient caregivers assume responsibility for maintaining this stabilization phase of treatment and continue to monitor and manage the patient's symptoms. Outpatient systems should avoid the immediate manipulation of dosages and drugs during the stabilization phase unless a medical emergency ensues.

BOX 17.8

Drug Profile: Risperidone (Risperdal; Consta, long-acting injectable)

DRUG CLASS: Atypical antipsychotic

RECEPTOR AFFINITY: Antagonist with high affinity for D_2 and 5-HT_2, also histamine (H_1) and α_1-, α_2-adrenergic receptors, weak affinity for D_1 and other serotonin receptor subtypes; no affinity for acetylcholine or β-adrenergic receptors.

INDICATIONS: Psychotic disorders, such as schizophrenia, schizoaffective illness, bipolar affective disorder, and major depression with psychotic features.

ROUTES AND DOSAGE: 1-, 2-, 3-, and 4-mg tablets and liquid concentrate (1mg/mL). 25, 50, and 75 mg long acting IM.

Adult Dosage: Initial dose typically 1 mg bid. Maximal effect at 6 mg/d. Safety not established above 16 mg/d. Use lowest possible dose to alleviate symptoms.

Geriatric: Initial dose, 0.5 mg/d, increase slowly as tolerated.

Children: Safety and efficacy with this age group have not been established.

INJECTION: Initiate 25 or 50 mg with oral supplementation for 2–3 weeks. Then injections only every 2–3 weeks. Given IM in gluteal area.

HALF-LIFE (peak effect): mean, 20 h (1 h, peak active metabolite = 3–17 h).

SELECT ADVERSE REACTIONS: Insomnia, agitation, anxiety, extrapyramidal symptoms, headache, rhinitis, somnolence, dizziness, headache, constipation, nausea, dyspepsia, vomiting, abdominal pain, hypersalivation, tachycardia, orthostatic hypotension, fever, chest pain, coughing, photosensitivity, weight gain.

WARNING: Rare development of neuroleptic malignant syndrome. Observe frequently for early signs of tardive dyskinesia. Use caution with individuals who have cardiovascular disease; risperidone can cause ECG changes. Avoid use during pregnancy or while breast-feeding. Hepatic or renal impairments increase plasma concentration.

Specific patient/family education

- Notify prescriber if tremor, motor restlessness, abnormal movements, chest pain, or other unusual symptoms develop.
- Avoid alcohol and other CNS depressant drugs.
- Notify prescriber if pregnancy is possible or planning to become pregnant. Do not breast-feed while taking this medication.
- Notify prescriber before taking any other prescription or OTC medication.
- May impair judgment, thinking, or motor skills; avoid driving or other hazardous tasks.
- During titration, the individual may experience orthostatic hypotension and should change positions slowly.
- Do not abruptly discontinue.

BOX 17.9

Drug Profile: Clozapine (Clozaril)

DRUG CLASS: Atypical antipsychotic

RECEPTOR AFFINITY: D_1 and D_2 blockade, antagonist for 5-HT_2, histamine (H_1), α-adrenergic, and acetylcholine. These additional antagonist effects may contribute to some of its therapeutic effects. Produces fewer extrapyramidal effects than standard antipsychotics with lower risk for tardive dyskinesia.

INDICATIONS: Severely ill individuals who have schizophrenia and have not responded to standard antipsychotic treatment. Unlabeled use for other psychotic disorders, such as schizoaffective disorder and bipolar affective disorder.

ROUTES AND DOSAGE: Available only in tablet form, 25- and 100-mg doses.

Adult Dosage: Initial dose 25 mg PO bid or qid, may gradually increase in 25–50 mg/d increments, if tolerated, to a dose of 300–450 mg/d by the end of the second week. Additional increases should occur no more than once or twice weekly. Do not exceed 900 mg/d. For maintenance, reduce dosage to lowest effective level.

Children: Safety and efficacy with children under 16 years have not been established.

HALF-LIFE (PEAK EFFECT): 12 h (1–6 h).

SELECT ADVERSE REACTIONS: Drowsiness, dizziness, headache, hypersalivation, tachycardia, hypo/hypertension, constipation, dry mouth, heartburn, nausea/vomiting, blurred vision, diaphoresis, fever, weight gain, hematologic changes, seizures, tremor, akathisia.

WARNING: Agranulocytosis, defined as a granulocyte count of <500 mm^3 occurs at about a cumulative 1-year incidence of 1.3%, most often within 4–10 weeks of exposure, but may occur at any time. Required registration with the clozapine.

Patient Management System, a WBC count before initiation, and weekly WBC counts while taking the drug and for 4 weeks after discontinuation. Rare development of neuroleptic malignant syndrome. No confirmed cases of tardive dyskinesia, but remains a possibility. Increased seizure risk at higher doses. Use caution with individuals who have cardiovascular disease; clozapine can cause ECG changes. Cases of sudden, unexplained death have been reported. Avoid use during pregnancy or while breast-feeding.

Specific patient/family education

- Need informed consent regarding risk for agranulocytosis. Weekly blood draws are required. Notify prescriber immediately if lethargy, weakness, sore throat, malaise, or other flu-like symptoms develop.
- Notify prescriber if pregnancy is possible or planning to become pregnant. Do not breast-feed while taking this medication.
- Notify prescriber before taking any other prescription or OTC medication. Avoid alcohol or other CNS depressant drugs.
- May cause drowsiness and seizures; avoid driving or other hazardous tasks.
- During titration, the individual may experience orthostatic hypotension and should change positions slowly.
- Do not abruptly discontinue.

Patients with schizophrenia generally face a lifetime of taking antipsychotic medications. Rarely is discontinuation of medications prescribed; however, many patients stop taking medications on their own. Some situations that require the cessation of medication use are neuroleptic malignant syndrome (see later) or agranulocytosis (dangerously low level of circulating neutrophils). Discontinuation is an option when tardive dyskinesia develops. Discontinuation of medications, other than in circumstances of a medical emergency, should be achieved by gradually lowering the dose over time. This diminishes the likelihood of withdrawal symptoms, which include withdrawal dyskinesias and withdrawal psychosis.

Monitoring Side Effects

EXTRAPYRAMIDAL SIDE EFFECTS. Parkinsonism that is caused by antipsychotic drugs is identical in appearance to Parkinson's disease and tends to occur in older patients. The symptoms are believed to be caused by the blockade of D_2 receptors in the basal ganglia, which throws off the normal balance between acetylcholine and dopamine in this area of the brain and effectively increases acetylcholine. The symptoms are managed by re-establishing the balance between acetylcholine and dopamine by reducing the dosage of the antipsychotic (increasing dopamine activity) or adding an anticholinergic drug (decrease acetylcholine activity), such as benztropine (Cogentin) or trihexyphenidyl (Artane). Discontinuation of the use of anticholinergic drugs should never be abrupt, which can cause a cholinergic rebound and result in withdrawal symptoms, such as vomiting, excessive sweating, and altered dreams and nightmares. Thus, the anticholinergic drug dosage should be reduced gradually (tapered) over several days. If a patient experiences akathisia (physical restlessness), an anticholinergic medication may not be particularly helpful. Table 17-4 lists anticholinergic side effects of antiparkinson drugs and several antipsychotic medications and interventions to manage them.

Dystonic reactions are also believed to result from the imbalance of dopamine and acetylcholine, with the latter dominant. Young men seem to be more vulnerable to this particular extrapyramidal side effect. This side effect, which develops rapidly and dramatically, can be very frightening for patients as their muscles tense and their body contorts. The experience often starts with oculogyric crisis, in which the muscles that control eye movements tense and pull the eyeball so that the patient is looking toward the ceiling. This may be followed rapidly by torticollis, in which the neck muscles pull the head to the side, or retrocollis, in which the head is pulled back, or orolaryngeal-pharyngeal hypertonus, in which the patient has extreme difficulty swallowing. The patient may also experience contorted extremities. These symptoms occur early in antipsychotic drug treatment, when the patient may still be experiencing psychotic symptoms. This compounds the patient's fear and anxiety and requires a quick response. The immediate treatment is to administer benztropine (Cogentin), 1 to 2 mg, or diphenhydramine (Benadryl), 25 to 50 mg, intramuscularly or intravenously. This is followed by daily administration of anticholinergic drugs and, possibly, by a decrease in antipsychotic medication (see Box 17-10 for more information about benztropine).

Akathisia appears to be caused by the same biologic mechanism as other extrapyramidal side effects. Patients are restless and report they feel driven to keep moving. They are very uncomfortable. Frequently, this response is misinterpreted as anxiety or increased psychotic symptoms, and the patient may be inappropriately given increased dosages of antipsychotic drug, which only perpetuates the side effect. If possible, the dose of antipsychotic drug should be reduced. A beta-adrenergic blocker such as propranolol (Inderal), 20 to 120 mg, may be required. Failure to manage this side effect is a leading cause of patients ceasing to take antipsychotic medications.

Tardive dyskinesia (impaired voluntary movement, resulting in fragmented or incomplete movements), tardive dystonia, and tardive akathisia are less likely to appear

Table 17.4	Nursing Interventions for Anticholinergic Side Effects	
Effect	**Intervention**
Dry mouth	Sips of water; hard candies and chewing gum (preferably sugar free)
Blurred vision	Avoid dangerous tasks; teach patient that this side effect will diminish in a few weeks
Decreased lacrimation	Artificial tears if necessary
Mydriasis	May aggravate glaucoma; teach patient to report eye pain
Photophobia	Sunglasses
Constipation	High-fiber diet; increased fluid intake; laxatives as prescribed
Urinary hesitancy	Privacy; run water in sink; warm water over perineum
Urinary retention	Regular voiding (at least every 2–3 h) and whenever urge is present; catheterize for residual; record intake and output; evaluate benign prostatic hypertrophy
Tachycardia	Evaluate for preexisting cardiovascular disease; sudden death has occurred with thioridazine (Mellaril)

BOX 17.10

Drug Profile: Benztropine mesylate (Cogentin)

DRUG CLASS: Antiparkinson agent

RECEPTOR AFFINITY: Blocks cholinergic (acetylcholine) activity, which is believed to restore acetylcholine/dopamine balance in the basal ganglia.

INDICATIONS: Used in psychiatry to reduce extrapyramidal symptoms (acute medication-related movement disorders), including pseudoparkinsonism, dystonia, and akathisia (not tardive syndromes) due to neuroleptic drugs such as haloperidol. Most effective with acute dystonia.

ROUTES AND DOSAGE: Available in tablet form, 0.5-, 1-, and 2-mg doses, also injectable 1 mg/mL.

Adult Dosage: For acute dystonia, 1–2 mg IM or IV usually provides rapid relief. No significant difference in onset of action after IM or IV injection. Treatment of emergent symptoms may be relieved in 1 or 2 days, with 1–2 mg orally 2–3 times/d. Maximum daily dose is 6 mg/d. After 1–2 weeks withdraw drug to see if continued treatment is needed. Medication-related movement disorders that develop slowly may not respond to this treatment.

Geriatric: Older adults and very thin patients cannot tolerate large doses.

Children: Do not use in children under 3. Use with caution in older children.

HALF-LIFE: 12–24 h, very little pharmacokinetic information is available.

SELECT ADVERSE REACTIONS: Dry mouth, blurred vision, tachycardia, nausea, constipation, flushing or elevated temperature, decreased sweating, muscular weakness or cramping, urinary retention, urinary hesitancy, dizziness, headache, disorientation, confusion, memory loss, hallucinations, psychoses, and agitation in toxic reactions, which are more pronounced in elderly people and occur at smaller doses.

WARNING: Avoid use during pregnancy or while breastfeeding. Give with caution in hot weather due to possible heatstroke. Contraindicated with angle-closure glaucoma, pyloric or duodenal obstruction, stenosing peptic ulcers, prostatic hypertrophy or bladder neck obstructions, myasthenia gravis, megacolon, or megaesophagus. May aggravate the symptoms of tardive dyskinesia or other chronic forms of medication-related movement disorder. Concomitant use of other anticholinergic drugs may increase side effects and risk for toxicity. Coadministration of haloperidol or phenothiazines may reduce serum levels of these drugs.

Specific patient/family education

- Take with meals to reduce dry mouth and gastric irritation.
- Dry mouth may be alleviated by sucking sugarless candies, adequate fluid intake, or good oral hygiene, increase fiber and fluids in diet to avoid constipation, stool softeners may be required. Notify prescriber if urinary hesitancy or constipation persists.
- Notify prescriber if rapid or pounding heartbeat, confusion, eye pain, rash, or other adverse symptoms develop.
- May cause drowsiness, dizziness, or blurred vision; use caution driving or performing other hazardous tasks requiring alertness. Avoid alcohol and other CNS depressants.
- Do not abruptly stop this medication because a flu-like syndrome may develop.
- Use caution in hot weather. Ensure adequate hydration. May increase susceptibility to heatstroke.

---

in individuals taking atypical, rather than conventional, antipsychotics. Table 17-5 describes these and associated motor abnormalities. Tardive dyskinesia is late-appearing abnormal involuntary movements (dyskinesia). It can be viewed as the opposite of parkinsonism both in observable movements and in etiology. Whereas muscle rigidity and absence of movement characterize parkinsonism, constant movement characterizes tardive dyskinesia. Typical movements involve the mouth, tongue, and jaw and include lip smacking, sucking, puckering, tongue protrusion, the bon-bon sign (where the tongue rolls around in the mouth and protrudes into the cheek as if the patient were sucking on a piece of hard candy), athetoid (worm-like) movements in the tongue, and chewing. Other facial movements, such as grimacing and eye blinking, also may be present.

Movements in the trunk and limbs are frequently observable. These include rocking from the hips, athetoid movements of the fingers and toes, jerking movements of the fingers and toes, guitar strumming movements of the fingers, and foot tapping. The long-term health problems for people with tardive dyskinesia are choking associated with loss of control of muscles used for swallowing and

compromised respiratory function leading to infections and possibly respiratory alkalosis.

Because the movements resemble the dyskinetic movements of some patients who have idiopathic Parkinson's disease and who have received long-term treatment with L-dopa (a direct-acting dopamine agonist that crosses the blood–brain barrier), the suggested hypothesis for tardive dyskinesia includes the supersensitivity of the dopamine receptor in the basal ganglia.

There is no consistently effective treatment; however, antipsychotic drugs mask the movements of tardive dyskinesia and have periodically been suggested as a treatment. This is counterintuitive because these are the drugs that cause the disorder. Newer antipsychotic drugs, such as clozapine, may be less likely to cause the disorder. The best management remains prevention through prescription of the lowest possible dose of antipsychotic drug over time that minimizes the symptoms of schizophrenia, prescription of these drugs for psychotic symptoms only, and early case finding by regular systematic screening of everyone receiving these drugs (see Table 17-5).

Table 17.5   Extrapyramidal Side Effects of Antipsychotic Drugs

Side Effect	Period of Onset	Symptoms
Acute Motor Abnormalities		
Parkinsonism or pseudoparkinsonism	5–30 d	Resting tremor, rigidity, bradykinesia/akinesia, mask-like face, shuffling gait, decreased arm swing
Acute dystonia	1–5 d	Intermittent or fixed abnormal postures of the eyes, face, tongue, neck, trunk, and extremities
Akathisia	1–30 d	Obvious motor restlessness evidenced by pacing, rocking, shifting from foot to foot; subjective sense of not being able to sit or be still; these symptoms may occur together or separately
Late-Appearing Motor Abnormalities		
Tardive dyskinesia	Months to years	Abnormal dyskinetic movements of the face, mouth, and jaw; choreothetoid movements of the legs, arms, and trunk
Tardive dystonia	Months to years	Persistent sustained abnormal postures in the face, eyes, tongue, neck, trunk, and limbs
Tardive akathisia	Months to years	Persisting, unabating sense of subjective and objective restlessness

Adapted from Casey, D. E. (1994). Schizophrenia: Psychopharmacology. In J. W. Jefferson & J. H. Greist (Eds.), *The Psychiatric Clinics of North America annual of drug therapy* (Vol. 1, pp. 81–100). Philadelphia: W. B. Saunders.

Orthostatic hypotension is another side effect of antipsychotic drugs. The primary antiadrenergic effect is decreased blood pressure, which may be general or orthostatic. Patients may be protected from falls by teaching them to rise slowly and by monitoring blood pressure before doses of drug. The nurse should monitor and document lying, sitting, and standing blood pressures when any antipsychotic drug therapy begins.

Hyperprolactinemica can occur. When dopamine is blocked in the tuberoinfundibular tract, it can no longer repress prolactin, the neurohormone that regulates lactation and mammary function. The prolactin level increases and, in some individuals, side effects appear. Gynecomastia (enlarged breasts) can occur among both sexes and is understandably distressing to individuals who may be experiencing delusional or hallucinatory body image disturbances. Galactorrhea (lactation) also may occur. Menstrual irregularities and sexual dysfunction are also possible. If these symptoms appear, the medication should be reduced or changed to another antipsychotic agent. Evidence for long-term consequences of hyperprolactinemia is lacking. Hyperprolactinemia is associated with the use of haloperidol and risperidone.

Weight gain is related to antipsychotic agents, especially olanzapine and clozapine, that have major antihistaminic properties. Patients may gain as much as 20 or 30 pounds within 1 year. Increased appetite and weight gain are often distressing to patients. Diet teaching and monitoring may have some effect on this side effect. Another solution is to increase the accessibility of healthful, easy-to-prepare food. Although nausea and vomiting can occur with the use of these drugs, most often, these drugs mask nausea.

Sedation is another possible side effect of antipsychotic medication. Patients should be monitored for the sedating effects of antipsychotic agents that are antihistaminic. In elderly patients, sedation can be associated with falls.

New-onset diabetes should be looked for in patients taking antipsychotic drugs. Recently, an association was made between new-onset diabetes mellitus and the administration of atypical antipsychotic agents, especially olanzapine and clozapine. Patients should be assessed and monitored for clinical symptoms of diabetes. Fasting blood glucose tests are commonly ordered for these individuals.

Cardiac arrhythmias may also occur. Prolongation of the QTc interval is associated with torsades de pointes (polymorphic ventricular tachycardia) or ventricular fibrillation. The potential for drug-induced prolonged QT interval is associated with many drugs. The newly approved antipsychotic agent ziprasidone (Geodon) may be more likely than other drugs to prolong the QT interval and change the heart rhythm. For these patients, baseline electrocardiograms may be ordered. Nurses should observe these patients for cardiac arrhythmias.

Agranulocytosis is a reduction in the number of circulating granulocytes and decreased production of granulocytes in the bone marrow that limits one's ability to fight infection. Agranulocytosis can develop with the use of all antipsychotic drugs, but it is most likely to develop with clozapine use. Although laboratory values below 500 cells/mm^3 are indicative of agranulocytosis, often granulocyte counts drop to below 200 cells/mm^3 with this syndrome.

Patients taking clozapine should have regular blood tests. White blood cell and granulocyte counts should be measured before treatment is initiated and at least weekly or twice weekly after treatment begins. Initial white blood cell counts should be above 3,500 cells/mm³ before treatment initiation; in patients with counts of 3,500 to 5,000 cells/mm³, cell counts should be monitored three times a week if clozapine is prescribed. Any time the white blood cell count drops below 3,500 cells/mm³ or granulocytes drop below 1,500 cells/mm³, use of clozapine should be stopped, and the patient should be monitored for infection.

However, a faithfully implemented program of blood monitoring should not replace careful observation of the patient. It is not unusual for blood cell counts to drop precipitously in a period of 2 to 3 days. This may not be discovered when the patient is on a strict weekly blood monitoring schedule. Any reported symptoms that are reminiscent of a bacterial infection (fever, pharyngitis, and weakness) should be cause for concern, and immediate evaluation of blood count status should be undertaken. Because patients are frequently discharged before the critical period of risk for agranulocytosis, patient education about these symptoms is also essential so that they will report these symptoms and obtain blood monitoring. In general, granulocytes return to normal within 2 to 4 weeks after discontinuation of use of the medication.

Drug–Drug Interactions

Several potential drug–drug interactions are possible when administering antipsychotic medications. One of the cytochrome P450 enzymes responsible for the metabolism of olanzapine and clozapine is 1A2. If either olanzapine or clozapine is given with another medication that inhibits this enzyme, such as fluvoxamine (Luvox), the antipsychotic blood level would increase and possibly become toxic. On the other hand, cigarette smoking can also induce 1A2 and lower concentration of drugs metabolized by this enzyme, such as olanzapine and clozapine. Smokers may require a higher dose of these medications than do nonsmokers (Stahl, 2000).

Several atypical antipsychotic agents, including clozapine, quetiapine, and ziprasidone, are metabolized by the 3A4 enzyme. Weak inhibitors of this enzyme include the antidepressants fluvoxamine, nefazodone, and norfluoxetine (an active metabolite of fluoxetine). Potent inhibitors of 3A4 enzyme include ketoconazole (antifungal), protease inhibitors, and erythromycin. If these drugs are given with clozapine, quetiapine, or ziprasidone, the antipsychotic level will rise. In addition, the mood stabilizer carbamazepine (Tegretol) is a 3A4 inducer. When this drug is given with clozapine, quetiapine, or ziprasidone, the antipsychotic dose should be increased to compensate for the 3A4 induction. If the use of carbamazepine is discontinued, dosage of the antipsychotic agent needs to be adjusted (Stahl, 2000).

Risperidone, clozapine, and olanzapine are substrates for the enzyme 2D6. Theoretically, antidepressants (fluoxetine and paroxetine) that inhibit this enzyme could increase these antipsychotics' levels. However, this is not usually clinically significant (Stahl, 2000).

Teaching Points

Nonadherence to the medication regimen is an important factor in relapse; the family must be made aware of the importance of the patient consistently taking medications. Medication education should cover the association between medications and the amelioration of symptoms (in general as well as individualized for the patient), side effects and their management, and interpersonal skills that help the patient and family report medication effects.

Emergency! Neuroleptic Malignant Syndrome

In neuroleptic malignant syndrome (NMS), severe muscle rigidity develops with elevated temperature and a rapidly accelerating cascade of symptoms (occurring during the next 48 to 72 hours), which can include two or more of the following: hypertension, tachycardia, tachypnea, prominent diaphoresis, incontinence, mutism, leukocytosis, changes in level of consciousness ranging from confusion to coma, and laboratory evidence of muscle injury (eg, elevated creatinine phosphokinase). NMS occurs in about 1% of those who receive antipsychotic drugs, especially the conventional antipsychotics such as haloperidol (and other drugs that block dopamine, such as metoclopramide) (Montoya, Ocampo, & Torres-Ruiz, 2003). As many as one third of these patients may die as a result of the syndrome. NMS is probably underreported and may account for unexplained emergency room deaths of patients taking these drugs who do not have diagnoses because their symptoms do not seem serious. The presenting symptom is a temperature greater than 37.5°C (usually between 38.3°C and 39.4°C) with no apparent cause.

The most important aspects of nursing care for patients with NMS relate to recognizing symptoms early, stopping the administration of any neuroleptic medications, and initiating supportive nursing care. In any patient with fever, fluctuating vital signs, abrupt changes in levels of consciousness, or any of the symptoms presented in Box 17-11, NMS should be suspected. The nurse should be especially alert for early signs and symptoms of NMS in high-risk patients, such as those who are agitated, physically exhausted, or dehydrated or who have an existing medical or neurologic illness. Patients receiving parenteral or higher doses of neuroleptic drugs or lithium concurrently must

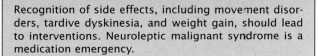

BOX 17.11

*Diagnostic Criteria for Neuroleptic Malignant Syndrome**

1. Treatment with neuroleptics within 7 days of onset (2–4 weeks for depot neuroleptic medications).
2. Hyperthermia
3. Muscle rigidity
4. Five of the following:
   - Change in mental status
   - Tachycardia
   - Hypertension or hypotension
   - Tachypnea or hypoxia
   - Diaphoresis or sialorrhea
   - Tremor
   - Incontinence
   - Creatinine phosphokinase elevation or myoglobinuria
   - Leukocytosis
   - Metabolic acidosis
5. Exclusion of other drug-induced, systemic, or neuropsychiatric illnesses

* All five items are required concurrently.
From Caroff, S., & Mann, S. (1993). Neuroleptic malignant syndrome. *Medical Clinics of North America, 77*, 185–202. Used with permission.

also be carefully assessed. The nurse should carefully monitor fluid intake and fluid and electrolyte status.

CRNE Note

Recognition of side effects, including movement disorders, tardive dyskinesia, and weight gain, should lead to interventions. Neuroleptic malignant syndrome is a medication emergency.

To prevent NMS from developing in a patient with signs or symptoms of the disorder, the nurse should immediately discontinue administration of any neuroleptic drugs and notify the physician. In addition, the nurse should "hold" any anticholinergic drugs that the patient may be taking. A common error made by nurses who fail to analyze the patient's total clinical picture (including vital signs, mental status changes, and laboratory values) is to continue the use of neuroleptic drugs. Figure 17-5 shows how to decide whether to withhold an antipsychotic medication. Medical treatment includes administering several medications. Dopamine agonist drugs, such as bromocriptine (modest success), and muscle relaxants, such as dantrolene or benzodiazepine, have been used. Antiparkinsonism drugs are not particularly useful. Some patients experience improvement with electroconvulsive therapy.

The vital signs of the patient with symptoms of NMS must be monitored frequently. In addition, it is important to check the results of the patient's laboratory tests for increased creatine phosphokinase, elevated white blood cell count, elevated liver enzymes, or myoglobinuria. The nurse must be prepared to initiate supportive measures or anticipate emergency transfer of the patient to a medical-surgical or an intensive care unit.

Treating high temperature (which frequently exceeds 39°C) is an important priority for these patients. High body temperature may be reduced with a cooling blanket and acetaminophen. Because many of these patients experience diaphoresis, temperature elevation, or dysphagia, it is important to monitor fluid hydration. Another important aspect of care for patients with NMS is safety. Joints and extremities that are rigid or spastic must be protected from injury. The treatment of these patients depends on the facility and availability of medical support services. In general, patients in psychiatric inpatient units that are separated from general hospitals are transferred to medical-surgical settings for treatment.

Emergency! Anticholinergic Crisis

There is also potential for abuse of anticholinergic drugs. Some patients may find the anticholinergic effects of these drugs on mood, memory, and perception pleasurable. Although at toxic dosages, patients may experience disorientation and hallucinations, lesser doses may cause patients to experience greater sociability and euphoria. Anticholinergic crisis is a potentially life-threatening medical emergency caused by an overdose of or sensitivity to drugs with anticholinergic properties. This syndrome (also called anticholinergic delirium) may result from an accidental or intentional overdose of antimuscarinic drugs, including atropine, scopolamine, or belladonna alkaloids, which are present in numerous prescription drugs and over-the-counter medicines. The syndrome may also occur in psychiatric patients who are receiving therapeutic doses of anticholinergic drugs, especially when such agents are combined with other psychotropic drugs that produce anticholinergic side effects. Numerous drugs commonly prescribed in psychiatric settings produce anticholinergic side effects, including tricyclic antidepressants and some antipsychotics. As a result of either drug overdose or sensitivity, these anticholinergic substances may produce an acute delirium or a psychotic reaction resembling schizophrenia. More severe anticholinergic effects may occur in older patients, even at therapeutic levels (Stahl, 2000).

The signs and symptoms of anticholinergic crisis are dramatic and physically uncomfortable (Box 17-12). This disorder is characterized by elevated temperature; parched mouth; burning thirst; hot, dry skin; decreased salivation; decreased bronchial and nasal secretions; widely dilated eyes (bright light is painful); decreased

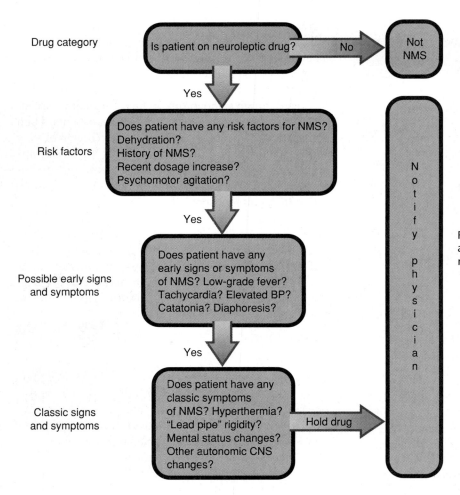

FIGURE 17.5   Action tree for "holding" a neuroleptic drug because of suspected neuroleptic malignant syndrome.

ability to accommodate visually; increased heart rate; constipation; difficulty urinating; and hypertension or hypotension. The face, neck, and upper arms may become flushed because of a reflex blood vessel dilation. In addition to peripheral symptoms, patients with anticholinergic psychosis may experience neuropsychiatric symptoms of anxiety, agitation, delirium, hyperactivity, confusion, hallucinations (especially visual), speech difficulties, psychotic symptoms, or seizures. The acute psychotic reaction that is produced resembles schizo-

phrenia. The classic description of anticholinergic crisis is summarized in the following mnemonic: "Hot as a hare, blind as a bat, mad as a hatter, dry as a bone."

In general, episodes of anticholinergic crisis are self-limiting, usually subsiding in 3 days. However, if untreated, the associated fever and delirium may progress to coma or cardiac and respiratory depression. Although rare, death is generally due to hyperpyrexia and brain-stem depression. Once use of the offending drug is discontinued, improvement usually occurs within 24 to 36 hours.

A specific and effective antidote, physostigmine, an inhibitor of anticholinesterase, is frequently used for treating and diagnosing anticholinergic crisis. Administration of this drug rapidly reduces both the behavioural and physiologic symptoms. However, the usual adult dose of physostigmine is 1 to 2 mg intravenously, given slowly during a period of 5 minutes because rapid injection of physostigmine may cause seizures, profound bradycardia, or heart block. Physostigmine is relatively short acting, so it may need to be given several times during the course of treatment. This drug provides relief from symptoms for a period of 2 to 3 hours. In addition to receiving physostigmine, patients who intentionally overdose on large amounts of anticholinergic drugs are treated by gastric

---

BOX 17.12

Signs and Symptoms of Anticholinergic Crisis

Neuropsychiatric signs: confusion; recent memory loss; agitation; dysarthria; incoherent speech; pressured speech; delusions; ataxia; periods of hyperactivity alternating with somnolence, paranoia, anxiety, or coma

Hallucinations accompanied by "picking," plucking, or grasping motions; delusions; or disorientation

Physical signs: unreactive dilated pupils; blurred vision; hot, dry, flushed skin; facial flushing; dry mucous membranes; difficulty swallowing; fever; tachycardia; hypertension; decreased bowel sounds; urinary retention; nausea; vomiting; seizures; or coma

lavage, administration of charcoal, and catharsis. The dose may be repeated after 20 or 30 minutes.

It is important for the nurse to be alert for signs and symptoms of anticholinergic crisis, especially in elderly people and children, who are much more sensitive to the anticholinergic effects of drugs, and in patients who are receiving multiple medications with anticholinergic effects. If signs and symptoms of the syndrome occur, the nurse should discontinue use of the offending drug and notify the physician immediately.

Other Somatic Interventions

Electroconvulsive therapy is suggested as a possible alternative when the patient's schizophrenia is not being successfully treated by medication alone. There are recent reports of electroconvulsive therapy as an augmentation to antipsychotic therapy (Ota et al., 2003; Tang & Ungvari, 2003). For the most part, this is not indicated unless the patient is catatonic or has a depression that is not treatable by other means.

Psychological Domain

Although schizophrenia is a brain disorder, the psychological manifestations are the most difficult to assess and treat. Many of these psychological manifestations improve with the use of medications, but they are not necessarily eliminated.

Psychological Assessment

Several assessment scales have been developed and received considerable reliability and validity testing to help evaluate positive and negative symptom clusters in schizophrenia. Box 17-13 lists standardized instruments used in assessing symptoms of patients with schizophrenia. These include the Scale for the Assessment of Positive Symptoms (SAPS) (Box 17-14), the Scale for the Assessment of Negative Symptoms (SANS) (Box 17-15), and the Positive and Negative Syndrome Scale (PANSS) (Kay, Fiszbein, & Opler, 1987), which assesses both symptom clusters in the same instrument. Tools that list symptoms, such as the Brief Psychiatric Rating Scale (see Appendix C), SANS, or SAPS can also be used to help patients self-monitor their symptoms.

Usually, information about prediagnosis experiences requires retrospective reporting by the patient or the family. This reporting is reliable for the frankly psychotic symptoms of delusions and hallucinations; however, negative symptoms are more difficult to date. In fact, negative symptoms vary from an imperceptive deviation from normal to a clear impairment. Negative symptoms probably occur earlier than positive symptoms and are less easily noted by the patient and significant others.

BOX 17.13

Rating Scales for Use With Schizophrenia

Scale for the Assessment of Negative Symptoms (SANS)

Available from Nancy C. Andreasen, MD, PhD, Department of Psychiatry, College of Medicine, The University of Iowa, Iowa City, IA 52242. Copyright 1984. *See Box 17-15.*

Scale for the Assessment of Positive Symptoms (SAPS)

Available from Nancy C. Andreasen (see above). *See Box 17-14.*

Abnormal Involuntary Movement Scale (AIMS)

Guy, W. (1976), *ECDEU: Assessment manual for psychopharmacology* (DHEW Publication No. 76-338). Washington, DC: Department of Health Education and Welfare, Psychopharmacology Branch.

Brief Psychiatric Rating Scale (BPRS)

Overall, J. E., & Gorham, D. R. (1988). The Brief Psychiatric Rating Scale (BPRS): Recent developments in ascertainment and scaling. *Psychopharmacology Bulletin, 24,* 97–99.

Dyskinesia Identification System: Condensed User Scale (DISCUS)

Sprague, R. L., & Kalachnik, J. E. (1991). Reliability, validity, and a total score cutoff for the Dyskinesia Identification Scale System: Condensed User Scale (DISCUS) with mentally ill and mentally retarded populations. *Psychopharmacology Bulletin, 27(1),* 51–58. *See Table 17-3.*

Simpson-Angus Rating Scale

Simpson, G. M., & Angus, J. W. S. L. (1970). A rating scale for extrapyramidal side effects. *Acta Psychiatrica Scandinavica (Suppl), 212,* 11–19. Copyright 1970 Munksgaard International Publishers, Ltd.

Responses to Mental Health Problems

Schizophrenia robs people of mental health and imposes social stigma. People with schizophrenia struggle to maintain control of their symptoms, which affect every aspect of their life. The person with schizophrenia displays a variety of interrelated symptoms and experiences deficits in several areas. More than half of patients report the following prodromal symptoms (in order of frequency): tension and nervousness, lack of interest in eating, difficulty concentrating, disturbed sleep, decreased enjoyment and loss of interest, restlessness, forgetfulness, depression, social withdrawal from friends, feeling laughed at, more religious thinking, feeling bad for no reason, feeling too excited, and hearing voices or seeing things.

Because schizophrenia is a disorder of thoughts, perceptions, and behaviour, it is sometimes not recognized as an illness by the person experiencing the symptoms. Many people with thought disorders do not believe that they have a mental illness. Their

BOX 17.14

Scale for the Assessment of Positive Symptoms (SAPS)

0 = None   1 = Questionable   2 = Mild   3 = Moderate
4 = Marked   5 = Severe

Hallucinations

1 *Auditory Hallucinations*   0 1 2 3 4 5
The patient reports voices, noises, or other sources that no one else hears.

2 *Voices Commenting*   0 1 2 3 4 5
The patient reports a voice that makes a running commentary on his behaviour or thoughts.

3 *Voices Conversing*   0 1 2 3 4 5
The patient reports hearing two or more voices conversing.

4 *Somatic or Tactile Hallucinations*   0 1 2 3 4 5
The patient reports experiencing peculiar physical sensations in the body.

5 *Olfactory Hallucinations*   0 1 2 3 4 5
The patient reports experiencing unusual smells that no one else notices.

6 *Visual Hallucinations*   0 1 2 3 4 5
The patient sees shapes or people that are not actually present.

7 *Global Rating of Hallucinations*   0 1 2 3 4 5
This rating should be based on the duration and severity of the hallucinations and their effect on the patient's life.

Delusions

8 *Persecutory Delusions*   0 1 2 3 4 5
The patient believes he is being conspired against or persecuted in some way.

9 *Delusions of Jealousy*   0 1 2 3 4 5
The patient believes his spouse is having an affair with someone.

10 *Delusions of Guilt or Sin*   0 1 2 3 4 5
The patient believes that he has committed some terrible sin or done something unforgivable.

11 *Grandiose Delusions*   0 1 2 3 4 5
The patient believes he has special powers or abilities.

12 *Religious Delusions*   0 1 2 3 4 5
The patient is preoccupied with false beliefs of a religious nature.

13 *Somatic Delusions*   0 1 2 3 4 5
The patient believes that somehow his body is diseased, abnormal, or changed.

14 *Delusions of Reference*   0 1 2 3 4 5
The patient believes that insignificant remarks or events refer to him or have some special meaning.

15 *Delusions of Being Controlled*   0 1 2 3 4 5
The patient feels that his feelings or actions are controlled by some outside force.

16 *Delusions of Mind Reading*   0 1 2 3 4 5
The patient feels that people can read his mind or know his thoughts.

17 *Thought Broadcasting*   0 1 2 3 4 5
The patient believes that his thoughts are broadcast so that he or others can hear them.

18 *Thought Insertion*   0 1 2 3 4 5
The patient believes that thoughts that are not his own have been inserted into his mind.

19 *Thought Withdrawal*   0 1 2 3 4 5
The patient believes that thoughts have been taken away from his mind.

20 *Global Rating of Delusions*   0 1 2 3 4 5
This rating should be based on the duration and persistence of the delusions and their effects on the patient's life.

Bizarre Behaviour

21 *Clothing and Appearance*   0 1 2 3 4 5
The patient dresses in an unusual manner or does other strange things to alter his appearance.

22 *Social and Sexual Behaviour*   0 1 2 3 4 5
The patient may do things considered inappropriate according to usual social norms (eg, masturbating in public).

23 *Aggressive and Agitated Behaviour*   0 1 2 3 4 5
The patient may behave in an aggressive, agitated manner, often unpredictably.

24 *Repetitive or Stereotyped Behaviour*   0 1 2 3 4 5
The patient develops a set of repetitive actions or rituals that he must perform over and over.

25 *Global Rating of Bizarre Behaviour*   0 1 2 3 4 5
This rating should reflect the type of behaviour and the extent to which it deviates from social norms.

Positive Formal Thought Disorder

26 *Derailment*   0 1 2 3 4 5
A pattern of speech in which ideas slip off track onto ideas obliquely related or unrelated.

27 *Tangentiality*   0 1 2 3 4 5
Replying to a question in an oblique or irrelevant manner.

28 *Incoherence*   0 1 2 3 4 5
A pattern of speech that is essentially incomprehensible at times.

29 *Illogicality*   0 1 2 3 4 5
A pattern of speech in which conclusions are reached that do not follow logically.

30 *Circumstantiality*   0 1 2 3 4 5
A pattern of speech that is very indirect and delayed in reaching its goal idea.

31 *Pressure of Speech*   0 1 2 3 4 5
The patient's speech is rapid and difficult to interrupt; the amount of speech produced is greater than that considered normal.

32 *Distractible Speech*   0 1 2 3 4 5
The patient is distracted by nearby stimuli that interrupt his flow of speech.

33 *Clanging*   0 1 2 3 4 5
A pattern of speech in which sounds rather than meaningful relationships govern word choice.

34 *Global Rating of Positive Formal Thought Disorder*   0 1 2 3 4 5
This rating should reflect the frequency of abnormality and degree to which it affects the patient's ability to communicate.

Inappropriate Affect

35 *Inappropriate Affect*   0 1 2 3 4 5
The patient's affect is inappropriate or incongruous, not simply flat or blunted.

BOX 17.15

Scale for the Assessment of Negative Symptoms (SANS)

0 = None 1 = Questionable 2 = Mild 3 = Moderate
4 = Marked 5 = Severe

Affective Flattening or Blunting

1 *Unchanging Facial Expression* 0 1 2 3 4 5
The patient's face appears wooden, changes less than expected as emotional content of discourse changes.

2 *Decreased Spontaneous Movements* 0 1 2 3 4 5
The patient shows few or no spontaneous movements, does not shift position, move extremities, etc.

3 *Paucity of Expressive Gestures* 0 1 2 3 4 5
The patient does not use hand gestures, body position, etc., as an aid to expressing ideas.

4 *Poor Eye Contact* 0 1 2 3 4 5
The patient avoids eye contact or "stares through" interviewer even when speaking.

5 *Affective Nonresponsivity* 0 1 2 3 4 5
The patient fails to smile or laugh when prompted.

6 *Lack of Vocal Inflections* 0 1 2 3 4 5
The patient fails to show normal vocal emphasis patterns; is often monotonic.

7 *Global Rating of Affective Flattening* 0 1 2 3 4 5
This rating should focus on overall severity of symptoms, especially unresponsiveness eye contact, facial expression, and vocal inflections.

Alogia

8 *Poverty of Speech* 0 1 2 3 4 5
The patient's replies to questions are restricted in amount; tend to be brief, concrete, and unelaborated.

9 *Poverty of Content of Speech* 0 1 2 3 4 5
The patient's replies are adequate in amount but tend to be vague, overconcrete, or overgeneralized, and convey little information.

10 *Blocking* 0 1 2 3 4 5
The patient indicates, either spontaneously or with prompting, that his train of thought was interrupted.

11 *Increased Latency of Response* 0 1 2 3 4 5
The patient takes a long time to reply to questions; prompting indicates that the patient is aware of the question.

12 *Global Rating of Alogia* 0 1 2 3 4 5
The core features of alogia are poverty of speech and poverty of content.

Avolition–Apathy

13 *Grooming and Hygiene* 0 1 2 3 4 5
The patient's clothes may be sloppy or soiled, and patient may have greasy hair, body odor, etc.

14 *Impersistence at Work or School* 0 1 2 3 4 5
The patient has difficulty seeking or maintaining employment, completing school work, keeping house, etc. If an inpatient, cannot persist at ward activities, such as OT, playing cards, etc.

15 *Physical Anergia* 0 1 2 3 4 5
The patient tends to be physically inert. May sit for hours and does not initiate spontaneous activity.

16 *Global Rating of Avolition–Apathy* 0 1 2 3 4 5
Strong weight may be given to one or two prominent symptoms if particularly striking.

Anhedonia–Asociality

17 *Recreational Interests and Activities* 0 1 2 3 4 5
The patient may have few or no interests. Both the quality and quantity of interests should be taken into account.

18 *Sexual Activity* 0 1 2 3 4 5
The patient may show a decrease in sexual interest and activity, or in enjoyment when active.

19 *Ability to Feel Intimacy and Closeness* 0 1 2 3 4 5
The patient may display an inability to form close or intimate relationships, especially with the opposite sex and family.

20 *Relationships With Friends and Peers* 0 1 2 3 4 5
The patient may have few or no friends and may prefer to spend all of time isolated.

21 *Global Rating of Anhedonia–Asociality* 0 1 2 3 4 5
This rating should reflect overall severity, taking into account the patient's age, family status, etc.

Attention

22 *Social Inattentiveness* 0 1 2 3 4 5
The patient appears uninvolved or unengaged. May seem "spacey."

23 *Inattentiveness During Mental Status Testing* 0 1 2 3 4 5
Tests of "serial 7s" (at least five subtractions) and spelling "world" backward: Score: 2 = 1 error; 3 = 2 errors; 4 = 3 errors.

24 *Global Rating of Attention* 0 1 2 3 4 5
This rating should assess the patient's overall concentration, clinically and on tests.

From Nancy C. Andreasen, MD, PhD, Department of Psychiatry, College of Medicine, The University of Iowa, Iowa City, IA 52242. Copyright 1984 Nancy C. Andreasen. Reprinted with permission.

denial of mental illness and the need for treatment poses problems for the family and clinicians. Ideally, in lucid moments, patients recognize that their thoughts are really delusions, that their perceptions are hallucinations, and that their behaviour is disorganized. In reality, many patients do not believe that they have a mental illness but agree to treatment to please family and clinicians.

Mental Status and Appearance
The patient may look eccentric or disheveled or have poor hygiene and bizarre dress. The patient's posture may suggest lethargy or stupor.

Mood and Affect
Patients with schizophrenia often display altered mood states. In some cases, they may show heightened emotional

activity; others may display severely limited emotional responses. Affect, the outward expression of mood, is categorized on a continuum: flat (emotional expression entirely absent), blunted (expression of emotions present but greatly diminished), and full range. Inappropriate affect is marked by incongruence between the emotional expression and the thoughts expressed. Other common emotional symptoms include the following:

- **Affective lability**—abrupt, dramatic, unprovoked changes in type of emotions expressed
- **Ambivalence**—the presence and expression of two opposing feelings, leading to inaction
- **Apathy**—reactions to stimuli are decreased, diminished interest and desire

Speech

Speech patterns may reflect obsessions, delusions, pressured thinking, loose associations, or flight of ideas and neologism. Speech is an indicator of thought content and other mental processes and is usually altered. An assessment of speech should note any difficulty articulating words (dysarthria) and difficulty swallowing (dysphagia) as indicators of medication side effects. In many instances, what an individual says is as important as how it is said. Both content and speech patterns should be noted.

Thought Processes and Delusions

Delusions can be distinguished from strongly held ideas by "the degree of conviction with which the belief is held despite clear contradictory evidence" (APA, 2000, p. 299). Culture must be considered when evaluating delusions. Delusional beliefs are those not sanctioned or held by a cultural or religious subgroup.

Bizarre delusions alone are sufficient to diagnose schizophrenia. It can often be difficult to distinguish between bizarre and nonbizarre delusions. Nonbizarre delusions generally have themes of jealousy and persecution and are derived from ordinary life experiences. For example, a woman believes that her husband, from whom she has recently separated, is trying to poison her, or a man believes that members of the Mafia are trying to kill him because, when he was in high school, he reported to the principal that several of his classmates were selling drugs at school (APA, 2000).

Bizarre delusions are those that are implausible, not understandable, and not derived from ordinary life experiences. Bizarre delusions often include delusions of control (that some outside force controls thoughts and actions), thought broadcasting (that others can read or hear one's thoughts), thought insertion (that someone has placed thoughts into one's mind), and thought withdrawal (that someone is removing thoughts from one's mind) (APA, 2000). For example, a patient who

has been with a hypnotist for 2 months reports that the hypnotist continued to read his mind and was "picking his brain away piece by piece." Another patient was convinced that a computer chip was placed in her vagina during a gynecologic examination and that this somehow directly influenced her physical movements and her thoughts.

Assessing and judging the content of the delusion and exploring other aspects of the delusional experience are helpful in understanding the significance of these false beliefs. The underlying feeling that accompanies the delusion should be identified. Other aspects to consider include the conviction with which the delusion is held; the extent other aspects of the individual's life are incorporated or affected by the delusion; the degree of internal consistency, organization, and logic evidenced in the delusion; and evaluating the amount of pressure (in terms of preoccupation and concern) individuals feel in their lives as a result of the delusion (see Box 17-16).

Hallucinations

Hallucinations are the most common example of disturbed sensory perception observed in patients with schizophrenia. Hallucinations can be experienced in all sensory modalities; however, auditory hallucinations are the most common in schizophrenia. Some specific hallucinations may be sufficient to diagnose schizophrenia, such as hearing voices conversing with each other or carrying on a discussion with someone who is not there. Because most individuals will not spontaneously share their hallucinatory experiences with an interviewer, the nurse may need to rely on indirect evidence in the patient's behaviour, such as (1) pauses during conversations in which the individual seems preoccupied or appears to be listening to someone other than the interviewer, (2) looking toward the perceived source of a voice, or (3) responding to the voices in some manner. Although patients may not spontaneously share their hallucinations, many validate observations of the examiner or admit to a history of hallucinations when asked (see Box 17-17).

Disorganized Communication

The other aspect of thought content and processes that may be altered in schizophrenia is the organization of expressed thoughts. Impaired verbal fluency (ability to produce spontaneous speech) is commonly present. Abrupt shifts in the focus of conversation are a typical symptom of disorganized thinking. The most severe shifts in focus may occur after only one or two words (word salad), after one or two phrases or sentences (flight of ideas or loose associations), or somewhat less severely as a shift that occurs when a new topic is repeatedly suggested and pursued from the current topic (tangentiality).

BOX 17.16

Therapeutic Dialogue: The Patient With Delusions

John joined the nurse in a game of pool. The following conversation occurred as they played.

Ineffective Approach

John: The RCMP put a transmitter in my molar, here (points to his right cheek).

Nurse: No one would put a transmitter in your tooth; come on, the RCMP isn't looking for you.

John: You get the striped ones. Yeah, they want to monitor me while I'm here. I know that they have the real Governor General here in the hospital. They are trying to get Paul Martin to intervene with the Ontario Police. Mark from Ottawa told me that.

Nurse: The Governor General can't possibly be here, I saw her on television this morning.

John: Maybe—she does have lighter hair and has different coloured contacts to disguise her eyes, but they're just trying to keep people from knowing what they're doing.

Nurse: John, Michaelle Jean isn't in the hospital; if she were, I would know it because I work here.

John: (With anger) You don't know anything! You are probably from the RCMP also. I have nothing else to say to you.

Effective Approach

John: The RCMP put a transmitter in my molar, here (points to his right cheek).

Nurse: Oh. Which balls are mine?

John: You get the striped ones. Yeah, they want to monitor me while I'm here. I know that they have the real Governor General here in the hospital. They are trying to get Paul Martin to intervene with the Ontario Police. Mark from Ottawa told me that.

Nurse: I suppose it could be Michaelle Jean, but do you suppose that it could just be someone who looks like her?

John: Maybe—she does have lighter hair and has different coloured contacts to disguise her eyes. But they're just trying to keep people from knowing what they're doing

Nurse: You sound a little overwhelmed with all the information you have.

John: No, no. I can handle it. The RCMP can't do anything to me, I'll never talk.

Nurse: I thought they could hear you when you talk to me.

John: Huh? Oh, that transmitter is so that they can send me misinformation. They send a tower of babble to my brain. They are trying to confuse me so that I stay away from the Governor General. They all think they can keep me from my mission.

Nurse: Who's they?

John: Everyone in the government. The RCMP, CSIS, CRA—all those alphabets.

Nurse: So everyone in the government is trying to get to you.

John: Well, maybe not everybody. Just the ones that care about money and the military. I don't think they care about me much in commerce or health and human services. Although they'd care too if they knew.

Nurse: I would think that's pretty frightening to have all these people out looking for you. You must be scared a lot.

John: It's scary but I can handle it. I've handled it all my life.

Nurse: You've been in scary situations all your life?

John: Yeah. I don't know. Maybe not scary, just hard. I never seemed to be able to do as well as my parents wanted—or as I wanted.

Critical Thinking Challenge

- How did the nurse's argumentative responses cause the patient to react in the first scenario?
- What effective communication techniques did the nurse use in the second scenario?

Cognitive Impairments

Although cognitive impairments in schizophrenia vary widely from patient to patient, several primary problems have been identified:

- attention may be increased and sustained on external stimuli over a period of time (hypervigilance)
- the ability to distinguish and focus on relevant stimuli may be diminished
- familiar cues may go unrecognized or be improperly encoded
- information processing may be diminished, leading to inappropriate or illogical conclusions from available observations and information (Cirillo & Seidman, 2003; Hartman, Steketee, Silva, Lanning, & Andersson, 2003).

Cognitive impairments are not easy to recognize. By relying only on clinical assessment, the nurse can miss the extent of the impairment. Using a standardized instrument such as the Mini-Mental Status Examination (MMSE), the Cognitive Assessment Screening Instrument (CASI), or the 7-Minute Screen can provide a screening measurement of cognitive function (see Chapter 10). If impairment exists, neuropsychological testing by a qualified psychologist may be necessary.

Memory and Orientation

Impairments in orientation, memory, and abstract thinking may be observed. Orientation to time, place, and person may remain relatively intact unless the patient is particularly preoccupied with delusions and hallucinations. Although all aspects of memory may be affected in schizophrenia, registration or the recall within seconds of newly learned information may be particularly diminished. This affects the individual's short-term and long-term memory. The ability to engage in abstract thinking may be impaired.

Insight and Judgment

Individuals display insight when they display evidence of knowing their own thoughts, the reality of external

BOX 17.17

Therapeutic Dialogue: The Patient With Hallucinations

The following conversation took place in a dayroom with several staff in the room. The patient was potentially very violent. Although it is a good example of dealing with someone who is hallucinating, it is not a situation that should be taken lightly. Always make certain that you have a means to leave a situation (ie, that you are not in the corner of a room), that the patient does not have a potential weapon, and that you have sufficient staff close by so that you are safe.

Jason approached the nurse and asked to play pool. The nurse debated about playing but chose to play because Jason appeared distracted, and the game might give him something to focus on.

Ineffective Approach

Nurse: Shall I break?

Jason: (Had been looking off to his right, but turns and looks directly at the nurse.) Yeah, go ahead. (Looks at the table briefly and then turns to look out the door and down the hallway.)

Nurse: (Breaking the pool balls without putting any in a pocket.) It's your turn. You can hit any that you'd like.

Jason: (Turning back to the table.) Huh? (Shaking his head as he stared at the table.) What?

Nurse: You know, Jason, you really should pay attention.

Jason: (Hits a ball in and moves to the other side of the table. Stops in line with the next shot but doesn't bend down to take aim. Stands very still, then shakes his head slightly and quickly. Leans down to take aim and then stands up again.)

Nurse: Jason. (Looks at nurse.) Jason! Are you going to play or not, I don't have all day.

Jason: Oh yeah. (Leans down, takes aim, and misses.)

Nurse: (Moves to where the next shot is. Position is near where Jason is standing. Nurse watches him carefully, moving closer to him.) Please move over, Jason.

Jason: No. (Doesn't move. In peripheral vision, nurse sees Jason's lips move and he again looks to his right and shakes his head in a staccato motion, as if trying to shake something out of his head.)

Effective Approach

Nurse: Shall I break?

Jason: (Had been looking off to his right, but turns and looks directly at the nurse.) Yeah, go ahead. (Looks at the table briefly and then turns to look out the door and down the hallway.)

Nurse: (Breaking the pool balls without putting any in a pocket.) Your turn; you can hit any that you'd like.

Jason: (Turning back to the table.) Huh? (Shakes his head as he stares at the table.) What?

Nurse: You can hit any ball you like. I didn't get any.

Jason: (Hits a ball in and moves to the other side of the table. Stops in line with the next shot but doesn't bend down to take aim. Stands very still, then shakes his head slightly and quickly. Leans down to take aim and then stands up again.)

Nurse: Jason. (He looks at nurse.) Are you aiming at the 10 ball?

Jason: Oh yeah. (Leans down, takes aim, and misses.)

Nurse: (Moving to where her next shot is. The position is very close to where Jason is standing. Nurse watches him carefully while moving closer to him.) Here, let me take this shot.

Jason: Oh. (Moves back. In peripheral vision nurse sees Jason's lips move and again he looks to his right and shakes his head in a staccato motion, as if trying to shake something out of his head.)

Nurse: I missed again. (Moves away from table and turns to Jason, who moves up to the table. He leans down and then stands up again. His lips move again as he turns his head to the right and then looks over his back toward the doorway.) Jason. Jason. (He looks at the nurse.) You have the striped ones.

Jason: (Nods and leans down to take a shot, which he makes. He then misses the next shot. He stands up and moves back from the table, again looking back toward the doorway. He shakes his head) "no".

Nurse: (Watches him closely and moves to the opposite side of the table, making the next shot. Lining up the next shot, Jason leans the pool cue against the table, looks past the nurse, and turns and walks away toward the door. Looks down the hallway, takes a few steps, stops for a minute or so, turns back into the room, and again looks past the nurse. Sits down and shakes his head again. Holds his head in his hands, with his hands covering his ears. The nurse picks up his pool cue and places both against the wall, out of the way. The nurse sits next to another staff member at a vantage point from which Jason can still be watched.)

Critical Thinking Challenge

- How did the nurse's impatience translate into Jason's behaviour in the first scenario?
- What effective communicating techniques did the nurse use in the second scenario?

objects, and their relationship to these. Judgment is the ability to decide or act on a situation. Insight and judgment are closely related to each other and depend on cognitive functions that are frequently impaired in people with schizophrenia.

Behavioural Responses

During periods of psychosis, unusual or bizarre behaviour often occurs. These behaviours can usually be understood within the context of the patient's disturbed thinking. The nurse needs to understand the significance of the behaviour to the individual. One patient moved the family furniture into the yard because he thought that evil spirits were hiding in the furniture. His bizarre behaviour was an attempt to protect his family. Another patient painted a sequence of numbers on his bedroom walls. He said that the numbers were the language of the angels. His bizarre thoughts were at the basis of his behaviour.

Because of the negative symptoms, specifically, avolition, patients may not seem interested or organized to complete normal daily activities. They may stay in bed most of the day or refuse to take a shower. Many times, they will agree to get up in the morning and go to work, but they never get around to it. Several specific behaviours are associated with schizophrenia, including stereotypy (idiosyncratic repetitive, purposeless movements), echopraxia (involuntary imitation of others' movements), and waxy flexibility (posture held in odd or unusual fixed position for extended periods). In some cases, certain behaviours need to be evaluated carefully to distinguish them from movements that are associated with medication side effects, such as grimacing, stereotypic behaviour, or agitation.

Self-Concept

In schizophrenia, self-concept is usually poor. Patients often are aware that they are hearing voices others do not hear. They recognize that they are different from others and are often scared of "going crazy." Many are aware of the loss of expectations for their future achievements. The pervasive stigma associated with having a mental illness contributes to the poor self-concept. Body image can be disturbed, especially during periods of hallucinations or delusions. One patient believed that her body was infected with germs and she could feel them eating away her insides.

Stress and Coping Patterns

Stressful events are often linked to psychiatric symptoms (see Chapter 7 for discussion of the diathesis-stress model). It is important to determine stresses from the patient's perspective because a stressful event for one may not be stressful for another (see Chapter 34). It is also important to determine typical coping patterns, especially negative coping strategies, such as the use of substances or aggressive behaviour.

SPIRITUALITY.   Many people with schizophrenia rely on their religious or spiritual beliefs for dealing with events interfering with their recovery journeys. Longo and Peterson (2002) made a distinction between religion and spirituality. Religion was defined as a set of beliefs, rituals, and practices that are prescribed by an organized religious institution, such as the Judeo-Christian, Islamic, or Hindu traditions. On the other hand, spirituality corresponded to the lived experience with the sacred (eg, supernatural power), which also relies on a system of beliefs and practices but in a broader and more personal approach than does religion. Religious or spiritual beliefs represent a valuable resource in coping with events interfering with recovery (Folkman & Greer, 2000). They may help to appraise difficult events into a positive light (eg, God gives us difficulties that we are able to handle). Religious or spiritual rituals, such as prayer, meditation, or worship activities, may also help to structure the daily lives of people with schizophrenia, which is an important rehabilitation goal. In addition, the relationship with the sacred or with God through prayer or other religious or spiritual activities may offer solace, peace, and serenity, sustaining individuals in their efforts toward recovery.

Risk Assessment

Because of high suicide and attempted suicide rates among patients with schizophrenia, the nurse needs to assess the patient's risk for self-injury: Does the patient speak of suicide, have delusional thinking that could lead to dangerous behaviour, have command hallucinations telling him or her to harm self or others? Does the patient have homicidal ideations? Does the patient lack social support and the skills to be meaningfully engaged with other people or a vocation? Substance-related disorders are also common among patients with schizophrenia, and nurses should assess for substance abuse.

Nursing Diagnoses for Psychological Domain

Many nursing diagnoses can be generated from data collected assessing the psychological domain. Disturbed thought processes can be used for delusions, confusion, and disorganized thinking. Disturbed sensory perception is appropriate for hallucinations or illusions. Other examples of diagnoses include disturbed body image, low self-esteem, disturbed personal identity, risk for violence, ineffective coping, and knowledge deficit.

Interventions for Psychological Domain

All the psychological interventions, such as counselling, conflict resolution, behaviour therapy, and cognitive interventions, are appropriate for patients with schizophrenia. The following discussion focuses on applying these interventions.

Special Issues in the Nurse–Patient Relationship

The development of the nurse–patient relationship with patients with schizophrenia centers on developing trust and accepting the person as a worthy human being. People with schizophrenia are often reluctant to engage in any relationship because of previous rejection and, in some instances, an underlying suspiciousness that is a part of the illness. If they are having hallucinations, their images of other people may be distorted and frightening. They are struggling to trust their own thoughts and perceptions, and engaging in an interaction with another human being may prove too overwhelming.

The nurse should approach the patient in a calm and caring manner. Engaging the patient in a relationship may take time. Short, time-limited interactions are best for a patient who is experiencing psychosis. Being consistent in interactions and following through on promises will help establish trust within the relationship.

Establishing a therapeutic relationship is crucial, especially with patients who deny that they are ill. Patients are more likely to agree to treatment if these recommendations are made within the context of a safe, trusting relationship. Even if some patients deny having mental illness, they may take medication and attend treatment activities because they trust the nurse.

Management of Disturbed Thoughts and Sensory Perceptions

Although antipsychotic medications may relieve positive symptoms, they do not always eliminate hallucinations and delusions. The nurse must continue helping the patient develop creative strategies for dealing with these sensory and thought disturbances. Information about the content of the hallucinations and delusions is needed, not only to determine whether the medications are effective, but also to assess safety and the meaning of these thoughts and perceptions to the patient. In caring for a patient who is experiencing hallucinations or delusions, nursing actions should be guided by three general patient outcomes:

- Decrease the frequency and intensity of hallucinations and delusions.
- Recognize that hallucinations and delusions are symptoms of a brain disorder.
- Develop strategies to manage the recurrence of hallucinations or delusions.

When interacting with a patient who is experiencing hallucinations or delusions, the nurse must remember that these experiences are real to the patient. The nurse should never tell a patient that these experiences are not real. Discounting the experiences blocks communication. It also is dishonest to tell the patient that you are having the same hallucinatory experience. It is best to validate the patient's experiences and identify the meaning of these thoughts and feelings to the patient. For example, a patient who believes that he or she is under surveillance by the RCMP probably feels frightened and suspicious of everyone. By acknowledging how frightening it must be to always feel like you are being watched, the nurse focuses on the feelings that are generated by the delusion, not the delusion itself. The nurse can then offer to help the patient feel safe within this environment. The patient, in turn, begins to feel that someone understands him or her.

Teaching Points

Teaching patients that hallucinations and delusions are part of the disorder becomes easier after the medication begins working. Once patients believe and acknowledge that they have a mental illness and that some of their thoughts are delusions and some of their perceptions are hallucinations, they can develop strategies to manage their symptoms.

Self-Monitoring and Relapse Prevention

Patients benefit greatly by learning techniques of self-regulation, symptom monitoring, and relapse prevention. By monitoring events, time, place, and stimuli surrounding the appearance of symptoms, the patient can begin to predict high-risk times for symptom recurrence. Cognitive behavioural therapy is often used in helping patients monitor and identify their emerging symptoms in order to prevent relapse (Gumley et al., 2003).

Another important nursing intervention is to help the patient identify who and where to talk about delusional or hallucinatory material. Because self-disclosure of these symptoms immediately labels someone as having a mental illness, patients should be encouraged to evaluate the environment for negative consequences of disclosing these symptoms. It may be fine to talk about it at home but not at the grocery store.

Enhancement of Cognitive Functioning

After identifying deficits in cognitive functioning, the nurse and patient can develop interventions that target specific deficits. The most effective interventions usually involve the whole treatment team. If the ability to focus or attend is an issue, patients can be encouraged to select activities that improve attention, such as computer games. For memory problems, patients can be encouraged to make lists and to write down important information.

Executive functioning problems are the most challenging for these patients. Patients who cannot manage daily problems may have planning and problem solving impairments. For these patients, developing interventions that closely simulate real-world problems may help. Through coaching, the nurse can teach and support the development of problem-solving skills. For example, during hospitalizations, patients are given medications and reminded to take them on time. They are often instructed in a classroom setting but rarely have an opportunity to practice self-medication and figure out what to do if their prescription expires, the medications are lost, or they forget their medications. Yet, when discharged, patients are expected to take medication at the prescribed dose at the prescribed time. Interventions designed to have patients actively engage in problem-solving behaviour with real problems are needed.

Another approach to helping patients solve problems and learn new strategies for dealing with problems is

BOX 17.18   RESEARCH FOR BEST PRACTICE

Might Within the Madness

THE QUESTION: This study used solution-focused therapy (SFT) to help thought-disordered patients better cope with some of their negative experiences and symptoms.

METHODS: The authors provided an overview of SFT, focussing on how these techniques might be used in an inpatient psychiatry setting with patients experiencing disordered thoughts.

Three patient cases were presented: a 26-year-old man admitted to an inpatient hospital psychiatric unit with intrusive auditory and visual hallucinations; a 67-year-old woman who lived most of her life on a farm and managed her symptoms well until a recent move to the city; and a 49-year-old woman who was experiencing paranoid delusions about bombers and airplanes.

FINDINGS: By using SFT, the nurses could see the individual as a person with hopes, dreams, and strengths. They also concluded that the SFT process was as important as the outcome.

IMPLICATIONS FOR NURSING: This study can have direct clinical application for those interested in developing solution-focussed techniques. Using some of the SFT techniques can help the nurse see past the disorder and view the patient as a human being with strengths.

From Hagen, B., & Mitchell, D. (2001). Might within the madness: Solution-focused therapy and thought-disordered clients. *Archives of Psychiatric Nursing, 15*(2), 86–93.

solution-focused therapy, which focuses on the strengths and positive attributes that exist within each person. This is a therapy that involves years of training to master, but there are techniques that can be used. For example, patients can be asked to identify the most important problem from their perspective. This focuses the patient on an important issue for that patient (Box 17-18).

Behavioural Interventions

Behavioural interventions can be very effective in helping patients improve motivation and organize routine, daily activities, such as maintaining a regular schedule and completing activities. Reinforcement of positive behaviours (getting up on time, completing hygiene, going to treatment activities) can easily be included in a treatment plan. In the hospital, patients gain ward privileges by following an agreed-on treatment plan.

Stress and Coping Skills

Developing skills to cope with personal, social, and environmental stresses is important to everyone, but particularly to those with a severe mental illness. Stresses can easily trigger symptoms that patients are trying to avoid. Establishing regular counselling sessions to support the development of positive coping skills is helpful for both the hospitalized patient and those in the community.

Patient Education

Cognitive deficits (difficulty in processing complex information, maintaining steady focus of attention, distinguishing between relevant and irrelevant stimuli, and forming abstractions), may challenge the nurse planning educational activities. Evidence indicates that people with schizophrenia may learn best in an errorless learning environment (O'Carroll, Russell, Lawrie, & Johnstone, 1999), that is, they are directly given correct information and then encouraged to write it down. Asking questions that encourage guessing is not as effective in helping them retain information. Trial-and-error learning is avoided. In one study, a group of people with schizophrenia who were taught using an errorless learning approach improved work skill in two entry-level job tasks (index card filing and toilet-tank assembly) and performed better than the group that was instructed with conventional trial-and-error instruction (Kern, Green, Mintz, & Liberman, 2003; Kern, Liberman, Kopelowicz, Mintz, & Green, 2002).

Teaching and explaining should occur in an environment with minimal distractions. Terminology should be clear and unambiguous. Visual aids can supplement verbal information, but these materials should have simple information stated in simple language. The nurse takes care not to overcrowd the visual material or incorporate images that draw attention away from important content. Teaching should occur in small segments with frequent reinforcement. Most important of all, teaching should occur when the patient is ready. Regular assessments of cognitive abilities with standardized instruments can help determine this readiness. These suggestions can be adapted for teaching during any phase of the illness.

Skill-training interventions should be designed to compensate for cognitive deficits. To help patients learn to process complex activities, such as catching a bus, preparing a meal, or shopping for food or clothing, nurses should break the activity into small parts or steps and list them for the patient's reference, for example:

- Leave apartment with keys in hand.
- Make sure you have correct bus fare in your pocket.
- Close the door.
- Walk to the corner.
- Turn right and walk 3 blocks to the bus stop.

Family Education

Because having a family member with schizophrenia is a life-changing event for the family and friends who provide care and support, educating patients and their families is crucial. It is a primary concern for the psychiatric–mental health nurse. Family support is crucial to help patients maintain treatment. Education should include information about the disease course, treatment

When caring for the patient with schizophrenia, be sure to include the caregiver as appropriate and address the following topic areas in the teaching plan:

☐ Psychopharmacologic agents, including drug action, dosage, frequency, and possible adverse effects. Stress importance of adherence to the prescribed regimen.

☐ Management of hallucinations

☐ Coping strategies such as self-talk, getting busy

☐ Management of the environment

☐ Use of contracts that detail expected behaviours, with goals and consequences

☐ Community resources

regimens, support systems, and life management skills (see Box 17-19). The most important factor to stress during patient and family education is the consistent taking of medication.

Social Domain

Social Assessment

Several difficulties with social functioning occur in schizophrenia. As the disorder progresses, individuals can become increasingly socially isolated. On a one-to-one basis, this occurs because the individual seems unable to connect with people in his or her environment. Several aspects of the symptoms already discussed can contribute to this, for example, emotional blunting and anhedonia (the inability to form emotional attachment and experience pleasure). Cognitive deficits that contribute to difficult social functioning include problems with face and affect recognition, deficiencies in recall of past interactions, problems with decision making and judgment in conflictual interactions, and poverty of speech and language. Poor functioning and the inability to complete activities of daily living are manifested in poor hygiene, malnutrition, and social isolation.

Functional Status

Functional status of patients with schizophrenia should be assessed initially and at regular periods. The usual assessment instrument is the Global Assessment of Functioning (GAF). If the GAF score is below 60, interventions should be designed to enhance social or occupational functioning.

Social Systems

In schizophrenia, support systems become very important in maintaining the patient in the community. The individual may become socially isolated if the treatment and management occur in long-term care facilities and group homes away from family and friends. One

challenge in treating schizophrenia is to identify and maintain the patient's links with family and significant others. Assessment of the formal support (eg, family, providers) and informal support (eg, neighbors, friends) should be conducted.

Quality of Life

People with schizophrenia often have a poor quality of life, especially older people, who may have spent many years in a long-term hospital. The nurse should assess the patient's quality of life and how it could be improved. Simple changes, such as arranging for a different roommate or improving access to social activities by meeting transportation needs, can greatly improve a patient's quality of life.

Family Assessment

The assessment of the family could take many forms, and the family assessment guide presented in Chapter 16 can be used. In some instances, the patient will be young and living with his or her parents. Often, the nurse's first contact with the patient and family is in the initial phases of the disorder. The family is dealing with the shock and disbelief of seeing a child with a mental illness that has lifelong consequences. In this instance, the assessment process may be extended over several sessions to provide the family with support and education about the disorder.

Because women with schizophrenia generally have better treatment outcomes than do men, many will marry and have children. These women experience the same life stresses as other women and may find themselves single parents, raising children in poverty-stricken conditions. Managing a psychiatric illness and trying to be an effective parent in a socially stigmatizing society is almost an impossibility because of the lack of financial resources and social support. This family will need an extensive assessment of financial need and social support. The family life cycle model presented in Chapter 16 can also be used as a framework for the assessment.

Nursing Diagnoses for Social Domain

The nursing diagnoses generated from the assessment of the social domain are typically Impaired Social Interaction, Ineffective Role Performance, Disabled Family Coping, or Interrupted Family Processes. Outcomes will depend on the specific diagnostic area.

Interventions for Social Domain

Promoting Patient Safety

Although violence is not a consistent behaviour of people with schizophrenia, it is always a concern during the initial phase when hallucinations or delusions may put patients at risk for harming themselves or others. Nonviolent patients who are experiencing hallucinations and delusions can also be at risk for victimization by more aggressive patients. The patient who is hallucinating needs to be protected. This protection may include increased staff monitoring and, if necessary, a safer environment in a secluded area.

The nurse's best approach to avoiding violence or aggression is to demonstrate respect for the patient and the patient's personal space, assess and monitor for signs of fear and agitation, and use preventive interventions before the patient loses control. Medications should be administered as ordered. Because most antipsychotic and antidepressant medications take 1 to 2 weeks to begin moderating behaviour, the nurse must be vigilant during the acute illness.

Reducing environmental stimulation is particularly important for individuals who are experiencing hallucinations but can be helpful for all patients when signs of fear and agitation are observed. Allowing patients to use private rooms or seclusion for brief periods can be an important preventive method.

Other techniques of managing the environment (milieu management) have been found to be helpful in inpatient settings. One researcher who examined aggression and violence in psychiatric hospitals found violent behaviour to be associated with the following predictors: history of violence, a coercive interaction style of using violence to obtain what is desired, and an environment in which violence is inadvertently rewarded, for example, by gaining staff attention (Morrison, 1992, 1993; Morrison et al., 2002). Morrison proposed the methods to help avoid acts of violence or aggression:

- Taking a thorough history that includes information about the patient's past use of violence
- Helping the patient to talk directly and constructively with those with whom they are angry, rather than venting anger to staff about a third person
- Setting limits with consistent and justly applied consequences
- Involving the patient in formulating a contract that outlines patient and staff behaviours, goals, and consequences
- Scheduling brief but regular time-outs to allow the patient some privacy without the attention of staff either before or after the time-out (these time-outs may be patient activated)

Staff need to have planned sessions after all incidents of violence or physical management in which the event is analyzed. These sessions allow staff to learn how better to manage these situations and evaluate patients' cues. With sensitive leadership, these sessions can help staff to learn more about the interaction of patient and staff characteristics that can contribute to these incidents.

Convening Support Groups

People with mental illness benefit from support groups that focus on daily problems and the stress of dealing with a mental illness. These groups are useful throughout the continuum of care and help reduce the risk for suicide. In the hospital setting, the focus of the group can be simply sharing the experience of living with a mental illness. In the community, a regular support group can provide interaction with people with similar problems and issues. Friendships often develop from these groups.

Implementing Milieu Therapy

Individuals with schizophrenia can be hospitalized or live in group homes for a long period of time. Expecting people who have an illness that interferes with their ability to live with family members to live with complete strangers in peace and harmony is unrealistic. Arranging the treatment environment to maximize therapy is crucial to the rehabilitation of the patient.

Developing Psychiatric Rehabilitation Strategies

Rehabilitation strategies are used to support the individual's recovery and integration into the community (see Chapter 18). Community-based psychosocial rehabilitation programs usually offer long-term intensive case management services to adults with schizophrenia. Programs provide a continuum of services to meet the changing needs of people with psychiatric disabilities. Patients set rehabilitation goals, and services are then provided to help "clients" (most programs do not use the term "patients") reach their goals. Services range from daily home visits to providing transportation, occupational training, and group support. Social skills training shows much promise for patients with schizophrenia, both individually and in groups. This is a method for teaching patients specific behaviours needed for social interactions. The skills are taught by lecture, demonstration, role playing, and homework assignments (see Chapters 12 and 15). Nurses may be team members and involved in case management or provision of services. These and other psychological treatment approaches, combined with breakthroughs in biologic therapy, continue to help improve the functioning and quality of life for patients with schizophrenia.

Family Interventions

When schizophrenia first becomes apparent, the patient and family must negotiate the mental health system for the first time (in most cases), a challenge that almost equals that of confronting the family member's illness. In most states, the mental health system is huge and is usually ignored unless an adult foster care home moves into a neighborhood or a family member becomes seriously mentally ill. The system includes private inpatient and outpatient clinics supported by insurance and public community mental health clinics and hospitals supported by public funds. Because mental health coverage in most insurance packages is insufficient for someone with schizophrenia, most families eventually deal with the public mental health system. If the patient is aggressive, many private facilities encourage hospitalization in a public sector facility even for the first admission.

Family members should be encouraged to participate in support groups that help family members deal with the realities of living with a loved one with a mental illness. Family members should be given information about local community and state resources and organizations such as mental health associations and those that can help families negotiate the complex provider systems.

EVALUATION AND TREATMENT OUTCOMES

Outcome research related to schizophrenia has redefined previous ways of thinking about the course of the disorder. Schizophrenia was once considered to have a progressively long-term and downward course, but it is now known that schizophrenia can be successfully treated and managed. In one older, but significant study, the researchers interviewed patients 20 to 25 years after diagnosis and found that 50% to 66% experienced significant improvement or recovery (Harding, Zubin, & Strauss, 1987). This study is important because it occurred before the development of atypical antipsychotic agents. Today, we can be hopeful that even more people can experience improvement or recover from schizophrenia.

CONTINUUM OF CARE

Continuity of care has been identified as a major goal of community mental health systems for patients with schizophrenia because they are at risk for becoming "lost" to services if left alone after discharge. Discharge planning encourages follow-up care in the community. In fact, many state mental health systems require an outpatient appointment before discharge. Treatment of schizophrenia occurs across a variety of settings. Not only inpatient hospitalization but also partial hospitalization, day treatment, and crisis stabilization can be used effectively.

Inpatient-Focussed Care

Much of the previous discussion concerns care in the inpatient setting. Today, inpatient hospitalizations are brief and focus on patient stabilization. Many times, patients are involuntarily admitted for a short period. During the stabilization period, the status is changed to voluntary admission, whereby the patient agrees to treatment.

Emergency Care

Emergency care ideally takes place in a hospital emergency room, but often the crisis occurs in the home. Patients are usually relapsing and do not recognize their bizarre or aggressive behaviours as symptoms. A specially trained crisis team is sent to assess the emergency and recommend further treatment. In the emergency room, patients are brought not only because of relapse but also because of medication side effects or water intoxication. Nurses should refer to the previous discussion for nursing management.

Community Care

Most of the care of patients with schizophrenia will be in the community through publicly supported mental health delivery systems. Community services include assertive community treatment, outpatient therapy, case management, and psychosocial rehabilitation, including clubhouse programs. For patients with a community treatment order (CTO) in effect that delineates the conditions required to live in the community, services must be congruent with those conditions (see Chapter 3). For all patients in the community, his or her health care should be integrated with physical health care. Nurses should be especially vigilant that patients with mental illnesses receive proper primary and medical health care.

CRNE Note

Priorities in the patient with acute symptoms of schizophrenia include managing psychosis and keeping the patient safe and free from harming self or others. In the community, the priorities are preventing relapse, maintain psychosocial functioning, psychoeducation, and improving quality of life.

Mental Health Promotion

In some cases, it is not the disorder itself that threatens the mental health of the person with schizophrenia but the stresses of trying to receive care and services. Health care systems are complex and are often at the mercy of a system rule that is outdated. Development of assertiveness and conflict resolution skills can help the person in negotiating access to systems that will provide

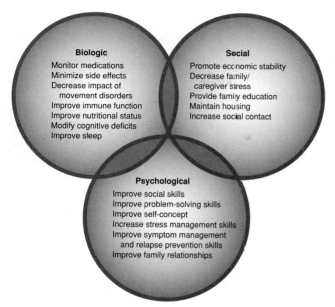

FIGURE 17.6 Biopsychosocial interventions for patients with schizophrenia.

services. Developing a positive support system for stressful periods will help promote a positive outcome (Fig. 17-6).

SUMMARY OF KEY POINTS

◘ The patient with schizophrenia displays a complex myriad of symptoms typically categorized as positive symptoms (those that exist but should not), such as delusions or hallucinations and disorganized thinking and behaviour, and negative symptoms (characteristics that should be there but are lacking), and these include alogia, avolition, anhedonia, and affective blunting.

◘ In the past, the diagnosis and treatment of schizophrenia focussed on the more observable and dramatic positive symptoms (ie, delusions and hallucinations), but recently scientists have shifted their focus to the disorganizing symptoms of cognition.

◘ The clinical presentation of schizophrenia occurs in three phases: phase 1 entails initial diagnosis and first treatment; phase 2 includes periods of relative calm between episodes of overt signs and symptoms but during which the patient needs sustained treatment; and phase 3 includes periods of exacerbation or relapse that require hospitalization or more frequent contacts with mental health professionals and increased use of resources.

◘ Biologic theories of what causes schizophrenia include genetic, infectious-autoimmune, neuroanatomic, and dopamine hypotheses. The last is supported by the advanced technology of positron emission tomography scan findings and the understanding of the mechanisms of antipsychotic medications.

◘ Biologic assessment of the patient with schizophrenia must include a thorough history and physical examination to rule out any medical illness or substance abuse problem that might be the cause of the patient's symptoms; assessment of risk for self-injury or injury to others; and creation of baseline health information before medications are administered. Several standardized assessment tools are available to help assess characteristic abnormal motor movements.

◘ Several nursing interventions address the biologic domain—promotion of self-care activities, activity, exercise, nutritional, thermoregulation, and fluid balance interventions. In general the antipsychotic drugs used to treat schizophrenia block dopamine transmission in the brain but also cause some troublesome and sometimes serious side effects, primarily anticholinergic side effects and extrapyramidal side effects (motor abnormalities). Newer antipsychotic agents block serotonin as well as dopamine. The nurse should be familiar with these drugs, their possible side effects, and the interventions required to manage or control side effects.

◘ The extrapyramidal side effects of antipsychotic drugs can appear early in drug treatment and include acute parkinsonism or pseudoparkinsonism, acute dystonia, and akathisia; or they can appear late in treatment after months or years. The primary example of late-appearing extrapyramidal side effects is tardive dyskinesia, which is a severe syndrome of abnormal motor movements of the mouth, tongue, and jaw.

◘ Psychological assessment must include equal attention to manifestations of both positive and negative symptoms and a concentrated focus on the cognitive impairments that make it so difficult for these patients to manage their disorder. Several standardized assessment tools assess for positive and negative symptoms. Development of the nurse–patient relationship becomes key in helping patients manage the disturbed thoughts and sensory perceptions. Interventions should be designed to enhance cognitive functioning. Patient and family education are critical interventions for the person with schizophrenia.

◘ Because schizophrenia is a lifetime disorder and patients require the continued support and care of mental health professionals and family or friends, one of the primary nursing interventions is ensuring that patients and families are properly educated regarding the course of the disorder, importance of drug maintenance, and need for consistent care and support. Research is demonstrating that interaction between patients and their families is key to the success of long-term treatments and outcomes.

CRITICAL THINKING CHALLENGES

1 Why are positive symptoms easier to track than negative symptoms?

2 Describe ways in which medical illness or substance abuse could cause a patient to show symptoms similar to schizophrenia.

3 Suggest reasons that a higher rate of schizophrenia is found in lower classes of people from urban, industrialized communities.

4 The physical environment is important to the patient with schizophrenia. Think of the typical hospital unit. What environmental factors could be stress producing or misleading to the person with schizophrenia?

5 Compare therapeutic and nontherapeutic communication skills when dealing with a person with schizophrenia who is actively hallucinating.

WEB LINKS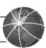

www.schizophrenia.ca   This is the site of the Schizophrenia Society of Canada, an organization committed to alleviating suffering caused by schizophrenia.

www.nami.org   This is the website of the National Alliance for the Mentally Ill in the United States.

www.nimh.nih.gov/publicat/schioph.htm   The U.S. National Institute of Mental Health website presents all aspects of the diagnosis and treatment of schizophrenia.

www.narsad.org   This is the site of the U.S. National Alliance for Research on Schizophrenia and Depression, which is a national organization that raises and distributes money for research.

www.schizophrenia.com   This is a not-for-profit information, support, and education center.

www.mentalhealth.com   This site of the Mental Health Network provides extensive information on schizophrenia.

MOVIES

Benny and Joon: 1993. Joon is a young woman with schizophrenia who lives with her overprotective brother. In an attempt to keep her safe, Joon's brother unsuccessfully hires one housekeeper after another. After winning a bet in a poker game, Joon's brother acquires Benny, played by Johnny Depp, who entertains and cares for Joon. A romance develops that results in Benny and Joon attempting to run away. Joon's symptoms reappear. After treatment, Joon struggles with becoming independent from both her brother and boyfriend.

VIEWING POINTS: How does Joon's brother's behaviour interfere with her normal growth and development? When Joon's symptoms appeared, how would you classify them according to the *DSM-IV-TR?* What advice would you like to give to Joon and her brother?

A Beautiful Mind: 2001. This academy award-winning movie starring Russell Crowe is based on the biography of the mathematician and Nobel Laureate John Nash by Sylvia Naasar. It presents the life and experiences of this man as he experienced schizophrenia. It shows how his life and work were altered and the effects on his relationships with family and colleagues. The movie depicts how this man came to terms with his illness.

VIEWING POINTS: How does the treatment John Nash received in the 1950s differ from treatment today? How would you classify his symptoms according to *DSM-IV-TR?* What is typical and/or problematic about Mr. Nash's relationship with the medications prescribed for him?

REFERENCES

Adityanjee, A. U. A., & Mathews, T. (1999). Epidemiology of neuroleptic malignant syndrome. *Clinical Neuropharmacology, 22*(3), 151–158.

Altamura, A. C., Bassetti, R., Bignotti, S., Pioli, R., & Mundo, E. (2003). Clinical variables related to suicide attempts in schizophrenic patients: A retrospective study. *Schizophrenia Research, 60,* 47–55.

American Psychiatric Association. (2000). *Diagnostic and statistical manual of mental disorders* (4th ed., Text revision). Washington, DC: Author.

Baldessarini, R. J. (2002). Clinical psychopharmacology: Overview and recent advances. Symposium conducted at Cape Cod Symposia, Eastham, Massachusetts.

Benes, F. M. (2000). Emerging principles of altered neural circuitry in schizophrenia. *Brain Research Developmental Brain Research, 31*(2–3), 251–269.

Boyd, M., & Lapierre, E. (1996). Fluid imbalance and water intoxication: The elusive syndrome. In A. McBride & J. Austin (Eds.), *Psychiatric mental health nursing: Integration of the biological into behavioural* (pp. 396–424). Philadelphia: WB Saunders.

Boyd, M. A., Williams, L., Evenson, R., Eckert, A., Beaman, M., & Carr, T. R. (1992). A target weight procedure for disordered water balance in long-term care facilities. *Journal of Psychosocial Nursing and Mental Health Services, 30*(12), 22–27.

Buchsbaum, M. (1990). The frontal lobes, basal ganglia, and temporal lobes as a site for schizophrenia. *Schizophrenia Bulletin, 16,* 377–387.

Byrne, M., Agerbo, E., Ewald, H., Eaton, W. W., & Mortensen, P. B. (2003). Parental age and risk of schizophrenia: A case-control study. *Archives of General Psychiatry, 60*(7), 673–678.

Caroff, S., & Mann, S. (1993). Neuroleptic malignant syndrome. *Medical Clinics of North America, 77,* 185–202.

Casey, D. E. (1994). Schizophrenia: Psychopharmacology. In J. W. Jefferson & J. H. Greist (Eds.), *The psychiatric clinics of North America annual of drug therapy* (Vol. 1, pp. 81–100). Philadelphia: WB Saunders.

Chou, Y. H., Halldin, C., & Farde, L. (2003). Occupancy of 5HT(1A) receptors in clozapine in the primate brain: A PET study. *Psychopharmacology, 166*(3), 234–240.

Ciompi, L. (1989). The dynamics of complex biological-psychosocial systems: Four fundamental psycho-biological mediators in the long-term evolution of schizophrenia. *British Journal of Psychiatry, 11*(Suppl, 5), 15–21.

Cirillo, M. A., & Seidman, L. J. (2003). Verbal declarative memory dysfunction in schizophrenia: From clinical assessment to genetics and brain mechanisms. *Neuropsychology Review, 13*(2), 43–77.

Csernansky, J. G. (2003). Treatment of schizophrenia: Preventing the progression of disease. *Psychiatric Clinics of North America, 26*(2), 367–379.

Davidson, L. L., & Heinrichs, R. W. (2003). Quantification of frontal and temporal lobe brain-imaging findings in schizophrenia: A meta-analysis. *Psychiatry Research, 122*(2), 69–87.

De Hert, M., McKenzie, K., & Peuskens, J. (2001). Risk factors for suicide in young people suffering from schizophrenia: A long-term follow-up study. *Schizophrenia Research, 47*(2–3), 127–134.

Dolder, C. R., Lacro, J. P., Dunn, L. B., & Jeste, D. V. (2002). Antipsychotic medication adherence: Is there a difference between typical and atypical agents? *American Journal of Psychiatry, 159*(1), 103–108.

Falkai, P., Schneider-Axmann, T., Honer, W. G., Vogeley, K., Schonell, H., Pfeiffer, U., Scherk, H., Block, W., Traber, F., Schild, H. H., Maier, W., & Tepest, R. (2003). Influence on genetic loading, obstetric complications, and premorbid adjustment on brain morphology in schizophrenia: A MRI study. *European Archives of Psychiatry and Clinical Neuroscience, 253*(2), 92–99.

Folkman, S., & Greer, S. (2000). Promoting psychological well-being in the face of serious illness: When theory, research and practice inform each other. *Psycho-Oncology, 9*, 11–19.

Franzen, G. (1970). Plasma free fatty acids before and after an intravenous insulin injection in acute schizophrenic men. *British Journal of Psychiatry, 116*(531), 173–177.

Ghose, S., Weickert, C. S., Colvin, S. M., Coyle, J. T., Herman, M. M., Hyde, T. M., & Kleinman, J. E. (2003). Glutamate carboxypeptidase II gene expression in the human frontal and temporal lobe in schizophrenia. *Neuropsychopharmacology, 29*(1), 117–125.

Goldman, L. S. (1999). Medical illness in patients with schizophrenia. *Journal of Clinical Psychiatry, 60*(Suppl 21), 1015.

Goldner, E. M., Hsu, L., Waraich, P., & Somers, J. M. (2002). Prevalence and incidence studies of schizophrenia disorders: A systematic review of the literature. *Canadian Journal of Psychiatry, 47*(9), 833–843.

Green, M. F., Kern, R. S., Braff, D. L., & Mintz, J. (2000). Neurocognitive deficits and functional outcome in schizophrenia: Are we measuring the "right stuff"? *Schizophrenia Bulletin, 26*(1), 119–137.

Gumley, A., O'Grady, M., McNay, L., Reilly, J., Power, K., & Norrie, J. (2003). Early intervention for relapse in schizophrenia: Results of a 12-month randomized controlled trial of cognitive behavioural therapy. *Psychological Medicine, 33*(3), 419–431.

Gur, R. E., & Gur, R. C. (2005). Neuroimaging in schizophrenia: Linking neuropsychiatric manifestations to neurobiology. In B. J. Sadock & V. A. Sadock (Eds.), *Comprehensive textbook of psychiatry* (pp. 1396–1408). Philadelphia: Lippincott Williams & Wilkins.

Gureje, O., & Bamidele, R. W. (1998). Gender and schizophrenia: Association of age at onset with antecedent, clinical and outcome features. *Australia New Zealand Journal of Psychiatry, 32*(3), 415–423.

Guy, W. (1976). *ECDEU: Assessment manual for psychopharmacology* (DHEW Publication No. 76-338). Washington, DC: Department of Health Education and Welfare, Psychopharmacology Branch.

Hafner, H. (2003). Gender differences in schizophrenia. *Psychoneuroendocrinology, 23*(Suppl 2), 17–54.

Hagen, B., & Mitchell, D. (2001). Might within the madness: Solution-focused therapy and thought-disordered clients. *Archives of Psychiatric Nursing, 15*(2), 86–93.

Harding, C., Zubin, J., & Strauss, J. (1987). Chronicity in schizophrenia: Fact, partial fact or artifact? *Hospital and Community Psychiatry, 38*(5), 477–486.

Harrison, G., Fouskakis, D., Rasmussen, F., Tynelius, P., Sipos, A., & Gunnell, D. (2003). Association between psychotic disorder and urban place of birth is not mediated by obstetric complications or childhood socioeconomic position: A cohort study. *Psychological Medicine, 33*(4), 723–731.

Hartman, M., Steketee, M. C., Silva, S., Lanning, K., & Andersson, C. (2003). Wisconsin Card Sorting Test performance in schizo-

phrenia: The role of working memory. *Schizophrenia Research, 63*(3), 201–217.

Health Canada. (2002). *A report on mental illnesses in Canada*. Retrieved August 31, 2005, from Government of Canada: http://www.phac-aspc.gc.ca/publicat/miic-mmac/pdf/chap_3_e.pdf.

Jibson, M. D., & Tandon, R. (2000). Treatment of schizophrenia. In D. L. Dunner & J. E. Rosenbaum (Eds.), *The psychiatric clinics of North America annual of drug therapy* (Vol. 7, pp. 83–113). Philadelphia: WB Saunders.

Kandel, E. R., Schwartz, J. H., & Jessell, T. M. (2000). *Principles of neural science* (4th ed.). New York: McGraw-Hill.

Kay, S. R., Fiszbein, A., & Opler, L. A. (1987). The Positive and Negative Syndrome Scale (PANSS) for schizophrenia. *Schizophrenia Bulletin, 13*, 261–276.

Kern, R. S., Green, M. V., Mintz, J., & Liberman, R. P. (2003). Does 'errorless learning' compensate for neurocognitive impairments in the work rehabilitation of persons with schizophrenia? *Psychological Medicine, 33*(3), 433–442.

Kern, R. S., Liberman, R. P., Kopelowicz, A., Mintz, J., & Green, M. F. (2002). Applications of errorless learning for improving work performance in persons with schizophrenia. *American Journal Psychiatry, 159*(11), 1921–1926.

Leucht, S., Barnes, T. R., Kissling, W., Engel, R. R., Correll, C., & Kane, J. M. (2003). Relapse prevention in schizophrenia with new-generation antipsychotics: A systematic review and exploratory meta-analysis of randomized, controlled trials. *American Journal of Psychiatry, 160*(7), 1209–1222.

Liberman, R. P., & Kopelowicz, A. (2005). Recovery from schizophrenia: A concept in search of research. *Psychiatric Services, 56*, 735–742.

Longo, D. A., & Peterson, S. M. (2002). The role of spirituality in psychosocial rehabilitation. *Psychiatric Rehabilitation Journal, 25*, 333–340.

Marengo, J. (1994). Classifying the courses of schizophrenia. *Schizophrenia Bulletin, 20*, 519–536.

McDonald, C., Grech, A., Toulopoulou, T., Schulze, K., Chapple, B., Sham, P., Walshe, M., Sharma, R., Sigmundsson, T., Chitnis, X., & Murray, R. M. (2003). Brain volumes in familial and non-familial schizophrenia probands and their unaffected relatives. *American Journal of Medical Genetics, 114*(6), 616–625.

McGlashan, T. H. (1994). Psychosocial treatments of schizophrenia: The potential relationships. In N. C. Andreasen (Ed.), *Schizophrenia: From mind to molecule* (pp. 189–215). Washington, DC: American Psychiatric Press.

Mercier-Guidez, E., & Loas, G. (2000). Polydipsia and water intoxication in 353 psychiatric inpatients: An epidemiological and psychopathological study. *European Psychiatry, 15*(5), 306–311.

Montoya, A., Ocampo, M., & Torres-Ruiz, A. (2003). Neuroleptic malignant syndrome in Mexico. *Canadian Journal of Clinical Pharmacology, 10*(3), 111–113.

Morrison, E. F. (1992). A coercive interactional style as an antecedent to aggression in psychiatric patients. *Research in Nursing and Health, 15*, 421–431.

Morrison, E. F. (1993). Toward a better understanding of violence in psychiatric settings: Debunking the myths. *Archives of Psychiatric Nursing, 7*, 328–335.

Morrison, E. F., & Carney Love, C. (2003). An evaluation of four programs for the management of aggression in psychiatric settings. *Archives in Psychiatric Nursing, 17*(4), 146–155.

Murray, R. M., & Bramon, E. (2005). Developmental model of schizophrenia. (2005). In B. J. Sadock & V. A. Sadock (Eds.), *Comprehensive textbook of psychiatry* (pp. 1381–1396). Philadelphia: Lippincott Williams & Wilkins.

New Freedom Commission on Mental Health. (2003). *Achieving the promise: Transforming mental health care in America: Final report.* Department of Health and Human Services (DHHS) Publication No. SMA-0303831. Rockville, MD: DHHS.

Niemi, L. T., Suvisaari, J. M., Tuulio-Henriksson, A., & Lonnqvist, J. K. (2003). Childhood developmental abnormalities in schizophrenia: Evidence from high-risk studies. *Schizophrenia Research, 60*(2–3), 239–258.

O'Carroll, R., Russell, H., Lawrie, S., & Johnstone, E. (1999). Errorless learning and the cognitive rehabilitation of memory-impaired schizophrenic patients. *Psychological Medicine, 29,* 105–112.

Ota, M., Mizukami, K., Katano, T., Sato, S., Takeda, T., & Asada, T. (2003). A case of delusional disorder, somatic type with remarkable improvement of clinical symptoms and single photon emission computed tomography findings following modified electroconvulsive therapy. *Progress in Neuro-Psychopharmacology & Biological Psychiatry, 27*(5), 881–884.

Overall, J. E., & Gorham, D. R. (1962). The Brief Psychiatric Rating Scale. *Psychological Reports, 10,* 799–812.

Overall, J. E., & Gorham, D. R. (1988). The Brief Psychiatric Rating Scale (BPRS): Recent developments in ascertainment and scaling. *Psychopharmacology Bulletin, 24,* 97–99.

Penn, A. A. (2001). Early brain wiring: Activity-dependent processes. *Schizophrenia Bulletin, 27*(3), 336–347.

Reeves, S., Stewart, R., & Howard, R. (2002). Service contact and psychopathology in very–late-onset schizophrenia-like psychosis: The effects of gender and ethnicity. *International Journal of Geriatric Psychiatry, 17*(5), 473–479.

Riggs, A., Dyksen, M., Kim, S., & Opsahl, J. (1991). A review of disorders of water homeostasis in psychiatric patients. *Psychosomatics, 32*(2), 133–148.

Ryan, M. C. M., Collins, P., & Thakore, J. H. (2003). Impaired fasting glucose tolerance in first-episode, drug-naive patients with schizophrenia. *American Journal of Psychiatry, 160,* 284–289.

Sallet, P. C., Elkis, H., Alves, T. M., Oliveira, J. R., Sassi, E., Campi de Castro, C., Busatto, F. G., & Gattaz, W. F. (2003). Reduced cortical folding in schizophrenia: An MRI morphometric study. *American Journal of Psychiatry, 160*(9), 1606–1613.

Schimmelbusch, W. H., Mueller, P. S., & Sheps, J. (1971). The positive correlation between insulin resistance and duration of hospitalization in untreated schizophrenia. *British Journal of Psychiatry, 118*(545), 42–36.

Sedvall, G. (1994). Positron-emission tomography as a metabolic and neurochemical probe. In N. C. Andreasen (Ed.), *Schizophrenia: From mind to molecule* (pp. 147–155). Washington, DC: American Psychiatric Press.

Simpson, G. M., & Angus, J. W. S. L. (1970). A rating scale for extrapyramidal side effects. *Acta Psychiatrica Scandinavica, 212*(Suppl), 11–19.

Snider, K., & Boyd, M. (1991). When they drink too much: Nursing interventions for patients with disordered water balance. *Journal of Psychosocial Nursing, 29*(7), 10–16.

Sprague, R. L., & Kalachnik, J. E. (1991). Reliability, validity, and a total score cutoff for the Dyskinesia Identification Scale System: Condensed User Scale (DISCUS) with mentally ill and mentally retarded populations. *Psychopharmacology Bulletin, 27,* 51–58.

Stahl, S. (2000). *Essential psychopharmacology: Neuroscientific basis and practical application* (2nd ed.). Cambridge, United Kingdom: Cambridge University Press.

Stahl, S. M. (2002). The metabolic syndrome: Psychopharmacologists should weigh the evidence for weighing the patient. *Journal of Clinical Psychiatry, 63,* 1094–1095.

Subotnik, K. L., Goldstein, M. J., Nuechterlein, K. H., Woo, S. M., & Mintz, J. (2002). Are communication deviance and expressed emotion related to family history of psychiatric disorders in schizophrenia? *Schizophrenia Bulletin, 28*(4), 719–729.

Tsuang, M. T., Stone, W. S., & Faraone, S. V. (2001). Genes, environment and schizophrenia. *British Journal of Psychiatry, 178*(Suppl 40), S18–S24.

United States Department of Health and Human Services (U.S. DHHS). (1999). *Mental health: A report of the Surgeon General.* Rockville, MD: Author.

United States Department of Health and Human Services (U.S. DHHS). (2001). *Mental health: Culture, race, and ethnicity—A supplement to mental health: A report of the Surgeon General.* Rockville, MD: Author.

van Meijel, B., van der Gaag, M., Kahn, R. S., & Grypdonck, M. H. (2003). Relapse prevention in patients with schizophrenia: The application of an intervention protocol in nursing practice. *Archives of Psychiatric Nursing, 17*(4), 165–172.

Walker, E., Kestler, L., Bollini, A., & Hochman, K. M. (2004). Schizophrenia: Etiology and course. *Annual Review of Psychology, 55,* 401–430.

Weisman, A. G., Gomes, L. G., & Lopez, S. R. (2003). Shifting blame away from ill relatives: Latino families' reactions to schizophrenia. *Journal of Nervous and Mental Disease, 191*(9), 574–581.

Westermeyer, J. F., & Harrow, M. (1988). Course and outcome in schizophrenia. In M. T. Tsuang & J. C. Simpson (Eds.), *Handbook of schizophrenia (vol. 3): Nosology, epidemiology, and genetics of schizophrenia* (pp. 205–244). New York: Elsevier.

Wing, J. K. (1988). Comments on the long-term term outcome of schizophrenia. *Schizophrenia Bulletin, 14,* 669–673.

Wuerker, A. K., Long, J. D., Haas, G. L., & Bellack, A. S. (2002). Interpersonal control, expressed emotion, and change in symptoms in families of persons with schizophrenia. *Schizophrenia Research, 58*(2–3), 281–292.

18

Schizoaffective, Delusional, and Other Psychotic Disorders

Nan Roberts, Roberta Stock, and Diana Clarke

LEARNING OBJECTIVES

After studying this chapter, you will be able to:

- Define schizoaffective disorder and distinguish the major differences among schizophrenia, schizoaffective, and mood disorders.
- Discuss the important epidemiologic findings related to schizoaffective disorder.
- Explain the primary etiologic factors regarding schizoaffective disorder.
- Explain the primary elements involved in assessment, nursing diagnoses, nursing interventions, and evaluation of patients with schizoaffective disorder.
- Define delusional disorder and explain the importance of nonbizarre delusions in diagnosis and treatment.
- Explain the important epidemiologic findings regarding delusional disorder.
- Discuss the primary etiologic factors of delusional disorder.
- Explain the various subtypes of delusional disorder.
- Explain the nursing care of patients with delusional disorder.

KEY TERMS

delusional disorder ▪ delusions ▪ erotomania ▪ misidentification ▪ nonbizarre delusions ▪ persecutory delusions ▪ psychosis ▪ schizoaffective disorder ▪ thymoleptic

Psychiatric and mental health nurses care for patients who have psychiatric disorders involving underlying psychoses other than schizophrenia and mood disorders. This chapter introduces other psychotic disorders and describes the associated nursing care. Central to understanding the problems of these patients is the concept of **psychosis**, a term used to describe a state in which an individual experiences positive symptoms, also known as psychotic symptoms (hallucinations, delusions, or disorganized thoughts, speech, or behaviour) (see Chapter 17). Other psychotic disorders defined by the presence of psychosis include schizophreniform, schizoaffective, delusional, brief psychotic, and shared psychotic disorders. Other psychotic disorders may be induced by drugs or alcohol.

Schizoaffective disorder is one of the more complex psychotic disorders but one of the more common diagnoses that the generalist nurse is likely to encounter. The person with delusional disorder is more likely to be treated in a medical-surgical setting and is rarely seen by a psychiatrist. This disorder often remains undiagnosed; therefore, for nurses practicing in nonpsychiatric settings, recognizing and understanding it are crucial to providing meaningful care.

Schizoaffective Disorder
CLINICAL COURSE

Schizoaffective disorder (SCA) is a complex and persistent psychiatric illness. This disorder was recognized in 1933 by Kasanin, who described varying degrees of symptoms of both schizophrenia and mood disorders, beginning in youth. All his patients were well adjusted before the sudden onset of symptoms that erupted after the occurrence of a specific environmental stressor. Since Kasanin's time, debate and controversy about the status of this disorder have been extensive, resulting in many different definitions and classifications that remain under consideration (Maj, Pirozzi, Formicola, Bartoli, & Bucci, 2000). Box 18-1 reflects the history of this debate.

SCA is characterized by intervals of intense symptoms alternating with quiescent periods, during which psychosocial functioning is adequate. The episodic nature of this disorder is characteristic. This disorder is at times marked by symptoms of schizophrenia; at other times, it appears to be a mood disorder. In other cases, both psychosis and pervasive mood changes occur concurrently.

In a recent Ontario study of early signs of schizophrenia spectrum disorders (schizophrenia, SCA, and schizophreniform disorder), it was found that greater psychobiologic changes (in appetite, sleep, energy, and restlessness) during the prepsychotic phase were associated with a more emotionally reactive form of schizophrenia (Norman, Scholten, Malla, & Ballageer, 2005).

BOX 18.1

History of the Diagnosis: Schizoaffective

- 1933: Kasanin first coined the phrase *schizoaffective psychosis.*
- 1980: *DSM-III* did not include diagnostic criteria for schizoaffective disorder.
- 1987: Schizoaffective disorder was first recognized as a separate diagnosis in the *DSM-III-R*; the definition included length of time in relationship to symptoms.
- 1994: Schizoaffective disorder was maintained as a separate disorder in the *DSM-IV.*
- 2000: Schizoaffective disorder was maintained as a separate disorder in the *DSM-IV-TR.*

CRNE Note

Patients with schizoaffective disorder have many similar responses to their disorder as people with schizophrenia, with one exception. These patients have many more "mood" responses and are very susceptible to suicide.

Patients with SCA are more likely to exhibit persistent psychosis, with or without mood symptoms, than are patients with a mood disorder. They feel that they are on a "chronic roller coaster ride" of symptoms that are often more difficult to cope with than the individual problem of either schizophrenia or mood disorder (Marneros, 2003). The diagnosis of this disorder is made only after these course-related characteristics are considered.

The long-term outcome of SCA is generally better than that of schizophrenia but worse than that of mood disorder (Moller et al., 2002). This group of patients resembles the mood disorder group in work function and the schizophrenia group in social function. In one study, compared with patients with a bipolar mood disorder, schizoaffective patients were less likely to recover and more likely to have persistent psychosis, with or without mood symptoms. Patients with SCA also have poorer executive function than do control subjects or patients with nonpsychotic bipolar disorder schizophrenia (Gooding & Tallent, 2002; Reichenberg et al., 2002).

DIAGNOSTIC CRITERIA

Mental health providers find SCA difficult to conceptualize, diagnose, and treat because the clinical picture varies. Patients often have misdiagnoses of schizophrenia. The difficulty in conceptualizing SCA is reflected in the controversy regarding the diagnostic criteria. For example, it has been argued that this disorder should be named either *schizophrenia with mood symptoms* or *mood disorder with schizophrenic symptoms.* More

Table 18.1 Key Diagnostic Characteristics of Schizoaffective Disorder 295.70

DSM IV

Diagnostic Criteria and Target Symptoms

- Uninterrupted period of illness with concurrent major depressive episode, manic episode, or mixed episode
- Bipolar type: manic or mixed episode or manic or mixed episode and major depressive episode
- Depressive type: only major depressive episode
- Characteristic symptoms of schizophrenia (two or more) during a 1-month period
  - Delusions
  - Hallucinations
  - Disorganized speech
  - Grossly disorganized or catatonic behaviour or negative symptoms
- Delusions or hallucinations for at least 2 weeks without prominent mood symptoms
- Symptoms of mood episode present for major portion of the active and residual periods of illness
- Not a direct physiologic effect of a substance or medical condition

Associated Findings

Associated Behavioural Findings
- Poor occupational functioning
- Restricted range of social contact
- Difficulties with self-care
- Increased risk for suicide

IN A LIFE

Louis Riel (1844–1885)
Metis Leader

Public Persona
Louis Riel, as leader of the Metis in Manitoba and Saskatchewan, has been remembered as the man who negotiated for the establishment of Manitoba as a province and who led the fight for the protection of Metis and aboriginal land and rights in Western Canada. Arrested for treason in 1884, he showed symptoms of grandiosity and paranoid delusions. He was declared "sane" by the superintendent of the Asylum for the Insane in Toronto, stood trial, and was hanged in 1885.

Personal Realities
Riel had numerous episodes of profound depression, apparent psychosis, and delusional thinking throughout his life. At times he believed he had been "substituted" for the real Louis Riel who had died. At other times, he talked about his "mission" to form a new religion and replace the Pope. He was hospitalized and committed to "insane asylums" on numerous occasions. He has, retrospectively, variably been "diagnosed" in the literature with paranoid schizophrenia, schizoaffective disorder, and bipolar disorder.

From Perr, I. N. (1992). Religion, political leadership, charisma and mental illness: The strange story of Louis Riel. *Journal of Forensic Science, 37*(2), 574–584; and Waite, P. (1987). Between three oceans: Challenges of a continental destiny. In C. Brown (Ed.), *The illustrated history of Canada* (pp. 279–373). Toronto: Lester & Orpen Dennys Ltd.

than 50 years after SCA was first described, the diagnosis was finally officially confirmed by the psychiatric community and included in the American Psychiatric Association's (APA, 1980) *Diagnostic and Statistical Manual of Mental Disorders*, 3rd edition, Revision (*DSM-III-R*) (Table 18-1).

To receive a diagnosis of SCA, a patient must have an uninterrupted period of illness when there is a major depressive, manic, or mixed episode, along with two of the following symptoms of schizophrenia: delusions, hallucinations, disorganized speech, disorganized or catatonic behaviour, or negative symptoms (eg, affective flattening, alogia, or avolition). In addition, although the person experiences problems with mood most of the time, the positive symptoms (delusions or hallucinations) must be present without the mood symptoms at some time during this period (for at least 2 weeks) (Table 18-1). Those with permanent delusions or auditory hallucinations report more basic symptoms (Fabisch et al., 2001). To clarify this disorder further, two related subtypes of SCA have been identified. In the bipolar type, the patient exhibits manic symptoms alone or a mix of manic and depressive symptoms. Patients with the depressive type display only symptoms of a major depressive episode (APA, 2000). The most common disorders from which SCA must be differentiated include mood disorders of manic, depressive, or mixed types and schizophrenia.

EPIDEMIOLOGY AND RISK FACTORS

The lifetime prevalence of SCA is estimated to be less than 1%, but there are no current studies (APA, 2000). This disorder occurs less commonly than does schizophrenia. The incidence of SCA is relatively constant across populations in varied geographic, climatic, industrial, and social environments. Environmental contributions are minimal.

Patients with schizoaffective disorder are at high risk for suicide. The risk for suicide in patients with psychosis is increased by the presence of depression. Risk for suicide is increased with the use of alcohol or substances, cigarette smoking, previous attempts at suicide, and previous hospitalizations (Potkin et al., 2003).

Lack of regular social contact may be a factor that confers a long-term risk for suicidal behaviour, which may be reduced by treatments designed to enhance social networks and contact (Radomsky, Haas, Mann, & Sweeney, 1999) and help patients to protect themselves against environmental stressors (Huxley, Rendall, & Sederer, 2000). Cognition is more impaired with SCA than with nonpsychotic mood disorder (Evans et al., 1999).

Age of Onset

SCA can affect children and the elderly. In children, the disorder is rare and is often indistinguishable from schizophrenia. In the elderly, this disorder becomes complicated because of frequent comorbid medical conditions. The typical age of onset for this disorder is early adulthood, and the most common type presented is bipolar. Other studies have reported a relatively late onset of SCA of mainly the depressive type (APA, 2000). Earlier age of onset is associated with longer illness, more severe illness, and worse outcomes (APA, 2000).

Gender

This disorder is more likely to occur in women than in men, which may be accounted for by a greater incidence of the depressive type in women (APA, 2000).

Ethnicity and Culture

Most patients with diagnoses of SCA are Caucasian. Although some reports have indicated a connection between SCA and social class, others support no specific association with race, geographic area, or class (Siris & Lavin, 1995).

Family

Some authorities support a familial association in SCA, but a clear familial pattern has not been established. Relatives of patients with diagnoses of SCA appear to be at increased risk for this disorder, schizophrenia, or both. There is some initial genome evidence that if there is a familial association, it is most likely related to the mother, not the father (DeLisi et al., 2002).

Comorbidity

SCA may be associated with substance abuse. Men may be likely to engage in antisocial behaviour. Twenty-five percent of patients with diagnoses of SCA experience postpsychotic depression and panic attacks (APA, 2000).

ETIOLOGY

Biologic Theories

Although the etiologies of schizophrenia and mood disorder have been investigated extensively, the etiology of SCA remains unresolved. Research to locate a biologic marker has been limited. Variables may be structural, as well as neurochemical.

Neuropathologic

Magnetic resonance imaging (MRI) and computed tomography scans have been used in the study of SCA for more than 10 years (Crow & Harrington, 1994; Lewine, Hudgins, Brown, Caudle, & Risch, 1995; Scott, Price, George, Brillman, & Rothfus, 1993). Midline brain abnormalities, especially in women, have been found. In SCA, changes in brain structure appear to be similar to those seen in bipolar disorder (Getz et al., 2002). Whether midline structural abnormality is directly causal, indirectly contributory, or an intriguing phenomenon in SCA is unclear.

Genetic

The etiology is believed to be primarily genetic. Results from family, twin, and adoption studies vary but suggest that SCA may consist of phenotypic variations or expressions of a genetic interform between schizophrenia and affective psychoses (DeLisi et al., 2002).

Biochemical

Before 1999, the prevailing neurochemical hypothesis was overactivity of dopamine pathways. Whether this disturbance of dopaminergic transmission is primary remains unclear (Rietschel et al., 2000). In studies of deficit symptoms in SCA, altered patterns of glucose metabolism have been found that might cause neurobiologic and neurophysiologic impairments (Regenold, Thapar, Marano, Gavirneni, & Kondapavuluru, 2002).

Psychological and Social Theories

Psychological, psychodynamic, environmental, and interpersonal factors may have a precipitating role when they coincide with a biomedical diathesis that creates vulnerability to this disorder (see Chapter 7 for explanation of the diathesis–stress theory). No current psychodynamic behavioural, cognitive, or developmental theories of causation explain SCA. Family dynamics do not appear to affect the development of this disorder, except for the strong genetic predisposition, which is virtually unexplained.

INTERDISCIPLINARY TREATMENT

Patients with SCA benefit from comprehensive treatment. Because this disorder is persistent, these individuals are constantly trying to manage complex symptoms. Ideally, most of the treatment occurs within the patient's natural environment, and hospitalizations are limited to times of symptom exacerbation, when symptoms are so severe or persistent that extended care in a protected environment is necessary.

Pharmacologic intervention is needed to stabilize the symptoms and presents specific challenges. Long-term atypical antipsychotic agents are as effective as the traditional combination of a standard antipsychotic agent and an antidepressant drug. Use of atypical antipsychotic agents has grown from 43% in 1995 to 70% in 1999 (Bartels et al., 2002). Mood stabilizers, such as lithium or valproic acid (see Chapter 13), may also be used. A combination of antipsychotic and antidepressant agents is sometimes used.

After the patient's condition has stabilized (ie, the patient exhibits a decrease in positive and negative symptoms), the treatment that led to remission of symptoms should be continued. Titrating antipsychotic agents to the lowest dose that provides suitable protection may enable optimal psychosocial functioning, while slowing recurrence of new episodes. Patients with SCA will likely need to remain on medication for the disorder. Electroconvulsive therapy is considered when symptoms are refractory to other interventions or when the patient's life is at risk and a rapid response is required (Swoboda, Conca, Konig, Waanders, & Hansen, 2001).

The treatment plan is revised regularly, and symptoms are monitored to guide medication management. Psychiatric nursing interventions in hospital and in community care are guided by the nursing diagnoses. Psychotherapy may help manage interpersonal relationships and mood changes. Social services are often needed to obtain disability benefits or services. Use of advanced practice clinicians helps to provide continuity of care (McCann & Baker, 2003).

PRIORITY CARE ISSUES

Patients with SCA may be at least as susceptible to suicide as those with mood disorder (Potkin et al., 2003). Living with a persistent psychotic disorder that has a mood component makes suicide a real risk.

NURSING MANAGEMENT: HUMAN RESPONSE TO DISORDER

Biologic Domain

Assessment

Assessment of patients with SCA is similar to assessment of those with schizophrenia and affective disorder. A careful history from the patient and family is crucial. The history should contain a description of the full range and duration of symptoms the patient has experienced and those observed by the family; this information is important for predicting outcomes. A patient who has had symptoms for a relatively long period of time has greater difficulty in overcoming effects of the psychosis, which may cause function to deteriorate.

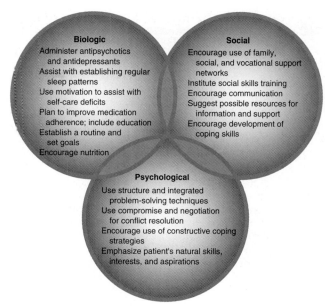

FIGURE 18.1 Biopsychosocial interventions for patients with schizoaffective disorders.

A thorough systems assessment is important to discover any physiologic problems the patient is experiencing, such as sleep pattern disturbances, difficulties with self-care, or poor nutritional habits.

Nursing Diagnoses for Biologic Domain

Common nursing diagnoses for the biologic domain are Disturbed Thought Process, Disturbed Sensory Perception, and Disturbed Sleep Patterns. Because of the variety of problems in patients with SCA, almost any nursing diagnosis could be generated. The persistent nature of this disorder lends itself to numerous and varied problems that must all be addressed (see Nursing Care Plan 18-1).

Interventions for Biologic Domain

Patient Education

Interventions are based on the needs identified in the biopsychosocial assessment (Fig. 18-1). Helping the patient to establish a regular sleep pattern by using a routine can promote or re-establish normal rest patterns. Focusing with the patient on the principles of good nutrition and identifying any barriers to healthy eating can improve nutritional status. Work with the patient to notice self-care deficits, especially those caused by lack of motivation. For deficits created by severe mood symptoms, establishing a routine and setting goals can be useful.

Pharmacologic Interventions

An in-depth history of the patient's medication is important in evaluating response to past medications

NURSING CARE PLAN 18.1

Patient With Schizoaffective Disorder

Ms. B is a 28-year-old divorced white woman with a 4-year-old daughter. They reside with Ms. B's parents. Ms. B is a hairdresser and tries to work, but she becomes stressed in the workplace, which results in her being fired. She has never applied for disability. Her parents are stressed because of the exacerbations of her illness and caring for her child.

Ms. B has had numerous hospitalizations for aggressive behaviour, noncompliance with medications, and receiving medications from various physicians, which results in inappropriate psychiatric management. She is medication seeking and is often prescribed benzodiazepines and diet pills by her primary care physician.

The patient has an ingrained delusional system that makes it hard to introduce reality orientation and feedback. She believes that her ex-husband has sexually abused

their child. She has gone to numerous attorneys to try to prosecute the ex-husband to no avail because of the lack of evidence to prove any abuse.

For the last 2 years, Ms. B has believed that a bank guard is in love with her. She is adamant about him protecting her and her child. She states that he watches over them. They have no contact other than speaking to each other when she enters the bank. She has been seeing a man the past 9 months, but states that she really does not care much for him and it is hard for her to move forward in the relationship because she loves the bank guard.

Medications have included antidepressants, neuroleptics (typical and atypical), mood stabilizers, benzodiazepines, sleep medications, and anticonvulsants. She often complains of being depressed and yet does not take the antidepressant medications when they are prescribed.

SETTING: INTENSIVE CARE PSYCHIATRIC UNIT IN A GENERAL HOSPITAL

Baseline Assessment: Ms. B is admitted to the hospital through the ER. She was hearing voices and was delusional. She has not been taking medications for several months. She is oriented in all spheres and well nourished but unkempt. She is verbalizing delusions about a man at the bank. She cannot sleep well and reportedly goes outdoors at night and yells at a bank guard. Reality feedback increases her agitation. She denies any problems.

Associated Psychiatric Diagnosis	Medications
Axis I: Schizoaffective disorder	None
Axis II: Deferred	
Axis III: None	
Axis: IV: Social problem (maintaining relationships)	
Economic problem (no income)	
Occupation problem (unemployed)	
Axis V: Current, 28	
Potential, 60	

NURSING DIAGNOSIS 1: INEFFECTIVE INDIVIDUAL COPING

Defining Characteristics	Related Factors
Inability to meet role expectations	Chronicity of the condition
Anxiety	Inadequate psychological resources secondary to delusions
Delusions	Inadequate coping skills
Inability to problem solve	Inadequate psychological resources to adapt to residential setting

Outcomes

Initial	Discharge
1. Identify coping patterns	5. Manage own behaviour
2. Identify stressors	6. Medication compliance
3. Identify personal strengths	7. Reduction of delusions
4. Accept support through the nursing relationship	

Interventions

Interventions	Rationale	Ongoing Assessment
Initiate a nurse–patient relationship to develop trust.	Through the use of the nurse–patient relationship, the patient will be able to maintain compliance with the treatment plan.	Determine whether patient is able to relate to the nurse.
Facilitate the identification of stressors in patient's environment.	To be able to cope with stressors, they need to be identified by the patient.	Assess whether patient is able to identify and verbalize stressors.

NURSING CARE PLAN 18.1 (Continued)

Interventions

Interventions	Rationale	Ongoing Assessment
Develop coping strategies to manage environmental stressors.	Patient needs to develop realistic strategies to handle environmental stressors.	Determine whether patient-identified strategies are realistic.
Help patient to identify personal strengths.	By identifying personal strengths, patient will increase confidence in using coping strategies.	Assess patient's ability to incorporate coping strategies into her daily routine.
Assist patient to understand the disorder and its management.	By understanding the disorder, patient can develop ways to manage her disorder.	Assess the patient's level of understanding of the disease.
Facilitate emotional support for the family.	Supported family is better equipped to support patient.	Assess family's ability to seek emotional support from the staff.
Teach coping skills.	By developing positive coping skills, anxiety and agitation will decrease.	Assess patient's ability to learn the skills to manage stressors.

Evaluation

Outcomes	Revised Outcomes	Interventions
Within the nursing relationship, Ms. B. was able to understand how coping skills can reduce stressors.	Support the patient's ability to recognize stressor and apply coping skills.	Discuss stressors and means of applying coping skills.
Increased insight into what behaviour is appropriate has helped the patient to decrease verbalization of delusions.	Provide ongoing support to maintain present level of functioning.	Discuss behaviour and provide reality feedback.

NURSING DIAGNOSIS 2: DISTURBED THOUGHT PROCESSES

Defining Characteristics	Related Factors
Delusions Impulsivity Medication noncompliance	Ingrained delusions Decreased ability to process secondary to delusions

Outcomes

Initial	Discharge
1. Maintain reality orientation. 2. Communicate clearly with others. 3. Expresses delusional material less frequently.	4. Identify situations that contribute to delusions. 5. Identify how delusions affect life situations. 6. Use coping strategies to deal with delusions. 7. Recognize changes in behaviour.

Interventions

Interventions	Rationale	Ongoing Assessment
Promote adherence to medication regimen.	Medication will reduce delusions.	Assess for side effects: heat intolerance, neuroleptic malignant syndrome, renal failure, constipation, dry mouth, increased appetite, salivation, nausea, vomiting, tardive dyskinesia, seizures, somnolence, agitation, insomnia, dizziness.
Teach actions, effects, and side effects of medications.	The more knowledgeable patients are about medication, the more likely they will comply.	Assess ability to understand information.
Support reality testing through helping patient to differentiate thoughts and feelings in relationship to situations.	When comparing thoughts with the situations, patients can develop skills to refute delusions.	Assess for medication compliance.

(continued)

NURSING CARE PLAN 18.1 (Continued)

Interventions

Interventions	Rationale	Ongoing Assessment
Monitor verbalization of delusional material. Identify stressors that promote delusions.	To determine whether medication is reducing delusional thoughts. If patient is able to identify stressors that promote dilusions, she can manage the stressors to effectively decrease delusions.	Assess verbalization of delusional material. Assess patient's ability to recognize stressors when they occur.
Assist patient in developing skills to deal with delusions (recognizing delusional themes can help the patient in distinguishing between reality- and nonreality-based patterns).	Even though medication can reduce the occurrence of delusions, they may continue in some people with decreased intensity. Cognitive-behavioural skills are important in dealing with these altered thoughts.	Monitor patient's ability to handle delusions.

Evaluation

Outcomes	Revised Outcomes	Interventions
Delusions will be less ingrained.	Continue to practice skills in reality orientation and communication.	Support verbalization of reality-based thoughts.
Patient verbalized action, effect, dosage, and side effects of medications.	Take prescribed medication regularly.	Give positive feedback for understanding of medication.
Medication compliance		Initiate pill counts to determine medication compliance.

Summary: Ms. B was discharged from the hospital. Verbalization of delusions had not decreased. She was less anxious. She is presently on Risperdal 2 mg AM and hs, Effexor XR 75 mg AM, Xanax 0.5 mg AM, and Seroquel 50 mg hs. Mother is helping by filling a weekly medication box. At times, Ms B. is questioning her delusions.

---

and predicting response to the present regimen. Investigate adherence to past treatment to determine the probability of successful intervention. Develop a plan to increase adherence based on any past problems or issues. For example, use medication boxes and calendars and get help from others in managing the medication. Recognizing medication side effects quickly and intervening promptly to alleviate them will help maintain adherence. Helping understand the need for medications is essential.

Mood and psychotic symptoms are equally important and should be evaluated throughout treatment. Atypical antipsychotic agents are generally prescribed because of their efficacy and safe side-effect profile. Clozapine, reported effective for SCA by several authorities, can reduce hospitalizations and risk for suicide (Potkin et al., 2003). A significant portion of patients whose symptoms have resisted other neuroleptic agents experience improvement with clozapine therapy (Volavka et al., 2002). Atypical antipsychotic agents may have **thymoleptic** (mood stabilizing), as well as antipsychotic, effects. Quetiapine has been found effective (Bech, 2001). Dosage is the same as that used for treating schizophrenia, but lower dosage ranges may also be effective.

CRNE Note

The medication regimen for patients with schizoaffective disorder will be complex and may include antipsychotics, mood stabilizers, antidepressants, and occasional antianxiety agents.

In many cases, symptoms of depression disappear when psychotic symptoms decrease. If depressive symptoms persist, adjunctive use of an antidepressant agent may be helpful. Successful use of anticonvulsant agents for this disorder has been documented in several clinical trials (Dietrich, Kropp, & Emrich, 2001). Mood stabilizers, which can decrease the frequency and intensity of episodes, may be an alternative adjunctive medication for mood states associated with the bipolar type.

Administering and Monitoring Medications

One of the greatest challenges in pharmacologic interventions is monitoring target symptoms and identifying changes in symptom pattern. Patients can switch from being relatively calm to being very emotional. Whether the patient is overreacting to an environmental event or mood symptoms have changed and the patient requires a medication change can be determined only through careful observation and documentation.

Adherence to medication regimens is critical to a successful outcome. Patients need an opportunity to discuss barriers to compliance.

MANAGING SIDE EFFECTS. Monitoring medication side effects in patients with SCA is similar to that in patients with schizophrenia. Extrapyramidal side effects, weight gain, and sedation should be assessed and documented.

MONITORING FOR DRUG INTERACTIONS. Avoid using lithium with antipsychotic medications. A few patients taking haloperidol and lithium have experienced an encephalopathic syndrome, followed by irreversible brain damage. Lithium may interact similarly with other antipsychotic agents. It may also prolong the effects of neuromuscular blocking agents. Use of nonsteroidal anti-inflammatory drugs may increase plasma lithium levels. Diuretics and angiotensin-converting enzyme inhibitors should be prescribed cautiously with lithium, which is excreted through the kidney (see Chapter 9 for more information).

Teaching Points

- Instruct patients to take medications as prescribed.
- Determine whether the patient has sufficient resources to purchase and obtain medications.
- Have the patient write down the prescribed medication and time of administration.
- Explain the target symptom for each medication (eg, psychosis and mood for atypical antipsychotic agents, mood for antidepressant and mood stabilizer drugs).
- Caution patients about orthostatic hypotension and instruct them to get up slowly from a lying or sitting position. Also advise them to maintain adequate fluid intake.
- Advise patients to contact their case coordinators or health care providers if they experience dramatic changes in body temperature (neuroleptic malignant syndrome [NMS]), inability to control motor movement (dystonia), or dizziness.
- Advise patients to avoid over-the-counter medications unless a prescriber is consulted.
- Advise patients taking olanzapine and clozapine to monitor body weight and report rapid weight gains.
- Advise patients to report symptoms of diabetes mellitus (frequent urination, excessive thirst, etc.).

Psychological Domain

Assessment

The patient's level of insight into his or her illness may play a role in the course and treatment of SCA. Patients with SCA tend to have better insight than those with schizophrenia (Pini, Cassano, Dell'Osso, & Amador, 2001). Stressors should be evaluated because they may trigger symptoms. Uncovering or exploratory techniques should generally be avoided. Mental status and reality contact may be compromised. Assessment of anxiety level or reactions to stressful situations is important because the combination of these symptoms with psychosis increases the patient's risk for suicide.

Nursing Diagnoses for Psychological Domain

In SCA, individuals vacillate between mood dysregulation and disturbed thinking. Typical nursing diagnoses for this domain include Hopelessness, Powerlessness, Ineffective Coping, and Low Self-esteem.

Interventions for Psychological Domain

Using appropriate interpersonal modalities is important to help the patient, family, and social and vocational support networks cope with the onslaught of acute episodes and recuperative periods. Patients with SCA have fewer awareness deficits than do patients with schizophrenia. Structured, integrated, and problem-solving psychotherapeutic interventions should be used to develop or increase the patient's insight. Psychoeducational interventions can help to decrease symptoms, enhance recognition of early regression, and hone psychosocial skills (see Boxes 18–2 and 18–3.)

Social Domain

Assessment

Social dysfunction is common in patients with diagnoses of SCA. Premorbid adjustment, such as marital

---

BOX 18.2

Psychoeducation Checklist: Schizoaffective Disorder

When caring for the patient with schizoaffective disorder, be sure to include the caregiver as appropriate and address the following topic areas in the teaching plan:
- ☐ Psychopharmacologic agents (antipsychotic or antidepressants), if used, including drug action, dosage, frequency, and possible adverse effects
- ☐ Methods to enhance adherence
- ☐ Sleep measures
- ☐ Consistent routines
- ☐ Goal setting
- ☐ Nutrition
- ☐ Support networks
- ☐ Problem solving
- ☐ Positive coping strategies
- ☐ Social and vocational skills training

BOX 18.3

Research for Best Practice Helping Women Living with Schizoprenia

THE QUESTION: What are women's perceptions of their experience with schizophrenia or schizoaffective disorder within the context of their life stages and corresponding health issues?

METHODS: Five focus groups totalling 28 women who self-identified as having schizophrenia or schizoaffective disorder and who were living in the community in Winnipeg, Manitoba met to discuss their health-related needs, ranging from parenting and reproductive health to relationships and aging.

FINDINGS: This group of women led marginalized, deprived lives in the face of multiple losses, social stigma, limited interpersonal contacts, and poverty. Although reasonably well educated, the majority of the group was unemployed and living on social assistance. Relationships were fraught with challenges. Making new friends or reestablishing connections with old friends was socially difficult and could be emotionally threatening, but not making friends resulted in isolation and loneliness. Intimate relationships created potential dangers of vulnerability and victimization. Women also struggled with their self-identity, whether to see themselves as women or as someone with a mental illness. Women felt, in many cases, that the health care system focussed on their illness and that they had become invisible as women. They struggled with medications that controlled their symptoms but resulted in side effects. They frequently did not feel comfortable sharing their concerns about side effects such as weight gain and amenorrhea with their health care providers. Nevertheless, they conveyed a persistent sense of wanting life to improve and hoping that it could. A sense of hope and, in many cases, spirituality, kept them going.

IMPLICATIONS FOR NURSING: The illness itself often takes precedence over other significant issues in women's lives, and practitioners may unwittingly contribute to diminished quality of life. Nurses can lessen the pain of a woman's dilemma by engaging her in discussions of options and providing support while she ponders which options are best for her; by monitoring her response to side effects of medications; by setting a climate that promotes discussion of sensitive subject matter; and by adopting an attitude of working with a woman in partnership.

From Chernomas, W. M., Clarke, D. E., & Chisholm, F. A. (2000). Perspectives of women living with schizophrenia. *Psychiatric Services, 51*(12),1517–1521.

status and adolescent social adjustment, may influence patients' level of functioning at the time of diagnosis and their prognoses. Assess for social skill deficits and problems with interpersonal conflicts, particularly in men. Assessment of an adult patient's childhood may give a clue to the patient's current level of social functioning. Assess the patient's use of fantasy and fighting as a means of coping. Patients who report the most severe peer rejection present with the angriest dispositions and display antisocial behaviours.

Nursing Diagnoses for Social Domain

Because of their mood and thought disturbances, these individuals will have significant problems in the social domain. Typical nursing diagnoses include Compromised Family Coping, Impaired Home Maintenance, and Social Isolation.

Interventions for Social Domain

Social skills training is useful for remediating social deficits and may result in positive social adjustment. Positive results include improved interpersonal competence and decreased symptom severity. Help in identifying feelings and in developing realistic goals, along with supportive therapy, can integrate insight into the disease process. Education focusing on conflict-resolution skills, promoting compromise, negotiation, and expression of negative feelings, can help the patient achieve positive social adjustment. Social skills can be improved through role playing and assertiveness training. Supportive, nurturing, and nonconfrontational interventions help to minimize anxiety and improve understanding (see Box 18-4).

Helping the patient to develop coping skills is essential. Teach communication skills to decrease conflicts and environmental negativity. Memory is linked with development of social skills; psychotic symptoms may interfere with retention of these skills, resulting in slower learning. These patients require long-term, intense social training.

Families are at risk for ineffective coping. Family members face many of the same issues faced by families of patients with schizophrenia and are often puzzled by the patient's emotional overreaction to normal daily stresses. Frequent arguments may lead to verbal and physical abuse.

EVALUATION AND TREATMENT OUTCOMES

Teaching skills to patients with SCA often takes longer than teaching other patients. When evaluating progress related to interventions, be patient if outcomes are not completely met. Psychoeducation results in increased knowledge of the illness and treatment, increased medication compliance, fewer relapses and hospitalizations, briefer inpatient stays, increased social function, decreased family tension, and lighter family burdens (Andres, Pfammatter, Garst, Teschner, & Brenner, 2000). Maintain realistic outcomes and praise small successes to promote positive outcomes (Fig. 18-2).

BOX 18.4

Therapeutic Dialog: Ms. B's "Delusions"

Ineffective Communication

Nurse: Hello, Ms. B, what has been happening?
Patient: The guy from the bank keeps me up all night.
Nurse: That's not possible.
Patient: He's there all the time to look after me.
Nurse: No, he's not. You just think that.
Patient: No, he really is. He is helping me.
Nurse: He does not even know who you are.

Effective Communication

Nurse: Hello, Ms. B. How have you been?
Patient: That guy from the bank is really bothering me.
Nurse: What is he doing?
Patient: He keeps me up all night. I go out in the street to yell at him.
Nurse: Have you actually seen him at night?
Patient: No, but I know he is there.

Nurse: How can he be there when you cannot see him.
Patient: He can't.
Nurse: Does it seem that the thoughts about him come from your mind?
Patient: This might be.
Nurse: Your illness often causes thoughts that are not reality based.
Patient: It seems real but yet so unreal. Those are sort of stupid thoughts.

Critical Thinking Challenge

- How could the nurse's approach in the first scenario have prevented development of a therapeutic relationship?
- How can the second scenario benefit the patient in developing insight into her delusions?
- Discuss the differences between the two approaches.

CONTINUUM OF CARE

Inpatient-Focussed Care

Hospitalization may be required during acute psychotic episodes or when suicidal ideations are present. This structured environment protects the patient from self-harm (ie, suicidal, assaultive, financial, legal, vocational, or social). During periods of acute psychosis, offering reassurance in a soft, nonthreatening voice and avoiding confrontational stances will help the patient begin to trust the staff and nursing care (see Chapter 8). Avoid seclusion and restraint and keep environmental stimulation to a minimum. Use the patient's coping capabilities to reinforce constructive aspects of functioning and enable a return to autonomy.

Emergency! Care

Emergency care is needed during symptom exacerbation. Psychosis, mood disturbance, and medication-related adverse effects account for most emergency situations. During an exacerbation of psychosis, patients may become agitated or aggressive. Assaultive behaviour can be managed by using therapeutic techniques (see Chapter 35) and pharmacologic management. If medications are used, benzodiazepines such as lorazepam are usually given. Patients are then evaluated for antipsychotic therapy. Possible medication-related adverse effects include NMS as a reaction to dopamine antagonists or serotonin intoxication, especially if the patient is taking an atypical antipsychotic agent and a selective serotonin reuptake inhibitor (see Chapter 17).

Family Intervention

Helping families support the patient in the home or a community placement is an integral part of nursing care. With patient permission, key family members can be included in home visits to learn about symptoms, medications, and side effects. By collaborating with family members, the nurse can strengthen the patient's willingness to follow treatment, monitor symptoms, and continue with rehabilitation and recovery.

Community Treatment

After the patient is released from the hospital, graduated levels of care (ie, partial hospitalization, day treatment,

Biologic
Improved sleep patterns
Increased participation in self-care activities
Improved nutrition
Increased compliance with medications
Decreased incidence of medication adverse effects

Social
Positive social adjustment
Improved conflict resolution
Improved communication skills
Increased use of community-related support systems
Improved home management

Psychological
Increased insight
Improved coping abilities
Decreased conflicts
Increased autonomy and self-esteem
Improved social and vocational skills
Increased awareness of personal strengths
Increased reality orientation
Decreased hallucinations and delusions

FIGURE 18.2 Biopsychosocial outcomes for patients with schizoaffective disorder.

group home) can help the patient to return to a more normal environment. Programs that foster building and practicing social and vocational skills are appropriate and should also incorporate the patient's natural skills, interests, and aspirations because they are as important as problems and deficits.

Because this illness is episodic, the person with SCA requires close and continued follow-up in the outpatient setting by psychiatrists, nurses, and therapists. These patients require ongoing medication management, supportive and cognitive therapy, and symptom management. If symptoms intensify, hospitalization may be required until they are brought under control.

Delusional Disorder
CLINICAL COURSE

Delusional disorder is a psychotic disorder characterized by nonbizarre, logical, stable, and well-systemized delusions that occur in the absence of other psychiatric disorders. **Delusions** are false, fixed beliefs unchanged by reasonable arguments. Although delusions are a symptom of many psychotic disorders, in delusional disorder, the delusions are **nonbizarre delusions;** that is, they are characterized by adherence to possible situations that could occur in real life and are plausible in the context of the person's ethnic and cultural background (APA, 2000).

Examples of real-life situations include being followed, poisoned, infected, loved at a distance, or deceived by a spouse or lover. A diagnosis of delusional disorder is based on the presence of one or more nonbizarre delusions for at least 1 month (APA, 2000). Delusions are the primary symptom of this disorder.

The course of delusional disorder is variable. Onset can be acute, or the disorder can occur gradually and become chronic. Patients with this disorder usually live with their delusions for years, rarely receiving psychiatric treatment. They are seldom brought to the attention of health care providers unless their delusion relates to their health (somatic delusion), or they act on the basis of their delusion and violate legal or social rules. Full remissions can be followed by relapses.

Apart from the direct impact of the delusion, psychosocial functioning is not markedly impaired. The person's clarity of thinking and behaviour and emotional responses are usually consistent with the delusional focus. In general, behaviour is not odd or bizarre. In fact, behaviour is remarkably normal, except when the patient focuses on the delusion. At that time, thinking, attitudes, and mood may change abruptly. Personality does not usually change, but the patient is gradually, progressively involved with the delusional concern (APA, 2000).

DIAGNOSTIC CRITERIA

Delusional disorder is characterized by the presence of nonbizarre delusions and includes several subtypes: erotomanic, grandiose, jealous, somatic, mixed, and unspecified (Table 18-2). These subtypes represent the prominent theme of the delusion. A patient who has met criteria A for schizophrenia does not receive a diagnosis of delusional disorder (see Chapter 17 for criteria A). Although hallucinations may be present, they are not prominent (APA, 2000).

If mood episodes occur with this disorder, the total duration of the mood episode is relatively brief compared with the total duration of the delusional period. The delusion is not caused by the direct physiologic effects of substances (ie, cocaine, amphetamines, marijuana) or a general medical condition (ie, Alzheimer's disease, systemic lupus erythematosus). Because delusional disorder is uncommon and possesses features that are characteristic of other illnesses, the differential diagnosis has clear-cut logic. It is a diagnosis of exclusion requiring careful evaluation. Distinguishing this

---

Table 18.2 Key Diagnostic Characteristics of Delusional Disorder 297.1 (DSM IV)

Diagnostic Criteria and Target Symptoms

- Nonbizarre delusions of at least 1 month's duration
- No presence of characteristic symptoms of schizophrenia
- Functioning not markedly impaired; behaviour not odd or bizarre
- If concurrent with delusions, mood disorders relatively brief in comparison with delusional periods
- Not a direct physiologic effect of substance or medical condition

Erotomanic type: delusions that another person of usually higher status is in love with the person

Grandiose type: delusions of inflated worth, power, knowledge, identity, or special relationship to a deity or famous person

Jealous type: delusions that the individual's sexual partner is unfaithful

Persecutory type: delusions that person or someone close to person is being malevolently treated in some way

Somatic type: delusion that person has some physical defect or general medical condition

Mixed type: delusions characteristic of more than one of the above types; no one theme predominates

Unspecified type: delusion cannot be clearly identified or described

Associated Findings

- Social, marital, or work problems
- Ideas of reference
- Irritable mood
- Marked anger and violent behaviour (especially with jealous type)

disorder from schizophrenia and mood disorders with psychotic features is difficult (APA, 2000).

The prevalence of delusion disorder is about 3 per 10,000 general population. It is a rare disease even in psychiatric samples (Meloy, 1999). Research data are limited because numbers of recorded case studies and participants are small, and the studies lack systematic description, assessment, and diagnosis.

Delusional disorder may be associated with dysfunction in the frontal-subcortical systems and with temporal dysfunction, particularly on the left side (Fujii, Ahmed, & Takeshita, 1999).

SUBTYPES

Erotomanic Delusions

The concept of **erotomania** dates to the 17th century. Erotomania rarely appears in the pure or primary form. Secondary erotomania, which occurs with other psychiatric conditions, is more common. Differential diagnosis is important for excluding other significant psychiatric disorders or histologic conditions.

The erotomanic subtype is characterized by the delusional belief that the patient is loved intensely by the "loved object," who is usually married, of a higher socioeconomic status, or otherwise unattainable. The patient believes that the loved object's position in life would be in jeopardy if his or her true feelings were known. In addition, the patient is convinced that he or she is in amorous communication with the loved object. The loved object is often a public figure (eg, movie star, politician) but may also be a common stranger. The patient believes that the loved object was the first to make advances and fall in love. The patient may entertain some delusional beliefs about a sexual relationship with the loved object, yet the beliefs are unfounded. The delusion, which often idealizes romantic love and spiritual union, rather than sexual attraction (APA, 2000), becomes the central focus of the patient's existence.

The patient may have minimal or no contact with the loved object and often keeps the delusion secret, but efforts to contact the loved object through letters, telephone calls, gifts, visits, surveillance, and stalking are also common. The patient may in many cases transfer his or her delusion to another loved object. There is some evidence that celebrity worship is associated with cognitive deficits (McCutcheon, Ashe, Houran, & Maltby, 2003).

Patients with erotomanic delusional disorder are generally unattractive; are often lower-level employees; lead withdrawn, lonely lives; are single with poor interpersonal relationships; and have limited sexual contacts or are sexually repressed. Clinical patients are mostly women, who do not usually act out their delusions. Forensic patients are mostly men, who tend to

be more aggressive and can become violent in pursuit of the loved object, although the loved object may not be the object of the aggression. Men in particular come into contact with the law in their pursuit of the loved object or in a misguided effort to rescue the loved object from some imagined danger. Orders of protection are generally ineffective, and criminal charges of stalking or harassment that lead to incarceration are ineffective as a long-term solution to the problem (Harmon, Rosner, & Owens, 1995; Munro, 1999). The result is repeated arrests and psychiatric examinations, followed by ineffective treatment. Patients are rarely motivated to seek psychiatric treatment. This disorder is difficult to control, contain, or treat. The patient seldom gives up the belief that he or she is loved by the loved object. Separation from the loved object is the only satisfactory means of intervention (APA, 2000). Cognitive rigidity arising from frontal-subcortical dysfunction may contribute to maintaining erotic delusions and result in inability to alter a belief system (Fujii et al., 1999).

Grandiose Delusions

Patients presenting with grandiose delusions are convinced they have a great, unrecognized talent or have made an important discovery. A less common presentation is the delusion of a special relationship with a prominent person (ie, an adviser to the President) or of actually being a prominent person (ie, the President). In the latter case, the person with the delusion may regard the actual prominent person as an impostor. Other grandiose delusions may be religious in nature, such as a delusional belief that he or she has a special message from a deity (APA, 2000; Munro, 1999).

Jealous Delusions

The central theme of the jealous subtype is the unfaithfulness or infidelity of a spouse or lover. The belief arises without cause and is based on incorrect inferences justified by "evidence" (ie, rumpled clothing, spots on sheets) the patient has collected. The patient usually confronts the spouse or lover with a host of such evidence. An associated feature is paranoia. The patient may attempt to intervene in the imagined infidelity by secretly following the spouse or lover or by investigating the imagined lover (APA, 2000; Munro, 1999).

Delusions of jealousy are difficult to treat and may diminish only with separation, divorce, or the death of the spouse or lover. Except in the elderly, such patients generally are male. Jealousy is a powerful, potentially dangerous emotion. Aggression, even violent behaviour, may result. Litigious behaviour is common, and symptoms with forensic aspects are often seen. Care is essential in determining how to work with this patient.

Somatic Delusions

Somatic delusions, a mix of psychotic and somatic symptoms, have been described for more than 100 years. The central theme of somatic delusions involves bodily functions or sensations. These patients believe they have physical ailments. Delusions of this nature are fixed, inarguable, and intense, with the patient totally convinced of the physical nature of the somatic complaint. The delusion occurs in the absence of other medical or psychiatric conditions. Medication can cause tactile hallucinations that result directly from the physiologic effects of the medication; when the medication or drug is removed, the symptoms disappear. Somatic delusions are manifested in the following beliefs (APA, 2000):

- A foul odor is coming from the skin, mouth (delusions of halitosis), rectum, or vagina
- Insects have infested the skin (delusional parasitosis)
- Internal parasites have infested the digestive system
- A certain body part is misshapen or ugly (contrary to visible evidence)
- Parts of the body are not functioning (eg, large intestine, bowels)

The delusion of infestation by insects cannot occur without sensory perceptions, which constitute tactile hallucinations. The patient vividly describes crawling, itching, burning, swarming, and jumping on the skin surface or below the skin. The patient maintains the conviction that he or she is infested with parasites in the absence of objective evidence to the contrary.

Patients with somatic delusions present a dilemma for health care systems because of their excessive use of health care resources. They seek repeated medical consultations with dermatologists, entomologists, infectious disease specialists, and general practitioners. They seek treatment from primary care physicians and refuse psychiatric referral. Even if they seek psychiatric help, these patients typically do not adhere to long-term psychiatric treatment. Patients often go through elaborate rituals to cleanse themselves or their surroundings of the perceived pests, collecting hair, scabs, and skin flakes as evidence of an infection. They insist on being given unnecessary medical tests and procedures and are consequently at risk for increased morbidity because of invasive evaluation. Anger and hostility are common among this group, and behavioural characteristics include shame, depression, and avoidance.

The somatic subtype is rare but may be underdiagnosed. Both genders are affected equally, but when onset occurs in late middle age, female patients tend to predominate. Studies of somatic delusions have been marred by methodologic uncertainties, and factors limiting investigation include rarity of the disease, lack of contact with psychiatrists, and noncompliance with the medication regimen. A variant of the somatic subtype is body dysmorphic disorder, which is classified under somatoform disorders in the *Diagnostic and Statistical Manual of Mental Disorders*, 4th edition, Text revision (*DSM-IV-TR*) (see Chapter 21).

Unspecified Delusions

In the mixed subtype, no one delusional theme predominates, and the patient presents with two or more types of delusions. In the unspecified subtype, the delusional beliefs cannot be clearly determined, or the predominant delusion is not described as a specific type. Patients are usually women who experience feelings of depersonalization and derealization and have negative-associated paranoid features. The delusions can be short-lived, recurrent, or persistent. This subtype also includes delusions of **misidentification** (ie, illusions of doubles), wherein a familiar person is replaced by an impostor. For example, the patient may believe that close family members have assumed the persona of strangers, or that people they know can change into other people at will. This type of delusion occurs rarely and is generally associated with schizophrenia, Alzheimer's disease, or other organic conditions (APA, 2000).

Persecutory delusions, the most common type seen, are not listed as a separate subtype in the *DSM-IV-TR*, but they are addressed as a subtype of delusional disorder in the text (APA, 2000). The central theme of persecutory delusions is the patient's belief that he or she is being conspired against, cheated, spied on, followed, poisoned, drugged, maliciously maligned, harassed, or obstructed in pursuit of long-term goals. The patient exaggerates small slights, which become the focus of the delusion.

The focus of persecutory delusions is often on some injustice that must be remedied by legal action (querulous paranoia). Patients often seek satisfaction by repeatedly appealing to courts and other government agencies (Harmon et al., 1995; Munro, 1999). These patients are often angry and resentful and may even behave violently toward the people the patient believes are persecuting him or her. The course may be chronic, although the patient's preoccupation with the delusional belief often waxes and wanes. The clarity, logic, and systematic elaboration of this delusional theme leaves a remarkable stamp on this condition (APA, 2000).

EPIDEMIOLOGY AND RISK FACTORS

Delusional disorder is relatively uncommon in clinical settings (APA, 2000). The best estimate of its prevalence in the population is about 0.03%, but precise information is lacking (APA, 2000). Lifetime morbidity is between 0.05% and 0.1% because of the late age of onset.

Few risk factors are associated with delusional disorder. Patients can live with their delusions without psychiatric intervention because their behaviour is normal, although if delusions are somatic, patients risk unnecessary medical interventions. Acting on delusions carries a risk for intervention by law enforcement agencies or the legal system. Suicide attempts are neither more nor less common than in the general population (Grunebaum et al., 2001).

Age of Onset

Delusional disorder can begin in adolescence and occurs in middle to later adulthood. Onset occurs at a later age than among patients with schizophrenia. A prevalence of 2% to 4% has been reported in the elderly (APA, 2000).

Gender

Gender does not appear to affect the overall frequency of most delusional disorders (APA, 2000). Patients with erotomanic delusions are generally women; in forensic settings, most people with this disorder are men. Men also tend to experience more jealous delusions, except in the elderly population, in which women outnumber men.

Ethnicity and Culture

A person's ethnic, cultural, and religious background must be considered in evaluating the presence of delusional disorder. The content of delusions varies between cultures and subcultures (APA, 2000).

Family

An increased familial risk and familial genetic factors are unknown.

COMORBIDITY

Mood disorders are frequently found in patients with delusional disorders, who typically have mild symptoms of depression such as irritable or dysphoric mood. Delusional disorder may also be associated with obsessive-compulsive disorder and paranoid, schizoid, or avoidant personality disorder (APA, 2000).

ETIOLOGY

The cause of delusional disorder is unknown. The only major feature of this condition is the formation and persistence of the delusions. Few have investigated possible neurophysiologic and neuropsychological causes of delusional disorder, and theories of causation are contradictory. No psychological or social theories of causation are addressed in the literature.

Biologic Theories

Neuropathologic

In patients with delusional disorder, MRI shows a degree of temporal lobe asymmetry. However, these differences are subtle, so delusional disorder may involve a neurodegenerative component (Ota et al., 2003). The tactile hallucinations of somatic delusions may arise from sensory alterations in the nervous system (Baker, Cook, & Winokur, 1995) or from sensory input that has been misinterpreted because of subtle cortical changes associated with aging.

Genetic and Biochemical

Delusional disorder is probably biologically distinct from other psychotic disorders, yet little or no attention has been paid to genetic factors. Delusions may involve faulty processing of essentially intact perceptions, whereby perceptions become linked with an interpretation that has deep emotional significance but no verifiable basis (Conway et al., 2002; McGuire et al., 2001). Alternately, a complex, malfunctioning dopaminergic system may lead to delusions (Morimoto et al., 2002). This explanation could lead to the argument that a particular delusion depends on the "circuit" that is malfunctioning. Denial of reality has been linked to right posterior cortical dysfunction. Some authors have proposed a combination of biologic and early life experiences as etiologic components (Bentall, Corcoran, Howard, Blackwood, & Kinderman, 2001).

INTERDISCIPLINARY TREATMENT

Few if any interdisciplinary treatments are associated with delusional disorder because patients rarely receive attention from health care providers. Pharmacologic intervention is often based on symptoms. For example, patients with somatic delusions are treated for the specific complaints with which they present. Use of benzodiazepines may be common with this disorder because complaints are vague.

PRIORITY CARE ISSUES

By the time a patient with a diagnosis of delusional disorder is seen in a psychiatric setting, he or she has generally had the delusion for a long time. It is deeply ingrained and many times unshakable, even with psychopharmacologic intervention. These patients rarely comply with medication regimens.

Male patients who have the erotomanic subtype are likely to require special care because they are more likely than other patients to act on their delusions (for example, by continued attempts to contact the loved object, or stalking). This group is generally seen in forensic settings.

NURSING MANAGEMENT: HUMAN RESPONSE TO DISORDER

Biologic Domain

Assessment

Body systems are assessed to evaluate any physical problems. In people with somatic delusional disorder, assessment may be difficult because of the number and variety of presenting symptoms. Complaints are explored to develop a complete symptom history and to determine whether symptoms have a physical basis or are delusional. Past history of each symptom should be determined because this information may affect outcome. The more recent the onset, the more favorable the prognosis.

CRNE Note

By definition, delusions are fixed, false beliefs that cannot be changed by reasonable arguments. The nurse should assess the patient's delusion to evaluate its significance to the patient and the patient's safety and the safety of others. The nurse should not dwell on the delusion or try to change it.

Most patients who receive diagnoses of delusional disorder do not experience functional difficulties or impairments. Self-care patterns may be disrupted in patients with the somatic subtype by the elaborate processes used to treat perceived illness (eg, bathing rituals, creams). Sleep may be disrupted because of the central and overpowering nature of the delusions.

A complete medication history, past and present, is also important to determine the patient's past response and what agents the individual perceives as effective. Examining the patient's records for tests and procedures may help to substantiate the individual's symptoms.

Nursing Diagnoses for the Biologic Domain

The nursing diagnoses for the biologic domain depend on the type of delusions that are manifested and the response to these symptoms. For example, for a woman with the somatic delusion that insects are crawling on her, Disturbed Sensory Perception (Tactile) would be

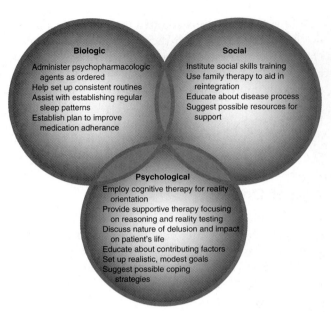

FIGURE 18.3 Biopsychosocial interventions for patients with delusional disorder.

appropriate. For others who are fearful of poisoning, Imbalanced Nutrition, Less Than Body Requirements, may be a useful diagnosis. Refusal of all medication may support a nursing diagnosis of Ineffective Therapeutic Regimen Management.

Interventions for Biologic Domain

Interventions are based on the problems identified during assessment (Fig. 18-3). Each is addressed individually. The nurse helps the patient to establish routines that can resolve problems and promote healthy functioning. A mechanism for managing the patient's medication regimen is developed.

Somatic Interventions

Delusional disorder has a reputation of being chronic and resistant to treatment. Treating somatic disorder is difficult because of the patient's insistence that the problem is not psychiatrically related. Many patients with delusional disorder are seen only by nonpsychiatric specialists, who use expensive and ineffective treatments. Patients with this disorder may adhere poorly to psychiatric pharmacotherapy, which may be directly related to the lack of insight about their illness (Nose, Barbui, & Tansella, 2003). Realistic and modest goals are most sensible. Establishing a therapeutic relationship is a goal for which to strive.

Pharmacologic Interventions

Sparse literature is available about using psychiatric medications in delusional disorder, and the available reports conflict. Antipsychotic agents are useful in improving acute symptoms by decreasing agitation and the intensity of the delusion. They may also be effective in the long term, but little formal information exists to support this theory.

Administering and Monitoring Medications

Patients often do not adhere to medication regimens and require monitoring of target symptoms. Look for an opportunity to discuss medications and to identify issues the patient may have with them.

Managing Side Effects

Management of side effects is similar to that in other disorders that have a delusional component. The nurse assesses for NMS, extrapyramidal side effects, weight gain, and sedation.

Monitoring for Drug Interactions

Interactions are similar to those seen with medications for other disorders. A detailed list of prior and current medications must be elicited from these patients, especially those with somatic delusions, because they may be receiving medications from many different practitioners.

Teaching Points

Patients may need help and information in order to take medication as prescribed. Determine whether the patient has sufficient resources to purchase and obtain medications, and explain target symptoms for each medication. Caution patients not to take over-the-counter medications without consulting their provider.

Psychological Domain

Assessment

Patients with delusional disorder show few if any psychological deficits, and those that do occur are generally related directly to the delusion. Use of the Minnesota Multiphasic Personality Inventory, a clinical scale that identifies paranoid symptom deviation, may be useful in substantiating the diagnosis.

Mental status is not generally affected. Thinking, orientation, affect, attention, memory, perception, and personality are generally intact. Presenting reality-based evidence in an attempt to change the person's delusion can be helpful in determining whether the belief can be altered with sufficient evidence. If mental status is altered, this fact is generally brought to the health professional's attention by a third party, such as police, family member, neighbour, physician, or attorney. In these cases, the person has usually acted in some manner to draw attention to himself or herself. Talk with the person to grasp the nature of the delusional thinking: theme, impact on the person's life, complexity, systematization, and related features.

Nursing Diagnosis for Psychological Domain

Numerous nursing diagnoses could be generated based on assessment of the psychological domain. Ineffective Denial, Impaired Verbal Communication, Deficient Knowledge, and Risk for Loneliness are some examples. The nursing diagnoses of Disturbed Self-concept, Disturbed Self-esteem, Anxiety, Fear, and Powerlessness may also be generated.

Interventions for Psychological Domain

Patients with delusional disorder are treated most effectively in outpatient settings with supportive therapy that allays the person's anxiety. Initiating discussion of the troubling experiences and consequences of the delusion and suggesting a means for coping may be successful. Assisting the person toward a more satisfying general adjustment is desirable (see Box 18-5).

Insight-oriented therapy is not useful because there is no benefit in trying to prove the delusion is not true, arguing the person out of the delusion, or telling the individual that the delusion is imaginary. Cognitive therapy with supportive therapy that focuses on reasoning or reality testing to decrease delusional thinking, or modifying the delusion itself, may be helpful. Educational interventions can aid the patient in understanding how factors such as sensory impairment, social and physical isolation, and stress contribute to the intensity of this disorder.

In certain instances, hospitalization is needed in response to dangerous behaviour that could include aggressiveness, poor impulse control, excessive psychological tension, unremitting anger, and threats. Suicide can be a concern, but most patients are not at risk. If hospitalization is required, the person needs to be approached tactfully, and legal assistance may be necessary.

BOX 18.5

Psychoeducation Checklist: Delusional Disorder

When caring for the patient with delusional disorder, be sure to include the caregiver, as appropriate, and address the following topic areas in the teaching plan:

☐ Psychopharmacologic agents (antipsychotic or antidepressants), if used, including drug action, dosage, frequency, and possible adverse effects
☐ Identification of troubling experiences
☐ Consequences of delusions
☐ Realistic goal setting
☐ Positive coping strategies
☐ Safety measures
☐ Social training skills
☐ Family participation in therapy

Social Domain

Assessment

A common characteristic of individuals with delusional disorder is normal behaviour and appearance unless their delusional ideas are being discussed or acted on. The cultural background of the person with delusional disorder has to be evaluated. Ethnic and cultural systems have different beliefs that are accepted within their individual context but not outside their group. Problems can occur in social, occupational, or interpersonal areas. In general, the person's social and marital functioning is more likely to be impaired than their intellectual or occupational functioning. Most are employed, although generally they hold low-paying jobs. Supportive family members and friends can mean a more positive outcome for the person living with a delusional disorder.

Life difficulties are often related to the delusion. Thus, assessing the person's capacity to act in response to the delusion is important. What is the person's level of impulsiveness (ie, related to behaviours of suicide, homicide, aggression, or violence)? Establishing as complete a picture of the person as possible, including the person's subjective private experiences and concrete psychopathologic symptoms, helps to reduce uncertainty in the assessment process.

Nursing Diagnoses for the Social Domain

Several nursing diagnoses can be generated from the assessment data for the social domain. Ineffective Coping, Interrupted Family Processes, and Ineffective Role Performance are examples.

Interventions for Social Domain

People with diagnoses of delusional disorder often become socially isolated. The secretiveness of their delusions and the importance the delusions have in their life are central to this phenomenon. Social skills training tailored to the patient's specific deficits can help to improve social adaptation. Family therapy can help the person reintegrate into the family; family education and patient education will enhance understanding of the patient and the disease process. However, group therapy is usually not beneficial because the patient lacks insight into the origin of the delusion. Families face many of the same issues as families of patients with other disorders involving delusions and are at risk for ineffective coping.

EVALUATION AND TREATMENT OUTCOMES

For patients with delusional disorders, the greater the lack of insight and the poorer the adherence to treatment

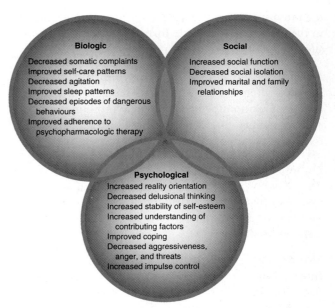

FIGURE 18.4 Biopsychosocial outcomes for patients with delusional disorder.

regimens, the more difficult it is to teach the individual. The patient rarely, if ever, develops full insight, and the symptoms related to the original diagnosis are not likely to disappear completely. In evaluating progress, the nurse must remember that outcomes are often not met completely. The nurse should maintain realistic outcomes and praise small successes to promote positive outcomes (Fig. 18-4).

CONTINUUM OF CARE

Inpatient-Focussed Care

Hospitalization rarely occurs and is usually initiated by the legal or social violations. Insight-oriented interventions help the patient to understand his or her situation. Avoid confrontational situations; use the patient's coping abilities to reinforce constructive aspects of functioning to enable a return to autonomy.

Emergency! Care

Emergency care is seldom required, unless the patient has had an incident with the law or legal system. The patient may be agitated or aggressive because the delusion, which is perceived as real, has been interrupted.

Family Intervention

Family therapy may be helpful. By helping the family to develop mechanisms to cope with the patient's delusions, nurses help the family to be more supportive and understanding of the patient.

Community Treatment

Patients with diagnoses of delusional disorder are treated most effectively in an outpatient setting. They should be encouraged to seek psychiatric treatment. Insight-oriented therapy to develop an understanding of the patient's delusion may be helpful. Medications are not often used with delusional disorder, but antipsychotic agents or benzodiazepines are helpful during exacerbations. Other treatments include supportive therapy, development of coping skills, cognitive therapy, and social skills training. Family therapy may be helpful.

Other Psychotic Disorders

Other disorders have psychoses as their defining features. The nursing care of patients with these disorders is not discussed specifically, but the generalist PMH nurse has the ability to apply care used with other disorders to the disorders presented here (Table 18-3).

SCHIZOPHRENIFORM DISORDER

The essential features of schizophreniform disorder are identical to those of criteria A for schizophrenia, with the exception of the duration of the illness, which can be less than 6 months (APA, 2000). However, symptoms must be present for at least 1 month to be classified as a schizophreniform disorder (Table 18-4). This diagnosis is also used as provisional if symptoms have lasted more than 1 month but it is uncertain whether the person will recover before the end of the 6-month period. Some research has suggested that this illness may be an early manifestation of schizophrenia (Iancu, Dannon, Ziv, & Lepkifker, 2002).

Altered social or occupational functioning may occur but is not necessary. Most patients experience interruption in one or more areas of daily functioning (APA, 2000).

BRIEF PSYCHOTIC DISORDER

In brief psychotic disorder, the length of the episode is at least 1 day but less than 1 month. The onset is sudden and includes at least one of the positive symptoms of criteria A for schizophrenia found in Chapter 17 (see also Table 18-4). Differentiating this illness from bipolar SCA is important (Marneros, Pillmann, Haring, Balzuweit, & Bloink, 2002).

The person generally experiences emotional turmoil or overwhelming confusion and rapid, intense shifts of affect (APA, 2000). Although episodes are brief, impairment can be severe, and supervision may be required to protect the person. Suicide is a risk, especially in younger patients. A predisposition to develop a brief psychotic disorder may include pre-existing personality disorders (APA, 2000). The person's ethnic and cultural background should also be considered in relation to the social or religious context of the symptoms presented.

Table 18.3	Other Psychotic Disorders
Disorder	**Definition**
Schizophreniform disorder	This disorder is identical to schizophrenia except the total duration of the illness can be less than 6 months (must be at least 1 month) and there may not be impaired social or occupational functioning.
Schizoaffective disorder	This disorder is characterized by an uninterrupted period of illness during which at some time there is a major depressive, manic, or mixed episode along with two of the following symptoms of schizophrenia: delusions, hallucinations, disorganized speech, disorganized or catatonic behaviour, or negative symptoms (affective flattening, alogia, or avolition).
Delusional disorder	This disorder is characterized by the presence of nonbizarre delusion and includes several subtypes: erotomanic, grandiose, jealous, somatic, mixed, and unspecified.
Brief psychotic disorder	In this disorder, there is a sudden onset of at least one positive psychotic symptom that lasts at least 1 day but less than 1 month. Eventually, the individual has a full return to normal.
Shared psychotic disorders (*folie à deux*)	In this disorder, one person who is in a close relationship with another person who already has a psychotic disorder with prominent delusions also develops the delusion.
Other psychotic disorders due to substances such as drugs and alcohol	The prominent hallucinations or delusions are judged to be due to the physiologic effects of substances (drugs, alcohol).

From American Psychiatric Association. (2000). *Diagnostic and statistical manual of mental disorders*, 4th ed., Text revision. Washington, DC: Author.

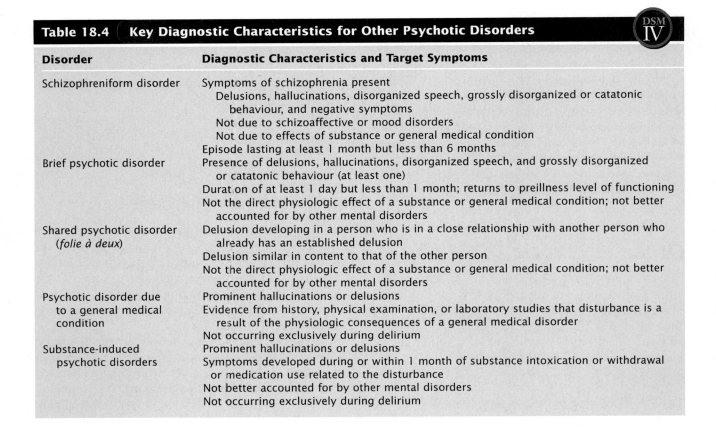

Table 18.4	Key Diagnostic Characteristics for Other Psychotic Disorders
Disorder	**Diagnostic Characteristics and Target Symptoms**

Schizophreniform disorder	Symptoms of schizophrenia present
	    Delusions, hallucinations, disorganized speech, grossly disorganized or catatonic
	      behaviour, and negative symptoms
	    Not due to schizoaffective or mood disorders
	    Not due to effects of substance or general medical condition
	Episode lasting at least 1 month but less than 6 months

Brief psychotic disorder	Presence of delusions, hallucinations, disorganized speech, and grossly disorganized
	    or catatonic behaviour (at least one)
	Duration of at least 1 day but less than 1 month; returns to preillness level of functioning
	Not the direct physiologic effect of a substance or general medical condition; not better
	    accounted for by other mental disorders

Shared psychotic disorder
  (folie à deux)
	Delusion developing in a person who is in a close relationship with another person who
	    already has an established delusion
	Delusion similar in content to that of the other person
	Not the direct physiologic effect of a substance or general medical condition; not better
	    accounted for by other mental disorders

Psychotic disorder due
  to a general medical
  condition
	Prominent hallucinations or delusions
	Evidence from history, physical examination, or laboratory studies that disturbance is a
	    result of the physiologic consequences of a general medical disorder
	Not occurring exclusively during delirium

Substance-induced
  psychotic disorders
	Prominent hallucinations or delusions
	Symptoms developed during or within 1 month of substance intoxication or withdrawal
	    or medication use related to the disturbance
	Not better accounted for by other mental disorders
	Not occurring exclusively during delirium

This disorder is uncommon but usually appears in early adulthood (APA, 2000).

SHARED PSYCHOTIC DISORDER

In shared psychotic disorder (*folie à deux*), a person develops a close relationship with another individual ("inducer" or "primary case") who has a psychotic disorder with prominent delusions (APA, 2000; Trabert, 1999) (see Table 18-4). With this disorder, the person believes and shares part or all of the inducer's delusional beliefs. The content of the delusions depends on the inducer, who is the dominant person in the relationship and imposes the delusions on the passive person (APA, 2000). This disorder is somewhat more common in women, and the age of onset is variable. Delusional beliefs are usually shared by people who have lived together for a long time in relative social isolation. However, family members rarely share the same delusional belief. When the relationship is interrupted, the passive person's delusional beliefs decrease or disappear (APA, 2000).

Treatment is sought infrequently (Trabert, 1999). When care is sought, the inducer usually brings the situation to clinical treatment (APA, 2000). When the passive person is removed from the setting, 93% have a favorable course even with no treatment (Trabert,

1999). If the inducer receives no intervention, the course is usually chronic.

PSYCHOTIC DISORDERS ATTRIBUTABLE TO SUBSTANCE

Patients with a psychotic disorder attributable to a substance present with prominent hallucinations or delusions that are the direct physiologic effects of a substance (eg, drug abuse, toxin exposure) (APA, 2000) (see Table 18-4). During intoxication, symptoms continue as long as the use of the substance continues. Withdrawal symptoms can occur for as long as 4 weeks. Differential diagnosis is recommended.

SUMMARY OF KEY POINTS

◘ Schizoaffective disorder has symptoms typical of both schizophrenia and mood disorders but is a separate disorder. Although these patients experience mood problems most of the time, the diagnosis of schizoaffective disorder depends on the presence of positive symptoms (ie, delusions or hallucinations) without mood symptoms at some time during the uninterrupted period of illness.

◘ Although controversy and discussion continue about whether schizoaffective disorder is truly a separate disorder, the *DSM-IV-TR* now identifies it as separate.

◘ Patients with schizoaffective disorder have fewer awareness deficits and appear to have more insight than do patients with true schizophrenia, a fact that can be used in teaching patients to control symptoms, recognize early regression, and develop psychosocial skills.

◘ Patients with schizoaffective disorder will likely never be medication free. Intermittent antipsychotic dosing is best for patients who can detect recurring symptoms and institute their own drug therapy.

◘ Nursing care for patients with schizoaffective disorder is focussed on minimizing psychiatric symptoms through promoting medication maintenance and on helping patients maintain optimal levels of functioning. Interventions centre on developing social and coping skills through supportive, nurturing, and nonconfrontational approaches. The nurse must be constantly attuned to the mood state of the patient and help the patient learn to solve problems, resolve conflict, and cope with social situations that trigger anxiety.

◘ Delusional disorder is characterized by stable, well-systematized, and logical nonbizarre delusions that could occur in real life and are plausible in the context of the patient's ethnic and cultural background. These delusions may or may not interfere with an individual's ability to function socially. Patients typically deny any psychiatric basis for their problem and refuse to seek psychiatric care. Patients whose delusions relate to somatic complaints are often seen on medical-surgical units of hospitals. Diagnosis otherwise is often made only when patients act on the basis of their delusions and violate the law or social rules.

◘ Delusional disorder is further classified as a particular subtype, depending on the nature and content of the patient's delusions, including erotomanic, grandiose, jealous, somatic, mixed, and unspecified.

◘ Patients with delusional disorder usually do not experience functional difficulties or mental status impairments. Their thinking, orientation, affect, attention, memory, perception, and personality generally remain intact.

◘ The therapeutic relationship is crucial to the successful treatment of the patient with delusional disorder. Nurses must be aware of the patient's fragile self-esteem and unusual sensitivities and anxieties and try to establish a trusting relationship through a flexible, nonjudgmental approach that promotes empathy, trust, and support while keeping physical and emotional detachment.

CRITICAL THINKING CHALLENGES

1 Mr. J. first received a diagnosis of schizophrenia, but after experiencing extreme mood disturbances, finally received a diagnosis of schizoaffective disorders. During a recent outpatient visit, he confides to a nurse that he just has stress and does not think that he really has any psychiatric problems. Identify assessment areas that should be pursued before the patient leaves his appointment. How would you confront the denial?

2 Ms. S. believed that she had bipolar disorder. At a recent clinic visit, she was told that she most probably had schizoaffective disorder. The patient asked the nurse how a bipolar disorder could turn into schizoaffective disorder. Identify three appropriate responses to her question.

3 A patient with schizoaffective disorder is prescribed an antipsychotic agent (Risperdal) and a mood stabilizer (Depakene). The patient asks you why both medications are needed. Develop the best response for this question. Be thorough.

4 At an interdisciplinary treatment team meeting, the nurse recommends that a woman with schizoaffective disorder attend an anger management group. The rest of the team believes that only a mood stabilizer is needed. Develop the rationale for attending the anger management group in addition to medication supplementation.

5 A patient was prescribed olanzapine (Zyprexa) and an antidepressant citalopram (Celexa) for the treatment of schizoaffective disorder. Since her last monthly visit, she gained 15 pounds. She is considering discontinuing her medication regimen because of the weight gain. Develop a plan to addresses her weight gain and her intention to discontinue her medication regimen.

6 A. has received a diagnosis of schizoaffective disorder, and B. has received a diagnosis of delusional disorder. How would the symptoms differ? Would there be any similarities? If so, what would they be?

7 Identify and explain each of the subtypes of delusional disorder.

8 An elderly person in a nursing home has a delusion that her husband is having an affair with her sister. Discuss nonpharmacologic nursing interventions that should be implemented with this patient. How would you explain her delusion to her husband? Choose one of the subtypes of delusion and develop a plan for clinical management, focusing on psychiatric nursing care, for a patient experiencing this condition.

9 A patient convincingly informs you that she is having an affair with a famous actor. They both attended the same college at about the same time. How would you determine whether this patient's belief is a delusion or reality? Is it important that the nurse understand whether the relationship is real? Explain the rationale for your answer.

10 A patient informs a student nurse that he is a member of the Secret Service and that he is undercover.

He asks the nurse to keep the secret. The student considers several possible responses, including redirecting the patient to a different topic and confronting him with the reality of his hospitalization. Discuss the best response to this patient's comment.

WEB LINKS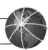

www.cmha.ca Web site for the Canadian Mental Health Association, which is a nationwide, charitable organization that promotes the resilience and recovery of people experiencing mental illness.

www.schizophrenia.ca Web site for the Schizophrenia Society of Canada, which provides support and education for individuals living with schizophrenia and their families.

www.mooddisorderscanada.ca Web site for the Mood Disorders Society of Canada, which is a volunteer organization designed to improve the lives of people living with mood disorders.

www.surgeongeneral.gov Web site for Healthy People 2010 and Report of the Surgeon General.

www.nami.org National Alliance for the Mentally Ill advocacy information.

www.mentalhealth.com Internet mental health web site that provides the American and European description of schizoaffective disorder and its treatment.

www.geocities.com/CollegePark/Classroom/6237 Learn from a registered psychiatric nurse about schizoaffective and other disorders and about what psychiatric nurses do.

www.mhinfosource.com Answers to questions about schizoaffective and other psychiatric disorders.

MOVIES

Misery. 1990. This movie stars James Caan as Paul Sheldon and Kathy Bates as Annie Wilkes. Sheldon is the writer of a popular mystery series who finishes his last novel in a secluded cabin in Colorado. After being rescued in a blizzard by Annie Wilkes, he becomes her prisoner when she prevents him from leaving his cabin. Annie is in love with him but is demanding and possessive. She identifies with the heroine in his latest novel, and is outraged at the conclusion of the novel.

SIGNIFICANCE: Annie demonstrates the thinking patterns associated with delusional disorder.

VIEWING POINTS: Identify the disturbed thinking that Annie demonstrates. Part of Annie's behaviour seems normal, and other behaviours are illogical. How are they linked?

REFERENCES

American Psychiatric Association (APA). (1980). *Diagnostic and statistical manual of mental disorders* (3rd ed.). Washington, DC: Author.

American Psychiatric Association (APA). (2000). *Diagnostic and statistical manual of mental disorders* (4th ed., Text revision). Washington, DC: Author.

Andres, K., Pfammatter, M., Garst, F., Teschner, C., & Brenner, H. D. (2000). Effects of a coping-oriented group therapy for schizophrenia and schizoaffective patients: A pilot study. *Acta Psychiatrica Scandinavica, 101*(4), 318–322.

Baker, P. B., Cook, B. L., & Winokur, G. (1995). Delusional infestation: The interference of delusions and hallucinations. *Psychiatric Clinics of North America, 18*(2), 345–361.

Bech, P. (2001). The significance of delusions in depressive disorders. *Current Opinions in Psychiatry, 14*(1), 47–49.

Bentall, R. P., Corcoran, R., Howard, R., Blackwood, N., & Kinderman, P. (2001). Persecutory delusions: A review and theoretical integration. *Clinical Psychology Review, 21*(8), 1143–1192.

Chernomas, W., Clarke, D., & Chisholm, F. (2000). Perspectives of women living with schizophrenia. *Psychiatric Services, 51,* 1517–1521.

Conway, C. R., Bollini, A. M., Graham, B. G., Keefe, R. S., Schiffman, S. S., & McEvoy, J. P. (2002). Sensory acuity and reasoning in delusional disorder. *Comprehensive Psychiatry, 43*(3), 175–178.

Crow, T. J., & Harrington, C. A. (1994). Etiopathogenesis and treatment of psychosis. *Annual Review of Medicine, 45,* 219–234.

DeLisi, L. E., Shaw, S. H., Crow, T. J., Shields, G., Smith, A. B., Larach, V. W., Wellman, N., Loftus, J., Nanthakumar, B., Razi, K., Stewart, J., Comazzi, M., Vita, A., Heffner, T., & Sherrington, R. (2002). A genome-wide scan for linkage to chromosomal regions in 382 sibling pairs with schizophrenia or schizoaffective disorder. *American Journal of Psychiatry, 159*(5), 803–812.

Dietrich, D. E., Kropp, S., & Emrich, H. M. (2001). Oxcarbazepine in affective and schizoaffective disorders. *Pharmacopsychiatry, 34*(6), 242–250.

Evans, J. D., Heaton, R. K., Paulsen, J. S., McAdams, L. A., Heaton, S. C., & Jeste, D. V. (1999). Schizoaffective disorder: A form of schizophrenia or affective disorder? *Journal of Clinical Psychiatry, 60*(12), 874–882.

Fabisch, K., Fabisch, H., Langs, G., Macheiner, H., Fitz, W., & Honigl, D. (2001). Basic symptoms and their contribution to the differential typology of acute schizophrenic and schizoaffective disorders. *Psychopathology, 34*(1), 15–22.

Fujii, D. E., Ahmed, I., & Takeshita, J. (1999). Neuropsychologic implications in erotomania: Two case studies. *Neuropsychiatry, Neuropsychology and Behavioral Management, 12*(2), 110–116.

Getz, G. E., DelBello, M. P., Fleck, D. E., Zimmerman, M. E., Schwiers, M. L., & Strakowski, S. M. (2002). Neuroanatomic characterization of schizoaffective disorder using MRI: A pilot study. *Schizophrenia Research, 55*(1–2), 55–59.

Gooding, D. C., & Tallent, K. A. (2002). Spatial working memory performance in patients with schizoaffective psychosis versus schizophrenia: A tale of two disorders? *Schizophrenia Research, 15*(3), 209–218.

Grunebaum, M. F., Oquendo, M. A., Harkavy-Friedman, J. M., Ellis, S. P., Li, S., Haas, G. L., Malone, K. M., & Mann, J. J. (2001). Delusions and suicidality. *American Journal of Psychiatry, 158*(5), 742–747.

Harmon, R. B., Rosner, R., & Owens, H. (1995). Obsessional harassment and erotomania in a criminal court population. *Journal of Forensic Science, 41*(2), 188–196.

Huxley, N. A., Rendall, M., & Sederer, L. (2000). Psychosocial treatments in schizophrenia: A review of the past 20 years. *Journal of Nervous and Mental Disease, 188*(4), 187–201.

Iancu, I., Dannon, P. N., Ziv, R., & Lepkifker, E. (2002). A follow-up study of patients with DSM-IV schizophreniform disorder. *Canadian Journal of Psychiatry, 47*(1), 56–60.

Kasanin, J. (1933). The acute schizo-affective psychoses. *American Journal of Psychiatry, 13*, 97–126.

Lewine, R. R., Hudgins, P., Brown, F., Caudle, J., & Risch, S. C. (1995). Differences in qualitative brain morphology findings in schizophrenia, major depression, bipolar disorder, and normal volunteers. *Schizophrenia Research, 15*(3), 253–259.

Maj, M., Pirozzi, R., Formicola, A. M., Bartoli, L., & Bucci, P. (2000). Reliability and validity of the *DSM-IV* diagnostic category of schizoaffective disorder: Preliminary data. *Journal of Affective Disorders, 57*(1–3), 95–98.

Marneros, A. (2003). The schizoaffective phenomenon: The state of the art. *Acta Psychiatrica Scandinavica Supplementum, 418*, 29–33.

Marneros, A., Pillmann, F., Haring, A., Balzuweit, S., & Bloink, R. (2002). The relation of 'acute and transient psychotic disorder' (ICD-10 F23) to bipolar schizoaffective disorder. *Journal of Psychiatric Research, 36*(3), 165–171.

McCann, T. V., & Baker, H. (2003). Models of mental health nurse–general practitioner liaison: Promoting continuity of care. *Journal of Advanced Nursing, 41*(5), 471–479.

McGuire, L., Junginger, J., Adams, S. G. Jr., Burright, R., & Donovick, P. (2001). Delusions and delusional reasoning. *Journal of Abnormal Psychology, 110*(2), 259–266.

McCutcheon, L. E., Ashe, D. D., Houran, J., & Maltby, J. (2003). A cognitive profile of individuals who tend to worship celebrities. *Journal of Psychology, 137*(4), 309–322.

Meloy, J. R. (1999). Erotomania, triangulation and homicide. *Journal of Forensic Science, 44*(2), 421–424.

Moller, H. J., Bottlender, R., Gross, A., Hoff, P., Wittmann, J., Wegner, U., & Strauss, A. (2002). The Kraepelinian dichotomy: Preliminary results of a 15-year follow-up study on functional psychoses: Focus on negative symptoms. *Schizophrenia Research, 56*(1–2), 878–894.

Morimoto, K., Miyatake, R., Nakamura, M., Watanabe, T., Hirao, T., & Suwaki, H. (2002). Delusional disorder: Molecular genetic evidence for dopamine psychosis. *Neuropsychopharmacology, 26*(6), 794–801.

Munro, A. (1999). *Delusional disorder*. Cambridge, MA: Cambridge University Press.

Norman, R., Scholten, D., Malla, A., & Ballageer, T. (2005). Early signs in schizophrenia spectrum disorders. *Journal of Nervous and Mental Disease, 193*, 17–23.

Nose, M., Barbui, C., & Tansella, M. (2003). How often do patients with psychosis fail to adhere to treatment programmes? A systematic review. *Psychological Medicine, 33*(7), 1149–1160.

Ota, M., Mizukami, K., Katano, T., Sato, S., Takeda, T., & Asada, T. (2003). A case of delusional disorder, somatic type with remarkable improvement of clinical symptoms and single photon emission computed tomography findings following modified electroconvulsive therapy. *Progress in Neuro-psychopharmacology & Biological Psychiatry, 27*(5), 881–884.

Perr, I. N. (1992). Religion, political leadership, charisma, and mental illness: The strange story of Louis Riel. *Journal of Forensic Sciences, 37*(2), 574–584.

Pini, S., Cassano, G. B., Dell'Osso, L., & Amador, X. F. (2001). Insight into illness in schizophrenia, schizoaffective disorder, and mood disorders with psychotic features. *American Journal of Psychiatry, 158*(1), 122–125.

Potkin, S. G., Alphs, L., Hsu, C., Krishnan, K., Anand, R., Young, F. K., Meltzer, H., & Green, A. (2003). Predicting suicidal risk in schizophrenic and schizoaffective patients in a prospective two-year trial. *Biological Psychiatry, 54*(4), 444–452.

Radomsky, E. D., Haas, G. L., Mann, J. J., & Sweeney, J. A. (1999). Suicidal behavior in patients with schizophrenia and other psychotic disorders. *American Journal of Psychiatry, 156*(10), 1590–1595.

Regenold, W. T., Thapar, R. K., Marano, C., Gavirneni, S., & Kondapavuluru, P. V. (2002). Increased prevalence of type 2 diabetes mellitus among psychiatric inpatients with bipolar I affective and schizoaffective disorders independent of psychotropic drug use. *Journal of Affective Disorders, 70*(1), 19–26.

Reichenberg, A., Weiser, M., Rabinowitz, J., Caspi, A., Schmeidler, J., Mark, M., Kaplan, Z., & Davidson, M. (2002). A population-based cohort study of premorbid intellectual, language, and behavioral functioning in patients with schizophrenia, schizoaffective disorder and nonpsychotic bipolar disorder. *American Journal of Psychiatry, 159*(12), 2027–2035.

Rietschel, M., Krauss, H., Muller, D. J., Schulze, T. G., Knapp, M., Marwinski, K., Marddt, A. O., Paus, S., Grunhage, F., Propping, P., Maier, W., Held, T., & Nothen, M. M. (2000). Dopamine d3 receptor variant and tardive dyskinesia. *European Archives of Psychiatry and Clinical Neuroscience, 250*(1), 31–35.

Scott, T. F., Price, T. R., George, M. S., Brillman, J., & Rothfus, W. (1993). Midline cerebral malformations and schizophrenia. *Journal of Neuropsychiatry and Clinical Neurosciences, 5*(3), 287–293.

Siris, S. G., & Lavin, M. R. (1995). Other psychotic disorders. In H. Kaplan & B. Sadock (Eds.), *Comprehensive textbook of psychiatry* (6th ed.). Baltimore: Williams & Wilkins.

Swoboda, E., Conca, A., Konig, P., Waanders, R., & Hansen, M. (2001). Maintenance electroconvulsive therapy in affective and schizoaffective disorder. *Neuropsychobiology, 43*(1)I, 23–28,

Trabert, W. (1999). Shared psychotic disorder in delusional parasitosis. *Psychopathology, 32*(1), 30–34.

Volavka, J., Czobor, P., Sheitman, B., Lindenmayer, J. P., Citrome, L., McEvoy, J. P., Cooper, T. B., Chakos, M., & Lieberman, J. A. (2002). Clozapine, olanzapine, risperidone, and haloperidol in the treatment of patients with chronic schizophrenia and schizoaffective disorder. *American Journal of Psychiatry, 159*(2), 255–262.

Waite, P. (1987). Between three oceans: Challenges of a continental destiny. In C. Brown (Ed.), *The illustrated history of Canada* (pp. 279–373). Toronto: Lester Orpen Denys Ltd.

CHAPTER 19

Mood Disorders

Sandra J. Wood and Yvonne M. Hayne, revised
from a chapter by Katharine P. Bailey

LEARNING OBJECTIVES

After studying this chapter, you will be able to:

- Describe the impact of underdiagnosed and untreated mood disorders as a major public health problem.
- Distinguish the clinical characteristics and course of depressive disorders and bipolar disorder.
- Analyze the prevailing biologic, psychological, and social theories that serve as a basis for caring for patients with mood disorders.
- Analyze the human responses to mood disorders with emphasis on concepts of mood, affect, depressed mood, and manic episode.
- Formulate nursing diagnoses based on a biopsychosocial assessment of patients with mood disorders.
- Formulate nursing interventions that address specific diagnoses based on a continuum of care.
- Identify expected outcomes and their evaluation.
- Analyze special concerns within the nurse–patient relationship common to treating people with mood disorders.

KEY TERMS

affect ▪ bipolar ▪ cyclothymic disorder ▪ depressive episode ▪ dysthymic disorder ▪ euphoria ▪ expansive mood ▪ hypomanic episode ▪ lability of mood ▪ manic episode ▪ mixed episode ▪ rapid cycling ▪ unipolar

KEY CONCEPTS

▪ mania ▪ mood ▪ mood disorders

The World Health Organization (WHO) predicts that mood disorders will be the number one public health problem in the 21st century. In Canada, new data from the Canadian Community Health Survey (CCHS) on mental health and well-being reports as many Canadians suffer from major depression as from other leading chronic medical conditions such as heart disease, diabetes, or a thyroid condition (Canadian Community Health Survey, 2004). In a 12-month period, 4.9% of the Canadian population, translating to approximately 1,600,000 of the total 32 million people in Canada (Today's News Releases, 2005), are estimated to have experienced either a major depressive or manic episode (Canadian Community Health Survey, 2004). Notable trends are to appreciable increases in these figures, such that escalating socioeconomic burdens to the nation can be anticipated. Latest figures pose costs for a 1-year period at $14.4 billion, nearly $500.00 for each Canadian (How Healthy Are Canadians, 2004, p. 6). At national and personal levels, mood disorders are associated with high levels of impairment in occupation, social, and physical functioning. Mood disorders often go undetected and untreated. Studies suggest that more than two thirds of people with bipolar disorder have their disease misdiagnosed (Hirschfeld, Lewis, & Vornik, 2003).

Federal-provincial initiatives in Canada have evolved varied collaborative approaches to mental health care such as that demonstrated in the "Shared Mental Health Care" model, which aims to more effectively diagnose, assess, and treat mental health patients in the context of the family physician's office (McElheran, Eaton, Rupcich, Basinger, & Johnston, 2004). Such collaborative endeavours are thought to increase efficiency in the utilization of health care resources by enhancing the prospects of astute identification of psychological and somatic complaints, making more apparent the correct diagnosis. Appropriate remedial care can then more readily be instituted to avert intensification of the illness. In mood disorders, the potential for suicide is significantly greater; therefore, these disorders affect premature mortality. Accurate diagnosing to establish efficacious pharmaceutical and psychological treatments is vital. Nurses practicing in any health care setting need to develop competence in assessing patients for the presence of a mood disorder and, if suspected, provide appropriate educational and clinical interventions or referral.

> ⬠ **KEY CONCEPT Mood** is a pervasive and sustained emotion that colors one's perception of the world and how one functions in it. Normal variations in mood occur as responses to specific life experiences. Normal mood variations, such as sadness, euphoria, and anxiety, are time limited and are not associated with significant functional impairment. The normal range of mood or affect varies considerably both within and between cultures.

> ⬠ **KEY CONCEPT Mood disorders**, as defined in the *Diagnostic and Statistical Manual of Mental Disorders*, 4th edition, text revision ([DSM-IV-TR]; American Psychiatric Association [APA], 2000), are recurrent disturbances or alterations in mood that cause psychological distress and behavioural impairment.

The primary alteration is in mood, rather than in thought or perception. Several terms describe observable expressions of mood (called **affect**) (APA, 2000), including the following:

- *Blunted*: significantly reduced intensity of emotional expression
- *Flat*: absent or nearly absent affective expression
- *Inappropriate*: discordant affective expression accompanying the content of speech or ideation
- *Labile*: varied, rapid, and abrupt shifts in affective expression
- *Restricted or constricted*: mildly reduced in the range and intensity of emotional expression

Primary mood disorders include both depressive (**unipolar**) and manic-depressive (**bipolar**) disorders. The *DSM-IV-TR* has established specific criteria for diagnostic classification of these disorders, including criteria for severity (a change from previous functioning), duration (at least 2 weeks), and clinically significant distress or impairment. Mood episodes are the "building blocks" for the mood disorder diagnoses. The *DSM-IV-TR* describes four categories of mood episodes: major depressive episode, manic episode, mixed episode, and hypomanic episode. This chapter focuses on the depressive disorders and bipolar disorder. The *DSM-IV-TR* categorizes mood disorders as follows:

- *Depressive disorders*: major depressive disorder, single or recurrent; dysthymic disorder; and depressive disorder not otherwise specified (NOS)
- *Bipolar disorders*: bipolar I disorder, bipolar II disorder, cyclothymic disorder, and bipolar disorder NOS
- *Mood disorder* caused by a general medical condition
- *Substance-induced mood disorder*
- *Mood disorder NOS*

In addition to the above, increased incidence of two diagnoses, within the category of mood disorders, warrants their mention. First, *postpartum onset specifier* is distinguished by onset of episode within 4 weeks postpartum. Second, *seasonal pattern specifier* is particularly notable in Canada, where weather patterns appear to dispose to the occurrence as well as remission of symptoms (APA Desk Reference, 2000, pp. 204–207).

Depressive Disorders
CLINICAL COURSE

The primary *DSM-IV-TR* criterion for major depressive disorder is one or more major depressive episodes.

In a major **depressive episode**, either a depressed mood or a loss of interest or pleasure in nearly all activities must be present for at least 2 weeks. Four of seven additional symptoms must be present: disruption in sleep, appetite (or weight), concentration, energy; psychomotor agitation or retardation; excessive guilt or feelings of worthlessness; and suicidal ideation (see Table 19-1). Individuals often describe themselves as depressed, hopeless, discouraged, or "down in the dumps." If individuals complain of feeling sad and empty, a depressed mood can sometimes be inferred from their facial expression and demeanor (APA, 2000; Health Canada, 2002).

Dysthymic disorder is a milder but more chronic form of major depressive disorder. The *DSM-IV-TR* criteria for dysthymic disorder are depressed mood for most days for at least 2 years and two or more of the following symptoms: poor appetite or overeating; insomnia or oversleeping; low energy or fatigue; low self-esteem; poor concentration or difficulty making decisions; and feelings of hopelessness. The NOS category includes disorders with depressive features that do not meet strict criteria for major depressive disorder.

Major depressive disorder is commonly a progressive, recurrent illness. With time, episodes tend to occur more frequently, become more severe, and are of a longer duration. About 25% of patients experience a recurrence during the first 6 months after a first episode, and about 50% to 75% have a recurrence within 5 years. The mean age of onset for major depressive disorder is about 40 years; 50% of all patients have an onset between the ages of 20 and 50 years. During a 20-year period, the mean number of episodes is five or six. Symptoms usually develop during a period of days to months. About 50% of patients have significant depressive symptoms before the first identified episode. An untreated episode typically lasts 6 to 13 months, regardless of the age of onset. Suicide is the most serious complication and occurs in 10% to 15% of those formerly hospitalized for depression (Angst, Angst, & Stassen, 1999).

DEPRESSIVE DISORDERS IN SPECIAL POPULATIONS

Children and Adolescents

Depressive disorders in children have manifestations similar to those seen in adults with a few exceptions. In major depressive disorder, children are less likely to experience psychosis, but when they do, auditory hallucinations are more common than delusions. They are

Table 19.1	Key Diagnostic Characteristics for Major Depressive Disorder 296.xx Major depressive disorder, single episode 296.2x Major depressive disorder, recurrent 296.3x	

Diagnostic Criteria and Target Symptoms	Associated Findings

■ Change from previous level of functioning during a 2-week period
  Depressed mood
  Markedly diminished interest or pleasure in all or almost all activities
  Significant weight loss when not dieting, or weight gain or change in appetite
  Insomnia or hypersomnia
  Psychomotor agitation or retardation
  Fatigue or loss of energy
  Feelings of worthlessness or excessive or inappropriate guilt
  Diminished ability to think or concentrate, or indecisiveness
  Recurrent thoughts of death, recurrent suicidal ideation without a specific plan, or a suicide attempt or specific plan for committing suicide
■ At least one symptom is depressed mood, or loss of interest or pleasure
■ Significant distress or impairment of social, occupational, or other important areas of functioning
■ Not a direct physiologic effect of substance or medical condition
■ Not better accounted for by bereavement, schizoaffective disorder; not superimposed on schizophrenia, schizophreniform disorder, delusional disorder, or psychotic disorder not otherwise specified
	Associated Behavioural Findings
	■ Tearfulness, irritability, brooding, obsessive rumination, anxiety, phobias, excessive worry over physical health, and complaints of pain
	■ Possible panic attacks
	■ Difficulty with intimate relationships
	■ Difficulties with sexual functioning
	■ Marital problems
	■ Occupational problems
	■ Substance abuse, such as alcohol
	■ High mortality rate; death by suicide
	■ Increased pain and physical illness
	■ Decreased physical, social, and role functioning
	■ May be preceded by dysthymic disorder

more likely to have anxiety symptoms, such as fear of separation, and somatic symptoms, such as stomach aches and headaches. Mood may be irritable, rather than sad, especially in adolescents. The risk for suicide, which peaks during the midadolescent years, is very real in children and adolescents. In Canada, the suicide rate since the 1980s (12.2 per 100,000 people in 1999) has remained fairly constant for teens aged 15 to 19; for both sexes, it is recorded as the second-leading cause of teen death, surpassed only by motor vehicle crashes (National Population Heath Survey [NPHS], 2004).

Elderly People

Most older patients with symptoms of depression do not meet the full criteria for major depression. However, it is estimated that 8% to 20% of older adults in the community and as many as 37% in primary care settings experience depressive symptoms. Treatment is successful in 60% to 80%, but response to treatment is slower than in younger adults. Depression in elderly people often is associated with chronic illnesses, such as heart disease, stroke, and cancer; symptoms may have a more somatic focus. Suicide is a very serious risk for the older adult, especially men. In Canada, people older than 80 years of age have the highest mortality rates due to suicide, of all age groups. Rates are the highest among men 85 years and older, at 31 suicides per 100,000 (Health Canada, 2002).

EPIDEMIOLOGY

Analysis of CCHS data reveals an estimated 3 million Canadians reported experiencing major depression at some point in their lifetime. Approximately 1.2 million Canadians aged 15 or over had a diagnosable major depressive episode in 2002 (Supplement to Health Reports, 2004). In Canada, major depressive disorders are seen to affect twice as many women as men. The risk for the disorder is noted to increase 1.5 to 3.0 times if a first-degree relative has the disorder. Further, the highest rates of first-onset depression occur in the young adult age group (12 to 24 years), with lower rates occurring in people 65 years of age and older (Remick, 2002). The U.S. picture is proportionately magnified, with approximately 7% of that nation experiencing a mood disorder in any given year. This percentage translates into an estimated 11 million people every year. It also appears that the chances of experiencing in the United States major depressive disorder are increasing in progressively younger age groups (U.S. DHHS, 1999). Major depressive disorder is twice as common in adolescent and adult women as in adolescent and adult men. Prepubertal boys and girls are equally affected. Major depressive disorders often co-occur with other psychiatric and substance-related disorders. Depression often is associated with a variety of medical conditions, particularly endocrine disorders, cardiovascular disease, neurologic disorders, autoimmune conditions, viral or other infectious diseases, certain cancers, and nutritional deficiencies, or as a direct physiologic effect of a substance (eg, a drug of abuse, a medication, other somatic treatment for depression, or toxin exposure) (APA, 2000).

Ethnic and Cultural Differences

Prevalence rates are unrelated to race. Culture can influence the experience and communication of symptoms of depression. Canada is a country of vast regional differences and numerous "microidentities" populated by indigenous and nonindigenous peoples. Many pockets of inhabitants such as Ukrainian and Asian cultures maintain "homeland" beliefs and ideologies that may influence individuals' experience and expression of emotional disturbances. Depressive symptoms evidenced in Canada's Aboriginal peoples may be quite

---

IN A LIFE

James Eugene Carrey (1962–)
Canadian-born Actor/Comedian

Public Persona

Jim Carrey grew up in Toronto, Canada. His notoriety as a comedian began with his earliest performance on *The Carol Burnett Show* at the age of 10. His stage talents ripened through stand-up comedy routines, done before classmates, throughout his school years. Carrey, a high school dropout, began his acting career in comedy clubs and with bit-part television and movie performances. Soon his unique on-screen characteristics caught the attention of film producers and movie goers alike, and he became a box-office success. Jim Carrey is well known for slapstick performances in such comedies as *Ace Ventura, The Mask,* and *Bruce Almighty.*

Personal Reality

Carrey publicly discussed his struggle with depression on *60 Minutes* (November 2004), exposing a serious, complicated side of himself as a person who was continually questioning himself and the world. Carrey has been candid about periods of desperation in his life: the poverty, deprivation, and anger that marked some of his early childhood and adolescence; the struggles through two failed marriages; the highs and the lows bordering on despair; and the extended use of Prozac that helped him "out of a jam." Through it all, Jim, described as using the mask of *comedy* to shield what remains a desperate kid, maintains "life is beautiful" and that he is committed to giving full expression to the "realness" of his being.

Source: *Jim Carrey* (2005). Retrieved August 29, 2005, from http://en.wikipedia.org/wiki/Jim_Carrey.

distinct coming from respective cultures, such as the Inuit, Metis, Blackfoot, Algonquian, Iroquoian, and so on (King Bood, 2005). Culture may dictate an iron resolve to keep feelings in check or unexpressed. Native spirituality, inherent to many First Nations peoples, may add a complexity to detecting *depression*, with each group expressing and coping with feelings differently. In some cultures, somatic symptoms, rather than sadness or guilt, may predominate. Complaints of "nerves" and headaches (in Ukrainian cultures); weakness, tiredness, or "imbalance" (in Chinese and Asian cultures); or problems of the "heart" (in Middle Eastern cultures) may be the way of expressing the depressive experience. Although culturally distinctive experiences must be distinguished from symptoms, it is also imperative not to dismiss a symptom routinely because it is viewed as the norm for a culture. The Canadian Nurses Association (CNA) recognizes that nurses must be equipped to care for an ever diverse population and value multiple ways of knowing, engaging, and expressing to be able to properly assess, accurately diagnose, and provide culturally sensitive care (Edmunds & Kinnaird-Iler, 2005).

Risk Factors

Depression is so common that it is sometimes difficult to identify risk factors. The generally agreed-on risk factors include the following:
- Prior episode of depression
- Family history of depressive disorder
- Lack of social support
- Stressful life event
- Current substance use
- Medical comorbidity
- Economic difficulties

ETIOLOGY

Genetics

Family, twin, and adoption studies demonstrate that genetic influences undoubtedly play a substantial role in the etiology of mood disorders. Major depressive disorder is more common among first-degree biologic relatives of people with this disorder than among the general population. Currently, a major research effort is focussing on developing a more accurate paradigm regarding the contribution of genetic factors to the development of mood disorders (Alda, 2001).

Neurobiologic Hypotheses

Neurobiologic theories of the etiology of depression emerged in the 1950s. These theories posit that major depression is caused by a deficiency or dysregulation in central nervous system (CNS) concentrations of the neurotransmitters norepinephrine, dopamine, and serotonin or in their receptor functions. These hypotheses arose in part from observations that some pharmacologic agents elevated mood, and subsequent studies identified their mechanisms of action. All antidepressants currently available have their therapeutic effects on these neurotransmitters or receptors. Current research focuses on the synthesis, storage, release, and uptake of these neurotransmitters, as well as on postsynaptic events (eg, second-messenger systems) (Donati & Rasenick, 2003).

Neuroendocrine and Neuropeptide Hypotheses

Major depressive disorder is associated with multiple endocrine alterations, specifically of the hypothalamic–pituitary–adrenal axis, the hypothalamic–pituitary–thyroid axis, the hypothalamic–growth hormone axis, and the hypothalamic–pituitary–gonadal axis. In addition, there is mounting evidence that components of neuroendocrine axes (eg, neuromodulatory peptides such as corticotropin-releasing factor) may themselves contribute to depressive symptoms. Evidence also suggests that the secretion of these hypothalamic and growth hormones is controlled by many of the neurotransmitters implicated in the pathophysiology of depression (Hanley & Van de Kar, 2003).

Psychoneuroimmunology

Psychoneuroimmunology is a recent area of research into a diverse group of proteins known as *chemical messengers* between immune cells. These messengers, called cytokines, signal the brain and serve as mediators between immune and nerve cells. The brain is capable of influencing immune processes, and conversely, immunologic response can result in changes in brain activity (Kronfol & Remick, 2000). The specific role of these mechanisms in psychiatric disease pathogenesis remains unknown.

Psychological Theories

Psychodynamic Factors

Most psychodynamic theorists acknowledge some debt to Freud's original conceptualization of the psychodynamics of depression, which ascribes etiology to an early lack of love, care, warmth, and protection and resultant anger, guilt, helplessness, and fear regarding the loss of love. The ensuing conflict between wanting to be loved and fear of rejection engenders pathologic self-punitiveness (also conceptualized as aggression turned inward), self-rejection, low self-esteem, and depressive symptoms (see Chapter 7).

Behavioural Factors

The behaviourists hold that depression occurs primarily as the result of a severe reduction in rewarding activities or an increase in unpleasant events in one's life. The resultant depression then leads to further restriction of activity, thereby decreasing the likelihood of experiencing pleasurable activities, which, in turn, intensifies the mood disturbance

Cognitive Factors

The cognitive approach maintains that irrational beliefs and negative distortions of thought about the self, the environment, and the future engender and perpetuate depressive affects (see Chapter 14).

Developmental Factors

Developmental theorists posit that depression may be the result of loss of a parent through death or separation or lack of emotionally adequate parenting. These factors may delay or prohibit the realization of appropriate developmental milestones.

Social Theories

Family Factors

Family theorists Wright and Leahey (2000) ascribe maladaptive "circular" patterns in family interactions as contributing to the onset of depression, particularly related to such factors as changes in family composition, losses related to serious illness or death of a family member, and disruption in the family dynamics related to abuse or violence. Their definition of family "is based on the family's beliefs about their conception of family rather than on who lives in the household" (pp. 70–71), and social and ethnic variants can affect the family's interpretation and experience of adversity (see Chapter 16).

Social Factors

Major depression may follow adverse or traumatic life events, especially those that involve the loss of an important human relationship or role in life. Social isolation, deprivation, and financial deprivation are risk factors (APA, 2002).

INTERDISCIPLINARY TREATMENT OF DISORDER

Although depressive disorders are the most commonly occurring mental disorders, they are usually treated within the primary care setting, not the psychiatric setting. Individuals with depression enter mental health settings when their symptoms become so severe that hospitalization is needed, usually for suicide attempts, or if they self-refer because of incapacitation. Interdisciplinary treatment of these disorders, which are often lifelong, needs to include a wide array of health professionals in all areas. The specific goals of treatment are:

- Reduce/control symptoms and, if possible, eliminate signs and symptoms of the depressive syndrome.
- Improve occupational and psychosocial function as much as possible.
- Reduce the likelihood of relapse and recurrence.

PRIORITY CARE ISSUES

The overriding concern for people with mood disorders is safety. In depressive disorders, suicide risk should always be considered, and suicide assessments should be routine (see Chapter 37).

Family Response to Disorder

Depression in one member affects the whole family. Spouses, children, parents, siblings, and friends experience frustration, guilt, and anger when the family member is immobilized and cannot function. It is often hard for others to understand the depth of the mood and how disabling it can be. Financial hardship can occur when the family member cannot go to work and spends days in bed. The lack of understanding and difficulty of living with a depressed person can lead to abuse. In Canada (1999/2000), women between the ages of 35 and 45 years have the greatest number of hospitalizations for major depressive disorder (Health Canada, 2002).

NURSING MANAGEMENT: HUMAN RESPONSE TO DISORDER

The diagnosis of major depressive disorder is made when *DSM-IV-TR* criteria are met. An awareness of the risk factors for depression, a comprehensive biopsychosocial assessment, history of illness, and past treatment are key to formulating a treatment plan and to evaluating outcomes. Interviewing a family member or close friend about the patient's day-to-day functioning and specific symptoms may be helpful in determining the course of the illness, current symptoms, and level of functioning.

Biologic Domain

Assessment

Because some symptoms of depression are similar to those of some medical problems or side effects of medication therapies, biologic assessment must include a physical systems review and thorough history of medical problems, with special attention to CNS function, endocrine function, anemia, chronic pain, autoimmune illness, diabetes, or menopause. Additional medical history includes surgeries; medical hospitalizations; head injuries; episodes of loss of consciousness; and pregnancies, childbirths, miscarriages, and abortions. A complete list of prescribed and over-the-counter medications should be compiled, including the reason a medication was prescribed or its use discontinued. A physical examination is recommended with baseline vital signs and baseline laboratory tests, including comprehensive blood chemistry panel, complete blood counts, liver function tests, thyroid function tests, urinalysis, and electrocardiograms. Biologic assessment also includes evaluating the patient for the characteristic neurovegetative symptoms listed below.

CRNE Note

In determining severity of depressive symptoms, nursing assessment should explore physical changes in appetite and sleep patterns and decreased energy. And considering the possibility of suicide should always be a priority with patients who are depressed. Assessment and documentation of suicide risk should always be included in patient care.

- *Appetite and weight changes*: In major depression, changes from baseline include decrease or increase in appetite with or without significant weight loss or gain (ie, a change of more than 5% of body weight in 1 month). Weight loss occurs when not dieting. Older adults with moderate to severe depression need to be assessed for dehydration as well as weight changes.
- *Sleep disturbance*: The most common sleep disturbance associated with major depression is insomnia. *DSM-IV-TR's* definitions of insomnia are divided into three categories: initial insomnia (difficulty falling asleep); middle insomnia (waking up during the night and having difficulty returning to sleep); or terminal insomnia (waking too early and being unable to return to sleep). Less frequently, the sleep disturbance is hypersomnia (prolonged sleep episodes at night or increased daytime sleep). The individual with either insomnia or hypersomnia complains of not feeling rested upon awakening.
- *Decreased energy, tiredness, and fatigue*: Fatigue associated with depression is a subjective experience of feeling tired regardless of how much sleep or physical activity a person has had. Even the smallest tasks require substantial effort.

CRNE Note

Remember the three major assessment categories listed above. A question may state several patient symptoms and expect the student to recognize that the patient being described is depressed.

In addition to a physical assessment including weight and appetite, sleep habits, and fatigue factors, an assessment of current medications should be completed. The frequency and dosage of prescribed and over-the-counter medications should be explored. In depression, the nurse must always assess the lethality of the medication the patient is taking. For example, if a patient has sleeping medications at home, the individual should be further queried about the number of pills in the bottle. Patients also need to be assessed for their use of alcohol, marijuana, and other mood-altering medications, as well as herbal substances because of the potential for drug–drug interactions. For example, patients taking antidepressants that affect serotonin regulation could also be taking St. John's wort (hypericum perforatum) to fight depression. The combined drug and herb could interact to cause serotonin syndrome (altered mental status, autonomic dysfunction, and neuromuscular abnormalities).

Nursing Diagnoses for Biologic Domain

There are several nursing diagnosis that could be formulated based on assessment data, including Disturbed Sleep Pattern, Imbalanced Nutrition, Fatigue, Self-Care Deficit, and Nausea. Other diagnoses that should be considered are Disturbed Thought Processes and Sexual Dysfunction.

Interventions for Biologic Domain

Because weeks or months of disturbed sleep patterns and nutritional imbalance only make depression worse, counselling and education should aim to establish normal sleep patterns and healthy nutrition.

Teaching Physical Care

Encouraging patients to practice positive sleep hygiene and eat well-balanced meals regularly helps the patient move toward remission or recovery. Activity and exercise are also important for improving depressed mood state. Most people find that regular exercise is hard to maintain. People who are depressed may find it impossible. When teaching about exercise, it is important to start with the current level of patient activity and increase slowly. For example, if the patient is spending most of the time in bed, encouraging the patient to get dressed every day and walk for 5 or 10 minutes may be all that patient can tolerate. Gradually, patients should be encouraged to have a regular exercise program and to slowly increase their food intake.

Pharmacologic Interventions

An antidepressant is selected based primarily on an individual patient's target symptoms and an individual agent's side-effect profile. Other factors that may influence choice include

- Prior medication response
- Drug interactions and contraindications
- Medication responses in family members
- Concurrent medical and psychiatric disorders
- Patient preference
- Patient age
- Cost of medication

Unlike many psychiatric disorders, depressive disorders may be time limited (they may end). As such, medication therapy should be reviewed periodically. The treatment and clinical management of psychiatric disorders are divided into the acute phase, continuation phase, maintenance phase, and, when indicated, discontinuation of medication use.

CRNE Note

Patients may be reluctant to take prescribed antidepressant medications or may self-treat depression. Continuing medication and emphasizing the potential drug–drug interactions should be included in the teaching plan.

- *Acute phase.* The primary goal of therapy for the acute phase is symptom reduction or remission. The objective is to choose the right match of medication and dosage for the patient. Careful monitoring and follow-up are essential during this phase to assess patient response to medications, adjust dosage if necessary, identify and address side effects, and provide patient support and education.
- *Continuation phase.* The goal of this treatment phase is to decrease the risk for relapse (a return of the current episode of depression). If a patient experiences a response to an adequate trial of medication, use of the medication generally is continued at the same dosage for at least 4 to 9 months after the patient returns to a clinically well state.
- *Maintenance phase.* For patients who are at high risk for recurrence (see Risk Factors), the optimal duration of maintenance treatment is unknown but is measured in years, and full-dose therapy is required for effective prophylaxis (Schatzberg, Cole, & DeBattista, 2003).
- *Discontinuation of medication use.* The decision to discontinue active treatment should be based on the

same factors considered in the decision to initiate maintenance treatment. These factors include the frequency and severity of past episodes, the persistence of dysthymic symptoms after recovery, the presence of comorbid disorders, and patient preference. Many patients continue taking medications for their lifetime.

Administering Antidepressant Medication Therapy

Antidepressant medications have proved effective in all forms of major depression. To date, controlled trials have shown no single antidepressant drug to have greater efficacy in the treatment of major depressive disorder. Antidepressant medications can be grouped as follows:

- cyclic antidepressants, which include the tricyclic antidepressants (TCAs), and maprotiline (a tetracyclic);
- selective serotonin reuptake inhibitors (SSRIs), which currently include escitalopram oxalate (Lexapro), fluoxetine (Prozac), sertraline (Zoloft), fluvoxamine (Luvox), paroxetine (Paxil), and citalopram (Celexa) (see Box 19-1 for more information);
- monoamine oxidase inhibitors (MAOIs), which include phenelzine (Nardil) and tranylcypromine (Parnate);
- "atypical" antidepressants, which include trazodone (Desyrel), bupropion (Wellbutrin), nefazodone (Serzone), venlafaxine (Effexor), and mirtazapine (Remeron). Table 13-9 in Chapter 13 lists antidepressant medications, usual dosage range, half-life, and therapeutic blood levels. For more information see Box 19-2.

The first-generation drugs, the TCAs and MAOIs, are being used less often than the second-generation drugs, the SSRIs and atypical antidepressants. Second-generation drugs selectively target the neurotransmitters and receptors thought to be associated with depression and to minimize side effects. The side-effect profiles of the two generations of drugs are significantly different as well (Table 19-2). The efficacy of the MAOIs is well established. Evidence suggests their distinct advantage in treating a specific subtype of depression, so-called atypical depression (characterized by increased appetite, reverse diurnal mood variation, and hypersomnia), depression with panic symptoms, or social phobia (Schatzberg et al., 2003). Given the complexity of their use, MAOIs usually are reserved for patients whose depression fails to respond to other antidepressants or patients who cannot tolerate typical antidepressants.

Monitoring Medications

Patients should be carefully observed when taking antidepressant medications, not only for the anticipated side effects generally associated with them (see Table 19-2) but also for their less common, sometimes even

---

BOX 19.1

Drug Profile: Escitalopram oxalate (Lexapro)

DRUG CLASS: Antidepressant

RECEPTOR AFFINITY: A highly selective serotonin reuptake inhibitor with low affinity for 5HT 1-7 or alpha and beta adrenergic, dopamine D1-5, histamine H1-3, muscarinic M1-5, and benzodiazepine receptors or for Na^+, K^+, Cl^-, and Ca^{++} ion channels that have been associated with various anticholinergic, sedative, and cardiovascular side effects.

INDICATIONS: Treatment of depression

ROUTES AND DOSAGES: Available as 5-, 10-, and 20-mg oral tablets.

Adults: Initially 10 mg once a day. May increase to 20 mg after a minimum of a week. Trials have not shown greater benefit at the 20-mg dose.

Geriatric: The 10-mg dose is recommended. Adjust dosage related to the drug's longer half-life and the slower liver metabolism of elderly patients.

Renal impairment: No dosage adjustment is necessary for mild to moderate renal impairment.

Children: Safety and efficacy not established in this population.

HALF LIFE (PEAK EFFECT): 27–32 h (4–7 h)

SELECTED ADVERSE REACTIONS: Most common adverse events include insomnia, diarrhea, nausea, increased sweating, dry mouth, somnolence, dizziness, and constipation. Most serious adverse events include ejaculation disorder in males; fetal abnormalities and decreased fetal weight in pregnant patients; serotonin syndrome if co-administered with MAOIs, St. John's Wort, or SSRIs, including citalopram (Celexa), of which escitalopram (Lexapro) is the active isomer.

SPECIFIC PATIENT/FAMILY EDUCATION:
- Do not take in combination with citalopram (Celexa) or other SSRIs or MAOIs. A 2-week washout period between escitalopram and SSRIs or MAOIs is recommended to avoid serotonin syndrome.
- Notify prescriber if pregnancy is possible or being planned. Do not breast-feed while taking this medication.
- Use caution driving or operating machinery until certain escitalopram does not alter physical abilities or mental alertness.
- Notify prescriber of any OTC medications, herbal supplements, or home remedies being used in combination with escitalopram.
- Ingestion of alcohol in combination with escitalopram is not recommended, although escitalopram does not seem to potentiate mental and motor impairments associated with alcohol.

Source: RX List available at http://www.rxlist.com/cgi/generic/lexapro.htm.

---

lethal possibilities. Although it is essential to know the valued benefits of antidepressants, it is equally important to be cognizant of the severe adverse effects these chemical agents can provoke. For example, some recent studies include evidence that both SSRIs and TCAs can induce the emergence of "medication activation syndrome" (extreme anxiety, hostility, agitation) and exacerbate suicidal ideation (Lam & Kennedy, 2005), the very things they are intended to avert. When observing patients taking antidepressants, nurses must be vigilant to the range of such possibilities, knowing also that in the depths of depression, saving medication for a later suicide attempt is quite common (Box 19-3). During antidepressant treatment, there is ongoing monitoring

---

BOX 19.2

Drug Profile: Mirtazapine (Remeron)

DRUG CLASS: Antidepressant

RECEPTOR AFFINITY: Believed to enhance central noradrenergic and serotonergic activity antagonizing central presynaptic α_2-adrenergic receptors. Mechanism of action unknown.

INDICATIONS: Treatment of depression.

ROUTES AND DOSAGE: Available as 15- and 30-mg tablets

Adults: Initially, 15 mg/d as a single dose preferably in the evening before sleeping. Maximum dosage is 45 mg/d.

Geriatric: Use with caution; reduced dosage may be needed.

Children: Safety and efficacy not established.

HALF-LIFE (PEAK EFFECT): 20–40 h (2 h)

SELECTED ADVERSE REACTIONS: Somnolence, dizziness, weight gain, elevated cholesterol/triglyceride and transaminase levels, malaise, abdominal pain, hypertension, vasodilation, vomiting, anorexia, thirst, myasthenia, arthralgia, hypoesthesia, apathy, depression, vertigo, twitching, agitation, anxiety, amnesia, increased cough, sinusitis, pruritus, rash, urinary tract infection, mania (rare), agranulocytosis (rare).

WARNING: Contraindicated in patients with known hypersensitivity. Use with caution in the elderly, patients who are breast-feeding, and those with impaired hepatic function. Avoid concomitant use with alcohol or diazepam, which can cause additive impairment of cognitive and motor skills.

SPECIFIC PATIENT/FAMILY EDUCATION:
- Take the dose once a day in the evening before sleep.
- Avoid driving or performing tasks requiring alertness.
- Notify prescriber before taking any OTC or other prescription drugs.
- Avoid alcohol or other CNS depressants.
- Notify prescriber if pregnancy is possible or planned.
- Monitor temperature and report any fever, lethargy, weakness, sore throat, malaise, or other "flu-like" symptoms.
- Maintain medical follow-up, including any appointments for blood counts and liver studies.

Table 19.2   Side Effects of Antidepressant Medications

Generic (Trade) Drug Name	Side Effects				
	Anticholinergic	Sedation	Orthostatic Hypotension	Gastrointestinal Distress	Weight Gain
Tricyclics: Tertiary Amines					
amitriptyline (Elavil)	+4	+4	+2	0	+4
clomipramine (Anafranil)	+3	+3	+2	+1	+4
doxepin (Sinequan)	+2	+3	+2	0	+3
imipramine (Tofranil)	+2	+2	+3	+1	+3
Tricyclics: Secondary Amines					
amoxapine (Asendin)	+3	+2	+1	0	+1
desipramine (Norpramin)	+1	+1	+1	0	+1
nortriptyline (Aventyl, Pamelor)	+2	+2	+1	0	+1
SSRIs					
fluoxetine (Prozac)	0/+1	0/+1	0/+1	+3	0
sertraline (Zoloft)	0	0/+1	0	+3	0
paroxetine (Paxil)	0	0/+1	0	+3	0
fluvoxamine (Luvox)	0/+1	0/+1	0/+1	+3	0
citalopram (Celexa)	0/+1	0/+1	0/+1	+3	0
escitalopram (Lexapro)	0/+1	0/+1	0/+1	+3	0
Atypical: Antidepressants					
venlafaxine (Effexor)	0	0	0	+3	0
trazodone (Desyrel)	0	+1	+3	+1	+1
nefazodone (Serzone)	0/+1	+1	+2	+2	0/+1
bupropion (Wellbutrin)	+2	+2	+1	0	0/+1
mirtazapine (Remeron)	+3	+4	+3	+3	+2

0 = absent or rare
0/+1 = lowest likelihood
+4 = highest likelihood

of vital signs, plasma drug levels as appropriate, liver and thyroid function tests, complete blood counts, and blood chemistry. Responsibilities include ensuring that patients are receiving a therapeutic dosage, helping in the evaluation of compliance, monitoring side effects, and helping to prevent toxicity. (Therapeutic blood levels for antidepressant medications are listed in Table 13-9 in Chapter 13.) Table 19-3 indicates various pharmacologic and nonpharmacologic interventions for the various side effects of antidepressant medications. Table 13-10 in Chapter 13 lists diet restrictions for those taking MAOIs.

Baseline orthostatic vital signs should be obtained before initiation of any medication, and in the case of medications known to have an impact on vital signs, such as TCAs, MAOIs, or venlafaxine, they should be

BOX 19.3

Guidelines: Monitoring and Administering Antidepressant Medications

Nurses should do the following in administering/monitoring antidepressant medications:

- Observe the patient for cheeking or saving medications for a later suicide attempt.
- Monitor vital signs: obtain baseline data before the initiation of medications (such as orthostatic vital signs and temperature).
- Monitor periodically liver and thyroid function tests, blood chemistry, and complete blood count as appropriate and compare with baseline values.
- Monitor patient symptoms for therapeutic response and report inadequate response to prescriber.
- Monitor patient for side effects and report to the prescriber serious side effects or those that are chronic

and problematic for the patient. (Table 19-3 indicates pharmacologic and nonpharmacologic interventions for common side effects.)

- Monitor drug levels as appropriate. (Therapeutic drug levels for antidepressants are listed in Table 13-9 in Chapter 13.)
- Monitor dietary intake as appropriate, especially with regard to MAOI antidepressants.
- Inquire about patient use of other medications, alcohol, "street" drugs, OTC medications, and/or herbal supplements that might alter the desired effects of prescribed antidepressants.

Table 19.3	Interventions to Relieve Side Effects of Antidepressants	
Side Effect	**Pharmacologic Intervention**	**Nonpharmacologic Intervention**
Dry mouth, caries, inflammation of the mouth	Bethanechol 10–30 mg tid Pilocarpine drops	Sugarless gum Sugarless lozenges 6–8 cups water per day Toothpaste for dry mouth
Nausea, vomiting	Cisapride 0.5 mg bid	Take medication with food Soda crackers, toast, tea
Weight gain	Change medication	Nutritionally balanced diet Daily exercise
Urinary hesitation Constipation	Bethanechol 10–30 mg tid Stool softener	6–8 cups water per day Bulk laxative Daily exercise 6–8 cups water per day Diet rich in fresh fruits and vegetables and grains
Diarrhea Orthostatic hypotension	OTC antidiarrheal	Maintain fluid intake Increase hydration Sit or stand up slowly
Drowsiness	Shift dosing time Lower medication dose Change medication	One caffeinated beverage at strategic time Do not drive when drowsy No alcohol or other recreational drugs Plan for rest time
Fatigue	Lower medication dose Change medication	Daily exercise
Blurred vision	Bethanechol 10–30 mg tid Pilocarpine eyedrops	Temporary use of magnifying lenses until body adjusts to medication
Flushing, sweating	Terazosin 1 mg qd Lower medication dose Change medication	Frequent bathing Lightweight clothing
Tremor	Beta-blockers Lower medication dose	Reassure patient that tremor may decrease as patient adjusts to medication. Notify caregiver if tremor interferes with daily functioning.

monitored on a regular basis. If these medications are administered to children or elderly patients, the dosage should be lowered to accommodate the physiologic state of the individual.

Tools for monitoring medication effects are objective observations, vital signs, the patient's subjective reports, and the administration of rating scales over the course of treatment. Responsibilities include ensuring that patients are receiving a therapeutic dosage (therapeutic blood levels for antidepressant medications are listed in Table 13-9 in Chapter 13), assessing adherence to the medication regimen, and evaluating compliance.

Individualizing dosages is essential for achieving optimal efficacy. When the newer antidepressants are used, this is usually done by fine-tuning medication dosage based on patient feedback. The TCAs, including imipramine (Tofranil), desipramine (Norpramin), amitriptyline (Elavil), and nortriptyline (Pamelor), have standardized valid plasma levels that can be useful in determining therapeutic dosages, although therapeutic plasma levels may vary from individual to individual. Blood samples should be drawn as close as possible to 12 hours away from the last dose. The newer antide-

pressants do not have established standardized ranges, and optimal dosing is based on efficacy and tolerability.

Monitoring and Managing Side Effects

FIRST-GENERATION ANTIDEPRESSANTS: TCAs AND MAOIs. The most common side effects associated with TCAs are the antihistaminic side effects (sedation and weight gain) and anticholinergic side effects (potentiation of CNS drugs, blurred vision, dry mouth, constipation, urinary retention, sinus tachycardia, and decreased memory).

Emergency!

If possible, TCAs should not be prescribed for patients at risk for suicide. Lethal doses of TCAs are only three to five times the therapeutic dose, and more than 1 g of a TCA is often toxic and may be fatal. Death may result from cardiac arrhythmia, hypotension, or uncontrollable seizures.

Serum TCA levels should be evaluated when overdose is suspected. In acute overdose, almost all symptoms develop within 12 hours. Anticholinergic effects are prominent: dry mucous membranes, warm and dry skin, blurred vision, decreased bowel motility, and urinary retention. CNS suppression (ranging from drowsiness to coma) or an agitated delirium may occur. Basic overdose treatment includes induction of emesis, gastric lavage, and cardiorespiratory supportive care. The most common side effects of MAOIs are headache, drowsiness, dry mouth, constipation, blurred vision, and orthostatic hypotension.

Emergency!

If co-administered with food or other substances containing tyramine (eg, aged cheese, beer, red wine), MAOIs can trigger a hypertensive crisis that may be life threatening. Symptoms include sudden, severe pounding or explosive headache in the back of the head or temples, racing pulse, flushing, stiff neck, chest pain, nausea and vomiting, and profuse sweating.

MAOIs are more lethal in overdose than are the newer antidepressants and thus should be prescribed with caution if the patient's suicide potential is elevated (see Chapter 13). An MAOI generally is given in divided doses to minimize side effects. These drugs are used cautiously in patients who are suicidal because of their relative lethality compared with the newer antidepressants.

Selected adverse effects of MAOIs include headache, drowsiness, dry mouth and throat, insomnia, nausea, agitation, dizziness, constipation, asthenia, blurred vision, weight loss, and postural hypotension. Although priapism was not reported during clinical trials, the MAOIs are structurally similar to trazodone, which has been associated with priapism (prolonged painful erection).

SECOND-GENERATION ANTIDEPRESSANTS: SSRIs AND ATYPICAL ANTIDEPRESSANTS. Serotonin syndrome is a potentially serious side effect caused by drug-induced excess of intrasynaptic serotonin (5-hydroxytryptamine [5-HT]). First reported in the 1950s, it was relatively rare until the introduction of the SSRIs. Serotonin syndrome is most often reported in patients taking two or more medications that increase CNS serotonin levels by different mechanisms (Nolan & Scoggin, 2001). The most common drug combinations associated with serotonin syndrome involve the MAOIs, the SSRIs, and the TCAs. Although serotonin syndrome can cause death, it is mild in most patients, who usually recover with supportive care alone. Unlike neuroleptic malignant syndrome, which develops within 3 to 9 days after the introduction of neuroleptic medications (see Chapter 17), serotonin syndrome tends to develop within hours or days after initiating or increasing the dose of serotoninergic medication or adding a drug with serotomimetic properties. The symptoms include altered

mental status, autonomic dysfunction, and neuromuscular abnormalities. At least three of the following must be present for a diagnosis: mental status changes, agitation, myoclonus, hyperreflexia, fever, shivering, diaphoresis, ataxia, and diarrhea. In patients who also have peripheral vascular disease or atherosclerosis, severe vasospasm and hypertension may occur in the presence of elevated serotonin levels. In addition, in a patient who is a slow metabolizer of SSRIs, higher-than-normal levels of these antidepressants may circulate in the blood. Medications that are not usually considered serotoninergic, such as dextromethorphan (Pertussin) and meperidine (Demerol), have been associated with the syndrome (Bernard & Bruera, 2000).

Emergency!

The most important emergency interventions are stopping use of the offending drug, notifying the physician, and providing necessary supportive care (eg, intravenous fluids, antipyretics, cooling blanket). Severe symptoms have been successfully treated with antiserotonergic agents, such as cyproheptadine (Sorenson, 2002).

Monitoring for Drug Interactions

Although SSRIs and newer atypical antidepressants produce fewer and generally milder side effects, which improves patient tolerability and compliance, there are some side effects to note. Among the most common are

- insomnia and activation
- headaches
- gastrointestinal symptoms
- weight gain

Sexual side effects, primarily diminished interest and performance, are also reported with some SSRIs, particularly sertraline. The most potentially harmful, but preventable, side effect/interaction of SSRIs is serotonin syndrome (Box 19-4).

The atypical antidepressant nefazodone (once a more popular medication) has been shown to raise hepatic enzyme levels in some patients, potentially leading to hepatic failure. Trazodone administration has been associated with erectile dysfunction and priapism. Bupropion can cause seizures, particularly in patients at risk for seizures. Bupropion has also been associated with the development of psychosis because it is dopaminergic, and its use should be avoided in patients with schizophrenia. Venlafaxine can cause increase in blood pressure, although this side effect appears to be dose related and can be controlled by lowering the dose (APA, 2002).

Potential drug interactions associated with agents that are metabolized by the cytochrome P-450 systems should be considered when children or elderly patients are treated (see Chapter 13). Five of the most important

BOX 19.4

Emergency: Serotonin Syndrome

CAUSE: Excessive intrasynaptic serotonin

HOW IT HAPPENS: Combining medications that increase CNS serotonin levels, such as SSRIs + MAOIs; SSRIs + St. John's Wort; or SSRIs + diet pills; dextromethorphan or alcohol, especially red wine; or SSRI + street drugs, such as LSD, MMDA, or Ecstasy.

SYMPTOMS: Mental status changes, agitation, ataxia, myoclonus, hyperreflexia, fever, shivering, diaphoresis, diarrhea

TREATMENT: Assess all medication, supplements, foods, and recreational drugs ingested to determine the offending substances.

Discontinue any substances that may be causative factors. If symptoms are mild, treat supportively on outpatient basis with propranolol and lorazepam and follow-up with prescriber.

If symptoms are moderate to severe, hospitalization may be needed with monitoring of vital signs and treatment with intravenous fluids, antipyretics, and cooling blankets.

FURTHER USE: Assess on a case-by-case basis and minimize risk factors for further medication therapy.

enzymes systems are 1A2, 2D6, 2C9, 2C19, and 3A4. The 1A2 system is inhibited by the SSRI fluvoxamine. Thus, other drugs that use the 1A2 system will no longer be metabolized as efficiently. For example, if fluvoxamine is given with theophylline, the theophylline dosage must be lowered, or else blood levels of theophylline will rise and cause possible side effects or toxic reactions, such as seizures. Fluvoxamine also affects the metabolism of atypical antipsychotics. On the other hand, smoking and caffeine can induce 1A2 system activity. This means that smokers may need to be given a higher dose of medications that are metabolized by this system (Stahl, 2000).

Fluoxetine (Prozac) and paroxetine (Paxil) are potent inhibitors of 2D6. One of the most significant drug interactions is caused by SSRI inhibition of 2D6 that in turn causes an increase in plasma levels of TCAs. If there is concomitant administration of an SSRI and a TCA, the plasma drug level of TCA should be monitored and probably reduced. In the 3A4 system, some SSRIs (fluoxetine, fluvoxamine, and nefazodone) will raise the levels of alprazolam (Xanax) or triazolam (Halcion) through enzyme inhibition, requiring reduction of dosage of the benzodiazepine. For more information see Table 19-4.

Teaching Points

If depression goes untreated or is inadequately treated, episodes can become more frequent, more severe, and of longer duration and can lead to suicide. Patient education involves explaining this pattern and the importance of continuing medication use after the acute phase of treatment to decrease the risk for future episodes. Patient concerns regarding long-term antidepressant therapy need to be assessed and addressed.

The risk for patients discontinuing their prescribed medication prematurely is not uncommon. It may be natural for patients to assume that their experience of symptom relief, after short-term medication use, means their disorder has resolved. It is important for the nurse to recognize this erroneous assumption and to make clear to patients that "response" is not the same thing as "remission." Although immediate relief of symptoms may signify response, remission is defined as the absence of symptoms for 1 year. Patients who discontinue their medications thinking their illness has resolved will be jeopardizing their state of health (Gutman, 2002).

Even after the first episode of major depression, medication should be continued for at least 6 months to 1 year after the patient achieves complete remission of symptoms. If the patient experiences a recurrence after tapering the first course of treatment, the regimen should be reinstituted for at least another year, and if the illness reoccurs, medication should be continued indefinitely (Schatzberg et al., 2003).

Teaching Points

Patients should be advised not to take the herbal substance St. John's wort if they are also taking prescribed antidepressants. St. John's wort also should not be taken if the patient is taking nasal decongestants, hay fever and asthma medications containing monoamines, amino acid supplements containing phenylalanine, or tyrosine. The combination may cause hypertension.

Other Somatic Therapies

ELECTROCONVULSIVE THERAPY. Although its therapeutic mechanism of action is unknown, electroconvulsive therapy (ECT) is an effective treatment for severe depression. It is generally reserved for patients whose disorder is refractory or intolerant to initial drug treatments and who are so severely ill that rapid treatment is required (eg, patients with malnutrition, catatonia, or suicidality).

ECT is contraindicated for patients with increased intracranial pressure. Other high-risk patients include those with recent myocardial infarction, recent cerebrovascular accident, retinal detachment, or pheochromocytoma (tumor on the adrenal cortex or other tumors) and those at risk for complications of anesthesia. Older age has been associated with a favourable response to ECT. Because depression can increase mortality risk in elderly people, in particular, and some elderly patients do not respond well to medication,

Table 19.4 Drug–Drug Interactions: Antidepressants

Antidepressant	Other Drug	Effect of Interaction/Treatment
Fluvoxamine	Theophylline	Increased theophylline level: seizures. Tx: Reduce theophylline levels when administering with fluvoxamine.
Fluoxetine, paroxetine	TCAs Benzodiazepines Phenothiazines	Increased in plasma levels of TCA. Tx: Reduce TCA levels when giving with fluoxetine or paroxetine.
Fluoxetine, fluvoxamine, nefazadone triazolam	Alprazolam Benzodiazepines	Increased plasma levels of alprazolam. Tx: Reduce dose of alprazolam when administered with benzodiazepines.
nefazodone	Digoxin Benzodiazepines Antihistamines	Increased levels of digoxin, antihistamines, and benzodiazepines. Tx: Reduce dose of nefazodone when giving with these medications.
Fluvoxamine	Caffeine Nicotine	Lowered levels of fluvoxamine. Tx: Increase dose of fluvoxamine in smokers or patients whose coffee, tea, or caffeinated drink intake is high.
SSRIs	Warfarin	Increased prothrombin time, bleeding. Tx: Monitor closely, decrease dose of warfarin if giving with SSRIs.
SSRIs	Lithium TCAs Barbiturates	Increased CNS effects of SSRIs. Tx: Adjust dosage of SSRI.
SSRIs	Phenytoin	Increased serum levels of phenytoin. Tx: Adjust dosage of phenytoin.

Data from McCuistion and Gutierrez, 2002; Stahl, 2000.

effective treatment is especially important for this age group (Blazer, Hybels, & Pieper, 2001).

Interventions for the Patient Undergoing ECT

The CNA supports standards and best practices that uphold and effectively regulate professional nursing care for patients (CNA, 2005). For those undergoing ECT, the role of the nurse includes providing educational and emotional support for the patient and family, assessing baseline or pretreatment level of function, preparing the patient for the ECT process, and monitoring and evaluating the patient's response to ECT, sharing it with the ECT team, and modifying treatment as needed (see Chapter 13). The actual procedure, possible therapeutic mechanisms of action, potential adverse effects, contraindications, and nursing interventions are described in detail in Chapter 13.

Light Therapy (Phototherapy)

Light therapy is described in Chapter 13. Given current research, light therapy is an option for well-documented mild to moderate seasonal, nonpsychotic, winter depressive episodes in patients with recurrent major depressive or bipolar II disorders, including children and adolescents (Glod & Baisden, 1999; Zahourek, 2000).

Psychological Domain

Assessment

The mental status examination is an effective clinical tool to evaluate the psychological aspects of major depression because the focus is on disturbances of mood and affect, thought processes and content, cognition, memory, and attention. The comprehensive mental status examination is described in detail in Chapter 10.

Mood and Affect

The person with depression has a sustained period of feeling depressed, sad, or hopeless and may experience anhedonia (loss of interest or pleasure). The patient may report "not caring anymore" or not feeling any enjoyment in activities that were previously considered pleasurable. In some individuals, this may include decrease in or loss of libido (sexual interest or desire) and sexual function. Depressed mood may be severe enough to provoke thoughts of suicide.

Numerous assessment scales are available for assessing depression. Easily administered self-report questionnaires can be valuable detection tools. These questionnaires cannot be the sole basis for making a diagnosis of major depressive episode, but they are sensitive to depressive symptoms. The following are six commonly used self-report scales:

- Edinburgh Postnatal Depression Scale (EPDS)
- General Health Questionnaire (GHQ)
- Center for Epidemiological Studies Depression Scale (CES-D)
- Beck Depression Inventory (BDI)
- Zung Self-Rating Depression Scale (ZSRDS)
- PRIME-MD (Pfizer)

Clinician-completed rating scales may be more sensitive to improvement in the course of treatment and may have a slightly greater specificity than do self-report questionnaires in detecting depression. These include the following:

- Hamilton Rating Scale for Depression (HAM-D) (see Appendix F)
- Montgomery-Asberg Depression Rating Scale (MADRS)
- National Institute of Mental Health Diagnostic Interview Schedule (DIS)

Thought Content

Depressed individuals often have an unrealistic negative evaluation of their worth or have guilty preoccupations or ruminations about minor past failings. Such individuals often misinterpret neutral or trivial day-to-day events as evidence of personal defects, and they have an exaggerated sense of responsibility for untoward events. As a result, they feel hopeless, helpless, worthless, and powerless. The possibility of disorganized thought processes (eg, tangential or circumstantial thinking) and perceptual disturbances (eg, hallucinations, delusions) should also be included in the assessment.

Suicidal Behaviour

Patients with major depression are at increased risk for suicide. Suicide risk should be assessed initially and throughout the course of treatment. Suicidal ideation includes thoughts that range from a belief that others would be better off if the person were dead or thoughts of death (passive suicidal ideation) to actual specific plans for committing suicide (active suicidal ideation). The frequency, intensity, and lethality of these thoughts can vary and can help to determine the seriousness of intent. The more specific the plan and the more accessible the means, the more serious the intent. Risk factors that must be carefully considered are the availability and adequacy of social supports, past history of suicidal ideation or behaviour, presence of psychosis or substance abuse, and decreased ability to control suicidal impulses.

Cognition and Memory

Many individuals with depression report impaired ability to think, concentrate, or make decisions. They may appear easily distracted or complain of memory difficulties. In older adults with major depression, memory difficulties may be the chief complaint and may be mistaken for early signs of a dementia (pseudodementia), complicating the diagnostic process (APA, 2000; Fischer, 2002). When the depression is fully treated, the memory problem often improves or fully resolves.

Nursing Diagnoses for Psychological Domain

Nursing diagnoses focussing on the psychological domain for the patient with a depressive disorder are numerous. If patient data lead to the diagnosis of Risk for Suicide, the patient should be further assessed for plan, intent, and accessibility of means. Other nursing diagnoses include Hopelessness, Low Self-Esteem, Ineffective Individual Coping, Decisional Conflict, Spiritual Distress, and Dysfunctional Grieving.

Interventions for Psychological Domain

Although pharmacotherapy is usually the primary treatment method for major depression, patients also can benefit from psychosocial and psychoeducational treatments. The most commonly used therapies are described. For patients with severe or recurrent major depressive disorder, the combination of psychotherapy (including interpersonal therapy, cognitive behavioural therapy, behaviour therapy, or brief dynamic therapy) and pharmacotherapy has been found to be superior to treatment with a single modality. Adding a course of cognitive behavioural therapy may be an effective strategy for preventing relapse in patients who have had only a partial response to pharmacotherapy alone (APA, 2000). Clinical practice guidelines suggest that the combination of medication and psychotherapy may be particularly useful in more complex situations (eg, depression in the context of concurrent, chronic general-medical or other psychiatric disorders, or in patients who fail to experience complete response to either treatment alone). Recent studies suggest that short-term cognitive and interpersonal therapies may be as effective as pharmacotherapy in milder depressions. Psychotherapy in combination with medication may also be used to address collateral issues, such as medication adherence or secondary psychosocial problems (Casacalenda, Perry, & Looper, 2002).

CRNE Note

A cognitive therapy approach is recommended for the acute phase of depression. This approach should be included in most nursing care plans for patients with depression.

Therapeutic Relationship

One of the most effective therapeutic tools for treating any psychiatric disorder is the therapeutic alliance, a helpful and trusting relationship between clinician and patient. The alliance is built from a number of activities, including the following:

- Establishment and maintenance of a supportive relationship
- Availability in times of crisis
- Vigilance regarding dangerousness to self and others
- Education about the illness and treatment goals
- Encouragement and feedback concerning progress
- Guidance regarding the patient's interactions with the personal and work environment
- Realistic goal setting and monitoring

Interacting with depressed individuals is challenging because they tend to be withdrawn and have difficulty expressing feelings and engaging in interpersonal interactions. The therapeutic alliance partly depends on winning the patient's trust through a warm and empathic stance within the context of firm professional boundaries (see Box 19-5).

CRNE Note

Establishing the patient–nurse relationship with a person who is depressed requires an empathic, quiet approach. Too much enthusiasm can block communication.

Cognitive Therapy

Cognitive therapy has been successful in reducing depressive symptoms during the acute phase of major depression (APA, 2002) (see Chapter 14). This therapy uses techniques, such as thought stopping and positive self-talk, to dispel irrational beliefs and distorted attitudes. In one study, remission rates after cognitive therapy were comparable to those after pharmacotherapy (Casacalenda et al., 2002). The use of cognitive therapy in the acute phase of treatment, combined with medication, has grown in the past few years and now may be considered first-line treatment for mildly to moderately depressed outpatients.

Behaviour Therapy

Behaviour therapy has been effective in the acute treatment of patients with mild to moderately severe depression, especially when combined with pharmacotherapy. Therapeutic techniques include activity scheduling, self-control therapy, social skills training, and problem solving. The efficacy of behaviour therapy in the continuation and maintenance phase of depression has not been subjected to controlled studies (APA, 2002). Behaviour therapy techniques are described in Chapter 12.

Interpersonal Therapy

Interpersonal therapy seeks to recognize, explore, and resolve the interpersonal losses, role confusion and transitions, social isolation, and deficits in social skills that may precipitate depressive states (APA, 2002). It maintains that losses must be mourned and related affects appreciated, that role confusion and transitions

BOX 19.5

Therapeutic Dialogue: Approaching the Depressed Patient

George Sadder is a 70-year-old retired businessman who has been admitted to a day treatment program because of complaints of stomach pains, insomnia, and hopelessness. He has withdrawn from social activities he previously enjoyed, such as golfing and going out to eat with his wife and friends. This morning he sits in a chair by himself, rather than joining a group activity.

Ineffective Approach

Nurse: "Hi, Mr. Sadder. My name is Sally. How are you feeling today?"
Mr. S: "Lousy, just lousy! I didn't sleep well last night, and my stomach is killing me!"
Nurse: "Oh, that is too bad! Have you had any breakfast?"
Mr. S: "No! Didn't I say that my stomach is killing me?"
Nurse: "Maybe eating breakfast would help your stomach pain."
Mr. S: "You don't know anything about my pain!" (gets up and walks away).

Effective Approach

Nurse: "Hi. My name is Sally."
Mr. S: "Hello, Sally. My name is George Sadder."

Nurse: "I'd like to sit down with you, if that is OK."
Mr. S: "If you want, but I am not much of a talker."
Nurse: "That's OK. We can talk or not, whatever you wish."
Mr. S: (Patient winces)
Nurse: "You just winced. Are you in pain?"
Mr. S: "Yes, my stomach has been killing me lately."
Nurse: "What do you usually do to ease the pain?"
Mr. S: "I usually take an antacid with my meals but forgot this morning."
Nurse: "I'll see if I can get some for you now."
Mr. S: "Thanks. When my stomach settles down, maybe we can talk."
Nurse: "That would be fine. I'll check back with you in a few minutes."

Critical Thinking Challenge

- What ineffective techniques did the nurse use in the first scenario and how did they impair communication?
- What effective techniques did the nurse use in the second scenario and how did they facilitate communication?

must be recognized and resolved, and that social skills deficits must be overcome to acquire social supports. Some evidence in controlled studies suggests that interpersonal therapy is more effective in reducing depressive symptoms with certain populations, such as depressed patients with human immunodeficiency virus infection, and less successful with patients who have personality disorders (APA, 2002) (see Chapter 24).

Family and Marital Therapy

Patients who perceive high family stress are at risk for greater future severity of illness, higher use of health services, and higher health care expense. Marital and family problems are common among patients with mood disorders; comprehensive treatment requires that these problems be assessed and addressed. They may be a consequence of major depression but may also increase vulnerability to depression and in some instances retard recovery. Research suggests that marital and family therapy may reduce depressive symptoms and the risk for relapse in patients with marital and family problems (Thase, 2000). The depressed spouse's mood has marked impact on the marital adjustment of the nondepressed spouse. It is recommended that treatment approaches be designed to help couples be supportive of each other, to adapt, and to cope with the depressive symptoms within the framework of their ongoing marital relations (Mead, 2002). Many family nursing interventions (discussed in detail in Chapter 16) may be used by the generalist psychiatric nurse in providing targeted family-centered care. These include

- Monitoring patient and family for indicators of stress.
- Teaching stress management techniques.
- Counselling family members on coping skills for their own use.
- Providing necessary knowledge of options and support services.
- Facilitating family routines and rituals.
- Assisting family to resolve feelings of guilt.
- Assisting family with conflict resolution.
- Identifying family strengths and resources with family members.
- Facilitating communication among family members.

Group Therapy

The role of group therapy in treating depression is based on clinical experience, rather than on systematic controlled studies. It may be particularly useful for depression associated with bereavement or chronic medical illness. Individuals may benefit from the example of others who have dealt successfully with similar losses or challenges. Survivors can gain self-esteem as successful role models for new group members. Medication support groups can provide information to the patient and to family members regarding prognosis and medication issues, thereby providing a psychoeducational forum.

Teaching Patients and Families

Patients with depression and their significant others often incorrectly believe that their illness is their own fault and that they should be able to "pull themselves up by their boot straps and snap out of it." It is vital to educate patients and their families about the nature, prognosis, and treatment of depression to dispel these false beliefs and the unnecessary guilt that ensues.

Patients need to know the full range of suitable treatment options before consenting to participate in treatment. The nurse can provide opportunities for them to question, discuss, and explore their feelings about past, current, and planned use of medications and other treatments (CNA, 2005). Developing strategies to enhance adherence and to raise awareness of early signs of relapse can be important aids to increasing treatment efficacy (see Box 19-6).

Social Domain

Assessment

Social assessment focuses on the individual's developmental history, family psychiatric history, patterns of relationships, quality of support system, education, work history, and impact of physical or sexual abuse on interpersonal function (see Chapter 10). Including a family member or close friend in the assessment process can be helpful. Changes in patterns of relating (especially social withdrawal) and changes in level of occupational functioning are commonly reported and may represent a significant deterioration from baseline behaviour. Increased use of "sick days" may occur. The family's

---

BOX 19.6

Psychoeducation Checklist: Major Depressive Disorder

When caring for the patient with a major depressive disorder, be sure to include the following topic areas in the teaching plan:
- ☐ Psychopharmacologic agents, including drug action, dosing frequency, and possible adverse effects
- ☐ Risk factors for recurrence, signs of recurrence
- ☐ Adherence to therapy and treatment program
- ☐ Nutrition
- ☐ Sleep measures
- ☐ Self-care management
- ☐ Goal setting and problem solving
- ☐ Social interaction skills
- ☐ Follow-up appointments
- ☐ Community support services

level of support and understanding of the disorder also need to be assessed.

Nursing Diagnoses for Social Domain

Nursing diagnoses common for the social domain include Ineffective Family Coping, Ineffective Role Performance, Interrupted Family Processes, and Caregiver Role Strain (if the patient is also a caregiver).

Interventions for Social Domain

Individuals experiencing depression have often withdrawn from daily activities, such as engaging in family activities, attending work, and participating in community activities. During hospitalization, patients often withdraw to their rooms and refuse to participate in unit activity. Nurses are challenged to help the patient balance the need for privacy with the need to return to normal social functioning. Depressed patients should never be approached in an overly enthusiastic manner; that approach will irritate them and block communication. On the other hand, patients should be encouraged to set realistic goals to reconnect with their families and communities. Explaining to patients that attending social activities, even though they do not feel like it, will promote the recovery process and helps patients achieve those goals.

Milieu Therapy

While hospitalized, milieu therapy (see Chapter 12) helps depressed patients maintain socialization skills and continue to interact with others. When depressed, people are often unaware of the environment and withdraw into themselves. On a psychiatric unit, depressed patients should be encouraged to attend and participate in unit activities. These individuals have a decreased energy level and thus may be moving more slowly than others; however, their efforts should be praised.

SAFETY. In many cases, patients are commonly admitted to the psychiatric hospital because of a suicide attempt. Suicidality should continually be evaluated, and the patient should be protected from self-harm (see Chapter 10). During the depths of depression, patients may not have the energy to complete a suicide. As patients begin to feel better and have increased energy, they may be at a greater risk for suicide. If a previously depressed patient appears to become energized overnight, he or she may have made a decision to commit suicide and thus may be relieved that the decision is finally made. The nurse may misinterpret the mood improvement as a positive move toward recovery; however, this patient may be very intent on suicide. These individuals should be carefully monitored to maintain their safety.

Other Interventions

Nurses are exceptionally well positioned to engage patients and their families in the active process of improving daily functioning, increasing knowledge and skill acquisition, and increasing independent living. Consumer-oriented support groups can help to enhance the self-esteem and the support network of participating patients and their families. Advice, encouragement, and the sense of group camaraderie may make an important contribution to recovery (CNA, 2005). Organizations providing support and information include the Canadian Mental Health Association (CMHA), Canadian Alliance on Mental Illness and Mental Health (CAMIMH), Mood Disorders Society of Canada, Native Mental Health Association of Canada, and the Organization for Bipolar Affective Disorders (OBAD).

Interventions for Family Members

The family needs education and support during and after the treatment of family members. Because major depressive disorder is a recurring disorder, the family needs information about specific antecedents to a family member's depression and what steps to take. For example, one patient may routinely become depressed during the fall of each year, with one of the first symptoms being excessive sleepiness. For another patient, a major loss, such as a child going to college or the death of a pet, may precipitate a depressive episode. Families of elderly patients need to be aware of the possibility of depression and related symptoms, often occurring after the deaths of friends and relatives. Families of children who are depressed often misinterpret depression as behaviour problems.

EVALUATION AND TREATMENT OUTCOMES

The major goals of treatment are to help the patient to be as independent as possible and to achieve stability, remission, and recovery from major depression. It is often a lifelong struggle for the individual. Ongoing evaluation of the patient's symptoms, functioning, and quality of life should be carefully documented in the patient's record in order to monitor outcomes of treatment.

CONTINUUM OF CARE

Individuals with depressive disorders may initially present in inpatient and outpatient medical and primary care settings, emergency rooms, and inpatient and outpatient mental health settings. Nurses should be able to recognize depression in these patients and make appropriate interventions or referrals. The continuum of care beyond these settings may include partial hospitalization or day treatment programs; individual, family, or group psychotherapy; home visits, and psychopharmacotherapy. Although most patients with major depression are treated in outpatient settings, brief hospitalization may be required if the patient is suicidal or psychotic.

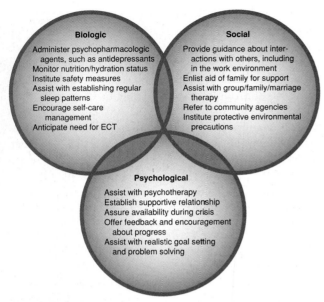

Biologic

Administer psychopharmacologic agents, such as antidepressants
Monitor nutrition/hydration status
Institute safety measures
Assist with establishing regular sleep patterns
Encourage self-care management
Anticipate need for ECT

Social

Provide guidance about inter-actions with others, including in the work environment
Enlist aid of family for support
Assist with group/family/marriage therapy
Refer to community agencies
Institute protective environmental precautions

Psychological

Assist with psychotherapy
Establish supportive relationship
Assure availability during crisis
Offer feedback and encouragement about progress
Assist with realistic goal setting and problem solving

FIGURE 19.1   Biopsychosocial interventions for patients with major depressive disorder (ECT, electroconvulsive therapy).

Nurses working on inpatient units provide a wide range of direct services, including administering and monitoring medications and target symptoms, conducting psychoeducational groups, and more generally, structuring and maintaining a therapeutic environment. Nurses providing home care have an excellent opportunity to detect undiagnosed depressive disorders and make appropriate referrals.

Nursing practice requires a coordinated, ongoing interaction among patients, families, and providers to deliver comprehensive services. This includes using the complementary skills of both psychiatric and medical care colleagues for forming overall goals, plans, and decisions and for providing continuity of care as needed (CNA, 2005). Collaborative care between the primary care provider and mental health specialist is also key to achieving remission of symptoms and physical well-being, restoring baseline occupational and psychosocial functioning, and reducing the likelihood of relapse or recurrence (Fig. 19-1).

Bipolar Disorders (Manic-Depressive Disorders)

DIAGNOSTIC CRITERIA

Bipolar disorder is distinguished from depressive disorders by the occurrence of manic or hypomanic (ie, mildly manic) episodes in addition to depressive episodes. The *DSM-IV-TR* divides bipolar disorders into three major groups: bipolar I (periods of major depressive, manic, or mixed episodes); bipolar II (periods of major depression and hypomania); and

cyclothymic disorder (periods of hypomanic episodes and depressive episodes that do not meet full criteria for a major depressive episode) (Table 19-5). These are described later. The specifiers describe either the most recent mood episode or the course of recurrent episodes; for example, "bipolar disorder I, most recent episode manic, severe with psychotic features."

> ● **KEY CONCEPT Mania** is primarily characterized by an abnormally and persistently elevated, expansive, or irritable mood for a duration of at least 1 week (or less, if hospitalized) (APA, 2000).

A **manic episode** is characterized by euphoria, a state of elation experienced as heightened sense of well-being. Osuji & Cullum (2005) elucidate the decreased inhibition, impulsivity, and distractibility, all of which negatively affect cognition in the areas of *attention* and *concentration*, and alter the individual's ability to learn and effectively solve problems. During a manic episode, the individual may manifest an expansive mood, manifesting inappropriate lack of restraint in expressing one's feelings and frequently overvaluing one's own importance. Expansive qualities include an unceasing and indiscriminate enthusiasm for interpersonal, sexual, or occupational interactions. Manic episodes can also consist of irritable mood, in which the person is easily annoyed and provoked to anger, particularly when the person's wishes are challenged or thwarted. In addition, manic episodes can consist of alterations between euphoria and irritability (**lability of mood**). To meet full *DSM-IV-TR* criteria, three (or four if the mood is irritable) of seven additional symptoms must be present: inflated self-esteem or grandiosity; decreased need for sleep; being more talkative or having pressured speech; flight of ideas or racing thoughts; distractibility; increase in goal-directed activity or psychomotor agitation; and excessive involvement in pleasurable activities that have a high potential for painful consequences. The disturbance must be severe enough to cause marked impairment in social activities, occupational functioning, and interpersonal relationships or to require hospitalization to prevent self-harm.

During a manic episode, decreased need to sleep is accompanied by increased energy and hyperactivity. The individual often remains awake for long periods at night or wakes up several times full of energy. Increased motor activity and agitation, which may be purposeful at first (eg, cleaning the house), may deteriorate into inappropriate or disorganized actions. The individual may get involved unrealistically in several new endeavours that may entail overspending or sexual encounters or drug or alcohol use, or high-risk activities such as driving too fast or taking up dangerous sports (see Box 19-7). The individual becomes overly talkative, feels pressured to continue talking, and at times is difficult to interrupt. Thoughts become disorganized and skip

| Table 19.5 | **Key Diagnostic Characteristics of Bipolar I Disorder 296.xx**
296.0x—Bipolar I, single manic episode
296.40—Bipolar I, most recent episode hypomanic
296.4x—Bipolar I, most recent episode manic
296.6x—Bipolar I, most recent episode mixed
296.5x—Bipolar I, most recent episode depressed
296.7—Bipolar I, most recent episode unspecified | 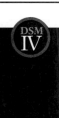 |

Diagnostic Criteria and Target Symptoms

- Presence of one or more manic episodes or mixed episodes, including one or more major depressive episodes

Manic episode
- Abnormally and persistently elevated, expansive, or irritable mood for at least 1 week
- Persistence of inflated self-esteem and grandiosity
- Decreased need for sleep
- More talkative than usual or pressure to keep talking
- Flight of ideas or racing thoughts
- Distractibility
- Increased goal-directed activity or psychomotor agitation
- Excessive involvement in pleasurable activities with high potential for painful results (such as unrestrained buying sprees, foolish business investments)
- Marked impairment in occupational functioning or in usual social activities or relationships; possible hospitalization to prevent harm; psychotic features

Major depressive episode (symptoms appear nearly every day)
- Depressed mood most of the day
- Markedly diminished interest or pleasure in all or most all activities for most of the day
- Significant weight loss when not dieting; weight gain or increase or decrease in appetite
- Insomnia or hypersomnia
- Psychomotor agitation or retardation
- Fatigue or loss of energy
- Feelings of worthlessness or excessive or inappropriate guilt
- Diminished ability to concentrate or indecisiveness
- Recurrent thoughts of death, suicidal ideation without a specific plan, suicide attempt or specific plan for committing suicide
- Not bereavement
- Clinically significant distress or impairment in social, occupational, or other important areas of functioning

Mixed episode
- Criteria for both manic and major depressive episodes nearly every day for at least 1 week
- Hospitalization to prevent harm; psychotic features

Hypomanic episode
- Distinct period of persistently elevated, expansive, or irritable mood through at least 4 days
- Clearly different from usual nondepressed mood
- Same symptoms as that for manic episode but does not cause impairment in social or occupational functioning or necessitate hospitalization
- Unequivocal change in function, uncharacteristic of person when asymptomatic
- Change observable by others

Associated Findings

Associated Behaviour Findings

Manic episode
- Resistive to efforts for treatment
- Disorganized or bizarre behaviour
- Change in dress or appearance
- Possible gambling and antisocial behaviour

Major depressive episode
- Tearfulness, irritability
- Obsessive rumination
- Anxiety
- Phobia
- Excessive worry over physical symptoms
- Complaints of pain
- Possible panic attacks
- Difficulty with intimate relationships
- Marital, occupational, or academic problems
- Substance abuse
- Increased use of medical services
- Attempted or complete suicide attempts

Mixed episode
- Similar to those for manic and depressive episodes

Hypomanic episodes
- Sudden onset with rapid escalation within 1–2 d
- Possibly precede or are followed by major depressive episode

Associated Physical Examination Findings

Manic episode
- Mean age of onset for first manic episode after age 21–30 yr
- Possible child abuse, spouse abuse, or other violent behaviour during severe manic episodes
- Associated problems involving school truancy, school failure, occupational failure, divorce, or episodic antisocial behaviour

Associated Laboratory Findings

Manic episodes
- Polysomnographic abnormalities
- Increased cortisol secretion

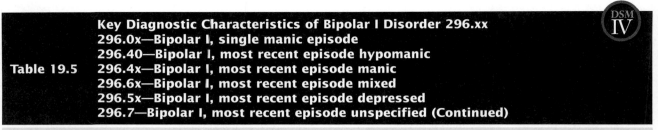

| Table 19.5 | **Key Diagnostic Characteristics of Bipolar I Disorder 296.xx**
 296.0x—Bipolar I, single manic episode
 296.40—Bipolar I, most recent episode hypomanic
 296.4x—Bipolar I, most recent episode manic
 296.6x—Bipolar I, most recent episode mixed
 296.5x—Bipolar I, most recent episode depressed
 296.7—Bipolar I, most recent episode unspecified (Continued) | DSM IV |

Diagnostic Criteria and Target Symptoms	Associated Findings
• Not severe enough to cause marked impairment in social or occupational functioning or to require hospitalization; no psychotic features • Episode not better accounted for by other disorders such as schizoaffective disorder and not superimposed on schizophrenia, schizophreniform, delusional, or psychotic disorders • Not a direct physiologic effect of substance or other medical condition	• Absence of dexamethasone nonsuppression • Possible abnormalities with norepinephrine, serotonin, acetylcholine, dopamine, or GABA neurotransmitter *Major depressive episode* • Sleep electroencephalogram abnormalities • Possible abnormalities with norepinephrine, serotonin, acetylcholine, dopamine, or GABA neurotransmitter systems

rapidly among topics that often have little relationship to each other. This decreased logical connection between thoughts is termed *flight of ideas*. Patients with mania have inflated self-esteem, which may range from unusual self-confidence to grandiose delusions. Other psychiatric disorders can have symptoms that mimic a manic episode. Schizophrenia, schizoaffective disorder, anxiety disorders, some personality disorders (borderline personality disorder and histrionic personality disorder), substance abuse involving stimulants, and adolescent conduct disorders should be ruled out when making a diagnosis of mania.

The *DSM-IV-TR* criteria for a **mixed episode** are met when the criteria for both a manic episode and a major depressive episode are met and are present for at least 1 week. Individuals who are having a mixed episode usually exhibit high anxiety, agitation, and irritability.

BOX 19.7

Clinical Vignette: The Manic Patient

Mr. Bell was a day trader on the stock market. Initially he was quite successful and, as a result, upgraded his lifestyle with a more expensive car, a larger and more luxurious house, and a boat. When the stock market declined dramatically, Mr. Bell continued to trade, saying that if he could just find the "right" stock he could earn back all of the money he had lost. He spent his days and nights in front of his computer screen, taking little or no time to eat or sleep. He defaulted on his mortgage and car and boat payments and was talking nonstop to his wife. She brought him to the hospital for evaluation

What Do You Think?
• What behavioural symptoms of mania does Mr. Bell exhibit?
• What cognitive symptoms of mania does Mr. Bell exhibit?

The criteria for a **hypomanic episode** are the same as for a manic episode, except that the time criterion is at least 4 days, rather than 1 week, and no marked impairment in social or occupational functioning is present.

The *DSM-IV-TR* criteria for **cyclothymic disorder** are the presence for at least 2 years of numerous periods with hypomanic symptoms and numerous periods with depressive symptoms that do not meet full criteria for a major depressive episode.

Secondary Mania

Mania can be caused by medical disorders or their treatments or by certain substances of abuse (eg, certain metabolic abnormalities, neurologic disorders, CNS tumors, and medications) (Strakowski & Sax, 2000).

Rapid Cycling Specifier

Rapid cycling can occur in both bipolar I and bipolar II disorders. In its most severe form, rapid cycling includes continuous cycling between subthreshold mania and depression or hypomania and depression (Suppes et al., 2001). The essential feature of rapid cycling is the occurrence of four or more mood episodes that meet criteria for manic, mixed, hypomanic, or depressive episode during the previous 12 months.

The *DSM-IV-TR* criteria for **cyclothymic disorder** are at least 2 years of numerous periods with hypomanic symptoms and numerous periods with depressive symptoms that do not meet full criteria for a major depressive episode.

CLINICAL COURSE

Bipolar disorder is a chronic, cyclic disorder. There is general agreement that later episodes of illness occur more frequently than earlier episodes, and increased frequency of episodes or more continuous symptoms have been reported in patients who experienced onset at an earlier age and who have a significant family history of illness. Some patients may have unpredictable and variable symptoms of the illness (Suppes et al., 2001). An additional feature of bipolar disorder is rapid cycling. Mixed states have been associated with increased suicidal ideation compared with pure mania (Maser et al., 2002). Bipolar disorder can lead to severe functional impairment as manifested by alienation from family, friends, and co-workers; indebtedness; job loss; divorce; and other problems of living (Rothbaum & Astin, 2000).

BIPOLAR DISORDER IN SPECIAL POPULATIONS

Children and Adolescents

Bipolar disorder in children has been recognized only recently. Although it is not well studied, depression usually appears first. Somewhat different than in adults, the hallmark of childhood bipolar disorder is intense rage. Children may display seemingly unprovoked rage episodes for as long as 2 to 3 hours. The symptoms of bipolar disorder reflect the developmental level of the child. Children younger than 9 years exhibit more irritability and emotional lability; older children exhibit more classic symptoms, such as euphoria and grandiosity. The first contact with the mental health system often occurs when the behaviour becomes disruptive, possibly 5 to 10 years after on its onset. These children often have other psychiatric disorders such as attention deficit hyperactivity disorder and conduct disorder (Kowatch & DelBello, 2005; Mohr, 2001) (see Chapter 27).

Elderly People

Tryssenaar, Chui, and Finch (2003) describe characteristic interferences in aspects of life's participation for the older adult accommodating serious mental illness. Unable to participate fully may affect such individuals' sense of life meaning and lead to feelings of loss regarding having a voice in life. Neurophysiologically, geriatric patients with mania demonstrate more abnormalities and cognitive disturbances (confusion and disorientation) than do younger patients. It generally was believed that the incidence of mania decreases with age because this population was thought to consist of only those individuals who had a diagnosis in younger years and managed to survive into old age. Recently, late-onset bipolar disorder was identified when researchers found evidence of an increased incidence of mania with age, especially in women after age 50 years and in men in the eighth and ninth decades. Late-onset bipolar disorder is

more likely related to secondary mania and consequently has a poorer prognosis because of comorbid medical conditions (McDonald, 2000).

EPIDEMIOLOGY

Distribution and Age of Onset

In Canada, the estimated 1-year prevalence for bipolar disorder (ie, the estimated percentage of the population who have the disorder during any 1-year period) is between 0.2% and 0.6% among adults in the general population (Health Canada, 2002). Most patients with bipolar disorder experience significant symptoms before age 25 years (Suppes et al., 2001). The estimated mean age of onset is between 21 and 30 years. Nearly 20% of patients with bipolar disorder diagnosed demonstrated symptoms before the age of 19 years (Mohr, 2001). Estimates of the prevalence of mania in elderly psychiatric patients are as high as 19%, with prevalence in nursing home patients estimated at about 10% (McDonald, 2000).

Gender, Ethnic, and Cultural Differences

Although no significant gender differences have been found in the incidence of bipolar I and II diagnoses, gender differences have been reported in phenomenology, course, and treatment response. In addition, some data show that female patients with bipolar disorder are at greater risk for depression and rapid cycling than are male patients, whereas male patients are at greater risk for manic episodes (Grunze, Amann, Dittmann, & Walden, 2002; Yildiz & Sachs, 2003). No significant differences have been found based on race or ethnicity (APA, 2000; CPA, 2005).

COMORBIDITY

The two most common comorbid conditions are anxiety disorders (most prevalent: panic disorder and social phobia) and substance use (most commonly alcohol and marijuana). Individuals with a comorbid anxiety disorder are more likely to experience a more severe course. A history of substance use further complicates the course of illness and results in less chance for remission and poorer treatment compliance (Goldberg et al., 1999).

ETIOLOGY

Current theories of the etiology of mood disorders are associated with chronic abnormalities of neurotransmission, which are thought to result in compensatory but maladaptive changes in brain regulation. In addition, use of controlled structural and functional imaging studies of patients with mood disorders have generated hypotheses that dysfunction of the CNS is associated with specific structural brain abnormalities and functional CNS alterations (Sheline, 2003).

Chronobiologic Theories

Sleep disturbance is an important aspect of depression and mania. Sleep patterns appear to be regulated by an internal biologic clock center in the hypothalamus. Artificially induced sleep deprivation is known to precipitate mania in some patients with bipolar disorder (Grunze et al., 2002). Because a number of neurotransmitter and hormone levels follow circadian patterns, sleep disruption may lead to biochemical abnormalities that affect mood. Seasonal changes in light exposure also trigger affective episodes in some patients, typically depression in winter and hypomania in the summer in the northern hemisphere (Cutler & Marcus, 1999).

Sensitization and Kindling Theory

Sensitization (increase in response with repetition of the same dose of drug) and the related phenomenon of kindling (subthreshold stimulation of a neuron generates an action potential; see Chapter 13) refer to animal models. Repeated chemical or electrical stimulation of certain regions of the brain produces stereotypical behavioural responses or seizures. The amount of the chemical or electricity required to evoke the response or seizure decreases with each experience. These phenomena have been used as models to explain why, over time, affective episodes, particularly those seen in patients with bipolar disorder, recur in shorter and shorter cycles and with less relation to environmental precipitants. It is hypothesized that repeated affective episodes might be accompanied by progressive alteration of brain synapses that lower the threshold for future episodes and increase the likelihood of illness. The kindling theory also helps explain the value of using antiseizure medication, such as carbamazepine and valproic acid, for mood stabilization.

Genetic Factors

The genetic basis for the development of bipolar disorder is only beginning to be explored. Results from family, adoption, and twin studies indicate that bipolar disorder is highly heritable (McCuffin et al., 2003). Such results show a 1% incidence rate in the general population compared with a 7% incidence rate for first-degree relatives of a patient with bipolar disorder, and 60% for a monozygotic twin of a bipolar patient (Payne, Potash, & DePaulo, 2005). Modes of genetic transmission and the cumulative effects of multiple genes interacting

IN A LIFE

Robert Norman Munsch (1945–)
Canadian Author of Children's Books

Public Persona
Robert Munsch has degrees in history and anthropology, studying to become a Jesuit priest until he realized he wanted to work with children. In 1975, he came to work at the preschool at the University of Guelph, where he was encouraged to publish the stories he was creating for the children. Munsch's meaningful stories are told with a "quirky" style of humour. In live performance, his expressions and voices endear him to audiences of all ages. A best-selling author, he has sold over 30 million books, more than any other Canadian author, and in 1999 Robert Munsch became a member of the Order of Canada.

Personal Reality
Of his childhood Munsch says he was friendless, dreadfully lonely, and "suicidally unhappy." For this he blames only a wrong set of genes. Munsch says he "dreamed" his way through school, recognizing the influence of all this on his writing. As a young adult, Munsch was brutally attacked by strangers and beaten so badly he suffered permanent memory loss. This, and the despair over his wife's two miscarriages, are incidents said to have been worked through in his story writing. He has bipolar affective disorder that is treated with medication. In speaking of his "manic-depression," he paints the depression as a black hole and the mania as being out of control, like driving a car too fast when you don't want to, being unable to slow down enough to even sleep, and hearing voices (Wong, 1999). His compelling stories draw on his own experience and help him capture the struggles with which children must contend.

Source: *Robert Munsch (2005)*. Retrieved September 4, 2005, from http://en.wikipedia.org/wiki/Robert_Munsch. Wong, J. (1999). Lunch with Robert Munsch. *The Globe and Mail*, May 26.

with environmental influences have yet to be definitively identified.

Psychological and Social Theories

Most psychological and social theories of mood disorders focus on loss as the cause of depression in genetically vulnerable individuals. Mania is considered to be a biologically rooted condition, but when viewed from a psychological perspective, mania is usually regarded as a condition that arises from an attempt to overcompensate for depressed feelings, rather than a disorder in its own right. It is now generally accepted that environmental conditions contribute to the timing of an episode of illness, rather than cause the illness (Johnson, Andersson-Lundman, Aberg-Wistedt, & Mathe, 2000).

INTERDISCIPLINARY TREATMENT OF DISORDERS

Patients with bipolar disorder have a complex set of issues and likely will be treated by an interdisciplinary team. Nurses, physicians, social workers, psychologists, and activity therapists all have valuable expertise for patients with bipolar disorder. For children with bipolar disorder, school teachers and counsellors are included in the team. For elderly patients, the primary care physician becomes part of the team. An important treatment goal is to minimize and prevent either manic or depressive episodes, which tend to accelerate over time. The fewer the episodes, the more likely the person can live a normal, productive life. Another important goal is to help the patient and family to learn about the disorder and manage it throughout a lifetime.

PRIORITY CARE ISSUES

During a manic episode, protection of the patient is a priority. It is during a manic episode that poor judgment and impulsivity result in risk-taking behaviours that can have dire consequences for the patient and family. For example, one patient withdrew all the family money from the bank and gambled it away. Risk for suicide is always a possibility. During a depressive episode, the patient may feel that life is not worth living. During a manic episode, the patient may believe that he or she has supernatural powers, such as the ability to fly. As patients recover from a manic episode, they may be so devastated by the consequences of impulsive behaviour and poor judgment during the episode that suicide seems like a reasonable option.

FAMILY RESPONSE TO DISORDER

Bipolar disorder can devastate families, who often feel that they are on an emotional merry-go-round, particularly if they have difficulty understanding the mood shifts. A major problem for family members is dealing with the consequences of impulsive behaviour during manic episodes, such as excessive debt, assault charges, and sexual infidelities.

NURSING MANAGEMENT: HUMAN RESPONSE TO DISORDER

The nursing care of patients with bipolar disorder is one of the most interesting yet greatest challenges in psychiatric nursing. In general, the behaviour of patients with bipolar disorder is normal between mood episodes. The ideal nursing care occurs during a period of time when the nurse can see the patient in the acute illness phase and in remission. Nursing care of bipolar depression should be approached in a manner similar to that used for major depressive disorder, as described previously.

BIOLOGIC DOMAIN
Assessment

With regard to the biologic domain, the assessment emphasis is on evaluating symptoms of mania and, most particularly, changes in sleep patterns. The assessment should follow the guidelines in Chapter 10. In the manic phase of bipolar disorder, the patient may not sleep, resulting in irritability and physical exhaustion. Because eating habits usually change during a manic or depressive episode, the nurse should assess changes in diet and body weight. Because patients with mania may experience malnutrition and fluid imbalance, laboratory studies, such as thyroid function, should be completed. Abnormal thyroid functioning can be responsible for the mood and behavioural disturbances. During a manic phase, patients often become hypersexual and engage in risky sexual practices. Changes in sexual practices should be explored.

Pharmacologic Assessment

When a patient is in a manic state, the previous use of antidepressants should be assessed because a manic episode may be triggered by antidepressant use. In such cases, use of antidepressants should be discontinued. Many times, manic or depressive episodes occur after patients stop taking their mood stabilizer, at which time the reason for stopping the medication should be explored. Patients may stop taking their medications because of side effects or because they no longer believe they have a mental disorder. Special attention should also focus on the use of alcohol and other substances. Usually, a drug screen is ordered to determine current use of substances.

Nursing Diagnoses for Biologic Domain

Among nursing diagnoses in this domain are Disturbed Sleep Pattern; Sleep Deprivation; Imbalanced Nutrition; Hypothermia, Deficient Fluid Volume; and Noncompliance if patients have stopped taking their medication. If patients are in the depressive phase of illness, the previously discussed diagnoses for depression should be considered.

Interventions for Biologic Domain
Physical Care

In a state of mania, the patient's physical needs are rest, adequate hydration and nutrition, and re-establishment of physical well-being. Self-care has usually deteriorated. For a patient who is unable to sit long enough to eat, snacks and high-energy foods should be provided that can be eaten while moving. Alcohol should be avoided. Sleep hygiene is a priority but may not be realistic until medications take effect. Limiting stimuli can be helpful in decreasing agitation and promoting sleep.

CRNE Note

Protection of patients with mania is always a priority. Ongoing assessment should focus on irritability, fatigue, and potential for harming self or others.

Teaching Points

Once the patient's mood stabilizes, the nurse should focus on monitoring changes in physical functioning in sleep or eating behaviour and teaching patients to identify antecedents to mood episodes. A regular sleep routine should be maintained if possible. High-risk times for manic episodes, such as changes in work schedule (day to night), should be avoided if possible. Patients should be taught to monitor the amount of their sleep each night and report decreases in sleep of more than 1 hour per night because this may be a precursor to a manic episode.

Intervention With Mood Stabilizers

Pharmacotherapy is essential in bipolar disorder to achieve two goals: rapid control of symptoms and prevention of future episodes or, at least, reduction in their severity and frequency. Pharmacotherapy continues through the various phases of bipolar disorder:

- *Acute phase.* The goal of treatment in the acute phase is symptom reduction and stabilization. Therefore, for the first few weeks of treatment,

mood stabilizers may need to be combined with antipsychotics or benzodiazepines, particularly if the patient has psychotic symptoms, agitation, or insomnia. If the clinical situation is not an emergency, patients usually start on a low dose and gradually increase the dose until maximum therapeutic benefits are achieved. Once stabilization is achieved, the frequency of serum level monitoring should be every 1 to 2 weeks during the first 2 months and every 3 to 6 months during long-term maintenance. Medications most commonly used for mood stabilization in bipolar disorder are discussed here and in Chapter 13.

- *Continuation phase.* The treatment goal in this phase is to prevent relapse of the current episode or cycling into the opposite pole. It lasts about 2 to 9 months after acute symptoms resolve. The usual pharmacologic procedure in this phase is to continue the mood stabilizer while closely monitoring the patient for signs or symptoms of relapse.
- *Maintenance phase.* The goal of treating this phase is to sustain remission and to prevent new episodes. The great weight of evidence favours long-term prophylaxis against recurrence after effective treatment of acute episodes. It is recommended that long-term or lifetime prophylaxis with a mood stabilizer be instituted after two manic episodes or after one severe manic episode or if there is a family history of bipolar disorder.
- *Discontinuation.* Like the course of major depressive disorder, the course of bipolar disorder typically is recurrent and progressive. Therefore, the same issues and principles regarding the decision to continue or discontinue pharmacotherapy apply (see Box 19-8).

The mainstays of somatic therapy are the mood-stabilizing drugs. The three agents that show significant efficacy in controlled trials are lithium carbonate

BOX 19.8 RESEARCH FOR BEST PRACTICE

Help for Families Affected by Bipolar Disorder

THE QUESTION: Is family-focussed treatment as effective or more or less effective than individual treatment for bipolar disorder?

METHODS: A qualitative study of families' responses to severe mental illness involved 29 participants representing 17 families who were interviewed three times in 2 years. Interviews were analyzed using a comparative technique that described families' responses to these mental illnesses. Living with ambiguity of mental illness was the central concern.

FINDINGS: These families attempted to live normally and sought to control the impact of the illness. The family goals included managing crises, containing and controlling symptoms, and crafting a notion of "normal." The strategies that the families used were being vigilant, setting limits on patients, invoking logic, dealing with sense of loss, seeing patients' strengths, and taking on roles. This study revealed that families were profoundly affected by the social contexts of mental illness.

IMPLICATIONS FOR NURSING: Families are the informal caregivers and develop their own strategies for dealing with family members with mental illnesses. Including families in psychoeducation programs can facilitate a partnership with the family and allow sharing of successful strategies.

From Rea, M. M., Tompson, M. C., Miklowitz, D. J., Goldstein, M. J., Hwang, S., & Mintz, J. (2003). Family-focused treatment versus individual treatment for bipolar disorder: results of a randomized clinical trial. *Journal of Consulting Clinical Psychology, 71*(3), 482–492.

Table 19.6   Mood Stabilizing Medications

Generic (Trade) Drug Name	Usual Dosage Range (daily)	Half-life (h)
lithium (Eskalith, Lithane)	600–1,800 mg	17–36
divalproex sodium (Depakote)	15–60 mg/kg	6–16
carbamazepine (Tegretol)	200–1,200 mg	25–65
olanzapine (Zyprexa)	5–20 mg	21–54
risperidone (Risperdol)	1–6 mg	20

(Lithium), divalproex sodium (Depakote), and carba-mazepine (Tegretol) (Table 19-6). Lithium, divalproex sodium, and the atypical antipsychotic olanzapine (Zyprexa) are approved by Health Canada, under the authority of the Food and Drugs Act, for treating acute mania.

LITHIUM CARBONATE. Lithium is the most widely used mood stabilizer (see Box 19-9). Combined response rates from five studies demonstrate that 70% of patients experienced at least partial improvement with lithium therapy. However, for most patients, lithium is not a fully adequate treatment for all phases of the illness, and particularly during the acute phase, supplemental use of antipsychotics and benzodiazepines is often beneficial. During acute depressive episodes, supplemental use of antidepressants is most often indicated (Keck et al., 2000). Because of its significant side-effect burden

(Table 19-7), lithium is poorly tolerated in at least one third of treated patients and has the narrowest gap between therapeutic and toxic concentrations of any routinely prescribed psychotropic agent (Belmaker & Yaroslavsky, 2000). Predictors of poor response to lithium in acute mania include a history of poor response, rapid cycling, dysphoric symptoms, mixed symptoms of depression and mania, psychiatric comorbidity, and medical comorbidity (Alda & Grof, 2000).

CRNE Note

Reviewing blood levels of lithium carbonate and dival-proex sodium are ongoing nursing assessments for patients receiving these medications. Side effects of mood stabilizers vary.

Lithium is a salt, and the interaction between lithium levels and sodium levels in the body and the relation-ship between lithium levels and fluid volume in the body remain crucial issues in its safe, effective use. The higher the sodium levels are in the body, the lower the lithium level will be, and vice versa. Thus, changes in dietary sodium intake can affect lithium blood levels that, in turn, may affect therapeutic results or increase the incidence of side effects. The same applies to fluid volume. If body fluid decreases significantly because of a hot climate, strenuous exercise, vomiting, diarrhea, or drastic reduction in fluid intake, then lithium levels can rise sharply, causing an increase in side effects,

BOX 19.9

Drug Profile: Lithium (Eskalith)

DRUG CLASS: Mood stabilizer

RECEPTOR AFFINITY: Alters sodium transport in nerve and muscle cells, increases norepinephrine uptake and sero-tonin receptor sensitivity, slightly increases intraneu-ronal stores of catecholamines, delays some second messenger systems. Mechanism of action is unknown.

INDICATIONS: Treatment and prevention of manic episodes in bipolar affective disorder. Used successfully in a num-ber of unlabelled uses such as prophylaxis of cluster headaches, premenstrual tension, bulimia, etc.

ROUTES AND DOSAGE: 150-, 300-, and 600-mg capsules. Lithobid, 300-mg slow-release tablets; Eskalith CR, 450-mg controlled-release tablets. Lithium citrate, 300-mg/5 mL liquid form.

Adult: In acute mania, optimal response is usually 600 mg tid or 900 mg bid. Obtain serum levels twice weekly in acute phase. Maintenance: Use lowest possible dose to alleviate symptoms and maintain serum level of 0.6–1.2 mEq/L. In uncomplicated maintenance obtain serum lev-els every 2–3 months. Do not rely on serum levels alone. Monitor patient side effects.

Geriatric: Increased risk for toxic effects, use lower doses, monitor frequently.

Children: Safety and efficacy in children younger than 12 y has not been established.

HALF-LIFE (PEAK EFFECT): mean, 24 h (peak serum levels in 1–4 h). Steady state reached in 5–7 d.

SELECT ADVERSE REACTIONS: Weight gain

WARNING: Avoid use during pregnancy or while breast-feeding. Hepatic or renal impairments increase plasma concentration.

SPECIFIC PATIENT/FAMILY EDUCATION:
- Avoid alcohol or other CNS depressant drugs.
- Notify prescriber if pregnancy is possible or planned. Do not breast-feed while taking this medication.
- Notify prescriber before taking any other prescription, OTC medication, or herbal supplements.
- May impair judgment, thinking, or motor skills; avoid driving or other hazardous tasks.
- Do not abruptly discontinue use.

Table 19.7	Lithium Blood Levels and Associated Side Effects
Plasma Level	**Side Effects or Symptoms of Toxicity**
<1.5 mEq/L Mild side effects	Metallic taste in mouth
	Fine hand tremor (resting)
	Nausea
	Polyuria
	Polydipsia
	Diarrhea or loose stools
	Muscular weakness or fatigue
	Weight gain
	Edema
	Memory impairments
1.5–2.5 mEq/L Moderate toxicity	Severe diarrhea
	Dry mouth
	Nausea and vomiting
	Mild to moderate ataxia
	Incoordination
	Dizziness, sluggishness, giddiness, vertigo
	Slurred speech
	Tinnitus
	Blurred vision
	Increasing tremor
	Muscle irritability or twitching
	Asymmetric deep tendon reflexes
	Increased muscle tone
>2.5 mEq/L Severe toxicity	Cardiac arrhythmias
	Blackouts
	Nystagmus
	Coarse tremor
	Fasciculations
	Visual or tactile hallucinations
	Oliguria, renal failure
	Peripheral vascular collapse
	Confusion
	Seizures
	Coma and death

progressing to lethal lithium toxicity. See Table 19-8 for lithium interactions with other drugs. See Chapter 13 for further discussion of lithium's possible mechanisms of action, pharmacokinetics, side effects, and toxicity.

Emergency!

If symptoms of moderate or severe toxicity (eg, cardiac arrhythmias, blackouts, tremors, seizures) are noted, withhold additional doses of lithium, immediately obtain a blood sample to analyze the lithium level, and push fluids if the patient can take fluids. Contact the physician for further direction about relieving the symptoms. Mild side effects tend to subside or can be managed by nursing measures (see Table 19-9).

DIVALPROEX SODIUM. Divalproex sodium (Depakote), an anticonvulsant, has a broader spectrum of efficacy and has about equal benefit for patients with pure mania as for those with other forms of bipolar disorder (ie, mixed mania, rapid cycling, comorbid substance abuse, and secondary mania). Moreover, in one large placebo-controlled study, patients taking divalproex sodium experienced a longer period of stable mood than did patients taking lithium or placebo (Bowden et al., 2000). Whereas divalproex is usually initiated at 250 mg twice a day or lower, in the inpatient setting it can be initiated in an oral loading dose using 20 to 30 mg/kg body weight (see Box 19-10). This may speed the reduction of manic symptoms and diminish the need for antipsychotics early in the course of therapy (Hirschfeld, Baker, Wozniak, Tracy, & Sommerville, 2003).

Baseline liver function tests and a complete blood count with platelets should be obtained before starting therapy, and patients with known liver disease should not be given divalproex sodium. Optimal blood levels appear to be in the range of 50 to 150 ng/mL. Levels may be obtained weekly until the patient is stable, and then every 6 months. Divalproex sodium is associated with increased risk for birth defects. Cases of life-threatening pancreatitis have been reported in adults and children receiving valproate, either initially or after several years of use. Some cases were described as hemorrhagic, with a rapid progression from onset to death. If pancreatitis is diagnosed, valproate use should be discontinued.

CARBAMAZEPINE. Carbamazepine, an anticonvulsant, also has mood-stabilizing effects. Data from various studies suggest that it may be effective in patients who experience no response to lithium. In addition, patients with secondary mania appear to be more responsive to carbamazepine than to lithium (Strakowski & Sax, 2000). The most common side effects of carbamazepine are dizziness, drowsiness, nausea, and vomiting, which may be avoided with slow incremental dosing. Carbamazepine has both benign and severe hematologic toxicities. Frequent clinically unimportant decreases in white blood cell counts occur. Estimates of the rate of severe blood dyscrasias vary from 1 in 10,000 patients treated to a more recent estimate of 1 in 125,000 (Schatzberg et al., 2003). Mild, nonprogressive elevations of liver function test results are relatively common. Carbamazepine is associated with increased risk for birth defects.

In patients older than 12 years, carbamazepine is begun at 200 mg once or twice a day. The dosage is increased by no more than 200 mg every 2 to 4 days, to 800 to 1,000 mg a day, or until therapeutic levels or effects are achieved. It is important to monitor for blood dyscrasias and liver damage. Liver function tests and complete blood counts with differential are minimal pretreatment laboratory tests and should be repeated about 1 month after initiating treatment, and at 3 months, 6 months, and yearly. Other yearly tests

Table 19.8   Lithium Interactions With Medications and Other Substances

Substance	Effect of Interaction
Angiotensin-converting enzyme inhibitors, such as: • Captopril • Lisinopril • Quinapril	Increases serum lithium; may cause toxicity and impaired kidney function
Acetazolamide	Increases renal excretion of lithium, decreases lithium levels
Alcohol	May increase serum lithium level
Caffeine	Increases lithium excretion, increases lithium tremor
Carbamazepine	Increases neurotoxicity, despite normal serum levels and dosage
Fluoxetine	Increases serum lithium levels
Haloperidol	Increases neurotoxicity, despite normal serum levels and dosage
Loop diuretics, such as furosemide	Increases lithium serum levels, but may be safer than thiazide diuretics; potassium-sparing diuretics (amiloride, spirolactone) are safest
Methyldopa	Increases neurotoxicity without increasing serum lithium levels
Nonsteroidal anti-inflammatory drugs, such as: • Diclofenac • Ibuprofen • Indomethacin • Piroxicam	Decreases renal clearance of lithium Increases serum lithium levels by 30%–60% in 3–10 d Aspirin and sulindac do not appear to have the same effect
Osmotic diuretics, such as: • Urea • Mannitol • Isosorbide	Increases renal excretion of lithium and decreases lithium levels
Sodium chloride	High sodium intake decreases lithium levels; low sodium diets may increase lithium levels and lead to toxicity
Thiazide diuretics, such as: • Chlorothiazide • Hydrochlorothiazide	Promotes sodium and potassium excretion; increases lithium serum levels; may produce cardiotoxicity and neurotoxicity
Tricyclic antidepressants	Increases tremor; potentiates pharmacologic effects of tricyclic antidepressants

should include electrolytes, blood urea nitrogen, thyroid function tests, urinalysis, and eye examinations. Carbamazepine levels are measured monthly until the patient is on a stable dosage. Studies suggest that blood levels in the range of 8 to 12 ng/mL correspond to therapeutic efficacy. See Table 19-10 for carbamazepine's interactions with other drugs. See Chapter 13 for further discussion of carbamazepine's possible mechanisms of action, pharmacokinetics, side effects, and toxicity.

Emergency!

Both valproate and carbamazepine may be lethal if high doses are ingested. Toxic symptoms appear in 1 to 3 hours and include neuromuscular disturbances, dizziness, stupor, agitation, disorientation, nystagmus, urinary retention, nausea and vomiting, tachycardia, hypotension or hypertension, cardiovascular shock, coma, and respiratory depression.

NEWER ANTICONVULSANTS. In small clinical trials, case reports, and anecdotal evidence, newer anticonvulsants also show promise as mood stabilizers. Lamotrigine (Lamictal) has efficacy in treating mania, both as a single agent and in combination with lithium or valproate (Bowden et al., 2003). Observations suggest that it may be particularly effective for rapid cycling and in the depressed phase of bipolar illness. Anecdotal evidence suggests that gabapentin (Neurontin) may be effective for acute mania, mood stabilization, and rapid cycling. Topiramate (Topamax) has been used mostly as add-on therapy in mixed patient samples with refractory mood disorders. A characteristic of topiramate is that it is more associated with weight loss than weight gain. Controlled trials are needed to evaluate further the efficacy of these and other anticonvulsants (Schatzberg et al., 2003).

Intervention With Antidepressants

Acute bipolar depression has received little scientific study in comparison with unipolar depression. Antidepressant drugs may cause either a switch to mania or a mixed state or may induce rapid cycling. Unfortunately, lithium or anticonvulsants are not as effective against depression as they are against mania. However, in a few patients, lithium or anticonvulsants can be used alone with good antidepressant effects. The most common treatment of bipolar depression is an antidepressant

Table 19.9   Interventions for Lithium Side Effects

Side Effect	Intervention
Edema of feet or hands	Monitor intake and output, check for possible decreased urinary output. Monitor sodium intake. Patient should elevate legs when sitting or lying. Monitor weight.
Fine hand tremor	Provide support and reassurance, if it does not interfere with daily activities. Tremor worsens with anxiety and intentional movements; minimize stressors. Notify prescriber if it interferes with patient's work and compliance will be an issue. More frequent smaller doses of lithium may also help.
Mild diarrhea	Take lithium with meals. Provide for fluid replacement. Notify prescriber if becomes severe; may need a change in medication preparation or may be early sign of toxicity.
Muscle weakness, fatigue, or memory and concentration difficulties	Provide support and reassurance; this side effect will usually pass after a few weeks of treatment. Short-term memory aids such as lists or reminder calls may be helpful. Notify prescriber if becomes severe or interferes with the patient's desire to continue treatment.
Metallic taste	Suggest sugarless candies or throat lozenges. Encourage frequent oral hygiene.
Nausea or abdominal discomfort	Consider dividing the medication into smaller doses, or give it at more frequent intervals. Give medication with meals.
Polydipsia	Reassure patient that this is a normal mechanism to cope with polyuria.
Polyuria	Monitor intake and output. Provide reassurance and explain nature of side effect. Also explain that this causes no physical damage to kidneys.
Toxicity	Withhold medication. Notify prescriber. Use symptomatic treatments.

combined with a mood stabilizer to "protect" the patient against a manic switch. The antidepressant agents are the same as those used in unipolar illness, although they are sometimes given in lower dosages and for shorter periods of time as a precaution.

Intervention With Antipsychotics

Antipsychotics are prescribed for patients who experience psychosis as a part of bipolar disorder. If patients cannot tolerate mood stabilizers, antipsychotics may be given, instead of antidepressants, to stabilize the moods.

BOX 19.10

Drug Profile: Divalproex Sodium (Depakote)

DRUG CLASS: Antimania agent
RECEPTOR AFFINITY: Thought to increase level of inhibitory neurotransmitter, GABA, to brain neurons. Mechanism of action is unknown.
INDICATIONS: Treatment of bipolar disorders.
ROUTES AND DOSAGE: Available in 125-mg delayed-release capsules, and 125-, 250-, and 500-mg enteric-coated tablets.
Adult dosage: Dosage depends on symptoms and clinical picture presented; initially, the dosage is low and gradually increased depending on the clinical presentation.
HALF-LIFE (PEAK EFFECT): 6–16 h (1–4 h)
SELECT ADVERSE REACTIONS: Sedation, tremor (may be dose related), nausea, vomiting, indigestion, abdominal cramps, anorexia with weight loss, slight elevations in liver enzymes, hepatic failure, thrombocytopenia, transient increases in hair loss.

WARNING: Use cautiously during pregnancy and lactation. Contraindicated in patients with hepatic disease or significant hepatic dysfunction. Administer cautiously with salicylates; may increase serum levels and result in toxicity.
SPECIFIC PATIENT/FAMILY EDUCATION:
- Take with food if gastrointestinal upset occurs.
- Swallow tablets or capsules whole to prevent local irritation of mouth and throat.
- Notify prescriber before taking any other prescription or OTC medications or herbal supplements.
- Avoid alcohol and sleep-inducing or OTC products.
- Avoid driving or performing activities that require alertness.
- Do not abruptly discontinue use.
- Keep appointments for follow-up, including blood tests to monitor response.

Table 19.10	Selected Medication Interactions With Carbamazepine
Interaction	**Drug Interacting With Carbamazepine**
Increased carbamazepine levels	Erythromycin Cimetidine Propoxyphene Isoniazid Calcium-channel blockers (Verapamil) Fluoxetine Danazol Diltiazem Nicotinamide
Decreased carbamazepine levels	Phenobarbital Primidone Phenytoin
Drugs whose levels are decreased by carbamazepine	Oral contraceptives Warfarin, oral anticoagulants Doxycycline Theophylline Haloperidol Divalproex sodium Tricyclic antidepressants Acetaminophen—increased metabolism, but also increased risk for hepatotoxicity

Generally, the antipsychotic dosage is lower than what is prescribed for patients with schizophrenia.

Administering and Monitoring Medication

During acute mania, patients may not believe that they have a psychiatric disorder and refuse to take medication. Because their energy is still high, they can be very creative in avoiding medication. Once patients begin to take medications, symptom improvement should be evident. If a patient is very agitated, a benzodiazepine may be given for a short period.

MONITORING AND MANAGING SIDE EFFECTS. It is unlikely that patients will take only one medication; they may receive several. In some instances, one agent will be used to augment the effects of another, such as supplemental thyroid hormone to boost antidepressant response in depression. Possible side effects for each medication should be listed and cross-referenced. When a side effect appears, the nurse should document the side effect and notify the prescriber so that further evaluation can be made. In some instances, medications should be changed.

MONITORING FOR DRUG INTERACTIONS. It is a well-established practice to combine mood stabilizers with antidepressants or antipsychotics. The previously discussed drug interactions should be considered when caring for a person with bipolar disorder. A big challenge is monitoring alcohol, drugs, over-the-counter medications, and herbal supplements. A complete list of all medications should be maintained and evaluated for any potential interaction (see Table 19-4 for specific drug interactions).

Teaching Points

For patients who are taking lithium, it is important to explain that a change in salt intake can affect the therapeutic blood level. If there is a reduction in salt intake, the body will naturally retain lithium to maintain homeostasis. This increase in lithium retention can lead to toxicity. Once stabilized on a lithium dose, salt intake should remain constant. This is fairly easy to do, except during the summer, when excessive perspiration can occur. Patients should increase salt intake during periods of perspiration, increased exercise, and dehydration. Most mood stabilizers and antidepressants can cause weight gain. Patients should be alerted to this potential side effect and should be instructed to monitor any changes in eating, appetite, or weight. Weight reduction techniques may need to be instituted. Patients also should be clearly instructed to check with the nurse or physician before taking any over-the-counter medication or herbal supplements.

Other Somatic Interventions: Electroconvulsive Therapy

ECT may be a treatment alternative for patients with severe mania who exhibit unremitting, frenzied physical activity. Other indications for ECT are acute mania that is unresponsive to antimanic agents or high suicide risk. ECT is safe and effective in patients receiving antipsychotic drugs. Use of valproate or carbamazepine will elevate the seizure threshold, requiring some adjustments in treatment.

Psychological Domain

Assessment

The assessment of the psychological domain should follow the process explained in Chapter 10. Individuals with bipolar disorder can usually participate fully in this part of the assessment.

Mood

By definition, bipolar disorder is a disturbance of mood. If the patient is depressed, using an assessment tool for depression may help determine the severity of depression. If mania predominates, evaluating the quality of the mood (elated, grandiose, irritated, or agitated) becomes important. Usually, mania is determined by clinical observation.

Cognition

In a depressive episode, the individual may not be able to concentrate enough to complete cognitive tasks, such as those called for in the Mini-Mental State Exam (MMSE). During the acute phase of a manic or depressive episode, mental status may be abnormal, and in a manic phase, judgment is impaired by extremely rapid, disjointed, and distorted thinking. Moreover, feelings such as grandiosity can interfere with normal executive functioning.

Thought Disturbances

Psychosis commonly occurs in patients with bipolar disorder, especially during acute episodes of mania. Auditory hallucinations and delusional thinking are part of the clinical picture. In children and adolescents, psychosis is not so easily disclosed.

Stress and Coping Factors

Stress and coping are critical assessment areas for a person with bipolar disorder. A stressful event often triggers a manic or depressive episode. In some instances, there are no particular stresses that preceded the episode, but it is important to discuss the possibility. Determining the patient's usual coping skills for stresses lays the groundwork for developing interventional strategies. Negative coping skills, such as substance use or aggression, should be identified because these skills need to be replaced with positive coping skills.

Risk Assessment

Patients with bipolar disorder are at high risk for injury to self (Dubovsky, 2005) and others, with 10% to 15% of patients completing suicide. Child abuse, spouse abuse, or other violent behaviours may occur during severe manic episodes; thus, patients should be assessed for suicidal or homicidal risk (APA, 2000). The risk for relapse and poorer treatment outcomes are associated with obesity. Preventing and treating obesity in patients with bipolar disorder could decrease the morbidity and mortality related to physical illness, enhance psychological well-being, and possibly improve the course of the disorder (Fagiolini, Kupfer, Houck, Novick, & Frank, 2003).

Nursing Diagnoses for Psychological Domain

Nursing diagnoses associated with the psychological domain of bipolar disorder include Disturbed Sensory Perception; Disturbed Thought Processes; Defensive Coping; Risk for Suicide; Risk for Violence; Ineffective Coping.

Interventions for Psychological Domain

Pharmacotherapy is the primary treatment for bipolar disorder but is often unsuccessful unless adjunctive psychosocial interventions are included in the treatment plan. Integration of psychotherapeutic techniques with pharmacotherapy is strongly recommended by clinicians *and* patients (Thase & Sachs, 2000). The most common psychotherapeutic approaches include psychoeducation, individual cognitive-behavioural therapy, individual interpersonal therapy, and adjunctive therapies, such as those for substance use (Rothbaum & Astin, 2000).

Several risk factors associated with bipolar disorders make patients more vulnerable to relapses and resistant to recovery. Among these are high rates of nonadherence to medication therapy, obesity, marital conflict, separation, divorce, unemployment, and underemployment. The goals of psychosocial interventions are to address risk factors and associated features that are difficult to address with pharmacotherapy alone. Particularly important are improving medication adherence, decreasing the number and length of hospitalizations and relapses, enhancing social and occupational functioning, improving quality of life, increasing the patient and family's acceptance of the disorder, and reducing the suicide risk (Rothbaum & Astin, 2000; Scott & Colom, 2005).

Psychoeducation

Psychoeducation is designed to provide information on bipolar disorder and successful treatment and recovery and usually focuses on medication adherence. The nurse can provide information about the illness and obstacles to recovery. Helping the patient to recognize warning signs and symptoms of relapse and to cope with residual symptoms and functional impairment are important interventions. Resistance to accepting the illness and to taking medication, the symbolic meaning of medication taking, and worries about the future can be discussed openly. In the interest of improved medication adherence, listening carefully to the patient's concerns about the medication, dosing schedules and dose changes, and side effects is helpful (see Box 19-11). Health teaching and weight management should be a component of any psychoeducation program. In addition to individual variations in body weight, many of the medications (divalproex sodium, lithium, antidepressants,

---

BOX 19.11

Psychoeducation Checklist: Bipolar I Disorder

When caring for the patient with a bipolar I disorder, be sure to include the following topic areas in the teaching plan:
- Psychopharmacologic agents, including drug action, dosage, frequency, and possible adverse effects
- Medication regimen adherence
- Strategies to decrease agitation and restlessness
- Safety measures
- Self-care management
- Follow-up laboratory testing
- Support services

olanzapine) are associated with weight gain. Monitoring weight and developing individual weight management plans can reduce the risk for relapse and increase the possibility of medication adherence.

Psychotherapy

Long-term psychotherapy may help prevent both mania and depression by reducing the stresses that trigger episodes and increasing the patient's acceptance of the need for medication. Patients should be encouraged to keep their appointments with the therapist, be honest and open, do the assigned homework, and give the therapist feedback on how the treatment is working (Kahn, Ross, Printz, & Sachs, 2000).

Social Domain

Assessment

One of the tragedies of bipolar disorder is its effect on social and occupational functioning. Cultural views of mental illness influence the patient's acceptance of the disorder. During illness episodes, patients often behave in ways that jeopardize their social relationships. Losing a job and going through a divorce are common events. When performing an assessment of social function, the nurse should identify changes resulting from a manic or depressive episode.

Nursing Diagnoses for Social Domain

Nursing diagnoses for adults can include Ineffective Role Performance; Interrupted Family Processes; Impaired Social Interaction; Impaired Parenting; and Compromised Family Coping. The diagnoses for children and adolescents can include Delayed Growth and Development and Caregiver Role Strain in family coping with a member with a bipolar disorder.

Interventions for Social Domain

Interventions focussing on the social domain are integral to nursing care for all ages. During mania, patients usually violate others' boundaries. Roommate selection for patients requiring hospital admittance needs to be carefully considered. If possible, a private room is ideal because patients with bipolar disorder tend to irritate others, who quickly tire of the intrusiveness. These patients may miss the cues indicating anger and aggression from others. The nurse should protect the manic patient from self-harm, as well as harm from other patients.

Support groups are helpful for people with this disorder. Participating in groups allows the person to meet others with the same disorder and learn management and preventive strategies. Support groups also are helpful in dealing with the stigma associated with mental illnesses.

Family Interventions

Marital and family interventions are often needed at different periods in the life of a person with bipolar disorder. For the family with a child with this disorder, additional parenting skills are needed to manage the behaviours. The goals of family interventions are to help the family understand and cope with the disorder. Interventions may range from occasional counselling sessions to intensive family therapy.

Family psychoeducation strategies have been shown to be particularly useful in decreasing the risk for relapse and hospitalization. In a study of 53 patients with mania, half were assigned to a 9-month family-focussed psychoeducational group and half to individually focussed treatment. Those in family-focussed treatment were less likely to be rehospitalized (Rea et al., 2003). For more information, see Box 19-8.

EVALUATION AND TREATMENT OUTCOMES

Desired treatment outcomes are stabilization of mood and enhanced quality of life. Primary tools for evaluating outcomes are nursing observation and patient self-report (see Nursing Care Plan 19-1).

CONTINUUM OF CARE

Inpatient Management

Inpatient admission is the treatment setting of choice for patients who are severely psychotic or who are an immediate threat to themselves or others. In acute mania, nursing interventions focus on patient safety because patients are prone to injury because of hyperactivity and often are unaware of injuries they sustain. Distraction may also be effective when a patient is talking or acting inappropriately. Removal to a quieter environment may be necessary if other interventions have not been successful, but the patient should be carefully monitored. Because during acute mania, patients are often impulsive, disinhibited, and interpersonally inappropriate, the nurse should avoid direct confrontations or challenges.

Medication management (Fig. 19-2), including control of side effects and promotion of self-care, is a major nursing responsibility during inpatient hospitalization. Nurses should be familiar with drug–drug interactions (Table 19-4) and with interventions to help control side effects.

Intensive Outpatient Programs

Intensive outpatient programs for several weeks of acute-phase care during a manic or depressive episode

NURSING CARE PLAN 19.1

The Patient With Bipolar Disorder

JR, a 43-year-old, single woman, lives in a metropolitan city and works for a large travel agency booking corporate business trips. She has a history of alcohol abuse that began when she was in high school. Initially, she relied on alcohol for stress reduction but gradually began abusing it. Her mother, grandfather, and sister all committed suicide within the past several years. JR's father has remarried and moved out of the area. JR has one brother whom she sees occasionally.

Three years ago, JR left her husband after 15 years of an unhappy marriage and moved into a small condominium in a less affluent neighbourhood. She began having symptoms of bipolar mixed disorder at that time, when she sold all her clothes, bleached her hair blonde, and began cruising the bars. She would consume excessive amounts of alcohol and often end up spending the night with a stranger. At first her behaviour was attributed to her recent divorce. When she began missing work and charging excessively on her credit cards, her friends and two children became concerned and convinced her to seek help for her behaviour.

JR received a diagnosis of manic episode, and treatment with lithium carbonate was initiated. Her mood stabilized briefly, but she had two more manic episodes within the next 18 months. Shortly after her last manic episode, she became severely depressed and attempted suicide. TCAs and MAOIs were tried, but she discontinued taking them after a significant weight gain. Once her depression lifted, her mood was stable for several months.

About 2 months ago, JR began missing work again because of depression. She refused to take any antidepressants and just wanted to "wait it out." She often boasted that her one success in life was helping people travel and have a good time. Last week she was told that her position was being eliminated because of a company issue. Now she believes that she is a failure as a wife, as an employee, and as a woman. She became despondent and finally took an overdose to "end it all."

SETTING: INTENSIVE CARE PSYCHIATRIC UNIT IN A GENERAL HOSPITAL

Baseline Assessment: Ms. R is a 43-year-old single woman transferred from ICU after a 3-day hospitalization following a suicide attempt with an overdose of multiple prescriptions and alcohol. She had her first manic episode 3 years before, and subsequently has had symptoms of a mixed bipolar mood disorder most of the time. Medication with lithium carbonate has not protected her from mood swings, and prior trials of TCAs and MAOIs have been unsuccessful. She is currently depressed, with pressured speech, agitation, irritability, sensory overload, inability to sleep, and anorexia.

Associated Psychiatric Diagnosis	*Medications*
Axis I: Bipolar I disorder, most recent episode mixed, severe, without psychotic features	Lithium carbonate 300 mg tid × 2 years
Axis II: Deferred (none apparent in her history, and she is currently too ill for personality disorder to be assessed)	L-Thyroxine 0.1 mg q AM × 1 d
	Clonazepam 0.5 mg bid for sleep and agitation
	Carbamazepine added on transfer to be titrated up to 400 mg tid
Axis III: Hypothyroidism	
Axis IV: Social problems (very poor marriage of 15 years, death by suicide of mother, grandfather, one sister)	
Axis V: GAF = Current 50	
Potential 85	

NURSING DIAGNOSIS 1: RISK SUICIDE

Defining Characteristics	*Related Factors*
Attempts to inflict life-threatening injury to self	Feelings of helplessness and hopelessness secondary to bipolar disorder
Expresses desire to die	Depression
Poor impulse control	Loss secondary to finances/job, divorce
Lack of support system	

OUTCOMES

Initial	*Discharge*
1. Develop a no self-harm contract.	5. Discuss the complexity of bipolar disorder.
2. Remain free from self-harm.	6. Identify the antecedents to depression.
3. Identify factors that led to suicidal intent and methods for managing suicidal impulses if they return.	
4. Accept treatment of depression by trying the SSRI antidepressants.	

(Continued)

NURSING CARE PLAN 19.1 (Continued)

INTERVENTIONS

Interventions	Rationale	Ongoing Assessment
Initiate a nurse–patient relationship by demonstrating an acceptance of Ms. R as a worthwhile human being through the use of nonjudgmental statements and behaviour.	A sense of worthlessness often underlies suicide ideation. The positive therapeutic relationship can maintain the patient's dignity.	Assess the stages of the relationship and determine whether a therapeutic relationship is actually being formed. Identify indicators of trust.
Initiate suicide precautions per hospital policy.	Safety of the individual is a priority with people who have suicide ideation. (See Chap. 37.)	Determine intent to harm self—plan and means.
Obtain a no self-harm contract.	A contract can help the patient resist suicide by providing a way of resisting impulses.	Determine patient's ability to commit to a contract.

Evaluation

Outcomes	Revised Outcomes	Interventions
Has not harmed self, denies suicidal thought/intent after realizing that she is still alive.	Absence of suicidal intent will continue.	Discontinue suicide precautions; maintain ongoing assessment for suicidality.
Made a no self-harm contract with nurse, agrees to keep it after discharge.	Maintain a no self-harm contract with outpatient mental health provider.	Support and reinforce this contract.
JR agreed to try to treat her depression by initiating treatment with Prozac.		

NURSING DIAGNOSIS 2: CHRONIC LOW SELF-ESTEEM

Defining Characteristics	Related Factors
Long-standing self-negating verbalizations Expressions of shame and guilt Evaluates self as unable to deal with events Frequent lack of success in work and relationships Poor body presentation (eye contact, posture, movements) Nonassertive/passive	Failure to stabilize mood Unmet dependency needs Feelings of abandonment secondary to separation from significant other Feelings of failure secondary to loss of job, relationship problems Unrealistic expectations of self

OUTCOMES

Initial	Discharge
1. Identify positive aspects of self. 2. Modify excessive and unrealistic expectations of self.	3. Verbalize acceptance of personal limitations. 4. Report freedom from most symptoms of depression. 5. Begin to take verbal and behavioural risks.

INTERVENTIONS

Interventions	Rationale	Ongoing Assessment
Enhance JR's sense of self by being attentive, validating your interpretation of what is being said or experienced, and helping her verbalize what she is expressing nonverbally.	By showing respect for the patient as a human being who is worth listening to, the nurse can support and help build the patient's sense of self.	Determine whether patient confirms interpretation of situation and if she can verbalize what she is expressing nonverbally.
Assist to reframe and redefine negative statements ("not a failure, but a setback").	Reframing an event positively rather than negatively can help the patient view the situation in an alternative way.	Assess whether the patient can actually view the world in a different way.
Problem-solve with patient about how to approach finding another job.	Work is very important to adults. Losing a job can decrease self-esteem. Focussing on the possibility of a future job will provide hope for the patient.	Assess the patient's ability to problem-solve. Determine whether she is realistic in her expectations.

NURSING CARE PLAN 19.1 (Continued)

Encourage positive physical habits (healthy food and eating patterns, exercise, proper sleep).	A healthy lifestyle promotes well-being, increasing self-esteem.	Determine JR's willingness to consider making lifestyle changes.
Teach patient to validate consensually with others.	Low self-esteem is generated by negative interpretations of the world. Through consensual validation, the patient can determine whether others view situations in the same way.	Assess JR's ability to participate in this process.
Teach esteem-building exercises (self-affirmations, imagery, use of humor, meditation/prayer, relaxation).	There are many different approaches that can be practiced to increase self-esteem.	Assess JR's energy level and ability to focus on learning new skills.
Assist in establishing appropriate personal boundaries.	In an attempt to meet their own needs, people with low self-esteem often violate other people's boundaries and allow others to take advantage of them. Helping patients establish their own boundaries will improve the likelihood of needs being met in an appropriate manner.	Assess JR's ability to understand the concept of boundary violation and its significance.
Provide an opportunity within the therapeutic relationship to express thoughts and feelings. Use open-ended statements and questions. Encourage expression of both positive and negative statements. Use movement, art, and music as means of expression.	The individual with low self-esteem may have difficulty expressing thoughts and feelings. Providing them with several different outlets for expression helps to develop skills for expressing thoughts and feelings.	Monitor thoughts and feelings that are expressed in order to help the patient examine them.
Explore opportunities for positive socialization.	Individuals with low self-esteem may be in social situations that reinforce negative valuation of self. Helping patient identify new positive situations will give other options.	Assess whether the new situations are potentially positive or are a re-creation of other negative situations.
JR began to identify positive aspects of self as she began to modify excessive and unrealistic expectations of self.	Strengthen ability to affirm positive aspects and examine expectations related to work and relationships.	Refer to mental health clinic for cognitive behavioural psychotherapy with a feminist perspective.
She verbalized that she would probably never work for the company again and that it would never be the same. She verbalized that she would need more assertiveness skills in her relationships.	Identify important aspects of job so that she can begin looking for a job that had those characteristics.	Attend a women's group that focuses on assertiveness skills.
As JR's mood improved, she was able to sleep through the night, and she began eating again—began feeling better about herself.	Maintain a stable mood to promote positive self-concept.	Monitor mood and identify antecedents to depression.

NURSING DIAGNOSIS 3: INEFFECTIVE INDIVIDUAL COPING

Defining Characteristics	*Related Factors*
Verbalization in inability to cope or ask for help	Altered mood (depression) caused by changes secondary to body chemistry (bipolar disorder)
Reported difficulty with life stressors	Altered mood caused by changes secondary to intake of mood-altering substance (alcohol)
Inability to problem solve	Unsatisfactory support system
Alteration in social participation	Sensory overload secondary to excessive activity
Destructive behaviour toward self	Inadequate psychological resources to adapt to changes in job status
Frequent illnesses	
Substance abuse	

(Continued)

NURSING CARE PLAN 19.1 (Continued)

OUTCOMES

Initial	Discharge
1. Accept support through the nurse–patient relationship.	6. Practice new coping skills.
2. Identify areas of ineffective coping.	7. Focus on strengths.
3. Examine the current efforts at coping.	
4. Identify areas of strength.	
5. Learn new coping skills.	

INTERVENTIONS

Interventions	Rationale	Ongoing Assessment
Identify current stresses in JR's life, including her suicide attempt and the bipolar disorder.	When areas of concern are verbalized by the patient, she will be able to focus on one issue at a time. If she identifies the mental disorder as a stressor, she will more likely be able to develop strategies to deal with it.	Determine whether JR is able to identify problem areas realistically. Continue to assess for suicidality.
Identify JR's strengths in dealing with past stressors.	By focussing on past successes, she can identify strengths and build on them in the future.	Assess if JR can identify any previous successes in her life.
Assess current level of depression using Beck's Depression Inventory or a similar one and intervene according to assessed level.	Severely depressed or suicidal individuals need assistance with decision making, grooming and hygiene, and nutrition.	Continue to assess for mood and suicidality.
Assist JR in discussing, selecting, and practicing positive coping skills (jogging, yoga, thought stopping).	New coping skills take a conscious effort to learn and will at first seem strange and unnatural. Practicing these skills will help the patient incorporate them into her coping strategy repertoire.	Assess whether JR follows through on learning new skills.
Educate regarding the use of alcohol and its relationship to depression.	Alcohol is an ineffective coping strategy because it actually exacerbates the depression.	Assess for the patient's willingness to address her drinking problem.
Assist patient in coping with bipolar disorder, beginning with education about it.	A mood disorder is a major stressor in a patient's life. To manage the stress, the patient needs a knowledge base.	Determine JR's knowledge about bipolar disorder.
Administer lithium as ordered (give with food or milk). Reinforce the action, dosage, and side effects. Review laboratory results to determine whether lithium is within therapeutic limits. Assess for toxicity. Recommend a normal diet with normal salt intake; maintenance of adequate fluid intake.	Lithium carbonate is effective in the treatment of bipolar disorder but must be managed. Patient should have a thorough knowledge of the medication and side effects.	Assess for target action, side effects, and toxicity.
Administer carbamazepine as ordered, to be titrated up to 400 mg tid. Observe for presence of hypersensitivity to the drug. Teach about action, dosage, and side effects. Emphasize the possibility of drug interaction with alcohol, some antibiotics, TCAs, and MAOIs.	Carbamazepine can be effective in bipolar disorder. However, it can increase CNS toxicity when given with lithium carbonate.	Assess for target action, side effects, and toxicity.
Administer thyroid supplement as ordered. Review laboratory results of thyroid functioning. Discuss the symptoms of hypothyroidism and how they are similar to depression. Emphasize the importance of taking lithium and L-thyroxine. Explain about the long-term effects of lithium on thyroid functioning.	Hypothyroidism can be a side effect of lithium carbonate and also mimics symptoms of depression.	Determine whether patient understands the relationship between thyroid dysfunction and lithium carbonate.

NURSING CARE PLAN 19.1 (Continued)

EVALUATION

Outcomes	Revised Outcomes	Interventions
Clonazepam 0.5 mg bid for sleep and agitation.		
JR easily engaged in a therapeutic relationship. She examined the areas in her life where she coped ineffectively.	Establish a therapeutic relationship with a therapist at the mental health clinic.	Refer to mental health clinic.
She identified her strengths and how she coped with stressors and especially her illness in the past. She is willing to try antidepressants again, in hopes of not having the weight gain.	Continue to view illness as a potential stressor that can disrupt life.	Seek advice immediately if there are any problems with medications.
She learned new problem-solving skills and reported that she learned a lot about her medication. She is committed to complying with her medication regimen. She identified new coping skills that she could realistically do. She will focus on strengths.	Continue to practice new coping skills as stressful situations arise.	Discuss with therapist the outcomes of using new coping skills. Attend Alcoholics Anonymous if alcohol is used as a stress reliever.

are used when hospitalization is not necessary or to prevent or shorten hospitalization. These programs are usually called *partial hospitalization* or *day hospitalization*. Close medication monitoring and milieu therapies that foster restoration of a patient's previous adaptive abilities are the major nursing responsibilities in these settings.

Setting up frequent office visits and crisis telephone calls are additional nursing interventions that can help to shorten or prevent hospitalization during the acute phase of a manic episode. Family sessions or psychoeducation that includes the patient are alternatives. Severely and persistently ill patients may need ongoing intensive treatment, but the frequency of visits can be decreased for patients whose conditions stabilize and who enter the continuation or the maintenance phase of treatment.

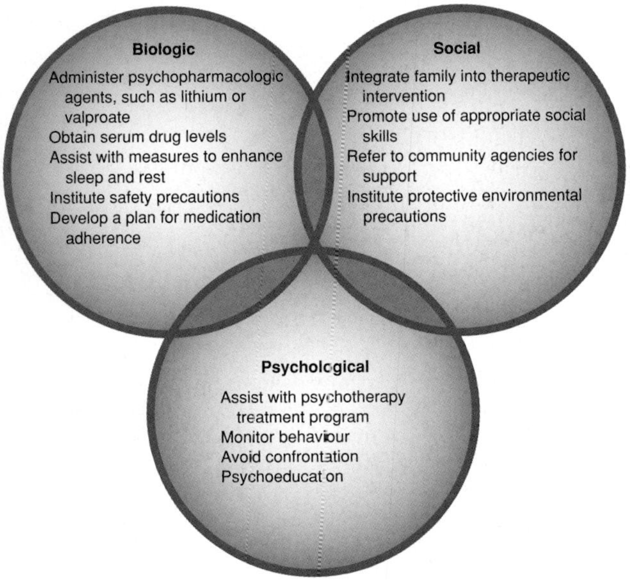

Spectrum of Care

In today's health care climate, with efforts to reduce hospitalization, most patients with bipolar disorder are treated as outpatients. Hospitalizations are usually brief, and treatment focuses on restabilization. Patients with mood disorders are likely to need long-term medication regimens and supportive psychotherapy to function in the community. Therefore, medication regimens and additional treatment planning need to be tailored to individual needs. Patients need extended and continued follow-up to monitor medication trials and side effects, reinforce self-care management, and provide continued psychosocial support.

Mental Health Promotion

Mental health promotion activities should be the focus during remissions. During this period, patients have an opportunity to learn new coping skills that promote positive mental health. Stress management and relaxation techniques can be practiced for use when needed. A plan for managing emerging symptoms can also be developed during this period.

Biologic
Administer psychopharmacologic agents, such as lithium or valproate
Obtain serum drug levels
Assist with measures to enhance sleep and rest
Institute safety precautions
Develop a plan for medication adherence

Social
Integrate family into therapeutic intervention
Promote use of appropriate social skills
Refer to community agencies for support
Institute protective environmental precautions

Psychological
Assist with psychotherapy treatment program
Monitor behaviour
Avoid confrontation
Psychoeducation

FIGURE 19.2 Biopsychosocial interventions for patients with bipolar I disorder.

SUMMARY OF KEY POINTS

◙ Mood disorders are characterized by persistent or recurring disturbances in mood that cause significant psychological distress and functional impairment. Moods can be broadly categorized as manic or dysphoric (typified by exaggerated feelings of elation or irritability) or depressive or dysthymic (typified by feelings of sadness, hopelessness, loss of interest, and fatigue).

◙ Primary mood disorders include both depressive disorders (unipolar depression) and manic-depressive disorders (bipolar disorders).

◙ Genetics undoubtedly play a role in the etiology of mood disorders. Risk factors include family history of mood disorders, prior mood episodes, lack of social support, stressful life events, substance use, and medical problems, particularly chronic or terminal illnesses.

◙ The recommended depression treatment guidelines include antidepressant medication, alone or with psychotherapeutic management or psychotherapy; electroconvulsive therapy for severe depression; or light therapy (phototherapy) for patients with seasonal depressive symptoms.

◙ Nurses must be knowledgeable regarding antidepressant medications, in particular therapeutic effects and associated side effects, toxicity, dosage ranges, and contraindications. Nurses must also be familiar with electroconvulsive therapy protocols and associated interventions. Patient education and the provision of emotional support during the course of treatment are also nursing responsibilities.

◙ Many symptoms of depression, such as weight and appetite changes, sleep disturbance, decreased energy, and fatigue, are similar to those of medical illnesses. Assessment includes a thorough medical history and physical examination to detect or rule out medical or psychiatric comorbidity.

◙ Biopsychosocial assessment includes assessing mood, speech patterns, thought processes and thought content, suicidal or homicidal thoughts, cognition and memory, and social factors, such as patterns of relationships, quality of support systems, and changes in occupational functioning. Several self-report scales are helpful in evaluating depressive symptoms.

◙ Establishing and maintaining a therapeutic nurse–patient relationship is key to successful outcomes. Nursing interventions that foster the therapeutic relationship include being available in times of crisis; providing understanding and education to patients and their families regarding goals of treatment; providing encouragement and feedback concerning the patient's progress; providing guidance in the patient's interpersonal interactions with others and work environment; and helping to set and monitor realistic goals.

◙ Psychosocial interventions for mood disorders include self-care management, cognitive therapy, behaviour therapy, interpersonal therapy, patient and family education regarding the nature of the disorder and treatment goals, marital and family therapy, and group therapy that includes medication maintenance support groups and other consumer-oriented support groups.

◙ Bipolar disorders are characterized by one or more manic episodes or mixed mania (co-occurrence of manic and depressive states) that cause marked impairment in social activities, occupational functioning, and interpersonal relationships and may require hospitalization to prevent self-harm.

◙ Manic episodes are periods in which the individual experiences abnormally and persistently elevated, expansive, or irritable mood characterized by inflated self-esteem, decreased need to sleep, excessive energy or hyperactivity, racing thoughts, easy distractibility, and inability to stay focussed. Other symptoms can include hypersexuality and impulsivity.

◙ Similar to treatment of major depressive disorder, pharmacotherapy is the cornerstone of treatment of bipolar illness, but adjunctive psychosocial interventions are needed as well. Pharmacologic therapy includes treatment with mood stabilizers alone or in combination with antipsychotics or benzodiazepines if psychosis, agitation, or insomnia is present and antidepressants for unremitted depression. Electroconvulsive therapy is a valuable alternative for patients with severe mania that does not respond to other treatment.

◙ Recent major advances in bipolar disorder treatment research validate the efficacy of integrated psychosocial and pharmacologic treatment involving family or couples therapies, psychoeducational programs, and individual cognitive-behavioural or interpersonal therapies.

CRITICAL THINKING CHALLENGES

1 Describe how you would do a suicide assessment on a patient in a physician's office who comes in distraught and expressing concerns about her ability to cope with her current situation.

2 Describe how you would approach the patient described in the previous thinking challenge if you determined that she was suicidal.

3 Discuss difficulties in the differential diagnosis of bipolar disorder in the manic phase and other medical and psychiatric disorders. List the information you would use to rule out the other diagnosis when dealing with a patient who appears to have mania.

4 Describe how you would approach a patient who is expressing concern that the diagnosis of bipolar

disorder will negatively affect his or her social and work relationships.

5 Your depressed patient does not seem inclined to talk about his/her depression. Describe the measures you would take to initiate a therapeutic relationship with him/her.

6 Your patient with mania is experiencing physical hyperactivity that is interfering with his or her sleep and nutrition. Describe the actions you would take to meet the patient's needs for nutrition and rest.

7 Prepare a hypothetical discussion with a patient with potential bipolar disorder concerning the advantages and disadvantages of lithium versus divalproex sodium for treatment of bipolar disorder.

8 Prepare a hypothetical discussion with a depressed patient with potential unipolar disorder concerning the advantages and disadvantages of each of the major classifications of antidepressants.

WEB LINKS

www.camimh.ca Canadian Alliance on Mental Illness and Mental Health (CAMIMH). This site displays the services of member mental health organizations that include health care practitioners, consumers, and their families. The alliance strives for mental illness prevention and mental health promotion. Accessibility to care and support for the mentally ill and their families is at the top of their agenda.

www.mooddisorderscanada.ca Mood Disorders Society of Canada (MDSC). This is a volunteer organization with a commitment to optimizing the quality of life for people with mood disorders. The MDSC gives a voice to consumers by establishing a national research agenda and developing strategies of care.

www.nnmh.ca National Network for Mental Health. The network functions as an advocate and educational resource for Canadian mental health consumers and their families and friends. The organization's goal is to unite to empower individuals.

www.cpa.ca Canadian Psychological Association. The Association takes an advisory role to people wanting to know about issues and care alternatives. Areas of focus include mental health problems related to mood disorders and the psychological factors necessary to maintain wellness in the context of such mood-related disorders.

www.cmha.ca Canadian Mental Health Association (CMHA). This organization uses a wellness model to approach such topics as mental fitness and how it is defined, acquired, and maintained across the life span.

www.suicideprevention.ca Canadian Association for Suicide Prevention. This site has information regarding suicide and the resources related to its prevention, for example, the location of crisis centers, survivor support groups, and related library materials. Guidelines to minimize the suicide risk of loved ones are available here.

obad@telusplanet.net Organization for Bipolar Affective Disorders (OBAD). This organization offers peer support for anyone affected by mood disorders, aiming to assist them to be active in their recovery and gain a sense of resolution in their lives.

www.nimh.nih.gov/practitioners/patinfo.cfm National Institutes of Mental Health (NIMH). This website of the National Institutes of Mental Health offers education information pamphlets on depression, bipolar disorder, and other mental illnesses that can be ordered or printed free of charge. These publications are in the public domain and can be reproduced without copyright infringement, as long as authorship is acknowledged.

www.bpkids.org Child and Adolescent Bipolar Foundation (CABF). This parent-led, not-for-profit membership organization maintains an extensive website of information and support for families and youth who have bipolar disorder. The organization has a large professional advisory board of experts in the field, including Kay Redfield Jamison, the author of *An Unquiet Mind*, a book about her own struggles with bipolar disorder. Most of the information is available to anyone visiting the website, but chat rooms, etc. are for members only. Membership is free for families, but there is a charge for professionals to belong to the organization.

www.psychguides.com A copy of the *Treatment of Bipolar Disorder: A Guide for Patients and Families* can be downloaded from this site.

MOVIES

About Schmidt. 2002. This movie is about a 67-year-old man, Warren Schmidt, played by Jack Nicholson, who retires from his job as an insurance company executive. He experiences work withdrawal and a lack of direction for his retirement. His wife, Helen, irritates him, and he has no idea what to do to fill his days. While watching television one day he is moved to sponsor a child in Africa with whom he begins a long, one-sided correspondence. When his wife dies unexpectedly, he is initially numb, then sad, and finally angry when he discovers that she had an affair with his best friend many years ago. He is estranged from his only daughter, Jeanie, whose wedding to Randall, a man he feels is beneath her, is imminent. The movie follows Warren as he searches for connection and meaning in his life.

SIGNIFICANCE: Warren Schmidt demonstrates a common phenomenon among the elderly when they retire. He also shows the impact of grief superimposed on initial dysthymia or depression.

VIEWING POINTS: Look for the changes in Schmidt's manifestations of depression in different situations. Note how he experiences the various stages of grieving. What do you think about Schmidt's search for significance and meaning in his life?

Mad Love. 1995. In this movie, Casey Roberts (Drew Barrymore), a pretty high school student, experiences bipolar disorder. Matt Leyland (Chris O'Donnell) is a fellow student who falls in love with her. Matt, unaware of Casey's medical condition and struggling with his own family issues, becomes enraptured with Casey and perceives her as a free spirit. When Casey attempts suicide and is admitted to a psychiatric unit, Matt helps her escape. To evade their parents, they embark on a trip to Mexico, a journey filled with misadventure. Despite Casey's erratic behaviour, Matt doesn't develop insight into Casey's illness until her behaviour becomes so disorganized that he must face it and try to help her get treatment and become well.

VIEWING POINTS: The euphoria, irritability, risk taking, poor judgment, and labile mood that are hallmarks of bipolar disorder are well illustrated in this movie, as is the depression that underlies mania. We can see the impact of bipolar disorder on loved ones. Look for Casey's inability to control her behaviour. Note her heightened perception of the sensory stimulation occurring around her. What other psychiatric diagnoses might resemble bipolar disorder? Consider the symptoms of borderline personality disorder, narcissistic disorder, and attention deficit hyperactivity disorder.

Mr. Jones. 1993. This film is about a musician, Mr. Jones, played by Richard Gere, and his psychiatrist. In his manic state, Mr. Jones is a charismatic, charming individual who persuades a contractor to hire him, proceeds to the roof of the building, and prepares to fly off the roof. He withdraws large sums of money from the bank. He knows that he has bipolar disorder but refuses to take his medication because of the side effects. He has episodes of depression during which he becomes suicidal. Once hospitalized, he struggles with trying to find a life on medication.

SIGNIFICANCE: Viewers can gain insight into the impact of mental illness on the promising career of a classical musician. This film illustrates the ways in which interpersonal relationships are affected by a psychiatric disorder. Unfortunately, the unethical romantic relationship between Mr. Jones and his psychiatrist detracts from the quality of the film's content.

VIEWING POINTS: Why does the diagnosis of paranoid schizophrenia not fit Mr. Jones' clinical picture in the admitting room? Identify the antecedents to the manic and depressive episodes. At what point is the physician–patient relationship first compromised? Are there early warning signs that should have alerted the psychiatrist that she was violating professional boundaries?

REFERENCES

Alda, M., & Grof, P. (2000). Genetics and lithium response in bipolar disorders. In J. C. Soares & S. Gershon (Eds.), *Bipolar disorders: Basic mechanisms and therapeutic implications* (pp. 529–543). New York: Marcel Dekker, Inc.

Alda, M. (2001). Genetic factors and treatment of mood disorders. *Bipolar Disorders, 3*(6), 318.

American Nurses Association. (2000). *Scope and standards of psychiatric–mental health clinical nursing practice.* Washington, DC: Author.

American Psychiatric Association (APA). (2000). *Diagnostic and statistical manual of mental disorders* (4th ed., Text revision). Washington, DC: Author.

American Psychiatric Association. (APA). (2000). *Desk reference to the diagnostic criteria from DSM-IV-TR.* Arlington, VA: Author.

American Psychiatric Association (APA). (2002). *Compendium of practice guideline for the treatment of psychiatric disorders.* Washington, DC: Author.

Angst, J., Angst, F., & Stassen, H. H. (1999). Suicide risk in patients with major depressive disorder. *Journal of Clinical Psychiatry, 60*(Suppl. 2), 57–62.

Arana, G. W., & Rosenbaum, J. F. (2000). *Handbook of psychiatric drug therapy* (4th ed.). Philadelphia: Lippincott Williams & Wilkins.

Belmaker, R. H., & Yaroslavsky, Y. (2000). Perspectives for new pharmacological interventions. In J. C. Soares & S. Gershon (Eds.), *Bipolar disorders: Basic mechanisms and therapeutic implications* (pp. 507–527). New York: Marcel Dekker, Inc.

Bernard, S. A., & Bruera, E. (2000). Drug interactions in palliative care. *Journal of Clinical Oncology, 18*(8), 1780–1799.

Blazer, D. G., Hybels, C. F., & Pieper, C. F. (2001). The association of depression and mortality in elderly persons: A case for multiple independent pathways. *Journal of Gerontology: Medical Sciences, 56A*(8), 505–509.

Bowden, C. L., Calabrese, J. R., McElroy S. L., Gyulai, L., Wassef, A., Petty, F., Pope, H. G., Chou, C. Y., Keck, P. E., Rhodes, L. J., Swann, A. C., Hirschfield, R. M. A., & Wozniak, P. J. (2000). A randomized placebo-controlled 12 month trial of divalproex and lithium in treatment of out patients with bipolar disorder. *Archives of General Psychiatry, 57,* 481–489.

Bowden, C. L., Calabrese, J. R., Sachs, G., Yatham, L. N., Asghar, S. A., Hompland, M., Montgomery, P., Earl, N., Smoot, T. M., & De-Veaugh-Geiss, J. (2003). A placebo-controlled 18-month trial of lamotrigine and lithium maintenance treatment in recently manic or hypomanic patients with bipolar 1 disorder. *Archives of General Psychiatry, 60*(4), 392–400.

Canadian Community Health Survey. (2004). Mental health and well-being (2004). Retrieved August 24, 2005, from http://www.statcan.ca/Daily/English/030903/d030903a.htm.

Canadian Nurses Association (CNA). (2005). Retrieved August 30, 2005, from http://cna-aiic.ca/CNA/practice/standards/default_ e.aspx.

Casacalenda, N., Perry, J. C., & Looper, K. (2002). Remission in major depressive disorder: A comparison of pharmacotherapy, psychotherapy, and control condition. *American Journal of Psychiatry, 159*(8), 1354–1360.

Cutler, J. L., & Marcus, E. R. (1999). Mood disorders. In *Psychiatry.* Philadelphia: WB Saunders.

Donati, R. J., & Rasenick, M. M. (2003). G protein signaling and the molecular basis of antidepressant action. *Life Science, 73*(1), 1–17.

Dubovsky, S. L. (2005). Treatment of bipolar depression. *Psychiatric Clinics of North America, 28*(2), 349–370.

Edmunds, K., & Kinnaird-Iler, E. (2005). In L. L. Stamler & L. Yiu (Eds.), *Community health nursing: A Canadian perspective* (pp. 247–264). Toronto: Pearson Prentice Hall.

Edinburgh Postnatal Depression Scale (1987). Retrieved August 28, 2005, from http://www.childbirthsolutions.com/articles/postpartum/epds/index.php.

Fagiolini, A., Kupfer, D. J., Houck, P. R., Novick, D. M., & Frank, E. (2003). Obesity as a correlate of outcome in patients with bipolar I disorder. *American Journal of Psychiatry, 160*(1), 112–117.

Fischer, C. E. (2002). A clinician's guide to interpreting cognitive measures in clinical trials for Alzheimer's disease. *Canadian Journal of Psychiatry.* Retrieved August 31, 2005, from http://cpa-apc.org/Publications/Archives/Bulletin/2002/june/geriatricPsych.asp.

Glod, C. A., & Baisden, N. (1999). Seasonal affective disorder in children and adolescents. *Journal of the American Psychiatric Nurses Association (Psychobiology Perspectives), 5*(1), 29–31.

Goldberg, J. F., Garno, J. L., Leon, A. C., et al. (1999). A history of substance abuse complicates remission from acute mania in bipolar disorder. *Journal of Clinical Psychiatry, 60,* 733–740.

Grunze, H., Amann, B., Dittmann, S., & Walden, J. (2002). Clinical relevance and possibilities of bipolar rapid cycling. *Neuropsychobiology, 45*(Suppl 1), 20–26.

Gutman, D. (2002). Remission in depression and the mind-body link. Retrieved August 23, 2005, from http://www.medscape.com/viewprogram/2067_pnt.

Hanley, N. R., & Van de Kar, L. D. (2003). Serotonin and the neuroendocrine regulation of the hypothalamic-pituitary-adrenal axis in health and disease. *Vitamins and Hormones: Advances in Research and Applications, 66,* 189–225.

Health Canada. (2002). *A Report on Mental Illness in Canada.* Ottawa: Author.

Hirschfeld, R. M., Baker, J. D., Wozniak, P., Tracy, K., & Sommerville, K. W. (2003). The safety and early efficacy of oral-loaded divalproex versus standard-titration divalproex, lithium, olanzapine, and placebo in the treatment of acute mania associated with bipolar disorder. *Journal of Clinical Psychiatry, 64*(7), 841–846.

Hirschfeld, R. M., Lewis, L., & Vornik, L. A. (2003). Perceptions and impact of bipolar disorder: How far have we really come? Results of the national depressive and manic-depressive association 2000 survey of individuals with bipolar disorders. *Journal of Clinical Psychiatry, 64*(2), 161–174.

How healthy are Canadians: Focus on mental health. (2004). Retrieved August 19, 2005, from http://www.statcan.ca/english/freepub/82-003-SIE/2004000/pdf/82-003-SIE2004000.pdf.

Jim Carrey. (2005). Retrieved August 29, 2005, from http://en.wikipedia.org/wiki/Jim_Carrey.

Johnson, L., Andersson-Lundman, G., Aberg-Wistedt, A., & Mathe, A. A. (2000). Age of onset in affective disorder: Its correlation with hereditary and psychosocial factors. *Journal of Affective Disorders, 59*(2), 139–148.

Kahn, D. A., Ross, R., Printz, D. J., & Sachs, G. S. (2000). Treatment of bipolar disorder: A guide for patients and families. In G. S. Sachs, D. J. Printz, D. A. Kahn, D. Carpenter, & J. P. Docherty (Eds.), The expert consensus guideline series: Medication treatment of bipolar disorder 2000. *Postgraduate Medicine Special Report,* April, pp. 1–8.

Keck, P. E., Mendlwicz, J., Calabrese, J. R., Fawcett, J., Suppes, T., Vestergaard, P. A., & Carbonell, C. (2000). A review of randomized controlled clinical trials in acute mania. *Journal of Affective Disorders, 59*(Suppl.1), 31–37.

King Blood, R. J. (2005). Aboriginal Canadians. In L. L. Stamler & L. Yiu (Eds.), *Community health nursing: A Canadian perspective* (pp. 239–246). Toronto: Pearson Prentice Hall.

Kowatch, R. A., & DelBello, M. P. (2005). Pharmacotherapy of children and adolescents with bipolar disorder. *Psychiatric Clinics of North America, 28*(2), 385–397.

Kronfol, Z., & Remick, D. G. (2000). Cytokines and the brain: Implications for clinical psychiatry. *American Journal of Psychiatry, 157*(5), 683–694.

Lam, R. W., & Kennedy, S. H. (2005). Prescribing antidepressants for depression in 2005: Recent concerns and recommendations. *Canadian Journal of Psychiatry, 49*(12).

Maser, J. D., Akiskal, H. S., Schettler, P., Scheftner, W., Mueller, T., Endicott, J., Solomon, D., & Clayton, P. (2002). Can temperament identify affectively ill patients who engage in lethal or near-lethal suicidal behaviour? A 14-year prospective study. *Suicide Life Threatening Behavior, 32*(1), 10–32.

McCuffin, P., Rijsdijk, F., Andrew, J., Sham, P., Katz, R., & Cardno, A. (2003). The heritability of bipolar affective disorder and the genetic relationship to unipolar depression. *Archives of General Psychiatry, 60*(5), 497–502.

McCuistion, L. E., & Gutierrez, K. J. (2002). *Real-world nursing survival guide: Pharmacology.* Philadelphia: WB Saunders.

McDonald, W. M. (2000). Epidemiology, etiology, and treatment of geriatric mania. *Journal of Clinical Psychiatry, 61*(Suppl. 13), 3–11.

McElheran, W., Eaton, P., Rupcich, C., Basinger, M., & Johnston, D. (2004). Shared mental health care: The Calgary model. *Families Systems, & Health, 22*(4), 424–438.

Mead, D. E. (2002). Marital distress, co-occurring depression, and marital therapy: Review. *Journal of Marital and Family Therapy, 28*(3), 299–314.

Mohr, W. (2001). Bipolar disorder in children. *Journal of Psychosocial Nursing, 39*(3), 12–23.

National Population Health Survey. (2004). The people: Major causes of death. Retrieved August 25, 2005, from http://142.206.72.67/02/02b/02b_003_e.htm.

Nolan, S., & Scoggin, J. A. (2001). Serotonin syndrome: Recognition and management. *US Pharmacist, 23*(2). www.uspharmacist.com.

Osuji, I. J., & Cullum, C. M. (2005). Cognition in bipolar disorder. *Psychiatric Clinics of North America, 28*(2), 427–441.

Payne, J. L., Potash, J. B., & DePaulo, J. R. (2005). Recent findings on the genetic basis of bipolar disorder. *Psychiatric Clinics of North America, 28*(2), 481–498.

Rea, M. M., Tompson, M. C., Miklowitz, D. J., Goldstein, M. J., Hwang, S., & Mintz, J. (2003). Family-focused treatment versus individual treatment for bipolar disorder: Results of a randomized clinical trial. *Journal of Consulting Clinical Psychology, 71*(3), 482–492.

Remick, R. A. (2002). Diagnosis and management of depression in primary care: A clinical update and review. *Canadian Medical Association, 167*(11).

Rothbaum, B. O., & Astin, M. C. (2000). Integration of pharmacotherapy and psychotherapy for bipolar disorder. *Journal of Clinical Psychiatry, 61*(Suppl. 9), 68–75.

Schatzberg, A. F., Cole, J. O., & DeBattista, C. (2003). *Manual of clinical psychopharmacology* (4th ed.). Washington, DC: American Psychiatric Publishing, Inc.

Scott, J., & Colom, F. (2005). Psychosocial treatments for bipolar disorders. *Psychiatric Clinics of North America, 28*(2), 371–384.

Sheline, Y. I. (2003). Neuroimaging studies of mood disorder effects on the brain. *Biological Psychiatry, 54*(3), 338–352.

Sorenson, S. (2002). Serotonin syndrome. *Utox Update, 4*(4), 1–2.

Stahl, S. (2000). *Essential psychopharmacology: Neuroscientific basis and practical applications.* Cambridge: Cambridge University Press.

Strakowski, S. M., & Sax, K. W. (2000). Secondary mania: A model of the pathophysiology of bipolar disorder. In J. C. Soares & S. Gershon (Eds.), *Bipolar disorders: Basic mechanisms and therapeutic implications.* New York: Marcel Dekker, Inc.

Suppes, T., Leverich, G. S., Keck, P. E, Nolan, W. A., Denicoff, K. D., Altschuler, L. L., McElroy, S. L., Rush, A. J., Kupka, R., Frye, M. A., Bickel, M., & Post, R. M. (2001, December). The Stanley Foundation for bipolar treatment outcome network: Demographics and illness characteristics of the first 261 patients. *Journal of Affective Disorders, 67*(1–3), 45–59.

Supplement to Health Reports. (2004). Bipolar disorder, social support and work. Retrieved August 24, 2005, from http://www.statcan.ca/Daily/English/030903/d030903a.htm.

Thase, M. E. (2000). Modulation of biological factors by psychotherapeutic interventions. In J. C. Soares & S. Gershon (Eds.), *Bipolar disorders: Basic mechanisms and therapeutic implications*. New York: Marcel Dekker, Inc.

Thase, M. E., & Sachs, G. S. (2000). Bipolar depression: Pharmacotherapy and related therapeutic strategies. *Biological Psychiatry, 48*, 558–572.

Today's News Releases From the Daily. (2005). Retrieved August 24, 2005, from http://www.statcan.ca/start.html.

Tryssenaar, J., Chui, A., & Finch, L. (2003). Growing older: The lived experience of older persons with serious mental illness. *Canadian Journal of Community Mental Health, 22*(1), 21–36.

United States Department of Health and Human Services (U.S. DHHS). (1999). *Mental Health: A report of the Surgeon General.* Rockville, MD: U.S. DHHS, Substance Abuse and Mental Health Services Administration, Center for Mental Health Services, National Institutes of Health, National Institute of Mental Health.

Wright, L. M., & Leahey, M. (2000). *Nurses and families: A guide to family assessment and intervention* (3rd ed.). Philadelphia: FA Davis.

Yildiz, A., & Sachs, G. S. (2003). Do antidepressants induce rapid cycling? A gender-specific association. *Journal of Clinical Psychiatry, 64*(7), 814–818.

Zahourek, R. (2000). Alternative, complementary or integrative approaches to treating depression. *Journal of the American Psychiatric Nurses Association, 6*(3), 77–86.

20

Anxiety Disorders

Robert B. Noud, Kathy Lee,
and Kathleen Hegadoren

LEARNING OBJECTIVES

After studying this chapter, you will be able to:

- Differentiate normal anxiety responses to stressors and fear from responses suggestive of an anxiety disorder.
- Discuss the epidemiology, etiology, symptomatology, and treatment of selected anxiety disorders.
- Discuss relevant theories and neurobiologic correlates of the anxiety disorders.
- Discuss biopsychosocial treatment approaches used for patients with anxiety disorders.
- Identify nursing diagnoses used in providing nursing care for patients with anxiety disorders.
- Develop a nursing care plan through the continuum of care for patients with panic disorder.
- Identify biopsychosocial indicators for four levels of anxiety and nursing interventions appropriate for each level.

KEY TERMS

agoraphobia ▪ allostasis ▪ anxiolytic ▪ depersonalization ▪ distraction ▪ exposure therapy ▪ flooding ▪ implosive therapy ▪ interoceptive conditioning ▪ panic attacks ▪ panic control treatment ▪ panicogenic ▪ phobia ▪ positive self-talk ▪ systematic desensitization

⬠ KEY CONCEPTS

anxiety ▪ compulsions ▪ obsessions ▪ panic

Anxiety is an uncomfortable feeling of apprehension or dread that occurs in response to internal or external stimuli and can result in physical, emotional, cognitive, and behavioural symptoms. All symptoms of anxiety disorders can be found in healthy individuals given particular circumstances.

Symptoms of anxiety that negatively affect the individual's ability to function in work or interpersonal relationships are considered symptomatic of an anxiety disorder. The anxiety disorders discussed in this chapter include panic disorder, obsessive-compulsive disorder (OCD), generalized anxiety disorder, phobias, posttraumatic stress disorder (PTSD), and acute stress disorder. Dissociative disorders are not classified as anxiety disorders; however, they are included as part of this chapter because overwhelming anxiety is a cardinal symptom of these disorders.

Panic disorder receives particular attention in this chapter, in part because of the frequency with which people experiencing panic symptoms seek emergency medical care. There is also significant overlap of symptoms and interventions applicable to other anxiety disorders. OCD is highlighted because patients with this disorder often do not seek medical attention and because diagnosing and treating this condition is difficult.

Normal Versus Abnormal Anxiety Response

Anxiety is an unavoidable human condition that takes many forms and serves different purposes. One's response to anxiety can be positive and motivate one to act, or it can produce paralyzing fear, causing inaction. Normal anxiety is described as being of realistic intensity and duration for the situation and is followed by relief behaviours intended to reduce or prevent more anxiety (Peplau, 1989). Normal anxiety response is appropriate to the situation, can be dealt with without repression, and can be used to help the patient identify what underlying problem has caused the anxiety.

McEwen (2005) conceptualizes normal responses as **allostasis**, the adaptive processes that maintain homeostasis through the production of various brain and peripheral stress-related chemicals. These mediators of our stress responses promote adaptation to perceived threat or stress. However, they also contribute to allostatic overload, the cumulative wear and tear on biological systems that can increase risk for stress-related disorders and physical health problems like cardiovascular and metabolic disorders (McEwen, 2005). During a perceived threat, rising anxiety levels cause physical and emotional changes in all individuals. A normal emotional response to anxiety consists of three parts: physiologic arousal, cognitive processes, and coping strategies. Physiologic arousal, or the fight-or-flight response, is the signal that an individual

is facing a threat. Cognitive processes decipher the situation and decide whether the perceived threat should be approached or avoided. Coping strategies are employed to resolve the threat. Table 20-1 summarizes many physical, affective, cognitive, and behavioural symptoms associated with anxiety. The factors that determine whether anxiety is a symptom of a mental disorder are the intensity of anxiety relative to the situation, the trigger for the anxiety, the particular symptom clusters that are associated with the anxiety, and the impact on day-to-day functioning.

Overview of Anxiety Disorders

Anxiety disorders are the most common of the psychiatric illnesses treated by health care providers. Direct and indirect costs of treating anxiety disorders are in the tens of billions of dollars. An estimated 19 million people are affected by anxiety disorders. Women experience anxiety disorders more often than do men (Dickstein, 2000). For example, the prevalence of generalized anxiety disorder is 3.6% in men and 6.6% in women, with increasing rates in both sexes by age (Wittchen et al., 1999). Posttraumatic stress disorder, panic disorder, and phobias are also overrepresented in women (Bland et al., 1988; Breslau et al., 1991). At high risk are smokers, individuals younger than 45 years, those separated or divorced, and survivors of abuse. Some anxiety disorders show evidence of genetic vulnerability, especially panic disorder, obsessive-compulsive disorder, and phobias (Hettema et al., 2001). Links have been shown between serotonin transporter and specific brain enzyme polymorphisms and anxiety-related personality in women (Enoch et al., 2003; Melke et al., 2001).

Anxiety disorders affect individuals of all ages. Edmonton studies have found prevalence rates of anxiety disorder in adults (18 years and older) to be 6.5% (Bland et al., 1988) and in elderly people (65 years and older) to be 3.1% (Newman et al., 1998). The lifetime prevalence rate of social anxiety disorder is reported to be about 10% (Sareen & Stein, 2000). Of depressed elderly patients, 35% will have at least one anxiety disorder diagnosis (Lenze et al., 2000). Anxiety disorders are the psychiatric disorders most frequently treated in children, with the percentage of children affected comparable to that of asthma (Castellanos & Hunter, 2000). Some evidence suggests a relationship between childhood separation anxiety disorder and atopic disorders (asthma, hives, hay fever, and eczema) and adult-onset panic disorder (Slattery et al., 2002). Indeed, symptoms of obsessive-compulsive disorder (OCD) and social anxiety disorder often begin in adolescence (Regier et al., 1998). Young patients with anxiety disorders often experience separation anxiety disorder, but this is often underacknowledged because fear of

Table 20.1   Symptoms of Anxiety

Physical

Cardiovascular

Sympathetic
Palpitations
Heart racing
Increased blood pressure

Parasympathetic
Actual fainting
Decreased blood pressure
Decreased pulse rate

Respiratory
Rapid breathing
Difficulty getting air
Shortness of breath
Pressure of chest
Shallow breathing
Lump in throat
Choking sensations
Gasping

Parasympathetic
Spasm of bronchi

Neuromuscular
Increased reflexes
Startle reaction
Eyelid twitching
Insomnia
Tremors
Rigidity
Spasm
Fidgeting
Pacing
Strained face
Unsteadiness
Generalized weakness
Wobbly legs
Clumsy motions

Skin
Face flushed
Face pale
Localized sweating (palm region)
Generalized sweating
Hot and cold spells
Itching

Gastrointestinal
Loss of appetite
Revulsion toward food
Abdominal discomfort
Diarrhea

Parasympathetic
Abdominal pain
Nausea
Heartburn
Vomiting

Eyes
Dilated pupils

Urinary Tract

Parasympathetic
Pressure to urinate
Increased frequency of urination

Affective

Edgy
Impatient
Uneasy
Nervous
Tense
Wound-up
Anxious
Apprehensive
Frightened
Alarmed
Terrified
Jittery

Cognitive

Sensory-Perceptual
Mind is hazy, cloudy, foggy, dazed
Objects seem blurred/distant
Environment seems different/unreal
Feelings of unreality/depersonalization
Self-consciousness
Hypervigilance

Thinking Difficulties
Cannot recall important things
Confused
Unable to control thinking
Difficulty concentrating
Difficulty focussing attention
Blocking
Loss of objectivity and perspective

Conceptual
Cognitive distortion
Fear of losing control
Fear of not being able to cope
Fear of physical injury or death
Fear of mental disorder
Fear of negative evaluations
Frightening visual images
Repetitive fearful ideation

Behavioural

Inhibited
Tonic immobility
Flight
Avoidance
Speech dysfluency
Impaired coordination
Restlessness
Postural collapse
Hyperventilation
Jumpy

Adapted from Beck, A. T., & Emery, C. (1985). *Anxiety disorders and phobias: A cognitive perspective* (pp. 23–27). New York: Basic Books.

strangers and other signs of anxiety are considered developmentally appropriate. Children and adolescents with anxiety disorders have higher rates of suicidal behaviour, early parenthood, drug and alcohol dependence, and educational underachievement later in life (Woodward, 2001).

Left untreated, anxiety symptoms persist, gradually worsen, and increase risk for other psychiatric disorders. Comorbidity is very common and shows some gender specificity, with substance use disorder more common in men. Major depressive disorder is a frequent comorbid diagnosis in both males and females.

Panic Disorder

Panic is an extreme, overwhelming form of anxiety often experienced when an individual is placed in a real or perceived life-threatening situation. Panic can be normal in response to a serious threat, but abnormal when it becomes more frequent and generalizes to situations that pose no real physical or psychological threat. Some people experience heightened anxiety because they fear experiencing another panic attack. This type of panic interferes with the individual's ability to function in everyday life and is characteristic of panic disorder.

> ⬟ **KEY CONCEPT Panic** can be a normal, but extreme, overwhelming form of anxiety often initiated when an individual is placed in a real or perceived life-threatening situation.

CLINICAL COURSE OF PANIC DISORDER

Panic disorder is a lifelong disorder that typically peaks in the teenage years and then again in the 30s, but can surface in childhood or after the fourth decade of life (American Psychiatric Association [APA], 2000). Six-month prevalence rates differ between men (0.4%) and women (1.0%) (Bland et al., 1988). Men and women show similar age of onset, but premorbid mood disorders and stressful life events are more common in women (Barzega et al., 2001). Panic disorder is treatable, but studies have shown that even after years of treatment, many cases remain symptomatic (APA, 2000; Gardos, 2000). In some cases, symptoms may even worsen.

Panic disorder is a chronic condition that has several exacerbations and remissions during the course of the disease. It is characterized by the appearance of disabling attacks of panic that often lead to other anxiety and mood disorders.

PANIC ATTACKS

Panic attacks are sudden, short periods of intense fear or discomfort that are accompanied by significant physical and cognitive symptoms. The physical symptoms are listed in Box 20-1 and reflect cardiorespiratory and gastrointestinal symptoms. Cognitive symptoms include disorganized thinking, irrational fears, depersonalization, and decreased ability to communicate. Feelings of impending doom or death, fear of going crazy or losing control, and desperation are common.

CRNE Note

Physical symptoms of panic attack are similar to cardiac emergencies. These symptoms are physically taxing and psychologically frightening to patients. Recognition of the seriousness of panic attacks should be communicated to the patient.

A panic attack usually peaks at 10 minutes, but the effects can last as long as 30 minutes, followed by a gradual return to normal functioning. Individuals with panic disorder experience recurrent, unexpected panic attacks followed by persistent concern about experiencing subsequent panic attacks. They fear implications of the attacks, and they have behavioural changes related to the attacks (APA, 2000).

Panic attacks cause fear of death because they mimic symptoms of a heart attack. Individuals often seek emergency medical care because they feel as if they are dying, but most will have a negative cardiac workup. People experiencing panic attacks may also believe that the attacks stem from an underlying major medical illness (APA, 2000). Even with sound medical testing and assurance of no underlying disease, these people often remain unconvinced. Panic attacks can occur in individuals first experiencing certain anxiety-provoking medical conditions, such as asthma, or in initial trials of illicit substance use. However, individuals with panic disorder continue to experience panic attacks with or without predisposing conditions (Box 20-2). Panic attacks can be either internally or externally driven. Externally driven panic attacks may result, for example, from actually seeing a feared object. An internally driven panic attack results from an

BOX 20.1

Panic Attacks

Discrete period of intense fear or discomfort with four (or more) of the following symptoms that develop abruptly and reach a peak within 10 minutes:

Palpitations, pounding heart, or accelerated heart rate	Sweating
Sensations of shortness of breath or smothering	Trembling or shaking
Feelings of choking	Nausea or vomiting
Chest pain or discomfort	Chills or hot flushes
Depersonalization (feeling detached from oneself)	Derealization (feeling of unreality)
Paresthesias (numbness or tingling sensations)	Fear of dying
Feeling dizzy, unsteady, light-headed, or faint	Fear of losing control or going crazy

M, a 22-year-old man, has experienced several life changes, including a recent engagement, loss of his father to cancer and heart disease, graduation from college, and entrance to the workforce as a computer engineer in a large inner-city company. Because of his active lifestyle, his sleep habits have been poor. He frequently uses sleeping aids at night and now drinks a full pot of coffee to start each day. He has started smoking to "relieve the stress." While sitting in heavy traffic on the way to work, he suddenly experienced chest tightness, sweating, shortness of breath, feelings of being "trapped," and foreboding that he was going to die. Fearing a heart attack, he went to an emergency room, where his discomfort subsided within a half hour. After several hours of testing, the doctor informed him that his heart was healthy. During the next few weeks, he experienced several episodes of feeling trapped and slight chest discomfort on his drive to work. He fears future "attacks" while sitting in traffic and while in his crowded office cubicle.

What Do You Think?

- What risk factors does M have that might contribute to the development of panic attacks?
- What lifestyle changes do you think would help M reduce stress?

Panic Disorder Without Agoraphobia

Recurrent unexpected panic attacks and 1 month or more (after an attack) of one of the following:
- Persistent concern about additional attacks
- Worry about the implications of the attack or its consequences
- Significant changes in behaviour related to the attacks

Not a direct physiologic effect of a substance or medical condition

Panic Disorder With Agoraphobia

Meets criteria for panic disorder, including panic attacks

Not better accounted for by any another mental disorder, such as a specific phobia or social phobia (eg, avoidance limited to social situations because of fear of embarrassment)

Agoraphobia:

Anxiety about being in places or situations from which escape might be difficult (or embarrassing) or in which help may not be available in the event of having an unexpected or situationally predisposed panic attack or panic-like symptoms

Fears typically involve characteristic clusters of situations that include being outside the home alone; being in a crowd or standing in a line; being on a bridge; and traveling in a bus, train, or automobile

Situations are avoided (eg, travel is restricted) or endured, with marked distress or anxiety about having a panic attack or panic-like symptoms; or the presence of a companion is required

uncomfortable, internal feeling. Sensations of being too hot or cramped in a small room might provoke panic attacks. APA (2000) defines these categories.

DIAGNOSTIC CRITERIA

Panic disorder is characterized by the onset of panic attacks. A person who has a diagnosis of panic attacks has periods of intense fear, at which time at least four physical or psychological symptoms are manifested. These symptoms include palpitations, sweating, shaking, shortness of breath or smothering, sensations of choking, chest pain, nausea or abdominal distress, dizziness, derealization or depersonalization, fear of going crazy, fear of dying, paresthesias, and chills or hot flashes (APA, 2000).

There are two types of panic disorder: with and without agoraphobia. Both types include recurrent and unexpected panic attacks, followed by 1 month or more of consistent concern about having another attack, worrying about the consequences of having another attack, or changing behaviour because of fear of the attacks (Box 20-3).

EPIDEMIOLOGY

Panic disorder can be found in almost 1.6% of the general population (2.9 million) at any given time, according to the Epidemiological Catchment Area survey. Six-month

prevalence rates were reported by an Edmonton group to be 0.4% in males and 1.0% in females (Bland et al., 1988), whereas others have found lifetime rates to be as high as 6.8% (Wang et al., 2000). It is highly associated with depression, medical conditions including hypertension, and cigarette smoking. Patients experiencing panic disorder with agoraphobia tend to have more coexisting anxiety disorders, anxiety attacks, and anticipatory anxiety than do patients who have panic disorder without agoraphobia. Women appear more likely to experience panic disorder with agoraphobia and more likely to experience panic symptoms after remission (Sheikh, Leskin, & Klein, 2002).

Agoraphobia and Other Phobias

Panic attacks can lead to the development of phobias, or persistent, unrealistic fears of situations, objects, or activities. People with phobias will go to great lengths to avoid the feared objects or situations to deter panic attacks. Box 20-4 presents examples of common phobias. Agoraphobia, fear of open spaces, often co-occurs

Phobia

Acrophobia (fear of heights)
Agoraphobia (fear of open spaces)
Ailurophobia (fear of cats)
Algophobia (fear of pain)
Arachnophobia (fear of spiders)
Brontophobia (fear of thunder)
Claustrophobia (fear of closed spaces)
Cynophobia (fear of dogs)
Entomophobia (fear of insects)
Hematophobia (fear of blood)
Microphobia (fear of germs)
Nyctophobia (fear of night or dark places)
Ophidiophobia (fear of snakes)
Phonophobia (fear of loud noises)
Photophobia (fear of light)
Pyrophobia (fear of fire)
Topophobia (stage fright)
Xenophobia (fear of strangers)
Zoophobia (fear of animal or animals)

with panic disorder. Agoraphobia can lead to avoidance behaviours. It begins with an intense, irrational fear of being in open spaces, being alone, or being in public places where escape might be difficult or embarrassing. The person fears that if a panic attack occurred, help would not be available, so he or she avoids such situations. Such avoidance interferes with routine functioning and eventually renders the person afraid to leave the safety of home. Some affected individuals continue to face feared situations, but with significant trepidation (ie, going in public only to pay bills, or to take children to school).

In many cases, agoraphobia develops quickly after a few panic attacks, but the resulting avoidance behaviours do not decrease the severity of the panic attacks (APA, 2000). Other patients can reduce panic attacks by dodging certain instances that precipitate attacks. Many of these individuals may be able to confront a situation if accompanied by someone else; for example, going out in public may be manageable with a friend.

ETIOLOGY

Genetic Theories

There appears to be a substantial familial predisposition to panic disorder. A meta-analysis of the genetic epidemiology of anxiety disorder found that genes account for 30% to 40% of the risk for panic disorder and that the risk for first-degree relatives is five times that of the general population (Hettema et al., 2001). If the family member manifests panic disorder before 20 years of age, the risk in family members jumps to 20 times that of the general population (APA, 2000). Twin studies have found the occurrence of panic attacks to be as much as five times more frequent in monozygotic than in dizygotic twins, suggesting that parenting and other environmental factors cannot wholly account for the development of panic disorder in adolescents. However, social conditioning may play a role in anxiety sensitivity or overestimating the degree of threat, both of which may increase risk for developing anxiety disorders.

Neuroanatomic Correlates

Certain neurologic abnormalities have been detected by magnetic resonance imaging in patients with panic disorder. The most common abnormalities are focal areas of abnormal activity in the fear network of the brain. This network includes the central nucleus of the amygdala, the hippocampus, and the periaqueductal gray area in the brain (Gorman, Kent, Sullivan, & Coplan, 2000). The amygdala and the hippocampus are integral parts of memory storage and emotion regulation. Abnormalities in these areas may indicate dysfunctional signalling between the various brain regions.

Biochemical Theories

Identification of neurotransmitter involvement in panic disorder has evolved from neurochemical studies with **panicogenic** substances known to produce panic attacks, such as yohimbine, norepinephrine, epinephrine, pentagastrin, sodium lactate, and carbon dioxide (CO_2). In addition, by knowing the pharmacodynamics of medications that reduce panic episodes, investigators have been able to hypothesize which neurotransmitters are involved in panic disorder.

Norepinephrine

Norepinephrine is implicated in panic disorders because of its effects on the systems most affected during a panic attack—the cardiovascular, respiratory, and gastrointestinal systems. Cell bodies of norepinephrine neurons in the brain are located in the locus ceruleus, which is one of the internal regulators of numerous biologic rhythms. The cell bodies make extensive projections to the cerebral cortex, cerebellum, limbic system, and spinal cord, as well as to the sympathetic nervous system. Electrical stimulation of the locus ceruleus in monkeys increases fear and anxiety. Norepinephrine effects are mediated by two types of receptors, alpha and beta, both having important subtypes, which contribute to the complexities of understanding the role of norepinephrine in panic disorder. Some drugs, such as propranolol, act primarily on beta-adrenergic receptors, reducing the peripheral symptoms of anxiety, but with limited effectiveness against panic disorder.

Accumulated evidence indicates that a dysregulation of the norepinephrine system may exist in panic disorder. Drugs that increase activity of the locus ceruleus often are panicogenic in individuals who have panic disorder but not in healthy subjects. For example, yohimbine, an alpha$_2$-receptor antagonist, increases the firing rate of norepinephrine neurons, which increases the release of norepinephrine and evokes increasing anxiety symptoms (Sallee, Sethuraman, Sine, & Liu, 2000).

Drugs that inhibit norepinephrine release are thought to be **anxiolytic**, meaning that they diminish anxiety symptoms. Medications such as propranolol and tricyclic antidepressants (TCAs) act on norepinephrine systems. However, only the TCAs have shown efficacy in the treatment of panic disorder.

Serotonin

Serotonin (5-HT) was indirectly implicated in the etiology of panic disorder when it was discovered that drugs that facilitate serotonergic neurotransmission were effective in relieving symptoms of panic disorder. Selective serotonin reuptake inhibitors (SSRIs) may impede the panic response by decreasing activity in the amygdala and interfering with transmission to extension sites in the hypothalamus (Gorman et al., 2000). These drugs can be activating and may initially increase anxiety symptoms. They produce symptom relief after 2 to 6 weeks of treatment.

Although serotonin may be involved in panic disorder, the responsible serotonin circuits and receptor subtypes are unknown. Serotonin systems and their multiple complex interactions with many other neurotransmitter systems make it difficult to identify any primary functional deficits. For example, serotonin and norepinephrine each can affect the release of the other from nerve terminals, suggesting reciprocal roles in regulating the interaction between these neurotransmitters and their respective receptors.

Gamma-Aminobutyric Acid

Gamma-aminobutyric acid (GABA) is the most abundant inhibitory neurotransmitter in the brain, and very small GABA neurons, called interneurons, affect the firing rates of neurons distributed throughout the brain, which explains why GABA has such global effects, such as overall electrical activity, memory processing, anxiety, and level of consciousness. Thus, depending on dose, activation of GABA neurons produces anticonvulsant, anxiolytic, or hypnotic actions, but, at the same time, can affect the creation of memory as events happen (called anterograde memory). Most of these effects are mediated through the GABA$_A$ receptor complex, a cell membrane ion channel specific to chloride ions. When GABA binds to this receptor, chloride ions flow into the cell, preventing that cell from firing. This receptor complex has binding sites for benzodiazepines, barbiturates, alcohol, and progesterone. These drugs and hormones potentiate GABA effects.

Although drugs that enhance GABA have anxiolytics properties, it has been difficult to tease out any abnormalities in GABA systems. However, newer neuroimaging techniques such as positron emission tomography, single-photon emission computed tomography, magnetic resonance imaging, and magnetic resonance spectroscopy may hold promise for providing more direct information about GABA and its role in anxiety and anxiety disorders.

Corticotropin-Releasing Factor

Corticotropin-releasing factor (CRF) is a neuropeptide that has widespread effects in the brain and in one of the major stress response systems, the hypothalamic-pituitary-adrenal (HPA) axis. CRF receptors are widely distributed in the hypothalamus, as well as the frontal cortex, amygdala, hippocampus, and locus ceruleus. Cortisol, the main output of the HPA axis, is significantly elevated during panic attacks (Bandelow et al., 2000). CRF and norepinephrine interact to regulate each other's release from nerve cells.

Cholecystokinin

Cholecystokinin (CCK) is another neuropeptide that has been implicated in the etiology of panic attacks. High concentrations of CCK are found in the cerebral cortex, the amygdala, and the hippocampus, areas implicated in fear and stress responses. Two subtypes of CCK receptors have been identified: CCK-A and CCK-B. CCK-A receptors are predominant in the peripheral systems; CCK-B receptors are widely distributed throughout the brain, particularly in the limbic system and cortex. When administered in challenge tests, CCK induces panic attacks in patients with panic disorder and, to a much lesser degree, in people without panic disorder (Bradwejn et al., 1992).

Other Neuropeptides

Evidence of altered growth hormone (GH) activity in patients with panic disorder provides additional support for the role of the hypothalamus in panic disorder. In healthy subjects, stimulating alpha-adrenergic receptors elevate GH. This process is blunted in individuals with panic disorder (Sallee et al., 2000). Another area of research implicates neuroactive steroids, including the various metabolites of progesterone, in the development of panic attacks (Strohle et al., 2003). This may contribute to the female gender bias observed in panic disorder.

Other Panicogenic Substances

In challenge tests, sodium bicarbonate, sodium lactate, and CO_2 induced panic attacks in people with panic disorders. CO_2 is the by-product of both sodium bicarbonate and lactate. It readily crosses the blood–brain barrier, producing transient cerebral hypercapnia. Hypercapnia stimulates CO_2 receptors, causing hyperventilation and, for vulnerable individuals, panic symptoms. Individuals with panic disorder may have hypersensitivity to CO_2 and subsequently experience a sensation of suffocation immediately before panic attacks. This effect may be directly related to the action of CO_2 on areas in the hypothalamus that regulate breathing and the interaction of these areas with noradrenergic pathways (Ben-Zion et al., 1999). Studies have been conducted in patients with panic disorder to detect cerebral blood flow abnormalities during panic attacks. Ponto and colleagues (2002) discovered abnormal patterns of cerebral blood flow in patients with symptomatic panic disorder after CO_2 inhalation. Patients who panic during intravenous challenges with sodium lactate have exhibited asymmetrical blood flow to various regions of the brain. However, hyperventilation is inherent in the panic process, which causes hypocapnia-induced vasoconstriction of blood vessels. Therefore, abnormal cerebral blood flow may be related to the hyperventilation, not directly to the panic attack, and measurements of accurate rates of blood flow may be distorted (Gorman et al., 2000).

Psychodynamic Theories

Psychodynamic theories contribute to the understanding of panic disorders by explaining the importance of the development of anxiety after separation and loss. Patients with panic disorder report greater numbers and severity of recent personal losses at symptom onset than do healthy control subjects. In a study of the background and personality traits of individuals with panic disorder, several commonalities were found, including being fearful or shy as a child; remembering their parents as angry, critical, or frightening; having feelings of discomfort with aggression; having long-term feelings of low self-esteem; and experiencing a stressful life event associated with frustration and resentment that preceded the initial onset of symptoms (Shear et al., 1993). These researchers proposed the following theory of causation. The child may begin with a neurophysiologic vulnerability that predisposes one to fearfulness. This fearfulness is enhanced by parental behaviour in some way, which results in disturbed parent–child relationships and causes the child to feel conflict about dependence and independence (separating from parent), self-doubt and confusion regarding self-identity, and personal control. These

negative feelings of low self-esteem and powerlessness appear to make the individual feel extremely vulnerable to the stress of normal life events, such as going to school, getting married, or becoming a parent. As the person attempts to ignore these negative feelings and seems powerless to control them, he or she continues to experience distress in repeated stressful events. The chronic, intense fear and dread culminate in the first panic attack. However, similar dynamics can also explain the emergence of depression. Factors that determine the specific clinical presentation and health outcomes related to chronic childhood psychological problems remain elusive.

Cognitive-Behavioural Theories

Learning theory underlies most cognitive-behavioural theories of panic disorder. Classic conditioning theory suggests that one learns a fear response by linking an adverse or fear-provoking event, such as a car accident, with a previously neutral event, such as crossing a bridge. One becomes conditioned to associate fear with crossing a bridge. Applying this theory to people with panic disorder has limitations. Phobic avoidance is not always developed secondary to an adverse event.

Further development of this theory led to an understanding of **interoceptive conditioning**, which pairs a somatic discomfort, such as dizziness or palpitations, with an impending panic attack. For example, during a car accident, the individual may experience rapid heartbeat, dizziness, shortness of breath, and panic. Subsequent experiences of dizziness or palpitations, unrelated to an anxiety-provoking situation, incite anxiety and panic. Many cognitive theorists further expound that people with panic disorder may misinterpret mild physical sensations (sweating, dizziness), causing panic as a result of learned fear (catastrophic interpretation). Some researchers hypothesize that individuals with a low sense of control over their environment or with a particular sensitivity to anxiety are vulnerable to misinterpreting normal stress. Controlled exposure to anxiety-provoking situations and cognitive countering techniques have proved successful in reducing the symptoms of panic.

RISK FACTORS

Several risk factors have been implicated in the development of panic disorder, including family history, substance and stimulant use or abuse, smoking tobacco, and undertaking severe stressors. In addition to contributing potential genetic predisposition, female gender has been implicated as a risk factor because females have more panic symptoms than do males. People who have several anxiety symptoms and those who experience separation anxiety during childhood often present with panic disorder later in life (Hayward, Killen, & Kraemer, 2000; Slattery et al., 2002). Other disorders that have been shown to precede panic disorder include social anxiety disorder and specific phobias (Barzega et al., 2001)

Because panic disorder manifests predominantly in young adults, determining which risk factors are highly associated with early life events would be prudent. Early life traumas, history of physical or sexual abuse, socioeconomic or personal disadvantages, and behavioural inhibition by adults have been associated with an increased risk for anxiety disorders in children (Castellanos & Hunter, 2000; Friedman et al., 2002; Marshall et al., 2000; Woodward, 2001).

Comorbidity

In addition to comorbid psychiatric disorders being common in those with panic disorder, certain physical health problems are also common. These include vertigo, cardiac disease, gastrointestinal disorders, and asthma. Patients with mitral valve prolapse, migraine headaches, and hypertension may also have an increased incidence of panic disorder. One might ponder whether these medical conditions produce similar somatic sensations to anxiety and over time increase risk for panic attacks and the development of panic disorder. The population with both physical health problems and panic symptoms report poorer quality of life than do those without such comorbidity.

PRIORITY CARE ISSUES

Panic disorder and depression are highly associated. Lenze and associates (2000) stated that 9.3% of patients with major depression have comorbid panic disorder. In addition, adolescents with panic disorder may be at higher risk for suicidal thoughts or attempt suicide more often than other adolescents (Valentiner, Gutierrez, & Blacker, 2002). Increased risk for suicide is more associated with PTSD than any other anxiety disorder; however, multiple health problems (including more than one psychiatric diagnosis) can increase suicide risk. Typically, individuals with panic disorder are treated as outpatients. Hospitalization is required when there are urgent additional psychiatric issues, such as comorbid depression that is not responsive to antidepressant therapies or increased suicide risk.

NURSING MANAGEMENT: HUMAN RESPONSE TO DISORDER

Because panic disorder encompasses the physical, psychological, and social spheres of the patient's world, assessment within a biopsychosocial framework is imper-

ative. Physiologic symptoms tend to be the impetus for patients to seek medical assistance. Often, patients are initially seen in emergency rooms because they seek treatment for their physical symptoms. Biologic, psychological, and social assessments unveil potential contributing factors and identify sources of strength that can guide the nurse to develop an individual action plan.

Biologic Domain

Assessment

Skillful assessment is required to rule out life-threatening causes, including primary or secondary cardiac or neurologic symptoms. Once it is determined that the patient has experienced a panic attack, the nurse should assess for any potential environmental triggers and obtain a detailed history of any previous similar experiences. Questions to ask the patient might include the following:

- What did you experience before and during the panic episode, including physical symptoms, feelings, and thoughts?
- When did you begin to feel that way? How long did it last?
- Have you ever experienced some of these symptoms before? If so, under what circumstances?
- Has anyone in your family ever had similar experiences?
- What do you do when you have these experiences that helps you to feel safe? Have the feelings and sensations ever gone away on their own?

Substance Use

Assessment for panicogenic substance use, such as sources of caffeine, pseudoephedrine, amphetamines, cocaine, or other stimulants, may rule out contributory issues either related or unrelated to panic disorder. The use of the recreational drug "Ecstasy" has also been linked with panic attacks. Tobacco use can also contribute to the risk for panic symptoms. Many individuals with panic disorder use alcohol or central nervous system (CNS) depressants in an effort to self-medicate anxiety symptoms, and withdrawal from CNS depressants may produce symptoms of panic.

Sleep Patterns

Sleep is often disturbed in patients with panic disorder. In fact, panic attacks can occur during sleep, and the patient may fear sleep for this reason. Nurses should closely assess the impact of sleep disturbance because it can increase the risk of further panic attacks and the development of depression.

Physical Activity

Active participation in a routine exercise program may help individuals reassess automatic thinking that relates increased heart rate and shortness of breathe to a physical crisis.

Interventions for Physiologic Domain

Panic disorder is characterized by phobic avoidance as the afflicted person attempts to avoid situations that increase panic. However, drastically changing lifestyle to avoid situations does not aid recovery. Interventions that focus on the physical aspects of anxiety and panic are particularly helpful in reducing the number and severity of the attacks, giving patients an increasing sense of accomplishment and control.

Breathing Control

Hyperventilation is common. Often, people are unaware that they take rapid, shallow breaths when they become anxious. Other common sensations are choking and pressure on the chest, restricting normal breathing.

Teaching Points

Teaching patients breathing control can be helpful. Focus on the breathing and help them to identify the rate, pattern, and depth. If the breathing is rapid and shallow, reassure the patient that exercise and breathing practice can help change this breathing pattern. Next, assist the patient in practicing abdominal breathing by performing the following exercises:

- Instruct the patient to breathe deeply by inhaling slowly through the nose. Have him or her place a hand on the abdomen just beneath the rib cage.
- Instruct the patient to observe that when one is breathing deeply, the hand on the abdomen will actually rise.
- After the patient understands this process, ask him or her to inhale slowly through the nose counting to five, pause, and then exhale slowly through pursed lips.
- While the patient exhales, direct attention to feeling the muscles relax, focussing on "letting go."
- Have the patient repeat the deep abdominal breathing for 10 breaths, pausing between each inhalation and exhalation. Count slowly. If the patient complains of feeling light-headed, instruct the patient to slow down the rate of his or her deep breathing.
- The patient should stop between each cycle of 10 breaths and monitor normal breathing for 30 seconds.
- This series of 10 slow abdominal breaths, followed by 30 seconds of normal breathing, should be repeated for 3 to 5 minutes.
- Help the patient to establish a time for daily practice of abdominal breathing.

Abdominal breathing may also be used to interrupt an episode of panic as it begins. Once patients have learned to identify their own early signs of panic, they can learn the four-square method of breathing, which helps divert or decrease the severity of the attack.

Patients should be instructed as follows:

- Advise the patient to practice during calm periods and to begin by inhaling slowly through the nose, count to four, then hold the breath for a count of four.
- Next, direct the patient to exhale slowly through pursed lips to a count of four and then rest for a count of four (no breath).
- Finally, the patient may take two normal breaths and repeat the sequence.

After patients practice the skill, the nurse should assist patients in identifying early physical cues that will alert them to use this calming technique. Some forms of yoga are especially helpful in teaching breathing relaxation techniques.

Nutritional Planning

Maintaining regular and balanced eating habits reduces the likelihood of hypoglycemic episodes, light-headedness, and fatigue.

Teaching Points

To help teach the patient about healthful eating and ways to minimize physical factors contributing to anxiety, the nurse may:

- Advise patients to plan to reduce caffeine consumption and then eliminate it from their diet. Many over-the-counter (OTC) remedies are now used to boost energy or increase mental performance, and some of these contain caffeine.
- Help patients develop a reasonable plan to decrease or eliminate all sources of caffeine from their diet.
- Assess for other potential sources of stimulants, such as some cold remedies and herbal products, and provide information about substitutes.

Relaxation Techniques

Teaching the patient relaxation techniques is another way to help individuals with panic and anxiety disorders. Some are unaware of the tension in their bodies and first need to learn to monitor their own tension. Isometric exercises and progressive muscle relaxation are helpful methods to learn to differentiate muscle tension from muscle relaxation. This method of relaxation is also helpful when patients have difficulty clearing the mind, focussing, or visualizing a scene, which are often required in other forms of relaxation, such as meditation. Box 20-5 provides one method of progressive muscle relaxation.

Selective Serotonin Reuptake Inhibitor Therapy

Several classes of pharmacologic agents are effective in treating panic disorder, including the SSRIs, TCAs, and benzodiazepines. However, the SSRIs are generally

BOX 20.5

Implementing Progressive Muscle Relaxation

Choose a quiet, comfortable location where you will not be disturbed for 20 to 30 minutes. Your position may be lying or sitting, but all parts of your body should be supported, including your head. Wear loose clothing, taking off restrictive items, such as glasses and shoes.

Begin by closing your eyes and clearing your mind. Moving from head to toe, focus on each part or your body and assess the level of tension. Visualize each group of muscles as heavy and relaxed.

Take two or three slow abdominal breaths, pausing briefly between each breath. Imagine the tension flowing from your body.

Each muscle group listed below should be tightened (or tensed isometrically) for 5 to 10 seconds and then abruptly released; visualize this group of muscles as heavy, limp, and relaxed for 15 to 20 seconds before tightening the next group of muscles. There are several methods to tighten each muscle group, and suggestions are provided below. Each muscle group may be tightened two to three times until relaxed. Do not overtighten or strain. You should not experience pain.

- Hands (tighten by making fists)
- Biceps (tighten by drawing forearms up and "making a muscle")
- Triceps (extend forearms straight, locking elbows)
- Face (grimace, tightly shutting mouth and eyes)
- Face (open mouth wide and raise eyebrows)
- Neck (pull head forward to chest and tighten neck muscles)
- Shoulders (raise shoulders toward ears)
- Shoulders (push shoulders back as if touching them together)
- Chest (take a deep breath and hold for 10 seconds)
- Stomach (suck in your abdominal muscles)
- Buttocks (pull buttocks together)
- Thighs (straighten legs and squeeze muscles in thighs and hips)
- Leg calves (pull toes carefully toward you, avoid cramps)
- Feet (curl toes downward and point toes away from your body)

Finally, repeat several deep abdominal breaths and mentally check your body for tension. Rest comfortably for several minutes, breathing normally, and visualize your body as warm and relaxed. Get up slowly when you are finished.

---

considered first-line treatment of panic disorder. Because of side effects and dietary restrictions, monoamine oxidase inhibitor (MAOI) antidepressants generally are used after all other options are exhausted.

SSRIs are used to treat many psychiatric conditions. Although not all SSRIs have received Health Canada approval for the treatment of panic disorder, some are used as "off-label" treatment of panic attacks. Sertraline (Zoloft), paroxetine (Paxil), and fluoxetine (Prozac) have all proved effective in the treatment of panic disorder in drug trials (Rapaport et al., 2001; Roy-Byrne et al., 2001; Wagstaff, Cheer, Matheson, Ormrod, & Goa, 2002). The initial increase in serotonergic activity from serotonin reuptake blockade may cause temporary increases in panic symptoms and even panic attacks, but this is usually short-lived and can be minimized by lower starting doses (Brauer, Nowicki, Catalano, & Catalano, 2002). Full clinical response is usually seen by 4 to 6 weeks of treatment.

CRNE Note

Psychopharmacologic treatment is almost always needed. Antidepressants are the medication of choice. Benzodiazepines should be used only for short periods of time. It is important to taper off benzodiazepines, if used for longer periods of time, to avoid any rebound anxiety or sleep disturbance.

ADMINISTERING AND MONITORING SSRIs. Overall, SSRIs produce fewer side effects than do other drugs, are safer to use, and are not lethal in the event of overdose. They may cause a temporary feeling of overstimulation when initiated, but slow titration can help to alleviate this feeling. Morning dosing decreases interference with sleep, but at higher doses, some patients find the medication sedating.

Paroxetine (Paxil) was the first of the SSRIs to be indicated for anxiety disorders. Dosing begins at 10 mg daily, usually in the morning, and then is increased by 10 mg per week at weekly intervals, not to exceed 60 mg daily. Controlled-release paroxetine (Paxil CR) dosing starts at 12.5 mg/d, increasing by 12.5 mg/d in intervals of not less than 1 week. Maximum dose is 75 mg/d. Sertraline (Zoloft) is usually started at 25 mg/d, increasing after 1 week to 50 mg/d. The maximum dose is 200 mg/d.

MONITORING SIDE EFFECTS. The most common side effects of the SSRIs are initial dizziness, restlessness, anxiety, and sexual dysfunction. Up to 50% of those taking SSRIs can experience some degree of sexual dysfunction and must be considered in treatment decisions for panic disorder. The nurse should ensure that the patient is aware of this before the drug is started and should initiate ongoing discussions about any emerging dysfunction during follow-up. Significant weight gain has also been observed in some patients. A withdrawal syndrome has been identified in individuals who suddenly stop taking SSRIs (Finfgeld, 2002). Patient education is an important preventative strategy to minimize withdrawal symptoms.

MONITORING FOR DRUG INTERACTIONS. Although the SSRIs as a class have well described properties that affect

BOX 20.6

Comparison of the Metabolic Inhibition Profiles and the Elimination Half Lives of the SSRIs

Drug	Specific CYP Enzymes				Half-Life*(hr)
	1A2	2C	2D6	3A4	
fluoxetine	NS	Moderate	Potent	Moderate	25–150 (parent); 180–230 (metabolite)
paroxetine	NS	NS	Potent	NS	10–65
fluvoxamine	Potent	Moderate	NS	Moderate	10–24
sertraline	NS	Moderate	NS	NS	20–36
citalopram	NS	NS	NS	NS	20–48

*Half-life is the time required to eliminate 50% of the drug from the body. The half-life for the metabolite is included for active metabolites. NS, not significant.

other drugs used at the same time, the relative risk of drug–drug interactions differs among the specific SSRIs (Box 20-6). The most common mechanism involved in SSRI–drug interaction is metabolic inhibition of key liver enzymes responsible for the metabolism of many other drugs. The SSRIs inhibit the metabolism of another drug, and thus, the level of that other drug would be increased. This increase in drug level would significantly increase the risk for serious side effects, as well as directly affecting adherence to a drug regime. Paroxetine and fluoxetine are the most potent of the SSRIs and thus carry the most risk for drug–drug interactions. Common drugs affected by this mechanism include thioridazine, digoxin, phenobarbital, TCAs, phenytoin, theophylline, and warfarin (for a more detailed listing, visit www.Drug-Interactions. com). Opposite metabolic interactions can also occur. For example, cimetidine (Tagamet) interferes with the metabolism of paroxetine, which might potentiate toxicity. Other potential drug–drug interactions come from interactions based on pharmacologic actions. For example, SSRIs must be used cautiously with MAOIs because there is risk for a serious hypertensive crises. Combinations of SSRI and tryptophan increase the risk for serotonin syndrome, an acute condition characterized by restlessness, blood pressure instability, and varying degrees of disorientation and cognitive impairment. The serotonin syndrome can also arise from combining SSRIs and such recreational drugs as Ecstasy and its analogues.

Teaching Points

Warn patients about using herbal products like St. John's wort because the similarity of action can increase the risk for serotonin syndrome. The sedative effects of the medications may impede attention and concentration; thus, sedative SSRIs like fluvoxamine are given at night. Other SSRIs like fluoxetine and paroxetine are taken in the morning because they are more stimulating and can interfere with sleep.

Tricyclic Antidepressant Therapy

The TCAs imipramine (Tofranil), nortriptyline (Pamelor), and clomipramine (Anafranil) reduce panic symptoms, probably by their dual action on serotonin and norepinephrine receptors. The therapeutic effects of TCAs usually occur after 3 to 4 weeks, but effects have been observed as early as 2 weeks after initiation. These drugs are "off-label" treatments because they are not approved by Health Canada for panic disorder.

ADMINISTERING AND MONITORING TCAs. The TCAs have a relatively long elimination half-life, and complaints of sedation are common. Therefore, single bedtime doses might be most helpful for patients. TCAs are highly bound to plasma proteins and are metabolized in the liver. These medications should be used with extreme caution in patients at risk for suicide. TCAs affect cardiac conduction, and overdoses can be fatal. An electrocardiogram is indicated before initiating therapy. In cross-tapering to different medications, sudden discontinuation of TCA use causes cholinergic rebound phenomenon, with flu-like symptoms of nausea, headache, and malaise. Assure patients that these effects do not indicate addiction to the medication.

TCAs may complicate underlying glaucoma, urinary retention, cardiovascular disorders, hepatic disease, and thyroid dysregulation because of their effects on various other neurotransmitter and hormone systems. They also lower the seizure threshold. Monitor closely if the patient has a seizure disorder. These medications have narrow therapeutic indexes and therefore require monitoring for toxicity at high doses.

MONITORING SIDE EFFECTS. Adverse effects of TCAs are very common and may compromise patients' willingness to continue using them, but side effects can be reduced by starting with a small dose and increasing slowly. Because patients with panic disorder usually require higher doses of antidepressant medication, anticholinergic side effects (dry mouth and eyes, blurred vision, photophobia, constipation, urinary hesitancy or retention, mydriasis, and tachycardia) are common and may necessitate a change in antidepressant type. Acetylcholine is involved with cognition, and anticholinergic side effects of TCAs may negatively affect cognition in elderly patients. In addition, many TCAs have alpha-adrenergic receptor effects on the body that lead to orthostatic hypotension, placing elderly individuals at increased risk for falls. Lying and standing blood pressure and pulse should be monitored frequently, especially during periods of increasing the dosage. Also observe for signs of dizziness or ataxia. Nortriptyline (Pamelor) has a lower risk for orthostatic hypotension and thus may be indicated if falls present a substantial risk.

The choice to initiate treatment with a TCA rather than an SSRI may be related to cost. TCAs have been on the market for a very long time and thus are very low in price compared with the newer SSRIs (pennies per day compared with dollars per day)

MONITORING FOR DRUG INTERACTIONS. TCAs interact with several medications, including MAOIs (severe hypertensive crises), SSRIs, and CNS depressants (enhanced CNS depression). Concomitant treatment with methylphenidate (Ritalin), cimetidine, and oral contraceptives may increase TCA serum levels. A consult to a psychiatrist is usually warranted if combination antidepressant therapy is required.

Teaching Points

Instruct the patient to take the medication exactly as prescribed and to be careful with any OTC medications or herbal products. Alcohol should be avoided. Warn the patient of the potential for sedation, especially at initiation of treatment, and, if appropriate, suggest taking the medication at bedtime. In addition, common and serious side effects of the medications should be discussed, as well as specific effects that require immediate attention.

Benzodiazepine Therapy
Specific benzodiazepines have produced antipanic effects, and their therapeutic onset is much faster (hours, not weeks) than that of antidepressants (Table 20-2).

Therefore, benzodiazepines are tremendously useful in treating intensely distressed patients. Alprazolam (Xanax), lorazepam (Ativan), and clonazepam (Rivotril) are widely used for panic disorder. They are well tolerated but carry the risk for withdrawal symptoms upon discontinuation of use (Box 20-7).

ADMINISTERING AND MONITORING BENZODIAZEPINES. Treatment may include administering benzodiazepines concurrently with antidepressants for the first 4 weeks, then tapering off the benzodiazepine. This strategy provides rapid symptom relief but avoids the complications of long-term benzodiazepine use. Benzodiazepines with short half-lives do not accumulate in the body, whereas benzodiazepines with half-lives of longer than 24 hours tend to accumulate with chronic treatment, are removed more slowly, and produce less intense symptoms on discontinuation of use (see Chapter 13).

Short-acting benzodiazepines, such as alprazolam and lorazepam, are associated with rebound anxiety, or anxiety that increases after the peak effects of the medication have decreased. Medications with short half-lives should be given in three or four small doses spaced throughout the day, with a higher dose at bedtime to allay anxiety-related insomnia. Clonazepam, a longer-acting benzodiazepine, requires less frequent dosing and has a lower risk for rebound anxiety. Rebound anxiety and insomnia are also common with abrupt cessation of benzodiazepine treatment. Symptoms associated with withdrawal of benzodiazepine therapy are more likely to occur after high doses and long-term therapy. They can also occur after short-term therapy. Withdrawal symptoms manifest in several ways, including psychological (apprehension, irritability, insomnia, and dysphoria), physiologic (tremor, palpitations, vertigo, sweating, muscle spasm, seizures), and perceptual (sensory hypersensitivity, depersonalization, feelings of motion, metallic taste).

Because of their depressive CNS effects, benzodiazepines should not be used to treat patients with comorbid sleep apnea. In fact, these drugs may actually decrease the rate and depth of respirations. Exercise caution in elderly patients for these reasons.

Table 20.2	Benzodiazepine Pharmacokinetics	
Drug	**Half-life (h)**	**Important Active Metabolites**
chlordiazepoxide (Librium)	10–20	Desmethylchlordiazepoxide, demoxepam, desmethyldiazepam
diazepam (Valium)	20–70	Desmethyldiazepam
clorazepate (Tranxene)	40–100	Desmethyldiazepam
temazepam (Restoril)	8–20	Desmethyldiazepam
clonazepam (Rivotril)	30–60	None
alprazolam (Xanax)	8–15	None
lorazepam (Ativan)	10–20	None
oxazepam (Serax)	30–120	None
triazolam (Halcion)	1.5–5	—

BOX 20.7

Drug Profile: Alprazolam (Xanax)

DRUG CLASS: Antianxiety agent with antidepressant properties.

RECEPTOR AFFINITY: High affinity to $GABA_A$ receptor, increases the ability of GABA to inhibit nerve cell firing.

INDICATIONS: Management of anxiety disorders, short-term relief of anxiety symptoms or depression-related anxiety, panic attacks with or without agoraphobia. Unlabelled uses for school phobia, premenstrual syndrome, and depression.

ROUTES AND DOSAGES: Available in 0.25-, 0.5-, 1-, and 2-mg scored tablets.

Adults: For anxiety: Initially, 0.25 to 0.5 mg PO tid titrated to a maximum daily dose of 4 mg in divided doses. For panic disorder: Initially, 0.5 mg PO tid increased at 3- to 4-d intervals in increments of no more than 1 mg/d. For school phobia: 2 to 8 mg/d PO. For premenstrual syndrome: 0.25 mg PO tid.

Geriatric patients: Initially, 0.25 mg bid to tid, increased gradually as needed and tolerated.

HALF-LIFE (PEAK EFFECT): 12 to 15 h (1–2 n)

SELECTED ADVERSE REACTIONS: Transient mild drowsiness, initially; sedation, depression, lethargy, apathy, fatigue, light-headedness, disorientation, anger, hostility, restlessness, headache, confusion, crying, constipation, diarrhoea, dry mouth, nausea, and possible drug dependence.

WARNINGS: Contraindicated in patients with psychosis, acute narrow angle glaucoma, shock, acute alcoholic intoxication with depressed vital signs, pregnancy, labour and delivery, and breast-feeding. Use cautiously in patients with impaired hepatic or renal function, and severe debilitating conditions. Risk for digitalis toxicity if given concurrently with digoxin. Increased CNS depression if taken with alcohol and other CNS depressants.

SPECIFIC PATIENT/FAMILY EDUCATION:

- Avoid using alcohol, or sleep-inducing or other OTC drugs.
- Take drug exactly as prescribed and do not abruptly stop taking the drug without consulting health care provider.
- Take drug with food if gastrointestinal upset occurs.
- Avoid driving a car or performing tasks that require alertness until aware of any drowsiness or dizziness.
- Report any signs and symptoms of adverse reactions, including short-term memory problems.

MONITORING SIDE EFFECTS. The side effects of benzodiazepine medications generally include headache, confusion, dizziness, disorientation, sedation, and visual disturbances. Sedation should be monitored after beginning medication use or increasing the dose. The patient should be cautious about activities that take significant attention and concentration when starting on benzodiazepines.

MONITORING FOR DRUG INTERACTIONS. Many benzodiazepines have active metabolites, so the pharmacologic effects can last for very long periods of time. The longer-acting drugs accumulate in fat stores, which means that women (who have higher percentage of body fat) and obese patients can continue to have drug effects long after the drug is discontinued. Drugs that interact with benzodiazepines include TCAs and digoxin; interaction may result in increased serum TCA or digoxin levels. Histamine-2 blockers (cimetidine) used with benzodiazepines may potentiate sedative effects. Monitor closely for effectiveness in patients who smoke; cigarette smoking may increase the clearance of benzodiazepines.

Teaching Points

Warn patients to avoid alcohol because of the additive effects on CNS depression. In addition, warn them not to engage in activities that require strict attention and concentration until the sedative effects of the medication are known.

Psychological Domain

Assessment

A complete assessment is necessary to determine patterns of panic attacks, characteristic symptoms in attacks, and the patient's emotional, cognitive, or behavioural responses (see Chapter 10). A comprehensive assessment includes any physical symptoms or conditions, such as cardiovascular or respiratory problems that may contribute to panic symptoms, overall mental status, suicidal tendencies and thoughts, cognitive thought patterns, avoidance behaviour patterns, and any comorbid depression symptoms. The patient's perceptions regarding his or her symptoms are discussed, as well as present and past coping strategies.

Self-Report Scales

Self-evaluation is difficult in panic disorder. Often specific triggers are no longer present, and the patient lives in fear of another panic attack with little sense of being able to control the attacks. Several tools are available to characterize and rate the patient's state of anxiety. Examples of these symptom and behavioural rating scales are provided in Box 20-8. All these tools are self-report measures and as such are limited by the individual's self-awareness and openness. However, the Hamilton Rating Scale for Anxiety (HAM-A), provided in Table 20-3, is an example of a scale rated by the clinician (Hamilton, 1959). This 14-item scale reflects both psychological and somatic aspects of anxiety.

BOX 20.8

Rating Scales for Assessment of Panic Disorder and Anxiety Disorders

Panic Symptoms

Panic-Associated Symptom Scale (PASS)
Argyle, N., Delito, J., Allerup, P., et al. (1991). The Panic-Associated Symptom Scale: Measuring the severity of panic disorder. *Acta Psychiatrica Scandinavica, 83,* 20–26.

Acute Panic Inventory
Dillon, D. J., Gorman, J. M., Liebowitz, M. R., et al. (1987). Measurement of lactate-induced panic and anxiety. *Psychiatry Research, 20,* 97–105.

National Institute of Mental Health Panic Questionnaire (NIMH PQ)
Scupi, B. S., Maser, J. D., & Uhde, T. W. (1992). The National Institute of Mental Health Panic Questionnaire: An instrument for assessing clinical characteristics of panic disorder. *Journal of Nervous and Mental Disease, 180,* 566–572.

Cognitions

Anxiety Sensitivity Index
Reiss, S., Peterson, R. A., & Gursky, D. M. (1986). Anxiety sensitivity, anxiety frequency, and the prediction of fearfulness. *Behaviour Research and Therapy, 24,* 1–8.

Agoraphobia Cognitions Questionnaire
Chambless, D. L., Caputo, G. C., Bright, P., & Gallagher, R. (1984). Assessment of fear in agoraphobics: The Body Sensations Questionnaire and the Agoraphobic Cognitions Questionnaire. *Journal of Consulting and Clinical Psychology, 52,* 1090–1097.

Body Sensations Questionnaire
Chambless, D. L., Caputo, G. C., Bright, P., & Gallagher, R. (1984). Assessment of fear in agoraphobics: The Body

Sensations Questionnaire and the Agoraphobic Cognitions Questionnaire. *Journal of Consulting and Clinical Psychology, 52,* 1090–1097.

Phobias

Mobility Inventory for Agoraphobia
Chambless, D. L., Caputo, G. C., Jasin, S. E., et al. (1985). The Mobility Inventory for Agoraphobia. *Behaviour Research and Therapy, 23,* 35–44.

Fear Questionnaire
Marks, I. M., & Matthews, A. M. (1979). Brief standard self-rating for phobic patients. *Behaviour Research and Therapy, 17,* 263–267.

Anxiety

State-Trait Anxiety Inventory (STAI)
Spielberger, C. D., Gorsuch, R. L., & Luchene, R. E. (1976). *Manual for the State-Trait Anxiety Inventory.* Palo Alto, CA: Consulting Psychologists Press.

Penn State Worry Questionnaire (PSWQ)
16-items developed to assess the trait of worry.
Meyer, T., Miller, M., Metzger, R., & Borkovec, T. (1990). Development and validation of the Penn State Worry Questionnaire. *Behaviour Research and Therapy, 28(6),* 487–495.

Beck Anxiety Inventory
21 items rating severity of symptoms on a 4-point scale.
Beck, A., Epstein, N., Brown, G., & Steer, R. (1988). An inventory for measuring clinical anxiety: The Beck Anxiety Inventory. *Journal of Consulting and Clinical Psychology, 56,* 893–897.

Mental Status Examination

During mental status examination, individuals with panic disorder may exhibit anxiety symptoms, including restlessness, irritability, poor concentration, and apprehensive behaviour. Assess by direct questioning if the patient is experiencing suicidal thoughts, especially if the person is abusing substances or is taking antidepressant medications.

Assessment of Cognitive Thought Patterns

Catastrophic misinterpretations of trivial physical symptoms can trigger panic symptoms. Once identified, these thoughts should serve as a basis for individualizing patient education to counter such false beliefs. Table 20-4 presents an example of a scale to assess catastrophic misinterpretations of the symptoms of panic. Several studies have found that individuals who feel a sense of control have less severe panic attacks. Individuals who fear loss of control during a panic attack often make the following types of statement:

- "I feel trapped."
- "I'm afraid others will know, or I'll hurt someone."
- "I feel alone. I can't help myself."
- "I'm losing control."

These individuals also tend to show low self-esteem, feelings of helplessness and demoralization, and overwhelming fears of experiencing panic attacks. They may have difficulty with assertiveness or expressing feelings.

Interventions for Psychological Domain

As with most anxiety disorders, panic disorder is usually treated in outpatient clinics and private physician practice. Hospitalization is usually limited to those with comorbid depression and increased suicide risk. Often panic disorder requires both pharmacotherapy and psychotherapeutic interventions. The outpatient nurse can assist the patient in identifying triggers to anxiety and countering these triggers with individualized psychological measures. Distraction techniques, positive self-talk, panic control treatment, exposure therapy, implosion therapy, and cognitive-behavioural therapy (CBT) can be useful.

Peplau devised general guidelines for nursing interventions that might be successful in treating patients with anxiety. These interventions help the patient attend to and react to input other than the subjective experience of anxiety. They are designed to help the

Table 20.3   Hamilton Rating Scale for Anxiety

Max Hamilton designed this scale to help clinicians gather information about anxiety states. The symptom inventory provides scaled information that classifies anxiety behaviour and assists the clinician in targeting behaviours and achieving outcome measures. Provide a rating for each indicator based on the following scale:

0 = None   1 = Mild   2 = Moderate
3 = Severe   4 = Severe, grossly disabling

Item	Symptoms	Rating
Anxious mood	Worries, anticipation of the worst, fearful anticipation, irritability	
Tension	Feelings of tension, fatigability, startle response, moved to tears easily, trembling, feelings of restlessness, inability to relax	
Fear	Of dark, strangers, being left alone, animals, traffic, crowds	
Insomnia	Difficulty in falling asleep, broken sleep, unsatisfying sleep and fatigue on waking, dreams, nightmares, night terrors	
Intellectual (cognitive)	Difficulty concentrating, poor memory	
Depressed mood	Loss of interest, lack of pleasure in hobbies, depression, early waking, diurnal swings	
Somatic (sensory)	Tinnitus, blurring of vision, hot and cold flushes, feelings of weakness, picking sensation	
Somatic (muscular)	Pains and aches, twitching, stiffness, myoclonic jerks, grinding of teeth, unsteady voice, increased muscular tone	
Cardiovascular symptoms	Tachycardia, palpitations, pain in chest, throbbing of vessels, fainting feelings, missing beat	
Respiratory symptoms	Pressure or constriction in chest, choking feelings, sighing, dyspnoea	
Gastrointestinal symptoms	Difficulty in swallowing, wind, abdominal pain, burning sensation, abdominal fullness, nausea, vomiting, borborygmi, looseness of bowels, loss of weight, constipation	
Genitourinary symptoms	Frequency of micturition, urgency of micturition, amenorrhoea, menorrhagic, development of frigidity, premature ejaculation, loss of libido, impotence	
Autonomic symptoms	Dry mouth, flushing, pallor, tendency to sweat, giddiness, tension headache, raising of hair	
Behaviour at interview	Fidgeting, restlessness or pacing, tremor of hands, furrowed brow, strained face, sighing or rapid respiration, facial pallor, swallowing, belching, brisk tendon jerks, dilated pupils, exophthalmos	

From Hamilton, M. (1959). The assessment of anxiety states by rating. *British Journal of Medical Psychology, 32,* 54.

patient focus on other stimuli and cope with anxiety in any form (Table 20-5). These general interventions apply to all anxiety disorders and therefore will not be reiterated in subsequent sections. Biopsychosocial interventions are addressed under the pertinent headings in Figure 20-1.

Distraction

Once patients can identify the early symptoms of panic, they may learn to implement **distraction** behaviours that take the focus off the physical sensations. Some distraction activities include initiating conversation with a nearby person or engaging in physical activity (e.g., walking, gardening, or house cleaning). Performing simple repetitive activities such as snapping a rubber band against the wrist, counting backward from 100 by 3s, or counting objects along the roadway might deter an attack.

Positive Self-Talk

During states of increased anxiety and panic, individuals can learn to counter fearful or negative thoughts by using planned and rehearsed positive coping statements,

called **positive self-talk**. "This is only anxiety, and it will pass," "I can handle these symptoms," and "I'll get through this" are examples of positive self-talk. These types of positive statements can give the individual a focal point and reduce fear when panic symptoms begin. Handheld cards that carry positive statements can be carried in a purse or wallet so that the person can retrieve them quickly when panic symptoms are felt. See Box 20-9 for an example of a therapeutic dialogue introducing such a technique.

Psychotherapies for Panic Disorder

Cognitive-behavioural therapy is a highly effective tool for treating panic disorder. It has been considered first-line treatment for panic and other anxiety disorders and is often used in conjunction with medications, including the SSRIs, in treating panic disorder (Kampman, Keijsers, Hoogduin, & Hendriks, 2002). The goals of CBT include helping the patient to manage his or her anxiety and correcting anxiety-provoking thoughts through interventions, including

Table 20.4	Panic Attack Cognitions Questionnaire			

Rate each of the following thoughts according to the degree to which you believe each thought contributes to your panic attack.

1 = Not at all   3 = Quite a lot
2 = Somewhat   4 = Very much

1. I'm going to die.	1	2	3	4
2. I'm going insane.	1	2	3	4
3. I'm losing control.	1	2	3	4
4. This will never end.	1	2	3	4
5. I'm really scared.	1	2	3	4
6. I'm having a heart attack.	1	2	3	4
7. I'm going to pass out.	1	2	3	4
8. I don't know what people will think.	1	2	3	4
9. I won't be able to get out of here.	1	2	3	4
10. I don't understand what is happening to me.	1	2	3	4
11. People will think I am crazy.	1	2	3	4
12. I'll always be this way.	1	2	3	4
13. I am going to throw up.	1	2	3	4
14. I must have a brain tumour.	1	2	3	4
15. I'll choke to death.	1	2	3	4
16. I'm going to act foolish.	1	2	3	4
17. I'm going blind.	1	2	3	4
18. I'll hurt someone.	1	2	3	4
19. I'm going to have a stroke.	1	2	3	4
20. I'm going to scream.	1	2	3	4
21. I'm going to babble or talk funny.	1	2	3	4
22. I'll be paralyzed by fear.	1	2	3	4
23. Something is physically wrong with me.	1	2	3	4
24. I won't be able to breathe.	1	2	3	4
25. Something terrible will happen.	1	2	3	4
26. I'm going to make a scene.	1	2	3	4

Adapted from Clum, G. A. (1990). Panic attack cognitions questionnaire. *Coping with panic: A drug-free approach to dealing with anxiety attacks.* Pacific Grove. CA: Brooks/Cole.

cognitive restructuring, breathing training, and psychoeducation.

Panic control treatment involves intentional exposure (through exercise) to panic-invoking sensations such as dizziness, hyperventilation, tightness in chest, and sweating. Identified patterns become targets for treatment. Patients are taught to use breathing training and cognitive restructuring to manage their responses and are instructed to practice these techniques between therapy sessions to adapt the skills to other situations.

Exposure therapy is the treatment of choice for agoraphobia. The patient is repeatedly exposed to real or simulated anxiety-provoking situations until he or she becomes desensitized and anxiety subsides.

Systematic desensitization, another exposure method used to desensitize patients, exposes the patient to a hierarchy of feared situations that the patient has rated from least to most feared. The patient is taught to use muscle relaxation as levels of anxiety increase through multisituational exposure. Planning and implementing exposure therapy requires special training. Because of the multitude of outpatients in treatment for agoraphobia, exposure therapy would be a useful tool for home health psychiatric nurses. Outcomes of home-based exposure treatment are similar to clinic-based treatment outcomes.

Implosive therapy is a provocative technique useful in treating agoraphobia in which the therapist identifies phobic stimuli for the patient and then presents highly anxiety-provoking imagery to the patient, describing the feared scene as dramatically and vividly as possible.

Flooding is a technique used to desensitize the patient to the fear associated with a particular anxiety-provoking stimulus. Desensitizing is done by presenting feared objects or situations repeatedly, without session breaks, until the anxiety dissipates. For example, a patient with ophidiophobia might be presented with a real snake repeatedly until his or her anxiety decreases.

Behaviour psychoeducation programs help to educate patients and families about the symptoms of panic. Individuals with panic disorder legitimately fear going crazy, losing control, or dying because of their physical symptoms. Attempting to convince a patient that such fears are groundless only heightens anxiety and impedes communication. Information and physical evidence, such as electrocardiogram results and laboratory test results, should be presented in a caring and open manner that demonstrates acceptance and understanding of their situation.

Box 20-10 suggests topics for individual or small-group discussion. It is especially important to cover such topics as the differences between panic attacks and heart attacks, the difference between panic disorder and other psychiatric disorders, and the effectiveness of various treatment methods.

Social Domain

Individuals with anxiety disorders, especially panic disorder and social phobias, often deteriorate socially as the disorder takes its toll on relationships with family and friends. If the disorder becomes severe enough, the person may become completely isolated. Therefore, it is an important area for assessment and active intervention, if necessary.

Assessment

During the assessment, the nurse needs to assess the patient's understanding of how panic disorder with or without severe avoidance behaviours has affected his or

Table 20.5	Nursing Interventions Based on Degrees of Anxiety
Degree of Anxiety	**Nursing Interventions**
Mild	Learning is possible. Nurse assists patient to use energy anxiety provides to encourage learning.
Moderate	Nurse to check own anxiety so patient does not empathize with it. Encourage patient to talk: to focus on one experience. to describe it fully, then to formulate the patient's generalizations about that experience.
Severe	Learning is less possible. Allow relief behaviours to be used but do not ask about them. Encourage the patient to talk: ventilation of random ideas is likely to reduce anxiety to moderate level. When this is observed by the nurse, proceed as above.
Panic	Learning is impossible. Thereness: Nurse to stay with the patient. Allow pacing and walk with the patient. No content inputs to the patient's thinking should be made by the nurse. (They burden the patient, who will distort them.) Pick up on what the patient says, eg, Pt: "What's happening to me—how did I get here?" N: "Say what you notice." Short phrases by the nurse—direct, to the point of the patient's comment, and investigative—match the current attention span of the patient in panic and therefore are more likely to be heard, grasped, and acted on, with the patient's responses gradually reducing the anxiety in a helpful way. Do not touch the patient; patients experiencing panic are very concerned about survival, are experiencing grave threat to self, and usually distort intentions of all invasions of their personal space.

From Peplau, H. (1989). Theoretical constructs: Anxiety, self, and hallucinations. In A. O'Toole & S. Welt (Eds.), *Interpersonal theory in nursing practice: Selected works of Hildegard E. Peplau.* New York: Springer.

her life along with that of the family. Pertinent questions include the following:

- How has the disorder affected your family's social life?
- What limitations related to travel has the disorder placed on you or your family?
- What coping strategies have you used to manage symptoms?
- How has the disorder affected your family members or others?

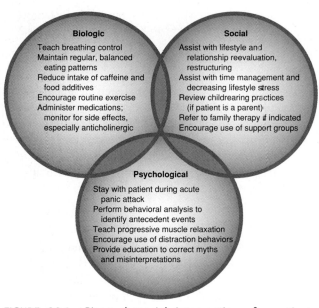

FIGURE 20.1 Biopsychosocial interventions for patients with panic disorder.

Cultural Factors

Cultural competence calls for the understanding of cultural knowledge, cultural awareness, cultural assessment skills, and cultural practice. Therefore, cultural differences must be considered in the assessment of panic disorder. Different cultures interpret sensations, feelings, or understandings differently. For example, symptoms of anxiety might be seen as witchcraft or magic (APA, 2000). Several cultures do not have a word to describe "anxiety" or "anxious" and instead may use words or meanings to suggest physical complaints. In addition, showing anxiety may be a sign of weakness in some cultures (Chen, Reich, & Chung, 2002). Many Asian OTC herbal remedies contain substances that may induce panic by increasing the heart rate, basal metabolic rate, blood pressure, and sweating (Chen et al., 2002). Diet pills and ginseng are two examples.

Interventions for Social Domain

Individuals with panic disorder, especially those with significant anxiety sensitivity, may need assistance in re-evaluating their lifestyle. Time management can be a useful tool. In the workplace or at home, underestimating the time needed to complete a chore or being overly involved in several activities at once increases stress and anxiety. Procrastination, lack of assertiveness, and difficulties with prioritizing or delegating tasks intensify these problems.

Writing a list of chores to be completed and estimating time to complete them provides concrete feedback

BOX 20.9

Therapeutic Dialogue: Panic Disorder With Agoraphobia

Panic Disorder With Agoraphobia

Mark, a 55-year-old Caucasian man was admitted 4 days ago to the psychiatric unit with exacerbation of anxiety symptoms and panic attacks during the last 3 weeks. He has a 30-year history of uncontrolled anxiety that is refractory to medications and psychotherapy. On admission, he stated that he feels suicidal at times because he thinks his life is not within his control. He feels embarrassed, angry, and "trapped" by his disorder. During the past 24 hours, Mark is seen crying at times; he also isolates himself in his room. Michelle, Mark's nurse, enters his room to make a supportive contact and to assess his current mental status.

Ineffective Approach

Nurse: Oh ... Why are you crying?

Patient: (Looks up, gives a nervous chuckle) Obviously, because I'm upset. I am tired of living this way. I just want to be normal again. I can't even remember what that feels like.

Nurse: You look normal to me. Everyone has bad days. It'll pass.

Patient: I've felt this way longer than you've been alive. I've tried everything and nothing works.

Nurse: You're not the first depressed person that I've taken care of. You just need to go to groups and stay out of your room more. You'll start feeling better.

Patient: (Angrily) Oh, it's just that easy. You have no idea what I'm going through! You don't know me! You're just a kid.

Nurse: I can help you if you help yourself. A group starts in 5 minutes, and I'd like to see you there.

Patient: I'm not going to no damn group! I want to be alone so I can think!

Nurse: (Looks about anxiously) Maybe I should come back after you've calmed down a little.

Effective Approach

Nurse: Mark, I noticed that you are staying in your room more today. What's troubling you?

Patient: (Looks up) I feel like I've lost complete control of my life. I'm so anxious and nothing helps. I'm tired of it.

Nurse: I see. That must be difficult. Can you tell me more about what you are feeling right now?

Patient: I feel like I'm going crazy. I worry all the time about having panic attacks. They make me scared I'm going to die. Sometimes I think I'd be better off dead.

Nurse: (Remains silent, continues to give eye contact)

Patient: Do you know what it's like to be a prisoner to your emotions? I can't even go out of the house sometimes and when I do, it's terrifying. I don't know what to think anymore.

Nurse: Mark, you have lived with this disorder for a long time. You say that the medications do not work to your liking, but what has helped you in the past?

Patient: Well, I learned in relaxation group that panic symptoms are probably caused by chemicals in my brain that are not working correctly. I learned that medications can help, but they don't work well for me. I tried an exposure plan and relaxation techniques to deal with my fears of leaving the house and my chronic anxiety. That did help some, but it's scary to do.

Nurse: It sounds like you have learned much about your illness, one that can be treated, so that you don't always have to feel this way.

Patient: This is easier to say right now when I'm here and can get help if I need it. It's hard to remember this when I'm in the middle of a panic attack and think I'm dying.

Nurse: It's harder when you're alone?

Patient: Much harder! And I'm alone so much of the time.

Nurse: Let's talk about some ways you can manage your panics when you're alone. Tell me some of the techniques you've learned.

Critical Thinking Challenge

- What tone is established by the nurse's opening question in the first scenario?
- Which therapeutic communication techniques did the nurse use in the second scenario to avoid the pitfalls encountered in the first scenario?
- What information was uncovered in the second scenario that was not touched on in the first?
- What predictions can you make about the interpersonal relationship likely to develop between the nurse and the patient in each scenario?

BOX 20.10

Psychoeducation Checklist

Panic Disorder

When caring for the patient with panic disorder, be sure to include the following topic areas in the teaching plan:

☐ Psychopharmacologic agents (anxiolytics or antidepressants) if ordered, including drug action, dosage, frequency, and possible adverse effects
☐ Breathing control measures
☐ Potential dietary triggers
☐ Exercise
☐ Progressive muscle relaxation
☐ Distraction behaviours
☐ Relevant psychotherapies and where they are available
☐ Time and specific stress management strategies
☐ Positive coping strategies

to the individual. Crossing out each activity as it is completed helps the patient to regain a sense of control and accomplishment. Large tasks should be broken into a series of smaller tasks to minimize stress and maximize sense of achievement. Rest, relaxation, and family time—frequently omitted from the daily schedule—must be included.

Family Response to Disorder

Families afflicted with panic disorder have difficulty with overall communication. Parents with agoraphobia may become discouraged and self-critical regarding their child-rearing abilities, which may cause their children to be overly dependent. Parents with panic disorder may inadvertently cause excessive fears, phobias, or excessive worry in their children. Individuals will need a tremendous amount of support and encouragement from significant others.

Pharmacologic treatment for panic disorder also affects the family in other ways. Medications used to treat panic disorder readily cross the placenta and are excreted in breast milk. Open discussions regarding the benefits of a healthy mother and available options for women who wish to breast-feed and recognition of a women's right to participate in decision making are all important in postpartum panic disorder. Pregnancy may actually protect against certain anxiety disorders, but postpartum onset of such disorders is not uncommon.

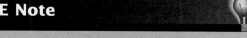

CRNE Note

Cognitive-behavioural therapy is the first-line psychotherapy for panic disorder, giving patients a sense of control over the recurring threats of panic and obsessions.

EVALUATION AND TREATMENT OUTCOMES

Patients can be assisted to keep a daily log of the severity of anxiety and the frequency, duration, and severity of panic episodes. This log will be a basic tool for monitoring progress as symptoms decrease. A number of self-help books can provide a rich source of reinforcement of simple interventions that can attenuate the intensity and frequency of panic symptoms. Rating scales may also be helpful to monitor changes in misinterpretations or other symptoms related to panic. Medications alone provide significant short-term improvement for many individuals, but a long-term combination of psychosocial and pharmacologic treatment is usually necessary.

Although many researchers consider panic disorder a chronic, long-term condition, the positive results from outcome studies should be shared with patients to provide encouragement and optimism that patients can learn to manage these symptoms. Outcome studies have demonstrated success with panic control treatment, CBT therapy, exposure therapy, and various medications specific to certain symptoms. Figure 20-2 illustrates a number of examples of biopsychosocial treatment outcomes for individuals with panic disorder.

CONTINUUM OF CARE

As with any disorder, continuum of patient care across multiple settings is crucial. Patients are treated in the least restrictive environment that will meet their safety needs. As the patient progresses through treatment, the environment of care changes from an emergency or

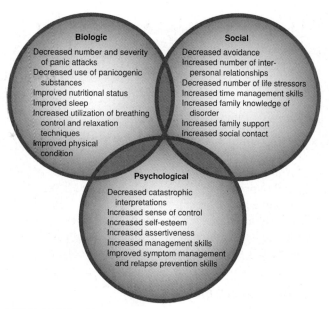

FIGURE 20.2   Biopsychosocial outcomes for patients with panic disorder.

inpatient setting to outpatient clinics or individual therapy sessions.

Inpatient-Focussed Care

Inpatient settings provide control for the individual with comorbid depression, increased risk for suicide, or poor treatment response to typical treatment strategies.

Emergency Care

Because individuals with panic disorder are likely to first present for treatment in an emergency room or primary care setting, nurses working in these settings should be involved in early recognition and referral. Consultation with a psychiatrist or mental health professional by the primary care physician can decrease both costs and overall patient symptoms (Katon, Roy-Byrne, Russo, & Cowley, 2002). Unnecessary emergency department visits cause soaring health care costs. Several interventions may be useful in reducing the number of emergency room visits related to panic symptoms. Psychiatric consultation and nursing education can be provided in the emergency department to explore other avenues of treatment. Remembering that the patient experiencing a panic attack is in crisis, nurses can take several measures to help alleviate symptoms, including the following:

- Stay with the patient and maintain a calm demeanour. (Anxiety often produces more anxiety, and a calm presence will help calm the patient.)

- Reassure the patient that you will not leave, that this episode will pass, and that he or she is in a safe place. (The patient often fears dying and cannot see beyond the panic attack.)
- Give clear, concise directions, using short sentences. Do not use medical jargon.
- Walk or pace with the patient to an environment with minimal stimulation. (The patient in panic has excessive energy.)
- Administer PRN anxiolytic medications as ordered and appropriate. (Pharmacotherapy is effective in treating acute panic.)

After the panic attack has resolved, allow the patient to vent his or her feelings. This often helps the patient in clarifying his or her feelings.

Family Interventions

In addition to learning the symptoms of panic disorder, nurses should have information sheets or pamphlets available concerning the disorder and any medications prescribed. Parents, especially single parents, will need assistance in child rearing and may benefit from services designed to provide some respite. Moreover, the entire family will need support in adjusting to the disorder. A referral for family therapy may be indicated. Involving the entire family in the therapy process is imperative. Families experience the symptoms, treatments, clinical setbacks, and recovery from chronic mental illnesses as a unit. Misunderstandings, misconceptions, false information, and stigma of mental illness, singly or collectively, impede recovery efforts.

Community Treatment

Most individuals with panic disorder will be treated on an outpatient basis. Referral lists of community resources and support groups are useful in this setting. Nurses can be directly involved in treatment, conducting psychoeducation groups on relaxation and breathing techniques, symptom management, and anger management. Advanced practice nurses conduct CBT and individual and family psychotherapy. In addition, medication monitoring groups re-emphasize the role of the medications, monitor for side effects, and enhance treatment compliance overall. See Nursing Care Plan 20-1.

Obsessive-Compulsive Disorder

Obsessive-compulsive disorder (OCD) is a psychiatric disorder characterized by severe obsessions, compulsions, or both that significantly interfere with normal daily routines. Affected patients feel chronically anxious

and that they have no control over the obsessions and compulsions, all of which have devastating consequences for patients.

Obsessions are characterized by excessive, unwanted thoughts or impulses that occur repetitively, causing severe anxiety and distress. Common obsessions include fears of contamination, pathologic doubt, the need for symmetry and completion, thoughts of hurting someone, and thoughts of sexual images (APA, 2000). Compulsions are repetitive actions or behaviours employed in an attempt to neutralize the anxiety felt from the obsession. For example, people with obsessive thoughts of becoming contaminated with dirt may wash their hands repeatedly to prevent contamination.

> **KEY CONCEPT Obsessions** are unwanted, intrusive, and persistent thoughts, impulses, or images that cause anxiety and distress. Obsessions create significant anxiety because they are not under the patient's control and are incongruent with the patient's usual thought patterns.

> **KEY CONCEPT Compulsions** are behaviours that are performed repeatedly, in a ritualistic fashion, with the goal of preventing or relieving anxiety and distress caused by obsessions.

Obsessive or compulsive behaviours are not necessarily signs of a psychiatric disorder if they do not persistently and significantly interfere with the person's ability to function. However, obsessions can consume a person's judgment to the degree that most of his or her day is spent performing actions in an attempt to minimize severe anxiety.

CLINICAL COURSE

The typical age of onset of OCD is in the early 20s to mid-30s, although symptoms of OCD can begin in childhood. Despite this early onset, it is often 7 to 10 years before individuals seek professional help because of the shame felt about the nature of their obsessions and compulsions (Hollander, 1997). Most common reasons that individuals with OCD seek professional help are relationship problems, generalized anxiety, alcohol or drug problems, and depression (Nestadt et al., 1998). The astute parent may notice that the child spends great amounts of time on trivial tasks or has failing grades because of poor concentration. Symptom onset of the disorder is gradual, and 15% of afflicted people show progressive decline in social and occupational functioning (APA, 2000). Men are affected more often as children and are most commonly affected by obsessions. Women have a higher incidence of checking and cleaning rituals,

NURSING CARE PLAN 20.1

Patient With Panic Disorder

Bill is a 65-year-old unmarried African American man who began having his first panic attacks after he retired from a post office position 2 years ago. He has been able to live alone until recently, when his daughter became concerned that he was isolating himself and refused to drive to pay bills or to go to the grocery store for food. He admitted to being fearful of leaving because of extreme nervousness and fear of a panic attack. His daughter convinced him to seek help, and he is now in a day treatment program at a local facility. He is able to attend the program most days.

SETTING: DAY TREATMENT PROGRAM, ADULT PSYCHIATRIC SERVICES

Baseline Assessment: Bill averages three or four panic attacks per week. His mental status is normal, with no cognitive impairment. MMSE is within normal limits. He has depressive symptoms but does not meet criteria for a mood disorder. He misses his job and feels as if part of his identity is lost. Vital signs are normal. He has a known 10-year history of hypertension, with a heart attack at the age of 57 years. He would like to "get rid of the feeling of nervousness" and be able to enjoy life like he did before retirement.

Associated Psychiatric Diagnosis	Medications
Axis I: Panic disorder with agoraphobia	Paroxetine CR (Paxil) 12.5 mg qd
Axis II: None	Lisinopril (Zestril) 20 mg daily
Axis III: History of hypertension	Lorazepam (Ativan) 1 mg every 6 hours PRN
Axis IV: Social problems (unable to leave home)	for extreme anxiety
GAF = Current 60	
Potential 90	

CARE PLAN FOR PANIC SYMPTOMS

Defining Characteristics	Related Factors
Trembling, increased pulse	Impending panic attacks
Fearful, irritable, scared, worried	Panic attacks
Apprehensive	

Outcomes

Initial	Long-term
Develop skills to decrease impact of panic attack	Carry out normal daily living and social activities outside of the house

Interventions

Interventions	Rationale
Meet daily with Bill to assess if he has had a panic attack within the last 24 hours.	Asking Bill to monitor panic attacks will provide data regarding potential antecedents to attacks.
Using a calm, reassuring approach, encourage verbalization of feelings, perceptions, and fears. Identify periods of time when anxiety level is at its highest.	Discussing the experience of anxiety will help the patient notice when his anxiety increases.
Teach Bill how to perform relaxation techniques.	Having strategies to deal with impending panic attack will decrease the intensity of the experience.
Teach Bill about the actions and side effects of paroxetine. Explain the purposes of each of the medications and track the use of PRN medications. Also, monitor for use of alcohol and herbal supplements.	Panic attacks are neurobiologic occurrences that respond to medications.

NURSING CARE PLAN 20.1 (Continued)

Ongoing Assessment

Determine whether Bill has had a panic attack.
Explore the antecedents and determine whether he was able to practice techniques from education programs.
Observe effectiveness of his technique and changes in anxiety/panic episodes.
Determine whether panic attacks decrease over time and whether there are side effects.
Determine his commitment to living a more normal life.

Evaluation

Outcomes	Revised Outcomes	Interventions
Bill's panic attacks decreased to once a week. Attended day treatment program every day. Able to go to grocery store.	Increase social activity outside of house.	Meet with Bill twice a week to monitor progress. Continue to reinforce the use of strategies in managing anticipatory anxiety.

with onset typically in the early 20s (Castle & Groves, 2000). This chronic disorder is characterized by episodes of symptom amelioration and exacerbation.

COMORBIDITY

Tourette's syndrome has an interesting relationship with OCD. There are similar alterations in brain functioning, and the two disorders often occur together (Johannes et al., 2003). Other psychiatric disorders co-occur as well. About two thirds of patients with OCD have a comorbid disorder, including depression (Overbeek, Schruers, Vermetten, & Greiz, 2002), social anxiety disorder, and panic disorder (Rasmussen & Eisen, 1990, 1992). Substance use disorder is common because individuals attempt to self-medicate their anxiety symptoms. A significant number of older depressed patients have OCD (Beekman, de Beurs, & von Balkom, 2000). Recent literature suggests that bipolar disorder and cyclothymic disorder may be comorbid with OCD (Kirkby, 2003; Perugi et al., 2002).

DIAGNOSTIC CRITERIA

The APA (2000) described five diagnostic criteria for OCD (see Table 20-6 for more detailed description of the symptom profile).

- Criterion A. The presence of obsessions or compulsions. Obsessions are defined as intrusive and inappropriate thoughts, images, or impulses causing marked anxiety, not simply excessive fretting over real-life situations. The person tries to ignore or suppress the thoughts or tries to neutralize them by some other thought or action, and understands that the thoughts are a product of his or her own mind. Compulsions are defined as repetitive behaviours that the person feels he or she must perform because of the thoughts or because of rules that must be rigidly followed, and actions performed to reduce stress or to prevent a catastrophe from occurring. The actions and thoughts are not realistically connected and are excessive to the situation.
- Criterion B. At some point in the disorder, the patient recognizes that the thoughts and actions are unreasonable or excessive. This criterion does not apply to children.
- Criterion C. The presence of the thoughts and rituals causes severe disturbance in daily routines, relationships, or occupational function and are time consuming, taking longer than 1 hour a day to complete.
- Criterion D. The thoughts or behaviours are not a result of another Axis I disorder.
- Criterion E. The thoughts or behaviours are not a result of the presence of a substance or a medical condition.

The specifier "With Poor Insight" is added if the patient does not see that the thoughts or behaviours are excessive or unreasonable.

OBSESSIVE-COMPULSIVE DISORDER IN SPECIAL POPULATIONS

Children

OCD affects between 1% and 2.3% or more of children and adolescents (APA, 2000). Because children subscribe to myths, superstition, and magical thinking, obsessive and ritualistic behaviours may go unnoticed. Behaviours such as touching every third tree, avoiding cracks in the sidewalk, or consistently verbalizing fears of losing a parent in an accident may have some underlying pathology but are common behaviours in childhood. However, it is increasing concerns about social, academic, and personal impairment that differentiate the common behaviours from OCD.

Table 20.6	Key Diagnostic Characteristics of Obsessive-Compulsive Disorder 300.3
Diagnostic Criteria and Target Symptoms	**Associated Findings**

Diagnostic Criteria and Target Symptoms	Associated Findings

• Recurrent obsession or compulsions
   Obsessions: inappropriate and intrusive recurrent and persistent thoughts, impulses, or images causing marked anxiety or distress that are not simply excessive worries
   Attempts to ignore, suppress, or neutralize obsessions with some other thought or action
   Recognizes them as a product of his or her own mind
   Compulsions: repetitive behaviours (such as handwashing, ordering, checking) or mental acts (such as praying, counting) person feels driven to perform in response to obsession or according to rigid rules
   Acts aimed at preventing or reducing the distress or preventing some dreaded event or situation
   Compulsions not connected realistically with what they are designed to neutralize or prevent or are clearly excessive
• Recognition by person that obsessions or compulsions are excessive or unrealistic (if not, specify with poor insight)
• Obsessions or compulsions are excessive or unrealistic
• Marked distress that is time-consuming or significantly interfering with normal routine and functioning
• If another psychiatric disorder present, content of obsessions or compulsions not restricted to it
• Not a direct physiologic effect of substance use or medical condition
	Associated Behavioural Findings
	• Avoidance of situations involving the content of the obsession or compulsion
	• Hypochondriacal concerns with frequent physician visits
	• Guilt
	• Sleep disturbances
	• Excessive use of alcohol or sedative, hypnotic, or anxiolytic medications
	• Compulsion performance a major life activity; may lead to serious marital, occupational, or social disability
	
	Associated Physical Examination Findings
	• Possible dermatologic problems caused by excessive washing with water or caustic cleaning agents
	
	Associated Laboratory Findings
	• Increase autonomic activity when confronted with circumstances that trigger obsession

EPIDEMIOLOGY

OCD has a 2.5% lifetime prevalence and a 1-year prevalence rate of 0.5% to 2.1% in the adult population. Rates are similar among women and men. First-degree relatives of people with OCD have a higher prevalence rate than the general population. Early-onset OCD increases the chances of OCD in relatives and predicts poorer treatment outcomes (Busatto, 2001). Other predictors of poor outcomes during life-long treatment include low social functioring and the presence of both obsessions and compulsions (Castle & Groves, 2000; Skoog & Skoog, 1999).

Many obsessive thoughts and compulsive acts are common in OCD. Checking rituals are common in this disorder. These patients must have objects in a certain order, perform motor activities in a rigid fashion, or arrange things in perfect symmetry. They may take a great deal of time to complete even the simplest task. These individuals tend to experience discontent, rather than anxiety, when things are not symmetrical or perfect. Other patients have magical thinking and perform compulsive rituals to ward off an imagined disaster. They use counting rituals to perform doing-and-undoing rituals (eg, repeatedly turning on and off the alarm clock) to help them feel that a disaster will not occur. Hoarders feel compelled to check their belongings

repeatedly to see that all is accounted for, and they may check the garbage to ensure that nothing of value was discarded.

Some patients have obsessions surrounding aggressive acts of hurting someone or themselves. After hitting a bump in the road, for example, these patients may obsess for hours over whether or not they hit a person. Parents may have recurrent intrusive thoughts that they may hurt their child.

Patients with religious obsessions obsess over the meaning of sins and whether they have followed the letter of the law. They tend to be hypermoral and have the need to confess. They may view their obsessions as a form of religious suffering. These patients are often resistant to treatment. Religious obsessions are most common where severe religious restrictions exist. Diagnosis is not made unless the thoughts or rituals clearly exceed cultural or religious norms, occur at inappropriate times as described by members of the same religion or culture, or interfere with social obligations (APA, 2000).

Some individuals with OCD have somatic fears and frequently seek medical treatment for physical symptoms, often just to get reassurance. Acquired immunodeficiency syndrome, cancer, heart attacks, and sexually transmitted diseases are some of the most common obsessional fears.

ETIOLOGY

During the 1990s, research evidence from neuroimaging studies, neurochemical studies, and treatment advances substantiated a predominantly neurobiologic basis for OCD. The following sections provide a brief overview of these findings and evidence pointing to genetic vulnerability. Psychological factors are also discussed because of their contributions to the disorder. Like most psychiatric disorders, the etiology of OCD is multifactorial, with genetic contributions, environmental factors, and psychosocial factors all playing interactive roles.

Biologic Research

Genetic, neuropathologic, and biochemical research, reviewed in this section, suggests that OCD has a biologic basis involving several neuroanatomic structures.

Genetic

OCD occurs more often in people who have first-degree relatives with OCD or with Tourette's disorder than it does in the general population. Some studies have also shown an increased prevalence of anxiety and mood disorders in relatives of individuals who have OCD. Twin studies have indicated that OCD occurs more frequently in siblings of monozygotic twins than of dizygotic twins. Furthermore, Mundo and colleagues (2000) discovered a link between the pathogenesis of OCD and $5\text{-HT}_{1D\beta}$ receptor gene. This discovery may lead to breakthroughs in pharmacologic treatments of OCD.

Neuropathologic

Structural neuroimaging studies using computed axial tomography and magnetic resonance imaging performed to find total-volume differences in brain structures have shown that a group of children with streptococcus-associated OCD, tics, or both have enlarged basal ganglia (caudate, putamen, and globus pallidus) compared with healthy children (Giedd et al., 2000). Basal ganglia structures are important in the control of fine motor movement.

Positron emission tomography and single-photon emission computed tomography reveal differences in cerebral glucose metabolism between patients with OCD and control subjects (see Chapter 9). Variation in methods of measurement produces some inconsistencies in the research findings. However, the most replicated results demonstrate increased glucose metabolism in the caudate nuclei (part of the basal ganglia), the orbitofrontal gyri (part of the frontal cortex involved in emotion), and the cingulate gyri (considered to be part of the limbic system, involved in connecting memory to emotion). Studies measuring cerebral blood flow and glucose metabolism in patients with OCD during exposure to feared stimuli and during relaxation have further implicated these regions of the brain (Baxter, 1992; Rauch et al., 1994).

Biochemical

There is pharmacologic evidence that serotonin plays a role in OCD. It has been studied through challenge tests in which serotonin agonists were administered to patients with OCD and control subjects. The most convincing evidence for serotonin's role is that serotonin-specific antidepressants relieve the symptoms of OCD for most patients. A single neurotransmitter is unlikely to be entirely responsible for OCD, but, to date, serotonin has been the most studied in relation to OCD. Conventional and novel antipsychotic medications and mood stabilizers have been used in conjunction with serotonin-targeting medications to treat refractory symptoms, suggesting that other brain pathways may be involved.

Infection

Interestingly, studies have found a link between infection with β-hemolytic streptococci and the subsequent emergence of OCD symptoms in children (Castle & Groves, 2000; Giedd et al., 2000).

Psychological Theories

Although psychological theories of OCD have not been empirically tested, the rich literature describing clinical examples and case histories helps us to understand the symptoms and behaviours related to OCD. A number of theories have been considered in the context of specific psychological frameworks. An example is in the context of a behavioural learning frame. Support for this theory comes from treatment success based on behavioural treatment of individuals with OCD.

Behavioural Explanations

Behavioural explanations for OCD stem from learning theory. From this viewpoint, obsessions are seen as conditioned stimuli. Through being associated with noxious events, stimuli that are usually considered neutral become anxiety provoking. The individual then engages in activities to escape or avoid the anxiety. Compulsions develop as the individual discovers behaviours that successfully reduce the obsessional anxiety. As the principles of operant conditioning indicate, the more the behaviours decrease the anxiety, the more likely the individual is to continue using them. However, the rituals or behaviours preserve the fear response because the person avoids the initial stimuli and thus never extinguishes the compulsion. Interrupting this cycle is the focus of behavioural therapy in treating an individual with OCD.

INTERDISCIPLINARY TREATMENT

Patients with OCD can be difficult to treat because of their symptoms and the pathology of the disease. The obsessions and compulsions consistently interfere with recovery efforts during the treatment course. Most patients with OCD are treated in specific outpatient programs and in private physician practice, but short-term hospitalization is often used for comorbid depression and for treatment of refractory symptoms. It is very important that all staff be consistent in their expectations and acceptance of the patient's behaviours, to keep these patients from becoming frustrated or confused regarding expectations during treatment (Box 20-11).

PRIORITY CARE ISSUES

As with any patient with a psychiatric disorder, a suicide assessment must be completed. Although patients with OCD do not usually become suicidal as a direct result of anxiety, the disorder greatly distresses the patient, who realizes the pointlessness and absurdity of the behaviours. Often, the patient has tolerated symptoms

---

BOX 20.11

Clinical Vignette: Obsessive-Compulsive Disorder

Robert, a 32-year-old man, is a new patient at a local psychiatric unit. He admitted himself to have his medicines evaluated because his obsessive thoughts and depression have worsened since his recent divorce. While in the hospital, he has quickly become viewed as a "problem patient" because he hoards linens and demands a new bar of soap for each of his five daily showers. He is compelled to open and close his door five times when he leaves or enters his room but does not know why. This behaviour has led to arguments with his roommate. In an effort to "help him," the staff locked his bathroom door to prevent him from showering so frequently. He tried to enter his bathroom to shower, and panicked when the staff refused to allow him to shower, telling him "You can live without it." After receiving PRN medication for extreme anxiety, Robert signed out of the hospital against medical advice because of embarrassment and anger toward the nursing staff.

What Do You Think?

- How could the staff have handled the situation differently so as to not disrupt Robert's or the unit's clinical care?
- What nursing interventions might be appropriate in providing Robert's care?

---

for quite some time before seeking treatment. The patient may feel a sense of hopelessness and helplessness and may contemplate suicide to end the suffering. An additional risk for suicide is created by the high probability of major depression, which often accompanies OCD. Patients may feel a need to punish themselves for their intrusive thoughts (e.g., religious coupled with sexual obsessions). Some patients have aggressive obsessions, and external limits may have to be imposed for protection of others (see Chapter 35).

NURSING MANAGEMENT: HUMAN RESPONSE TO DISORDER

Obsessions create tremendous anxiety, and patients perform compulsions to relieve the anxiety temporarily. If the compensatory ritual is not performed, the person feels increased anxiety and distress. Common compulsions include washing, cleaning, checking, counting, repeating actions, ordering (eg, insisting that items be stored in a particular manner), confessing (eg, repeatedly describing past misconduct), and requesting assurances.

Individuals with OCD do not consider their compulsions pleasurable. Often they recognize them as odd and may initially try to resist them. Resistance eventually fails, and patients incorporate repetitive behaviours into daily routines, performing activities in a specific, ritual order. If this sequence is disturbed, the person experiences extreme anxiety until the process can be repeated in the correct sequence (see Table 20-6). Interpersonal relationships suffer, and the patient may actively isolate himself or herself. Indeed, individuals with OCD are more likely to be young, separated or divorced, and unemployed.

Biologic Domain

Assessment

Patients with OCD do not have a higher prevalence of physical disease. However, they may complain of multiple physical symptoms. With late-onset OCD (after 35 years of age) and with symptoms in children that occur after a febrile illness, cerebral pathology should be excluded. Each patient with OCD should be assessed for dermatologic lesions caused by repetitive hand washing, excessive cleaning with caustic agents, or bathing. Osteoarthritic joint damage secondary to cleaning rituals may be observed.

Interventions for Biologic Domain

Psychopharmacologic Treatment

The SSRIs are considered to be first-line treatment agents used for OCD. Clomipramine (a serotonin-selective TCA) was the first drug to produce significant advances in treating OCD. Other drugs may be used to treat refractory OCD symptoms, including lithium, risperidone (Risperdal), quetiapine (Seroquel), olanzapine (Zyprexa), and haloperidol (Haldol). An Expert Consensus Panel has developed detailed guidelines for the treatment of OCD (http://www.psychguides.com/ocgl.html).

ADMINISTERING AND MONITORING MEDICATIONS. Antidepressants used to treat OCD are often given in higher doses than those normally used to treat depression. Aggressive treatment may be indicated to bring the symptoms under control. Thus, medication effects, including signs of toxicity, must be closely monitored to provide safe and adequate care. These medications often take several weeks or months to relieve compulsions, and even longer to decrease obsessions.

Clomipramine pharmacotherapy should begin at 25 mg daily, taken at night, with gradual titration during a period of 2 weeks, to 150 mg to 250 mg daily, in divided doses. The maximum dose for children is 200 mg daily. This drug is not approved for children younger than 10 years.

The general rule for SSRI treatment is to start at lower doses to minimize any initial side effects like gastrointestinal upset and restlessness. Weekly increases are given with ongoing monitoring. Although not all the SSRIs are approved specifically for OCD or are all approved for children with OCD, the choice of the specific SSRI is usually based on individual response.

MONITORING SIDE EFFECTS. Side effects pose a particular problem for some individuals who are preoccupied with somatic concerns. Unwanted physical symptoms from the medications can become the focus of obsessions. These individuals particularly need frequent reassurance that they are not becoming physically ill and that most side effects are transient. To ignore or minimize these concerns will only heighten the patient's anxiety and potentially interfere with the desire to continue treatment.

Common side effects of clomipramine include significant sedation, anticholinergic side effects, and an increased risk for seizures. Dizziness, tremulousness, and headache are frequent complaints. Administration at night minimizes complaints of sedation and fatigue. Research is being conducted to compare responses to clomipramine and venlafaxine, a serotonin-norepinephrine reuptake inhibitor (SNRI) in the treatment of OCD. One preliminary study shows that venlafaxine may be as efficacious as clomipramine but with less harsh side effects (Albert, Aguglia, Maina, & Bogetto, 2002).

SSRIs can cause sedation, dizziness, somnolence, and headache. In addition, sexual dysfunction is a common complaint in patients, which may necessitate a change of medication. The SSRIs can cause gastrointestinal upset and restlessness when first started. Monitor patients for insomnia and adjust the dosing time if needed. Weight gain can occur with SSRIs but is relatively rare (Van Ameringen, Mancini, Pipe, Campbell, & Oakman, 2002).

MONITORING FOR DRUG INTERACTIONS. See earlier section regarding potential drug interactions with SSRIs.

ELECTROCONVULSIVE THERAPY. The effect of electroconvulsive therapy (ECT) on decreasing obsessions and compulsions has not been extensively studied. However, it may be helpful in treating severe depressive symptoms in patients who have not experienced response to other treatments and who are at significant risk for suicide. Nursing's role in caring for the patient undergoing ECT is outlined in Chapter 19.

Psychosurgery

Although rare, psychosurgery has been used to treat extremely severe OCD that has not responded to prolonged and intensive drug treatment, behavioural therapy, or a combination of the two. Modern stereotactic surgical techniques that produce lesions of the cingulum (a bundle of connective pathways between the two hemispheres) or anterior limb of the internal capsule (a region near the thalamus and part of the circuit connecting to the cortex) may bring about substantial clinical benefit in some patients without causing significant morbidity (Kim et al., 2003). Other treatment options include radiotherapy and deep brain stimulation in which electrical current is applied through an electrode inserted into the brain (Nuttin, Cosyn, Demeulemeester, Gybels, & Meyerson, 1999).

Maintaining Skin Integrity

For the patient with cleaning or hand-washing compulsions, attention to skin condition is necessary. Encourage the patient to use tepid water when washing and hand cream after washing. Remove harsh, abrasive soaps and replace with moisturizing soaps. The treatment team should work with the patient to decrease the frequency of washing by structuring time schedules and time-limited washing.

Teaching Points

Nurses play an important interdisciplinary role in managing medication for patients with OCD, which includes educating patients and families about medications. Because patients may become discouraged with perceived lack of effect, they should be informed that these medications may take several weeks before their effects are felt. All patients should be warned not to stop taking prescribed medications abruptly.

Patients should be instructed to avoid alcohol and not to operate heavy machinery while taking these medications until the sedative effects are known. Instruct patients to inform their providers about any OTC medications or herbal products they are taking because some will interact with these medications.

Psychological Domain

Assessment

The nurse should assess the type and severity of the patient's obsessions and compulsions. Most individuals will appear neatly dressed and groomed, cooperative, and eager to answer questions. Orientation and memory are not usually impaired, but patients may be distracted by obsessional thoughts. Individuals with severe symptoms may be preoccupied with fears or with discussing their obsessions, but in most instances, direct questions must be asked to reveal symptoms. For example, the nurse may begin indirectly by asking how long it takes the individual to dress in the morning or leave the house, but usually needs to ask follow-up questions, such as: Do you find yourself frequently returning to the house to make sure that you have turned off the lights or the stove, even when you know that you have already checked this? Does this happen every day? Are you ever late for work or for important appointments?

Speech will be of normal rate and volume, but often, individuals with an obsessional style of thinking will exhibit circumferential speech. This speech is loaded with irrelevant details but eventually addresses the question. Listening may be frustrating and require considerable patience, but you must remember that such speech is part of the disorder and may be beyond the patient's awareness. Continually interrupting and redirecting them can interfere with establishing a therapeutic relationship, especially in the initial assessment. Redirection should be done in a gentle and noncritical manner to allow the patient to refocus.

Identifying the degree to which the OCD symptoms interfere with the patient's daily functioning is important. Several rating scales can be used to identify symptoms and monitor improvement. Examples of these scales are provided in Box 20-12. The Yale-Brown Obsessive Compulsive Scale (Y-BOCS) is a popular,

---

BOX 20.12

Rating Scales for Assessing Obsessive-Compulsive Symptoms

Yale-Brown Obsessive Compulsive Scale (Y-BOCS)
Goodman, W., Price, L., Rasmussen, S., et al. (1989). The Yale-Brown Obsessive Compulsive Scale (Y-BOCS): Part I. Development, use and reliability. *Archives of General Psychiatry, 46*, 1006–1011.

The Maudsley Obsessional-Compulsive Inventory (MOC)
Rachman, S., & Hodgson, R. (1980). *Obsessions and Compulsions.* New York: Prentice-Hall.

The Leyton Obsessional Inventory
Cooper, J. (1970). The Leyton Obsessional Inventory. *Psychiatric Medicine, 1*, 48.

---

clinician-rated 16-item scale that obtains separate subtotals for severity of obsessions and compulsions. The Maudsley Obsessive-Compulsive Inventory is a 30-item, true–false, self-assessment tool that may help the individual to recognize individual symptoms.

Interventions for Psychological Domain

The nurse's interpersonal skills are crucial to successful intervention with the patient who has OCD. Nurses must control their own anxiety. The nurse should interact with the patient in a calm, nonauthoritarian fashion without exhibiting any disapproval of the patient or the patient's behaviours, while demonstrating empathy about the distress that the disorder has caused. This approach is one of the most effective means available for communicating appreciation for the individual, as separate from the illness.

Response Prevention

An effective behavioural intervention for patients with OCD who perform rituals is exposure with response prevention. The patient is exposed to situations or objects that are known to induce anxiety but is asked to refrain from performing the ritualistic behaviours. One goal of this procedure is to help the patient understand that resisting the rituals while exposed to the object of anxiety is less stressful and time-consuming than performing the rituals. Another goal is to confound the expectation of distressing outcomes and eventually extinguish the compulsive behaviours. Most patients improve with exposure and response prevention, but few become completely symptom free.

Thought Stopping

Thought stopping is used with patients who have obsessional thoughts. The patient is taught to interrupt obsessional thoughts by saying "Stop!" either aloud or subvocally. This activity interrupts and delays the uncontrollable spiral of obsessional thoughts. Research supporting this technique is scant; however, practitioners have found it useful in multimodal treatment with exposure and response prevention, relaxation, and cognitive restructuring.

Relaxation Techniques

Patients with OCD experience insomnia because of their heightened anxiety levels. Relaxation exercises may be helpful in improving sleep patterns. These exercises do not affect OCD symptoms, but they may be used to decrease anxiety. The nurse may also teach the patient other relaxation measures, such as deep breathing, taking warm baths, meditation, music therapy, or other quiet activities.

Cognitive Restructuring

Cognitive restructuring is a method of teaching the patient to restructure dysfunctional thought processes by defining and testing them (Beck & Emery, 1985). Its goal is to alter the patient's immediate, dysfunctional appraisal of a situation and perception of long-term consequences. The patient is taught to monitor automatic thoughts, then to recognize the connection between thoughts, emotional response, and behaviours. The distorted thoughts are examined and tested by for-or-against evidence presented by the therapist, which helps the patient to realistically assess the likelihood that the feared event will happen if the compulsive behaviour is not performed. The patient begins to analyze his or her thoughts as incongruent with reality. For example, even if the alarm clock is not checked 30 times before going to bed, it will still go off in the morning, and the patient will not be disciplined for tardiness at work. Maybe it needs to be checked only once or twice.

Cue Cards

Cue cards are tools used to help the patient restructure thought patterns. They contain statements that are positively oriented and pertain to the patient's specific obsessions and compulsions. Cue cards use information from the patient's symptom hierarchy, an organizational system that breaks down the obsessions and compulsions from least to most anxiety provoking. These cards can help reinforce the belief that the patient is safe and can tolerate the anxiety caused by delaying or controlling compulsive rituals. Examples of cue cards are in Box 20-13.

Psychoeducation

Psychoeducation is a crucial addition to all forms of therapy for the patient with OCD. Education is also important for the family, as are opportunities to openly discuss the frustration of living with someone with this disorder.

Teaching Points

The patient should be given information about all aspects of OCD, its impact on the individual, and the typical longitudinal course. Knowing that this is a chronic disorder

---

BOX 20.13

Examples of Cue Card Statements

- It's the OCD, not me.
- These are only OC thoughts; OC thoughts don't mean action; I will not act on the thoughts.
- My anxiety level goes up but will always go down. I never sat with the anxiety long enough to see that it would not harm me.
- Trust myself.
- I did it right the first time.
- Checking the locks again won't keep me safe. I really am safe in the world.

BOX 20.14

Psychoeducation Checklist

Obsessive-Compulsive Disorder
When caring for the patient with OCD, be sure to include the patient's caregiver, if appropriate, and address the following topic areas in the teaching plan:
☐ Psychopharmacologic agents (SSRIs, MAOIs, lithium, or anxiolytics) if ordered, including drug action, dosage, frequency, and possible adverse effects
☐ Skin care measures
☐ Ritualistic behaviours and alternative activities
☐ Thought stopping
☐ Relaxation techniques
☐ Cognitive restructuring
☐ Community resources

---

with remissions and exacerbations may help to lessen discouragement during times when symptoms have increased. Treatment is a shared responsibility between the patient, his or her family, and the professional treatment team. The patient should be included in all aspects of treatment decision making. If local support groups are available, the patient should be referred to reduce feelings of uniqueness and embarrassment about the disease. Family education will help the patient practice behavioural homework (Box 20-14).

Social Domain

Assessment

Nurses must consider sociocultural factors when evaluating OCD. At times, cultural or religious beliefs may be misunderstood and mistaken for obsessions or compulsions. Shame and embarrassment over the irrational thoughts and behaviours often lead to social isolation and relational difficulties. The time demands related to the compulsions often lead to decreased occupational success. Thus, assessment of current level of functioning in social, occupational, and personal spheres is important.

Interventions for Social Domain

- For the hospitalized patient, unit routines must be carefully and clearly explained to decrease fear of the unknown. Initially providing a private room may decrease the fear and anxiety related to explaining one's behaviour to other patients.
- Help the patient choose relaxation or recreational activities that can be interrupted and later continued, to minimize frustration.
- Assist the patient in arranging a schedule of activities that incorporates some private time but also integrates the patient into normal unit activities.

Family Response to Disorder

Those with more severe symptoms are more likely to be more impaired in social skills and to have more difficulties with intimacy, and, consequently, are less likely to marry. Some studies have also shown higher divorce rates for individuals with OCD (Grabe et al., 2000). They also have higher rates of celibacy, possibly because they fear being dirty or becoming contaminated.

OCD often diminishes the quality of family relationships. Individuals with this disorder may ask family members to become involved in their rituals of checking or providing repeated reassurance (Koran, 2000). Those with OCD can become very angry and frustrated with family members for failing to comply with their requests for help with rituals. These feelings can result in verbal and even physical altercations. Many family members find themselves modifying routines to suit a patient's symptoms and report this to be at least moderately distressing for them (Calvocoressi et al., 1999). The most troublesome symptoms of OCD for families to cope with include the patient's ruminations, long-standing unemployment, rituals, noncompliance with medication, depression, withdrawal from social and family contact, lack of motivation, and excessive arguing (Cooper, 1996). Spouses report a variety of issues such as sexual difficulties; overwhelming feelings of frustration, anger, guilt, and fatigue; and disrupted family and social life. Other relatives reported moderate to severe burden in coping with an individual with OCD. They stated they had difficulty going on holidays, poor social relationships, and neglected their hobbies due to their relative's illness (Magliano, Tosini, & Guarneri, 1996).

EVALUATION AND TREATMENT OUTCOMES

Several methods can be used to measure the response to treatment, including changes in Y-BOCS scores or other rating scales, self-reports regarding decreases in frequency and duration of rituals, increasing sense of self-efficacy, and the ability to complete activities of daily living in a timely manner. The patient should be able to participate in family and social activities with minimal anxiety. Both the patient and his or her family should also have knowledge about OCD and know about additional sources of information and support in their community.

CONTINUUM OF CARE

Inpatient-Focussed Care

These patients require a significant amount of staff time. They may monopolize bathrooms or showers or have disruptive rituals involving eating. The nurse should help the patient perform activities of daily living to ensure that they are completed. Monitoring medication effects, teaching psychoeducation groups, ensuring adequate caloric intake, and providing individual patient counselling are additional inpatient interventions.

Emergency Care

Individuals with OCD frequently use medical services long before they seek psychiatric treatment. Therefore, early recognition of symptoms and referral are important concerns for nurses working in primary care and other medical settings. Once individuals are referred, most psychiatric treatment of OCD occurs on an outpatient basis. Although only individuals with severely debilitating symptoms or self-harming thoughts and actions are hospitalized, patients may experience intense anxiety symptoms to the point of panic. In such an emergency, benzodiazepines and other anxiolytics can be used.

Family Interventions

The families of patients with OCD will need to be educated about the etiology of the disorder. Understanding the biologic basis of the disorder should decrease some of the stigma and embarrassment they may feel about the bizarre nature of the patient's obsessions and compulsions. Education about both biologic and psychological treatment approaches should be provided. Family assistance in monitoring symptom remission and medication side effects is invaluable. Family members can also assist the patient with behavioural and cognitive interventions. When caring for the patient with OCD, be sure to include the patient's caregiver, if appropriate, and address the following topic areas in the teaching plan:

- Medications: drug action, dosage, frequency, and possible adverse effects
- Skin care measures
- Ritualistic behaviours and alternative activities
- Thought stopping
- Relaxation techniques
- Cognitive restructuring
- Community resources

Community Treatment

Partial hospitalization programs and day treatment programs care for most patients with OCD. They allow patients to maintain significant independence, while beginning medications and behavioural therapies. Specific day-treatment psychotherapy programs for OCD are available in some larger urban centres. Specific outpatient clinics may also be available. Self-help groups and self-help books can also help patients keep symptoms under control.

Generalized Anxiety Disorder

Generalized anxiety disorder (GAD) is characterized by long-standing, excessive worry and anxiety (apprehensive expectation). Individuals with this disorder experience excessive worry and anxiety almost daily for extended periods. The anxiety does not usually pertain to a specific situation; rather, it concerns a number of real-life activities or events. Ultimately, the excessive worry and anxiety cause great distress and must significantly interfere with the patient's daily personal or social life.

CLINICAL COURSE

The onset of GAD is insidious. Many patients complain of being chronic worriers. GAD affects individuals of all ages. About half the individuals presenting for treatment report onset in childhood or adolescence, although onset after 20 years of age is also common. Adults with GAD often worry about matters such as their job, household finances, health of family members, or simple matters, such as household chores or being late for appointments. The intensity of the worry fluctuates, and stress tends to intensify the worry and anxiety symptoms (APA, 2000).

Patients with GAD often have mood symptoms, from mild depressive symptoms, such as dysphoria, to comorbid, major depressive disorder. They are also highly somatic, with complaints of multiple clusters of physical symptoms, including muscle aches, soreness, and gastrointestinal ailments (APA, 2000). In addition to physical complaints, patients with GAD often experience poor sleep habits, irritability, trembling, twitching, poor concentration, and an exaggerated startle response.

Transient anxiety is an integral part of the human condition and serves as a powerful behavioural motivator. However, if anxiety is excessive and disproportionate to identifiable stressors in terms of severity, persistence, and disability, then it requires professional attention and likely some treatment (Rickels & Schweitzer, 1998). Generally, patients with GAD feel frustrated, disgusted with life, demoralized, and hopeless. They may state that they cannot remember a time that they did not feel anxious. They experience a sense of ill-being and uneasiness and a fear of imminent disaster. Over time, they may recognize that their chronic tension and anxiety are unreasonable.

COMORBIDITY

Patients with GAD often have other psychiatric disorders. Roughly three fourths of patients with GAD have at least one additional current or lifetime psychiatric diagnosis. The most common comorbid disorders are major depressive disorder, social phobia, specific phobia, panic disorder, and dysthymia. Lenze and colleagues (2000) found that 27.5% of depressed elderly patients have a comorbid anxiety disorder; Beekman and associates (2000) found that 30.3% of patients with GAD also had major depressive disorder.

Substance use disorder is a significant problem associated with GAD. Patients with GAD may use alcohol, anxiolytics, or herbal or OTC products to relieve anxiety symptoms, but these self-medication strategies often lead to further despondency and self-criticism. The individual ends up with multiple psychiatric problems, rather than one.

DIAGNOSTIC CRITERIA

The APA (2000) describes several diagnostic features of GAD: excessive worry and anxiety about several issues that occurs more days than not for a period of at least 6 months (Criterion A). The patient has little or no control over the worry (Criterion B). The anxiety and worry are accompanied by at least three of the following symptoms for at least 6 months: sleep disturbance, becoming easily fatigued, restlessness, poor concentration, irritability, and muscle tension (Criterion C). The worry and anxiety focuses are not limited to the qualities of another psychiatric diagnosis, including panic disorder, social phobia, OCD, separation anxiety disorder, anorexia nervosa, somatization disorder, or hypochondriasis and do not exclusively occur with PTSD (Criterion D). The worry and anxiety cause significant impairment in social, occupational, or other significant area of functioning (Criterion E). Finally, the disturbance is not substance induced or caused by a general medical condition and does not occur exclusively with a mood, psychotic, or pervasive developmental disorder (Criterion F) (Table 20-7).

GENERALIZED ANXIETY DISORDER IN SPECIAL POPULATIONS

The lowest lifetime and 12-month prevalence rates for GAD occur in younger age groups, and the highest rates are found in those older than 35 years of age. The disorder has a gender bias, with more women having GAD than men (Wittchen & Hoyer, 2001). Children with GAD may manifest their symptoms through worry about their performance in school or sports and often excel in these areas (Castellanos & Hunter, 2000).

Elderly people also experience GAD, although anxiety in old age has not received much attention. Nonetheless, many elderly patients in depression and anxiety studies meet the criteria for GAD or have significant anxiety symptoms (Beekman et al., 2000; Lenze et al., 2000; Wang et al., 2000). Benzodiazepines should be used with

Table 20.7	Key Diagnostic Characteristics of General Anxiety Disorder	

Diagnostic Criteria and Target Symptoms	Associated Findings
<ul><li>Excessive anxiety and worry (apprehensive expectation) occurring for more days than not for at least 6 months involving a number of events or activities Restlessness or feeling keyed up or on edge Being easily fatigued Difficulty concentrating or mind going blank Irritability Muscle tension Sleep disturbance</li><li>Difficulty controlling the worry</li><li>Focus of anxiety and worry not confined to another psychiatric disorder</li><li>Clinically significant distress or impairment of functioning resulting from anxiety, worry, or physical symptoms</li><li>Not a direct physiologic effect of a substance or medical condition</li><li>Does not occur exclusively during a mood disorder, psychotic disorder, or pervasive developmental disorder</li></ul>	*Associated Behavioural Findings* <ul><li>Possible depressive symptoms</li></ul>*Associated Physical Examination Findings* <ul><li>Muscle tension with twitching, trembling, feeling shaky, and muscle aches and soreness</li><li>Clammy cold hands, dry mouth, sweating, nausea or diarrhoea, "lump in the throat"</li></ul>

caution in elderly patients with GAD because these drugs can produce memory and motor impairment.

EPIDEMIOLOGY

Because comorbid psychiatric diagnoses are common, assessing the true prevalence of this disorder is difficult. However, GAD is common, affecting nearly 4% of the population at any given time. Large community-based population studies show that the lifetime prevalence rate is nearly 10% (Fifer et al., 1994). Of those presenting at anxiety disorder clinics, 25% have GAD and a primary or comorbid diagnosis (APA, 2000). Epidemiologic studies of clinical populations are difficult because most individuals with GAD present in primary care with somatic and sleeping problems.

ETIOLOGY

In addition to GAD being associated with increasing age and being female, other correlates have been identified. These include being previously married, being unemployed, and working within the home, suggesting that psychosocial and environmental factors are involved in the development of GAD. Biologic theories of causation for GAD have focussed on broader issues of allostasis and the effect of persistent anxiety on physical and mental health. Although no direct etiologic theory has emerged, most researchers in the area recognize GAD is a chronic debilitating disorder that requires further investigation.

Neurochemical Theories

Symptoms suggesting activation of the sympathetic nervous system are common in GAD, and studies have found evidence of norepinephrine system dysregulation. Venlafaxine, an SNRI, is approved for the treatment of GAD. Medications that act on serotonin, such as the SSRIs, are also effective in treating anxiety. Although more research is needed to understand the underlying pathophysiology, treatments affecting serotonin and norepinephrine systems or the $GABA_A$ receptor complex suggest areas of research exploration.

Genetic Theories

Few studies have examined genetic factors in the etiology of GAD. One study of twins revealed that GAD is a moderately inheritable disorder. Individuals with GAD may have a genetic vulnerability that predisposes them to anxiety sensitivity. However, the epidemiologic data that show that the prevalence of GAD increases with age suggest that environmental factors play a significant role in the development of GAD.

Psychological Theories

Cognitive-behavioural theory regarding the etiology of GAD proposes that the disorder results because of inaccurate assessment of perceived environmental dangers. These inaccuracies result from selective focus on negative details, distorted information processing, and an overly pessimistic view of one's coping ability. Sources of anxiety change over different developmental stages and include such conflicts as fear of separation, fear of failure, and fear of loss of love.

Sociologic Theories

The family environment might also play an important role because one may become anxious through learned behaviour or parental modeling. Although there are no specific sociocultural theories related to the development of GAD, a high-stress lifestyle and multiple stressful life events may be contributors. Individuals with GAD are hypersensitive to stress and anxiety-provoking events.

RISK FACTORS

Unresolved conflicts, cognitive misinterpretations, and life stressors (previous failed relationships, not working or working at home) are examples of potential contributors to the development of the disorder. Behavioural inhibition, characterized by shyness, fear, or becoming withdrawn in unfamiliar situations, may be a risk factor for GAD and other anxiety disorders (Castellanos & Hunter, 2000).

NURSING MANAGEMENT: HUMAN RESPONSE TO DISORDER

Nursing assessment and intervention for individuals with GAD include many of the same biopsychosocial considerations that apply to panic disorder. Assessment of the patient's anxiety symptoms should include the following questions; answers are used to tailor individual approaches:

- How do you experience anxiety symptoms?
- Are you aware when you are becoming anxious?
- Are you aware of any connection between your anxiety and any physical symptoms?
- What coping mechanisms have you used in the past and what has been successful? Why do you think they are not working for you now?
- What life stressors add to these symptoms? What changes can you make to reduce these stressors?

Biologic Domain

Assessment

Diet and Nutrition

Some ordinary food stimulants, such as caffeine, are known to induce anxiety symptoms, and patients with GAD may be hypersensitive to them. Many OTC medications can alter mood and may increase anxiety symptoms. A concrete step that patients with GAD can take to reduce anxiety is to eliminate caffeine from their diets. Nurses can help patients achieve a caffeine-free state through education and dietary management, while assisting with pain relief for the headache that often accompanies caffeine withdrawal. Additional substances that can provoke anxiety are diet pills, amphetamines, ginseng, and ma huang (Chen et al., 2002).

Sleep Patterns

Sleep disturbance is a common symptom for individuals with GAD, so the patient's sleep pattern should be assessed closely. Alcohol should be avoided because it disturbs the sleep cycle. Conscientious sleep hygiene is important. Avoiding such things as alcohol and coffee (even tea for those very sensitive to caffeine) in the evening, eating late in the evening, working on difficult work-related or personal issues in the evening, and initiating night time discussion about sensitive issues with family members all may decrease sleep disturbance. Having bedtime routines that include a warm bath, quiet reading, and relaxation techniques also promote sleep.

Interventions for Biologic Domain

The physical symptoms of anxiety and the neurotransmitter systems involved suggest that several medications can be effective in treating GAD. Benzodiazepines are commonly used, but long-term use is not recommended. Other drug treatments include antidepressants, such as paroxetine, imipramine, buspirone, and venlafaxine.

Administering and Monitoring Medications

Although widely used in patients with GAD, benzodiazepine treatment remains somewhat controversial. If the patient self-medicates, benzodiazepines may complicate treatment because of their addictive qualities. However, many people with GAD are reluctant to take prescribed medications, and most do not seek treatment until their level of suffering is substantial. Benzodiazepines offer quick relief from anxiety symptoms until the antidepressant therapeutic effects are felt, which may take a few weeks. Hydroxyzine (a histamine receptor antagonist) shows promise for treating GAD and may provide an alternative to benzodiazepines (Llorca et al., 2002).

Buspirone. Buspirone (BuSpar) is an antidepressant with anxiolytic properties. It acts by inhibiting spontaneous firing of serotonergic neurons in the dorsal raphe and by antagonism of 5-HT1a receptors in the dorsal raphe, hippocampus, and parts of the frontal cortex. These actions in serotonin pathways may increase brain noradrenergic and dopaminergic activity (see Chapter 13 for additional information). Buspirone must be taken for 3 to 4 weeks before its anxiolytic effects are felt. This delay may be difficult for patients to tolerate and may need a short course of benzodiazepines during the initiation phase of treatment with buspirone.

Antidepressants. Venlafaxine, paroxetine, and imipramine have proven effective in treating GAD. They have serotonergic and noradrenergic effects, which are believed to reduce anxiety symptoms (Rickels et al., 2000; Rickels, Pollack, Sheehan, & Haskins, 2000).

Monitoring Side Effects

TCAs (imipramine) and benzodiazepines cause significant side effects and drug interactions that require ongoing monitoring. (See the discussions of these medications in the section on treatment of panic disorder.)

Buspirone side effects include dizziness, insomnia, drowsiness, and nervousness. Dry mouth, blurred vision, and abdominal distress can occur but are uncommon.

Venlafaxine has a relatively benign side-effect profile. Anticholinergic effects, including dry mouth and constipation, are common but much less problematic compared with TCAs. This drug also causes dizziness, nervousness, and insomnia. Transient hypertension occurs in some patients; therefore, blood pressure should be monitored. Gastrointestinal effects (nausea and vomiting) can occur as well.

Monitoring for Drug Interactions. Venlafaxine and buspirone both interact with MAOIs, and neither should be initiated within 14 days of treatment of each other unless under a specialist's care. Although buspirone does not increase alcohol-induced impairment, it is prudent to avoid use of alcohol because it depresses the CNS.

Teaching Points

Teaching points for venlafaxine and buspirone include informing the patient that the anxiolytic effects of the medication will not be felt for several weeks. Warn patients against operating heavy machinery until they know the effects of the medication. If benzodiazepine therapy is being tapered and buspirone therapy started, instructions to the patient should include a warning not to discontinue use of the benzodiazepine suddenly because of the risks for withdrawal symptoms, rebound anxiety, and seizures.

Psychological and Social Domains

Psychological and social assessment and intervention strategies for GAD are similar to those for panic disorder; refer to the section on panic disorder. Cognitive and behavioural therapies, effective treatments for GAD, are generally underused. Outcome studies indicate that cognitive treatment achieves significant reductions in the severity of somatic and anxiety symptoms, with many patients regaining normal function. Combining relaxation and supportive and cognitive therapies may potentiate therapeutic effects.

EVALUATION AND TREATMENT OUTCOMES

Treatment outcomes for patients with GAD include reducing the frequency and intensity of anxiety and controlling the factors that stimulate or provoke this uncomfortable state. Specifically, evaluation can focus on the individual's ability and skills in using techniques that control anxiety, such as relaxation, positive self-talk, and stress management. Reducing personal and environmental stress; eliminating certain foods and drinks, such as caffeine, in the diet; and developing strategies to deal with stressful family situations are outcome successes.

CONTINUUM OF CARE

Like patients with panic disorder, patients with GAD often seek treatment in emergency rooms or from medical internists because of the physical symptoms associated with the illness. Only about one third of patients with GAD seek psychiatric treatment (APA, 2000), and many patients do not seek any treatment. Many patients with GAD who do seek treatment consult internists, cardiologists, or neurologists for their physiologic symptoms. Nurses in these settings must be aware of the disorder and able to provide necessary assessment and intervention. Nurses in home health settings have an excellent opportunity to identify symptoms of undiagnosed GAD and make appropriate referrals.

Whether treatment is home or clinic based, both the patient and the health professional must actively participate in monitoring and managing environmental stress levels. Patients need a relaxing and quiet environment. Reducing noise and lowering lights induces relaxation; methods such as breathing control exercises, progressive muscle relaxation, and other interventions discussed previously in this chapter may also be helpful (Box 20-15).

SPECIFIC PHOBIA

Specific phobia (formally simple phobia) is a disorder marked by persistent fear of clearly discernible, circumscribed objects or situations, which often leads to

---

BOX 20.15

Psychoeducation Checklist

Generalized Anxiety Disorder
When caring for the patient with generalized anxiety disorder, be sure to include the following topic areas in the teaching plan:
□ Psychopharmacologic agents (benzodiazepines, antidepressants, nonbenzodiazepine anxiolytics) if ordered, including drug action, dosage, frequency, and possible adverse effects
□ Breathing control
□ Nutrition and diet restriction
□ Sleep measures
□ Progressive muscle relaxation
□ Time management
□ Positive coping strategies

avoidance behaviours. The lifetime prevalence rates range from 7% to 11%, and the disorder generally affects women twice as much as men. It has a bimodal distribution, peaking in childhood and then again in the 20s. The focus of the fear in specific phobia may result from the anticipation of being harmed by the phobic object. For example, dogs are feared because of the chance of being bitten, or automobiles are feared because of the potential of crashing. The focus of fear may likewise be associated with concerns about losing control, panicking, or fainting on exposure to the phobic object.

Anxiety is usually felt immediately on exposure to the phobic object, and the level of anxiety is usually related to both the proximity of the object and the degree to which escape is possible. For example, anxiety heightens as a cat approaches a person who fears cats and lessens when the cat moves away. At times, the level of anxiety escalates to a full panic attack, particularly when the person must remain in a situation from which escape is deemed to be impossible. Fear of specific objects is fairly common, and the diagnosis of specific phobia is not made unless the fear significantly interferes with functioning or causes marked distress. Assessment differentiates simple phobia from other diagnoses with overlapping symptoms. Box 20-2 lists a number of specific phobias. Among adult patients who are seen in clinical settings, the most to least common phobias are situational phobias, natural environment phobias, blood–injection–injury phobia, and animal phobias. The most common phobias among community samples are of heights, mice, spiders, and insects (APA, 2000).

Blood–injection–injury type phobia merits special consideration because the phobia surrounds medical treatments. The physiologic processes that are exhibited during phobic exposure include a strong vasovagal response, which significantly increases blood pressure and pulse, followed by deceleration of the pulse and lowering of blood pressure in the patient. Monitor closely when giving required injections or medical treatments.

About 75% of patients with blood–injection–injury phobia report fainting on exposure. Factors that may predispose individuals to specific phobias may include traumatic events, unexpected panic attacks in the presence of the phobic object or situation, observation of others experiencing a trauma, or repeated exposure to information warning of dangers, such as parents repeatedly warning young children that dogs bite.

Phobic content must be evaluated from an ethnic or cultural background. In many cultures, fears of spirits or magic is common and should be considered part of a disorder only if the fear is excessive in the context of the culture, causes the individual significant distress, or impairs the ability to function.

Psychotropic drugs have not been effective in the treatment of specific phobia. Anxiolytics may give short-term relief of phobic anxiety, but there is no evidence that they affect the course of the disorder. The treatment of choice for specific phobia is exposure therapy. Patients who are highly motivated can experience success with treatment (Newman, Erickson, Przeworski, & Dzus, 2003).

SOCIAL PHOBIA

Social phobia (social anxiety disorder) involves a persistent fear of social or performance situations in which embarrassment may occur. It is a common anxiety disorder with lifetime prevalence rates of 10% to 13% (Magee et al., 1996), although most who meet criteria do not get diagnosed (Ballenger et al., 1998). Exposure to a feared social or performance situation nearly always provokes immediate anxiety and may trigger panic attacks. People with social phobias fear that others will scrutinize their behaviour and judge them negatively. They often do not speak up in crowds out of fear of embarrassment. They will go to great lengths to avoid feared situations. If avoidance is not possible, they will suffer through the situation with visible anxiety.

People with social phobia appear to be highly sensitive to disapproval or criticism, tend to evaluate themselves negatively, and have poor self-esteem and a distorted view of personal strengths and weaknesses. They may magnify personal flaws and underrate any talents. They often believe others would act with more assertiveness in a given social situation. Men and women with social phobia tend to have difficulties with dating and with sexual relationships (Bodinger et al., 2002). Children tend to underachieve in school because of test-taking anxiety. This is an important area that should be assessed in all patients.

Onset is usually in early adolescence. There are two subtypes of this disorder. Generalized social phobia is diagnosed when the individual experiences fears related to most social situations, including public performances and social interactions. These individuals are likely to demonstrate deficiencies in social skills, and their phobias interfere with their ability to function. Individuals with specific social phobias fear and avoid only one or two social situations. Classic examples of such situations are eating, writing, or speaking in public or using public bathrooms.

Social phobias, like panic disorder and specific other phobias, are linked to a number of key neurotransmitter systems. Recent evidence links low dopamine receptor binding to social anxiety disorder (Schneier et al., 2000).

Pharmacotherapy for social phobia can include the MAOIs, SSRIs (in particular, fluvoxamine, sertraline, and paroxetine), and more recently gabapentin. Open trials (where the experimental design does not include the researcher's blindness to treatment and the drug's noncomparison to placebo) of nefazodone and venlafaxine show promise (Stein et al., 1999; Stein, Versiani, Hair, & Kumar, 2002; Van Ameringen et al., 1999).

POST-TRAUMATIC STRESS DISORDER

PTSD affects roughly 8% of the general population, and women are more likely than men to be affected. However, the prevalence of PTSD in clinical populations varies significantly by type of trauma, ranging from about 20% after motor vehicle crash to more than 80% after a prisoner of war experience. PTSD is defined by characteristic symptoms that develop after a traumatic event involving a personal experience of threatened death, injury, or threat to physical integrity. It may also include witnessing such an event happening to another person or learning that a family member or close friend has experienced such an event. Examples of traumatic events are experiencing interpersonal trauma (physical or sexual assault as a child or adult), military combat, natural disasters, or terrorist attack; being taken hostage; undergoing incarceration as a prisoner of war; enduring torture; participating in a motor vehicle crash; or being diagnosed with a life-threatening illness.

Individuals with PTSD have three core symptom clusters: re-experiencing, avoidance, and heightened arousal. They re-experience the event through distressing images, thoughts, or perceptions and may have recurrent nightmares. In addition, the patient may experience flashbacks and exhibit extreme stress upon exposure to an event or image that resembles the traumatic event (e.g., fireworks may bring back memories of war). Patients will avoid discussing the event altogether or avoid people and places that remind them of the traumatic event. Increased arousal is evidenced by difficulty sleeping, irritability, poor concentration, exaggerated startle response, or hypervigilance (APA, 2000).

Risk factors for PTSD include a prior diagnosis of depression or acute stress disorder (Brewin, Andrews, Rose, & Kirk, 1999). Other factors include being female, pre-existing personality, the duration, and intensity of trauma involved, environmental issues, coping style, low self-esteem, and previous traumatic events.

IN A LIFE

Lieutenant-General Romeo Dallaire
Commander of UN Peacekeeping Force, Rwanda, 1994

Public Personna
Romeo Dallaire, a former Canadian General, is well known for his service in Rwanda. He was given the task of enforcing a peace agreement between the largely Hutu-led government and Tutsi rebels. However, the circumstances of the situation turned out to be much more complex. The Hutu extremists were preparing for genocide against the minority Tutsis. Discovering the gravity of the problem, General Dallaire requested more forces, but was denied. Thus, when the massacre began, Dallaire and his 500 remaining men were left to try and stop a genocide that resulted in 800,000 Tutsi casualties in 100 days. Dallaire's hands were tied by the UN's strict rules of engagement and his repeatedly denied requests for more resources. The personal consequences of the tragic situation continue to haunt Dallaire and others who witnessed the horrific human carnage.

Personal Realities
Upon his return to Canada, Dallaire was faced with another difficult task: dealing with the horror he had experienced in Rwanda. He was diagnosed with PTSD, *which at the time was underacknowledged by National Defence.* Dallaire describes the challenge of being diagnosed with PTSD: "Sometimes I wish I had lost a leg instead of having all those brain cells screwed up. You lose a leg, it's obvious; you've got therapy, all kinds of stuff. You lose your marbles; very very difficult to explain, very difficult to gain that support that you need."

Dallaire began pharmacologic and psychological therapies, but he battled severe depression, attempting suicide several times. Dallaire's struggle became public shortly after he was medically released from the Armed Forces. In June 2000, Dallaire was found partially clothed, drunk, and near comatose on a park bench in Hull, Quebec. This incident gained national attention and sparked debate over PTSD. The experience also prompted Dallaire to begin writing his novel, *Shake Hands With the Devil: The Failure of Humanity in Rwanda,* a task he feels has helped him toward recovery.

Although Dallaire continues to struggle with PTSD, he is now a spokesperson and advocate. He has been acknowledged with the Dr. Samuel Henry Prince Humanitarian Award "For Exemplary Leadership of the Canadian Forces and the People of Canada in Advancing Understanding of Traumatic Stress and the Need for Compassionate Response" (http://www.ctsn-rcst.ca). He has received numerous other humanitarian awards and has helped the Canadian military create the video, *Witness the Evil,* to encourage traumatized soldiers of peacekeeping operations to seek help. On March 25, 2005, Dallaire was appointed as a member of the Canadian Senate.

From The National. *The unseen scars post traumatic stress disorder.* Available from CBC News, The National website, http://www.tv. cbc.ca/national; Wikipedia: The Free Encyclopedia. (2005). *Romeo Dallaire.* Available from Wikipedia: The Free Encyclopedia website, http://en.wikipedia.org; CBC News Indepth. (2005). *Romeo Dallaire.* Available from CBC News Online website, http://www.cbc/ca; Heer, J. (2004). Romeo Dallaire: Haunted by genocide. *Boston Globe-Ideas,* April 4.

Clinical treatment guidelines have been established for PTSD and include pharmacologic therapies, such antidepressants (TCAs and SSRIs) and mood stabilizers (carbamazepine and valproate). Minipress, an antihypertensive agent, has been found to decrease recurrent nightmares in patients with PTSD (Raskind et al., 2002). This is an area for future research. Most individuals with PTSD benefit from a combination of pharmacotherapy and specific psychotherapies, such as CBT and prolonged exposure techniques (Foa et al., 1997).

ACUTE STRESS DISORDER

Acute stress disorder shares the same three symptom clusters as PTSD, but differs in duration (symptoms emerging 2 to 4 days after exposure to a traumatic stressor and lasting up to 1 month) and in the necessity of experiencing dissociative symptoms (numbing, detachment, a reduction of awareness to one's surroundings, derealization, depersonalization, or dissociative amnesia). Controversy continues regarding whether acute stress disorder should be more accurately considered early PTSD and whether early dissociation is necessary for diagnosis. Both of these disorders are the topic of intense research activity, and leading experts are theorizing that these disorders are the result of failed recovery, rather than immediate psychopathologic processes. Most individuals show some level of re-experiencing, avoidance, and hyperarousal in the aftermath of a traumatic event, but will recover over time. For those who develop stress disorders, the recovery processes are overwhelmed by internal and external factors that lead to persistent and debilitating symptoms. It should also be noted that for women and children, depression is the most common response to a serious stressor.

SUMMARY OF KEY POINTS

■ Anxiety-related disorders are the most common of all psychiatric disorders and comprise a wide range of disorders, including panic disorder, obsessive-compulsive disorder, generalized anxiety disorder, phobias, acute stress disorder, and post-traumatic stress disorder.

■ The anxiety disorders share the common symptom of recurring anxiety but differ in symptom profiles. Panic attacks occur in many of the disorders. Those experiencing anxiety disorders have high levels of physical and emotional symptoms and often experience dual diagnoses with other anxiety disorders, substance use disorder, or depression. These disorders often significantly impair an individual's ability to function socially, occupationally and personally. For example, patients with panic disorder are often seen in a number of health care settings, including hospital emergency rooms or clinics, presenting with a confusing array of physical and emotional symptoms. Skillful intervention is required to eliminate possible life-threatening causes and to support individuals to reinterpret their symptoms and seek professional help for panic disorder.

■ Current research points to a combination of biologic and psychosocial factors that cause persistent anxiety. Other research demonstrates that there are also personality traits that predispose individuals to anxiety disorders, including low-self esteem, external locus of control, some negative family influences, and some traumatic or stressful precipitating event. These biologic and psychosocial components combine to yield a true biopsychosocial theory of causation.

■ Treatment approaches for all anxiety-related disorders are somewhat similar, including pharmacotherapy, psychological treatments, or often a combination of both.

■ Nurses at the generalist level use interventions from each of the dimensions—biologic, psychological, and social. Approaching these patients with knowledge of the disorder, understanding, and calm is crucial. Nurses can be instrumental in crisis intervention, medication management, and psychoeducation. Psychoeducation is essential in the management of anxiety disorders and includes methods to help patients control and cope with the anxiety reactions (ie, control of breathing, stress reduction, and relaxation techniques), education regarding medication side effects and management, and education of family members to understand these disorders.

CRITICAL THINKING CHALLENGES

1 How does patient culture affect the assessment of anxiety?

2 How might one differentiate shyness from social anxiety disorder?

3 How might the etiology of depression and anxiety be similar, as antidepressant medications are used to treat both?

4 What are some of the barriers in assessing pathologic anxiety in children? Are anxiety disorders underdiagnosed or overdiagnosed in children? Explain.

5 What role might parents, aside from genetics, play in contributing to the development of anxiety disorders in their offspring?

6 What are the risks and benefits of treating anxiety disorders with benzodiazepine medications in persons with substance abuse?

7 Pregnancy appears to protect against the development of some anxiety disorders, and postpartum onset of anxiety disorders is not uncommon. What biopsychosocial dynamics may be involved?

WEB LINKS

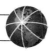

www.anxietycanada.ca This is the website of the Anxiety Disorders Association of Canada. It has information regarding anxiety disorders, including 10 educational brochures, each focussed on a particular anxiety disorder.

www.cmha.ca The Canadian Mental Health Association has information about anxiety disorders on their website.

www.nimh.nih.gov/anxiety/anxietymenu.cfm This is the National Institute of Mental Health's anxiety disorder website. An anxiety disorders education program is available.

www.anxman.org This Anxiety Panic Internet Resource site has self-help resources for those with panic disorder.

www.psych.org/public_info/anxiety_day.cfm This site is offered by the American Psychiatric Association and provides resources, articles, and valuable information on all anxiety disorders.

www.healingwell.com/anxiety/ This website on anxiety disorders provides articles and other resources for anxiety disorders. On-line ordering of resources is also available.

MOVIES

As Good As It Gets: 1997. Novelist Melvin Udall, played by Jack Nicholson, lives in his own world of obsessive-compulsive behaviour patterns, avoiding cracks in sidewalks and rigidly adhering to a regimen of daily breakfasts in the café, where single mom Carol Connelly, played by Helen Hunt, works. Udall's world is changed when he unwillingly becomes a sitter for his next-door neighbour's dog.

VIEWING POINTS: Identify the behaviours that indicate that Udall has an anxiety disorder. Observe feelings that are generated in you by Udall's behaviour. How are Udall's friends able to tolerate his behaviour?

REFERENCES

Albert, U., Aguglia, E., Maina, G., & Bogetto, F. (2002). Venlafaxine versus clomipramine in the treatment of obsessive-compulsive disorder: A preliminary single-blind, 12 week, controlled study. *Journal of Clinical Psychiatry, 63*(11), 1004–1009.

American Psychiatric Association (APA). (2000). *Diagnostic and statistical manual of mental disorders* (4th ed., Text revision). Washington, DC: Author.

Argyle, N., Delito, J., Allerup, P., et al. (1991). The Panic-Associated Symptom Scale: Measuring the severity of panic disorder. *Acta Psychiatrica Scandinavica, 83*, 20–26.

Allgulander, C., Bandelow, B., Hollander, E., Montgomery, S. A., Nutt, D. J., Okasha, A., et al. (2003). WCA-recommendations for the long-term treatment of generalized anxiety disorder. *CNS Spectrums, 8*(8), 53–61.

Bailey, J. E., Argyropoulos, S. V., Lightman, S. L., & Nutt, D. J. (2003). Does the brain noradrenaline network mediate the effects of the CO2 challenge? *Journal of Psychopharmacology, 17*(3), 252–259.

Ballenger, J. C. (1999). Current treatments of the anxiety disorders in adults. *Biological Psychiatry, 46*(11), 1579–1594.

Bandelow, B., Wedekind, D., Pauls, J., Brooks, A., Hajak, G., & Ruther, E. (2000). Salivary cortisol in panic attacks. *American Journal of Psychiatry, 157*, 454–456.

Barzega, G., Maina, G., Venturello, S., & Bogetto, F. (2001). Gender-related differences in the onset of panic disorder. *Acta Psychiatrica Scandinavica, 103*(3), 189–195.

Baxter, L. (1992). Neuroimaging studies of obsessive compulsive disorder. *Psychiatric Clinics of North America, 15*(4), 871–883.

Beck, A., & Emery, G. (1985). *Anxiety disorders and phobias: A cognitive perspective.* New York: Basic Books.

Beck, A., Epstein, N., Brown, G., & Steer, R. (1988). An inventory for measuring clinical anxiety: The Beck Anxiety Inventory. *Journal of Consulting and Clinical Psychology, 56*, 893–897.

Beekman, A., de Beurs, E., von Balkom, A., et al. (2000). Anxiety and depression in later life: Co-occurrence and communality of risk factors. *American Journal of Psychiatry, 157*, 89–95.

Ben-Zion, I., Meiri, G., Greenberg, B., et al. (1999). Enhancement of CO_2-induced anxiety in healthy volunteers with the serotonin agonist metergoline. *American Journal of Psychiatry, 156*, 1635–1637.

Blanco, C., Schneier, F. R., Schmidt, A., Blanco-Jerez, C. R., Marshall, R. D., Sanchez-Lacay, A., et al. (2003). Pharmacological treatment of social anxiety disorder: A meta-analysis. *Depression and Anxiety, 18*(1), 29–40.

Bland, R. C., Newman, S. C., & Orn H., (1988). Period prevalence of psychiatric disorders in Edmonton. *Acta Psychiatrica Scandinavica Supplement, 338*, 33–42.

Bodinger, L., Hermesh, H., Aizenberg, D., et al. (2002). Sexual function and behaviour in social phobia. *Journal of Clinical Psychiatry, 63*(10), 874–879.

Breslau, N., Davis, G.C., Andreski, P., & Peterson, E. (1991). Traumatic events and posttraumatic stress disorder in an urban population of young adults. *Archives of General Psychiatry, 48*, 216–222.

Bradwejn, J., Koszycki, D., du Tertre, A., et al. (1992). The cholecystokinin hypothesis of panic and anxiety disorders: A review. *Journal of Psychopharmacology, 6*, 345–351.

Brauer, H., Nowicki, P., Catalano, G., & Catalano, M. (2002). Panic attacks associated with citalopram. *Southern Medical Journal, 95*(9), 1088–1089.

Brewin, C., Andrews, B., Rose, S., & Kirk, M. (1999). Acute stress disorder and posttraumatic stress disorder in victims of violent crime. *American Journal of Psychiatry, 156*(3), 360–366.

Busatto, G. (2001). Regional cerebral blood flow abnormalities in early-onset obsessive-compulsive disorder: An exploratory SPECT study. *Journal of the American Academy of Child and Adolescent Psychiatry, 40*(3), 347–354.

Cagnacci, A., Arangino, S., Renzi, A., Zanni, A. L., Malmusi, S., & Volpe, A. (2003). Kava-kava administration reduces anxiety in peri-menopausal women. *Maturitas, 44*(2), 103–109.

Calvocoressi, L., Mazure, C.M., Kasl, S.V., Skolnick, J., Fisk, D., Vegso, S.J., Van Noppen, B.L., & Price, L.H. (1999). Family accommodation of obsessive-compulsive symptoms: Instrument development and assessment of family behavior. *Journal of Nervous and Mental Disorders. 187*, 636–642.

Castle, D., & Groves, A. (2000). The internal and external boundaries of obsessive-compulsive disorder. *Australian and New Zealand Journal of Psychiatry, 34*, 249–255.

Castellanos, D., & Hunter, T. (2000). Anxiety disorders in children and adolescents. *Southern Medical Journal, 92*(10), 946–954.

Chambless, D. L., Caputo, G. C., Bright, P., & Gallagher, R. (1984). Assessment of fear in agoraphobics: The Body Sensations Questionnaire and the Agoraphobic Cognitions Questionnaire. *Journal of Consulting and Clinical Psychology, 52*, 1090–1097.

Chambless, D. L., Caputo, G. C., Jasin, S. E., et al. (1985). The Mobility Inventory for Agoraphobia. *Behaviour Research and Therapy, 23*, 35–44.

Chen, J-P., Reich, L., & Chung, H. (2002). Anxiety disorders. *Western Journal of Medicine, 176*(4), 249–253.

Clum, G. A. (1990). Panic Attack Cognitions Questionnaire. *Coping with panic: A drug-free approach to dealing with anxiety attacks.* Pacific Grove, CA: Brooks/Cole.

Cooper, J. (1970). The Leyton Obsessional Inventory. *Psychiatric Medicine, 1*, 48.

Cooper, M. (1996). Obsessive-compulsive disorder: Effects on family members. *Orthopsychiatry, 66*, 296–304.

Dannon, P. N., Iancu I., & Grunhaus L. (2002). Psychoeducation in panic disorder patients: effect of a self-information booklet in a randomized, masked-rater study. *Depression and Anxiety, 16*(2), 71–76.

Dickstein, L. (2000). Gender differences in mood and anxiety disorders. From bench to bedside: American Psychiatric Press Review of Psychiatry (vol. 18). *American Journal of Psychiatry, 157*(7), 1186–1187.

Dillon, D. J., Gorman, J. M., Liebowitz, M. R., et al. (1987). Measurement of lactate-induced panic and anxiety. *Psychiatry Research, 20*, 97–105.

Emmanuel, J., Simmonds, S., & Tyrer, P. (1998). Systematic review of the outcome of anxiety and depressive disorders. *British Journal of Psychiatry Supplement, 34*, 35–41.

Enoch, M. A., Xu, K., Ferro, E., Harris, C. R., & Goldman, D. (2003). Genetic origins of anxiety in women: A role for a functional catechol-O-methyltransferase polymorphism. *Psychiatric Genetics, 13*(1), 33–41.

Fifer, S.K., Mathias, S.D., Patrick, D.L., Mazonson, P.D., Lubeck, D.P., & Buesching, D.P. (1994). Untreated anxiety among adult primary care patients in a Health Maintenance Organization. *Archives of General Psychiatry, 51*, 740–750.

Finfgeld, D. L. (2002). Selective reuptake inhibitor. Discontinuation syndrome. *Journal of Psychosocial Nursing and Mental Health Services, 40*(12), 18.

Flint, A. J. (2005). Generalised anxiety disorder in elderly patients: Epidemiology, diagnosis and treatment options. *Drugs & Aging, 22*(2), 101–114.

Foa, E.B. (1997). Psychological processes related to recovery from a trauma and the effective treatment for PTSD. *Annals of the New York Academy of Science, 821*, 410–424.

Friedman, S., Smith, L., Fogel, D., et al. (2002). The incidence and influence of early traumatic life events in patients with panic disorder: A comparison with other psychiatric outpatients. *Journal of Anxiety Disorders, 16*(3), 259–272.

Gardos, G. (2000). Long-term treatment of panic disorder with agoraphobia in private practice. *Journal of Psychiatric Practice, 6*, 140–146.

Giedd, J., Rapaport, J., Garvey, M., et al. (2000). MRI assessment of children with obsessive compulsive disorder or tics associated with streptococcal infection. *American Journal of Psychiatry, 157*(2), 281–283.

Goodman, W., Price, L., Rasmussen, S., et al. (1989). The Yale-Brown Obsessive Compulsive Scale (Y-BOCS): Part 1. Development, use and reliability. *Archives of General Psychiatry, 46*, 1006–1011.

Gorman, J., Kent, J., Sullivan, G., & Coplan, J. (2000). Neuroanatomical hypothesis of panic disorder, revised. *American Journal of Psychiatry, 157*(4), 493–505.

Grabe, H. J., Meyer, C., Hapke, U., Rumpf, H.-J., Freyberger, H. J., Dilling, H., et al. (2000). Prevalence, quality of life and psychosocial function in obsessive-compulsive disorder and subclinical obsessive-compulsive disorder in northern Germany. *European Archives of Psychiatry & Clinical Neuroscience, 250*, 262–268.

Halbreich, U. (2003). Anxiety disorders in women: A developmental and lifecycle perspective. *Depression and Anxiety, 17*(3), 107–110.

Hamilton, M. (1959). The assessment of anxiety states by rating. *British Journal of Medical Psychology, 32*, 54.

Hamilton, M., & White, J.M. (1959). Clinical syndromes in depressive states. *Journal of Mental Sciences, 105*, 985–998.

Hayward, C., Killen, J., & Kraemer, H. (2000). Predictors of panic attacks in adolescents. *Journal of the American Academy of Child and Adolescent Psychiatry, 39*(2), 207–214.

Hettema, J. M., Neale, M. C., & Kendler, K. S. (2001). A review and meta-analysis of the genetic epidemiology of anxiety disorders. *American Journal of Psychiatry, 158*(10), 1568–1578.

Hollander, E. (1997). Obsessive-compulsive disorder: The hidden epidemic. *Journal of Clinical Psychiatry, 58*, 3–6.

Howell, H. B., Brawman-Mintzer, O., Monnier, J., & Yonkers, K. A. (2001). Generalized anxiety disorder in women. *Psychiatric Clinics of North America, 24*(1), 165.

Hoyer, J., Becker, E. S., & Margraf, J. (2002). Generalized anxiety disorder and clinical worry episodes in young women. *Psychological Medicine, 32*(7), 1227–1237.

Johannes, S., Wieringa, B. M., Nager, W., Rada, D., Muller-Vahl, K. R., Emrish, H. M., Dengler, R., Munte, R. F., & Dietrich, D. (2003). Tourette syndrome and obsessive-compulsive disorder: Event-related brain potentials show similar mechanisms of frontal inhibition but dissimilar target evaluation processes. *Behaviour Neurology, 14*(1–2), 9–17.

Judd, L. L., Kessler, R. C., Paulus, M. P., Zeller, P. V., Wittchen, H. U., & Kunovac, J. L. (1998). Comorbidity as a fundamental feature of generalized anxiety disorders: Results from the National Comorbidity Study (NCS). *Acta Psychiatrica Scandinavica Supplement, 393*, 6–11.

Kampman, M., Keijsers, G., Hoogduin, C., & Hendriks, G. (2002). A randomized, double-blind, placebo-controlled study of the effects of adjunctive paroxetine in panic disorder patients unsuccessfully treated with cognitive-behavioral therapy alone. *Journal of Clinical Psychiatry, 63*(9), 772–777.

Katon, W., Roy-Byrne, P., Russo, J., & Cowley, D. (2002). Cost-effectiveness and cost offset of a collaborative care intervention for primary care patients with panic disorder. *Archives of General Psychiatry, 59*(12), 1098–1104.

Kent, J. M., Coplan, J. D., & Gorman, J. M. (1998). Clinical utility of the selective serotonin reuptake inhibitors in the spectrum of anxiety. *Biological Psychiatry, 44*(9), 812–824.

Kessler, R. C. (2002). *National Comorbidity Survey, 1990–1992.* (Computer file). Conducted by University of Michigan, Survey Research Center. 2nd ed. ICPSR. Ann Arbor, MI: Inter-University Consortium for Political and Social Research (producer and distributor).

Kessler, R. C., Berglund, P. A., Dewit, D. J., Ustun, T. B., Wang, P. S., & Wittchen, H. U. (2002). Distinguishing generalized anxiety disorder from major depression: Prevalence and impairment from current pure and comorbid disorders in the US and Ontario. *International Journal of Methods in Psychiatric Research, 11*(3), 99–111.

Kim, C. H., Chang, J. W., Koo, M. S., Kim, J. W., Suh, H. S., Park, I. H., & Lee, H. S. (2003). Anterior cingulotomy for refractory obsessive-compulsive disorder. *Acta Psychiatrica Scandinavica, 107*(4), 241–243.

Kirkby, K. (2003). Obsessive-compulsive disorder: Towards better understanding and outcomes. *Current Opinion in Psychiatry, 16*(1), 49–55.

Koran, L. M. (2000). Quality of life in obsessive-compulsive disorder. *Psychiatric Clinics of North America, 23*, 509–517.

Lader, M. H., & Bond, A. J. (1998). Interaction of pharmacological and psychological treatments of anxiety. *British Journal of Psychiatry Supplement, 34*, 42–48.

Lauria-Horner, B. A., & Pohl, R. B. (2003). Pregabalin: A new anxiolytic. *Expert Opinion on Investigational Drugs, 12*(4), 663–672.

Lenze, E., Mulsant, B., Shear, M., et al. (2000). Comorbid anxiety disorders in depressed elderly patients. *American Journal of Psychiatry, 157*(5), 722–728.

Llorca, P., Spadone, C., Sol, O., et al. (2002). Efficacy and safety of hydroxyzine in the treatment of generalized anxiety disorder: A 3 month double-blind study. *Journal of Clinical Psychiatry, 63*(11), 1020–1027.

Lydiard, R. B. (2003). The role of GABA in anxiety disorders. *Journal of Clinical Psychiatry, 64,* 21–27.

Magee, W.J., Eaton, W.W., Wittchen, H.U., McGonagle, K.A., & Kessler, R.C. (1996). Agoraphobia, simple phobia and social phobia in the national Comorbidity Survey. *Archives of General Psychiatry, 53,* 159–168.

Magliano, L., Guarneri, M., Marasco, C., Tosini, P., Morosini, P.L., & Maj, M. (1996). A new questionnaire assessing coping strategies in relatives of patients with schizophrenia: Development and factor analysis. *Acta Psychiatrica Scandinavia, 94,* 224–228.

Marks, I. M., & Matthews, A. M. (1979). Brief standard self-rating for phobic patients. *Behaviour Research and Therapy, 17,* 263–267.

Marshall, R., Schneier, F., Lin, S. H., et al. (2000). Childhood trauma and dissociative symptoms in panic disorder. *American Journal of Psychiatry, 157*(3), 451–453.

McEwen, B. (2005). Stressed or stressed out: What is the difference? *Journal of Psychiatry and Neuroscience, 30,* 315–318.

Melke, J., M., Landen, Baghei, F., Rosmond, R., Holm, G., Bjorntorp, P., Westberg, L., Hellstrand, M., & Eriksson, E. (2001). Serotonin transporter gene polymorphisms are associated with anxiety-related personality traits in women. *American Journal of Medical Genetics, 105*(5), 458–463.

Meyer, T., Miller, M., Metzger, R., & Borkovec, T. (1990). Development and validation of the Penn State Worry Questionnaire. *Behaviour Research and Therapy, 28*(6), 487–495.

Mundo, E., Ritcher, M., Sam, F., et al. (2000). Is the 5-HT (1D beta) receptor gene implicated in the pathogenesis of obsessive compulsive disorder? *American Journal of Psychiatry, 157*(7), 1160–1161.

Nestadt, G., Bienvenu, O. J., Cai, G., Samuels, J., & Eaton, W. W. (1998). Incidence of obsessive-compulsive disorder in adults. *Journal of Nervous and Mental Disease, 186*(7), 401–406

Newman, M., Erickson, T., Przeworski, A., & Dzus, E. (2003). Self-help and minimal contact therapies for anxiety disorders: Is human contact necessary for therapeutic efficacy? *Journal of Clinical Psychology, 59*(3), 251–274.

Newman, S. C., Bland, R. C., & Orn, H. T. (1998). The prevalence of mental disorders in the elderly in Edmonton: A community survey using GMS-AGECAT. Geriatric Mental State-Automated Geriatric Examination for Computer Assisted Taxonomy. *Canadian Journal of Psychiatry, 43*(9), 910–914.

Nuttin, B., Cosyn, P., Demeulemeester, H., Gybels, J., & Meyerson, B. (1999). Electrical stimulation in anterior limbs of internal capsules in patients with obsessive-compulsive disorder. *Lancet, 354*(9189), 1526.

Overbeek, T., Schruers, K., Vermetten, E., & Greiz, E. (2002). Comorbidity of obsessive-compulsive disorder and depression: Prevalence, symptom severity, and treatment effect. *Journal of Clinical Psychiatry, 63*(12), 1106–1112.

Peplau, H. (1989). Theoretic constructs: Anxiety, self, and hallucinations. In A. O'Toole & S. Welt (Eds.), *Interpersonal theory in nursing practice: Selected works of Hildegard E. Peplau.* New York: Springer.

Perugi, G., Toni, C., Frare, F., Travierso, M., Hantouche, E., & Akiskal, H. (2002). Obsessive-compulsive-bipolar comorbidity: A systematic exploration of clinical features and treatment outcome. *Journal of Clinical Psychiatry, 63*(12), 1129–1134.

Pohjavaara, P., Telaranta, T., & Vaisanen, E. (2003). The role of the sympathetic nervous system in anxiety: Is it possible to relieve anxiety with endoscopic sympathetic block? *Nordic Journal of Psychiatry, 57*(1), 55–60.

Ponto, L., Kathol, R., Kettelkamp, R., et al. (2002). Global cerebral blood flow after CO_2 inhalation in normal subjects and patients with panic disorder determined with [^{15}O] water and PET. *Journal of Anxiety Disorders, 16*(3). 247–258.

Rachman, S., & Hodgson, R. (1980). *Obsessions and compulsions.* New York: Prentice-Hall.

Rapaport, M. H., Wolkow, R., Rubin, A., Hackett, E., Pollack, M., & Ota, K. U. (2001). Sertraline treatment of panic disorder: Results of a long-term study. *Acta Psychiatrica Scandinavica, 104*(4), 289–298.

Raskind, M., Thompson, C., Petrie, E., et al. (2002). Prazosin reduces nightmares in combat veterans with posttraumatic stress disorder. *Journal of Clinical Psychiatry, 63*(7), 565–568.

Rasmussen, S. A., & Eisen, J. L. (1990). Epidemiology of obsessive-compulsive disorder. *Journal of Clinical Psychiatry, 51,* 10–13.

Rasmussen, S. A., & Eisen, J. L. (1992). The epidemiology and clinical features of obsessive-compulsive disorder. *Psychiatric Clinics of North America, 15,* 743–758.

Rauch, S., Jenike, M., Alpert, N., et al. (1994). Regional cerebral blood flow measured during symptom provocation in obsessive-compulsive disorder using oxygen 15-labelled carbon dioxide and positron emission tomography. *Archives of General Psychiatry, 51,* 62–70.

Regier, D. A., Rae, D. S., Narrow, W. E., Kaelber, C. T., & Schatzberg, A. F. (1998). Prevalence of anxiety disorders and their comorbidity with mood and addictive disorders. *British Journal of Psychiatry Supplement, 34,* 24–28.

Reiss, S., Peterson, R. A., & Gursky, D. M. (1986). Anxiety sensitivity, anxiety frequency, and the prediction of fearfulness. *Behaviour Research and Therapy, 24,* 1–8.

Rickels, K., & Schweizer, E. (1998). The spectrum of generalised anxiety in clinical practice: the role of short-term, intermittent treatment. *British Journal of Psychiatry, 173,* 49–54.

Rickels, K., DeMartinis, N., Garcia-Espana, F., et al. (2000). Imipramine and buspirone in treatment of patients with generalized anxiety disorder who are discontinuing long-term benzodiazepine therapy. *American Journal of Psychiatry, 157*(12), 1973–1979.

Rickels, K., Pollack, M., Sheehan, D., & Haskins, J. (2000). Efficacy of extended-release venlafaxine in nondepressed outpatients with generalized anxiety disorder. *American Journal of Psychiatry, 157*(6), 968–974.

Roy-Byrne, P. P., Clary, C. M., Miceli, R. J., Colucci, S. V., Xu, Y., & Grundzinski, A. N. (2001). The effect of selective serotonin reuptake inhibitor treatment of panic disorder on emergency room and laboratory resource utilization. *Journal of Clinical Psychiatry, 62*(9), 678–682.

Sallee, F., Sethuraman, G., Sine, L., & Liu, H. (2000). Yohimbine challenge in children with anxiety disorders. *American Journal of Psychiatry, 157,* 1236–1242.

Sareen, J., & Stein., M. (2000). A review of the epidemiology and approaches to the treatment of social anxiety disorder. *Drugs, 59*(3), 497–509.

Sareen, J., Houlahan, T., Cox, B. J., & Asmundson, G. J. (2005). Anxiety disorders associated with suicidal ideation and suicide attempts in the National Comorbidity Survey. *Journal of Nervous and Mental Disease, 193*(7), 450–454.

Schneier, F., Liebowitz, M., Abi-Dargham, A., et al. (2000). Low dopamine D2 receptor binding potential in social phobia. *American Journal of Psychiatry, 157*(3), 457–459.

Scupi, B. S., Maser, J. D., & Uhde, T. W. (1992). The National Institute of Mental Health Panic Questionnaire: An instrument for assessing clinical characteristics of panic disorder. *Journal of Nervous and Mental Disease, 180,* 566–572.

Shear, M. K., Cooper, A. M., Klerman, G. L., et al. (1993). A psychodynamic model of panic disorder. *American Journal of Psychiatry, 150,* 859–866.

Sheikh, J. I., Leskin, G. A., & Klein, D. F. (2002). Gender differences in panic disorder: Findings from the National Comorbidity Survey. *American Journal of Psychiatry, 159*(8), 1438.

Singh, Y. N., & Singh, N. N. (2002). Therapeutic potential of kava in the treatment of anxiety disorders. *CNS Drugs, 16*(11), 731–743.

Skoog, G., & Skoog, I. (1999). A 40-year follow-up of patients with obsessive-compulsive disorder. *Archives of General Psychiatry, 56,* 121–127.

Slattery, M., Klein, D., Mannuzza, S., et al. (2002). Relationship between separation anxiety disorder, parental panic disorder, and atopic disorders in children: A controlled high-risk study (Statistical data included). *Journal of the American Academy of Child and Adolescent Psychiatry, 41*(8), 947–954.

Spielberger, C. D., Gorsuch, R. L., & Luchene, R. E. (1976). *Manual for the state-trait anxiety inventory.* Palo Alto, CA: Consulting Psychologists Press.

Stein, M., Fryer, A., Davidson, J., et al. (1999). Fluvoxamine treatment of social phobia (social anxiety disorder): A double-blind, placebo-controlled trial. *American Journal of Psychiatry, 156*(5), 756–760.

Stein, D., Versiani, M., Hair, T., & Kumar, R. (2002). Efficacy of paroxetine for relapse prevention in social anxiety disorder: A 24-week study. *Archives in General Psychiatry, 59*(12), 1111–1118.

Strohle, A., Romeo, E., Di Michele, F., Pasini, A., et al. (2003). Induced panic attacks shift gamma-aminobutyric acid type A receptor modulatory neuroactive steroid composition in patients with panic disorder: Preliminary results. *Archives in General Psychiatry, 60*(2), 161–168.

Valentiner, D., Gutierrez, P., & Blacker, D. (2002). Anxiety measures and their relationship to adolescent suicidal ideation and behavior. *Journal of Anxiety Disorders, 16*(1), 11–32.

Van Ameringen, M., Mancini, C., Pipe, B., Campbell, M., & Oakman, J. (2002). Topiramate treatment for SSRI-induced weight gain in anxiety disorders. *Journal of Clinical Psychiatry, 63*(11), 981–984.

Vertue, F. M. (2003). From adaptive emotion to dysfunction: An attachment perspective on social anxiety disorder. *Personality and Social Psychology Review, 7*(2), 170–191.

Wagstaff, A. F., Cheer, S. M., Matheson, A. F., Ormrod, D., & Goa, K. L. (2002). Spotlight on paroxetine in psychiatric disorders in adults. *CNS Drugs, 16*(6), 425–434.

Wang, P., Berglund, P., & Kessler, R. (2000). Recent care of common mental disorders in the United States: Prevalence and conformance with evidenced-based recommendations. *Journal of General Internal Medicine, 15,* 284–292.

Wittchen, H.U., Usten, T.B., & Kessler, R.C. (1999). Diagnosing mental disorders in the community. A difference that matters? *Psychological Medicine, 29,* 1021–1027.

Wittchen, H. U. and Hoyer, J. (2001). Generalized anxiety disorder: nature and course. *Journal of Clinical Psychiatry, 62*(Suppl 11), 15–19.

Wittchen, H. U. (2002). Generalized anxiety disorder: prevalence, burden, and cost to society. *Depression and Anxiety, 16*(4), 162–171.

Woodward, L. (2001). Life course outcomes of young people with anxiety disorders in adolescence. *Journal of the American Academy of Child and Adolescent Psychiatry, 40*(9), 1086–1093.

Yonkers, K. A., Dyck, I. R., & Keller, M. B. (2001). An eight-year longitudinal comparison of clinical course and characteristics of social phobia among men and women. *Psychiatric Services, 52*(5), 637–643.

Yonkers, K. A., Bruce, S. E., Dyck, I. R., & Keller, M. B. (2003). Chronicity, relapse, and illness. Course of panic disorder, social phobia, and generalized anxiety disorder: Findings in men and women from 8 years of follow-up. *Depression and Anxiety, 17*(3), 173–179.

21

Somatoform and Related Disorders

Mary Ann Boyd and L. Elizabeth Hood

LEARNING OBJECTIVES

After studying this chapter, you will be able to:

- Explain the concept of somatization and its occurrence in people with mental health problems.
- Discuss the epidemiologic factors related to somatic problems.
- Compare the etiologic theories of somatization disorder from a biopsychosocial perspective.
- Contrast the major differences between somatoform and factitious disorders.
- Discuss human responses to somatization disorder.
- Apply the elements of nursing management to a patient with somatization disorder.

KEY TERMS

alexithymia ▪ factitious disorders ▪ malingering ▪ pseudologia fantastica ▪ pseudoneurologic symptoms ▪ psychosomatic ▪ somatization disorder ▪ somatoform disorders

⬟ KEY CONCEPT

- somatization

The connection between the "mind" and "body" has been hypothesized and described for centuries. The term **psychosomatic** describes conditions in which a psychological state contributes to the development of physical illness. For example, the connection between stress and heart disease is well documented and serves as the rationale for stress management interventions for heart attack victims. The term somatization is used when unexplained physical symptoms are present that are related to psychological distress. This chapter explores the concept of somatization and explains the care of patients whose psychiatric disorder has as its primary characteristic the manifestation of unexplained physical symptoms related to psychological distress.

> ⬢ **KEY CONCEPT Somatization** is the term used when unexplained physical symptoms are present that are related to psychological distress.

Although somatization is common in many psychiatric disorders, including depression, anxiety, and psychosis, it is the primary symptom of somatoform and factitious disorders. A **somatoform disorder** is one in which the patient experiences physical symptoms as a result of psychological stress. A **factitious disorder** is one in which the patient self-inflicts injury as a result of psychological stress to seek medical treatment. The major difference between the two diagnostic categories is that in the somatoform disorders, the physical symptoms are not deliberately produced by the patient. The somatoform disorders are clustered into six different clinical syndromes:

1. Somatization disorder
2. Undifferentiated somatoform disorder
3. Conversion disorder
4. Pain disorder
5. Hypochondriasis
6. Body dysmorphic disorder

The factitious disorders include factitious disorder and factitious disorder not specified. This chapter presents the nursing care of patients experiencing a somatoform disorder and factitious disorder. Somatization disorder is explained in detail because symptoms of all the other somatoform disorders are present.

Somatization

Anyone who feels the pain of a sore throat or the ache of influenza has a somatic symptom (from *soma*, meaning body), but it is not considered to be somatization unless the physical symptoms are an expression of emotional stress. Previously known as "hysteria" or "Briquet's syndrome," the cluster of symptoms associated with dysfunctional preoccupation with physical malady is now called somatization disorder (Mai, 2004). There

may or may not be an identifiable physiologic cause of the medical problems, but chronic stress is obvious. With somatization, physical sensations are amplified, and the individual seeks medical care for the symptoms. People who somatize view their personal problems in physical terms, rather than in psychosocial terms. For example, a woman quits her job complaining of being chronically tired, rather than recognizing that she is emotionally stressed from the constant harassment of a coworker. These individuals internalize their stress or cope with life problems and stressors by expressing anxiety, stress, and frustration through their own physical symptoms.

CULTURAL DIFFERENCES IN SOMATIZATION

A high correlation exists between somatization and ethnicity (Kirmayer & Young, 1998). Because norms, values, and expectations about illness are culturally based, physical sensations are experienced according to culturally defined expectations. In cultures in which the expression of physical discomfort is more acceptable than psychological distress, the disruption of routine body cycles, such as digestive or menstrual cycles, sleep, physical balance, and orientation, are commonly the focus of patient concern, instead of problems with interpersonal relationships, economic crises, death of a spouse, adjustment to marriage, and inability to become pregnant.

GENDER AND SOMATIZATION

Although the actual somatic experience appears to be different in men than in women (Kroenke & Spitzer, 1998), one group of researchers showed that women were more likely to be diversified somatizers, who have frequent, brief sickness with a variety of complaints. Men were more likely to be asthenic somatizers, with fewer diverse complaints but more chronically disabled by fatigue, weakness, or common minor illnesses. As well, spouses of men incarcerated with antisocial or addictive traits have a higher incidence of somatoform disorders (Cloninger, Martin, Guze, & Clayton, 1986; Cloninger, von Knorring, Sigvardsson, & Bohman, 1986).

Somatization Disorder

Somatization disorder is a chronic relapsing condition characterized by multiple physical symptoms that typically develop during times of emotional distress. The disorder can change with time and can vary from person to person (American Psychiatric Association [APA], 2000).

Somatization disorder can be defined as "a polysymptomatic disorder that begins before age 30 years, extends over a period of several years, and is characterized by a combination of pain, gastrointestinal, sexual, and psychoneurological symptoms" (APA, 2000).

CLINICAL COURSE

In somatization disorder, patients have recurring, multiple, and clinically significant somatic problems that involve several body systems. Other somatoform disorders are characterized by only one set of complaints, such as conversion disorder (see later discussion) or pain disorder. Physical problems in somatization disorder cut across all body systems, such as gastrointestinal (nausea, vomiting, diarrhea), neurologic (headache, backache), or musculoskeletal (aching legs). The physical illness may last 6 to 9 months. These individuals perceive themselves as being "sicker than the sick" and report all aspects of their health as poor. They are often disabled and cannot work. They quickly become frustrated with their primary health care providers, who do not seem to appreciate the seriousness of their symptoms and who are unable to verify a particular problem that accounts for their extreme discomfort. Consequently, they "provider-shop," moving from one to another until they find one who will give them new medication, hospitalize them, or perform surgery. Characteristically, these individuals undergo multiple surgeries. People with somatization disorder evoke negative subjective responses in health care providers, who usually wish that the patient would go to someone else.

CRNE Note

Patients with somatoform disorders will seek health care from multiple providers but will avoid mental health specialists.

Because a psychiatric diagnosis of somatization disorder is made only after numerous unexplained physical problems, psychiatric and mental health (PMH) nurses do not usually care for these individuals early in the disorder. Instead, nurses in primary care and medical-surgical settings are more likely to encounter these patients.

DIAGNOSTIC CRITERIA

The diagnosis is made when there is a pattern of multiple, recurring, "significant" somatic complaints. Table 21-1 lists the key diagnostic criteria and target symptoms. A significant complaint is one that received medical treatment or for which the symptoms cause impairment in social, occupational, or other areas of functioning (APA, 2000).

SOMATIZATION DISORDER IN SPECIAL POPULATIONS

Evidence suggests that this disorder occurs in all populations and cultures. The type and frequency of somatic symptoms may differ across cultures.

Children

Although many children experience unexplained medical symptoms, somatization disorder is not usually diagnosed until adolescence. Menstrual difficulties may be one of the first symptoms. More research is needed to identify risk factors and treatment outcomes (Lieb, Pfister, Mastaler, & Wittchen, 2000).

Elderly People

Somatization disorder occurs in the elderly, but there is little research specific to this population. Subjective non–well-being (never feeling good), rather than objective health measures, may be an indicator of somatization (Schneider et al., 2003). One of the nursing challenges is to differentiate the somatic symptoms of this disorder from other medical problems that should be diagnosed and treated. In the elderly, somatic symptoms can represent many things, such as depression or bereavement. Recognizing the complexity of physical manifestations and assessing the symptom pattern are important.

EPIDEMIOLOGY

The estimated prevalence of somatization disorder ranges from 0.2% to 2% of the general population (APA, 2000; Grabe et al., 2003). Because these individuals see themselves as medically sick and may never see a mental health provider, these estimates may underrepresent the true prevalence. Some estimates are as high as 11% of the population. Thus, in many people, somatization disorder is unrecognized, undiagnosed, and mismanaged in primary care settings (Yates, 2002). Recent World Health Organization (WHO, 2004) statistics indicate that mortality rates for somatoform disorder are low in Canada and the United States (0.03 deaths per million population); as compared with some European countries (eg, 2.13 deaths per million population in Luxembourg).

Age of Onset

Somatization disorder, by definition, occurs before the age of 30 years, usually during adolescence. The individual may not receive a diagnosis before the age of 30 years, but one unexplained somatic symptom must be present before this age. This disorder typically has its

Table 21.1	Key Diagnostic Characteristics of Somatization Disorder 300.81	

Diagnostic Criteria and Target Symptoms	Associated Findings
<ul><li>History of many physical complaints beginning before age 30 and occurring over a period of several years</li><li>Complaints requiring treatment or causing significant impairment in social, occupational, or other important area of functioning<ul><li>History of pain related to at least four different sites or functions, such as head, abdomen, back, joints, extremities, chest, rectum, during menstruation, during sexual intercourse, or during urination</li><li>History of at least two gastrointestinal symptoms, such as nausea, bloating, vomiting (other than during pregnancy), diarrhea, or intolerance of several different foods</li><li>History of at least one sexual or reproductive symptom, such as sexual indifference, erectile or ejaculatory dysfunction, irregular menses, excessive menstrual bleeding, vomiting throughout pregnancy</li><li>History of one pseudoneurologic symptom or deficit suggesting a neurologic condition not limited to pain, such as conversion symptoms (impaired coordination or balance, paralysis or localized weakness, difficulty swallowing or lump in throat, aphonia, urinary retention, hallucinations, loss of touch or pain sensation, double vision, blindness, deafness, seizures; dissociative symptoms, for example, amnesia, or loss of consciousness other than fainting)</li></ul></li><li>Symptoms cannot be explained by a known general medical condition or direct effects of a substance<ul><li>Symptoms unexplainable or excessive</li><li>When a general medical condition exists, the physical complaints or resulting impairments are in excess of what would be expected from the history, physical examination, or laboratory findings</li></ul></li><li>Symptoms are not intentionally produced or feigned</li></ul>	*Associated Behavioural Findings*<ul><li>Colorful, exaggerated complaints lacking specific factual information</li><li>Inconsistent historians</li><li>Treatment sought from several physicians with numerous medical examinations, diagnostic procedures, surgeries, and hospitalizations</li><li>Anxiety and depressed mood</li><li>Impulsive with antisocial behaviour, suicide threats and attempts, and marital discord</li></ul>*Associated Physical Findings*<ul><li>Absence of objective findings to fully explain subjective complaints</li><li>Possible diagnosis of functional disorders, such as irritable bowel syndrome</li></ul>

onset in childhood or adolescence and is remarkably stable, lasting many years into adulthood (Lieb et al., 2002; Mullick, 2002).

Getting older does not increase the likelihood of receiving a diagnosis of somatization disorder; epidemiologic data indicate that the prevalence of somatization among people younger than 45 years is similar to the rate among those older than 45 years. However, patients who begin to have symptoms after 30 years are not likely to have enough symptoms to meet the criteria in the *Diagnostic and Statistical Manual of Mental Disorders*, 4th ed., text revision (*DSM-IV-TR*; APA, 2000) for somatization disorder and are more likely to have a diagnosable medical problem (Gureje, et al., 1997).

Gender, Ethnic, and Cultural Differences

Somatization disorder occurs primarily in women, particularly those in lower socioeconomic status and with high emotional distress (Ladwig, Marten-Mittag, Erazo, & Gundel, 2001). The prevalence in men in the United States and Canada is less than 0.2%. Reports of greater prevalence among men from other countries, such as Greece and Puerto Rico, suggest that cultural factors contribute to the appearance of the disorder.

Comorbidity

Somatization disorder frequently coexists with other psychiatric disorders, most commonly depression. Others include panic disorder, mania, phobic disorder, obsessive-compulsive disorder, psychotic disorders, and personality disorders (Garyfallos et al., 1999). Nurses rarely see patients who have only somatization disorder.

Ultimately, numerous unexplained medical problems also coexist with this disorder because many patients have received medical and surgical treatments, often unnecessarily, and are plagued with side effects. A disproportionately high number of women who eventually receive diagnoses of somatization disorder have been treated for irritable bowel syndrome, polycystic ovary disease, and chronic pain. It is estimated that as many as 94% of people with irritable bowel syndrome have psychiatric disorders, especially major depression, anxiety, and somatization disorder (Whitehead, Palsson, & Jones, 2002). Many also have had non–cancer-related hysterectomies. Even after the patient is treated by mental health providers and develops some understanding of the disorder, the physical problems do not disappear.

ETIOLOGY

The cause of somatization disorder is unknown. The following are theories regarding the development of the disorder.

Biologic Theories

Neuropathologic Theory

The neuropathology of somatization disorder is unknown. Evidence suggests that there is decreased activity in certain brain areas, such as the caudate nuclei, left putamen, and right precentral gyrus in somatization disorder (Garcia-Campayo, Sanz-Carrillo, Baringo, & Ceballos, 2001; Hakala et al., 2002). These findings indicate that a hypometabolism may be associated with somatization disorder.

Genetic

Although somatization disorder has been shown to run in families, the exact transmission mechanism is unclear. Strong evidence suggests an increased risk for somatization disorder in first-degree relatives, indicating a familial or genetic effect (APA, 2000). Because many women with somatization disorder live in chaotic families, environmental influence could explain the high prevalence in first-degree relatives. Males in these families show high risk for antisocial personality disorder and substance abuse.

Biochemical Changes

Research is as yet insufficient to identify specific biochemical changes. However, because these patients experience other psychiatric problems, such as depression or panic, clearly many neurobiologic changes occur. Women with this disorder often have numerous menstrual problems and often undergo hysterectomies. Because of these symptoms, studies are needed to determine the involvement of the hypothalamic–pituitary–gonadal axis, which regulates estrogen and testosterone secretion.

Psychological Theories

Somatization has been explained as a form of social or emotional communication, meaning the bodily symptoms express an emotion that cannot be verbalized. The adolescent who experiences severe abdominal pain after her parents' argument or the wife who receives nurturing from her husband only when she has back pain are two examples. From this perspective, somatization may be a way of maintaining relationships. Following this line of reasoning, as an individual's physical problems become a way of controlling relationships, so somatization becomes a learned behaviour pattern. With time, physical symptoms develop automatically in response to perceived threats. Finally, somatization disorder develops when somatizing becomes a way of life.

Social Theories

Somatization disorders occur everywhere, but the symptoms may vary from culture to culture. In addition, the conceptualization of somatization disorder is primarily Western. In non-Western societies, where the mind–body distinction is not made and symptoms have different meanings and explanations, these physical manifestations are not labeled as a psychiatric disorder (Box 21-1). For example, within Chinese culture as well as Latin American countries, depression is more likely

---

BOX 21-1

Somatization in Chinese Culture

In Chinese tradition, the health of the individual reflects a balance between positive and negative forces within the body. Five elements at work in nature and in the body control conditions (fire, water, wood, earth, metal); five viscera (liver, heart, spleen, kidneys, lungs); five emotions (anger, joy, worry, sorrow, fear); and five climatic conditions (wind, heat, humidity, dryness, cold). All illness is explained by imbalances among these elements. Because emotion is related to the circulation of vital air within the body, anger is believed to result from an adverse current of vital air to the liver. Emotional outbursts are seen as results of imbalances among the natural elements, rather than the results of behaviour of the person.

The stigma of mental illness in the Chinese culture is so great that it can have an adverse effect on a family for many generations. If problems can be attributed to natural causes, the individual and family are less responsible, and stigma is minimized. The Chinese have a culturally acceptable term for symptoms of mental distress—the closest translation of which would be *neurasthenia*—which comprises somatic complaints of headaches, insomnia, dizziness, aches and pains, poor memory, anxiety, weakness, and loss of energy.

described in somatic symptoms, such as headaches, gastrointestinal disturbances, or complaints of "nerves," rather than the sadness or guilt associated with major depression (Jorge, 2003; Yick, Shibusawa, & Agbayani-Siewert, 2003).

RISK FACTORS

This disorder tends to run in families, and children of mothers with multiple unexplained somatic complaints are more likely to have somatic problems. Adults are at higher risk for unexplained medical symptoms if they experienced unexplained symptoms as children or if their parents were in poor health when the patient was about 15 years old (Hotopf, Mayou, Wadsworth, & Wessely, 1999). Female gender, substance use, and anxiety disorder seem to be risk factors, and women with somatization disorder appear more likely to have been sexually abused as children than those with other psychiatric conditions, such as mood disorders (Lieb et al., 2002). Individuals with depression are especially likely to experience somatization (Gureje & Simon, 1999).

INTERDISCIPLINARY TREATMENT

The care of patients with somatization disorders involves three approaches:
- Providing long-term general management of the chronic condition;
- Conservatively treating symptoms of comorbid psychiatric and physical problems;
- Providing care in special settings, including group treatment (Huibers, Beurskens, Bleijenberg, & van Schayck, 2003).

The cornerstone of management is trust. Ideally, the patient sees only one health care provider at regularly scheduled visits. During each primary care visit, the provider should conduct a partial physical examination of the organ system in which the patient has complaints. Physical symptoms are treated conservatively using the least intrusive approach. In the mental health setting, the use of cognitive behaviour therapy (CBT) produced better results than antidepressant or supportive psychotherapy (Mai, 2004). In a review of 31 clinical trials, patients treated with CBT improved more than did control subjects in 71% of the studies. Benefits were observed whether or not psychological distress was ameliorated (Kroenke & Swindle, 2000).

NURSING MANAGEMENT: HUMAN RESPONSE TO DISORDER

Somatization is the primary response to this disorder. The defining characteristics, depicted in the biopsychosocial model (Fig. 21-1), are so well integrated that

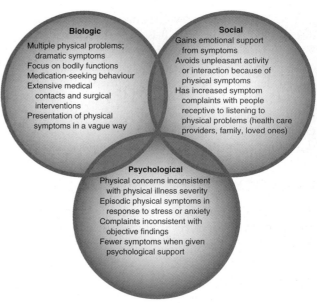

FIGURE 21.1 Biopsychosocial characteristics of patients with somatization disorder.

separating the psychological and social dimensions is difficult. The most common characteristics follow:
- Reporting the same symptoms repeatedly;
- Receiving support from the environment that otherwise might not be forthcoming (such as gaining a spouse's attention because of severe back pain);
- Expressing concern about the physical problems inconsistent with the severity of the illness (being "sicker than the sick").

Biologic Domain

During the assessment interview, allow enough time for the patient to explain all medical problems; a hurried assessment interview blocks communication.

Assessment

Past medical treatment has been ineffective because it did not address the underlying psychiatric disorder. However, PMH nurses typically see these patients for problems related to the coexisting psychiatric disorder, such as depression, not because of the somatization disorder. While taking the patient's history, the nurse will discover that the individual has had multiple surgeries or medical problems and realize that somatization disorder is a strong possibility. If the patient has not already received a diagnosis of somatization disorder, the nurse should screen for it by determining the presence of the most commonly reported problems associated with this disorder, which include dysmenorrhea, lump in throat, vomiting, shortness of breath, burning in sex organs, painful extremities, and amnesia. If the patient has these symptoms, he or she should be seen by a mental health

BOX 21-2

Health Attitude Survey

On a scale of 1 to 5, please indicate the extent to which you agree (5) or disagree (1).

Dissatisfaction With Care

1. I have been satisfied with the medical care I have received. (R)
2. Doctors have done the best they could to diagnose and treat my health problems. (R)
3. Doctors have taken my health problems seriously.
4. My health problems have been thoroughly evaluated. (R)
5. Doctors do not seem to know much about the health problems I have had.
6. My health problems have been completely explained. (R)
7. Doctors seem to think I am exaggerating my health problems.
8. My response to treatment has not been satisfactory.
9. My response to treatment is usually excellent. (R)

Frustration With Ill Health

10. I am tired of feeling sick and would like to get to the bottom of my health problems.
11. I have felt ill for quite a while now.
12. I am going to keep searching for an answer to my health problems.
13. I do not think there is anything seriously wrong with my body. (R)

High Utilization of Care

14. I have seen many different doctors over the years
15. I have taken a lot of medicine recently.
16. I do not go to the doctor often. (R)
17. I have had relatively good health over the years.

Excessive Health Worry

18. I sometimes worry too much about my health.
19. I often fear the worst when I develop symptoms.
20. I have trouble getting my mind off my health.

Psychological Distress

21. Sometimes I feel depressed and cannot seem to shake it off.
22. I have sought help for emotional or stress-related problems.
23. It is easy to relax and stay calm. (R)
24. I believe the stress I am under may be affecting my health.

Discordant Communication of Distress

25. Some people think that I am capable of more work than I feel able to do.
26. Some people think that I have been sick just to gain attention.
27. It is difficult for me to find the right words for my feelings.

(R) indicates items reversed for scoring purposes. Scoring—The higher the score, the more likely somatization is a problem.
From Noyes, R. Jr., Langbehn, D., Happel, R., Sieren L., & Muller, B. (1999). Health Attitude Survey: A scale for assessing somatizing patients. *Psychosomatics*, 40(6), 470–478.

provider qualified to make the diagnosis. Box 21-2 presents the Health Attitude Survey, which can be used as a screening test for somatization.

Review of Systems

Although these patients' symptoms have usually received considerable attention from the medical community, a careful review of systems is important because the appearance of physical problems is usually related to psychosocial problems. Even as the nurse continues to see the patient for mental health problems, an ongoing awareness of biologic symptoms is important, particularly because these symptoms are de-emphasized in the overall management.

Pain is the most common problem in people with this disorder. Because the pain is usually related to symptoms of all the major body systems, it is unlikely that a somatic intervention such as an analgesic will be effective on a long-term basis. The nurse must remember that although there is no medical explanation for the pain, the patient's pain is real and has serious psychosocial implications. A careful assessment should include the following questions:

- What is the pain like?
- What is the extent of the pain?
- What helps the pain get better?
- When is the pain at its worst?
- What has worked in the past to relieve the pain?

Physical Functioning

The actual physical functioning of these individuals is often marginal. They usually have problems with sleep, fatigue, activity, and sexual functioning. Assessment of these areas will generate data to be used in establishing a nursing diagnosis. The amount and quality of sleep are important, as are the times when the individual sleeps. For example, an individual may sleep a total of 6 hours each diurnal cycle, but only from 2:00 to 6:00 AM, plus an afternoon nap.

Fatigue is a constant problem, and a variety of physical problems interfere with normal activity. These patients report overwhelming lack of energy, which makes maintaining usual routines or accomplishing daily tasks impossible. Fatigue is accompanied by the inability to concentrate on simple functions, leading to decreased performance and disinterest in surroundings. Patients tend to be lethargic and listless and often have little energy (Box 21-3).

Female patients with this disorder usually have had multiple gynecologic problems. The reason is not known,

Clinical Vignette: Somatization Disorder and Stress

Ms. J, age 42 years, has been coming to the mental health clinic for 2 years for her nerves. She has seen only the physician for medication, but now has been referred to the nurse's new stress management group because she is experiencing side effects to all the medications that have been tried. The psychiatrist has diagnosed somatization disorder and wants her to learn to manage her "nerves" without medication.

At the first meeting with the nurse, Ms. J was preoccupied with chest pain and bloating that had lasted for the past 6 months. Her chest pain is constant and sharp at times. The pain does not prevent her from going to her job as a waitress but does interfere with meal preparation at night for her family and her ability to have sexual intercourse. She has numerous other physical problems, including allergies to certain perfumes, dysmenorrhea, ovarian polycystic disease (ovarian cysts), chronic urinary tract infections, and rashes. She is constantly fatigued and has frequent leg cramps. She states that she is too tired to fix dinner for her family. On days off from work, she takes a nap in the afternoon, sleeping until evening. She is unable to fall asleep at night.

She believes that she will soon have to have her gallbladder removed because of occasional referred pain to her back and nausea that occurs a couple hours after eating. She is not enthusiastic about a stress management group and does not believe that it will help her problems. However, she has agreed to consider it, insisting that the psychiatrist will continue prescribing diazepam (Valium).

What Do You Think?

How would you prioritize Ms. J's physical symptoms? What strategies would you use in the group to help Ms. J explore the roots of her stress and fatigue?

but symptoms of dysmenorrhea, painful intercourse, and pain in the "sex organs" suggests involvement of the hypothalamic–pituitary–gonadal axis. Physiologic indicators, such as those produced by laboratory tests, are not available. However, a careful assessment of the patient's menstrual history, gynecologic problems, and sexual functioning is important. The physical manifestations of somatization disorder often lead to altered sexual behaviour.

Pharmacologic Assessment

A psychopharmacologic assessment of these patients is challenging. Patients with somatization disorder frequently provider-shop, perhaps seeing seven or eight different providers within a year. Because they often receive medications from each provider, they are usually taking a large number of drugs. They tend to protect their sources and may not be truthful in identifying the actual number of medications they are ingesting. A pharmacologic assessment is needed not only because of the number of medications but also because these individuals frequently have unusual side effects. Because of their somatic sensitivity, they often overreact to medication.

These patients spend much of their life trying to find out what is wrong with them. When one provider after another can find little if any explanation for their symptoms, many become anxious. To alleviate their anxiety, they either self-medicate with over-the-counter medications and substances of abuse (eg, alcohol, marijuana) or find a provider who prescribes an anxiolytic. Because the anxiety of their disorder cannot be treated within a few weeks with an anxiolytic, they become dependent on medication that should not have been prescribed in the first place.

Although anxiolytics have a place in therapeutics, most are addictive. Therefore, they are not recommended for long-term use. Usually, anxiolytics complicate the treatment of somatoform disorders. Unfortunately, by the time individuals experiencing somatoform disorder see a mental health provider, they have often already begun taking one of the benzodiazepines. Many times, the reason they agree to see a mental health provider is because their primary health provider refused to continue prescribing an anxiolytic without a psychiatric evaluation.

Nursing Diagnoses for the Biologic Domain

Because somatization disorder is a chronic illness, patients could have almost any one of the nursing diagnoses at some time in their life. At least one nursing diagnosis likely will be related to the individual's physical state. Fatigue, Pain, and Disturbed Sleep Patterns are usually supported by the assessment data. The challenge in devising outcomes for these problems is to avoid focusing on the biologic aspects and instead help the patient overcome the fatigue, pain, or sleep problem through biopsychosocial approaches.

Interventions for the Biologic Domain

Nursing interventions that focus on the biologic dimension become especially important because medical treatment must be conservative, and aggressive pharmacologic treatment must be avoided. Each time a nurse sees the patient, time spent on the physical complaints should be limited. Several biologic interventions, including pain management, activity enhancement, nutrition regulation, relaxation, and pharmacologic interventions, may be useful in caring for patients with somatization disorder.

Pain Management

In pain management, a single approach rarely works. Pain is a primary issue. After a careful assessment of the pain, the nurse should develop nonpharmacologic strategies to reduce it (see Caudill-Slosberg, 2002). If gastrointestinal pain is frequent, eating and bowel habits should be explored and modified. For back pain, exercises and consultation from a physical therapist may be useful. Headaches are a challenge. Self-monitoring and tracking them engages the patient in the therapeutic process and helps to identify psychosocial triggers.

Activity Enhancement

Helping the patient establish a daily routine, especially during times when the patient does not work, may alleviate some of the difficulty with sleeping. Encouraging the patient to get up in the morning and go to bed at night at specific times can help the patient to establish a routine. Regular exercise is important to improve overall physical state, but patients often use numerous reasons to avoid activity. The nurse needs to work with the patient to foster adequate movement for healthier living.

Nutrition Regulation

Patients with somatization disorder often have gastrointestinal problems and may have special nutritional needs. The nurse discusses with the patient the nutritional value of foods. Because these individuals often take medications that lead to weight gain, weight control strategies may be discussed (see Chapter 12). For overweight individuals, suggest healthy, low-calorie food choices. Teach patients about balancing dietary intake with activity levels to increase their awareness of food choices.

Relaxation

Patients taking anxiolytic medication for stress reduction can be taught relaxation techniques. The challenge for the nurse is to help a patient develop strategies for routine practice and evaluation of effect. The nurse should consider a variety of techniques, including simple relaxation techniques, distraction, and guided imagery (see Chapter 12).

Psychopharmacologic Interventions

No medication is particularly recommended for somatization disorder. Psychiatric symptoms of comorbid disorders, such as depression and anxiety, are treated pharmacologically as appropriate. Often, these patients are depressed and are taking an antidepressant. Depressed mood itself is not an indication for initiation of antidepressant treatment. If depressed mood persists and insomnia, decreased appetite, decreased libido, and anhedonia are also present, aggressive psychopharmacologic management is indicated (Fallon et al., 2003). A wide variety of drugs are available, including the selective serotonin reuptake inhibitors (SSRIs), tricyclic antidepressants, and monoamine oxidase inhibitors (MAOIs) (see Chapters 13 and 19). Patients with somatization disorder usually take several different antidepressants throughout the course of the disorder. Seek evidence that the depressive symptoms are cleared before discontinuing use of the medication (see Box 21-4).

Phenelzine (Nardil) is one of the MAOIs that is effective in treating not just depression but also the chronic pain and headaches common in people with somatization disorder. Depression is usually successfully treated with antidepressants (see Chapters 13 and 19). Food–drug interactions are the most serious side effects of MAOIs; while taking such agents, patients should avoid foods high in tyramine (see Chapter 13).

Anxiety associated with a somatization disorder is more difficult to treat pharmacologically than depression. Nonpharmacologic approaches such as biofeedback or relaxation should be used. Benzodiazepines should be avoided because of the psychological dependence associated with these medications. Buspirone (BuSpar), a non-benzodiazepine, does not lead to tolerance or withdrawal and may be useful for relief of anxiety.

Monitoring and Administering Medications

In somatization disorder, patients are usually treated in the community, where they often engage in self-medication. The nurse should carefully question patients about self-administered medicine and determine which medicines they are currently taking (including over-the-counter and herbal supplements). The nurse should listen carefully to determine effects the patient attributes to the medication. This information should be documented and reported to the rest of the team. If medication is being taken from multiple providers, an evaluation of possible drug–drug interaction needs to be completed. The nurse needs to work with the patient, and the patient should be encouraged to continue taking only prescribed medication.

Monitoring and Managing Side Effects

These individuals often have idiosyncratic reactions to their medications. Side effects should be assessed, but the patient should be encouraged to compare the benefits of the medication with any problems related to side effects.

Monitoring Drug Interactions

In working with patients with somatization disorder, the nurse must always be on the lookout for drug–drug interactions. Medications these patients take for physical problems could interact with psychiatric medications. Patients may be taking alternative medicines, such as herbal supplements, that need to be evaluated for possible adverse interactions (Garcia-Campayo & Sanz-Carrillo, 2000). The patient should be encouraged to use the same pharmacy for filling all prescriptions so that possible reactions can be checked.

Psychological Domain

The cognitive functioning of individuals with somatization disorder is usually within normal limits. What is

BOX 21-4

Drug Profile: phenelzine (Nardil)

DRUG CLASS: Monoamine oxidase inhibitor

RECEPTOR AFFINITY: Inhibits MAO, an enzyme responsible for breaking down biogenic amines, such as epinephrine, nor-epinephrine, and serotonin, allowing them to accumulate in neuronal storage sites throughout the central and peripheral nervous systems.

INDICATIONS: Treatment of depression characterized as "atypical, nonendogenous," or "neurotic" or nonresponsive to other antidepressant therapy or in situations in which other antidepressant therapy is contraindicated

ROUTE AND DOSAGE: Available as 15-mg tablets.

Adults: Initially, 15 mg PO tid, increasing to at least 60 mg/d at a fairly rapid pace consistent with patient tolerance. Therapy at 60 mg/d may be necessary for at least 4 weeks before response occurs. After maximum benefit is achieved, dosage is reduced gradually over several weeks. Maintenance dose may be 15 mg/d or every other day.

Geriatric: Adjust dosage accordingly because patients over 60 years of age are more prone to develop adverse effects.

Pediatric: Not recommended for children under 16 years of age.

HALF-LIFE (PEAK EFFECTS): Unknown (48–96 h).

SELECTED ADVERSE REACTIONS: Dizziness, vertigo, headache, overactivity, hyperreflexia, tremors, muscle twitching, mania, hypomania, jitteriness, confusion, memory impairment, insomnia, weakness, fatigue, overstimulation, restlessness, increased anxiety, agitation, blurred vision, sweating, constipation, diarrhea, nausea, abdominal pain, edema, dry mouth, anorexia, weight changes, hypertensive crisis, orthostatic hypotension, and disturbed cardiac rate and rhythm.

WARNINGS: Contraindicated in patients with pheochromocytoma, congestive heart failure, hepatic dysfunction, severe renal impairment, cardiovascular disease, history of headache, and myelography within previous 24 h or scheduled within next 48 h. Use cautiously in patients with seizure disorders, hyperthyroidism, pregnancy, or lactation, and those scheduled for elective surgery. Possible hypertensive crisis, coma, and severe convulsions may occur if administered with tricyclic antidepressants; possible hypertensive crisis when taken with foods containing tyramine. Increased risk for adverse interaction is possible when given with meperidine. Additive hypoglycemic effect can occur when taken with insulin and oral sulfonylureas.

SPECIFIC PATIENT/FAMILY EDUCATION:

- Take drug exactly as prescribed; do not stop taking abruptly or without consulting your health care provider.
- Avoid consuming any foods containing tyramine while taking this drug and for 2 weeks afterward.
- Avoid alcohol, sleep-inducing drugs, over-the-counter drugs such as cold and hay fever remedies and appetite suppressants—all of which may cause serious or life-threatening problems.
- Report any signs and symptoms of adverse reactions.
- Maintain appointments for follow-up blood tests.
- Report any complaints of unusual or severe headache or yellowing of eyes or skin.
- Avoid driving a car or performing any activities that require alertness.
- Change position slowly when going from a lying to sitting or standing position to minimize dizziness or weakness.

---

most noticeable about their mental status is their flamboyant appearance and exaggerated speech. They are often dressed in attention-getting clothes, with bright colours, flashy shoes, or an outrageous hairstyle. Their language is colourful and can be entertaining. However, these individuals seem preoccupied with personal illnesses and may even keep a record of symptoms. They have a constant focus on bodily functions, and "living with diseases" truly becomes a way of life.

Individuals with somatization disorder usually have intense emotional reactions to life stressors. These patients usually have a series of personal crises beginning at an early age. Typically, a new symptom or medical problem develops during times of emotional stress. It is critical that the physical assessment data be linked to psychological and social events. A history of major psychological events should be compared with the chronology of physical problems. Special attention should be paid to any history of sexual abuse or trauma in the patient's younger years. Early sexual abuse also may interfere with sexual fulfillment in adulthood.

The individual's mood is usually labile, often shifting from extremely excited to depressed. Response to physical symptoms is usually exaggerated, such as interpreting a simple cold as pneumonia or a brief chest pain as a heart attack. Family members may not believe the physical symptoms are real and may view them as attention-seeking behaviour because symptoms often improve when the patient receives attention. For example, a woman who has been in bed for 3 weeks with severe back pain may suddenly feel much better once her children visit her.

There is emerging evidence that some people with somatic symptoms have alexithymia, difficulty identifying and expressing feelings in words (De Gucht & Heiser, 2003; Mai, 2004). Researchers in Toronto studying alexithymia in patients with somatoform pain disorder found that they were more descriptive of the location and severity of pain (Cox, Kuch, Parker, Shulman, & Evans, 1994). Researchers continue to search for illness patterns in people who have difficulty identifying and expressing emotion (Kojima, Senda, Nagaya, Tokudome, & Furukawa, 2003; Porcelli et al., 2003).

CRNE Note

Encourage patients with somatoform disorder to discuss and explore physical problems as well as psychosocial issues.

Nursing Diagnoses for the Psychological Domain

Nursing diagnoses that target responses to somatization disorder typical of the psychological domain include the following: Anxiety, Ineffective Sexuality Patterns, Impaired Social Interactions, Ineffective Coping, and Ineffective Therapeutic Regimen Management.

Interventions for the Psychological Domain

The choice of psychological intervention depends on the specific problem the patient is experiencing. The most important and ongoing intervention is the maintenance of a therapeutic relationship.

Development of a Therapeutic Relationship

The most difficult aspect of nursing care is developing a sound, positive nurse–patient relationship, yet this relationship is crucial. Without it, the nurse is just one more provider who fails to meet the patient's expectations. Developing this relationship requires time and patience.

Therapeutic communication techniques should be used to refocus the patient on psychosocial problems related to the physical manifestations (see Box 21-5).

During periods when symptoms of other psychiatric disorders surface, additional interventions are needed (see Chapter 8). For example, if depression occurs, additional supportive or cognitive approaches may be needed.

Counselling

Counselling, with a focus on problem solving, is needed from time to time. These patients have chaotic lives and need support through the multitude of crises. Although they sometimes appear flamboyant and self-assured, their constant complaints may irritate others. The consequences of their impaired social interaction with others must be examined within a counselling framework. The nurse helps the patient identify stressors, explore related thoughts and feelings, and develop more positive coping responses to deal with a chaotic lifestyle.

Patient Education: Health

Health teaching is useful throughout the nurse–patient relationship. These patients have many questions about illnesses, symptoms, and treatments. Emphasize positive health care practices and minimize the effects of serious illness. Because of problems in managing medications and treatment, the therapeutic regimen needs constant monitoring, resulting in ample opportunities for teaching. One area that might require special health

---

BOX 21-5

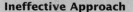

Therapeutic Dialogue: Establishing a Relationship

Ineffective Approach

Nurse: Good morning Ms. C.
Patient: I'm in so much pain. Take that breakfast away.
Nurse: You don't want your breakfast?
Patient: Can't you see? I hurt! When I hurt, I can't eat!
Nurse: If you don't eat now, you probably won't be able to have anything until lunch.
Patient: Who cares. I have no intention of being here at lunchtime. I don't belong here.
Nurse: Ms. C, I don't think that your doctor would have admitted you unless there is a problem. I would like to talk to you about why you are here.
Patient: Nurse, I'm just here. It's none of your business.
Nurse: Oh.
Patient: Please leave me alone.
Nurse: Sure, I will see you later.

Effective Approach

Nurse: Good morning, Ms. C.
Patient: I'm in so much pain. Take that breakfast away.
Nurse: (Silently removes tray. Pulls up chair and sits down.)
Patient: My back hurts.
Nurse: Oh, when did the back pain start?
Patient: Last night. It's this bed. I couldn't get comfortable.

Nurse: These beds can be pretty uncomfortable.
Patient: My back pain is shooting down my leg.
Nurse: Does anything help it?
Patient: Sometimes if I straighten out my leg it helps.
Nurse: Can I help you straighten out your leg?
Patient: Oh, it's OK. The pain is going away. What did you say your name is?
Nurse: I'm Susan Miller, your nurse while you are here.
Patient: I won't be here long. I don't belong in a psychiatric unit.
Nurse: While you are here, I would like to spend time with you.
Patient: OK, but you understand, I do not have any psychiatric problems.
Nurse: We can talk about whatever you want. But, since you want to get out of here, we might want to focus on what it will take to get you ready for discharge.

Critical Thinking Challenge

- What communication mistakes did the nurse in the first scenario make?
- What communication strategies helped the patient feel comfortable with the nurse in the second scenario? How is the first scenario different from the second?

teaching is impaired sexuality. Because of their long history of physical problems related to the reproductive tract, these patients may have difficulty carrying out normal sexual activity, such as intercourse, reaching orgasm, and so forth. Basic teaching about normal sexual function is often needed (see Box 21-6).

Social Domain

People with somatization disorder spend excessive time seeking medical care and attending to their multiple illnesses. Most are unemployed. Because they believe themselves to be very sick, they also believe that they are disabled and cannot work. These individuals are rarely satisfied with health care providers, who can find no basis for a medical diagnosis. However, their social network often consists of a series of providers, rather than peers. Identifying a support network requires sorting out the health care providers from family and friends.

Assessment

Family members may become weary of the individual's constant complaints of physical problems. These individuals usually live in chaotic families with multiple problems. In assessing the family structure, other members with psychiatric disorders must be identified. Women may be married to abusive men who have antisocial personality disorders; alcoholism is common. Identifying the positive and negative aspects of relationships within the family is important.

Symptoms of somatization disorder usually disrupt the family's social life. Changes in routine or major life events often precipitate the appearance of a symptom. For example, a patient may be planning a vacation with the family, but at the last minute decides she cannot go because her back pain has returned and she will not be able to sit in the car. These family disruptions are common.

Nursing Diagnoses for the Social Domain

Some of the nursing diagnoses related to the social domain that are typical of people with somatization disorder include the following: Risk for Caregiver Role Strain, Ineffective Community Coping, Disabled Family Coping, and Social Isolation.

Interventions for the Social Domain

Patients with somatic disorders are usually isolated from their families and communities. Strengthening social relationships and activities often becomes the focus of the nursing care. The nurse should help the patient identify individuals with whom contact is desired, ask for a commitment to contact them, and encourage them to reinitiate a relationship. The nurse should counsel the patient about talking too much about their symptoms with these individuals and emphasize that medical information should be shared with the nurse. The nurse must also ensure that the patient knows when the next appointment is scheduled.

Group Interventions

Although these patients may not be good candidates for insight group psychotherapy, they do benefit from cognitive–behavioural groups that focus on developing coping skills for everyday life (Lidbeck, 2003). Because most of the patients are women, participation in groups that address feminist issues should be encouraged to strengthen their assertiveness skills and improve their generally low self-esteem (Fig. 21-2).

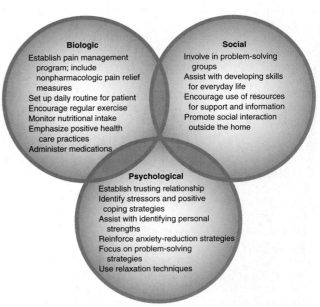

FIGURE 21.2 Biopsychosocial interventions for patients with somatization disorder.

When leading a group that has members with this disorder, redirection can keep the group from giving too much attention to a person's illness. However, these individuals need reassurance and support while in a group. They may verbalize that they do not fit in or belong in the group. In reality, they are feeling insecure and threatened in the situation. The group leader needs to show patience and understanding in order to engage the individual effectively in meaningful group interaction.

Family Interventions

The results of a family assessment often reveal that families of these individuals need education about the disorder, helpful strategies for dealing with the multiple complaints of the patient, and usually, help in developing more effective communication patterns. Because of the chaotic nature of their families and the lack of healthy problem solving, physical and psychological abuse may be evident. The nurse should be particularly sensitive to any evidence of physical or sexual abuse (see Chapter 36).

Evaluation and Treatment Outcomes

The outcomes for patients with somatization disorder should be realistic. Because this is a lifelong disorder, small successes should be expected. Specific outcomes should be identified, such as gradually increasing social contact. Over time, there should be a gradual reduction in the number of health care providers the individual contacts and gradual improvement in the ability to cope with stresses (Fig. 21-3).

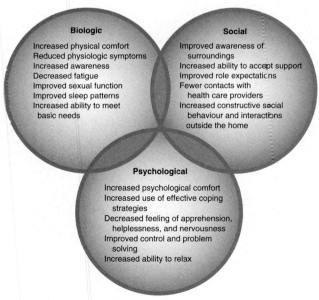

Biologic
Increased physical comfort
Reduced physiologic symptoms
Increased awareness
Decreased fatigue
Improved sexual function
Improved sleep patterns
Increased ability to meet
  basic needs

Social
Improved awareness of
  surroundings
Increased ability to accept support
Improved role expectations
Fewer contacts with
  health care providers
Increased constructive social
  behaviour and interactions
  outside the home

Psychological
Increased psychological comfort
Increased use of effective coping
  strategies
Decreased feeling of apprehension,
  helplessness, and nervousness
Improved control and problem
  solving
Increased ability to relax

FIGURE 21.3   Biopsychosocial outcomes for patients with somatization disorder.

CONTINUUM OF CARE

Inpatient Care

Ideally, these individuals will spend minimal time in the hospital. Inpatient stays occur when their comorbid disorders become symptomatic. While an inpatient, the patient should be the responsibility of one primary nurse who provides or oversees all the nursing care. The inpatient nurse must establish a relationship with the patient (and family) and consult other nursing staff members about this disorder.

Emergency Care

The emergencies these individuals experience may be physical (eg, chest pain, back pain, gastrointestinal symptoms) or stress responses related to a psychosocial crisis. Occasionally, these individuals become suicidal and require an intensive level of care. Generally speaking, nonpharmacologic interventions should be tried first, with very conservative use of antianxiety medications. All attempts should be made to retrieve records from other facilities.

Community Treatment

These patients can spend a lifetime in the health care system and still have little continuity of care. Switching from provider to provider is detrimental to their long-term care. Most are outpatients. When they are hospitalized, it is usually for evaluation of medical problems. When their comorbid psychiatric disorders, such as depression, become symptomatic, these patients may also be hospitalized for a short time. See Nursing Care Plan 21-1.

MENTAL HEALTH PROMOTION

Patients with somatization disorder should focus on "staying healthy," instead of focusing on their illness. For these individuals, approaching the topic of health promotion usually has to be within the context of preventing further problems. Setting aside time for themselves and identifying activities that meet their psychological and spiritual needs, such as connecting with their faith group, are important in maintaining a healthy balance.

Other Somatoform Disorders

The other somatoform disorders have many symptoms that are similar to those of somatization disorder but are often not as debilitating. The following discussion summarizes the other somatoform disorders and highlights the primary focus of nursing management.

NURSING CARE PLAN 21.1

Nursing Care Plan for a Patient With Somatization Disorder

SC is a 48-year-old woman who is making her weekly visit to her primary care physician for unexplained multiple somatic problems. This week, her concern is reoccurring abdominal pain that fits no symptom pattern. Upon physical examination, a cause of her abdominal pain could not be found. She is requesting a refill of alprazolam (Xanax), which is the only medication that relieves her pain. She is in the process of applying for disability income because of being completely disabled by neck and shoulder pain. The physician and office staff avoid her whenever possible. The physician will not refill the prescription until SC is evaluated by the consulting mental health team that provides weekly evaluations and services.

SETTING: PRIMARY CARE OFFICE

Baseline Assessment: 48-year-old Caucasian, obese woman who appears very angry. She resents being forced to see a psychiatric clinician for the only medication that works. She denies any psychiatric problems or emotional distress. SC is wearing a short, black top and too tight slacks. Her hair is in curlers and she says that it is too much trouble to comb her hair. Cognitive aspects of mental status appear normal, but she admits to being slightly depressed and takes the alprazolam for her nerves. She says she has nothing to live for, but denies any thoughts of suicide. She is dependent on her children for everything and feels very guilty about it. She spends most of her waking hours going to various doctors and taking combinations of medications to relieve her pains. She has no friends or nonfamily social contacts.

Associated Psychiatric Diagnosis	*Medications*
Axis I: R/O depression	Premarin, 1.2 mg qd
Axis II: Somatization disorder	Alprazolam (Xanax), 25 mg tid
Axis III: S/P hysterectomy	Ranitidine HCL (Zantac), 150 mg with meals
S/P gastric bypass	Simethicone, 1,235 mg qid with meals
S/P carpel tunnel release	Calcium carbonate, 1,200 mg qd
Chronic shoulder, neck pain, vertigo	Multiple vitamin, qd
Axis IV: Social problems (father died 6 months ago,	Zolpidem tartrate (Ambien), 10 mg at hs PRN
divorced 9 months)	Ibuprofen, 600 mg q4h PRN pain
Economic problems (small pension)	Maalox, PRN
Occupational problems (potential disability)	Preparation H suppositories
GAF = Current, 60	
Potential, 75	

NURSING DIAGNOSIS 1: CHRONIC LOW SELF-ESTEEM

Defining Characteristics	*Related Factors*
Self-negating verbalizations (long-standing)	Feeling unimportant to family
Hesitant to try new things	Feeling rejected by ex-husband
Expresses guilt	Constant physical problems interfering with normal
Evaluates self as being unable to deal with events	social activities

OUTCOMES

Initial	*Long-term*
Identify need to increase self-esteem	Participate in individual or group therapy for esteem building

INTERVENTIONS

Interventions	*Rationale*	*Ongoing Assessment*
Establish rapport with patient.	Individuals with low self-esteem feel vulnerable and may be reluctant to discuss true feelings.	Ask patient for her perceptions of care and the helping relationship.
Encourage patient to spend time dressing and grooming appropriately.	Confidence and self-esteem improve when a person looks well groomed.	Monitor responses.

NURSING CARE PLAN 21.1 (Continued)

Nursing Care Plan for a Patient With Somatization Disorder

Interventions	Rationale	Ongoing Assessment
Encourage patient to discuss various somatic problems, as well as psychological and interpersonal issues.	Patients with somatization disorder need time to express their physical problems. It helps them feel valued. The best way to build a relationship is to acknowledge physical symptoms.	Monitor time that patient spends explaining physical symptoms.
Explore opportunities for SC to meet other people with similar, nonmedical interests.	Focusing SC on meeting others will improve the possibilities of increasing contacts.	Observe willingness to identify other interests besides physical problems.

EVALUATION

Outcomes	Revised Outcomes	Interventions
SC admitted to having low self-esteem, but was very reluctant to consider meeting new people.	Focus on building self-esteem.	Identify activities that will enhance personal self-esteem.

NURSING DIAGNOSIS 2: INEFFECTIVE THERAPEUTIC REGIMEN MANAGEMENT

Defining Characteristics	Related Factors
Choices of daily living ineffective for meeting health care goal Verbalizes difficulty with prescribed regimens	Inappropriate use of benzodiazepines for nerves

OUTCOMES

Initial	Long-term
Openly discuss the use of medications.	Use nonpharmacologic means for stress reduction especially antianxiety medications.

INTERVENTIONS

Interventions	Rationale	Ongoing Assessment
Clarify the frequency and purpose of taking alprazolam.	Unsupervised polypharmacy is very common with these patients. Further clarification is usually needed.	Carefully track self-report of medication use; determine whether patient is disclosing the use of all medications.
Educate patient about the effects of combining medications, emphasizing negative effects.	Education about combining medication is the beginning of helping patient become effective in medication regimen.	Observe patient's ability and willingness to consider negative effects.
Explore ways to gradually reduce number of medications, including other means of managing physical symptoms.	Assisting patients to identify appropriate ways and means to manage health care regimens	Evaluate patient's ability to problem solve.

EVALUATION

Outcomes	Revised Outcomes	Interventions
Patient disclosed use of medications, but was unwilling to consider changing ineffective use of medication.	Identify next step if primary care physician does not refill prescription.	Discuss the possibility of not being able to obtain alprazolam. Refer patient to mental health clinic for further evaluation.

UNDIFFERENTIATED SOMATOFORM DISORDER

Patients who complain of only one type of physical problem, that lasts at least 6 months without adequate explanation, may be diagnosed with undifferentiated somatoform disorder. This disorder is different from somatization disorder in that prior to 30 years of age, these patients do not have multiple, unexplained physical problems; instead, they may have just one. Fatigue, loss of appetite, and gastrointestinal or genitourinary problems are the most common complaints. This disorder is most frequently seen in women of lower socioeconomic status. The course of the disorder is unpredictable, and often another mental or physical disorder is diagnosed. For this disorder, nursing care is similar to that for somatization disorder.

CONVERSION DISORDER

In conversion disorder, the somatic symptoms pertain specifically to neurologic conditions affecting voluntary motor or sensory function, called **pseudoneurologic symptoms**. Patients with conversion disorder present with symptoms of impaired coordination or balance, paralysis, aphonia (inability to produce sound), difficulty swallowing or a sensation of a lump in the throat, and urinary retention. They also may have loss of sensation, vision problems, blindness, deafness, and hallucinations. In some instances, they may have seizures (APA, 2000). These symptoms do not follow neurologic paths, but rather follow the individual's conceptualization of the problem. If only the pseudoneurologic symptoms are present, the patient receives a diagnosis of conversion disorder. The nurse must understand that the physical sensation is real for the patient. There is evidence of a relationship between childhood trauma (such as sexual abuse) and conversion disorder (Roelofs, Keijsers, Hoogduin, Naring, & Moene, 2002). In approaching this patient, the nurse treats the conversion symptom as a real symptom that may have distressing psychological aspects. The nurse intervenes by acknowledging the pain and helps the patient deal with it. As trust develops within the nurse–patient relationship, the nurse can help the patient develop problem-solving approaches to everyday problems.

PAIN DISORDER

In pain disorder, pain severe enough for the patient to seek medical attention interferes with social and occupational functioning. The onset of the pain is associated with psychological factors, such as a traumatic or humiliating experience. Because of the pain, the individual cannot return to work or school. Unemploy-

ment, disability, and family problems frequently follow. Pain disorder is believed to be relatively common. From 10% to 15% of adults in the United States within a given year are disabled by back pain (APA, 2000). Pain disorder may occur at any age. Women experience headaches and musculoskeletal pain more often than do men. Acute pain tends to resolve within a short time; chronic pain may persist for many years. Pain medication should be prescribed conservatively. If mood disorders are also present, mood stabilizers not only treat the depression but also may treat the pain (Maurer, Volz, & Sauer, 1999). Nursing care focuses on helping patients identify strategies to relieve pain (Caudill-Slosberg, 2002) and to examine stressors in their lives.

HYPOCHONDRIASIS

The difference between hypochondriasis and the other somatoform disorders is that patients with hypochondriasis are preoccupied with their fears about developing a serious illness based on their misinterpretation of body sensations. In hypochondriasis, the fear of having an illness continues despite medical reassurance and interferes with psychosocial functioning. These individuals spend time and money on repeated examinations looking for feared illnesses. For example, an occasional cough or the appearance of a small sore results in the person making an appointment with an oncologist. Hypochondriasis sometimes appears if the patient had a serious childhood illness or if a family member has a serious illness. The prevalence of hypochondriasis in general medical practice is estimated to be between 2% and 7% (APA, 2000). These patients are most likely seen in medical-surgical settings, unless they have a coexisting psychiatric disorder.

Several interventions have been effective in reducing patients' fears of experiencing serious illnesses. CBT, stress management, and group interventions lead to a decrease in intensity and increase in control of symptoms (Fava, Grandi, Rafanelli, Fabbri, & Cazzaro, 2000; Walker, Vincent, Furer, Cox, & Kjemisted, 1999). Whether the positive outcomes result from the intervention itself, or from the symptom validation and increased attention given to the patient, is unknown. However, based on these studies, nursing management should include listening to the patient's report of symptoms and fears, validating it by acknowledging that the fears may be real, asking the patient to monitor symptoms in a journal, and encouraging the patient to bring the journal to the next visit. By actually seeing the symptom pattern, the nurse can continue to assess and help the patient better understand the significance and implications of symptoms. The outcome of this approach should be a decrease in fears and better control of the symptoms.

Emily Carr (1871–1945)
Canadian Painter and Writer

Public Personna
Emily Carr was an accomplished artist and writer best known for her vivid depictions of Native culture and Canadian West Coast nature. Influenced by early educational sojourns to San Francisco, England, and France, and later encouraged by the Group of Seven, Carr developed her unique impressionistic style in both painting and writing. Embellished with dramatizations and idealism, works like *Growing Pains* autobiographically depicted the struggle of her life. Raised in a strict Victorian home, Carr has been described as rebellious, yet overweight, irritable, and socially insecure.

Personal Realities
Carr's career was interrupted many times with bouts of poor health. Just over 100 years ago, Carr was treated in an English sanatorium. Many of the symptoms she described were representative of what today is called hypochondriasis, clinical depression, and/or conversion disorder.

BODY DYSMORPHIC DISORDER

Patients with body dysmorphic disorder (BDD) focus on real (but slight) or imagined defects in appearance, such as a large nose, thinning hair, or small genitals. Preoccupation with the defect causes significant distress and interferes with their ability to function socially. They feel so self-conscious that they avoid work or public situations. Some fear that their "ugly" body part will malfunction. This disorder occurs equally in men and women, but few epidemiologic data are available. In anxiety disorders and depression, BDD is estimated to occur in 5% to 40% of patients (APA, 2000). BDD may be present in 25% of patients with anorexia nervosa (Rabe-Jablonska & Tomasz, 2000). In patients receiving dermatology care and cosmetic surgery, the estimate is 6% to 15% (Phillips, Dufresne, Wilkel, & Vittorio 2000; Uzun et al., 2003).

BDD usually begins in adolescence and continues throughout adulthood. These individuals are not usually seen in psychiatric settings unless they have a coexisting psychiatric disorder or a family member insists on psychiatric attention. BDD is an extremely debilitating disorder and can significantly impair an individual's quality of life (Box 21-7). The obvious nursing diagnosis is Impaired Body Image. While developing a therapeutic relationship, the nurse should respect these patients' preoccupation and avoid challenging their beliefs. However, the nurse should also assess the extent of preoccupation with the body part. If the patient is actually disfigured, the preoccupation may take on a phobic quality (Newell, 1999). If so, referral to a mental health specialist should be considered. The generalist nurse can help the patient by developing interventions for other nursing diagnoses that may be present, such as Social Isolation, Low Self-Esteem, and Ineffective Coping. These patients will often be treated with an antidepressant (Phillips & Najjar, 2003).

Factitious Disorders

The other type of psychiatric disorders characterized by somatization is factitious disorders; patients with these disorders intentionally cause an illness or injury to receive the attention of health care workers. These individuals are motivated solely by the desire to become a patient and develop a dependent relationship with a

---

BOX 21-7

Clinical Vignette: Body Dysmorphic Disorder

K, a 16-year-old girl, for about 6 months has believed that her pubic bone is becoming increasingly dislocated and prominent. She believes that everyone stares at and talks about it. She does not remember a particular event related to the appearance of the symptom, but is absolutely convinced that she can be helped only by a surgical correction of her pubic bone.

She was treated recently for anorexia nervosa with marginal success. Although her weight is nearly normal, she continues to be preoccupied with the looks of her body. She spends almost the entire day in her bedroom, wearing excessively large pajamas, and she refuses to leave the house. Once or twice a day, she lowers herself to the ground and measures, with her fingers, the distance between her pelvic girdle and the ground in order to check the position of the pubic bone.

In desperation, her parents called the clinic for help. The family was referred to a home health agency and a psychiatric home health nurse who arranged for an assessment visit.

What Do You Think?
- How should the nurse approach K? Should an assessment begin immediately?
- From the vignette, identify nursing diagnoses, outcomes, and interventions.

Adapted from Sobanski, E., & Schmidt, M. H. (2000). "Everybody looks at my pubic bone"—A case report of an adolescent patient with body dysmorphic disorder. *Acta Psychiatric Scandinavia*, 101, 80–82.

health care provider. There are two classes of factitious disorders: factitious disorder and factitious disorder, not otherwise specified.

FACTITIOUS DISORDER

Although feigned illnesses have been described for centuries, it was not until 1951 that the term *Münchausen's syndrome* was used to describe the most severe form of this disorder, which was characterized by fabricating a physical illness, having recurrent hospitalizations, and going from one provider to another (Asher, 1951). Today, this disorder is called factitious disorder and is differentiated from **malingering,** in which the individual who intentionally produces illness symptoms is motivated by another specific self-serving goal, such as being classified as disabled or avoiding work.

Unlike people with borderline personality disorder, who typically injure themselves overtly and readily admit to self-harm, patients with factitious disorder injure themselves covertly. The illnesses are produced in such a manner that the health care provider is tricked into believing that a true physical or psychiatric disorder is present. The *DSM-IV-TR* identifies three subtypes of factitious disorder: (1) one that has predominantly psychological symptoms, (2) one that has predominately physical symptoms (Münchausen's syndrome), and (3) one that has a combination of physical and psychological manifestations, with neither one predominating (APA, 2000).

The self-produced physical symptoms appear as medical illnesses and cut across all body systems. They include seizure disorders, wound-healing disorders, the abscess processes (introduction of infectious material below the skin surface), and feigned fever (rubbing the thermometer). In one study of 42 children and adolescents who falsify chronic illness, most patients were female, and the most commonly reported falsified or induced conditions were fevers, ketoacidosis, purpura, and infections (Libow, 2000).

These patients are extremely creative in simulating illnesses, and they tell fascinating, but false, stories of personal triumph. These tales are referred to as **pseudologia fantastica** and are a core symptom of the disorder. Pseudologia fantastica are stories that are not entirely improbable and often contain a matrix of truth and falsehood. These patients falsify blood, urine, and other samples by contaminating them with protein or fecal material. They self-inject anticoagulants to receive diagnoses of "bleeding of undetermined origin" or ingest thyroid hormones to produce thyrotoxicosis. They also inflict injury on themselves by inserting objects or feces into body orifices, such as the urinary tract and open wounds. They produce their own surgical scars, especially abdominal, and when treated surgi-

cally, they delay wound healing through scratching, rubbing, or manipulating the wound and introducing bacteria into the wound. These patients put themselves in life-threatening situations through actions such as ingesting allergens known to produce an anaphylactic reaction.

Patients who manifest primarily psychological symptoms produce psychotic symptoms such as hallucinations and delusions, cognitive deficits such as memory loss, dissociative symptoms such as amnesia, and conversion symptoms such as pseudoblindness or pseudoparalysis. These individuals often appear psychotic, depressed, or suicidal after an unconfirmed tragedy. When questioned about details, they become defensive and uncooperative. Sometimes, these individuals have a combination of both physical and psychiatric symptoms.

EPIDEMIOLOGY

The prevalence of this disorder is unknown because diagnosing it and obtaining reliable data are difficult. Prevalence was reported to be high when researchers were actually looking for the disorder in specific populations. Within large general hospitals, factitious disorders are diagnosed in about 1% of patients with whom mental health professionals consult. The age range of patients with the disorder is between 19 and 64 years. The median age of onset is the early 20s. Once thought to occur predominantly in men, this disorder is now reported predominantly in women. No genetic pattern has been identified, but it does seem to run in families. Many of these people have comorbid psychiatric disorders, such as mood disorders, personality disorders, and substance-related disorders.

ETIOLOGY

The etiology of factitious disorders is believed to have a psychodynamic basis. The theory is that these individuals, who were often abused as children, received nurturance only during times of illness; thus, they try to recreate illness or injury in a desperate attempt to receive love and attention. During the actual self-injury, the individual is reported to be in a trancelike, dissociative state. Many patients report having an intimate relationship with a health care provider, either as a child or as an adult, and then experiencing rejection when the relationship ended. The self-injury and subsequent attention is an attempt by the individual to re-enact those experiences and gain control over the situation and the other person. Often, the patients exhibit aggression after being discovered, allowing them to express revenge on their perceived tormentor (Feldman, 2004).

These patients are usually discovered in medical-surgical settings. They are hostile and distance themselves from others. Their network is void of friends and family and usually consists only of health care providers, who change at regular intervals. In factitious disorder, the patients fabricate a detailed and exaggerated medical history. When the interventions do not work and the fabrication is discovered, the health care team feels manipulated and angry. When the patient is confronted with the evidence, he or she becomes enraged and often leaves that health care system, only to enter another. Eventually, the person is referred for mental health treatment. The course of the disorder usually consists of intermittent episodes (APA, 2000).

NURSING MANAGEMENT: HUMAN RESPONSE TO DISORDER

The overall goal of treatment is for the patient to replace the dysfunctional, attention-seeking behaviours with positive behaviours. To begin treatment, the patient must acknowledge the deception, but confrontation does not appear to lead to acknowledgment (Krahn, Li, & O'Connor, 2003). The mental health team has to accept and value the patient as a human being who needs help. The pattern of self-injury is well established and meets overwhelming psychological needs, so giving up the behaviours is difficult. The treatment is long-term psychotherapy. The generalist psychiatric–mental health nurse will most likely care for the patient during or after periods of feigned illnesses. More is known about the treatment of individuals with factitious physical disorders than of those with psychological disorders.

Assessment

A nursing assessment should focus on obtaining a history of medical and psychological illnesses. Physical disabilities should be identified. Early childhood experiences, particularly instances of abuse, neglect, or abandonment, should be identified to understand the underlying psychological dynamics of the individual and the role of self-injury. Family relationships become strained as the members become aware of the self-inflicted nature of this disorder. Family assessment is important.

Nursing Diagnoses

The nursing diagnoses could include almost any diagnosis: Risk for Trauma, Risk for Self-Mutilation, Ineffective Individual Coping, or Low Self-Esteem.

Desired outcomes include decreased self-injurious behaviour and increased positive coping behaviours. Any nursing intervention must be implemented within the context of a strong nurse–patient relationship (Moffatt, 2000).

Nursing Interventions

Nurses must continually examine their own feelings about these patients. The fabrications and deceits may provoke anger and a sense of betrayal in the nurse. To be effective with these patients, the nurse must be aware of these feelings and resolve them by developing a better understanding of the underlying psychodynamic issues. Therapeutic confrontation in the context of a helping relationship can be effective if the patient feels supported and accepted and if there is clear communication among the patient, the mental health care team, and family members. All care should be centralized within one facility, and the patient should see providers regularly, even when not in active crisis. Offering the patient a face-saving way of giving up the factitious disorder is often crucial. The treatment goal is recovery, not confession. Behavioural techniques that shape new behaviours help the patient move forward toward a new life.

The goal is for care to be given within the context of one system. A team that knows the patient, agrees on a treatment approach, and follows through is crucial to the patient's eventual recovery. For this to happen, the medical, psychiatric, inpatient, and outpatient teams need to communicate with each other on a regular basis. Family members must also be aware of the need for consistent treatment.

FACTITIOUS DISORDER, NOT OTHERWISE SPECIFIED

The diagnosis factitious disorder, not otherwise specified is reserved for people who do not quite meet all the diagnostic criteria of factitious disorder (Table 21-2). Within the category of factitious disorder, not otherwise specified, the *DSM-IV-TR* (APA, 2000) includes a rare, but dramatic disorder, factitious disorder by proxy, or *Münchausen's by proxy*, which involves another person, usually the mother, who inflicts injuries on her child to gain the attention of the health care provider through her child's injuries. These actions include inducing seizures, poisoning, or smothering. This most severe form of child abuse is usually identified in the emergency room or by critical care nurses (Hughes & Corbo-Richert, 1999). The mother rarely admits injuring the child and thus is not amenable to treatment; the child is removed from the mother's care. This form of child abuse is distinguished from other forms by routine, unwitting involvement of health care workers, who subject the child to physical harm and emotional distress through tests, procedures, and medication trials. Some researchers suspect that children who are abused in this way may later experience factitious disorder (Libow, 2000).

Table 21.2	**Key Diagnostic Characteristics of Factitious Disorder** **300.16 With predominantly psychological signs and symptoms** **300.19 With predominantly physical signs and symptoms** **300.19 With combined psychological and physical signs and symptoms**

Diagnostic Criteria and Target Symptoms	**Associated Findings**

▪ Intentionally producing psychological or physical signs and symptoms
    Subjective complaints, such as pain in absence of pain
    Self-inflicted conditions
    Exaggeration or exacerbation of pre-existing medical conditions
    Any combination or variation
▪ Motivated by need to assume sick role
▪ Absence of external incentives for behaviour
	Associated Behavioural Findings
	▪ Very dramatic, but vague, inconsistent history
	▪ Pathologic lying about history to intrigue listener
	▪ Extensive knowledge of medical terminology and hospital routines
	▪ Repeated hospitalizations in numerous hospitals, in many locations
	▪ Complaints of pain and requests for analgesics common
	▪ Eagerly undergo extensive workups with invasive procedures and operations
	▪ Deny allegations that symptoms are factitious once revealed, usually followed by rapid discharge against medical advice.
	(With predominantly psychological signs and symptoms)
	▪ Claims of depression, suicidal ideation, auditory and visual hallucinations, recent and remote memory loss, and dissociative symptoms
	▪ Extremely suggestible
	▪ Negativistic and uncooperative when questioned
	
	Associated Physical Examination
	▪ Severe right lower quadrant pain with nausea and vomiting, massive hemoptysis, generalized rashes and abscesses, fever of unknown origin, bleeding secondary to ingestion of anticoagulants, and "lupus-like" syndromes
	▪ Symptoms limited to person's knowledge, sophistication, and imagination

SUMMARY OF KEY POINTS

◘ Somatization is psychological stress that is manifested in physical symptoms and is the chief characteristic of somatoform disorders and factitious disorders. The difference between these two types of disorders is that in somatoform disorders, the individuals experience unexplained physical symptoms but do not self-inflict injuries, whereas in factitious disorders, individuals self-inflict injuries to gain medical attention.

◘ Somatization is affected by sociocultural and gender factors. It occurs more frequently in women than men; in those less educated; in those living in urban areas; and in those who are older, separated, widowed, or divorced.

◘ The somatoform disorders are clustered into six different clinical syndromes: (1) somatization disorder, (2) undifferentiated somatoform disorder, (3) conversion disorder, (4) pain disorder, (5) hypochondriasis, and (6) body dysmorphic disorder. The person with somatization disorder suffers multiple physical problems and symptoms, in contrast to those with other clinical subtypes, in which one major symptom recurs.

◘ Somatization disorder, the most complex of the somatoform disorders, is a chronic relapsing condition characterized by multiple physical symptoms that develop during times of emotional distress and occur primarily in women.

◘ Factitious disorders include two subtypes: (1) factitious disorder and (2) factitious disorder, not otherwise specified. In factitious disorder, physical or psychological symptoms (or both) are fabricated to assume the sick role. Factitious disorder, not otherwise specified includes factitious disorder by proxy, the intentional production of symptoms in others, usually children.

◘ Identifying and diagnosing somatoform and factitious disorders is very complex because patients with the disorders refuse to accept any psychiatric basis to their problems and often go for years moving from one health care provider to another to receive medical attention and avoid psychiatric assessment.

◘ These patients are often seen on the medical-surgical units of hospitals and go years without receiving a correct diagnosis. In most cases, they finally receive mental health treatment because of comorbid conditions, such as depression and panic.

◨ The development of the nurse–patient relationship is crucial to assessing these patients and identifying appropriate nursing diagnoses and interventions. Because these patients deny any psychiatric basis to their problem and continue to focus on their symptoms as being medically based, the nurse must take a nonjudgmental, open approach that acknowledges the symptoms and that helps the patient explore, understand behaviour, and focus on new ways of coping with stress.

◨ Health teaching is important in helping the individual develop positive lifestyle changes in place of somatization responses. Identifying personal strengths and supporting the development of positive skills improve self-esteem and personal confidence. Teaching the use of biofeedback and relaxation provides the patient with positive coping skills.

CRITICAL THINKING CHALLENGES

1 A depressed young white woman is admitted to a psychiatric unit in a state of agitation. She reports extreme abdominal pain. Her admitting provider tells you that she has a classic case of somatization disorder and to de-emphasize her physical symptoms. Under no circumstances is she to have any pain medication. Conceptualize how to approach, assess, and intervene with this patient.

2 Compare and contrast somatoform disorders with factitious disorders.

3 Develop a motivation continuum of "self-injury" for patients with borderline personality disorder, somatization disorder, factitious disorder, and factitious disorder by proxy.

4 Develop a teaching plan for an individual who has a long history of somatization disorder but who recently received a diagnosis of breast cancer. How will the patient be able to differentiate the physical symptoms of somatization disorder from those associated with the treatment of her breast cancer?

5 A woman of Chinese origin was admitted for panic attacks and numerous somatic problems, ranging from dysmenorrhea to painful joints. Results of all medical examinations have been negative. She truly believes that her panic attacks are caused by a weak heart. What approaches should the nurse use in providing culturally sensitive nursing care?

6 A person experiencing depression with somatic features is started on a regimen of Nardil, 15 mg tid. She believes that she is allergic to most foods but insists on having wine in the evenings because it helps digest her food. Develop a teaching plan that provides the knowledge that she needs to prevent a hypertensive crisis caused by excessive tyramine but that is sensitive to the patient's food preferences.

WEB LINKS

www.athealth.com Somatization and somatoform disorders. Friday's Progress Notes, July 14, 2000, *Mental Health Information*, Volume 4, Issue 21.

www.intelihealth.com InteliHealth provides health information. Somatization disorder can be found through a search on this website.

www.mental-health-matters.com/disorders. A website for consumers and professionals. Describes several psychiatric disorders, including somatization disorders.

MOVIES

The Piano: 1992. This is a thought-provoking account of the life of an English colonial settler who encounters isolation, repression, exploitation, and abuse. The traumatic origin and functional limitations indicative of conversion disorder are poignantly depicted in this movie. Experiencing nonorganic habitual dysphonia (mutism), the main character asserts and expresses herself with others mainly through music.

SIGNIFICANCE: Somatoform and related disorders are rarely clearly depicted in films. *The Piano* exemplifies the functional physical, interpersonal, and occupational effects of symptoms associated with conversion disorder.

VIEWING POINTS: Identify the symptoms and related behaviour associated with somatoform disorder. Consider the effects of emotional and physical trauma.

REFERENCES

American Psychiatric Association. (2000). *Diagnostic and statistical manual of mental disorders* (4th ed., Text revision). Washington, DC: Author.

Asher, R. (1951). Münchausen's syndrome. *Lancet, 1*, 339–341.

Caudill-Slosberg, M. A. (2002). *Managing pain before it manages you* (revised ed.). New York: Guilford Press.

Cloninger, C., Martin, R., Guze, S., & Clayton, P. (1986). A prospective follow-up and family study of somatization in men and women. *American Journal of Psychiatry, 143*(7), 873–878.

Cloninger, C., von Knorring, A., Sigvardsson, S., & Bohman, M. (1986). Symptom patterns and causes of somatization in men. II. Genetic and environmental independence from somatization in women. *Genetic Epidemiology, 3*(3), 171–185.

Cox, B. J., Kuch, K., Parker, J. D, Shulman, I. D., & Evans, R. J. (1994). Alexithymia in somatoform disorder patients with chronic pain. *Journal of Psychosomatic Research, 38*(6), 523–527.

De Gucht, V., & Heiser, W. (2003). Alexithymia and somatization: A quantitative review of the literature. *Journal of Psychosomatic Research, 54*, 425–434.

Fallon, B. A., Qureshi, A. I., Schneier, F. R., Sanchez-Lacay, A., Vermes, D., Feinstein, R., Connelly, J., & Liebowitz, M. R. (2003).

An open trial of fluvoxamine for hypochondriasis. *Psychosomatics, 44*(4), 298–303.

Fava, G., Grandi, S., Rafanelli, C., Fabbri, S., & Cazzaro, M. (2000). Explanatory therapy in hypochondriasis. *Journal of Clinical Psychiatry, 61*(4), 317–322.

Feldman, M. D. (2004). Playing sick? Untangling the web of Munchausen syndrome, Munchausen by proxy, malingering factitious disorders. Philadelphia: Brunner Rutledge. Taylor & Francis.

Garcia-Campayo, J., & Sanz-Carrillo, C. (2000). The use of alternative medicines by somatoform disorder patients in Spain. *British Journal of General Practice, 50*(455), 487–488.

Garcia-Campayo, J., Sanz-Carrillo, C., Baringo, T., & Ceballos, C. (2001). A SPECT scan in somatization disorder patients: An exploratory study of eleven cases. *Australian and New Zealand Journal of Psychiatry, 35*(3), 359–363.

Garyfallos, G., Adamopoulou, A., Karastergiou, A., Voikli, M., Ikonomidis, N., Donias, S., Giouzepas, J., & Dimitriou, E. (1999). Somatoform disorders: Comorbidity with other *DSM-III-R* psychiatric diagnoses in Greece. *Comprehensive Psychiatry, 40*(4), 299–307.

Grabe, H. J., Meyer, C., Hapke, U., Rumpf, H. J., Freyberger, H. J., Dilling, H., & John, U. (2003). Specific somatoform disorder in the general population. *Psychosomatics, 44*(4), 304–311.

Gureje, O., & Simon, G. E. (1999). The natural history of somatization in primary care. *Psychological Medicine, 29*(3), 669–676.

Gureje, O., Simon, G. E., Ustun, T. B., & Goldberg, D. P. (1997). Somatization in cross-cultural perspective: A World Health Organization study in primary care. *American Journal of Psychiatry, 154*(7), 989–995.

Hakala, M., Karlsson, H., Ruotsalainen, U., Koponen, S., Bergman, J., Stenman, H., Kelavuori, J. P., Aalto, S., Kuuki, T., & Niemi, P. (2002). Severe somatization in women is associated with altered cerebral glucose metabolism. *Psychological Medicine, 32*(8), 1379–1385.

Hotopf, M., Mayou, R., Wadsworth, M., & Wessely, S. (1999). Childhood risk factors for adults with medically unexplained symptoms: Results from a national birth cohort study. *American Journal of Psychiatry, 156*(11), 1796–1800.

Hughes, L. M., & Corbo-Richert, B. (1999). Munchausen syndrome by proxy: Literature review and implications for critical care nurses.

Huibers, M. J., Beurskens, A. J., Bleijenberg, G., & van Schayck, C. P. (2003). The effectiveness of psychosocial interventions delivered by general practitioners. *Cochrane Database of Systematic Reviews, (2),* CD 3494.

Jorge, J. R. (2003). Depression in Brazil and other Latin American countries. *Seishin Shinkeigaku Zasshi, 105*(1), 9–16.

Kirmayer, L. J., & Young, A. (1998). Culture and somatization: Clinical, epidemiological correlates. *Psychosomatic Medicine, 60,* 420–430.

Kojima, M., Senda, Y., Nagaya, T., Tokudome, S., & Furukawa, T. A. (2003). Alexithymia, depression and social support among Japanese workers. *Psychotherapy and Psychosomatics, 72*(6), 307–314.

Krahn, L. E., Li, H., & O'Connor, M. K. (2003). Patients who strive to be ill: Factitious disorder with physical symptoms. *American Journal of Psychiatry, 160*(6), 1163–1168.

Kroenke, K., & Swindle, R. (2000). Cognitive-behavioral therapy for somatization and symptom syndromes: A critical review of controlled clinical trials. *Psychotherapy Psychosomatics, 69*(4), 205–215.

Kroenke, K., & Spitzer, R. (1998). Gender differences in the reporting of physical and somatoform symptoms. *Psychosomatic Medicine, 60,* 150–155.

Ladwig, K. H., Marten-Mittag, B., Erazo, N., & Gundel, H. (2001). Identifying somatization disorder in a population-based health examination survey: Psychosocial burden and gender differences. *Psychosomatics, 42*(6), 511–518.

Libow, J. A. (2000). Child and adolescent illness falsification. *Pediatrics, 105*(2), 336–342.

Lidbeck, M. (2003). Group therapy for somatization disorders in primary care: Maintenance of treatment goals of short cognitive-behavioural treatment one-and-a half-year follow-up. *Acta Psychiatrica Scandinavica, 107*(5), 449–456.

Lieb, R., Pfister, H., Mastaler, M., & Wittchen, H. U. (2000). Somatoform syndromes and disorders in a representative population sample of adolescents and young adults: Prevalence, comorbidity and impairments. *Acta Psychiatrica Scandinavica, 101*(3), 194–208.

Lieb, R., Zimmermann, P., Friis, R. H., Hofler, M., Tholen, S., & Wittchen, H. U. (2002). The natural course of DSM-IV somatoform disorders and syndromes among adolescents and young adults: A prospective-longitudinal community study. *European Psychiatry, 17*(6), 321–331.

Mai, F. (2004). Somatization disorder: A practical review. *Canadian Journal of Psychiatry, 49,* 652–662.

Maurer, I., Volz, H. P., & Sauer, H. (1999). Gabapentin leads to remission of somatoform pain disorder with major depression. *Pharmacopsychiatry, 32*(6), 255–257.

Moffatt, C. (2000). Self-inflicted wounding: Identification, assessment and management. *British Journal of Community Nursing, 5*(1), 34–40.

Mullick, M. S. (2002). Somatoform disorders in children and adolescents. *Bangladesh Medical Research Council Bulletin, 28*(3), 112–122.

Newell, R. J. (1999). Altered body image: A fear-avoidance model of psychosocial difficulties following disfigurement. *Journal of Advanced Nursing, 30*(5), 1230–1238.

Phillips, K. A., Dufresne, R. J., Wilkel, C. S., & Vittorio, C. C. (2000). Rate of body dysmorphic disorder in dermatology patients. *Journal of American Academy of Dermatology, 42*(3), 436–441.

Phillips, K. A., & Najjar, F. (2003). An open-label study of citalopram in body dysmorphic disorder. *Journal of Clinical Psychiatry, 64*(6), 715–720.

Porcelli, P., Bagby, R. M., Taylor, G. J., DeCarne, M., Leandro, G., & Todarello, O. (2003). Alexithymia as predictor of treatment outcome in patients with functional gastrointestinal disorders. *Psychosomatic Medicine, 65*(5), 911–918.

Rabe-Jablonska, J. J., & Tomasz, M. (2000). The links between body dysmorphic disorder and eating disorders. *European Psychiatry, 15*(5), 302–305.

Roelofs, K., Keijsers, G. P., Hoogduin, K. A., Naring, G. W., & Moene, F. C. (2002). Childhood abuse in patients with conversion disorders. *American Journal of Psychiatry, 159*(11), 1908–1913.

Schneider, G., Wachter, M., Driesch, G., Kruse, A., Nehen, H. G., & Heuft, G. (2003). Subjective body complaint as an indicator of somatization in elderly patients. *Psychosomatics, 44*(2), 91–99.

Sobanski, E., & Schmidt, M. H. (2000). 'Everybody looks at my pubic bone'—A case report of an adolescent patient with body dysmorphic disorder. *Acta Psychiatrica Scandinavica, 101,* 80–82.

Uzun, O., Basoglu, C., Akar, A., Cansever, A., Ozsahin, A., Cetil, M., & Ebrinc, S. (2003). Body dysmorphic disorder in patients with acne. *Comprehensive Psychiatry, 44*(5), 415–419.

Walker, J., Vincent, N., Furer, P., Cox, B., & Kjemisted, K. (1999). Treatment preference in hypochondriasis. *Journal of Behavior Therapy & Experimental Psychiatry, 30*(4), 251–258.

Whitehead, W. E., Palsson, O., & Jones, K. R. (2002). Systematic review of the comorbidity of irritable bowel syndrome with other disorders: What are the causes and implications? *Gastroenterology, 122*(4), 1140–1156.

Yates, W. R. (2002). Somatoform disorders. Available at: www.emedicing.com/MED/topic3527.htm. Accessed: June 10, 2003.

Yick, A. G., Shibusawa, T., & Agbayani-Siewert, (p. 2003). Partner violence, depression, and practice implications with families of Chinese descent. *Journal of Cultural Diversity, 10*(3), 96–104.

For challenges, please refer to the **CD-ROM** in this book.

22

Eating Disorders

Kate Weaver

LEARNING OBJECTIVES

After studying this chapter, you will be able to:

- Distinguish the signs and symptoms of anorexia nervosa from those of bulimia nervosa.
- Describe two etiologic theories of both anorexia nervosa and bulimia nervosa.
- Explain the importance of body image, body dissatisfaction, and gender identity in developmental theories that explain etiology of eating disorders.
- Describe the neurobiology and neurochemistry in both anorexia nervosa and bulimia nervosa.
- Explain the impact of sociocultural norms on the development of eating disorders.
- Describe the risk factors and protective factors associated with the development of eating disorders.
- Formulate nursing diagnoses for individuals with eating disorders.
- Describe nursing interventions for individuals with anorexia nervosa and bulimia nervosa.
- Differentiate binge eating disorder from bulimia nervosa.
- Analyze special concerns within the nurse–client relationship for the nursing care of individuals with eating disorders.
- Identify strategies for prevention and early detection of eating disorders.

KEY TERMS

anorexia nervosa ▪ binge eating ▪ binge eating disorder ▪ body image ▪ bulimia nervosa ▪ cue ▪ elimination ▪ self-monitoring

⬟ KEY CONCEPTS

body dissatisfaction ▪ body image distortion/disturbed body experience ▪ dietary restraint ▪ drive for thinness ▪ enmeshment ▪ interoceptive awareness

The first Canadian publication about eating disorders was a detailed clinical case report in the *Maritime Medical News* of April 1895 by Dr. Peter Inches, a registered physician in the province of New Brunswick. Inches described the following characteristics that he observed in a 17-year-old patient separated from her family while attending boarding school: low weight, loss of menses, and "almost complete refusal of food of any kind" (p. 74). This 19th century publication was for the most part ignored in subsequent reviews.

Only since the 1970s have eating disorders received national attention because several high-profile personalities and athletes with these disorders have received front-page news coverage and because increasingly more individuals, families, and communities were affected. The increased incidence of anorexia nervosa and bulimia nervosa has prompted mental health professionals to understand their causes and devise effective treatments. Moreover, there has been a concomitant increase in research studies addressing the intense obsession with being thin and the dissatisfaction with one's body that underlie these potentially life-threatening disorders. Thus, mental health professionals are crucial to prevention, early diagnosis, and treatment of both anorexia nervosa and bulimia nervosa.

This chapter focuses on anorexia nervosa and bulimia nervosa. In addition, binge eating disorder (BED), a newly identified eating disorder in its infancy relative to research, is briefly considered. Symptoms of these disorders, such as dieting, binge eating, and preoccupation with weight and shape, overlap significantly. Experts view these symptoms along a continuum of normal to pathologic eating behaviours (White, 2000a) (Fig. 22-1), an approach that helps to identify partial-syndrome or subclinical cases.

Many individuals with anorexia nervosa have bulimic symptoms, and many with bulimia nervosa have anorexic symptoms. For this reason, types of anorexia, such as the purging type, and types of bulimia, such as the restricting type, are differentiated based on the predominant symptom the individual uses to restrict food and weight. These disorders differ in definition, clinical course, etiologies, and interventions and are considered separately in this chapter. However, because their risk factors and prevention strategies are similar, they are discussed together, under one heading.

Anorexia Nervosa

CLINICAL COURSE

The onset of **anorexia nervosa** is usually in early adolescence. Onset can be slow, in that serious dieting can be present long before an emaciated body—the result of starvation—is noticed. This discovery often prompts diagnosis. Because the incidence of subclinical or partial-

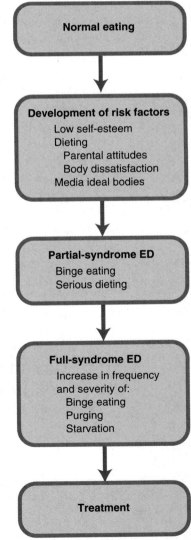

FIGURE 22.1 Continuum of dieting disorders with symptoms. ED, eating disorder.

syndrome cases, in which most of the symptoms are present (eg, female may continue to menstruate), is higher than that of full-syndrome anorexia nervosa, many affected individuals may not receive early treatment of their symptoms, or in some cases, they receive no treatment (see Fig. 22-1). Partial-syndrome cases are described in the American Psychiatric Association's (APA) *Diagnostic and Statistical Manual of Mental Disorders*, 4th ed., Text revision (*DSM-IV-TR*) as Eating Disorder Not Otherwise Specified (APA, 2000). Full-syndrome eating disorders fully meet stringent medical diagnostic criteria.

The long-term outcome of anorexia nervosa has improved during the past 15 to 20 years because awareness of the disease has increased, resulting in early detection. It can be considered a chronic condition, with relapses characterized by significant weight loss. However, unlike most mental illnesses, eating disorders are curable (Anderson, 2001). Reporting conclusive outcomes for anorexia nervosa is difficult because of the variety of definitions used to determine recovery. Although individuals who have recovered have restored normal weight, menses, and eating behaviours, some continue to have distorted body images and be preoccupied with weight and food, many develop bulimia nervosa, and many continue to have symptoms of other psychiatric illnesses. Conclusions from a review of 119 outcome studies revealed that, on average, less than half of individuals recovered (Steinhausen, 2002). In these and other studies, about 10% to 25% of individuals go on to experience bulimia nervosa (White, 2000b). A poor outcome has been related to an initial lower minimum weight, the presence of purging (vomiting), and a later age of onset. Duration of treatment predicts positive outcome; the longer treatment continues, the better the outcome (Fichter & Quadflieg, 1999; Steinhausen, 2002).

DIAGNOSTIC CRITERIA

The diagnostic criteria for anorexia nervosa have been refined in each edition of the *DSM-IV-TR* (APA, 2000). For example, the amount of weight loss or lack of weight gain required for the diagnosis of anorexia nervosa has changed over time. In the third edition of the *DSM* (APA, 1987), a weight 75% of that appropriate to age and height is required, whereas in the *DSM-IV-TR* (2000), a weight 85% of the appropriate weight is specified. Research on core symptoms has resulted in very specific criteria (Table 22-1). It is important to note that the *DSM-IV-TR*

Table 22.1	Key Diagnostic Characteristics for Anorexia Nervosa	

Diagnostic Criteria	Target Symptoms and Associated Findings
<ul><li>Refusal to maintain body weight at or above a minimally normal weight for age and height</li><li>Intense fear of gaining weight or becoming fat, even though underweight</li><li>Disturbance in way person experiences body shape or weight</li><li>Undue influence of body weight or shape on self-evaluation or denial of seriousness of current low body weight</li><li>Absence of at least three consecutive menstrual cycles (in postmenarchal females)</li><li>Restricting type: not regularly engaged in binge eating or purging behaviour (such as self-induced vomiting or misuse of laxatives, diuretics, or enemas)</li><li>Binge eating and purging type: regularly engaging in binge eating or purging behaviour</li></ul>	<ul><li>Depressive symptoms such as depressed mood, social withdrawal, irritability, insomnia, and diminished interest in sex</li><li>Obsessive-compulsive features related and unrelated to food</li><li>Preoccupation with thought of food</li><li>Concerns about eating in public</li><li>Feelings of ineffectiveness</li><li>Strong need to control one's environment</li><li>Inflexible thinking</li><li>Limited social spontaneity and overly restrained initiative and emotional expression</li></ul>*Associated Physical Examination Findings*<ul><li>Complaints of constipation, abdominal pain</li><li>Cold intolerance</li><li>Lethargy and excess energy</li><li>Emaciation</li><li>Significant hypotension, hypothermia, and skin dryness</li><li>Bradycardia and possible peripheral edema</li><li>Hypertrophy of salivary glands, particularly the parotid gland</li><li>Dental enamel erosion related to induced vomiting</li><li>Scars or calluses on dorsum of hand from contact with teeth for inducing vomiting</li></ul>*Associated Laboratory Findings*<ul><li>Leukopenia and mild anemia</li><li>Elevated blood urea nitrogen</li><li>Hypercholesterolemia</li><li>Elevated liver function studies</li><li>Electrolyte imbalances, metabolic alkalosis, or metabolic acidosis</li><li>Low normal serum thyroxine levels; decreased serum triiodothyronine levels</li><li>Low serum estrogen levels</li><li>Sinus bradycardia</li><li>Metabolic encephalopathy</li><li>Significantly reduced resting energy expenditure</li><li>Increased ventricular/brain ratio secondary to starvation</li></ul>

Table 22.2   Complications of Eating Disorders

Body System	Symptoms
From Starvation to Weight Loss	
Musculoskeletal	Loss of muscle mass, loss of fat (emaciation)
	Osteopenia (*bone mineral* deficiency) and less frequently osteoporosis
Metabolic	Hypothyroidism (symptoms include lack of energy, weakness, intolerance to cold, and bradycardia)
	Hypoglycemia, decreased insulin sensitivity
Cardiac	Bradycardia, hypotension, loss of cardiac muscle, small heart, cardiac arrhythmias including atrial and ventricular premature contractions, prolonged QT interval, ventricular tachycardia, sudden death
Gastrointestinal	Delayed gastric emptying, bloating, constipation, abdominal pain, gas, diarrhea
Reproductive	Amenorrhea, low levels of luteinizing hormone and follicle-stimulating hormone, irregular periods
Dermatologic	Dry, cracking skin and brittle nails due to dehydration, lanugo (fine baby-like hair over body), edema, acrocyanosis (bluish hands and feet); hair thinning
Hematologic	Leukopenia, anemia, thrombocytopenia, hypercholesterolemia, hypercarotenemia
Neuropsychiatric	Abnormal taste sensation (possible zinc deficiency)
	Neurologic deficits in cognitive processing of new information; decreased total brain volume; increased brain ventricular size
	Apathetic depression, mild organic mental symptoms, sleep disturbances, fatigue
Related to Purging (Vomiting and Laxative Abuse)	
Metabolic	Electrolyte abnormalities, particularly hypokalemia, hypochloremic alkalosis; hypomagnesemia; increased blood urea nitrogen
Gastrointestinal	Salivary gland and pancreatic inflammation and enlargement with increase in serum amylase; esophageal and gastric erosion (esophagitis) rupture; dysfunctional bowel with haustral dilation; superior mesenteric artery syndrome
Dental	Erosion of dental enamel (perimyolysis), particularly frontal teeth with decreased decay
Neuropsychiatric	Seizures (related to large fluid shifts and electrolyte disturbances), mild neuropathies, fatigue, weakness, mild organic mental symptoms
Cardiac	Ipecac cardiomyopathy arrhythmias

still requires amenorrhea as a criterion (see Table 22-1), thereby excluding men from the diagnosis of anorexia nervosa. The World Health Organization diagnostic criteria (1993) include widespread endocrine disorder that manifests in men as loss of sexual interest and potency.

Anorexia nervosa is categorized into two major types: restricting and binge eating or purging. We now understand more clearly that many of the clinical features associated with anorexia nervosa may result from malnutrition or semistarvation. For example, classic research on volunteers who have been semistarved and observations of prisoners of war and conscientious objectors have demonstrated that these states are characterized by symptoms of food preoccupation, binge eating, depression, obsession, and apathy. Drastic measures to resist overeating persist long after the semistarvation experience, even when food is plentiful. Table 22-2 presents the medical complications, signs, and symptoms of eating disorders that result from starving or binge eating and purging. Many somatic systems are compromised in individuals with eating disorders.

Originally, the central feature of the disorder was thought to be a distorted body image (Bruch, 1973). Body image refers to a mental picture of one's own body.

Body image disturbance occurs when there is extreme discrepancy between one's own mental picture of his or her body and the perception of the outside world.

To adolescents, body image is important because it has a complex psychological impact on overall self-concept and is a crucial factor in determining how adolescents interact with others and think society will respond to them. For most individuals, body image is consistent with how others view them. However, those with anorexia nervosa may have a body image distortion in that they may "see" themselves as obese and undesirable, even when they are emaciated.

> **KEY CONCEPT Body image distortion** occurs when the individual perceives his or her body disparately from how the world or society views it.

Why do individuals with anorexia nervosa see themselves differently? Investigators and clinicians have recently determined that anorexia nervosa is not always associated with body image distortion (Andersen & Yager, 2005). Rather, individuals with anorexia nervosa may suffer disturbance in how they experience their bodies, which contributes to body dissatisfaction. They

BOX 22.1

Psychological Characteristics Related to Eating Disorders

Anorexia Nervosa
Decreased interoceptive awareness
Sexuality conflict/fears
Maturity fears
Ritualistic behaviours

Bulimia Nervosa
Impulsivity
Boundary problems
Limit-setting difficulties

Anorexia Nervosa and Bulimia Nervosa
Difficulty expressing anger
Low self-esteem
Body dissatisfaction
Powerlessness
Ineffectiveness
Perfectionism
Dietary restraint
Obsessiveness
Compulsiveness
Nonassertiveness
Cognitive distortions

"see that they are thin"; however, they may cling to slenderness as protection against a body that they loathe" (Massey-Stokes, 2001, p. 292).

Essential to the diagnosis of anorexia nervosa are self-induced starvation behaviours, relentless drive for thinness or a morbid fear of becoming fat, and signs and symptoms resulting from the starvation. Box 22-1 lists the common psychological characteristics of eating disorders.

Individuals with anorexia nervosa have an intense drive for thinness. They see themselves as fat, fear becoming fatter, and are "driven" to work toward "undoing" this fear.

> **KEY CONCEPT Drive for thinness** is an intense physical and emotional process that overrides all physiologic body cues.

The individual with anorexia nervosa ignores body cues, such as hunger and weakness, and concentrates all efforts on controlling food intake. The entire mental focus of the individual with anorexia nervosa narrows to only one goal: weight loss. Typical thought patterns are: "If I gain a kilo, I'll keep gaining." This all-or-nothing thinking keeps these individuals on rigid regimens for weight loss.

The behaviour of individuals with anorexia nervosa becomes organized around food-related activities, such as preparing food, counting calories, and reading cookbooks. Much behaviour concerning what, when, and how they eat is ritualistic. Food combinations and the order in which foods may be eaten, and under which circumstances, can seem bizarre. One individual, for example, would eat only cantaloupe, carrying it with her to all meals outside of her home, and consuming it only if it were cut in smaller than bite-sized pieces and only if she could use chopsticks, which she also carried with her.

Feelings of inadequacy and a fear of maturity are characteristic of the individual with anorexia nervosa. Weight loss becomes a way for these individuals to experience some sense of control and combat feelings of inadequacy and ineffectiveness. Every lost pound is viewed as a success, and weight loss often confers a feeling of virtuousness. Because these individuals feel inadequate, they fear emotional maturation and the unknown challenges the next developmental stages will bring. For some, remaining physically small is believed to symbolize remaining childlike. Perfectionism is an important characteristic of women with anorexia nervosa (Halmi et al., 2000). Individuals with anorexia nervosa may also have difficulty defining feelings because they are confused about or unsure of emotions and visceral cues, such as hunger. This uncertainty is called a lack of interoceptive awareness.

> **KEY CONCEPT Interoceptive awareness** is a term used to describe the sensory response to emotional and visceral cues, such as hunger.

Those with anorexia nervosa are confused about sensations; therefore, their responses to cues are inaccurate and inappropriate. Often they cannot name feelings they are experiencing, such as anxiety. This profound lack of interoceptive awareness is thought to be partially responsible for developing and maintaining this disorder and some instances of bulimia nervosa.

In addition, individuals with anorexia nervosa may avoid conflict and have difficulty expressing negative emotions, especially anger (Geller, Cockell, & Goldner, 2000). They may have an overwhelming sense of guilt. Because of the ritualistic behaviours, all-encompassing focus on food and weight, and feelings of inadequacy that accompany anorexia nervosa, social contacts are gradually reduced, and the patient becomes isolated. With more severe weight loss comes others symptoms, such as apathy, depression, and even mistrust of others.

EPIDEMIOLOGY

An Ontario study found that 0.66% of women and 0.16% of men aged 15 to 64 had full-syndrome anorexia nervosa (Woodside et al., 2001). An additional 1.15% of women and 0.76% of men had partial-syndrome. The lifetime prevalence of anorexia nervosa is reported to be 0.5% to 1%. Anorexia nervosa is less common than bulimia nervosa. A similar prevalence is found in most Western countries; the disorder is also more prevalent within U.S. ethnic minorities and those in other countries than previously recognized. Cultural change itself may be associated with increased vulnerability to eating disorders, especially when values about physical aesthetics are involved (Miller & Pumariega, 2001). For example, eating disorders have increased among Chinese women in Hong Kong who are exposed to Western views of ideal body types. Chinese-American men and women living in the United States have higher rates of eating disorders than do those living in their native country (Davis & Katzman, 1999).

Age of Onset

The age of onset is typically between 14 and 16 years. Adolescents are vulnerable because of stressors associated with their development, especially concerns about body image, autonomy, and peer pressure, and their susceptibility to such influences as the media, which extols an ideal body type. Unhealthy dieting behaviours are prevalent in Canadian girls as young as 10 years of age (McVey, Tweed, & Blackmore, 2004) and in boys at 13 years (Jonat & Birmingham, 2004). An important predictor of anorexia nervosa is early-onset menses, as early as 10 or 11 years of age.

Gender Differences

In treatment settings, females are 10 times more likely than males to have anorexia nervosa. This disparity has been attributed to society's influence on females to achieve an ideal body type. Box 22-2 highlights some of the findings about eating disorders in males.

Ethnic and Cultural Differences

In the United States, eating disorders are slightly more common among Hispanic and Caucasian populations and less common among African Americans and Asians (Fitzgibbon et al., 1998). In the past 15 to 20 years, the incidence among various ethnic groups has increased. Contextual variables that may influence eating disorders in women of color are level of acculturation, socioeconomic status, peer socialization, family structure, and immigration status (Kuba & Harris, 2001).

In Canada, cultural beliefs have been identified as significant contributing factors in eating disorder development (Farrales & Chapman, 1999). However, Canadian research on eating disorders and ethnicity is limited.

Familial Predisposition

First-degree relatives of people with anorexia nervosa have higher rates of this disorder. Rates of partial syn-

---

BOX 22.2

Boys and Men With Eating Disorders

Eating disorders in boys and men are becoming more prevalent. Men are more likely to have a later onset than women, at about age 20.5 years. Boys and men are also more likely to be involved in an occupation or sport in which weight control influences performance, such as wrestling (Braun, Sunday, Huang, & Halmi, 1999).

Men with anorexia nervosa of the restricting type were found to have lower testosterone levels. In studies comparing men and women on psychological characteristics, men had lower drive for thinness and body dissatisfaction scores, but higher perfectionism scores (Joiner, Katz, & Heatherton, 2000).

In another investigation, predictors of binge eating were different for men compared with women. Anger and depression preceded binges in men, whereas dieting failure was the most significant predictor of a binge in women (Costanzo et al., 1999). Men and women did not differ with regard to comorbid conditions, such as depression and substance abuse, but men had less reported sexual abuse than did women with eating disorders. In one study, men had prevalence ratios of 1 male case for every 3 female cases when partial-syndrome cases were considered (Woodside et al., 2001). More recently, Health Canada (2003) reported a ratio of male to female cases of approximately 1:5 in a survey of more than 30,000 people conducted in 2001 and 2002. This higher ratio is related to only full-syndrome cases. Eating disorders are undiagnosed in males, so prevalence rates may seem much higher in women than they actually are.

---

drome or subthreshold cases among female family members of individuals with anorexia nervosa are even higher (Strober et al., 2000; Woodside, Field, Garfinkel, & Heinmaa, 1998). Female relatives also have high rates of depression, leading researchers to hypothesize that a shared genetic factor may influence development of both disorders.

Comorbidity

Comorbid major depression and dysthymia are common in individuals with anorexia nervosa (North & Gowers, 1999; Toner, Garfinkel, & Garner, 1988), as are obsessive-compulsive disorder (OCD) and anxiety disorders such as phobias and panic disorder. In many individuals with anorexia nervosa, OCD symptoms predate the anorexia nervosa diagnosis by about 5 years, leading many researchers to consider OCD a causative or risk factor for anorexia nervosa (Anderluk et al., 2003; Milos et al., 2002). Cluster C personality disorders are also associated with anorexia nervosa (Kaye, Klump, Frank, & Strober, 2000). These comorbid conditions often resolve when anorexia nervosa has been treated successfully. In other cases, symptoms of a premorbid condition, such as OCD, remain even though an individual has recovered from anorexia nervosa. This finding has influenced many experts to believe that many of the characteristics of anorexia nervosa, such as perfectionism and making sure that everything is symmetric or that objects are placed the same distance from each other and the like (symmetry-seeking) are trait, rather than state, characteristics and may actually influence the development of the disorder.

ETIOLOGY

Some of the risk factors and the etiologic factors for eating disorders overlap. For example, dieting is a risk factor for the development of anorexia nervosa, but it is also a biologic etiologic factor, and in its most serious form—starving—it is also a symptom. This overlap of risk factors, causes, and symptoms must be kept in mind. Viewing them along a continuum from less to more severe helps with this conceptualization (see Fig. 22-1). Most experts agree that anorexia nervosa (as well as bulimia nervosa) is multidimensional and multidetermined. Figure 22-2 depicts the biopsychosocial etiologic factors for anorexia nervosa.

Biologic Theories

Most of what is known about the etiology of anorexia nervosa is focused on psychological factors. There is little conclusive evidence regarding biologic theories of causation. Part of this difficulty stems from the many comorbid conditions, such as depression and OCD, associated with a diagnosis of anorexia nervosa, which some researchers view as having a shared etiology. In addition, many of the biologic changes noted in

anorexia nervosa have been determined to be the result of starvation and are considered state, rather than trait or causative, factors. Little evidence exists to substantiate that dysregulations in appetite-satiety systems cause anorexia nervosa, as some have suggested. Appetite dysregulation is best viewed as the end product or result of an interaction between the environment and physiology. The biopsychosocial model of this interaction best explains the etiology (see Fig. 22-2).

Neuropathologic Theories

Magnetic resonance imaging (MRI) and computed tomography (CT) disclose changes in the brain of individuals with anorexia nervosa who have significant weight loss (eg, changes such as cerebral ventricular enlargement, in particular dilation of the third and lateral ventricles, and enlargement of the cortical sulci and the interhemispheric fusion have been found). This neuropathy and deficits in white matter reverse with weight gain. Yet, grey matter changes resulting from starvation may not fully return to normal after months of weight restoration (Katzman, Zipursky, Lambe, & Mikulis, 1997; Lambe, Katzman, Miluluis, Kennedy, & Zipursky, 1997). To date, evidence supports that brain structure changes follow rather than cause anorexia nervosa.

Genetic Theories

Genetic research on eating disorders is in its infancy. There is little evidence to suggest that a specific gene influences anorexia nervosa (Bulik, Sullivan, Wade, & Kendler, 2000). The existence of comorbid conditions makes it difficult to determine the influence of genetics on anorexia nervosa. Separating genetic influences from environmental influences when twins share a similar family environment is difficult, but investigators reviewing data from twin studies recently demonstrated that the concordance rate for monozygotic twins is higher (44%) than for dizygotic twins (12.5%). Thus, a genetic factor may be involved in the etiology of anorexia nervosa (Bulik et al., 1998).

Biochemical Theories

Studies of neuroendocrine, neuropeptide, vasopressin, oxytocin, and neurotransmitter functioning in patients with eating disorders indicate that these systems may be related to maintaining anorexia nervosa. Endogenous opioids may contribute to denial of hunger in patients with the disorder. Some studies have shown weight gain after patients received opiate antagonists. Thyroid function is also decreased in patients with this disorder. However, most research has established that these neurotransmitter and neuroendocrine

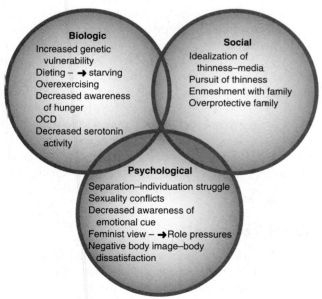

FIGURE 22.2 Biopsychosocial etiologies for patients with anorexia nervosa. OCD, obsessive-compulsive disorder.

abnormalities, such as blunted serotonergic function in low-weight patients, must be viewed with caution as causative factors because these disturbances are state related and tend to normalize after symptom remission and weight gain (Bailer & Kaye, 2003). At best, these changes may be viewed as indicating vulnerability in some individuals, who under certain psychological and environmental conditions, such as cultural pressures, starve themselves. In these individuals, effects on central serotonergic function may result from starvation, rather than triggering it (Ward, Tiller, Treasure, & Russell, 2000).

Psychological Theories

The most widely accepted theory of anorexia nervosa is psychoanalytic. In this theory, key tasks of separation-individuation and autonomy are interrupted. Struggles around identity and role, body image formation, and sexuality fears predominate as a result of developmental arrests. Because anorexia nervosa is usually diagnosed between 14 and 18 years of age, developmental struggles of adolescence have long been an acceptable theory of causation (Bruch, 1973).

During early adolescence, when individuals begin to establish their independence and autonomy, some girls may feel inadequate or ineffective. Dieting and weight control are viewed as a means to defend against these feelings. In later adolescence, when separation-individuation is a developmental task, similar conflicts arise when the adolescent is ill prepared for this stage and feels inadequate and ineffective in going forward emotionally.

Gender identity has been hypothesized to explain the significant difference between the numbers of females and males who experience anorexia nervosa and bulimia nervosa. Studies have shown that girls and boys do not differ dramatically in self-esteem until just before adolescence. At the time self-doubt increases in girls, pubertal weight gain can also occur, resulting in a rounded, mature shape. Thus, normal occurrences can add to confusion about one's identity. Other researchers believe that confusion and self-doubt are aided by conflicting messages that young women receive from society about their roles in life. Young girls may interpret expectations about how they should look, what roles they should perform, and what they should achieve in society as pressures to achieve "all." Young women who aspire to their interpretation of these expectations often try to please others to avoid conflicts around perceived expectations. Feminists have focused on this role pressure as one part of an explanation for the significant increase in eating disorders and for the greater prevalence in females. Box 22-3 outlines some feminist assumptions regarding role, feminism, and the development of eating disorders.

BOX 22.3

Feminist Ideology and Eating Disorders

Since the 1970s, proponents of the feminist cultural model of eating disorders have advanced a position to explain the higher prevalence of these disorders in women. Feminists believe there is a struggle women have today similar to ones they believe women have had in history. They believe that during the Victorian era, "hysteria," a well-known emotional illness, developed as a result of oppression when women were not allowed to express their feelings and opinions and were "silenced" by a male-dominated society. Feminist scholars claim that women today are socialized to avoid self-expression in the face of conflict, seek attachment through putting others first, judge self by external standards, and present an outward compliant self while the inner self grows angry. They believe that the development of an eating disorder is a reaction against these expectations and norms of society (Gutwill, 1994).

Feminists have taken issue with what they call the biomedical model of explanation for the development of eating disorders, seeing it as limiting and patriarchal. It is the recovery of society that must take place to decrease the prevalence of eating disorders. Feminists believe that this will occur only when women are emancipated, given a voice, and socialized differently. They call for more research in which women are coresearchers as well as "subjects," helping to provide the investigators with their own stories and perspectives.

⬤ **KEY CONCEPT Sexuality fears** are often underlying issues for patients with anorexia nervosa. Starvation is viewed as a response to these fears.

In females, anorexia nervosa usually develops during adolescence, when dating begins. Female adolescents usually experience dating as more stressful than males do because intimacy is more important to females. Thus, they tend to attribute the failure of a relationship to an inadequacy in themselves (Streigel-Moore, 1993). During the past several years, females have become involved sexually at increasingly younger ages. Although they are often ill prepared, they can experience a great deal of pressure from peers to do so. Parents may be unprepared to address sexual activity with daughters at younger ages than expected. If parents are not available to help with decisions, anxiety about them can increase. Bruch (1973) has described self-starvation as the female adolescent's response to her fear of adult sexuality. Sexual anxieties may promote binge eating as well.

Social Theories

More than with any other psychiatric condition, society plays a significant role in the development of eating disorders. Theories about social norms and expectations explain some of the causes of eating disorders (Brumberg, 1988). The media, the fashion industry, and peer pressure are significant social influences. Magazines and television shows depict young girls and adolescents, with thin and often emaciated bodies, as glamorous (Tiggerman & Pickering, 1996). Wanting to be like these models both in character and appearance, female adolescents diet. Two of the most common adolescent dieting methods—restricting calories and taking diet pills—have been shown to be influenced by women's beauty and fashion magazines (Thomsen, Weber, & Brown, 2002). For young girls, dolls such as Barbie® have been found to negatively influence their views of normal body types (Brownell & Napolitano, 1995) (see Box 22-4). In addition, many types of media discuss dieting and exercise as ways to achieve success, popularity, power, and the like. Comparing one's own body to the bodies of models may produce significant body dissatisfaction, a key characteristic associated with dieting, low self-esteem, and development of an eating disorder.

> **KEY CONCEPT** In **body dissatisfaction**, the body becomes overvalued as a way of determining one's worth. Body dissatisfaction has been related to low self-esteem, depression, dieting, bingeing, and purging.

Once the body is considered all-important, the individual begins to compare her body with others, such as those of celebrities. Images from television and fashion magazines are particularly powerful for young girls and adolescents struggling with the tasks of identity and body image formation (Andrist, 2003). Body dissatisfaction resulting from this comparison, in which one's own body is perceived to fall short of an ideal, may be dissatisfaction about one's weight, shape, size, or even a certain body part. Even in the absence of overweight, most adolescents surveyed in numerous studies were dissatisfied with their bodies. Many adolescents act to overcome this dissatisfaction through dieting and overexercising. In those who have other risk factors and are thus more vulnerable, eating disorder symptoms may develop.

Family Responses

Early family theories and studies have classically labelled the family of the individual with anorexia nervosa as overprotective, enmeshed, unable to resolve conflicts, and rigid. In an enmeshed family, boundaries that define individual autonomy are weak. One member may relay communication from another to a third. Excessive togetherness may intrude on privacy (Minuchin, Rossman, & Baker, 1978).

> **KEY CONCEPT** **Enmeshment** refers to an extreme form of intensity in family interactions.

Overprotectiveness is defined as a high degree of concern for one another. The parents' overprotectiveness may retard the child's development of autonomy and competence (Minuchin et al., 1978). *Rigidity* refers to families who are heavily committed to maintain the status quo and find change difficult. Conflict is avoided, and a strong moral code or religious orientation is usually the rationale. In a recent study of 30 mother and daughter dyads, Ogden and Steward (2000) found high body dissatisfaction and dietary restraint for daughters when both mothers and daughters believed that boundaries between each other were unclear and that each should live up to the others' expectations. While this study tends to amplify the earlier understanding of the family's impact on the development of anorexia, the findings must be interpreted cautiously because no one etiologic factor is predominant in the development of anorexia nervosa. Rather, biopsychosocial factors converge to contribute to its development.

RISK FACTORS

Risk factors for developing eating disorders are well known. Similar factors put women at risk for both anorexia nervosa and bulimia nervosa. Risk factors are often classified in the same way as the etiologic categories: biologic, psychological, and social (Fig. 22-3).

Biologic

Dieting despite weight loss and an increase in basal metabolic rate (BMR) are the most significant biologic risk factors studied. Overexercising is also a risk factor. Girls begin to diet at an early age because of body dissatisfaction, a need for control, or a prepubertal weight increase, making both actual weight gain and the fear of weight gain risk factors (Taylor et al., 1998). Restricting food can lead to starvation, in the case of anorexia nervosa, or to binge eating and purging. High-level exercise and compulsive physical activity can precipitate and maintain such eating disorder symptoms as food obsessing, poor concentration, and binge eating (Davis et al., 1997).

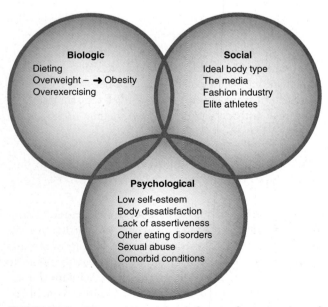

FIGURE 22.3 Biopsychosocial risk factors for anorexia and bulimia nervosa.

Psychological

Results of numerous studies have shown that low self-esteem, body dissatisfaction, and feelings of ineffectiveness also put individuals at risk for an eating disorder. Much of the recent research on these factors has demonstrated that resilience or protective factors, such as academic achievement, family connectedness, emotional well-being, and positive self-esteem, can mediate these risk factors and prevent development of an eating disorder (Croll, Neumark-Sztainer, Story, & Ireland, 2002).

Sociocultural

The media, the fashion industry, and society's focus on the ideal body type are risk factors for eating disorders. In addition, peer pressure and attitudes influence eating behaviours. Some adolescents have reported that dieting, binge eating, and purging were learned behaviours, resulting from peer pressure and a need to conform.

Athletes are at greater risk for developing eating disorders because excessive exercise and perfectionism are thought to precipitate symptoms (Davis, Katzman, & Kirsch, 1999). Pressure from coaches and parents, along with the actual physical demands of a sport, can also contribute. Elite athletes training for national and international competition are particularly at risk (Garner, Rosen, & Barry, 1998). Ballet dancers are at high risk because of the need to maintain a particular appearance (see Box 22-5).

Family

Individuals with eating disorders are more likely to perceive their families as having excessive appearance and achievement concerns and to be more critical of the family's functioning than their parents (Vandereyken, 2002). Parental attitudes about weight have been found to influence body dissatisfaction and dieting; parental comments about weight or shape, or even parents' worrying about their own weight, can influence adolescents in much the same way as the media does (Smolak, Levine, & Schermer, 1999). In investigations on attitudes, parents of daughters with eating disorders were found to have often teased these daughters about their weight, and mothers had overestimated their daughters' weight, but not their sons' (Schwartz, Phares, Tantleff-Dunn, & Thompson, 1999). Low levels of paternal affection, communication, and time spent with daughters and sons during their childhood has been associated with high rates of eating and weight problems and eating disorders during their adolescence or early adulthood (Johnson, Cohen, Kasen, & Brook, 2002). As well, middle school females who were teased about their appearance or about being heavy by older siblings demonstrated significantly higher levels of body

BOX 22.5   RESEARCH FOR BEST PRACTICE

Females and Athletics

THE QUESTION: Many investigations have highlighted that there are certain groups at risk for eating disorders, such as ballet dancers and gymnasts. Some of these investigations have found conflicting results on which groups are at risk. This is because factors such as the type of sport (eg, gymnastics), whether the athlete is an elite one, and whether the sport requires a lean look for competition, were considered in only some studies.

METHODS: Researchers conducted a comprehensive review and analysis of all of the studies on athletics, dance, and eating disorder symptoms from 1975 to 1999.

FINDINGS: Ballet dancers are one of the most at-risk groups. Contrary to previous assumptions, especially by the popular press, running, swimming, and gymnastics were not as risky as ballet dancing. Although elite versus high school athletes were more at risk than nonathletes, this was not true for elite runners, swimmers, or gymnasts.

Findings from this study are important because healthy athletic competition, which increases confidence, at the middle school and high school levels has been shown to be a protective factor in preventing risk factors such as body dissatisfaction from developing into an eating disorder. However, there is a growing body of research on the female athlete triad (amenorrhea, osteoporosis, and disordered eating), especially because of the dramatic increase in women participating in organized sports during the past 30 years. This triad is associated with an imbalance between energy intake and energy expenditure. Therefore, the benefits of athletic achievement as a protective factor must be weighed against medical morbidity.

IMPLICATIONS FOR NURSING: Assessing high-risk groups such as ballet dancers and athletes for the development of eating disorders is important in working in the community and for school health nurses. Teaching parents and adolescents about the value of healthy athletic competition as a protective factor and as a means of intervening in obesity may or may not outweigh potential risks. An accurate assessment of each young woman is important before assuming athletics are "protective."

From Smolak, L., Murnen, S. K. & Ruble, A. (2000). Female athletes and eating problems: A meta analysis. *International Journal of Eating Disorders, 27*(4), 371–380.

dissatisfaction, thin-idealization, dietary restriction, bulimic behaviours, and depression, and lower levels of self-esteem than females who were not teased (Keery, Boutelle, van den Berg & Thompson, 2005).

Concurrent Disorders

Comorbidity is related to the etiology of eating disorders. Anorexia nervosa puts women at risk for bulimia nervosa. An estimated 25% to 30% of women with anorexia nervosa go on to experience binge eating and purging (White, 2000b). This relationship has been explained as incomplete recovery that eventually turns to purging when restricting food intake is no longer effective.

Sexual Abuse

Childhood sexual abuse has been suggested as a risk factor for eating disorders. Many investigations have supported the notion that, although childhood sexual abuse has occurred in a larger percentage of women with bulimia nervosa than in the general population, this percentage may not be larger than the percentage of women with other psychiatric disorders who have experienced such abuse (Perkins & Luster, 1999). In comparing rates and parameters of abuse in women with anorexia nervosa and borderline personality disorder, Laporte and Guttman (2001) found that women with anorexia nervosa experienced less multiple abuse and at an older age than the women with personality disorder. Nonetheless, sexual or physical abuse occurred in one fifth and verbal abuse in one third of the women with anorexia nervosa studied. Therefore, inquiring about history of sexual, physical, and verbal victimization in assessing a person with an eating disorder is necessary to identify deleterious effects that can be addressed in treatment.

INTERDISCIPLINARY TREATMENT

Treatment of the patient with anorexia nervosa focuses on initiating nutritional rehabilitation, resolving conflicts around body image disturbance, increasing effective coping, addressing the underlying conflicts related to maturity fears and role conflict, and assisting the family with healthy functioning and communication. Several methods are used to accomplish these goals during the stages of illness and recovery.

When selecting the type of treatment (ie, inpatient, day hospitalization, or outpatient) for anorexia nervosa and bulimia nervosa, clinicians rely on criteria that have been developed to assist them. Typically, the medical complications presented in Table 22-2 influence the decision to hospitalize an individual with an eating disorder. Suicidality is another reason for hospitalization. The criteria for hospital admission are outlined in Table 22-3.

In most instances, an individual with anorexia nervosa must be hospitalized to restore weight. The individual may be admitted to a specialized eating disorder unit or program, or to a general psychiatric medical or pediatric unit. Because these individuals are often intelligent

Table 22.3	Criteria for Hospitalization of Patients With Eating Disorders

Medical	Psychiatric
• Weight loss, <75% below ideal • Heart rate, <40 beats/min; children <20 beats/min • Temperature, <36°C • Blood pressure, <90/60 mmHg; children, <80/50 mmHg • Glucose, <60 mg/dL • Serum potassium, <3 mEq/L • Severe dehydration • Electrolyte imbalance	• Risk for suicide • Severe depression • Failure to comply with treatment • Inadequate response to treatment at another level of care (outpatient)

Adapted from Yager, J., & Workgroup in Eating Disorders. (2000). *Practice guideline for the treatment of patients with eating disorders*, 2nd ed: American Psychiatric Association. Retrieved August 16, 2005, from http://www.psych.org.

and engaging and (with the exception of their emaciated state) appear nonimpaired, the severity of the disorder and distress may be underestimated. Particularly in a busy unit where other patients' symptoms of mental illness may be more overt, the needs of individuals with eating disorders are at risk for being secondary to those of others because they may be erroneously perceived as less sick (Wolfe & Gimby, 2003). Thus, it is important to remember the high rates of mortality and medical complications among individuals with eating disorders. If these individuals' somatic systems are seriously compromised, a medical unit might be the choice for this initial intensive refeeding phase. In most psychiatric units, all members of the team participate in a weight-gain protocol. Dietitians plan this weight-increasing program; physicians, nurses, psychologists, and social workers monitor the refeeding process and its effects on the individual and establish the intensive therapies that must be instituted after the refeeding phase.

Individuals with anorexia nervosa must be monitored closely because at the time of admission they are severely malnourished (see Table 22-2). They usually are placed on a privilege-earning program in which privileges, such as having visitors and receiving passes to go outside the hospital, are earned based on weight gain.

After an acceptable weight (at least 85% of ideal) is established, the patient may be discharged to a partial hospitalization program or an intensive outpatient program. The intensive therapies needed to help patients with their underlying issues (eg, body satisfaction and self-esteem) and to help families with communication usually begin after refeeding because concentration is usually impaired in the severely undernourished individual with anorexia. Family therapy typically begins while the individual is still hospitalized. Art therapy and psychodrama have been demonstrated to be more effective than traditional group therapy for adolescents with eating disorders, especially during the acute phases, when the concentration required for verbal therapy may be impaired (Diamond-Raab & Orrell-Valente, 2002).

PHARMACOLOGIC INTERVENTIONS

Research demonstrates that selective serotonin reuptake inhibitors (SSRIs) are not effective for individuals who are in the acute phase of this disorder or hospitalized, as initially believed (Strober, Pataki, Freeman, & DeAntonio, 1999), possibly because patients' low body weights cause low protein stores, and protein is needed for SSRI metabolism. Other experts claim that the symptoms of anorexia nervosa, such as body distortion, hyperkinesis, and apathy, are primarily the result of starvation, which causes changes in brain chemistry. Thus, restoring weight influences symptom remission more significantly than does psychopharmacology. Of course, comorbid conditions such as depression should be treated with appropriate antidepressant medication (see Chapter 19). Some clinical experts who work with these patients have found that the SSRIs can be effective later, during outpatient treatment and after weight restoration. Target symptoms such as obsessiveness, ritualistic behaviours, and perfectionism can remit with these medications. SSRIs must be used with caution, and the patient's weight must be constantly monitored because, during the initiation phase, some of the SSRIs may cause weight loss. Recently, olanzapine has been used for severe anorexia, resulting in weight gain, less resistance to treatment, and reduced agitation (Jensen & Mejlhede, 2000; LaVia, Grey, & Kaye, 2000). However, the use of this drug and others in this category needs to be explored further.

PRIORITY CARE ISSUES

Mortality is high among patients with anorexia nervosa; the crude rate has been determined to be between 5% and 7% (Crow, Praus, & Thuras, 1999). Some studies report that mortality rates for women aged 15 to 24 years with anorexia nervosa may be 12 times higher than the mortality rates from all other causes of death for age-matched community-comparison groups of women and twice as high as for other female psychiatric populations (Eckert, Halmi, Marchi, Grove, & Crosby, 1995; Sullivan, 1995). Factors that correlate with death are illness of long duration, bingeing and purging, and comorbid illnesses (Herzog et al., 2000). Substance abuse, particularly severe alcohol use, predicts mortality in patients with anorexia nervosa (Keel et al., 2003; Korndorfer et al., 2003).

Another issue to consider with this population is stigma. Many young girls are avoided, especially in their emaciated state. Peers do not know how to approach them because they may appear both frightening and fragile (Gowers & Shore, 1999). A recent university study supported this theory and found that most men would feel uncomfortable dating a woman with an eating disorder. Males in the study who had experienced dating someone with an eating disorder expressed even stronger uncomfortable feelings, stating that conflict was the predominant issue in the relationship (Sobol & Bursztyn, 1998).

NURSING MANAGEMENT: HUMAN RESPONSE TO DISORDER

Therapeutic Relationship

Establishing a therapeutic relationship with individuals with anorexia nervosa may be difficult initially because they are suspicious and mistrustful. They often express fear of adults, especially health care professionals, whom they believe want to "make them fat." By the time they are hospitalized, mistrust can almost reach a state of paranoia. Because of their low body weight and starvation, they are often impatient and irritable. A firm, accepting, and patient approach is important in working with these individuals. Providing a rationale for all interventions helps build trust, as does a consistently nonreactive approach. Power struggles over eating are common, and remaining nonreactive is a challenge. During such power struggles, the nurse should always think about his or her own feelings of frustration and need for control (see Box 22-6).

Biologic Domain

Assessment

A thorough evaluation of body systems is important because many systems can be compromised by starvation. A careful history from both the individual with anorexia nervosa and the family, including the length and duration of symptoms, such as fasting, avoiding meals, and overexercising, is necessary to assess altered nutrition. The longer the duration of these behaviours typically means more difficult and prolonged recovery periods. Nursing management involves various biopsychosocial assessment and interventions (see Nursing Care Plan 22-1).

CRNE Note

Eating disorders are serious psychiatric disorders that threaten life. Careful assessment and referral for treatment are important nursing interventions.

The individual's weight is determined using the BMI and a scale. Currently, criteria for discharge require

---

BOX 22.6

Therapeutic Dialogue: The Client With an Eating Disorder

Ineffective Approach

NURSE: You haven't eaten your lunch yet.
CLIENT: I can't. I'm already fat.
NURSE: Look at you, you're skin and bones.
CLIENT: I'll eat when I go out this afternoon on pass.
NURSE: You can't go on pass. You have to start realizing that you are sick. Because you can't take care of yourself, we are in charge.
CLIENT: You're trying to control me.
NURSE: We are trying to be responsible.
CLIENT: I won't eat!
NURSE: We have set up punishments for not eating.
CLIENT: Then I won't go out! At least I won't get fatter.

Effective Approach

NURSE: You haven't eaten your lunch.
CLIENT: I can't. I'm already fat.
NURSE: You're uncomfortable with how you see yourself and with eating?
CLIENT: I'll eat when I go out on pass.
NURSE: You and I, and the other members who are part of your treatment team, wrote your behavioural plan together, and you know you will not be able to go out because your pass is dependent on eating both breakfast and lunch. Here!
CLIENT: You're trying to control me.
NURSE: The intent of the plan is to help you learn to take control over the eating disorder. It sure does mean a lot of hard work for you. How can I help you now with this meal?
CLIENT: What if I eat half?
NURSE: No, you must eat all of it. Why don't I sit here while you eat? Eating is scary for you. We can talk about other choices you have on the unit; tonight, you can choose the movie or board games.
CLIENT: Okay, at least I have some choices.

Critical Thinking Challenge

- What effect did the first interaction have on the client's behaviour? Why?
- In the second interaction, what theories and interventions regarding eating disorders did the nurse use in her approach to the client?

NURSING CARE PLAN 22.1

Nursing Care Plan for a Patient With Anorexia Nervosa

JS is a 16-year-old female adolescent who appears much younger. She is 165 cm (5'5") and weighs 42 kilograms (92 pounds). She has been treated unsuccessfully in an outpatient clinic and now is being admitted to stabilize her weight. She does not believe that she is too thin and resents being forced to be hospitalized. Hospitalization was precipitated by being asked to leave the gymnastics team because of low body weight.

SETTING: INPATIENT PSYCHIATRIC UNIT

Baseline assessment: JS appears frail, pale, and dressed in oversized clothes. She is tearful, states that she is depressed and angry and that she has no friends. Physical examination results: bradycardiapulse = 58, hypotension (88/60), constipation, amenorrhea, dry skin patches, and cold intolerance. BMI = 15.3, Hypokalemia (K+ = 3.5); leukopenia (WBCs <5,000). Dehydration, temperature elevation, 99°F, elevated BUN, abnormal thyroid functioning, bone density of one standard deviation below mean age-adjusted scores.

Associated Psychiatric Diagnosis	Medications

Axis I: Anorexia nervosa
    Binge-eating/purging type
Axis II: None
Axis III: None
Axis IV: Social support (social withdrawal)
GAF = Current 55
    Potential 75
	Fluoxetine (Prozac), 20 mg in AM

NURSING DIAGNOSIS 1: IMBALANCED NUTRITION: LESS THAN BODY REQUIREMENTS

Defining Characteristics	Related Factors
Unable to increase food intake Weight more than 20% below ideal weight	Believes she cannot eat most foods Purges by vomiting "occasionally" Exercises 6–8 h daily Sleep pattern disturbed by exercise

Outcomes

Initial	Long-term
Maintains daily intake of 1,500 calories Eliminates exercising while in hospital Ceases purging for 1 week	Gains .5–1.5 kg (1–3 pounds) per week until weight is at least 85% of ideal weight. Develops strategies to maintain weight.

Interventions

Interventions	Rationale	Ongoing Assessment
Allow JS to verbalize feelings such as anxiety related to food and weight gain—develop a therapeutic relationship.	Through a relationship and examining her feelings, she may be more likely to cooperate with nutritional regimen.	Determine anxiety level when discussing food and weight gain.
Monitor meals and snacks, record amount eaten.	Severe anorexia is life threatening. Aggressive interventions are needed to ensure adequate intake.	Monitor intake. Assess JS's ability to complete meals on time and without supplements.
Do not substitute other foods for food on meal trays. Limit caffeine intake to 1 cup coffee (soda) daily.	People with anorexia usually "play games" with food. By prohibiting substitution, a more positive approach is encouraged. Caffeine is an appetite suppressant and has a diuretic effect.	Determine how willing JS is to follow nutritional regimen.
Monitor 1 h after meals for purging. Weigh daily in hospital gown after she has voided. Monitor vital signs daily, electrolytes.	Physical signs of impending complications include evidence of purging, decreasing body weight, hypotension, hyperthermia, and hypokalemia.	Monitor vital signs, weight, and electrolytes, especially potassium.
Provide psychoeducational intervention. Teach risks of osteopenia and role of fat-soluable vitamins.	Increase awareness.	Observe comprehension of material. Repeat teaching after refeeding if concentration initially impaired.

NURSING CARE PLAN 22.1 (Continued)

Evaluation

Outcomes	Revised Outcomes	Interventions
JS gains 2 kg (5 pounds) at the end of 1½ weeks. Has been cooperative with meal regimen.	Ceases binge–purge episodes for 1 week. Continues to increase her weight 0.5–1.5 kg/week (1–3 pounds/week).	Daily weights while on unsupervised meals. Praise her for her successes. Arrange or discharge to outpatient clinic or day hospital program.
She has begun to acknowledge the seriousness of her illness and the life-threatening aspects of severe dieting and purging.	Establish and maintain regular, adequate nutritional eating habits.	Participation in relapse-prevention classes.

NURSING DIAGNOSIS 2: DISTURBED BODY IMAGE/BODY EXPERIENCE

Defining Characteristics	Related Factors
Verbalizes that she is too fat Perceives herself as unattractive Hides body in large, baggy clothing	Inaccurate perceptions of physical appearance secondary to anorexia nervosa Believes that "one can never be too rich or too thin" Equates physical fitness and attractiveness with thinness

Outcomes

Initial	Long-term
Verbalizes feelings related to changing body shape and weight Identifies beliefs about controlling body size	Acknowledges negative consequences of too little fat on body Identifies positive aspects of her body and its ability to function

Interventions

Interventions	Rationale	Ongoing Assessment
Explore JS's beliefs and feelings about body. Maintain a nonjudgmental approach.	To help JS gain a more positive body image, an understanding of her own views is important.	Monitor for statements that identify perceptions of her body. Is her view *distorted* or *dissatisfied?*
Assist JS in identifying positive physical characteristics.	In anorexia, the body is viewed negatively. By focusing on parts of the body that are positive, such as eyes or hands, JS can begin to experience a positive image of her body.	Observe for patient's reaction to her body. Which areas are viewed positively? Observe for negative statements related to body size and self-esteem.
Clarify JS's views about an ideal body.	Many societal cues idealize an unrealistically thin female body.	Monitor for statements indicating external pressures to lose weight, experiences of teasing about body changes, or evidence of sexual abuse from others.
Provide education related to normal growth of women's bodies and role of fat in protection of body.	Providing education will help in reinforcing a broader view of the importance of a healthy body.	Assess patient's willingness to learn information

Evaluation

Outcomes	Revised Outcomes	Interventions
JS revealed that she believes that she is too fat but does have positive physical traits—eyes. She believes that those who are overweight have lost control of their lives. She knows some models who are 6' and weigh barely 45 kg (100 lb).	Accept alternative beliefs related to her own body.	Gradually, focus on other positive physical aspects of JS's body. Discuss grooming that encourages a more attractive look. Challenge her beliefs about body weights of models.
Willing to read information about normal body functioning.	Accept a new view of body functioning as a complex phenomenon.	Discuss the biologic aspect of the development of body weight. Emphasize multiple factors that determine body weight.

patients to be at least 85% of ideal weight according to height and weight tables. BMI, thought to reflect weight most accurately because exact height is used, is calculated by dividing weight in kilograms squared by height in meters. An acceptable BMI is between about 19 and 25.

Nursing Diagnoses for Biologic Domain

A primary nursing diagnosis is Imbalanced Nutrition: Less Than Body Requirements.

Interventions for Biologic Domain

Refeeding, the most important intervention during the hospital or initial stage of treatment (Fig. 22-4), is also the most challenging. The nurse will encounter resistance to weight gain and refusal to eat and must monitor and record all intake carefully as part of the weight gain protocol.

The refeeding protocol typically starts with 1,500 calories a day and is increased slowly until the individuals with anorexia nervosa is consuming about 3,500 calories a day in several meals. The usual plan for individuals with very low weights is a weight gain of between .5 and 1.0 kg (1 and 2 pounds) a week.

Weight-increasing protocols usually take the form of a behavioural plan, using positive reinforcements (ie, outings or passes) and negative reinforcements (ie, returning to bed rest) to encourage weight gain. The reinforcements are incremental and based on progress. For example, phone calls, walks arround the unit, and walks outside the hospital occur before day passes and weekend passes. When all staff members agree on a clear protocol for behaviours related to eating and weight gain, reactivity of the staff to the individual with anorexia nervosa is

greatly reduced. These protocols provide ready-made, consistent responses to food-refusal behaviours and should be carried out in a caring and supportive context. When negative reinforcements are implemented, the individual must be helped to see that these actions are not punitive. On rare occasions when the individual is unable to recognize or accept the eating disorder as harmful, nasogastric tube feedings may be necessary.

Menses history also must be explored. Most individuals with anorexia nervosa have reached menarche but have experienced amenorrhea for some months because of starvation. A return to regular menses signifies substantial body fat restoration. Sleep disturbance is also common, and these individuals are viewed as hyperkinetic. They sleep little, but usually awaken in an energized state. A structured, healthy sleep routine must be established immediately to conserve energy and calorie expenditure because of low weight. To further conserve energy, individuals are often relegated to bed rest until a certain amount of weight is regained. Exercise is generally not permitted during refeeding and only with caution after this phase. Inpatients must be closely supervised because they are often found exercising in their rooms, running in place and doing calisthenics.

Psychological Domain

Assessment

The psychological symptoms that individuals with anorexia experience are listed in Box 22-1. The classic symptoms—fear of weight gain, unrealistic expectations and thinking, and ritualistic behaviours—are easily noted during a clinical interview. Often, people with anorexia nervosa avoid conflict and have difficulty expressing negative emotions, such as anger. Other conflicts, such as sexuality fears and feelings of ineffectiveness, may underlie this disorder. These symptoms may not be apparent during a clinical interview; however, a variety of instruments are available to clinicians and researchers for determining the presence and severity of symptoms. Box 22-7 lists well-known instruments used to assess psychological symptoms associated with eating disorders. The Eating Attitude Test is frequently used in community and clinical samples (Box 22-8). There is an abbreviated 26-item version of this test, EAT26, and also a child version, the CHEAT. The results of these paper-and-pencil tests can help identify the most significant symptoms for an individual and indicate a focus for interventions, especially therapy.

Nursing Diagnosis for Psychological Domain

Two common nursing diagnoses in anorexia nervosa are Anxiety and Disturbed Body Image.

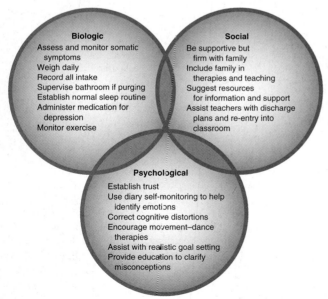

FIGURE 22.4 Biopsychosocial interventions for individuals with anorexia nervosa.

BOX 22.7

Assessment Instruments

1. Tests for Disordered Eating (Symptoms)

Compulsive Eating Scale
Dunn, P. K., & Ondercin, P. (1981). Personality variables related to compulsive eating in college women. *Journal of Clinical Psychology, 31,* 43–49

Eating Attitude Tests
Garner, D. M., & Garfinkel, P. E. (1979). The Eating Attitude Test: An index of the symptoms of anorexia nervosa. *Psychological Medicine, 9,* 273–279

Garner, D. M., Olmsted, M. P., Bohr, Y., & Garfinkel, P. E. (1982). The Eating Attitude Test: Psychometric features and clinical correlates. *Psychological Medicine, 12,* 871–878

Children's Eating Attitude Test (CHEAT)
Maloney, M., McGuire, J., & Daniels, S. R. (1988). Reliability testing of a children's version of the Eating Attitude Test. *Journal of the American Academy of Child and Adolescent Psychiatry, 27,* 541–543

Eating Disorder Examination-Questionnaire (EDE-Q)
Carolyn Black, Rutgers University Eating Disorders Clinic, 41C Gordon Road, Piscataway, NJ 08854

Eating Disorder Inventory-2 (EDI-2) and EDI-2 Symptom Checklist (EDI-2-SC)
Garner, D. M. (1991). *Eating disorder inventory—2 professional manual.* Odessa, FL: Psychological Assessment Resources

Garner, D. M. (1991). *Eating disorder inventory—C.* Lutz, FL: Psychological Assessment Resources

Eating Habits Questionnaire (Restraint Scale)
Herman, C. P., & Mack, D. (1975). Restrained and unrestrained eating. *Journal of Personality, 43,* 647–660

Yale-Brown-Cornell Eating Disorder Scale (YBC-EDS)
Mazure, C. M., Halmi, K. A., Sunday, S. R., Romano, S. J., & Einhorn, A. M. (1994). Yale-Brown-Cornell Eating Disorder Scale: Development, use, reliability, and validity. *Journal of Psychiatric Research, 28,* 425–445

2. Tests of Body Dissatisfaction/Body Image

Body Shape Questionnaire (BSQ)
Cooper, P., Taylor, M., Cooper, Z., & Fairburn, C. (1987). The development and validation of the BSQ. *International Journal of Eating Disorders, 6,* 485–494

Color-a-Person Test
Wooley, S. C., & Kearney-Cooke, A. (1986). Intensive treatment of bulimia and body image disturbance. In K. D. Brownell & J. P. Foreyt (Eds.), *Handbook of eating disorders: Physiology, psychology and treatment of obesity, anorexia, and bulimia* (pp. 476–502). New York: Basic Books

3. Tests of Emotional and Cognitive Components

Cognitive Behavioral Dieting Scale
Martz, D. M., Sturgis, E. T., & Gustafson, S. B. (1996) Development and preliminary validation of the Cognitive Behavioral Dieting Scale. *International Journal of Eating Disorders, 19,* 297–309

Emotional Eating Scale
Arrow, B., Kenardy, J., & Agras, W. S. (1995). The emotional eating scale: The development of a measure to assess coping with negative affect by eating. *Internationl Journal of Eating Disorders, 18,* 79–90

4. Risk Factors Identification

The McKnight Risk Factor Survey
Shisslak, C. M., Renger, R., Sharpe, T., et al. (1999). Development and evaluation of the McKnight Risk Factor Survey for assessing potential risk and protective factors for disordered eating in preadolescent and adolescent girls. *International Journal of Eating Disorders, 25,* 195–214 (Versions available for younger and older children)

Interventions for Psychological Domain

For interoceptive awareness problems (inability to experience visceral cues and emotions), the nurse can encourage individuals with anorexia nervosa to keep a journal. Most of these individuals use a somatic complaint such as "I feel bloated" or "I'm fat" to replace a negative emotion such as guilt or anger. Although refeeding following a state of starvation may cause bloating in some cases, bloating often is perceived and part of body dissatisfaction. Help individuals to identify these feelings by having them write a description of the "fat feeling" and list possible underlying emotions and troublesome situations next to this description.

Understanding Feelings

Identifying feelings, such as anxiety and fear, and especially negative emotions, such as anger, is the first step in helping individuals to decrease conflict avoidance and develop effective strategies for coping with these feelings.

Do not attempt to change distorted body image by merely pointing out that the individual is actually too thin. This symptom is often the last to resolve itself, and some individuals may take years to see their bodies realistically. However, although this symptom is difficult to abate, individuals can continue to fear becoming fat but not be driven to act on the distortion by starving. The fear of becoming fat eventually lessens with time.

The nurse can help individuals with eating disorders to restructure the way they view the world, especially relative to food, eating, weight, and shape. Faulty ways of viewing these situations result in ineffective coping. Table 22-4 lists some cognitive distortions commonly experienced by individuals with eating disorders and some typical restructuring responses or statements that challenge the distortion, which the nurse can present as more realistic ways of perceiving situations. Other therapies, such as movement and dance therapy, can help the individual experience pleasure from his or her body, although dance should be used cautiously during refeeding because of energy-expenditure concerns. Imagery

BOX 22.8

Eating Attitude Test

Please place an (x) under the column that applies best to each of the numbered statements. All the results will be strictly confidential. Most of the questions relate to food or eating, although other types of questions have been included. Please answer each question carefully. Thank you.

	Always	Very Often	Often	Sometimes	Rarely	Never
1. Like eating with other people	—	—	—	—	—	×
2. Prepare foods for others but do not eat what I cook	×	—	—	—	—	—
3. Become anxious before eating	×	—	—	—	—	—
4. Am terrified about being overweight	×	—	—	—	—	—
5. Avoid eating when I am hungry	×	—	—	—	—	—
6. Find myself preoccupied with food	×	—	—	—	—	—
7. Have gone on eating binges in which I feel that I may not be able to stop	×	—	—	—	—	—
8. Cut my food into small pieces	×	—	—	—	—	—
9. Am aware of the calorie content of foods that I eat	×	—	—	—	—	—
10. Particularly avoid foods with a high carbohydrate content (eg, bread, potatoes, rice)	×	—	—	—	—	—
11. Feel bloated after meals	×	—	—	—	—	—
12. Feel that others would prefer I ate more	×	—	—	—	—	—
13. Vomit after I have eaten	×	—	—	—	—	—
14. Feel extremely guilty after eating	×	—	—	—	—	—
15. Am preoccupied with a desire to be thinner	×	—	—	—	—	—
16. Exercise strenuously to burn off calories	×	—	—	—	—	—
17. Weigh myself several times a day	×	—	—	—	—	—
18. Like my clothes to fit tightly	—	—	—	—	—	×
19. Enjoy eating meat	—	—	—	—	—	×
20. Wake up early in the morning	×	—	—	—	—	—
21. Eat the same foods day after day	×	—	—	—	—	—
22. Think about burning up calories when I exercise	×	—	—	—	—	—
23. Have regular menstrual periods	—	—	—	—	—	×
24. Am aware that other people think I am too thin	×	—	—	—	—	—
25. Am preoccupied with the thought of having fat on my body	×	—	—	—	—	—
26. Take longer than others to eat	×	—	—	—	—	—
27. Enjoy eating at restaurants	—	—	—	—	—	×
28. Take laxatives	×	—	—	—	—	—
29. Avoid foods with sugar in them	×	—	—	—	—	—
30. Eat diet foods	×	—	—	—	—	—
31. Feel that food controls my life	×	—	—	—	—	—
32. Display self-control around food	×	—	—	—	—	—
33. Feel that others pressure me to eat	×	—	—	—	—	—
34. Give too much time and thought to food	×	—	—	—	—	—
35. Suffer from constipation	—	×	—	—	—	—
36. Feel uncomfortable after eating sweets	×	—	—	—	—	—
37. Engage in dieting behaviour	×	—	—	—	—	—
38. Like my stomach to be empty	×	—	—	—	—	—
39. Enjoy trying new rich foods	—	—	—	—	—	×
40. Have the impulse to vomit after meals	×	—	—	—	—	—

Scoring: The patient is given the questionnaire without the X's, just blank. 3 points are assigned to endorsements that coincide with the X's; the adjacent alternatives are weighted as 2 points and 1 point, respectively. A total score of more than 30 indicates significant concerns with eating behaviour.
From Garner, D., & Garfinkel, P. (1979). The Eating Attitude Test: An index of the symptoms of anorexia nervosa. *Psychological Medicine, 9,* 273–279.

Table 22.4	Cognitive Distortions Typical of Patients With Eating Disorders, With Restructuring Statements	
Distortion	**Clarification or Restructuring**
Dichotomous or all-or-nothing thinking "I've gained 1 kilo (2 pounds), so I'll be up by 50 kilos (100 pounds) soon."	"You have never gained 50 kilos (100 pounds), but I understand that gaining 1 kilo (2 pounds) is scary."
Magnification "I binged last night, so I can't go out with anyone."	"Feeling bad and guilty about a binge are difficult feelings, but you are in treatment and you have been monitoring and changing your eating."
Selective abstraction "I can only be happy 5 kilos (10 pounds) lighter."	"When you were 5 kilos (10 pounds) lighter, you were hospitalized. You can choose to be happy about many things in your life."
Overgeneralization "I didn't eat anything yesterday and did okay, so I don't think *not* eating for a week or two will harm me."	"Any starvation harms the body, whether or not outward signs were apparent to you. The more you starve, the more problems your body will encounter."
Catastrophizing "I purged last night for the first time in 4 months—I'll never recover."	"Recovery includes ups and downs, and it is expected you will still have some mild but infrequent symptoms."

and relaxation are often used to overcome distortions and to decrease anxiety.

While in the hospital, individuals usually are evaluated for discharge to day hospitalization or to intensive outpatient therapy, depending on the resources available, the extent of family support, and comorbidity. In both instances, the individual and family will participate in a combination of individual and family therapy.

Interpersonal Therapy

Interpersonal therapy (IPT) is a type of treatment that focuses on uncovering and resolving the developmental and psychological issues underlying the disorder. Role transitions, control, and ineffective feelings typically are the focus (McIntosh et al., 2000). Cognitive therapy may also be incorporated to continue to address and change distortions about food and interactions with others.

Family therapy is usually initiated in the hospital and continued more intensively after discharge. The section on Etiology: Family discusses some of the family concerns, which are the focus of the therapy.

Patient Education

When weight is restored and concentration is improved, individuals with anorexia nervosa can maximally benefit from psychoeducation. Although these individuals have a wealth of knowledge about food and calories, they also have misinformation that needs clarifying. For example, they are often unclear about the role of "fats" in a healthy diet and try to be as "fat free" as possible. A thorough assessment of their knowledge is important because they seem to be "walking calorie books" with little information on the role of all of the nutrients and the importance of including them in a healthy diet.

CRNE Note

Setting realistic eating goals is one of the most helpful interventions for individuals with eating disorders. Because those with anorexia nervosa are often perfectionistic, they often set unrealistic goals.

Teaching Points

One of the most helpful skills the nurse can teach is to set realistic goals around food and also around other activities or tasks. Because of perfectionism, individuals with anorexia often set unrealistic goals and end up frustrated. The nurse can help them consider essential topic areas pertinent to their recovery (see Box 22-9) and teach them to establish smaller, more realistic, attainable goals.

BOX 22.9

Psychoeducation Checklist: Anorexia Nervosa

When caring for the patient with anorexia nervosa, be sure to include the following topic areas in the teaching plan:
- ☐ Psychopharmacologic agents, if used, including drug, action, dosage, frequency, and possible adverse effects
- ☐ Nutrition and eating patterns
- ☐ Effect of restrictive eating or dieting
- ☐ Weight monitoring
- ☐ Safety and comfort measures
- ☐ Avoidance of triggers
- ☐ Self-monitoring techniques
- ☐ Trust
- ☐ Realistic goal setting
- ☐ Resources

Families and friends are eager to help the individual with anorexia but often need direction. Box 22-10 provides a list of strategies and suggested readings that may assist them.

Social Domain

Nursing Diagnosis for Social Domain

Ineffective Coping is a predominant nursing diagnosis with regard to the social domain.

Interventions for Social Domain

Younger individuals with anorexia nervosa may have lost some school time because of hospitalization. Integrating back into a school and classroom setting is difficult for most. Shame and guilt about having an eating disorder and being hospitalized must be addressed. Because these patients typically have isolated themselves before hospitalization and treatment, renewing friendships and relationships with peers may provoke anxiety. Involving school nurses and teachers in the re-entry process may help.

Denial, guilt, and fear are common reactions of the family (Sharkey-Orgnero, 1999). Family therapy is important if the individual still lives at home. Skilled therapists are able to help family members with their feelings, increase effective communication, decrease protectiveness, and resolve guilt. Often, siblings become resentful of the individual with an eating disorder because of the significant amount of attention they get from the parents. Having siblings attend family sessions to discuss these feelings and the effect the illness has had on them is helpful.

EVALUATION AND TREATMENT OUTCOMES

Several factors influence the outcome of treatment for anorexia nervosa. Particularly, long duration of symptoms and low weight when treatment begins predict poor outcomes, whereas family support and involvement generally improve outcomes. Comorbid conditions and their severity will also influence recovery. Although individuals are discharged from the hospital when their weight has reached 85% of what is considered ideal, restoration of healthy eating and changes in maladaptive thinking may not have yet occurred. Recovery from anorexia nervosa is a complex process of self-development that occurs across phases (see Box 22-11). Individuals who are in the process of recovering from anorexia nervosa may continue to restrict foods and to have cognitive distortions in the beginning phases of recovery. Therefore, without intensive outpatient treatment, including nutritional counselling and support, they are unlikely to recover fully. Distorted thinking and eating patterns can set the stage for a relapse and later for the possible development of bulimia nervosa. Many of the instruments used to assess eating disorder symptoms (see Box 22-7) can be used throughout the individual's treatment to evaluate attitudes and thinking processes that continue to prevent full recovery. Nurses are ideally positioned within hospital and community health treatment settings to help individuals with anorexia nervosa to facilitate their recovery.

CONTINUUM OF CARE

Hospitalization

Hospitalization is required based on criteria noted in Table 22-3. Anorexia nervosa in its acute stage is unlikely to be manageable in outpatient settings.

Emergency Care

Death may result from cardiac problems associated with starvation and suicide. However, emergency care is not usually needed for individuals with anorexia nervosa. Family members and peers usually notice the weight loss and emaciation before the individual's systems are compromised to the degree that they require emergency treatment. If systems are compromised enough to warrant emergency treatment, or the individual is suicidal, she or he usually is admitted immediately for inpatient care.

Family Assessment and Intervention

The family of the person with anorexia will need extensive treatment and follow-up. The therapist, psychologist,

BOX 22.11

Research for Best Practice Recovering from Anorexia Nervosa

BACKGROUND: Anorexia nervosa (AN) erodes the health of individual women, families, and communities. We lack theoretical understanding of women's subjective experiences of recovery within social context.

QUESTION: How do women recover from AN within the same sociopolitical environment in which the eating disorders developed in the first place?

METHOD: Using grounded theory through a feminist lens, the perceptions of 12 Canadian women who considered themselves recovered or recovering from AN were explored. Analysis of data from in-depth individual interviews with the women generated a conceptualization of recovering that was confirmed by the women.

FINDINGS: Recovering from AN is a journey of self-development from the *perilous self-soothing* of devastating weight loss to the *informed self-care* of healthy eating and problem-solving practices.

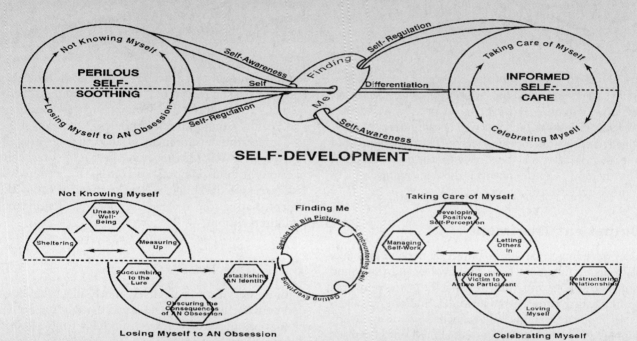

Women recover by creating learning paths of increased *self-awareness* (acknowledging own feelings and perspectives), *self-differentiation* (maintaining sense of self while in relationships with others), and *self-regulation* (managing uncomfortable affective states). They overcome the predicament of *not knowing myself* (being controlled, suffering uneasy well-being, and relentlessly comparing selves to others) and *losing myself to the AN obsession* (succumbing to the lure of AN, establishing anorectic identities, and hiding the eating disorder from others). At a cutting point called *finding me,* women begin to see the eating disorder as problematic, to identify their unique identity, and to accept responsibility for recovering. They learn to take care of themselves by resolving eating and noneating (eg, working through grief, anger) issues, developing a positive sense of self, and acquiring support from others. They fully recover by celebrating myself: overcoming the initial vulnerabilities that fostered the development of the eating disorder, restructuring relationships to invest in relationships that meet their needs and detach from those that do not, and adopting a compassionate approach of acceptance toward self and the world.

IMPLICATIONS FOR NURSING: Women may be reluctant to relinquish AN because it serves as comfort and the means for negotiating difficult developmental and situational transitions. Nurses can help women recognize their actions of perilous self-soothing as information depicting their experiences of health. Subsequent interventions can be designed to help women get in touch with their inner experiences, evaluate their role in relationships, and learn to manage stress and painful affective responses.

From Weaver, K. D., Wuest, J., & Ciliska, D. (2005). Understanding women's journey of recovering from anorexia nervosa. *Qualitative Health Research, 15*(2), 188–206.

advanced practice nurse, or social worker meets regularly, at least once a week, with the individual and the family. This method has been demonstrated to be more effective than family therapy without the individual or individual therapy alone (Robin et al., 1999). The family therapy focuses on such issues as separation-individuation, auton-

omy, ineffective communication, and practical issues, such as how parents can help their daughters or sons to effectively monitor food intake. Many family theorists believe that eating disorders develop because of family dysfunction and therefore have some unrealized meaning for each family. For example, the individual may be

Table 22.5	Prevention Strategies for Parents and Children

Parents	Children
Education	**Education**
Real vs. ideal weight	Peer pressure regarding eating, weight
Influence of attitudes, behaviours, teasing	Menses, puberty, normal weight gain
Ways to increase self-esteem	Strategies for obesity
Role of media: TV, magazines	Ways to develop or improve self-esteem
Signs and symptoms	Body image traps: media, retail clothing
Interventions for obesity	Adapting and coping with problems
Boys at risk also	Reporting friends with signs of eating disorders
Observe for rituals	**Screening** for risk factors
Supervision of eating and exercise	**Assessment** for treatment
	Follow-up: monitor for relapse

attempting to keep a splitting, divorcing, or estranged family together with the eating disorder. In other instances, parents may be trying to prevent a daughter from separating and individuating because they are emotionally unprepared for this process. The development of an eating disorder may be a reaction to these situations. The therapy helps to uncover these meanings and to improve effective parenting.

Outpatient Treatment

After refeeding, treatment of anorexia nervosa may take place on an outpatient basis and involves individual and family therapy, nutrition counselling to reinforce healthy eating patterns and attitudes, and physician visits to monitor weight and evaluate somatic recovery. Support groups, often suggested, should not be substituted for therapy. In fact, some self-directed support groups that lack professional leadership can actually delay or prevent needed professional treatment. The role of support groups to maintain recovery requires further study.

PREVENTION

Eating disorders are among the most preventable mental disorders. Instruments such as the McKnight Risk Factor Survey (Shisslak et al., 1999), which measure the presence and degree of risk factors, can be used to plan prevention or treatment (see Box 22-7). National eating disorder awareness and advocacy groups work toward educating the general public, those at risk, and those who work with groups at risk, such as teachers and coaches. They also monitor the media and work to remove unhealthy advertisements and articles that appear in magazines appealing to vulnerable individuals. A list of on-line resources and some programs and their purposes is found in the Web Links section at the end of this chapter.

Prevention and early detection strategies for parents and schoolteachers are often the focus of school nurses and mental health nurses who work in the community. Some of these strategies appear in Table 22-5 and are based on research of risk factors and protective factors. These protective factors, such as confidence and healthy competition in athletics, have been shown to prevent the development of an eating disorder for individuals at risk (Taylor et al., 1998). Dieting, being overweight, and body dissatisfaction are examples of risk factors underlying the development of eating disorders that can be reversed with early identification and intervention.

Bulimia Nervosa

Bulimia nervosa is a relatively newly identified disorder; until about 25 years ago, it was thought to be a type of anorexia nervosa. However, findings from extensive investigations have identified its characteristics as a separate entity. It is more prevalent than anorexia nervosa. Individuals with bulimia nervosa are usually older at onset than are those with anorexia nervosa. The disorder generally is not as life threatening as anorexia nervosa. The usual treatment is outpatient therapy. Outcomes are better for bulimia nervosa than for anorexia nervosa, and mortality rates are lower.

CLINICAL COURSE

There are few outward signs associated with bulimia nervosa. Individuals binge and purge in secret and are typically of normal weight; therefore, it does not come to the attention of parents and peers as readily as does anorexia nervosa. Treatment consequently can be delayed for years as individuals attempt on their own to get their eating under control. These individuals usually initiate their own treatment when control of their eating becomes impossible. Once treatment is undertaken and completed, they typically recover completely, except in cases in which personality disorders and comorbid serious depression are also present.

Individuals with bulimia nervosa may present as overwhelmed and overly committed individuals who

Table 22.6   Key Diagnostic Characteristics for Bulimia Nervosa

Diagnostic Criteria	Target Symptoms and Associated Findings
<ul><li>Recurrent episodes of binge eating</li><li>Characterized by both of the following: eating in a discrete period of time an amount larger than most people would eat during a similar period of time and under similar circumstances; sense of lack of control over eating during the episode</li><li>Recurrent inappropriate compensatory behaviour to; prevent weight gain, such as self-induced vomiting, misuse of laxatives, diuretics, enemas, or other medications; fasting; or excessive exercise</li><li>Binge eating and inappropriate compensatory behaviours occurring on average at least twice a week for 3 months</li><li>Self-evaluation unduly influenced by body shape and weight</li><li>Not occurring exclusively during episodes of anorexia nervosa</li><li>*Purging type:* regular engagement in self-induced vomiting or misuse of diuretics, laxatives, or enemas</li><li>*Nonpurging type:* use of other inappropriate compensatory behaviours, such as fasting or excessive exercise without regular engagement in self-induced vomiting, or misuse of laxatives, diuretics, or enemas</li></ul>	<ul><li>Usually within normal weight range, possible overweight or underweight</li><li>Restriction of total calorie consumption between binges, selecting low-calorie foods while avoiding foods perceived to be fattening or likely to trigger a binge</li><li>Increased frequency of depressive symptoms and anxiety symptoms</li><li>Possible substance abuse or dependence involving alcohol or stimulants</li></ul>*Associated Physical Examination Findings*<ul><li>Loss of dental enamel</li><li>Chipped, ragged, or moth-eaten teeth appearance</li><li>Increased incidence of dental caries</li><li>Scars on dorsum of hand from manually inducing vomiting</li><li>Cardiac and skeletal myopathies from use of syrup of ipecac for vomiting</li><li>Menstrual irregularities</li><li>Dependence on laxatives</li><li>Esophageal tears</li></ul>*Associate Laboratory Findings*<ul><li>Fluid and electrolyte abnormalities</li><li>Metabolic alkalosis (from vomiting) or metabolic acidosis (from diarrhea)</li><li>Mildly elevated serum amylase levels</li></ul>

have difficulty with setting limits and establishing appropriate boundaries. They have an enormous number of rules regarding food and food restriction, and they feel shame, guilt, and disgust about their binge eating and purging. They may also be impulsive in other areas of their lives, such as spending.

DIAGNOSTIC CRITERIA

The key characteristics for the diagnosis of bulimia nervosa appear in Table 22-6 (also see Box 22-1). There are two types of bulimia nervosa: purging type and restricting type. Individuals with the restricting type are similar to those with anorexia nervosa. However, in bulimia, restricting is followed by binge eating, which is then followed by another period of restricting. In the purging type, binge eating is followed by purging. The difference between purging in the individual with anorexia and purging in the individual with bulimia is the severe weight loss and amenorrhea that accompanies anorexia nervosa. Bulimia nervosa involves engaging in recurrent episodes of binge eating and compensatory purging in the form of vomiting or using laxatives, diuretics, or emetics, or in nonpurging compensatory behaviours, such as fasting or overexercising in order to avoid weight gain. These episodes must occur at least twice a week for a period of at least 3 months in order to meet

the *DSM-IV-TR* criteria (APA, 2000). People with this disorder may binge and purge as many as several times a day.

Binge eating is defined as rapid, episodic, impulsive, and uncontrollable ingestion of a large amount of food during a short period of time, usually 1 to 2 hours. Eating is followed by feelings of guilt, remorse, and often self-contempt, leading to purging. To assuage the out-of-control feeling, severe dieting is instituted, and these restrictions, referred to as *dietary restraint*, precipitate the next binge. The restrictions are viewed as "rules," such as no sweets, no fats, and so forth. Each binge seems to influence stricter and stricter rules about what cannot be consumed, leading to more frequent binge eating. This cycle has prompted clinicians to focus treatment on interventions related to dietary restraint, or purging behaviours. When dietary restraint is resolved, or purging is prevented, binge eating is decreased.

> ⬟ **KEY CONCEPT Dietary restraint** has been described by researchers in the field of eating disorders as a way to explain the relationship between dieting and binge eating (Polivy & Herman, 1993).

Dieters' deprivation, or restraint, whether real or imagined, contributes to overeating and bingeing. Deprivation may operate in a straightforward fashion by instigating a drive toward repletion. Another possibility is that deprivation alters one's perceptual reactivation to attractive food cues, making them more irresistible. Attempted deprivation may make dieters more prone to feel distress over their dietary "failures," especially if dieting has become a way to overcome body dissatisfaction and to compensate for distress through binge eating. Whether the eating is influenced by the attraction of forbidden foods or by internal needs to assuage failure, there is significant evidence that restraining one's intake is a precondition for bouts of overeating.

A number of studies have uncovered a group of individuals who binge in the same way as those with bulimia nervosa but who do not purge or compensate for binges through other behaviours. This disorder is now classified in a temporary way in the *DSM-IV-TR* as binge eating disorder (BED). These individuals also differ in that most of them are also obese. Box 22-12 describes BED and the current understanding about this disorder. Because this is a newly recognized disorder, until additional research clarifies its symptoms, etiology, and treatment, it is now described in the Appendix of the *DSM-IV-TR* (APA, 2000). Clinicians classify BED as an "eating disorder not otherwise specified" until it has been researched further for inclusion as a separate diagnosis in the *DSM-IV-TR*. Its etiology is believed to be similar to that of bulimia nervosa. Yet understanding and treating of binge eating disorder are still in the

---

BOX 22.12

Binge Eating Disorder

Binge eating disorder (BED), although still in the research stage to refine its characteristics for inclusion in the *DSM-IV-TR* (APA, 2000) as a separate entity, is estimated to affect 3% to 4% of the population. The criteria for BED consist of binge eating, which includes both the ingestion of a large amount of food in a short period of time and a sense of loss of control during the binge; distress regarding the binge; eating until uncomfortably full; and feelings of guilt or depression following the binge. Purging does not occur with BED, and this differentiates it from bulimia nervosa. In addition, investigators have shown that individuals with BED have lower dietary restraint and are higher in weight, even though many are not obese, than those with bulimia nervosa. It has been estimated that 10% to 30% of obese individuals have BED. Some women with bulimia nervosa have reported that they binged without purging for several years before developing bulimia nervosa at as young as age 10 years (Bulik et al., 1998).

Cognitive behaviour therapy has not been as effective for BED as it is for bulimia nervosa. Investigations have shown that sertraline has been effective in reducing binges. Topiramate, used for epilepsy, has been studied for use for BED and was found to decrease binge eating and appetite. Some weight loss was also a result of treatment with this medication. More studies are needed to confirm its effectiveness (Shapira, Goldsmith, & McElroy, 2000).

---

investigative stages, and at this point most experts use interventions similar to those used for bulimia nervosa.

BULIMIA NERVOSA IN SPECIAL POPULATIONS

Bulimia nervosa occurs in all age groups. It is not as common in children as in adolescents and adults; children appear more likely to have binge eating disorder (BED) (APA, 2000). This finding has only recently been reported, and more data are needed to substantiate this theory.

EPIDEMIOLOGY

Lifetime prevalence of bulimia nervosa is reported to be 3% to 8%, depending on whether clinical or community populations are sampled. Stricter criteria are used when clinical groups are studied, making the prevalence rate lower. An Ontario study found that 0.13% of men and 1.46% of women had full-syndrome bulimia nervosa, with an additional 0.95% of men and 1.70% of women having partial-syndrome (Woodside et al., 2001). The occurrence is more common than that of anorexia nervosa (APA, 2000).

Age of Onset

Typically, the age of onset is between 18 and 24 years. The incidence of bulimia nervosa is increasing among women between 25 and 45 years but has been relatively stable in the typical age group (Pawluck & Gorey, 1998).

Gender Differences

A ratio of 3 to 5 females to 1 male experiences bulimia nervosa (Health Canada, 2003; Woodside et al., 2001). Box 22-2 highlights differences in males with eating disorders.

Ethnic and Cultural Differences

Bulimia nervosa is related to culture in the same way as anorexia nervosa. In Western cultures and those becoming westernized in their norms, the focus on achieving a thin body ideal underlies the dieting and dietary restraint that sets up the trajectory toward a diagnosable eating disorder. Hispanic and white women have higher rates than do Asian and African American women.

Familial Differences

There is some support for a familial link for bulimia nervosa. First-degree relatives of women with bulimia nervosa are more likely than control subjects and women with other psychiatric disorders to have bulimia nervosa, and when subclinical symptoms are considered, the prevalence in first-degree relatives is even higher (Lilenfeld et al., 1998).

Comorbidity

The most common comorbid conditions are substance abuse and dependence, depression, and OCD. In one study, women continued having OCD after remission of their bulimic symptoms, underlining the notion that some comorbid conditions may occur before the eating disorder, are trait-related features, and may actually have a role in precipitating the disorder (von Ranson, Kaye, Weltzin, Rao, & Matsunaga, 1999).

Cluster B, Axis II disorders, such as borderline personality disorder, are also found frequently in these individuals (Matsunaga et al., 2000), and many women with bulimia nervosa have had anorexia nervosa previously.

ETIOLOGY

Some of the predisposing or risk factors for anorexia nervosa and bulimia nervosa overlap with theories of causality (see Fig. 22-3). For example, dieting puts an individual at risk for the development of bulimia nervosa. The dieting can turn into dietary restraint, a symptom that leads to binge eating and purging. However, not all individuals who diet experience bulimia nervosa. The interplay of other risk factors (eg, body dissatisfaction and separation-individuation issues) most likely explains the development of this disorder.

Biologic Theories

Some progress has been made in understanding the biologic causes of bulimia nervosa. Dieting, one of the most important causative factors, occurs in the United States in girls as young as 8 years of age. Canadian children in grades three and four say they'd rather lose a parent, get cancer, or live through nuclear war than be fat (National Eating Disorder Information Centre, 1998). Dieting is believed to affect serotonergic regulation. As in anorexia nervosa, overexercising has also contributed to some of the symptoms of bulimia nervosa, especially in individuals with the restricting type of this disorder.

Neuropathologic

The changes noted in the brain by MRI are the result of eating dysregulation, rather than the cause. As with anorexia nervosa, these changes disappear when symptoms such as dietary restraint, binge eating, and purging remit.

Genetic

A specific gene responsible for bulimia nervosa has not been identified. Recently, twin studies have been reviewed to determine the role genetics might play in the development of bulimia nervosa. Whereas it has been widely recognized that environment also plays a role, in several twin studies, genetic influences outweighed environmental ones (Bulik et al., 2000). Findings continue to be treated with caution because sorting out environmental and genetic influences is difficult when twins live in the same environment.

Biochemical

The most frequently studied biochemical theory in bulimia nervosa relates to lowered brain serotonin neurotransmission. People with bulimia nervosa are believed to have altered modulation of central serotonin neuronal systems (Kaye, Gendall, et al., 2000).

Studies have typically looked to tryptophan, an amino acid and serotonin precursor, to explain this mechanism. Findings from several studies have demonstrated that women with bulimia nervosa experience symptoms of depressed mood, a desire to binge, and an increase in weight and shape concerns when tryptophan is depleted through dieting (Smith, Fairburn, & Cowen, 1999). To further advance these findings, in another study, women who had recovered from bulimia nervosa (ie, symptoms had remitted) were examined after ingestion of a formula to deplete tryptophan. They returned to symptoms of a desire to binge, preoccupation with shape, and depressed mood (Wolfe et al., 2000). Chronic depletion of plasma tryptophan is thought to be one of the major mechanisms whereby persistent dieting can lead to the development of eating disorders in vulnerable individuals.

Psychological and Social Theories

Psychological factors in the etiology of bulimia nervosa have been studied extensively, and most experts believe that these factors converge with environmental or sociocultural factors within individuals with a biologic predisposition, causing symptoms to develop. As with anorexia nervosa, psychoanalytic developmental theories that explain separation-individuation are important in causality. Because the age of onset for bulimia nervosa is late adolescence, going away to college, for example, may represent the first physical separation for some adolescents, who are unprepared for the emotional separation. In addition, an inability to set limits and develop healthy boundaries leads to a sense of being overwhelmed and "drained." In most instances, women with bulimia nervosa are not assertive and have difficulty saying no, fearing that they will not be liked. Overwhelming feelings often lead to binge eating, either to avoid or to distract oneself from feelings such as resentment, or binge eating can serve to assuage emptiness, or to fill up a "drained" self with food.

Cognitive Theory

Many experts view cognitive theory as influential in eating disorder symptoms. It explains the distorted thinking present in people with bulimia nervosa. This explanation is similar for depression, in which a particular thought pattern is learned (see Chapter 14 for an explanation of cognitive theory). Many experts view bulimia nervosa as a disorder of thinking, in that distortions are the basis of behaviours such as binge eating and purging. Psychological triggering mechanism models explain that cues such as stress, negative emotions, and even environmental cues (eg, the presence of attractive food) play a role in etiology. However, today these cognitive and triggering theories are viewed as an explanation for maintaining the binge eating once it has been established, rather than an explanation of causality.

The same sociocultural factors that underlie anorexia nervosa play a significant role in the development of bulimia nervosa.

Family

The families of individuals who experience bulimia nervosa have been primarily studied from the "outsider" perspectives of researchers and clinicians, and are reported to be chaotic, with few rules and unclear boundaries.

The families' "insider" perspectives have received little attention from researchers. Thus, as with anorexia nervosa, theories of causation do not individually explain the development of bulimia nervosa. Rather, the convergence of many of these factors at a vulnerable stage of individual development helps explain causality.

RISK FACTORS

The risk or predisposing factors for bulimia nervosa are similar to those for anorexia nervosa (see Fig. 22-3). Society's influences, such as the media and peer pressure, underlie the desire to achieve an ideal thin body type. Comparing oneself to these ideal body types leads to body dissatisfaction. These factors influence behaviours such as dietary restraint and overexercising. Dietary restraint leads to binge eating, and purging ensues because of a fear of becoming fat.

INTERDISCIPLINARY TREATMENT

Individuals with bulimia nervosa benefit from a comprehensive multifaceted treatment approach. The goals for treatment for individuals with bulimia nervosa focus on stabilizing and then normalizing eating, which means stopping the binge–purge cycles; restructuring dysfunctional thought patterns and attitudes, especially about eating, weight, and shape; teaching healthy boundary setting; and resolving conflicts about separation-individuation. Treatment usually takes place in an outpatient setting,

except when the patient is suicidal or when past outpatient treatment has failed (Table 22-3).

In addition to intensive psychotherapy, cognitive behavioural therapy (CBT) or IPT and pharmacologic interventions are usually also necessary. The SSRIs demonstrated effectiveness in treating binge eating and purging, even without comorbid depression. Nutrition counselling is an important part of outpatient treatment to stabilize and normalize eating. Some mental health professionals, psychologists, advanced practice psychiatric nurses, and social workers specialize in treating eating disorders, often working with nutritionists who also have expertise in working with this population. Group psychotherapy and support groups are also used. Family therapy is not usually a part of the treatment because many people with bulimia nervosa live on college campuses away from home or are older and on their own. Usually, treatment becomes less intensive as symptoms remit. Therapy focuses on psychological issues, such as boundary setting and separation-individuation conflicts and on changing problematic behaviours and dysfunctional thinking using CBT.

CRNE Note

Therapeutic relationships and cognitive interventions are priority in the nursing care of individuals with eating disorders.

PRIORITY CARE ISSUES

Because of the comorbid conditions of depression and borderline personality disorder, some individuals with bulimia nervosa may become suicidal. They are also often at risk for self-mutilation. Because they display high levels of impulsivity, shoplifting, and overspending, financial and legal difficulties have been associated with bulimia nervosa.

NURSING MANAGEMENT: HUMAN RESPONSE TO DISORDER

The primary nursing diagnoses for patients with bulimia nervosa are Imbalanced Nutrition: Less Than Body Requirements, Powerlessness, Anxiety, and Ineffective Coping. Establishing a therapeutic relationship precedes biopsychosocial assessment and interventions.

Therapeutic Relationship

Individuals with bulimia nervosa experience a great deal of shame and guilt. They also often have an intense need to please and be liked and may approach the nurse–patient relationship in a superficial manner. They are too ashamed to discuss their symptoms but do not want to disappoint others, so they may discuss more social or unrelated issues in an attempt to engage the nurse. A nonjudgmental, accepting approach, stressing the importance of the relationship and outlining its purpose, are important at the outset. Explaining the nature of the relationship and the goals of therapy will help clarify the boundaries.

Biologic Domain

Despite that most individuals with bulimia nervosa maintain normal weights, the physical ramifications of this disorder may be similar to those of anorexia nervosa. Hypokalemia can contribute to muscle weakness and fatigability, as well as to the development of cardiac arrhythmias, palpitations, and cardiac conduction defects. Patients who purge risk fluid and electrolyte abnormalities that can further compromise cardiac status. Neuropsychiatric disturbances, such as poor concentration and attention, and sleep disturbances are common.

Assessment

The nurse should assess current eating patterns, determine the number of times a day the individual binges and purges, and note dietary restraint practices. Sleep patterns and exercise habits are also important.

Nursing Diagnoses for Biologic Domain

Imbalanced Nutrition: Less Than Body Requirements and Disturbed Sleep Pattern are typical nursing diagnoses for the biologic domain.

Interventions for Biologic Domain

If the patient is admitted to the hospital, meals and all food intake must be strictly monitored to normalize eating. Bathroom visits should also be supervised to prevent purging. Outpatients are asked to record their intake, binges, and purges to form a foundation for changing behaviours with CBT (see Chapter 14 for a description of CBT). Because individuals with bulimia nervosa have chaotic lifestyles and are often overcommitted, sleep may be a low priority. Sleep-deprived individuals may assume that food would be helpful, and they begin to eat, triggering a binge. To encourage regular sleep patterns, individuals should go to bed and rise at about the same time every day.

Pharmacologic Interventions

Whereas pharmacologic intervention is effective for symptom remission in bulimia nervosa, experts agree that the combination of CBT and medication has had the best results (Wilson et al., 1999). Fluoxetine (Prozac) has been the most studied for bulimia nervosa in clinical trials (see Box 22-13). Effective doses are usually 60 mg per day, a higher dosage than that used to treat depression. Sertraline (Zoloft) has also been used effectively. These medications, prescribed for binge eating and purging, are effective even when depression is not present (Goldstein, Wilson, Arscroft, & Al-Banna, 1999). The most important concern in using these medications is decreased appetite and weight loss during the first few weeks of administration. Weight should be monitored, especially during this period.

BOX 22.13

Drug Profile: Fluoxetine Hydrochloride (Prozac)

DRUG CLASS: Selective serotonin reuptake inhibitor

RECEPTOR AFFINITY: Inhibits central nervous system neuronal uptake of serotonin with little effect on norepinephrine; thought to antagonize muscarinic, histaminergic, and α adrenergic receptors.

INDICATIONS: Treatment of depressive disorders, most effective in major depression, obesity, bulimia, and obsessive-compulsive disorder

ROUTES AND DOSAGE: Available in 10- and 20-mg pulvules and 20 mg/5 mL oral solution

Adults: 20 mg/d in the morning, not to exceed 80 mg/d. Full antidepressant effect may not be seen for up to 4 weeks. If no improvement, dosage is increased after several weeks. Dosages >20 mg/d are administered twice daily. For eating disorders: typically 40 mg to 60 mg/d recommended.

Geriatric: Administer at lower or less-frequent doses; monitor responses to guide dosage.

Children: Safety and efficacy have not been established.

HALF-LIFE (PEAK EFFECT): 2 to 3 d (6–8 h)

SELECTED ADVERSE REACTIONS: Headache, nervousness, insomnia, drowsiness, anxiety, tremors, dizziness, lightheadedness, nausea, vomiting, diarrhea, dry mouth, anorexia, dyspepsia, constipation, taste changes, upper respiratory infections, pharyngitis, painful menstruation, sexual dysfunction, urinary frequency, sweating, rash, pruritus, weight loss, asthenia, and fever

WARNINGS: Avoid use in pregnancy and while breast-feeding. Use with caution in patients with impaired hepatic or renal function and diabetes mellitus. Possible risk for toxicity if taken with tricyclic antidepressants.

SPECIAL PATIENT AND FAMILY EDUCATION:
- Be aware that drug may take up to 4 weeks to get full antidepressant effect.
- Take drug in the morning or divided doses, if necessary.
- Report any adverse reactions.
- Avoid driving a car or performing hazardous activities because the drug may cause drowsiness or dizziness.
- Eat small, frequent meals to help with complaints of nausea and vomiting.

Monitoring and Administration of Medication

The intake of medication must be monitored for possible purging after administration. The effect of the medication will depend on whether it has had time to absorb.

Teaching Points

Individuals should be instructed to take medication as prescribed. SSRIs must be taken in the morning because they can cause insomnia. Persons taking SSRIs should be informed that any weight loss they initially experience is temporary and is usually regained after a few weeks, when the medication dosage has stabilized.

Psychosocial Domain

Assessment

For the individual with bulimia nervosa, psychological assessment focuses on cognitive distortions—cues or stimuli that lead to dysfunctional behaviour affecting symptom development—and knowledge deficits. The psychological characteristics typical of individuals with bulimia nervosa are presented in Box 22-1.

Individuals with bulimia nervosa display a significant number of cognitive distortions, examples of which are found in Table 22-4. These thought patterns form the basis for "rules" and lead the way to destructive eating patterns. During routine history taking, individuals may relate many of these erroneous assumptions. Situations that produce feelings of being overwhelmed and powerless need to be explored, as does the individual's ability to set boundaries, control impulsivity, and maintain quality relationships. These underlying issues may precipitate binge eating. Body dissatisfaction should be openly explored. Several assessment tools are available to gauge such characteristics as body dissatisfaction and impulsivity (see Box 22-8). Mood is an important area for evaluation because many people with bulimia nervosa also have depression. Symptoms of depression, especially the vegetative signs, should be thoroughly explored (see Chapter 19).

Nursing Diagnoses for Psychosocial Domain

Deficient Knowledge, Disturbed Thought Processes, and Powerlessness are among the common diagnoses for the social domain.

Interventions for Psychosocial Domain

Both CBT and IPT have been used for individuals with bulimia nervosa. The combination of CBT and pharma-cologic interventions is best for producing an initial decrease in symptoms (Leung, Waller, & Thomas, 2000; Mitchell, Peterson, Meyers, & Wunderlich, 2001). Behavioural therapy alone has not been as effective as CBT. IPT has had positive outcomes but may take longer to change binge eating and purging symptoms. While binge eating may persist, little work can be done on underlying interpersonal issues, such as boundary setting, because the patient is intent on feeling out of control with eating. Therefore, cognitive therapy is begun first, to address the distorted thinking processes influencing dietary restraint, binge eating, and purging. Decreasing these symptoms will eliminate the out-of-control feelings.

CBT is usually conducted in a group, with one or two sessions a week. A series of sessions is instituted to change dysfunctional thinking, rigid rules about eating, and impulsive behaviours. The cognitive interventions focus on distorted or dysfunctional thought patterns.

Behavioural Techniques

The behavioural techniques, such as **cue elimination** and response prevention, require self-monitoring to individualize the therapy. **Self-monitoring** is accomplished using a diary, in which the individual records binges and purges and precipitating emotions and environmental cues. Emotional and environmental cues are identified, and alternative responses are suggested, tried, and reinforced. When a cue or stimulus leads to a dysfunctional or unhealthy response, the response can be eliminated, or an alternate, healthier response to the cue can be substituted, tried, and then reinforced. Figure 22-5 gives two examples of behavioural interventions. In example 1, for the individual with anorexia nervosa, the response is modified or altered to a healthier one; in example 2, for the individual with bulimia nervosa, the cue is changed to produce a different, healthier response. Other techniques, such as postponing binges and purges through distraction, a technique to interrupt the cycle, are also effective.

Psychoeducation

In addition to cognitive and behavioural techniques, educational strategies are also incorporated into CBT during weekly sessions.

Teaching Points

For individuals with bulimia nervosa, psychoeducation focuses on setting boundaries and healthy limits, developing assertiveness, learning nutritional concepts related to healthy eating, and clarifying misconceptions about food (White, 1999). Rules that result from dichotomous thinking also must be addressed because of their role in dietary restraint and resulting binge eating.

Family Assessment and Intervention. Families caring for members with bulimia nervosa report

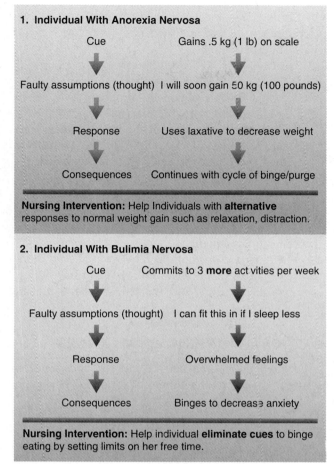

1. Individual With Anorexia Nervosa

Cue	Gains .5 kg (1 lb) on scale
↓	↓
Faulty assumptions (thought)	I will soon gain 50 kg (100 pounds)
↓	↓
Response	Uses laxative to decrease weight
↓	↓
Consequences	Continues with cycle of binge/purge

Nursing Intervention: Help Individuals with **alternative** responses to normal weight gain such as relaxation, distraction.

2. Individual With Bulimia Nervosa

Cue	Commits to 3 **more** activities per week
↓	↓
Faulty assumptions (thought)	I can fit this in if I sleep less
↓	↓
Response	Overwhelmed feelings
↓	↓
Consequences	Binges to decrease anxiety

Nursing Intervention: Help individual **eliminate cues** to binge eating by setting limits on her free time.

FIGURE 22.5 Examples of the relationship of cues, thoughts, responses: behavioural interventions.

experiencing intense emotions, including guilt, feelings of helplessness, anger, fear, and self-blame (Perkins, Winn, Murray, Murphy, & Schmidt, 2004). The nurse must explore with families the negative impact of giving care to assess its physical and psychosocial toll and to evaluate coping capacity. Perkins and colleagues identified a number of strategies families use to manage the difficulties associated with the eating disorder: thinking positively, using humour, maintaining their own interests, and actively obtaining information about bulimia nervosa.

Group Therapy

Group therapy is cost-effective and increases learning more effectively than does individual treatment because individuals learn from each other as well as from the nurse, therapist, or leader. Some experts have recommended 12-step programs for treating bulimia nervosa. However, many clinicians who work in this specialty have noted that these programs, with their strict rules, can be counterproductive for individuals with bulimia nervosa, who already have rigid rules and are "abstinent" in many ways that lead to binge eating. Broad parameters regarding food choices (eg, all foods allowed in

moderation), in combination with knowledge about healthy eating, should be encouraged instead.

After symptoms subside, individuals can concentrate on interpersonal issues in therapy, such as feelings of inadequacy and low self-esteem, which often underlie their lack of assertiveness.

The nurse can assist these individuals to understand the binge–purge cycle and the role of rigid rules in contributing to this cycle. The value of eating meals regularly to ward off hunger and reduce the possibility of a binge is also important. Individuals who abuse laxatives must be taught that, although these drugs produce water-weight loss, they are ineffective for true, lasting weight loss. Moreover, laxative-dependent bowel may result (Garner, 1997). Individuals also need information about potassium depletion, electrolyte imbalances, dehydration, and the medical consequences of binge eating and purging. Other topics for psychoeducation are included in Box 22-14.

EVALUATION AND TREATMENT OUTCOMES

Individuals with bulimia nervosa have better recovery outcomes than do those with anorexia nervosa. Outcomes have improved since the early 1990s, partially because of earlier detection, research on what treatments are most effective, and neuropharmacologic research and advances. Experts in the field of eating disorders report a 69% to 70% recovery rate with CBT and medication (Keel et al., 1999). Other studies comparing various methods (such as supportive therapy) have also demonstrated that CBT produces the best results (Wilson et al., 1999). Because CBT requires a specialist's care, current treatment research is exploring the use of self-help models, including manuals that can be combined

---

BOX 22.14

Psychoeducation Checklist: Bulimia Nervosa

When caring for the individual with bulimia nervosa, be sure to include the following topic areas in the teaching plan:

☐ Psychopharmacologic agents, if used, including drug, action, dosage, frequency, and possible adverse effects
☐ Binge–purge cycle and effects on body
☐ Nutrition and eating patterns
☐ Hydration
☐ Avoidance of cues
☐ Cognitive distortions
☐ Limit setting
☐ Appropriate boundary setting
☐ Assertiveness
☐ Resources
☐ Self-monitoring and behavioural interventions
☐ Realistic goal setting

with psychopharmacology (Mitchell et al., 2001). Frequency of binge eating and purging and severity of dietary restraint at initial treatment, depression, and borderline personality disorder predict a poor outcome after treatment (Bulik et al., 1998; Keel et al., 1999). Good outcome has been associated with a shorter duration of illness; receiving treatment within the first few years of illness is associated with an 80% recovery rate (Reas, Williamson, Martin, & Zucker, 2000).

CONTINUUM OF CARE

Although individuals with bulimia nervosa are less likely than those with anorexia nervosa to require hospitalization, those with extreme dehydration and electrolyte imbalance, depression and suicidality, or symptoms that have not remitted with outpatient treatment need hospitalization.

However, most treatment takes place in outpatient settings. After treatment, referrals to recovery groups and support groups are important to prevent relapse.

PREVENTION

As with anorexia nervosa, preventing bulimia nervosa requires effort on the part of teachers, school nurses, parents, and society as a whole. Because many of the risk factors are seen early in children attending elementary school, educating school nurses and teachers is an important focus for psychiatric–mental health nurses working in the community. Protective factors that mediate between risk factors and the development of an eating disorder must be emphasized and developed. Table 22-5 covers important prevention strategies for parents and their children or adolescents.

Society has begun to engage in an effort to help young individuals resist developing eating disorders. Many of the Web links listed at the end of this chapter have on-line help and resources for young individuals, families, teachers, and health care professionals.

SUMMARY OF KEY POINTS

- Anorexia nervosa and bulimia nervosa have some common symptoms but are classified as discrete disorders in the *DSM-IV-TR*.
- Eating disorders are best viewed along a continuum that includes subclinical or partial-syndrome disorders; because these disorders occur more frequently than full syndromes, they are often overlooked but, once identified, can be prevented from worsening.
- Similar factors predispose individuals to the development of anorexia nervosa and bulimia nervosa, and these factors represent a biopsychosocial model of risk. These disorders are preventable, and identifying risk factors assists with prevention strategies.

- Etiologic factors contribute in combination to the development of eating disorders; no one factor provides an explanation.
- Treatment of anorexia nervosa almost always includes hospitalization for refeeding; bulimia nervosa is treated primarily on an outpatient basis.
- For individuals with bulimia nervosa, cognitive behavioural therapy improves symptoms sooner than does interpersonal therapy, and CBT is most effective when combined with medication. For individuals with anorexia, family therapy plus individual interpersonal therapy is the most effective.
- Pharmacotherapy can be effective for bulimia nervosa but not for anorexia nervosa, especially during acute malnourishment.
- The outcomes for bulimia nervosa are better than those for anorexia nervosa. The type and severity of comorbid conditions and the length of the illness influence outcomes.

CRITICAL THINKING CHALLENGES

1 Discuss the potential difficulties and risks in attempting to treat a client with anorexia nervosa in an outpatient setting.
2 A client in the clinic is seen for bulimia nervosa and is prescribed fluoxetine. She reports great success immediately and attributes this to weight lost. What are your concerns and interventions?
3 Parents are often in need of support and suggestions for how to help prevent eating disorders. Develop a teaching program and include the topics and rationale for suggestions chosen.
4 Identify the important nursing management components of a refeeding program for a hospitalized individual with anorexia nervosa.
5 Bulimia nervosa is often described as a closet disorder with secretive binge eating and purging. Identify the signs and symptoms of each system involved for someone with this disorder.
6 Positive outcomes for the recovery of bulimia nervosa and anorexia nervosa are dependent on many factors. Identify the factors that promote positive outcomes and those related to poorer outcomes and prognosis.

WEB LINKS

www.nedic.ca   National Eating Disorder Information Centre (NEDIC), CW 1-211, 200 Elizabeth Street, Toronto, ON, M5G 2C4. This site provides information and resources for individuals, families, friends, and teachers on eating disorders and weight preoccupation. It offers an information and support telephone line at (416) 340-4156.

www.bana.ca Bulimia Anorexia Nervosa Association (BANA), University of Windsor, Windsor ON. The BANA site has information on specialized treatment education, support services for individuals affected directly and indirectly by eating disorders, and prevention of eating disorders, negative body image, and low self-esteem.

www.sheenasplace.org Sheena's Place, 87 Spadina Road, Toronto, ON, M5R 2T1. This site describes Sheena's Place, Canada's first community-based centre to offer services at no cost to people affected by severe eating and body image issues. The site provides information and support to parents, siblings, friends, spouses, partners, teachers, and other care providers.

www.something-fishy.org A Web site about Eating Disorders that is dedicated to raising awareness, emphasizing that Eating Disorders are NOT about food and weight; they are just the symptoms of something deeper going on, inside.

www.disorderedeating.ca The Eating Disorder Resource Centre of British Columbia provides educational, referral and research services to people struggling with disordered eating, their support networks, community-based organizations, students, educators, and professionals.

kidshelp.sympatico.ca (1-800-668-6868) This Kids Help Phone site offers a toll-free, national telephone counselling service for Canadian children and youth experiencing violence, alcohol or drug abuse, issues related to suicide, or suffering from an eating disorder. It features tips for parents and others.

MOVIES

Killing Us Softly 3: Advertising's Image of Women. 2000

This short documentary (32 minutes) illustrates and critiques over 160 ads and TV commercials that portray women in narrowly defined and marginalized ways. Themes include body image, objectification of women, trivialization of women's power, sexuality, pornography, and violence. Although the film is mainly about women, it suggests the effects of a media culture that limits men's emotion.

VIEWING POINTS: Corporations' and their advertisers' use images of girls and women to sell products. How does this contribute to eating disorders? What is the possible impact on older women and women considered overweight who do not measure up to media images of beauty? Do advertisers have a responsibility to society regarding the attitudes that their images support?

Slim Hopes: Advertising & the Obsession with Thinness. 1995

This award-winning short film deconstructs the way female bodies are depicted in advertising images and the negative effects of these images on women's health. There are 6 themes entitled: Impossible beauty, Waif look, Constructed bodies, Food & sex, Food & control, Weight loss industry, and Freeing imaginations.

VIEWING POINTS: The thin ideal for women portrayed in the media fosters body dissatisfaction because it is unobtainable by most women. What are the costs of this dissatisfaction to health and society? What cultural expectations for women and for men underlie media messages? What effect do the media messages and associated expectations have on how boys and men view and relate to girls and women, and to themselves? What is the effect on how girls and women view and relate to boys and men, and to themselves? What can nurses do to help clients resist these harmful media messages? What can nurses do to help themselves?

Thin Dreams. 1986. This is a National Film Board of Canada documentary exploring how young women in high school feel about their bodies and how their self-images are affected by North American society's obsession with thinness. There are three dramas dealing with shopping, dieting, and dating and boyfriends. The young women are shown to worry about their weight, talk endlessly about it, and either diet or plan to diet. It is an excellent introduction to female adolescent self image and body image, but is slightly dated.

VIEWING POINTS: How do adolescent body images and societal values contribute to the development of eating disorders? How might male students feel about their bodies, and what factors help to shape those self-images? What topics and approaches suggested by Thin Dreams would you include if you were developing a program for prevention of eating disorders?

REFERENCES

Addolorato, G., Taranto, C., DeRossi, G., & Gasbarinni, G. (1997). Neuroimaging of cerebral and cerebella atrophy in anorexia nervosa. *Psychiatry Research*, 76(2–3), 105–110.

American Psychiatric Association. (1987). *Diagnostic and statistical manual of mental disorders (DSM-III)* (3rd ed.). Washington, DC: Author.

American Psychiatric Association (APA). (2000). *Diagnostic and statistical manual of mental disorders* (4th edition, Text revision). Washington, DC: Author.

Anderluk, M. B., Tchanturia, K., Rabe-Hesketh, S., & Treasure, J. (2003). Childhood obsessive-compulsive personality traits in adult women with eating disorders: Defining a broader eating disorder phenotype. *American Journal of Psychiatry*, 160(2), 242–247.

Andersen, A., & Yager, J. (2005). Eating disorders. In B. J. Saddock & V. A. Saddock (Eds.), *Kaplan & Saddock's comprehensive textbook of psychiatry* (8th ed., pp. 2002–2021). Philadelphia: Lippincott Williams & Wilkins.

Anderson, A. (2001). Progress in eating disorder research. *American Journal of Psychiatry, 158*, 515–517.

Andrist, L. (2003). Media images, body dissatisfaction, and disordered eating in adolescent women. *American Journal of Maternal/Child Nursing, 28*(2), 119–123.

Arrow, B., Kenardy, J., & Agras, W. S. (1995). The Emotional Eating Scale: The development of a measure to assess coping with negative affect by eating. *International Journal of Eating Disorders, 18,* 79–90.

Bailer, U. F., & Kaye, W. H. (2003). A review of neuropeptide and neuroendocrine dysregulation in anorexia and bulimia nervosa. *Current Drug Targets CNS Neuronal Disorders, 2*(1), 53–59.

Berghold, K. M., & Lock, J. (2002). Assessing guilt in adolescents with anorexia nervosa. *American Journal of Psychotherapy, 56*(3), 378–390.

Braun, D. L., Sunday, S. R., Huang, A., & Halmi, K. A. (1999). More males seek treatment for eating disorders. *International Journal of Eating Disorders, 25*(4), 415–424.

Brownell, K., & Napolitano, M. A. (1995). Distorting reality for children: Body size proportions of Barbie and Ken dolls. *International Journal of Eating Disorders, 18,* 295–298.

Bruch, H. (1973). *Eating disorders: Obesity, anorexia nervosa and the person within.* New York: Basic Books.

Brumberg, J. (1988). *Fasting girls: The emergence of anorexia nervosa as a modern disease.* Cambridge: Harvard University Press.

Bulik, C. M., Sullivan, P. F., Joyce, P. M., et al. (1998). Prediction of one-year outcome in bulimia nervosa. *Comprehensive Psychiatry, 39*(4), 206–254.

Bulik, C. M., Sullivan, P., Wade, T., & Kendler, K. (2000). Twin studies of eating disorders: A review. *International Journal of Eating Disorders, 27,* 1–20.

Casper, R. C., & Lyubomorisky, S. (1997). Individual psychopathology relative to reports of unwanted sexual experiences as predictors of a bulimic eating pattern. *International Journal of Eating Disorders, 21,* 229–236.

Cooper, P., Taylor, M., Cooper, Z., & Fairburn, C. (1987). The development and validation of the BSQ. *International Journal of Eating Disorders, 6,* 485–494.

Costanzo, P. R., Musante, G. J., Friedman, K. E., et al. (1999). The gender specificity of emotional, situational, and behavioral indicators of binge eating in a diet-seeking obese population. *International Journal of Eating Disorders, 26*(2), 205–210.

Croll, J., Neumark-Sztainer, D., Story, M., & Ireland, M. (2002). Prevalence and risk and protective factors related to disordered eating behaviors among adolescents: Relationship to gender and ethnicity. *Journal of Adolescent Health, 13*(2), 166–175.

Crow, S., Praus, B., & Thuras, P. (1999). Mortality from eating disorders: A 5–10 year record limiting study. *International Journal of Eating Disorders, 26,* 97–101.

Davis, C., & Katzman, M. A. (1999). Perfection as acculturation: Psychological correlates of eating problems in Chinese male and female students living in the United States. *International Journal of Eating Disorders, 25,* 65–70.

Davis, C., Katzman, D. K., Kaptein, S., et al. (1997). The prevalence of high-level exercise in the eating disorders: Etiological implications. *Comprehensive Psychiatry, 38*(6), 321–326.

Davis, C., Katzman, D. K., & Kirsch, C. (1999). Compulsive physical activity with anorexia nervosa: A psycho-behavioural spiral of pathology. *Journal of Nervous and Mental Diseases, 187*(6), 336–342.

Diamond-Raab, L., & Orrell-Valente, J. K. (2002) Art therapy, psychodrama and verbal therapy: An integrative model of group therapy in the treatment of adolescents with anorexia nervosa and bulimia nervosa. *Child and Adolescent Psychiatric Clinics of North America, 11*(2), 343–364.

Dunn, P. K., & Ondercin, P. (1981). Personality variables related to compulsive eating in college women. *Journal of Clinical Psychology, 31,* 43–49.

Eckert, E. D., Halmi, K. A., Marchi, P., Grove, W., & Crosby, R. (1995). Ten-year follow-up of anorexia nervosa: Clinical course and outcome. *Psychological Medicine, 25,* 143–156.

Farrales, L., & Chapman, G. E. (1999). Filipino women living in Canada: Constructing meaning of body, food and health. *Health Care for Women International, 20,* 179–194.

Fichter, M. M., & Quadflieg, N. (1999). Six-year course and outcome of anorexia nervosa. *International Journal of Eating Disorders, 26*(4), 359–385.

Fitzgibbon, M. L., Spring, B., Avellone, M. E., et al. (1998). Correlates of binge eating in Hispanic black and white women. *International Journal of Eating Disorders, 24,* 43–52.

Garner, D. (1997). Psychoeducational principles in treatment. In D. M. Garner & P. E. Garfinkel (Eds.), *Handbook of treatment for eating disorders* (2nd ed., pp. 145–177). New York: Guilford Press.

Garner, D. M. (1991a). *Eating disorder inventory—2 professional manual.* Odessa, FL: Psychological Assessment Resources.

Garner, D. M. (1991b). *Eating disorder inventory—C.* Lutz, FL: Psychological Assessment Resources.

Garner, D. M., & Garfinkel, P. E. (1979). The Eating Attitude Test: An index of the symptoms of anorexia nervosa. *Psychosomatic Medicine, 10,* 647–656.

Garner, D. M., Olmsted, M. P., Bohr, Y., & Garfinkel, P. E. (1982). The Eating Attitude Test: Psychometric features and clinical correlates. *Psychological Medicine, 12,* 871–878.

Garner, D. M., Rosen, L. W., & Barry, D. (1998). Eating disorders among athletes: Research and recommendations. *Child and Adolescent Psychiatric Clinics of North America, 7,* 839–857.

Geller, J., Cockell, S., & Goldner, E. (2000). Inhibited expression of negative emotions and interpersonal orientation in anorexia nervosa. *International Journal of Eating Disorders, 28,* 8–19.

Golden, N. H., Ashtari, M., Kohn, M. R., et al. (1996). Reversibility of cerebral ventricular enlargement in anorexia nervosa, demonstrated by quantitative magnetic resonance imaging. *Journal of Pediatrics, 128*(2), 296–301.

Goldstein, D. J., Wilson, M. G., Arscroft, R. C., & Al-Banna, M. (1999). Effectiveness of fluoxetine therapy in bulimia nervosa regardless of comorbid depression. *International Journal of Eating Disorders, 25,* 19–28.

Gowers, S. G., & Shore, A. (1999). The stigma of eating disorders. *International Journal of Clinical Practice, 53*(5), 386–388.

Gutwill, S. (1994). Women's eating problems: Social context and the internalization of culture. In C. Bloom, A. Gitter, S. Gutwill, et al. (Eds.), *Eating problems: A feminist psychoanalytic treatment model* (pp. 1–27). New York: Basic Books.

Halmi, K. A., Sunday, S. R., Strober, M., et al. (2000). Perfectionism in anorexia nervosa: Variation by clinical subtype, obsessionality, and pathological eating behavior. *American Journal of Psychiatry, 157,* 1799–1805.

Health Canada. (2003). *Canadian community health survey.* Ottawa, ON: Statistics Canada.

Herman, C. P., & Mack, D. (1975). Restrained and unrestrained eating. *Journal of Personality, 43,* 647–660.

Herzog, D. B., Greenwood, D. N., Dorer, D. J., et al. (2000). Mortality in eating disorders: A descriptive study. *International Journal of Eating Disorders, 28,* 20–26.

Inches, P. R. (1895). Anorexia nervosa. *Maritime Medical News, 7,* 73–75.

Jensen, V. S., & Mejlhede, A. (2000). Anorexia nervosa treatment with olanzapine. *British Journal of Psychiatry, 177*(2), 87.

Johnson, J. G., Cohen, P., Kasen, S., & Brook, J. S. (2002). Childhood adversities associated with risk for eating disorders or weight problems during adolescence or early adulthood. *American Journal of Psychiatry, 159,* 394–400.

Joiner, T. E., Katz, J., & Heatherton, T. F. (2000). Personality factors differentiate late adolescent females and males with chronic bulimic symptoms. *International Journal of Eating Disorders, 27,* 191–197.

Jonat, L. M., & Birmingham, C. L. (2004). Disordered eating attitudes and behaviours in the high-school students of a rural Canadian community. *Eating & Weight Disorders, 9*(4), 306–308.

Katzman, D. K., Zipursky, R. B., Lambe, E. K., & Mikulis, D. J. (1997). A longitudinal magnetic resonance imaging study of brain changes in adolescents with anorexia nervosa. *Archives of Pediatrics & Adolescent Medicine, 151*(8), 793–797.

Kaye, W. H., Gendall, K. A., Fernstrom, M. H., et al. (2000). Effects of acute tryptophan depletion on mood in bulimia nervosa. *Biological Psychiatry, 47*(2), 151–157.

Kaye, W. H., Klump, K. L., Frank, G. K., & Strober, M. (2000). Anorexia and bulimia. *Annual Review of Medicine, 51*, 299–313.

Keel, P. K., Dorer, D. J., Eddy, K. T., et al. (2003). Predictors of mortality in eating disorders. *Archives of General Psychiatry, 60*, 179–183.

Keel, P. K., Mitchell, J. E., Milre, K. B., et al. (1999). Long-term outcome of bulimia nervosa. *Archives of General Psychiatry, 56*, 63–69.

Keery, H., Boutelle, K., van den Berg, P., & Thompson, K. (2005). The impact of appearance-related teasing by family members. *Journal of Adolescent Health, 37*, 120–127.

Korndorfer, S. R., Lucas, A. R., Suman, V. J., et al. (2003). Long-term survival of patients with anorexia nervosa: A population based study in Rochester, MN. *Mayo Clinic Proceedings, 78*(3), 278–284.

Kuba, S. A., & Harris, D. J. (2001). Eating disturbances in women of color: An exploratory study of contextual factors in the development of disordered eating in Mexican-American women. *Health Care for Women International, 22*(3), 281–298.

Lambe, E., Katzman, D. K., Miluluis, D., Kennedy, S., & Zipursky, R. (1997). Cerebral grey matter volume deficits after weight recovery from anorexia nervosa. *Archives of General Psychiatry, 54*, 537–542.

Laporte, L., & Guttman, H. (2001). Abusive relationships in families of women with borderline personality disorder, anorexia nervosa and a control group. *Journal of Nervous and Mental Disease, 180*, 522–531.

LaVia, M. C., Grey, M., & Kaye, W. H. (2000). Case reports of olanzapine treatment of anorexia nervosa. *International Journal of Eating Disorders, 27*, 363–366.

Leung, N., Waller, G., & Thomas, G. (2000). Outcome of group cognitive-behavioral therapy for bulimia nervosa: The role of core beliefs. *Behaviour Research and Therapy, 38*(2), 145–156.

Lilenfeld, L. R., Kaye, W. H., Greeno, C. G., et al. (1998). A controlled family study of anorexia nervosa and bulimia nervosa: Psychiatric disorders in first-degree relatives and effects of proband comorbidity. *Archives of General Psychiatry, 55*(7), 603–610.

Maloney, M., McGuire, J., & Daniels, S. R. (1988). Reliability testing of a children's version of the Eating Attitude Test. *Journal of the American Academy of Child and Adolescent Psychiatry, 27*, 541–543.

Martz, D. M., Sturgis, E. T., & Gustafson, S. B. (1996). Development and preliminary validation of the Cognitive Behavioral Dieting Scale. *International Journal of Eating Disorders, 19*, 297–309.

Massey-Stokes, M. (2001). Communication, expressing feelings, and creative problem solving. In J. J. Robert-McComb (Ed.), *Eating disorders in women and children: Prevention, stress management, and treatment* (pp. 291–307). Boca Raton, FL: CRC Press.

Matsunaga, H., Kaye, W. H., McConaha, C., et al. (2000). Personality disorders among subjects recovered from eating disorders. *International Journal of Eating Disorders, 27*, 353–357.

Mazure, C. M., Halmi, K., A., Sunday, S. R., Romano, S. J., & Einhorn, A. M. (1994). Yale-Brown-Cornell Eating Disorder Scale: Development, use, reliability, and validity. *Journal of Psychiatric Research, 28*, 425–445.

McIntosh, V. V., Bulik, C. M., McKenzie, J. M., et al. (2000). Interpersonal psychotherapy for anorexia nervosa. *International Journal of Eating Disorders, 27*, 125–139.

McVey, G., Tweed, S., & Blackmore, E. (2004). Dieting among preadolescent and young adolescent females. *Canadian Medical Association Journal, 170*, 1559–1561.

Miller, M. N., & Pumariega, A. J. (2001). Culture and eating disorders: a historical and cross-cultural review. *Psychiatry, 64*(2), 93–110.

Milos, G., Spindler, A., Ruggiero, G., Klaghofer, R., Schnyder, V. (2002). Comorbidity of obsessive-compulsive disorders and duration of eating disorders. *International Journal of Eating Disorders, 26*(3), 284–289.

Minuchin, S., Rossman, B. L., & Baker, L. (1978). *Psychosomatic families.* Cambridge: Harvard University Press.

Mitchell, J. E., Peterson, C. B., Meyers, T., & Wunderlich, S. (2001). Combining pharmacotherapy in the treatment of patients with eating disorders. *Psychiatric Clinics of North America, 24*(2), 315–323.

National Eating Disorder Information Centre. (1998). *Canadian children in grade three and four say they'd rather lose a parent, get cancer or live through nuclear war than be fat* [Online.] Retrieved from *http://www.nedic.ca/.*

North, C., & Gowers, S. (1999). Anorexia nervosa, psychopathology and outcome. *International Journal of Eating Disorders, 26*, 386–391.

Ogden, J., & Steward, J. (2000). The role of the mother–daughter relationship in explaining weight concern. *International Journal of Eating Disorders, 28*(11), 78–83.

Patel, P., Wheatcroft, R., Park, R. J., & Stein, A. (2002). The children of mothers with eating disorders. *Clinical Child and Family Psychological Review, 5*(1), 1–19.

Pawluck, D. E., & Gorey, K. M. (1998). Secular trends in the incidence of anorexia nervosa: Integrative review of population based studies. *International Journal of Eating Disorders, 23*, 347–352.

Perkins, D. F., & Luster, T. (1999). The relationship between sexual abuse and purging: Findings from a community wide survey of female adolescents. *Child Abuse and Neglect, 23*, 371–382.

Perkins, S., Winn, S., Murray, J., Murphy, R., & Schmidt, U. (2004). A qualitative study of the experiences of caring for a person with bulimia nervosa. Part 1: The emotional impact of caring. *International Journal of Eating Disorders, 36*(3), 256–268.

Polivy, J., & Herman, C. P. (1993). Etiology of binge eating: Psychological mechanisms. In C. G. Fairburn & G. T. Wilson (Eds.), *Binge eating: Nature, assessment and treatment* (pp. 173–205). New York: Guilford.

Reas, D. L., Williamson, D. A., Martin, C. K., & Zucker, N. L. (2000). Duration of illness predicts outcome for bulimia nervosa: A long term follow up study. *International Journal of Eating Disorders, 27*, 428–434.

Robin, A. L., Siegel, P. T., Moye, A. W., et al. (1999). A controlled comparison of family versus individual therapy for adolescents with anorexia nervosa. *Journal of the American Academy of Child and Adolescent Psychiatry, 38*(12), 1482–1489.

Schwarz, D., Phares, V., Tantleff-Dunn, S., & Thompson, J. K. (1999). Body image, psychological functioning, and parental feedback regarding physical appearance. *International Journal of Eating Disorders, 18*, 339–344.

Shapira, N. A., Goldsmith, T. D., & McElroy, S. L. (2000). Treatment of binge eating disorder with topiramate: A clinical case series. *Journal of Clinical Psychiatry, 61*(5), 368–372.

Sharkey-Orgnero, M. I. (1999). Anorexia nervosa: A qualitative analysis of parents' perspectives on recovery. *Eating Disorders, 7*, 123–141.

Shisslak, C., Renger, R., Sharpe, T., et al. (1999). Development and evaluation of the McKnight Risk Factor Survey for assessing potential risk and protective factors for disordered eating in preadolescent and adolescent girls. *International Journal of Eating Disorders, 25*, 195–214.

Smith, K. A., Fairburn, C. G., & Cowen, P. J. (1999). Symptomatic relapse in bulimia nervosa following acute tryptophan depletion. *Archives of General Psychiatry, 56*(2), 171–176.

Smolak, L., Levine, M. P., & Schermer, F. (1999). Parental input and weight concern among elementary school children. *International Journal of Eating Disorders, 25*, 263–271.

Smolak, L., Murnen, S. K., & Ruble, A. (2000). Female athletes and eating problems: A meta analysis. *International Journal of Eating Disorders, 27*(4), 371–380.

Sobol, J., & Bursztyn, M. (1998). Dating people with anorexia nervosa and bulimia nervosa: Attitudes and beliefs of university students. *Women & Health, 27*(3), 73–85.

Steinhausen, H. C. (2002). The outcome of anorexia nervosa in the 20th century. *American Journal of Psychiatry, 159*, 1284–1293.

Streigel-Moore, R. (1993). Etiology of binge eating: A developmental perspective. In C. G. Fairburn & G. T. Wilson (Eds.), *Binge eating, nature, assessment and treatment* (pp. 144–172). New York: Guilford.

Strobel. (2002, February 2, 2002).

Strober, M., Freeman, R., Lampert, C., et al. (2000). Controlled family study of anorexia nervosa and bulimia nervosa: Evidence of shared liability and transmission of partial syndromes. *American Journal of Psychiatry, 157*(3), 393–401.

Strober, M., Pataki, C., Freeman, R., & DeAntonio, M. (1999). No effect of adjunctive fluoxetine on eating behavior or weight phobia during the inpatient treatment of anorexia nervosa: An historical case controlled study. *Journal of Child and Adolescent Psychopharmacology, 9*(3), 195–201.

Sullivan, P. (1995). Mortality in anorexia nervosa. *American Journal of Psychiatry, 152*, 1073–1074.

Taylor, C. B., Sharpe, T., Shisslak, C., et al. (1998). Factors associated with weight loss in adolescent girls. *International Journal of Eating Disorders, 24*, 31–42.

Thomsen, S. R., Weber, M. M., & Brown, L. B. (2002). The relationship between reading beauty and fashion magazines and the use of pathogenic dieting methods among adolescent females. *Adolescence, 37*(145), 1–18.

Tiggerman, M., & Pickering, A. (1996). The role of television in adolescent women's body dissatisfaction and drive for thinness. *International Journal of Eating Disorders, 20*, 199–203.

Toner, B., Garfinkel, P., & Garner, D. (1988). Affective and anxiety disorders in the long-term follow-up of anorexia nervosa. *International Journal of Psychiatry and Medicine, 18*, 357–364.

Tranquada, D. (2000). The hunger that kills.

Vandereyken, W. (2002). Families of patients with eating disorders. In C. G. Fairburn & K. D. Brownell (Eds.), *Eating disorders and obesity* (2nd ed., pp. 215–220). New York: Guilford.

von Ranson, K. M., Kaye, W. H., Weltzin, T. E., Rao, R., & Matsunaga, H. (1999). Obsessive-compulsive disorder symptoms before and after recovery from bulimia nervosa. *American Journal of Psychiatry, 156*(11), 1703–1708.

Ward, A., Tiller, J., Treasure, J., & Russell, G. (2000). Eating disorders: Psyche or soma. *International Journal of Eating Disorders, 27*, 279–287.

Weaver, K. D., Wuest, J., & Ciliska, D. (2005). Understanding women's journey of recovering from anorexia nervosa. *Qualitative Health Research, 15*(2), 188–206.

White, J. H. (1999). The development and clinical testing of an outpatient program for women with bulimia nervosa. *Archives of Psychiatric Nursing, 13*(4), 179–191.

White, J. H. (2000a). Eating disorders in elementary and middle school children: Risk factors, early detection and prevention. *Journal of School Nursing, 16*(2), 26–35.

White, J. H. (2000b). Symptom development in bulimia nervosa: A comparison of women with and without a history of anorexia nervosa. *Archives of Psychiatric Nursing, 14*(2), 81–92.

Wiederman, M., & Pryor, T. (2000). Body dissatisfaction, bulimia, and depression among women: The mediating role of drive for thinness. *International Journal of Eating Disorders, 27*, 90–95.

Wilson, G. T., Loeb, K. L., Walsh, B. T., et al. (1999). Psychological versus pharmacological treatments of bulimia nervosa: Predictors and processes of change. *Journal of Consulting and Clinical Psychology, 67*(4), 451–459.

Wolfe, B. E., & Gimby, L. B. (2003). Caring for the hospitalized patient with an eating disorder. *Nursing Clinics of North America, 38*, 75–99.

Wolfe, B. E., Metzger, E. D., Levine, J. M., et al. (2000). Serotonin function following remission from bulimia nervosa. *Neuropsychopharmacology, 22*(3), 257–263.

Woodside, B., Field, L. L., Garfinkel, P., & Heinmaa, M. (1998). Specificity of eating disorders diagnoses in families of probands with anorexia nervosa and bulimia nervosa. *Comprehensive Psychiatry, 39*(5), 261–264.

Woodside, B., Garfinkel, P., Lin, E., Goering, P., Kaplan, A., Goldbloom, D. S., & Kennedy, S. H. (2001). Comparisons of men with full or partial eating disorders, men without eating disorders, and women with eating disorders in the community. *American Journal of Psychiatry, 158*(4), 570–574.

Wooley, S. C., & Kearney-Cooke, A. (1986). Intensive treatment of bulimia and body image disturbance. In K. D. Brownell & J. P. Foreyt (Eds.), *Handbook of eating disorders: Physiology, psychology and treatment of obesity, anorexia, and bulimia* (pp. 476–502). New York: Basic Books.

World Health Organization. (1993). *The ICD-10 classification of mental and behavioural disorders: Diagnostic criteria for research.* Geneva: Author.

Yager, J., & Workgroup in Eating Disorders. (2000). *Practice guideline for the treatment of patients with eating disorders* (2nd ed.). American Psychiatric Association. Retrieved August 16, 2005 from http://www.psych.org.

For challenges, please refer to the **CD-ROM** in this book.

23

Substance Use Disorders

Barbara G. Faltz, Richard V. Wing, and Jean Robinson Hughes

LEARNING OBJECTIVES

After studying this chapter, you will be able to:

- Distinguish among the actions, effects, and withdrawal symptoms (if any) of alcohol, marijuana, stimulants, sedatives, hallucinogens, phencyclidine, opiates, nicotine, solvents, and caffeine.
- Describe the biologic, psychological, and social theories that attempt to explain substance use, dependence, and addiction.
- Compare the strengths and limitations of several intervention approaches to substance use disorders.
- Describe the effects of alcohol and other drug classes on pregnancy and infants.
- Describe appropriate nursing diagnoses and treatment interventions for clients who are not ready to accept (deny) problematic substance use.
- Formulate nursing diagnoses based on a biopsychosocial assessment of people with substance use disorders.
- Formulate nursing interventions that address specific diagnoses related to substance use disorders.
- Discuss the influence of culture on our understanding and treatment approaches when working with people with substance use disorders.

KEY TERMS

- abuse ▪ addiction ▪ alcohol withdrawal syndrome ▪ Alcoholics Anonymous ▪ anhedonia ▪ anxiolytic ▪ codependence ▪ countertransference ▪ craving ▪ delirium tremens ▪ denial ▪ dependence ▪ detoxification ▪ hallucinogen ▪ harm reduction ▪ inhalants ▪ Korsakoff's psychosis ▪ methadone maintenance ▪ narcotics ▪ opiates ▪ reality confrontation ▪ relapse ▪ sedative-hypnotic drugs ▪ substance-related disorders ▪ tolerance ▪ use ▪ Wernicke's syndrome ▪ withdrawal

⬟ KEY CONCEPTS

- confronting reality ▪ enhancing motivation for change

Ancient and modern history chronicles the negative impact of alcohol and drug dependence on various cultures and civilizations. The human use and abuse of alcohol and other drugs has been around since the beginning of history; so too have the subsequent social and emotional problems that accompany substance dependence. Today, alcohol and other drug problems have reached epidemic proportions in Canada, with incidence rising in younger age groups, particularly among adolescents and young adults. What used to be a problem primarily of older adolescents and young adults now appears to be a problem affecting younger and younger children and older and older adults. Exposure to illegal drugs, which 25 years ago was primarily an issue only in certain areas of major cities, is now a threat in almost every local neighbourhood, community, and school—from the most urban centre to the most rural and remote setting. Substance dependence has been identified by Canada's Drug Strategy (Government of Canada, 1998) as one of the major health issues in our nation and is the focus of much social and political concern. The connection between substance dependence and addiction and related social and health issues is critical. For example, the rise in violence associated with the sale and distribution of illicit drugs in neighbourhoods and schools jeopardizes the health and well-being of communities. At the same time, the criminalization of illicit drug users under current drug control legislation in Canada contradicts the objectives of public health and may even contribute to the drug-related problems (prevention of infectious disease transmission among illicit drug users) that harm reduction tries to alleviate (Fischer, 2005).

Statistics show that children are being exposed to, and experiment with, drugs at younger ages (Government of Canada, 1998). There is an increased risk for spread of human immunodeficiency virus (HIV) infection, hepatitis B and C, tuberculosis, and other communicable diseases among alcohol and other drug users; the number of premature deaths or traumatic injuries has risen as the result of drug overdoses or other unsafe activities or practices engaged in while under the influence of alcohol or drugs (eg, motor vehicle crashes); and there is an enormous increase in domestic violence and abuse and neglect (in children and seniors) resulting from substance dependence. The medical and social implications are profound as we face a new generation of children who are at risk for serious medical, developmental, learning, and psychological problems. In addition, the ensuing substance use problems associated with, or stemming from, perinatal and childhood exposure to drugs and alcohol are also profound. Indeed, the evidence that being hung-over while engaged in activities of significant responsibility (work, school, or taking care of children) is a common occurrence reported by adults (26%) who are dependent on alcohol (Statistics Canada, 2004) and highlights the pervasive nature of the substance abuse problem.

Substance dependence exacts a heavy toll on the health of individuals and communities. According to the recent Canadian Addiction Survey (Canadian Centre on Substance Abuse [CCSA], 2004), nearly one fourth of former and current drinkers report that, at some point in their lives, their drinking has caused harm to themselves (eg, physical health, friendships, financial, work, legal, learning, housing) and to others (humiliated/verbal/physical abuse, family/marriage problems). The cost of this toll to society is enormous (estimated at nearly $9 billion in 1992), in areas related to health care (eg, hospitalization, treatment services), the workplace (eg, Employee Assistance programs, drug testing), transfer payments (eg, social welfare, workers' compensation), crime and law enforcement (eg, police, courts), and lost productivity (eg, reduced output, sick time) (Single, Robson, Xie, & Rehm, 1996). Substance dependence threatens to affect the overall welfare of our nation and our health care system. Nurses and mental health professionals are well positioned on the frontlines of the health care system for providing sound promotion and prevention strategies as well as assessment, early diagnosis, and treatment approaches. Nurses play a vital role in helping to educate individuals, families, and communities.

This chapter reviews types of substance use, their biologic and psychological effects on individuals, current theories regarding the etiology of substance use disorders, and interventions available for treatment. The role of the nurse is discussed in terms of assessment and planning interventions to help meet the needs of clients and family members who seek treatment. Professional issues regarding chemical dependency within the nursing profession are also examined.

DEFINITIONS AND TERMS

Perceptions of substance use, misuse, abuse, and dependence change over time. For example, alcoholism, viewed as moral corruption during prohibition times, gradually has become understood as a disease (addiction), and then as a multidimensional problem with biologic and physiological mechanisms, psychological processes (learning, conditioning, modelling, and coping with stress), and social and environmental processes (interpersonal relationships and broader culture) (Health Canada, 2003a). Accordingly, new terminology has also emerged to describe a range of drinking problems, such as "problem use" generally referred to as "continued use despite negative consequences," (Fingerhood, 2000) and "binge drinker" referring to someone who does not necessarily drink regularly but drinks excessively (the equivalent of four drinks or more) (Blow, Walton, Barry, Coyne, Mudd, & Copeland, 2000). The problem with these changing views and terms regarding drinking is that they allow for subjective interpretation and create a lack of consistency in accurately defining what is being observed: is it alcohol abuse, alcohol dependence, alcoholism, heavy drinking, or a drinking problem? (Fingerhood, 2000, p. 985).

The following are some common terms used to describe behaviour patterns along the continuum of substance use risk (Health Canada, 2000):

- **No use**—the person does not use alcohol or other drugs.
- **Use**—the person drinks alcohol or swallows, smokes, sniffs, or injects a mind-altering substance.
- **Experimental use**—the person tries a drug out of curiosity and may or may not use the drug again.
- **Social/occasional use**—the person uses the drug in an amount or frequency that is not harmful.
- **Medication use as directed**—the person uses drugs as prescribed, under medical supervision. The risk of harm is minimized.
- **Harmful use** (sometimes called **abuse**)—the person experiences negative consequences of drugs (eg, health problems, family, school, work, or legal problems).
- **Dependence**—the person continues to use alcohol or drugs despite adverse consequences to one's physical, social, and psychological well-being.
- **Addiction**—the person experiences severe psychological and behavioural dependence on drugs or alcohol.
- **Withdrawal**—the person experiences adverse physical and psychological symptoms that occur when use of a substance ceases.
- **Detoxification**—the person experiences the process of being safely and effectively withdrawn from an addictive substance, usually under medical supervision.
- **Harm reduction**—the person experiences the process of pragmatically and effectively minimizing use-related harms (Fischer, 2005).
- **Relapse**—the person experiences the recurrence of alcohol- or drug-dependent behaviour, having previously achieved and maintained abstinence for a significant time beyond the period of detoxification.

DIAGNOSTIC CRITERIA

The American Psychiatric Association's (APA, 2000) *Diagnostic and Statistical Manual of Mental Disorders*, 4th edition, text revision (*DSM-IV-TR*) classifies **substance-related disorders** as disorders related to taking a drug of abuse, including alcohol, amphetamines, cannabis (marijuana), cocaine, hallucinogens, inhalants, nicotine, opioids, phencyclidine, sedatives-hypnotics, anxiolytics, caffeine, and other unknown substances. These disorders are further categorized as those related to the harmful use or abuse of a substance, those related to dependence on a substance, or those induced by intoxication or withdrawal. The *DSM-IV-TR* outlines diagnostic criteria for both harmful use or abuse of substance and dependence (Table 23-1).

EPIDEMIOLOGY AND CULTURAL ISSUES

Epidemiologic data on alcohol and other drugs causing dependence come from several sources. Surveys, such as the Canadian Community Health Survey: Mental Health and Well-Being (CCHS) and the National Population Health Survey (NPHS), examine prevalence in selected populations during a given time period or for a period of years. The Canadian Community Epidemiology Network on Drug Use (CCENDU) serves as a surveillance system and provides comparative data about the nature, extent, and consequences of harmful use or abuse of substances. In addition, given that many of the national surveys do not identify Aboriginal people who are living in mainstream Canada or include those living in designated communities (on reserves), the National Native Addictions Partnership Foundation's Treatment Activity Reporting System (TARS) has been created to track substance use among these populations.

The frequency and danger of drugs and behaviours associated with drug use are generally underestimated by the public and health care professionals alike. Further, recent reviews of the literature have found significant variability in the reported prevalence rates of alcohol and substance use disorders among different countries and even among regions within the same country. There are a number of possible methodologic (eg, definition of terms, how information is collected) and cultural (eg, legal status of the substance, community norms) reasons for this variability, rendering the statistical picture somewhat tentative or vague (Somers, Goldner, Waraich, & Hsu, 2004). Keeping these limitations in mind, estimates show that in 2002 about 641,000 Canadians, or 2.6% of the household population aged 15 years or older, were dependent on alcohol, and 194,000 (0.8%) were dependent on illicit drugs, rates fairly similar to those in Australia and the United States (Statistics Canada, 2004). Further, the Canadian Addiction Survey (CCSA, 2004) showed that among those who drank during the previous year, 17% (13.6% of all Canadians) were considered high-risk drinkers (25% men, 9% women). Both binge drinking (60%) and heavy illicit drug use (37%) occurred most frequently during the early adult years (20 to 24 years of age) and fell with advancing age (5%). The pattern of alcohol use was fairly consistent across the country, with about 1 in 10 Canadians having engaged in heavier drinking (CCSA, 2004). However, significantly higher percentages were found in the four Atlantic Provinces and in Alberta.

Table 23.1 *DSM-IV* Substance-Related Disorders	
Substance Disorder	**Diagnostic Criteria**
Substance Dependence Alcohol dependence Amphetamine dependence Cannabis dependence Cocaine dependence Hallucinogen dependence Inhalant dependence Nicotine dependence Opioid dependence Phencyclidine dependence Sedative, hypnotic, or anxiolytic dependence Polysubstance dependence	Maladaptive pattern of substance use leading to clinically significant impairment or distress ■ Impairment manifested by three or more of the following: tolerance (need for markedly increased amounts of the substance to reach intoxication or desired effect), withdrawal, substance often taken in large amounts or over a longer period than was intended, persistent desire or unsuccessful efforts to cut down or control use, much time spent in activities necessary to obtain the substance or use it, reduction or cessation of important social, occupational, or recreational activities, use continued despite knowledge of having persistent or recurrent physical or psychological problem likely to have been caused or exacerbated by the substance

Substance Abuse
Alcohol abuse
Amphetamine abuse
Cannabis abuse
Cocaine abuse
Hallucinogen abuse
Inhalant abuse
Opioid abuse
Phencyclidine abuse
Sedative, hypnotic, or anxiolytic abuse
	■ Maladaptive pattern of substance use leading to clinically significant impairment or distress
	■ Impairment manifested by three or more of the following occurring within a 12-month period:
	   Recurrent use, resulting in failure to fulfill major role obligations at work, school, or home
	   Recurrent use in situations that are physically hazardous
	   Recurrent substance-related legal problems
	   Continued use despite feeling persistent or recurrent effects of the substance
	■ Symptoms never met criteria for substance dependence

Substance Intoxication Alcohol intoxication Alcohol intoxication delirium Amphetamine intoxication Amphetamine intoxication delirium Caffeine intoxication Cannabis intoxication Cannabis intoxication delirium Cocaine intoxication Cocaine intoxication delirium Hallucinogen intoxication Hallucinogen intoxication delirium Opioid intoxication Opioid intoxication delirium Inhalant intoxication Inhalant intoxication delirium Phencyclidine intoxication, delirium Sedative, hypnotic, or anxiolytic intoxication	■ Reversible substance-specific syndrome due to recent ingestion or exposure to a substance ■ Clinically significant maladaptive behavioural or psychological changes due to effect of substance on central nervous system, developing during or shortly after use of substance ■ Symptoms not due to general medical condition, nor better accounted for by another mental disorder
Substance Withdrawal Alcohol withdrawal, delirium Amphetamine withdrawal Cocaine withdrawal Opioid withdrawal Sedative, hypnotic, or anxiolytic withdrawal, delirium	■ Development of substance-specific syndrome due to cessation or reduction in substance use, previously heavy and prolonged ■ Syndrome causing significant distress or impairment in social, occupational, or other important areas of functioning

An examination of trends of alcohol consumption indicates that use decreased in the 1980s and early 1990s as attitudes became less tolerant of drinking, legal and social pressures and actions against drinking and driving increased, and concerns about health increased. However, the trend has recently reversed (CCSA, 2004). Current figures show that approximately 6,700 Canadians die each year from alcohol use (mostly from accidents and suicides), and another 86,000 are hospitalized (CCSA, 2005).

Gender Differences

Recent study results have revealed that while men (47%) generally engage in heavy drinking more frequently than women (24%) and are more likely than women to be dependent on alcohol (3.9% vs. 1.1%) and drugs (1.1% vs. 0.5%), gender differences vary with substance and age (Statistics Canada, 2004). For example, women still outnumber men in the frequency of harmful use of prescribed psychoactive medications (Health Canada, 2001a). In addition, according to the Canadian Tobacco Use Monitoring Survey (Health Canada, 2004), although male tobacco smokers continue to outnumber women tobacco smokers at every age, the difference is marginal among teens (boys 21% vs. girls 19%). Drug and alcohol use patterns also vary within the female gender according to certain demographic factors (age, education, marital status, employment, race and ethnicity), and her partner's substance use pattern (Gomberg, 1999). These patterns can result in numerous health effects (Health Canada, 2001a, p. 11), such as the following:

- Physical health problems (tend to be more severe and immediate)
- Reproductive problems (disruptions in menstrual cycle, fetal development, child birth, menopause, and sexual responsiveness and dysfunction)
- Associated mental health disorders (anxiety, depression, phobias, panic, and eating disorders)
- Increased risk for suicide ideation and completion

In addition, a large number of women who engage in harmful use of substances have also endured childhood sexual abuse and prior victimization (including physical violence) (Health Canada, 2001a).

Successful treatment of women who engage in harmful use of alcohol or other drugs is dependent on services that are gender specific, ethnically and culturally sensitive, and linked to a comprehensive array of related supports. Unfortunately, many women who desire treatment for alcohol and other drug dependencies also endure a number of other problems that act as barriers or impinge on their recovery (Box 23-1) (Health Canada, 2001a; Marion, 1995).

BOX 23.1

Barriers to Recovery

Personal Barriers
- Functioning as a single parent
- Fear of being isolated
- Living in abusive or unstable environments

Interpersonal Barriers
- Fear of losing children
- Lack of family support

Community/Societal Barriers
- Social stigma

Program/Structural Barriers
- Lack of transportation, child care, and finances needed for treatment-related activities
- Lack of available, accessible (psychological, geographic), flexible, and appropriate treatment services

---

Age Differences

The prevalence of alcohol use continues to grow rapidly among the youngest (Adlaf, Paglia, & Ivis, 1999) and oldest (Tyas & Rush, 1994) populations in Canada. Problematic alcohol use constitutes approximately one third of the emergency room population (Stewart & Richards, 2000), 20% of the outpatient population, and between 20% and 40% of the inpatient population (Isaacson & Schorling, 1999).

Youth

Given that adolescence itself is characterized by change (separation from family, establishment of autonomy and identity, trend toward unconventionality), it is difficult to define what constitutes a substance use problem among youth when some involvement with alcohol, drugs, and tobacco is statistically normative (Health Canada, 2001b, 2001c). There is some evidence that use patterns in adolescence may not be predictive of long-term substance use problems, and current thinking suggests that only a small number of adolescent heavy drinkers are likely to progress to alcohol dependence (Health Canada, 2001c). Although drinking appears to be starting at a later age than in the past (13% of 7th-grade youth), attitudes have grown increasingly tolerant of experimentation (less disapproving and more unaware of the risk), and harmful use has increased (eg, multiple substances, larger amount consumed, and more frequent use) (Health Canada, 2001c). Close to 68% of Canadian adolescents in grades 7 to 13 report drinking alcohol during the previous year, and 11% report drinking at hazardous or harmful levels (Adlaf et al., 1999). Current patterns show that the prevalence of drug use increases with age throughout adolescence, and on average, only about one third to one fourth of youth (12 to 19 years of age) do not use drugs. Alcohol remains the most commonly used substance, followed by tobacco and cannabis, and 3% to 10% of mainstream youth engage in the nonmedical use of inhalants, stimulants, cocaine, tranquilizers, and barbiturates. Among those youth who engage in illegal substance use (about one third), a striking number report problematic use (eg, attending school or playing a sport while high, or using drugs in the morning), which often results in physical injury, property damage, or engaging in unprotected sexual activity. Indeed, about one in four youth aged 15 to 19 years reports some type of harm connected to their drinking—more than double the rate for the population as a whole (Johnston, O'Malley, & Bachman, 2000). Yet, only 1% of students report having received treatment for their substance use problems in the past year.

Alcohol continues as the drug used most frequently in rural and smaller towns, and the drug use patterns remain similar to those in more urban communities, as do the reasons for using drugs (a way of coping with negative experiences). However, although it is difficult to describe the substance use patterns of youth who are on the margins of society (eg, homeless, not in school), they appear to be much higher than those for mainstream youth (Health Canada, 2001c). Indeed, evidence suggests that somewhere between 66% and more than 88% of the street youth in Canada consume alcohol or a combination of drugs (including injection).

Seniors

As harmful substance use patterns grow steadily among the young, evidence also suggests that substance use is an increasing problem among seniors (Fleming, Manwell, Barry, Adams, & Stauffacher, 1999; Health Canada, 2003b). A rapidly growing percentage of the population in Canada (19% of the population by 2021), with a growing representation of women (53% in 2000) (Statistics Canada, 2002), seniors are more susceptible to the effects of alcohol than younger adults. This is because of the physiologic changes associated with aging: an increase in the percentage of body fat, a reduction in lean body mass, and a reduction in the total volume of water in the body (less body water to dilute the alcohol) (Dufour & Fuller, 1995; Smith, 1995). Recent revisions in the recommendations about alcohol intake propose no more than one drink a day for both men and women older than 65 years (Blow et al., 2000). However, evidence suggests that approximately 11% of men and 9% of women older than 75 years exceed these recommendations (Adams, Barry, & Fleming, 1996).

Added to the problem of alcohol use is that involving prescription drug use, which is more prevalent among those older than 64 years than among younger adults (Bergob, 1994; Government of Canada, 1998). Indeed, some evidence shows that in a given month, approximately 18% of senior women and 14% of senior men commonly use three or more prescription drugs (compared with 2% of younger women and 8% of younger men) (Bergob, 1994). Less than 1% of Canadian seniors report using illegal drugs, such as marijuana, cocaine, and heroin (Health Canada, 2003b).

Adding to the problem of substance use is the evidence that seniors are less likely than younger adults to perceive their drug use as problematic (Nemes, Rao, Zeiler, Munly, Holtz, & Hoffman, 2004), possibly because individuals have not engaged in the harmful use of substances during their younger years, or because the effects of harmful use patterns, which vary somewhat for seniors, are often misattributed to aging: confusion, forgetfulness, anxiety, depression, sleep problems, injury from falls, reduction in the effectiveness of medications, conflict or withdrawal from family and friends, and improper eating habits accompanied by weight loss (Addiction Research Foundation, 1993). In addition, a number of seniors who have coped well in the past using positive strategies find themselves using substances in later years to manage the loss, or the overwhelming caregiving responsibilities, of their partners (Fleming et al., 1999). Research suggests that elders who abuse substances are at greater risk for self-neglect and may be more easily exploited and abused by others (Health Canada, 2003b). Research also indicates that victims of abuse may choose to self-medicate with drugs and alcohol.

To ensure effective treatment and rehabilitation services for seniors, the characteristics and prevalence of their substance use problems need to be carefully identified. However, health care professionals are less likely to screen seniors than younger adults for drug or alcohol abuse, which perpetuates the underdiagnosis of substance abuse in elders (Statistics Canada, 2000).

The Workplace

Two main factors make addiction a critical workplace issue. First, addiction usually strikes younger workers, and second, addictions are often chronic and cyclical in nature, requiring treatment on and off for many years (CCSA, 1999b). During a 30-day period, about 1.2% of the Canadian workforce experiences a substance abuse

---

IN A LIFE

John Alexander Macdonald (1815–1891)
Prime Minister of Canada

Public Personna
Sir John A. Macdonald, the first Prime Minister of Canada, is known as the "Father of Confederation." Emigrating to the Province of Canada from Glasgow, Scotland, he studied law in Kingston and was admitted to the Bar in 1836. As a politician, he used his diplomatic talents to create the alliances necessary for Canada to become a nation. He was the Liberal Conservative party leader (1867–1891), accomplishing the initiation of an intercolonial railway, the creation of the Northwest Mounted Police in 1873, and the creation of Canada's first National Park (Banff, Alberta) in 1885. He was knighted in 1867. John A. Macdonald died while in office, 3 months after winning his fourth consecutive election, in June 1891.

Personal Realities
John A. Macdonald married Isabella Clark in 1843. They had two sons, one who died in infancy. Isabella became an invalid, dying in 1856. In 1867 he married again to Susan Bernard. They had a daughter who suffered from "hydrocephaly" which resulted in mental and physical handicaps. He suffered from a well-publicized drinking problem as well as depression. He was known for drinking throughout meetings and parliamentary proceedings, causing him to be forgetful and at times inefficient while in office.

disorder, and a further 0.8% has a comorbid mental disorder (Dewa, Lesage, Goering, & Caveen, 2004). About one in five Canadian workers drinks at some time in the workplace, and close to 1% have used illicit drugs at work (CCSA, 1999b). Substance abuse causes workplace problems (in judgment, alertness, perception, motor coordination, and emotional state) and is a major cause of unemployment, absenteeism, and a significant number of workplace accidents (Coambs, & McAndrews, 1994)

Lower-status workers, young people, and males, along with workers in particular industries (eg, domestic work, construction, materials handling, transport, seafaring, food and beverage, brewery, journalism, mining, sales, small business, and armed forces), are particularly prone to substance use problems (Martin, Kraft, & Roman, 1994). It seems that characteristics of the work environment (eg, stress), organizational and coworker norms, and ready availability influence substance use on the job. Annual productivity losses in Canada amount to $6 billion as a result of harmful alcohol and drug use, representing 1.7% of the gross domestic product (GDP), or $414 per capita (CCSA, 1999b). Aside from the obvious health, safety, and productivity concerns, a number of other factors have prompted workplaces to view substance use as an indicator of organizational problems to take action. Government legislation (eg, labour codes) has become stronger, employers have become increasingly concerned about liability (eg, around related substance use accidents) and high-quality output and ethical standards, and workplace insurance programs have increasingly required substance abuse policy (CCSA, 1999b).

The Health Professional With Dependence Problems

Even nurses are victims of substance use problems. Although there are no accurate statistics, the prevalence of alcoholism or alcohol problems within the profession is estimated to be between 6% and 20% of the practicing population and between 3% and 5% for drug abuse (Markey & Stone, 1997). Further, nearly 70% of all disciplinary cases heard by state boards in the United States involve substance abuse (Wennerstrom & Rooda, 1996). Yet, despite these figures, the nursing literature and nursing curricula direct only minimal attention to this serious health care matter.

One of the most sensitive, and most stigmatized, aspects of substance use involves acknowledging the fact that nurses and other health professionals are not exempt from the problem (Ludwig, Marecki, Wooldridge, & Sherman, 1996). Nurses need to be alert to the indicators (absenteeism, reduced output, and accidents) that account for the billions of dollars each year in lost productivity in the Canadian workplace (Single, Robson, Xie, & Rehm, 1996). There are many opportunities for

nurses to maintain their substance use habits in the workplace. They may actively "use" before coming to work, or steal medications prescribed for clients (eg, give only half dose to clients, take the reserve from deliberately damaged narcotic vials) (Hughes, Hanscom, & Broom, 2001; Wennerstrom & Rooda, 1996).

Nurses need to reconcile the ethical dilemmas associated with confronting a colleague in need and fulfilling their professional responsibility of reporting the colleague to workplace administration or their professional regulatory body to ensure that client care is protected. In addition, nurses need to know how to assist a colleague in accessing appropriate supports (eg, confidential employee assistance programs are available in many workplaces throughout Canada). See Box 23-2 for an example of the way a colleague might be confronted.

Aboriginal Populations

Although accurate and complete data are limited regarding the prevalence of alcohol and drug consumption among the Aboriginal communities, there is a consensus among authorities that they suffer significantly higher rates of addictions than the rest of the population (Kirby

---

BOX 23.2

Confronting a Colleague

A nurse who observes performance deterioration in a colleague's practice and suspects that she has come to work under the influence of alcohol might confront the colleague with statements such as the following (Hughes et al., 2001):

I've noticed that your nursing practice has been slipping lately—and you don't seem to be as alert to client needs. In fact, you just don't seem to be yourself.... You've told me that things at home haven't been going well. I'm worried about you.... Sometimes, when *I* get to the end of my rope I find it difficult to leave my worries at home. I'm wondering if *your* worries followed *you* to work today? ... And I'm also sensing that alcohol came with you too—perhaps you hoped that it might calm your nerves enough to get through the day.... The alcohol tells me that you're not managing at all well right now and need some help. *I* am here for you.... There are also some services here at work that provide confidential help for staff. I would be willing to help you contact them—if you want.... I know you care about the clients and wouldn't purposely put them at risk—but your drinking does create a threat to their well-being. You also know, just as I do, that administration needs to be notified.... These are going to be tough calls ... but they must be made ... and if *you* are the one to make the contacts, then *you* are the one taking control, and you will be taking a first step in solving the problem. I have to make a call, but you can make your own call first, and I would be willing to support you if that would help.

& Keon, 2004). Further, the rates of fetal alcohol syndrome (and its effects) are higher among the Aboriginal community. Experts agree that although the causes of these addiction problems in Aboriginal and non-Aboriginal communities may be similar, Aboriginal communities have added cultural factors that affect individual decision making.

Addictions have been implicated as both the cause and effect of the relatively poor health of Canada's Aboriginal people since their contact began with Europeans (National Native Addictions Partnership Foundation, 2000). "The indigenous cultures simply had no protective social norms in place to moderate or set limits on the amount of alcohol consumed or to define the limits of safe, socially acceptable behaviour to accompany its use". Over the years, as their once powerful role in the economic exchange systems of early Canada was displaced through economic developments, the Aboriginal people lost their traditional economies and became particularly vulnerable to the health and social problems so characteristic of economically marginalized members of all industrialized societies—crippling alcohol and harmful substance use patterns (solvents, street drugs, prescription drugs).

In 2001, just over 1.3 million people (4.4% of the Canadian population) reported some Aboriginal ancestry (including Indian, Inuit, and Métis) (Statistics Canada, 2003). The Aboriginal community is generally younger (average age, 25 years) than their non-Aboriginal counterparts (average age, 38 years), with one third younger than the age of 15 years. Although some Aboriginal people live on designated reserves and settlements, many are integrated into non-Aboriginal communities, with about one half living in urban areas located in Northern and Prairie communities (8% in Winnipeg).

Current thinking argues that, although improving, the health of Aboriginal people in Canada is significantly poorer than that of the rest of Canadians (Health Canada, 1999a, 1999b). Further, of all the health problems seen in Aboriginal peoples, those related to substance abuse may be most reflective of the health of the community at large—a general alienation from its customs and traditions.

Although a fully accurate account of the prevalence of harmful substance use is not known, available research evidence, using both provider observations and user self-report methods, suggests that the relative numbers of alcohol users in First Nations and Inuit communities has declined substantially in recent decades, with levels well below national averages (National Native Addictions Partnership Foundation, 2000). However, among those who do abuse substances, the harmful effects have been enormous and commonplace, particularly among the youth.

Aboriginal people are significantly more likely than non-Aboriginal people to be hospitalized, four times more likely to be injured or poisoned, nearly twice as likely to die, and six to eight times more likely to complete suicide—all due to closely related impairments from alcohol or other psychoactive drugs (Single, Robson, & Scott, 1997). In addition, substance abuse plays a significant role in their criminal behaviour, both in terms of incarceration (more than 75% of Aboriginals in jail have alcohol problems) and homicide (10 times higher than the non-Aboriginal population) (Health Canada, 1999b). Although alcohol remains the primary substance of choice for 58% of Aboriginal substance users, about 20% of users choose other drugs (from which they are three times more likely to die than non-Aboriginals), and compared with the general population, Aboriginals are significantly more likely to use multiple drugs (46% of substance users in treatment centres in Saskatchewan).

Concurrent Disorders

Many substance-dependent people have concurrent mental disorders. Also known as dual disorders, dual diagnosis, and comorbid substance abuse disorders and mental disorders (Centre for Addiction and Mental Health, 2005), the term concurrent mental disorder can be defined as the coexistence of at least one mental disorder and at least one substance of abuse or dependence, as defined by the *DSM-IV-TR* (Health Canada, 2002a). Some disorders are in part a by-product of long-term substance dependence; others predispose the individual to alcohol or drug abuse. For example, alcohol dependence is 21 times more likely to occur among people with antisocial personality disorders and 4 times more likely among people with schizophrenia; and among those treated for alcohol-related disorders, up to 70% to 80% may have a mental disorder (Health Canada, 2002a). Whatever the reason, nurses should be aware that clients with substance dependence often have anxiety disorders, phobias, or obsessive-compulsive and affective disorders, such as major depression and dysthymia (Fu et al., 2002). Other coexisting mental disorders include attention-deficit hyperactivity disorder and personality disorders (Rosenthal & Westreich, 1999). These are discussed in detail in Chapters 24 and 27. Nurses need to remember that clients do not compartmentalize their problems, so health professionals should not either (Health Canada, 2002a).

Alcohol, and drug-dependent individuals are at high risk for death caused by drug overdose but are also at increased risk for death by other causes, including homicide, suicide, and opportunistic infections, such as HIV, secondary to drug injection practices (Selwyn & Merino, 1997). Studies have documented the connection between alcohol dependence and increased risk for a variety of other illnesses (Health Canada, 1996), including for example, diabetes mellitus, gastrointestinal problems, hypertension, liver disease, and stroke (U.S. DHHS, 1997b); cocaine use and increased risk for cardiovascular complications; and intoxication and increased risk for traumatic injury from vehicular crashes or other injuries (Caulker-Burnett, 1994).

ETIOLOGY

Researchers have long asked what causes addictive behaviour and why some people feel compelled to keep using substances they know are harmful. Growing evidence suggests both psychological and biologic bases of addiction, which may explain this apparently self-destructive behaviour. Although genetic evidence indicates that there is a familial predisposition toward addiction (Fu et al., 2002), a common genetic marker has not been found. Evidence of neurochemical, neurophysiologic, and psychopharmacologic mechanisms common to alcohol and other drug addiction have been found (Fig. 23-1).

Genetic Factors

Most of the data regarding substance dependence are from the alcoholism studies and suggest the influence of genetic factors in its development. Genetic studies primarily focus on families, twins, and adoption and seek a baseline trait marker of alcoholism. The reported prevalence of substance abuse among biologic family members differs from study to study. However, the likelihood of addiction is associated with biologic relatedness, and this association decreases as biologic distance increases (Hesselbrock, Hesselbrock, & Epstein, 1999).

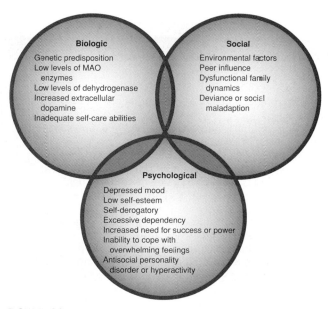

FIGURE 23.1 Biopsychosocial etiologies for clients with substance abuse.

Other important studies in determining genetic predisposition are adoption studies in which rates of alcoholism were evaluated in children of parents with alcoholism who were raised by adoptive parents. One landmark study evaluated individuals raised apart from their biologic parents, comparing those who had a biologic parent with alcoholism with those who were raised by an adoptive parent with alcoholism. Those who had a biologic parent with severe alcoholism were significantly more likely to experience alcoholism than were those being raised by an adoptive parent with alcoholism (Schuckit, Goodwin, & Winokur, 1972). Another early adoption study in Denmark found that sons of parents with alcoholism were about four times more likely to experience alcoholism than were control subjects (sons of parents without alcoholism), regardless of who raised them (Goodwin, 1979). Recently Fu and colleagues (2002) explored the possibility that the risks for alcohol dependence, marijuana dependence, depression, and antisocial personality disorder might share a genetic basis.

Controversy surrounding the search for a specific gene that could cause alcoholism and other drug dependencies centers on an allele of dopamine receptor D2 that appeared to be implicated in severe cases of alcoholism and some other substance use disorders (Anthenelli & Schuckit, 1997). Although some data suggest nonspecific genetic markers in alcoholism risk, these data are not conclusive (Vanyukov, 1999).

Neurobiologic Theories

Some studies suggest that drugs of abuse reinforce dependence by stimulating future use through a biologic brain reward mechanism, whereby the regions in the brain that primarily are stimulated are responsible for drug dependencies (Schuckit, 1999). Often, a compelling urge to use alcohol or other drugs dominates an addict's thoughts and affects the addict's mood and behaviour (Goldstein & Volkow, 2002). This urge is defined as **craving**.

Intoxication with drugs, such as cocaine, phencyclidine, alcohol, nicotine, and various opiates, increases extracellular levels of dopamine. This dopamine-related "high" becomes the reinforcement mechanism in the brain. The neurochemical status in the brain readjusts to these increased levels of dopamine as being the "normal" neurochemical state; the user then requires increased amounts of substances to produce the same dopamine-related effects (Goldstein & Volkow, 2002). This need for increased amounts of a substance to achieve the same results is termed **tolerance**. This readjustment of the "normal" neurochemical homeostasis may explain the **anhedonia** (diminished enjoyment of life) that occurs in long-term cocaine users when they discontinue use.

These neurobiologic theories are further substantiated by animal behavioural studies indicating that both animals and humans self-administer substances in similar patterns, producing addictive behaviour. Animals prefer to self-administer drugs, rather than eat, drink water, or rest, even to the point of death (Gardner, 1997). Another study showed that animals will work for injections of alcohol and other drugs that are administered to specific areas in the brain that cause craving but not for drugs administered to areas of the brain unrelated to craving (Miller & Gold, 1994).

Psychological Theories

The psychological theories support the notion that some individuals are born with personality traits that make them more susceptible to substance abuse; some call it an "addictive personality." One researcher identified five psychosocial needs common to those who become addicted: need to feel self-worth, need to have control over the environment, need to feel intimate contact with others, need to accomplish something valuable, and need to eliminate pain or other powerful negative feelings (Peele, 1985). Another identified six psychodynamic issues that often lead to substance abuse: excessive dependency needs, need for success or power, inability to care for self adequately, gender identity problems, inability to cope with overwhelming painful feelings, and dysfunctional family dynamics (Kaufman, 1994). See Table 23-2.

Behavioural Theories

Many investigators have turned their attention to the behavioural characteristics of childhood and adolescence that might predispose a person to substance abuse. Some have postulated that conduct problems of childhood,

such as deviance, misbehaviour, and aggression, might be important behavioural risk factors for later substance abuse, particularly for boys. A few convincing studies demonstrate a strong connection between childhood conduct problems, hyperactivity, impulsivity, and future substance abuse (Brehm & Khantzian, 1997). A history of general deviance or social maladaption in the form of police trouble or long-standing behavioural problems has been linked to risk for developing drug dependence.

Social Theories

Many studies focussed on peer drug use and affiliation with troubled peers as strong determinants of teenage drug involvement (Chassin et al., 1993; Hawkins, Catalano, & Miller, 1992). Peer interaction is a crucial influencing factor in determining adolescents' exposure to alcohol and drugs (Hesselbrock et al., 1999). The proportion of users versus non users (peers) (Health Canada, 2001b) and peers' perceptions of alcohol use as being a useful way of reducing tension and other alleged positive attributes contribute to their increased use (Segal & Stewart, 1996).

Certain neighbourhood characteristics may also be factors in increased drug abuse, including high population density, physical deterioration, high levels of crime, and illegal drug trafficking (Hesselbrock et al., 1999). These social factors may increase an individual's feeling of alienation, leading to escapist and other deviant behaviour (Segal & Stewart, 1996).

Summary of Etiologic Theories

The modern disease model of substance abuse is truly a biopsychosocial one—it encompasses the body, the

Table 23.2	Psychological Issues Leading to Substance Abuse
Issue	**Psychodynamics**
Excessive dependence needs	Excessive dependence needs lead to rejection and a sense of failure. Resulting anxiety is relieved by substance abuse.
Need for success or power	Excessive fear of success or failure or appearing weak or challenged. Substance abuse can provide temporary illusion of adequacy and power.
Inadequate self-care abilities	Individual has inadequate abilities to self-regulate or self-soothe, or has low self-esteem. Substance abuse provides temporary resolution of psychological pain.
Gender identity issues	Males more socialized to externalize stress and feelings by drinking alcohol and using drugs. Women are more socialized to "treat" feelings of low self-esteem with alcohol or other drugs.
Affect intolerance	Overwhelming painful feelings from childhood that cannot be tolerated or discussed. Individual may be able to express these feelings when intoxicated.
Family systems	Symbolic fusion with parent, failure to separate from parent and develop own self-identity during adolescence can lead to a too rigid or too flexible bonding with substance-abusing peers, leaving individual vulnerable to peer pressure to drink and use drugs.

Adapted from Kaufman, F. (1994). *Psychotherapy of addicted persons*. New York: Guilford Press.

mind, and social and environmental influences in studying the disease and formulating treatment (Health Canada, 2003a; Wallace, 1990). Recent biologic studies in humans and animals have confirmed a genetic predisposition underpinning drinking behaviours and significant genetic differences in self-administration for several other drugs, yet no precise genetic marker has been established. Recent evidence from genetics, neurochemistry, and pharmacology has revealed the essential biologic component of alcoholism—that it is a chronic and progressive disease that must be treated. This disease is influenced not just by the biologic components but also by the individual's temperament and feelings about self (psychological components) and environmental factors, such as parental and family relationships as well as peer pressure in the school or workplace (social components). To understand and treat substance-dependent people, nurses must understand and treat all facets of this illness.

ALCOHOL

Most Canadians drink alcohol. Reliable surveys indicate that 90% of adult Canadians have had a drink. According to the most comprehensive data, only about 17% of the population are high-risk drinkers, yet 80% or more of the alcohol consumed in Canada is consumed by these high-risk drinkers (Statistics Canada, 2004). Alcohol (or ethanol) is a sedative anaesthetic found in various proportions in liquor, wine, and beer. Alcohol produces a sedative effect by depressing the central nervous system (CNS). This effect causes the individual to experience relaxed inhibitions, heightened emotions, mood swings that can range from bouts of gaiety to angry outbursts, and cognitive impairments such as reduced concentration or attention span, and impaired judgment and memory. Depending on the amount of alcohol ingested, the effects can range from feelings of mild sedation and relaxation, to confusion and serious impairment of motor functions and speech, to severe intoxication that can result in coma, respiratory failure, and death. See Table 23-3 for a summary of the effects of abused substances.

The intensity of CNS impairments depends on how much alcohol is consumed in a given period of time and how rapidly the body metabolizes it. Intoxication is determined by the level of alcohol in the blood, called *blood alcohol level* (BAL). The body can metabolize 1 oz of liquor, a 5-oz glass of wine, or a 12-oz can of beer per hour without intoxication.

Excessive or long-term abuse of alcohol can adversely affect all body systems, and the effects can be serious and permanent. Years of alcohol abuse can cause cerebellar degeneration from increased levels of acetaldehyde, a toxic by-product of alcohol metabolism, and can result in impaired coordination, a broad-based

unsteady gait, and fine tremors. Sedative-hypnotic long-term effects include disturbances in rapid-eye-movement (REM) sleep and chronic sleep disorders. Although certain alcohol-related cognitive impairment is reversible with abstinence, long-term alcohol abuse can cause specific neurologic complications that lead to organic brain disorders, known as alcohol-induced amnestic disorders (discussed later).

People who abuse alcohol can exhibit various patterns of use. Some engage in heavy drinking on a regular or daily basis; others may abstain from drinking during the week and engage in heavy drinking on the weekends; still others can experience longer periods of sobriety interspersed with bouts of binge drinking (several days of intoxication).

Thus, all clients should be screened not only for alcohol use disorders, but also for drinking patterns or behaviours that may place them at increased risk for experiencing adverse health effects or alcoholism. Risky (binge) drinkers who have not yet become alcohol dependent often can be treated successfully within a primary care setting (Ballesteros, Gonzalez-Pinto, Querajeta, & Cerino, 2004). According to Canada's Drug Strategy (Government of Canada, 1998), to be effective, prevention, treatment, and rehabilitation programs must consider the determinants of health and address the underlying factors associated with alcohol abuse.

Biologic Responses to Alcohol

Alcohol makes the neuronal membranes more permeable to potassium (K^+) and chloride (Cl^-) and closes sodium (Na^+) and calcium (Ca^{++}) channels. This increased permeability depresses the CNS, and adrenergic activity raises blood pressure and heart rate. Alcohol is metabolized in the liver as a carbohydrate into carbon dioxide and water. The breakdown process (oxidation) of the compound ethanol (CH_3CH_2OH) is: ethanol → acetaldehyde + water → acetic acid → carbon dioxide + water. Acetaldehyde is toxic and is usually broken down by acetaldehyde dehydrogenase. Rapid alcohol intake can cause an accumulation of acetaldehyde, which then combines with the neurotransmitters dopamine and serotonin to produce tetrahydroisoquinolines and β-carbolines. Physical dependence on alcohol becomes a problem when CNS cells require alcohol to function normally (Moak & Anton, 1999).

People who have abused alcohol for long periods of time often experience alcohol tolerance, a phenomenon producing a more rapid metabolism of alcohol and decreased response to sedating, motor, and anxiolytic effects. These individuals may demonstrate higher blood alcohol levels than normal before they experience symptoms of intoxication. The locus ceruleus, a brain structure that normally inhibits the action of ethanol, is

Table 23.3 Summary of Effects of Abused Substances, Overdose, Withdrawal Syndromes, and Prolonged Use

Substance	Route	Effects (E) and Overdose (O)	Withdrawal Syndrome	Prolonged Use
Alcohol	Oral	E: Sedation, decreased inhibitions, relaxation, decreased coordination, slurred speech, nausea O: Respiratory depression, cardiac arrest	Tremors; seizures, increased temperature; pulse, and blood pressure; delirium tremens	Affects all systems of the body. Can lead to other dependencies.
Stimulants (amphetamines, cocaine)	Oral, IV, inhalation, smoking	E: Euphoria, initial CNS stimulation then depression, wakefulness, decreased appetite, insomnia, paranoia, aggressiveness, dilated pupils, tremors O: Cardiac arrhythmias/arrest, increased or lowered blood pressure, respiratory depression, chest pain, vomiting, seizures, psychosis, confusion, seizures, dyskinesias, dystonias, coma	Depression: psychomotor retardation at first, then agitation; fatigue then insomnia; severe dysphoria and anxiety; cravings, vivid, unpleasant dreams; increased appetite. Amphetamine withdrawal is not as pronounced as cocaine withdrawal.	Is often alternated with depressants. Weight loss and resulting malnutrition and increased susceptibility to infectious diseases. May produce schizophrenia-like syndrome with paranoid ideation, thought disturbance, hallucinations, and stereotyped movements
Cannabis (marijuana, hashish, THC)	Smoking, oral	E: Euphoria or dysphoria, relaxation and drowsiness, heightened perception of colour and sound, poor coordination, spatial perception and time distortion, unusual body sensations (weightlessness, tingling, etc.), dry mouth, dysarthria, and food cravings O: Increased heart rate, reddened eyes, dysphoria, lability, disorientation		Can decrease motivation and cause cognitive deficits (inability to concentrate, memory impairment).
Hallucinogens (LSD, MDMA)	Oral	E: Euphoria or dysphoria, altered body image, distorted or sharpened visual and auditory perception, depersonalization, bizarre behaviour, confusion, incoordination, impaired judgment and memory, signs of sympathetic and parasympathetic stimulation, palpitations (blurred vision, dilated pupils, sweating) O: Paranoia, ideas of reference, fear of losing one's mind, depersonalization, derealization, illusions, hallucinations, synesthesia, self-destructive/aggressive behaviour, tremors		"Flashbacks" or HPPD may occur after termination of use.
Phencyclidine (PCP)	Oral, inhalation, smoking	E: Feeling superhuman, decreased awareness of and detachment from the environment, stimulation of the respiratory and cardiovascular system, ataxia, dysarthria, decreased pain perception O: Hallucinations, paranoia, psychosis, aggression, adrenergic crisis (cardiac failure, CVA, malignant hyperthermia, status epilepticus, severe muscle contractions)		"Flashbacks," HPPD, organic brain syndromes with recurrent psychotic behaviour, which can last up to 6 months after not using the drug, numerous psychiatric hospitalizations and police arrests.
Opiates (heroin, codeine)	Oral, injection, smoking	E: Euphoria, sedation, reduced libido, memory and concentration difficulties, analgesia, constipation, constricted pupils O: Respiratory depression, stupor, coma	Abdominal cramps, rhinorrhea, watery eyes, dilated pupils, yawning, "goose flesh," diaphoresis, nausea, diarrhea, anorexia, insomnia, fever	Can lead to criminal behaviour to get money for drugs, risk for infection related to needle use (eg, HIV, endocarditis, hepatitis).

Substance	Route	Effects	Withdrawal	Consequences
Sedatives, hypnotics, anxiolytics	Oral, injection	E: Euphoria, sedation, reduced libido, emotional lability, impaired judgment O: Respiratory depression, cardiac arrest	Anxiety rebound and agitation, hypertension, tachycardia, sweating, hyperpyrexia, sensory excitement, motor excitation, insomnia, possible tonic–clonic convulsions, nightmares, delirium, depersonalization, hallucinations	Often alternated with stimulants, use with alcohol enhances chance of overdose, risk for infection related to needle use.
Inhalants (glue, lighter fluid)	Inhalation	E: Euphoria, giddiness, excitation O: CNS depression: ataxia, nystagmus, dysarthria, coma and convulsions	Similar to alcohol but milder, with anxiety, tremors, hallucinations, and sleep disturbance as the primary symptoms	Long-term use can lead to liver and renal failure, blood dyscrasias, damage to the lungs. CNS damage (OBS, peripheral neuropathies, cerebral and optic atrophy, parkinsonism).
Nicotine	Smoking	E: Stimulation, enhanced performance and alertness, and appetite suppression O: Anxiety	Mood changes (craving, anxiety) and physiologic changes (poor concentration, sleep disturbances, headaches, gastric distress, and increased appetite)	Increased chance for cardiac disease and lung disease.
Caffeine	Oral	E: Stimulation, increased mental acuity, inexhaustability O: Restlessness, nervousness, excitement, insomnia, flushing, diuresis, gastrointestinal distress, muscle twitching, rambling flow of thought and speech, tachycardia or cardiac arrhythmia, agitation	Headache, drowsiness, fatigue, craving, impaired psychomotor performance, difficulty concentrating, yawning, nausea	Physical consequences are under investigation.

CNS, central nervous system; CVA, cerebrovascular accident; GI, gastrointestinal; HIV, human immunodeficiency virus; HPPD, hallucinogen persisting perceptual disorder; OBS, organic brain syndrome.

believed to be instrumental in the development of alcohol tolerance.

Alcohol Withdrawal Syndrome

Alcohol withdrawal syndrome, which occurs after alcohol consumption is reduced or when abstaining from alcohol after prolonged use, causes changes in vital signs, diaphoresis, and gastrointestinal and CNS adverse effects. The severity of withdrawal symptoms ranges from mild to severe, depending on the length and amount of alcohol use. Symptoms include increased heart rate and blood pressure, diaphoresis, mild anxiety, restlessness, and hand tremors (Table 23-4). In clients with alcoholism or in chronic drinkers, the alcohol withdrawal syndrome usually begins within 12 hours after abrupt discontinuation or attempt to decrease consumption. Only 5% of individuals with alcohol dependence ever experience severe complications of withdrawal, such as **delirium tremens** or grand mal (tonic–clonic) seizures (Miller, Gold, & Smith, 1997).

CRNE Note

Alcohol abuse continues to require nursing assessment and interventions in all settings (home, community, ambulatory, inpatient, and long-term settings alike). Nurses who are open to the possibility that no client is too young or too old, too healthy or too infirm, or too poor or too wealthy to have substance use problems (smoking, alcohol, prescription drugs, licit and illicit drugs) are well positioned to detect areas of potential or actual need. Clients who abuse alcohol for long periods of time are at high risk for delirium tremens. Observing for signs of seizure activity is a priority nursing intervention.

Alcohol-Induced Amnesic Disorders

Alcohol is directly toxic to the brain, causing atrophy of the frontal cortex and eventually chronic brain syndrome. Clients with alcohol-induced amnesic disorders usually have a history of many years of heavy alcohol use and are generally older than 40 years. Symptom onset can be gradual or develop over many years. Impairment can be severe, and once the disorder is established, it can persist indefinitely.

Wernicke's syndrome is caused by thiamine deficiency and is not exclusive to alcoholism. Wernicke's encephalopathy manifests with oculomotor dysfunctions (bilateral abducens nerve palsy), ataxia, and confusion. Glucose administration can precipitate Wernicke's encephalopathy. Encephalopathy often evolves when thiamine deficiency is chronic and untreated. **Korsakoff's psychosis,** also known as alcohol amnestic disorder, is characterized by both retrograde and anterograde amnesia with sparing of intellectual function. Confabulation is a key feature. As many as one half of clients with Korsakoff's psychosis do not experience significant improvement even if alcohol is no longer used (Miller et al., 1997).

Psychopharmacology

Several medications can help an individual overcome the symptoms of alcohol withdrawal: benzodiazepines; long-acting CNS depressants, which produce sedation and reduce anxiety symptoms; and neuroleptic drugs, such as risperidone (Risperdal) or other antipsychotic agents, if hallucinations or disorientation should occur. Antianxiety and sedating drugs, such benzodiazepines, are useful when substituted for the shorter-acting drug alcohol. Benzodiazepines usually are administered based on elevations in heart rate, blood pressure, and temperature

Table 23.4	Alcohol Withdrawal Syndrome		
	Stage I: Mild	**Stage II: Moderate**	**Stage III: Severe**
Vital signs	Heart rate elevated, temperature elevated, normal or slightly elevated systolic blood pressure	Heart rate 100–120 bpm; elevated systolic blood pressure and temperature	Heart rate, 120–140 bpm; elevated systolic and diastolic blood pressures; elevated temperature
Diaphoresis	Slightly	Usually obvious	Marked
Central nervous system	Oriented, no confusion, no hallucinations	Intermittent confusion; transient visual and auditory hallucinations and illusions, mostly at night	Marked disorientation, confusion, disturbing visual and auditory hallucinations, misidentification of objects, delusions related to the hallucinations, delirium tremens, disturbances in consciousness
	Mild anxiety and restlessness	Painful anxiety and motor restlessness	Agitation, extreme restlessness, and panic states
	Restless sleep	Insomnia and nightmares	Unable to sleep
	Hand tremors, "shakes," no convulsions	Visible tremulousness, rare convulsions	Gross uncontrollable tremors, convulsions common
Gastrointestinal system	Impaired appetite, nausea	Anorexia, nausea, and vomiting	Rejecting all fluid and food

and on the presence of tremors. Clients can be given 5 to 10 mg of diazepam (Valium) every 2 to 4 hours, or 25 to 100 mg of chlordiazepoxide hydrochloride (Librium) every 4 hours. Medication given early in the course of withdrawal and in sufficient dosages can prevent the development of delirium tremens. Should withdrawal delirium occur, higher doses are used, with careful monitoring of the client to prevent overdose. These drugs are also extremely effective during withdrawal as anticonvulsants because they act more rapidly than phenytoin (Dilantin), which can take 7 to 10 days to reach therapeutic levels. Seizures, if they occur, usually do so within the first 48 hours of withdrawal.

Disulfiram is not a treatment or cure for alcoholism, but it can be used as adjunct therapy to help deter some individuals from drinking while using other treatment modalities to teach new coping skills to alter abuse behaviours. Disulfiram prevents alcohol use by causing an adverse reaction (including flushing, nausea, vomiting, and diarrhoea) to alcohol consumption, which is mediated by inhibition of acetaldehyde dehydrogenase. However, in a Veterans Administration multisite study, abstinence rates were no better in the disulfiram group than in control subjects, although a subgroup of socially stable older clients who relapsed drank less if they were assigned to the disulfiram group (Kristenson, 1995). Because other evidence supports its efficacy in decreasing alcohol intake, disulfiram may be useful in carefully selected clients provided with appropriate counselling, although adverse effects, such as hepatotoxicity and neuropathy, and potentially severe interactions with alcohol limit its widespread use (O'Connor & Schottenfeld, 1998).

Naltrexone was originally used as a treatment for heroin abuse, but it has been approved for treatment of alcohol dependence and targets alcohol's effects on the brain. One study has shown that high doses of naltrexone and alcohol produced the greatest decreases in liking alcohol. The findings support the role of endogenous opioids as determinants of alcohol's effects and suggest that naltrexone may be particularly useful in clients who continue to drink heavily (McCaul, Wand, Eissenberg, Rohde, & Cheskin, 2000).

In various treatment programs, naltrexone decreased drinking rates, prolonged abstinence, and hindered relapse to uncontrolled drinking among abstinent clients with alcoholism who sampled alcohol during treatment. Targeted use of naltrexone also may be effective for decreasing alcohol consumption levels among problem drinkers who do not have alcoholism (NIAAA, 2002b).

Adequate Nutrition and Supplemental Vitamins

Poor nutrition and vitamin deficiencies are often symptoms of alcohol dependence. Multivitamins and adequate nutrition are essential for clients who are severely malnourished, but other vitamin replacements may be necessary for certain individuals. Thiamine (vitamin B_1) may be needed when a client is in withdrawal, to decrease ataxia and other symptoms of deficiency. It is usually given orally, 100 mg four times daily, but can be given intramuscularly or by intravenous infusion with glucose. Folic acid deficiency is corrected with administration of 1.0 mg orally, four times daily. Magnesium deficiency also is found in those with long-term alcohol dependence. Magnesium sulfate, which enhances the body's response to thiamine and reduces seizures, is given prophylactically for clients with histories of withdrawal seizures. The usual dose is 1.0 g intramuscularly, four times daily for 2 days.

COCAINE

Cocaine is a powerful stimulant; its use in Canada had dropped to 0.7% in 1994 from 1.4% in 1989 (Government of Canada, 1998). Cocaine is an alkaloid found in the leaves of the *Erythroxylon coca* plant that is native to western South America, where for hundreds of years natives have known the powerful intoxicating effects of chewing the coca leaves. Cocaine is made from the leaves into a coca paste that is refined into cocaine hydrochloride, a crystalline form (white powder appearance), which is commonly inhaled or "snorted" in the nose, injected intravenously (with water), or smoked. The smokable form of cocaine, often called *free-base cocaine*, can be made by mixing the crystalline cocaine with ether or sodium hydroxide.

After cocaine is inhaled or injected, the user experiences a sudden burst of mental alertness and energy ("cocaine rush") and feelings of self-confidence, being in control, and sociability, which last 10 to 20 minutes. This high is followed by an intense let-down effect ("cocaine crash"), in which the person feels irritable, depressed, and tired, and craves more of the drug. Although it has not been proved that cocaine is physically addictive, it is clear that users experience a serious psychological addiction and pattern of abuse. Although cocaine users typically report that the drug enhances their feelings of well-being and reduces anxiety, cocaine also is known to bring on panic attacks in some individuals. Studies have also shown that long-term cocaine use leads to increased anxiety. Severe anxiety, along with restlessness and agitation, are also among the major symptoms of cocaine withdrawal. Research also suggests that there could be a different aspect to anxiety, and stress may be among the factors that lead to cocaine use (Bowersox, 1996). Users quickly seek more cocaine or other drugs, such as alcohol, marijuana, or sleeping pills, to rid themselves of the terrible effects of crashing. Withdrawal causes intense depression, craving, and drug-seeking behaviour that may last for weeks. Individuals who discontinue cocaine use often relapse.

Crack cocaine, often called "crack," is a form of free-base cocaine produced by mixing the crystal with water and baking soda or sodium bicarbonate and boiling it until a rock precipitant remains. The hardened crystal is then broken into pieces ("cracked") and smoked in cigarettes or water pipes. This extremely potent form produces a rapid high and intense euphoria and an even more dramatic crash. It is extremely addictive because of the intense and rapid onset of euphoric effects, which leave users craving more.

Cocaine emerged as the popular drug of the 1990s and was characterized as the drug of the wealthy, the young and upwardly mobile professionals or celebrities, and those in high-profile social circles. Then crack cocaine emerged as a cheap street drug, and it became available to all socioeconomic circles. Crack quickly became one of the leading addictive drugs of the 1990s, causing serious national health concerns.

Biologic Responses to Cocaine

Cocaine is absorbed rapidly through the blood–brain barrier and is readily absorbed through the skin and mucous membranes. Cocaine acts as a potent local anaesthetic when applied directly to tissue, preventing both the generation and conduction of nerve impulses by inhibiting the rapid influx of sodium ions through the nerve membrane. Peak intoxication occurs rapidly with intravenous injection or inhalation. Injecting releases the drug directly into the bloodstream and heightens the intensity of its effects. Smoking entails inhalation of cocaine vapour or smoke into the lungs, where absorption into the bloodstream is as rapid as by injection (NIDA, 1999). The resulting increased levels of dopamine in the synaptic cleft cause euphoria and, in excess, psychotic symptoms. Dopamine and dopamine metabolite levels are depleted by prolonged cocaine use. This absence of dopamine (which normally inhibits prolactin secretion) increases prolactin levels in the blood. Cocaine use increases norepinephrine levels in the blood, causing tachycardia, hypertension, dilated pupils, and rising body temperatures. Dopamine and dopamine metabolite levels are depleted by prolonged cocaine use. Serotonin excess contributes to sleep disturbances and anorexia.

New research shows that even a single injection of cocaine induces a long-acting increase in excitatory synaptic transmission in the ventral tegmental area of the brain in rats and mice. This increase has many similarities to the changes in neural activity involved in learning and memory processes in many areas of the brain. This single dose of cocaine "usurped" a cellular mechanism normally involved in an adaptive learning process, which could help explain cocaine's ability to take control of incentive-motivational systems in the brain and produce compulsive drug-seeking behaviour (NIDA, 2001).

Cocaine Intoxication

Intoxication causes CNS stimulation, the length of which depends on the dose and route of administration. With steadily increasing doses, restlessness proceeds to tremors and agitation, followed by convulsions and CNS depression. In lethal overdose, death generally results from respiratory failure. A toxic psychosis is also possible and may be accompanied by physical signs of CNS stimulation (tachycardia, hypertension, cardiac arrhythmias, sweating, hyperpyrexia, and convulsions) (NIDA, 1999).

Research has revealed a potential dangerous interaction between cocaine and alcohol. Taken in combination, the two drugs are converted by the body to cocaethylene, which has a longer duration of action in the brain and is more toxic than either drug alone. Notably, this mixture of cocaine and alcohol is the most common two-drug combination that results in drug-related death (NIDA, 2002).

Cocaine Withdrawal

Long-term cocaine use depletes norepinephrine, resulting in the "crash" when use of the drug is discontinued and causing the user to sleep 12 to 18 hours. Upon awakening, withdrawal symptoms may occur, characterized by sleep disturbances with rebound REM sleep, anergia (lack of energy), decreased libido, depression with possible suicidality, anhedonia, poor concentration, and cocaine craving (Weaver & Schnoll, 1999). Treating cocaine addiction is complex and involves assessing the psychobiological, social, and pharmacologic aspects of abuse. Several new drugs are being investigated for treating cocaine addiction. One of the most promising, selegiline, was in multisite phase III clinical trials during 1999, administered by both transdermal patch and a time-release pill. However, after a review of the studies to date, there is no current evidence supporting the clinical use of antidepressants, carbamazepine, disulfiram, or lithium in treating cocaine dependence (DeLima, deOlivera Soceres, Reisser, & Farrell, 2002).

CRNE Note

In cocaine withdrawal, clients are excessively sleepy because of the norepinephrine depletion. Recovery is difficult because of the intense cravings. Nursing interventions should focus on helping clients use practical strategies to solve problems related to managing these cravings.

AMPHETAMINES AND OTHER STIMULANTS

Amphetamines were first synthesized for medical use in the 1880s. Amphetamines (eg, Biphetamine, Delcobase,

Dexedrine, Obetrol) and other stimulants, such as phenmetrazine (Preludin) and methylphenidate (Ritalin), act on the CNS and peripheral nervous system. They are used to treat attention-deficit hyperactivity disorder in children, narcolepsy, depression, and obesity (on a short-term basis). Some people engage in harmful use of these drugs to achieve the effects of alertness, increased concentration, a sense of increased energy, euphoria, and appetite suppression. Amphetamines are indirect catecholamine agonists and cause the release of newly synthesized norepinephrine. Like cocaine, they block the reuptake of norepinephrine and dopamine, but they do not affect the serotonergic system as strongly. They also affect the peripheral nervous system and are powerful sympathomimetics, stimulating both α and β receptors. This stimulation results in tachycardia, arrhythmias, increased systolic and diastolic blood pressures, and peripheral hyperthermia (Weaver & Schnoll, 1999). The effects of amphetamine use and the clinical course of an overdose are similar to those of cocaine. Amphetamine abuse may be treated with pharmacologic agents similar to those used for cocaine, such as antidepressants and dopaminergic agonists. Amphetamine withdrawal symptoms are not as pronounced as those of cocaine withdrawal.

CANNABIS (MARIJUANA)

Marijuana is often classified as a hallucinogenic drug, but its effects are usually not as dramatic or as intense as those of other hallucinogens. Marijuana is usually smoked and causes relaxation, euphoria, at times dyscoria (abnormal pupillary reaction or shape), spatial misperception, time distortion, and food cravings. It causes relaxation and drowsiness, unlike other hallucinogens, and is often associated with decreased motivation after long-term use. Effects begin immediately after the drug enters the brain and last from 1 to 3 hours.

Marijuana is a legal drug in Canada governed by the Controlled Substances Act (2001), available for those who have a terminal illness or serious medical condition, and for symptoms associated with certain serious medical conditions (Health Canada, 2003a). It remains the most commonly used drug of all drugs that are used illegally (Health Canada, 2000). According to Canada's Addiction Survey (Statistics Canada, 2004), marijuana use has generally remained fairly stable: approximately 44.5% for lifetime use and approximately 14% for past year use—with 1 in 20 Canadians reporting a cannabis-related concern. Student surveys reflect higher marijuana use rates: rates of past year use vary from 16% to 38%, but near 70% for lifetime use among 18- to 24-year-old youth. Marijuana cultivation continues to spread throughout the country, and the exportation of Canadian marijuana to the United States is increasing (RCMP, 2003).

A drug is addicting if it causes compulsive, often uncontrollable drug craving, seeking, and use, even in the face of negative health and social consequences. Marijuana meets this criterion. In addition, animal studies suggest marijuana causes physical dependence, and according to the 2000 National Household Survey on Drug Abuse (NHSDA) report, some people report withdrawal symptoms, including irritability, difficulty sleeping, and increased anxiety. They also display increased aggression, which peaks about 1 week after last use.

Marijuana's active ingredient is D-9-tetrahydrocannabinol (THC). Marijuana is the common name for the plant *Cannabis sativae*, also known as hemp. Hashish, the resin found in flowers of the mature *C. sativae* plant, is its strongest form, containing 10% to 30% THC. Marijuana is fat soluble and is absorbed rapidly after being smoked or taken orally. After ingestion, THC binds with an opioid receptor in the brain—the μ receptor. This action engages endogenous brain opioid receptors, which are associated with enhanced dopamine activity because THC blocks dopamine reuptake (Stephens, 1999). THC can be stored for weeks in fat tissue and in the brain and is released extremely slowly. Long-term use leads to the accumulation of cannabinoids in the body, primarily the frontal cortex, the limbic areas, and the brain's auditory and visual perception centres. In other areas of the brain, it exerts cardiovascular effects, results in ataxia, and causes increased psychotropic effects. Marijuana use impairs the ability to form memories, recall events, and shift attention from one thing to another. It disrupts coordination of movement, balance, and reaction time. Studies show that 6% to 11% of fatal accident victims have positive THC test results (NIDA, 2000).

Controversy surrounds the use and effects of marijuana both in the medical world and in legal circles. Some evidence suggests that marijuana can be useful in the medical treatment of certain disorders. Marijuana has been used successfully to treat epilepsy, postoperative pain, headache and other types of pain, asthma, glaucoma, muscle spasms in people with cerebral palsy, and poor appetite in clients with cancer and weight loss or chemotherapy-related nausea and vomiting. Some believe that legitimizing the use of marijuana for medical reasons in Canada has legitimized its use for recreational purposes as well.

Supporters actively engage in research around the medicinal effects of marijuana (eg, investigating its effects on pain associated with multiple sclerosis and other forms of severe pain). However, others are busy trying to document its alleged negative effects. For example, some believe that marijuana produces amotivational syndrome, described as changes in personality involving, for example, motivation, personality, and cognition (NIDA, 2002). Marijuana likely does not directly cause motivational problems: rather, it may interact with predisposing personality characteristics in some individuals to produce this clinical phenomenon (Stephens, 1999). Some researchers attribute this syndrome to the long-term effects of THC on the brain and to the slow release of stored THC in fat tissue. Others maintain that heavy marijuana use has no effect on motivation, learning, or perception and that these characteristics are not the result of marijuana use but rather are part of the causes.

HALLUCINOGENS

The term **hallucinogen** refers to drugs that produce euphoria or dysphoria, altered body image, distorted or sharpened visual and auditory perception, confusion, incoordination, and impaired judgment and memory. Severe reactions may cause paranoia, fear of losing one's mind, depersonalization, illusions, delusions, and hallucinations. Hallucinogens typically affect the autonomic and regulatory nervous systems first, increasing heart rate and body temperature and slightly elevating blood pressure. The individual may experience dry mouth, dizziness, and subjective feelings of being hot or cold. Gradually, the physiologic changes fade, and perceptual distortions and hallucinations become prominent (Stephens, 1999). Intense mood and sexual behaviour changes may occur; the user may feel unusually close to others or distant and isolated. The true content of hallucinogenic drugs purchased on the street is always in doubt; they are often misidentified or adulterated with other drugs.

There are more than 100 different hallucinogens with substantially different molecular structures. Psilocybin, D-lysergic acid diethylamide (LSD), mescaline, and numerous amphetamine derivatives are just a few hallucinogens (Stephens, 1999). During the 1960s, LSD became a popular recreational drug associated with the antiestablishment movement of peace, free love, and sex that characterized the "hippies" and the "Woodstock generation." Acute LSD psychological toxicity, so-called bad trips during which users feel extreme anxiety or fear and experience frightening hallucinations, were often reported or experienced by users. These experiences are characteristically panic reactions that develop when individuals feel that the hallucinogenic experience will never end or when they have difficulty distinguishing drug effects from reality (Stephens, 1999).

LSD binds to and activates a specific receptor for the neurotransmitter serotonin. Normally, serotonin binds to and activates its receptors and then is taken back up into the neuron that released it. LSD binds very tightly to the serotonin receptor, causing a greater than normal activation of the receptor. Because serotonin has a role in many of the brain's functions, activation of its receptors by LSD produces widespread effects, including

rapid emotional swings, altered perceptions, and, if taken in a large enough dose, delusions and visual hallucinations.

According to the Canadian Addiction Survey (CCSA, 2004) 11% of the population reports a lifetime use of hallucinogens, 11% for cocaine, 6% for speed, and 4% for Ecstasy. In addition, the lifetime use of drugs such as inhalants, heroin, steroids, and intravenous drugs is about 1% in Canada. Other than marijuana, all other illicit drug use across provinces remains relatively low, with past-year use levels at 3% or less. Lower levels are reported in the Atlantic region and higher levels in Quebec, Alberta, and most notably British Columbia.

CLUB DRUGS

MDMA (3,4-methlyendioxymethamphetamine), or Ecstasy, along with GHB (γ-hydroxybutyrate), flunitrazepam (Rohypnol), and ketamine, are among drugs used by teens and young adults as part of the nightclub, bar, and rave scene and thus are known as "club drugs." Sadly, accidental deaths due to hypothermia and dehydration have been documented from such drug use (Health Canada, 2000).

MDMA, which is similar in structure to methamphetamine, causes serotonin to be released from neurons in greater amounts than normal. Once released, this serotonin can excessively activate serotonin receptors. Scientists have also shown that MDMA causes excess dopamine to be released from dopamine-containing neurons. Alarmingly, research in animals has demonstrated that MDMA can damage and destroy serotonin-containing neurons. MDMA can cause hallucinations, confusion, depression, sleep problems, drug craving, severe anxiety, and paranoia. In high doses, MDMA can cause a sharp increase in body temperature (malignant hyperthermia), leading to muscle breakdown, kidney and cardiovascular failure, and death.

Rohypnol, ketamine, and GHB are predominately CNS depressants. Often colourless, tasteless, and odourless, the drugs can be ingested unknowingly. Known also as "date rape" drugs when mixed with alcohol, they can be incapacitating, causing a euphoric, sedative-like effect and producing an "anterograde amnesia," which means individuals may not remember events they experience while under the influence of these drugs.

Phencyclidine (PCP), which is not a true hallucinogen, can affect many neurotransmitter systems. It interferes with the functioning of the neurotransmitter glutamate, which is found in neurons throughout the brain. Like many other drugs, it also causes dopamine to be released from neurons into the synapse. At low to moderate doses, PCP causes altered perception of body image but rarely produces visual hallucinations. PCP can also cause effects that mimic the primary symptoms of schizophrenia, such as delusions and mental turmoil.

People who use PCP for long periods of time have memory loss and speech difficulties (NIDA, 2000).

Nursing interventions depend on presenting behaviours and anticipated complications. Often, clients can present at psychiatric emergency departments in acute states of intoxication or in dissociated states, and they may be combative. Intoxication can last 4 to 6 hours, with an extensive period of de-escalation. The primary goals of intervention are to reduce stimuli, maintain a safe environment for the client and others, manage behaviour, and observe the client carefully for medical and psychiatric complications. Instructions to the client should be clear, short, and simple, and delivered in a firm but nonthreatening tone.

OPIATES

Derived from poppies, **opiates** are powerful drugs that have been used for centuries to relieve pain. They include opium, heroin, morphine, and codeine. Even centuries after their discovery, opiates are still the most effective pain relievers. Although heroin has no medicinal use, other opiates, such as morphine and codeine, are used to treat pain related to illnesses (eg, cancer) and medical and dental procedures. When used as directed by a physician, opiates are safe and generally do not produce addiction. However, opiates also possess very strong reinforcing properties and can quickly trigger addiction when used improperly (NIDA, 2000).

The term *opiate* refers to any substance that binds to an opioid receptor in the brain to produce an agonist action. Opiates cause CNS depression, sleep or stupor, and analgesia. Major opiates used today are heroin, codeine, and meperidine. Opiates are commonly referred to as **narcotics,** although in legal terms, narcotics is a catch-all term for all illegal drugs. According to the Canadian Addiction Survey (CCSA, 2004), 16.5% of adult Canadians have used any one of five drugs (cocaine or crack, hallucinogens, PCP or LSD,

speed or amphetamines, heroine, Ecstasy), during their lifetime and 3% used at least one of the drugs during the past 12 months. There has been an increasing spread to middle-class users, and the proportion of people seeking treatment has continued to increase.

There are three types of opiate-related drugs: agonists, antagonists, and mixed agonist-antagonists. Opiate agonists increase the CNS effects, and antagonists block these effects. Opiates elicit their powerful effects by activating opiate receptors that are widely distributed throughout the brain and body. The effect produced by activated receptors in the brain correlates with the area of the brain involved. Two important effects produced by opiates are pleasure (or reward) and pain relief. The brain itself also produces substances known as endorphins that activate the opiate receptors. Research indicates that endorphins are involved in many functions, including respiration, nausea, vomiting, pain modulation, and hormonal regulation (NIDA, 2000).

Opiates cause tolerance and physical dependence that appear to be specific for each receptor subtype. Tolerance develops particularly to the analgesic, respiratory depression, and sedative actions of opiates. Often, a 100% increase in dose is used to achieve the same physical effects when tolerance exists. Physical dependence can develop rapidly. When use of the drug is discontinued, after a period of continuous use, a rebound hyperexcitability withdrawal syndrome usually occurs. Table 23-5 describes the onset, duration, and symptoms of mild, moderate, and severe withdrawal symptoms.

Heroin

Heroin, processed from morphine, a naturally occurring substance extracted from the seed pod of certain varieties of the poppy plant, is an illegal, highly addictive drug that is the most abused and most rapidly acting of the opiates. Typically sold as a white or brownish powder or as the black sticky substance known as "black tar heroin" on the

Table 23.5	Severity of Opiate Withdrawal Syndrome		
Initial Onset and Duration	**Mild Withdrawal**	**Moderate Withdrawal**	**Severe Withdrawal**
Onset: 8–12 h after last use of short-acting opiates. 1–3 d after last use for longer-acting opiates, such as methadone	Physical: yawning, rhinorrhea, perspiration, restlessness, lacrimation, sleep disturbance	Physical: dilated pupils, bone and muscle aches, sensation of "goose flesh," hot and cold flashes	Physical: nausea, vomiting, stomach cramps, diarrhea, weight loss, insomnia, twitching of muscles and kicking movements of legs, increased blood pressure, pulse, and respirations
Duration: Severe symptoms peak between 48 and 72 h. Symptoms abate in 7–10 d for short-acting opiates. Methadone withdrawal symptoms can last several weeks.	Emotional: increased craving, anxiety, dysphoria	Emotional: irritability, increased anxiety, and craving	Emotional: depression, increased anxiety, dysphoria, subjective sense of feeling "wretched"

streets, it is frequently "cut" with other substances, such as sugar, starch, powdered milk, quinine, and strychnine or other poisons. It can be sniffed, snorted, and smoked but is most frequently injected, which poses risks for transmission of HIV and other diseases from the sharing of needles or other injection equipment. Evidence shows that the number of Canadians using an injectable drug at some point in their lifetime rose from 1.7 million in 1994 to 4.1 million in 2004 (CCSA, 2004). Vancouver has the dubious distinction of having the highest prevalence rate (25%) and incidence (18.6 per 100) of HIV among injection drug users in North America (Government of Canada, 1998). In addition, there was a 40% increase in known cases of HIV/AIDS in federal correctional institutions between 1994 and 1995, largely associated with injection drug use.

One of the most detrimental long-term effects of heroin is addiction itself, which causes neurochemical and molecular changes in the brain. Heroin also produces profound degrees of tolerance and physical dependence, which are powerful motivating factors for compulsive use and abuse. Once addicted, heroin users gradually spend more and more time and energy obtaining and using the drug, until these activities become their primary purpose in life (NIDA, 2002). In response to this complex substance problem, Canada joined Switzerland, the Netherlands, Germany, Spain, and the United Kingdom in early 2005 to undertake a drug trial to determine whether prescribing pharmaceutical heroin to addicted people can help reduce the death, disease, crime, and suffering associated with illicit heroin use (Canadian Institutes of Health Research, 2005).

Naltrexone (Trexan)

Naltrexone has been used successfully to treat opiate addiction. It binds to opiate receptors in the CNS and competitively inhibits the action of opioid drugs, including those with mixed narcotic agonist-antagonist properties, thereby blocking the intoxicating effects. It is contraindicated in pregnant clients and in clients with allergy to narcotic antagonists. If a client should require analgesia while taking naltrexone, a nonopioid agent is recommended. If opioid analgesia is necessary, such as for surgery or severe pain, it must be administered cautiously because the amount required for analgesia may result in respiratory depression. Clients should be informed that taking opiates while taking naltrexone is extremely dangerous because the interaction can cause respiratory depression and death. Should an opiate-dependent individual take naltrexone before he or she is fully detoxified from opiates, withdrawal symptoms may result.

Opiate Detoxification

Opiate detoxification is achieved by gradually reducing an opiate dose over several days or weeks. Many treatment programs include administering low doses of a substitute drug that can help satisfy the drug craving without providing the same subjective high, such as methadone.

Methadone Maintenance Treatment

Methadone maintenance is the treatment of opiate addiction with a daily, stabilized dose of methadone. Methadone is used because of its long half-life of 15 to 30 hours. Methadone is a potent opiate and is physiologically addicting, but it satisfies the opiate craving without producing the subjective high of heroin.

Detoxification is accomplished by setting the beginning methadone dose and then slowly reducing it during the next 21 days. Treatment programs determine the dose of methadone that will block subjective feelings of craving and will not cause somnolence or intoxication in clients. The initial dose of methadone is determined by the severity of withdrawal symptoms and is usually 20 to 30 mg orally. If, after 1 to 2 hours, symptoms persist, the dosage can be raised and then should be re-evaluated daily during the first few days of treatment. Initial doses of greater than 40 mg can cause severe discomfort as the detoxification proceeds.

Clients receive this dose daily in conjunction with regular drug abuse counselling focussed on the elimination of illicit drug use; on lifestyle changes, such as finding friends who do not use drugs or achieving stability in one's living situation; strengthening social supports; and structuring time for pursuits that do not involve drug use. After illicit drug use ceases for a period of time, major lifestyle changes have been made, and social supports are in place, clients may gradually detoxify from methadone with continuing support through community support groups, such as Narcotics Anonymous.

The length of methadone treatment varies for each client. When to begin detoxification from methadone varies widely, depending on the client's commitment to abstinence, lifestyle changes that have occurred, and strong peer group support, all of which are needed to sustain the client during methadone detoxification, when increased cravings often occur.

Methadone treatment, combined with behavioural therapy and counselling, has been used effectively and safely to treat opioid addiction for more than 30 years (NIDA, 1997). Combined with behavioural therapy and counselling, methadone enables clients to stop using heroin.

Like methadone, L-acetyl-α-methadol (LAAM) is a synthetic opiate that can be used to treat heroin addiction. LAAM, taken orally, can block the effects of heroin for as long as 72 hours with minimal side effects. It has a longer duration of action than methadone, permitting dosing just three times per week, thereby eliminating the need to take doses home over weekends (NIDA, 1997).

In recent clinical trials, buprenorphine taken three times a week has proven to be effective in treating opioid addiction (Zickler, 2001). An inexpensive drug, buprenorphine could lower costs to the health care system while providing treatment for many more clients with addiction (McNicholas, 2002/2003). Discontinuing buprenorphine use does not require tapering, as does methadone, which makes it easier to stop treatment (NIDA, 1997).

SEDATIVE-HYPNOTICS AND ANXIOLYTICS

Sedative-hypnotic drugs and anxiolytic (antianxiety) agents are medications that induce sleep and reduce anxiety. Table 23-6 lists sedative-hypnotic and anxiolytic medications, their generic and trade names, and common indications for use. This class of substances is essentially one of prescription drugs but can include alcohol and marijuana because of their sedative-hypnotic properties.

Table 23.6	Sedative-Hypnotic, Anxiolytic Agents and Their Effects	
Generic Name	**Trade Name**	**Effects**
Benzodiazepines		
Alprazolam	Xanax	S, A
Chlordiazepoxide	Librium	S, A
Clonazepam	Klonopin	anticonvulsant
Clorazepate	Tranxene	S, A
Diazepam	Valium	S, A, anticonvulsant
Estazolam	ProSom	H
Flurazepam	Dalmane	H
Halazepam	Paxipam	S, A
Lorazepam	Ativan	S, A
Oxazepam	Serax	S, A
Prazepam	Centrax	S, A
Quazepam	Doral	H
Temazepam	Restoril	H
Triazolam	Halcion	H
Barbiturates		
Amobarbital	Amytal	S
Butabarbital	Butisol	S
Butalbital	Fiorinal	S, analgesic
Pentobarbital	Nembutal	H
Phenobarbital	Barbita, Luminol	S, anticonvulsant
Secobarbital	Seconal	H
Others		
Buspirone	BuSpar	S, A
Chloral hydrate	Noctec, Somnos	H
Ethchlorvynol	Placidyl	H
Glutethimide	Doriden	H
Meprobamate	Miltown, Equanil	S, A
Methylprylon	Noludar	H

S, sedative; H, hypnotic; A, antianxiety.

Sedative-hypnotic and anxiolytic agent abuse is complex. Use of these drugs is often controversial because of society's ambivalence regarding the proper or ethical use of medications to treat anxiety and insomnia, and physicians and mental health professionals often face ethical questions in treating them. More than 8% of Canadians 65 years and older use prescribed tranquilizers and sleeping pills (Government of Canada, 1998). Prescription drug dependency, particularly for sedatives, pain killers, and anxiety-reducing compounds, has consistently been widespread among Aboriginal populations, most notably among women (NNADAP, 2000). Indeed, Health Canada was warned in 1997 by the Auditor General that its Aboriginal populations were overusing prescription drugs.

If both physician and client consider carefully the risks of these drugs, they can be a useful, safe, and appropriate treatment (Brady, Myrick, & Malcolm, 1999). Clients who abuse prescription medications are often somnolent, have a clouded mental state, or may feel hyperactive or anxious after using the medication yet continue to use it without reporting its distressing side effects. They often take the next dose ahead of time, may exceed the prescribed daily dosage, may lobby for a higher dose or a stronger medication, may supplement medication with alcohol or other drugs, or may obtain prescriptions for the same medication from several physicians.

Biologic Reactions for Benzodiazepines

Barbiturates were the first class of drugs used to treat sleep disturbances and anxiety, but benzodiazepines have largely replaced barbiturates because of their comparative safety with regard to potential toxicity and addictive qualities. Benzodiazepines modulate γ-aminobutyric acid (GABA) transmission and interact with specific receptor sites in the brain. GABA is the most abundant inhibitory neurotransmitter in the brain. Benzodiazepines, by displacing an endogenous binding inhibitor, increase GABA's affinity for its receptor and thus enhance GABA function (Brady et al., 1999). Benzodiazepines act in a manner similar to alcohol and other sedative hypnotics, making neuronal membranes more permeable to K^+ and Cl^- and closing Na^+ and Ca^{++} channels, which causes CNS depression. Although benzodiazepines increase total sleep time, they decrease the duration of REM sleep.

Benzodiazepine Withdrawal

The severity of symptoms during benzodiazepine withdrawal depends on the duration and dosage of regular use; symptoms include the following:

- Anxiety rebound—tension, agitation, tremulousness, insomnia, anorexia

- Autonomic rebound—hypertension, tachycardia, sweating, hyperpyrexia
- Sensory excitement—paresthesias, photophobia, hyperacusis (sensitivity to sound), illusions
- Motor excitation—hyperreflexia, tremors, myoclonus, fasciculation (visible muscle contraction), myalgia, muscle weakness, tonic–clonic convulsions
- Cognitive excitation—nightmares, delirium, depersonalization, hallucinations

Two methods of withdrawal are currently used. The first is to use the same medication in decreasing doses, and the second is to substitute an equivalent dose of phenobarbital and reduce the dose slowly (Brady et al., 1999).

Nursing interventions for withdrawal states are similar to those for alcohol withdrawal. Symptoms may begin to emerge as long as 8 days after cessation of a long-acting benzodiazepine. Often, clients combine these drugs with alcohol, which is extremely dangerous and can put clients at risk for overdose, causing coma or death. The combination of benzodiazepines and alcohol also complicates withdrawal treatment because the client may seem to improve after the alcohol withdrawal syndrome subsides, only to have similar symptoms emerge as the benzodiazepine withdrawal syndrome appears.

INHALANTS

Inhalants are organic solvents, also known as *volatile substances*, that are CNS depressants. When inhaled, they cause euphoria, sedation, emotional lability, and impaired judgment. Intoxication can result in respiratory depression, stupor, and coma. Inhalants typically are used by young individuals; low cost, universal availability, ease of access, and local custom are probably important factors in promoting their use (Pandina & Hendren, 1999). Solvent use is a particular challenge in the Aboriginal communities of Canada. For example, one study reported that 20% of the youth in Manitoba and 15% of those in Quebec had tried solvent sniffing (Health Canada, 1999b). Among the youth who had tried, 3% of the Manitoba sample and 2% of the Quebec sample were regular users. Typically, these youth started sniffing between the ages of 4 and 11 years, and lived in homes with significant disadvantage (substance abuse, family conflict, unemployment, malnutrition, financial hardship, and physical abuse). In response to the solvent use problem, the Federal Government has established the National Youth Solvent Abuse Program (NYSAP) and funded inpatient centres that require the removal of children from their home communities (NNADAP, 2000 p. 8).

Most inhalants are common household products that give off mind-altering chemical fumes when sniffed. They include the following:

- *Adhesives*: airplane glue, polyvinyl chloride cement, rubber cement
- *Aerosols*: paint, hair spray, analgesics, asthma sprays, deodorants, air fresheners
- *Anaesthetics*: nitrous oxide, halothane, enflurane, isoflurane, ethyl chloride
- *Solvents*: paint and nail polish removers, paint thinners, correction fluids, lighter fluid, petroleum
- *Cleaning agents*: dry cleaning fluid, spot removers, degreasers, computer cleaners
- *Food products*: whipped cream and cooking oil sprays
- *Nitrites*: amyl, butyl, isopropyl nitrite

The chemical structure of the various types of inhalants is diverse, making it difficult to generalize about their effects. However, the vaporous fumes can change brain chemistry and may permanently damage the brain and CNS (NIDA, 2000). Magnetic resonance imaging scans of users demonstrate severe changes in cerebral white matter (NIDA, 2002).

Neurotoxicity

Inhalants are easily absorbed through the lungs and are widely distributed in the body, reaching the highest concentrations in fat tissue and the nervous system, where the most profound effects are exhibited. Mild intoxication occurs within minutes and can last as long as 30 minutes. Often, the drugs are inhaled repeatedly to maintain an intoxicated state for hours. Initially, the person experiences a sense of euphoria, but as the dose increases, confusion, perceptual distortions, and severe CNS depression appear. Inhalant users are also at risk for *sudden sniffing death*, which can occur when the inhaled fumes take the place of oxygen in the lungs and CNS, causing the user to suffocate. Inhalants can also cause death by disrupting the normal heart rhythm, which can lead to cardiac arrest (NIDA, 2000).

Chronic neurologic syndromes can result from long-term use. Long-term inhalant use is linked to widespread brain damage and cognitive abnormalities that can range from mild impairment to severe dementia. In recent studies, considerably more inhalant users than cocaine users had brain abnormalities, and their damage was more extensive. Inhalant users also performed significantly worse on tests of working memory and of the ability to focus attention, plan, and solve problems (NIDA, 2002). A withdrawal syndrome is reported, similar to alcohol withdrawal but milder, with primary symptoms of anxiety, tremors, hallucinations, and sleep disturbance.

NICOTINE

Nicotine, the addictive chemical mainly responsible for the high prevalence of tobacco use, is the primary reason tobacco is named a public health menace (Slade, 1999). Smoking is more prevalent among people with alcoholism, polysubstance users, and psychiatric clients than among the general population (Health Canada, 1997). Nicotine stimulates the central, peripheral, and autonomic nervous systems, causing increased alertness, concentration, attention, and appetite suppression. It is readily absorbed and is carried in the bloodstream to the liver, where it is partially metabolized. It is also metabolized by the kidneys and is excreted in the urine.

Nicotine acts as an agonist of the nicotinic cholinergic receptor sites and stimulates autonomic ganglia in both the parasympathetic and sympathetic nervous systems, resulting in increased release of norepinephrine or acetylcholine. The release of epinephrine by nicotine from the adrenal medulla increases fatty acids, glycerol, and lactate levels in the blood, thereby increasing the risk for atherosclerosis and cardiac muscle pathology (Slade, 1999).

Other medical complications of nicotine use are numerous. Smoking either cigarettes or cigars can cause respiratory problems, lung cancer, emphysema, heart problems, and peripheral vascular disease. In fact, smoking is the largest preventable cause of premature death and disability. In addition, recent research has shown that nicotine addiction is extremely powerful and is at least as strong as addictions to other drugs, such as heroin and cocaine; 70% of those who quit relapse within a year (NIDA, 2000).

According to the summary results of the Canadian Tobacco Use Monitoring Survey (Health Canada, 2004), just over 5 million people older than 14 years (20% of the population) currently smoke (23% men, 17% women) in Canada. The general trend in the number of cigarettes smoked daily continues to decline (Health Canada, 2004). However, smoking rates vary according to geography. More rural than urban dwellers smoke (24% vs. 19%), and fewer rural than urban dwellers have smoking restrictions in the workplace (55% vs. 70%). Likewise, smoking rates vary according to ethnicity. Aboriginal people are between 2 and 2.5 times more likely to be regular smokers compared with the non-Aboriginal population (NNADAP, 2000).

Nicotine Withdrawal and Replacement Therapy

Nicotine withdrawal is marked by mood changes (craving, anxiety, irritability, depression) and physiologic changes (difficulty in concentrating, sleep disturbances, headaches, gastric distress, and increased appetite) (Slade, 1999). Nicotine replacements such as transdermal patches, nicotine gum, nasal spray, and inhalers have been used successfully to assist in withdrawal by reducing the craving for tobacco. Patches are rotated on skin sites and help maintain a steady blood level of nicotine. Products such as Habitrol, Nicoderm, and ProStep are used daily, with the decrease in strength of nicotine occurring during a period of 6 to 12 weeks.

The use of this medication should be accompanied by social support and education to enhance the commitment to abstain from tobacco. Symptoms of excessive nicotine released by the patches can resemble withdrawal symptoms. People with cardiovascular disease and peripheral vascular disease may not be candidates for this therapy because increased cardiac stimulation and peripheral vasoconstriction are common side effects. Smoking while using transdermal patches will enhance negative cardiovascular side effects. Clients who do smoke during therapy should not use patches.

CAFFEINE

Caffeine is a stimulant found in many drinks (coffee, tea, cocoa, soft drinks), chocolate, and over-the-counter medications, including analgesics, stimulants, appetite suppressants, and cold relief preparations. Currently, regular daily consumption of behaviourally active doses is widespread throughout the world, with use by more than 80% of the adults in the United States (Griffiths, 2000). Studies sponsored by Coca-Cola, done by psychologist Hollingsworth in 1912, showed that in doses of 65 to 130 mg, caffeine exerts beneficial effects on both mental and motor performance; these results hold true today. However, at a dose of 300 mg, caffeine can cause tremors, poor motor performance, and insomnia (Bolton, 1981). If caffeine is overused, it can cause physical side effects and precipitate a withdrawal syndrome marked by headaches, drowsiness, and craving (APA, 2000).

Symptoms of caffeine intoxication can include five or more of the following: restlessness, nervousness, excitement, insomnia, flushed face, diuresis, gastrointestinal disturbance, muscle twitching, rambling flow of thought and speech, tachycardia or cardiac arrhythmia, periods of inexhaustibility, and psychomotor agitation (APA, 2000).

Caffeine is an alkaloid and a xanthine derivative. Doses of less than 200 mg, found in 1 to 2 cups of percolated coffee, stimulate the cerebral cortex and increase mental acuity. Doses exceeding 500 mg (more than 5 cups of coffee) increase the heart rate; stimulate respiratory, vasomotor, and vagal centres and cardiac muscles, resulting in increased force of cardiac contraction; dilate pulmonary and coronary blood vessels; and constrict blood flow to the cerebral vascular system. Psychiatric symptoms such as panic, schizophrenia, or manic-depressive symptoms can be exacerbated by caffeine in higher doses.

Caffeine withdrawal syndrome has been described as headache, drowsiness, and fatigue, sometimes with impaired psychomotor performance, difficulty concentrating, craving, and psychophysiologic complaints, such as yawning or nausea. Clients with caffeine dependence can be supported in their efforts at withdrawal by learning about the caffeine contents of beverages and medication, using decaffeinated beverages, and managing individual withdrawal symptoms.

PRESCRIPTION DRUGS

Abuse of and addiction to prescription drugs are a problem for some clients. Three classes of prescription drugs are most commonly abused: (1) opioids, which are prescribed most often to treat pain; (2) CNS depressants, which are used to treat anxiety and sleep disorders; and (3) stimulants, which are prescribed to treat the sleep disorder narcolepsy, attention-deficit hyperactivity disorder, and obesity. The risk for addiction exists when these medications are used in ways other than as prescribed.

The misuse of prescription drugs may be most common among elderly people, who use prescription medications approximately three times more frequently than the general population and have the poorest rates of compliance with directions for taking medications (Government of Canada, 1998).

No single type of treatment is appropriate for all individuals addicted to prescription medications, and a combination of behavioural and pharmacologic interventions may be needed. All health care providers should be aware of the potential for prescription drug misuse and should continually assess for it.

STEROIDS

Anabolic steroids are synthetic substances related to the male sex hormones (androgens). Developed in the late 1930s to treat hypogonadism, they are also used to treat delayed puberty, some types of impotence, and wasting of the body caused by HIV infection or other diseases. They promote growth of skeletal muscle and the development of male sexual characteristics. There are more than 100 different types; to be used legally, all require a prescription. Some dietary supplements, such as dehydroepiandrosterone (DHEA) and androstenedione (Andro), can be purchased in commercial health stores. They are often used in the belief that large doses can convert into testosterone or a similar compound in the body that will promote muscle growth, but this belief has not been proven. The 1999 NIDA-funded Monitoring the Future survey estimates that 2.7% of 8th and 10th graders and 2.9% of 12th graders in the United States have taken anabolic steroids at least once in their lives. Although use among men is higher than among women, use among women is growing (NIDA, 2002).

Individuals are motivated by a desire to build muscles and improve sports performance, so the temptation to use is great among athletes at all levels. Unannounced testing seems to have had an impact on the use of performance-enhancing drugs in Olympic sports in Canada. Evidence shows that the number of positive tests has declined from 2.5% in 1993 to 1.1% in 1996. However, the situation was much worse among power-lifters and body builders (25% positive tests) (Government of Canada, 1998).

The agents are available orally under a variety of names (Anadrol, Oxandrin, and Dianabol) and by injection (Deca-Durabolin, Depo-Testosterone) or ointment preparations, and users frequently take as much as 100 times more than the doses used for treating medical conditions. "Stacking," or taking two or more steroids together, is practiced in the belief that interaction will produce a greater effect on muscle size. In cyclic dosage regimens, a practice called "pyramiding" is used by starting with low doses in a stacking combination, increasing the dosage during a period of weeks, and then tapering to zero dose in the belief that the drug-free cycle allows time for the body's hormonal system to recuperate. As with stacking, the perceived benefits of pyramiding have not been substantiated scientifically.

Case reports and small studies indicate that anabolic steroids, in high doses, increase irritability and aggression. Some steroid users report that they have committed aggressive acts, such as physical fighting, armed robbery or using force to obtain something, committing property damage, stealing from stores, or breaking into a house or building, and that they engage in these behaviours more often when they take steroids than when they are drug free. Other behavioural effects include euphoria, increased energy, sexual arousal, mood swings, distractibility, forgetfulness, and confusion.

With time, anabolic steroid use is associated with increased risk for heart attack and stroke, blood clotting, cholesterol changes, hypertension, depressed mood, fatigue, restlessness, loss of appetite, insomnia, reduced libido, muscle and joint pain, and severe liver problems, including hepatic cancer. Males can have reduced sperm production, shrinking of the testes, and difficulty or pain in urinating. There can be undesirable body changes—breast enlargement in men and masculinization of women's bodies. Both sexes can experience hair loss and acne. Intravenous or intramuscular use of the drug and needle sharing puts users at risk for HIV, hepatitis B and C, and infective endocarditis, as well as bacterial infections at injection sites.

Few studies have been conducted of anabolic steroid use. Current knowledge is based largely on the experiences of a few physicians who have worked with clients undergoing steroid withdrawal. They have found that supportive therapy, including education about what clients may experience during withdrawal, and evaluation for depression and suicidal thoughts, is sufficient in some cases.

If symptoms are severe or prolonged, medications or hospitalization may be required. Behavioural therapies may be indicated, as well as medications to restore the hormonal system after its disruption by steroid use (NIDA, 2002).

NURSING MANAGEMENT: HUMAN RESPONSE TO DISORDER

In psychiatric and substance-dependence treatment programs, the assessment process is, in part, a treatment intervention. Often, clients are not ready to acknowledge (are in denial about) the severity of the problem and about the emotional, social, legal, vocational, or other consequences of it.

Assessment Issues

The assessment is crucial to understanding level of use, abuse, or dependence and to determining the client's denial or acceptance of treatment. Assessment is often detailed and may involve family members and loved ones. Box 23-3 gives examples of typical behaviours exhibited by individuals in each level of use, abuse, dependence, and addiction. Box 23-4 is an example of a nursing assessment guide that can be used to obtain information about an individual's substance use history. Usually, nurses encounter individuals during crisis when they seek professional help. These situations offer an opportunity to explore the fear of acknowledging their addiction that keeps it thriving. By referring to

this as "fear" rather than "denial," as many professionals do, nurses can engage with the client as a supportive partner rather than a confrontational authority. The nurse's approach should be caring, matter-of-fact, gentle, direct, and aimed to enhance strengths. Approaches that are punitive or attempt to elicit feelings of guilt or shame are destructive to the therapeutic relationship. See Nursing Care Plan 23-1.

Fear of Acknowledgment (Denial of a Problem)

Fear of acknowledgment (denial) is the client's fear of accepting his or her loss of control over substance use or the severity of the consequences associated with the substance dependence. The fear can be expressed in a variety of behaviours and attitudes and may not be expressed as an overt denial of the problem. For example, clients may admit to a problem, even thank you for helping them to realize they have a problem, but insist they can overcome the problem on their own and do not need outside help.

People who fear acknowledgement are in the pre-contemplation stage (no intention to change) according to the *Transtheoretical Model of Self-Change* (Prochaska, Norcross, & DiClemente, 1994). The model views change on a continuum from *pre-contemplation*, to *contemplation*, *preparation*, *action*, and finally *maintenance*. Using this model, nurses refrain from the urge to either

---

BOX 23.3

Behaviours in Substance Use, Abuse, Dependence, and Addiction

Substance Use
- Does not have possible danger or potential legal problems
- Engages in use to enhance social situations and interaction
- Is not intended to result in intoxication
- Has control of the amount and frequency of use
- Exhibits socially acceptable behaviour while using

Prescription Medication Use
- Use is for the dose, frequency, and indications prescribed
- Use is for the particular episode of the condition for which it was prescribed
- Use is coordinated among prescribing physicians

Substance Abuse
- Use for intoxication or feeling of being "high"
- Use that interferes with normal life functions (eg, producing sleep when inappropriate, excitability or irritability interfering with social interaction)
- Potential harm to self or others (eg, driving while intoxicated, use of injection drug equipment)
- Use that has legal consequences (ie, all use of illicit drugs)
- Use resulting in socially unacceptable behaviour (eg, public drunkenness, verbal or physical abuse)

- Use to alter normal feeling states such as sadness or anxiety

Prescription Medication—Harmful Use (Abuse)
- Use is at a higher dose and greater frequency than prescribed
- Use is for indications other than prescribed or for self-diagnosed condition
- Use results in feeling tired or having a clouded mental state or feeling "hyperactive" or nervous

Substance Dependence
- Supplementing medication with alcohol or drugs
- Soliciting more than one physician for the same medication
- Inability to control the amount and frequency of use
- Tolerance to larger amounts of the substance
- Withdrawal symptoms when stopping use
- Severe consequences from alcohol or drug use

Substance Addiction
- Drug craving
- Compulsive use
- Presence of aberrant drug-related behaviours
- Repeated relapse into drug use after withdrawal

BOX 23.4

Substance/Harmful Use (Abuse) Evaluation

Drug/Last Use   **Pattern of Use (Amount, route, first use, frequency, and length of use)**

Alcohol:
Stimulants:
Opiates:
Sedative-hypnotics and anxiolytic agents:
Hallucinogens:
Marijuana:
Inhalants:
Nicotine:
Caffeine:

Dependency Indicators

1. Tolerance (increasing use of drug or alcohol with the same level of intoxication): _____
2. Withdrawal symptoms: a. Shakes? Tremors? _____ b. Cramps, diarrhea, or rapid pulse? _____
   c. Feeling paranoid, fearful? _____ d. Difficulty sleeping? _____
3. Consequences of use (presenting problems, persistent or recurrent emotional, social, legal, or other problems):
   _____
4. Loss of control of amount, frequency, or duration of use: _____
5. Desire or efforts to decrease use or control use: _____
6. Preoccupation (increasing focus or time spent on use and obtaining substances): _____
7. Social, vocational, recreational activities affected by use: _____
8. Previous alcohol/drug abuse treatment: _____

Nursing Diagnoses:

---

rescue or badger the client into acknowledgement and, instead, begin their work with strategies that raise consciousness and build relationships. Nurses present themselves as honest, direct, informed partners and, in turn, can be viewed as non-threatening, 'safe' professionals (Hughes, et al., 2001). They confront issues directly but do not judge (e.g., "Yes, 5 drinks over 2 hours would affect your decision-making and render you unsafe to drive. That is why the police stopped your car."). They do not invest in nurse-outcomes, and, instead, let clients know that they care *about*, and are willing to work *with*, them. They also provide choice (e.g., "Let's think about the options you have in this situation"), draw on client strengths (e.g., "So you cut down on your drinking/using when you found out you were pregnant. That's a big step!"), and focus more on solutions than problems (e.g., "In the past when you've managed something well, what worked?").

Enhancing Motivation for Change

Evidence suggests that the most effective philosophical principles of helping (Dunst, Trivette, & Deal, 1994) are grounded in such models of nursing as the McGill Model of Nursing (Gottlieb & Rowat, 1987). Effective helping models incorporate certain fundamental beliefs about clients, as follow:

- All people aspire to and are motivated toward better health and well-being.
- All people have the potential to develop and reach this end.

- People learn best how to use this potential through active participation.
- When people do not participate, the environmental supports must be strengthened.
- For change to take a lasting hold, people must believe that their participation is critical to the change process.

Nurses need to reflect on their performance and ensure that it includes proven help-giving behaviours. Current thinking (Dunst, Trivette, & Deal, 1994) suggests that helping works best when it involves principles that achieve the following:

- Enable individuals (create opportunities to promote competent, self-sustaining individuals with respect to their abilities to mobilize their social networks to get needs met and attain desired goals).
- Empower individuals (carry out interventions in a manner in which individuals acquire a sense of control over their lives as a result of an effort to meet their needs.
- Strengthen individuals and their natural support networks and neither usurp decision making nor supplant their support networks with professional services (ie, use professionals prudently)
- Enhance individual's acquisition of a wide variety of competencies that permit them to mobilize their support to meet their needs.

Longitudinal studies show that motivation is a key predictor of whether individuals will change their substance use behaviour (U.S. DHHS, 1999).

NURSING CARE PLAN 23.1

Client With Alcoholism

JG is a 55-year-old mechanic with a 25-year history of alcohol dependence. He is the youngest of three children born of "blue-collar" parents who valued hard work. His mother is still living with JG's older sister, but his father died of cirrhosis, a complication of years of alcohol abuse. JG has two children who are married with children, living in other provinces. He rarely sees them. He has been drinking as much as 2 litres of vodka per day for 3 years since sustaining a work-related back injury. He has a history of binge drinking on weekends. He denies other drug use.

Recently, his wife moved out of the house after 28 years of marriage. An argument about his drinking ended in a physical fight. She had to be treated in the emergency room for a broken arm. Their relationship had progressively deteriorated over the years. JG was sexually impotent due to excessive drinking, and she had moved into the spare bedroom. He was admitted to the hospital through the emergency department 2 weeks after his wife left him, with a gash above his right eye from a fall he sustained while intoxicated. His wife returned to care for him.

JG began to have symptoms of alcohol withdrawal and became anxious shortly after admission. He requested hospital admission for alcohol detoxification and was transferred to a detoxification and brief treatment unit.

SETTING: INPATIENT DETOXIFICATION UNIT, PSYCHIATRIC HOSPITAL

Baseline Assessment: First admission, last drink 7 PM. Admission vital signs: T 99.2°F, HR 98, R 20, BP 140/88 on admission to the ER. He has a history of withdrawal seizures and hallucinosis. He had a blood alcohol level (BAL) of 0.15 mg%, becoming increasingly anxious and restless. He was given diazepam, 10 mg PO at that time.

Four hours after admission, vital signs were T 99.8°F, HR 110, R 22, BP 152/100. He continued to be anxious and was tremulous, diaphoretic, and nauseous. Diazepam 20 mg PO stat was given.

Associated Psychiatric Diagnosis	Medications
Axis I: Alcohol withdrawal with hallucinations; alcohol abuse	Thiamine
Axis II: None	Folic acid
Axis III: Unspecified back injury	Multivitamins
Axis IV: Social problems (social withdrawal); occupational problems (work-related injury)	Diazepam, 10 mg q2h, for elevated BP, HR, and tremors
Axis V: GAF = Current 60; Potential 75	Haloperidol, 5.0 mg IM PRN, for hallucinations or agitation

NURSING DIAGNOSIS 1: RISK FOR INJURY

Defining Characteristics	Related Factors
Sensory deficits	Altered cerebral function secondary to alcohol withdrawal
Balance and equilibrium deficits	Potential withdrawal seizures resulting from magnesium deficiency or hypoglycaemia
Lack of awareness of hazards	Anxiety

Outcomes

Initial	Discharge
1. Prevent falls and other physical injuries.	2. Relate an intent to practice selected prevention harm reduction measures such as at least reducing substance use, maintaining adequate nutrition, removing loose throw rugs, using adequate lighting.

Interventions

Interventions	Rationale	Ongoing Assessment
Identify stage of alcohol withdrawal and severity of symptoms. Monitor gait and motor coordination, presence of tremors, mental status, electrolyte balance, and seizure activity.	The more severe the reactions, the more likely that disorientation, confusion, and restlessness increase. As the client moves from stage I to III, he becomes at higher risk for a fall or injury.	Determine whether JG is becoming more disoriented, increasing his risk for injury.
Institute seizure precautions (bed in low position, padded side rails).	Withdrawal seizures usually occur within 48 hours after last drink.	Monitor for seizure activity.

(continued)

NURSING CARE PLAN 23.1 (Continued)

Interventions

Interventions	Rationale	Ongoing Assessment
Orient patient to surroundings and call light, maintain consistent physical environment. Avoid sudden moves, loud noises, discussion of patient at bedside, and lighting that casts shadows downward.	Disorientation often occurs as blood alcohol level drops. These symptoms can last several days. Decreased environmental stimulation helps calm the patient, which in turn promotes optimal CNS responses.	Determine JG's level of orientation to surroundings. Determine whether he can use call light. Observe reactions to loud noises and monitor room environment.

Evaluation

Outcomes (at 3 days)	Revised Outcomes	Interventions
Gait steady, patient hydrated. No seizure activity. Client oriented.	Maintain current level of orientation.	Continue to monitor for any signs of disorientation.

NURSING DIAGNOSIS 2: DISTURBED THOUGHT PROCESSES

Defining Characteristics	Related Factors
Hallucinations (auditory, visual, and tactile) Inaccurate interpretation of stimuli Confusion and disorientation	Physiologic changes secondary to alcohol withdrawal

Outcomes

Initial	Discharge
1. Recognize changes in thinking/behaviour. 2. Identify situations that occur before hallucinations/delusions.	3. Maintain reality orientation.

Interventions

Interventions	Rationale	Ongoing Assessment
Encourage communication that enhances the development of the nurse–client partnership and relationship and promotes JG's sense of integrity (eg, empathy, practical information, choices).	The therapeutic relationship is important to individuals with alcohol withdrawal because of their fear of withdrawal symptoms and need for reassurance and support.	Monitor the development of the nurse–client relationship—the client's willingness to trust
Assess for the presence of any hallucinations through observation and interview. Provide support.	Hallucinations can occur when clients are withdrawing from alcohol. If hallucinations are severe, client may experience delirium tremens.	Assess client frequently to determine the presence of hallucinations.
Administer haloperidol, 5.0 mg IM PRN, for hallucinations or agitation.	Administering an antipsychotic eliminates or reduces the occurrence of hallucinations.	Observe for hypotension. Instruct client to avoid getting out of bed quickly to prevent falling.
JG had one episode of hallucinations. It occurred 8 hours after admission with no identifiable precipitating event.	Continue to maintain reality orientation. Provide empathy around fears and support/encouragement for JG's strengths (eg, perseverance).	Continue to monitor for hallucinations.

NURSING DIAGNOSIS 3: ANXIETY

Defining Characteristics	Related Factors
Physiologic: increased heart rate, elevated blood pressure, increased respiratory rate, diaphoresis, trembling, nausea Emotional: apprehension about alcohol withdrawal, nervousness, losing control after back injury Cognitive inability to concentrate, lack of awareness of surroundings	Physiologic changes secondary to alcohol withdrawal

NURSING CARE PLAN 23.1 (Continued)

Outcomes

Initial	Discharge
1. Identify an increase in physiologic and psychological comfort. 2. Maintain stable vital signs.	3. Describe anxiety as it relates to fear of detoxification comfort process and use of alcohol. Identify strategies to combat/cope with anxiety.

Interventions

Interventions	Rationale	Ongoing Assessment
Demonstrate an empathic, accepting attitude by being calm and informing JG of any treatment.	A calm attitude of the nurse can help relax a client.	Observe JG's reaction to the explanations and initiation of any treatments.
Include the client in decision making regarding his care. Offer choices.	Empowering the client in decision making helps him gain control over his situation.	Monitor decisions in terms of feasibility.
Administer diazepam, 10 mg q2h for elevated BP, HR, and tremulousness PRN.	Diazepam can reduce the physiologic impact of alcohol withdrawal.	Monitor vital signs, level of anxiety, and client's sense of control.
Explain that anxiety is a symptom of withdrawal and is usually time limited. Teach practical coping strategies	Knowledge that the anxiety will decrease will help client deal with the current anxiety.	Monitor whether or not JG understands that his discomfort will disappear and his ability to use/experience relief from coping strategies
Observe sleeping behaviour.	Sleep is often disturbed. Sleep deprivation contributes to anxiety.	Monitor quality of sleep.

Evaluation

Outcomes	Revised Outcomes	Interventions
JG was able to refocus and redirect attention when exhibiting mild anxiety. Sleeping about 6 hours.	None	None
Identified an increase in apprehension as his BP increased. Given diazepam as ordered.	Relate an increase in apprehension when it occurs.	Assess client and teach him about apprehension and a change in vital signs.
JG discussed his fears of the detoxification process. Expressed mixed feelings about continuing treatment.	Comply with treatment regimen.	Discuss concrete strategies with JG for following up with treatment once he is detoxified, including ways to enlist support. Praise and build on observed strengths.

CRNE Note

Motivational approaches are priority interventions for clients with substance use disorders. They help clients recognize a problem and develop change strategies.

KEY CONCEPT Enhancing motivation for change involves recognizing a problem, searching for a way to change, and then beginning and sticking with the change strategy (Miller, 1995). Ambivalence about substance use is normal and can be resolved by working with clients' own concerns about their use of alcohol and other drugs. Motivation is fluid and can be modified. Counselling is client centred, empathic, and built on reflective listening (Brown & Graves, 2005). The client is accepted and viewed as having the resources and motivation for change; the counsellor's task is to foster that motivation. Experiences such as increased distress levels, critical life events, a period of evaluation or appraisal of one's life, recognizing negative consequences of use, and positive and negative external incentives for change can all influence a client's commitment to change (U.S. DHHS, 1999).

Motivation is a cost-effective intervention for substance users and compares well with much longer, more costly treatments (Brown & Graves, 2005). Techniques that enhance motivation are associated with increased success in treatment, higher rates of abstinence, and successful follow-up treatment (U.S. DHHS, 1999). Motivational interviewing is a method of therapeutic intervention that seeks to elicit self-motivational statements from clients, supports behavioural change, and creates a discrepancy between the client's goals and their continued alcohol and other drug use (Miller & Rollnick, 1991). The acronym FRAMES (*f*eedback, *r*esponsibility, *a*dvice, *m*enu, empathy, *s*elf-efficacy) was

BOX 23.5

F.R.A.M.E.S.—Effective Elements of Brief Intervention

Feedback

Provide clients with personal feedback regarding their individual status, such as personal alcohol and other drug consumption relative to norms, information about elevated liver enzyme values, and so forth.

Responsibility

Emphasize the individual's freedom of choice and personal responsibility for change. General themes are as follows:
1. It's up to you; you're free to decide to change or not.
2. No one else can decide for you or force you to change.
3. You're the one who has to do it if it's going to happen.

Advice

Include a clear recommendation or advice on the need for change, typically in a supportive and concerned, rather than in a judgmental, manner.

Menu

Provide a menu of treatment options, from which clients may pick those that seem more suitable or appealing.

Empathic Counselling

Show warmth, support, respect, and understanding in communication with clients.

Self-efficacy

Reinforce self-efficacy, or an optimistic feeling that he or she can change

---

coined by Miller and Sanchez in 1994 to summarize elements of brief interventions with clients using motivational interviewing (Box 23-5).

Confronting Reality

The issue of confrontation is complex in addiction treatment.

> **KEY CONCEPT Confronting reality** has many different meanings and is often emotionally charged. Moffett (1999) defined confronting reality as "a therapeutic strategy that promotes the person's experience of the natural consequences of one's behaviour; e.g., thoughts, feelings, and actions [Box 23-6]. Feedback [from others] is a form of confrontation, i.e., information about the [discrepancies and] the impact of one's behaviour on oneself or others."

Learning from previous behaviour and its consequences is how change occurs. The nurse should be aware of these levels of confrontation and should support the client in using the reality feedback received to grow in the recovery process.

There are several general guidelines for establishing therapeutic interactions (see Box 23-7) with clients in chemical dependence treatment programs:
- Encourage honest expression of feelings.
- Listen to what the individual is really saying.
- Express empathy and caring *about* (not simply caring *for*) the individual.
- Hold the individual responsible for behaviour.
- Provide choices.
- Provide clear and consistent feedback.
- Maintain an attitude of active helping.
- Be true to your own values or nursing practice.
- Communicate the treatment plan to the client and to others on the treatment team.
- Monitor your own reactions to the client.

Countertransference

Countertransference is the total emotional reaction of the treatment provider to the client (see Chapter 7).

BOX 23.6

Levels of Reality Confrontation

I. Inform
   A. To inform someone about the general consequences of an anticipated behaviour (eg, warning nonsmokers about the health risks of smoking)
   B. To inform someone about the general consequences of their behaviour (eg, educating drinkers about the health consequences of drinking)
   C. To inform someone about the personal consequences of their behaviour (eg, to give feedback on their liver function tests; other health consequences)
   D. To inform someone emphatically about the consequences of either behaviour (eg, attack therapy). This

form of confrontation is used much less today in treatment settings because it can have a negative effect on the therapeutic relationship and can be abusive.

II. Experience
   A. To experience the consequences of their behaviour in their natural environment (eg, loss, job loss, separation, family disaffection legal fees, and sentences)
   B. To experience the consequences of their behaviour in a designed environment that generates those consequences immediately and dramatically (eg, a therapeutic community or interactional group therapy)

BOX 23.7

Therapeutic Dialogue: The Client With Alcoholism

Ineffective Approach

Nurse: I would like to talk with you about alcoholism.

Client: Alcoholism! It's not that bad. Everyone gets loaded.

Nurse: You tell why you were drinking. Your wife left you. You drink a couple of litres of vodka a day. Your blood alcohol level was 0.15% when you were admitted.

Client: So what! I do have some problems, or I wouldn't be here. But, I'm not an alcoholic. (fear of acknowledgment—denial)

Nurse: Do you know what alcoholism is?

Client: Sure I do. My father was one. He was a useless bum. I'm not anything like him.

Nurse: It sounds like you are a lot like him.

Client: I think I need to rest now. My back is killing me. (avoidance)

Effective Approach

Nurse: I would like to talk with you about what happens when you drink.

Client: It's not that bad. Everyone gets loaded!

Nurse: So you're hoping that you are no different than everyone else . . . and you're hoping that will mean you don't have a problem. What concerns do you have about your drinking?

Client: I'm not really concerned. My wife is. She thinks I drink too much. I even quit once for her.

Nurse: You cared enough about your wife to give up drinking for a while. What does she tell you about that?

Client: Well, she nags me a lot, and says it costs too much money, but I can stop whenever I want. Her nagging only made me drink again.

Nurse: It sounds as if she is really worried about you and about your drinking, but you have your doubts about how serious it is....It's pretty frightening to think about what it means if your wife is right....and that you really might have done serious harm to yourself with your drinking.

Client: I have a lot of problems besides alcohol. I never use drugs. I only drink because it relaxes me and makes it easier to deal with stress.

Nurse: Many people drink to help them cope with stress. Stress can be unbearable—no matter how hard you try to get rid of it, it can leave you feeling helpless. Drinking can seem like the only alternative. But eventually the drinking itself causes stress. While you are here, do you think it would be useful to look at the stress in your life and how it relates to your drinking?

Client: Yes. But I only drink when things get too out of hand. My health is pretty good.

Nurse: We can provide information about your health and alcohol use. In order to evaluate what information may be helpful, I would like to get a little more information about your drinking. Your wife might also feel better if she were able to learn more about alcoholism and its effects on you and the family. We have a family education group so that she can learn about alcohol abuse. Family therapy is also available.

Critical Thinking Challenge

- What effect did the nurse have on the client in using the word *alcoholism* in the first interaction?
- Discuss what communication approaches the nurse used in the second scenario to engage the client in disclosing problems with alcohol and his relationship with his wife. How does this nurse's approach vary from the one in the first interaction?

Clients with substance abuse disorders can generate strong feelings and reactions in nurses and other health care providers (Table 23-7). These feelings can be generated by overt unpleasant behaviours of the substance-dependent persons, such as lying, deceit, manipulation, or hostility. Alternatively, these feelings may be more subconscious and stem from past experiences with people with alcoholism or addicts or even from dealing with situations in the care provider's own family, or from feeling overwhelmed by the apparent pervasiveness and chronicity of the substance use problems and their own perceived inability to help.

Codependence

Codependence is a maladaptive coping pattern of family members or others closely related to the addict or person with alcoholism that results from prolonged exposure to the behaviours associated with substance dependence and is characterized by boundary distortions, poor relationship and friendship skills, compulsive and obsessive behaviours, inappropriate anger, sexual maladjustment, and resistance to change (Kitchens, 1991).

The development of codependence from childhood to adulthood, characterized by Kitchens (1991), is depicted in Figure 23-2. During years of coping with the addiction-related behaviours, family members become "locked into" certain roles and behaviours and are unable to readjust their behaviour patterns for new situations and relationships. They may learn to use some of the same maladaptive behaviour patterns and defence mechanisms as the substance-dependent family member, such as denial or escape mechanisms, and may even abuse substances themselves.

The codependency label, described by Whitfield (1997), is controversial and is viewed by many as an oversimplification of complex emotions and behaviours of family members. Mental health professionals should be careful not to use it as a catch-all diagnosis and to take special care to assess and plan interventions that address each person's particular situation, problems, and needs.

Table 23.7 (Client Behaviours and Countertransference Reactions

Client Behaviour	Common Nursing Reaction
Behaves as a victim	Feels a sense of helplessness, increased need to give advice and "fix" the situation and the client; shows anger toward the client for not being able to take care of the situation himself or herself
Is intrusive, hostile, belittling	Can be frightened, withdraw from client, express anger overtly, or be passive-aggressive (ie, suggesting discharge to the team or ignoring legitimate requests)
Does everything right, is insightful, pleasant, and so forth	Congratulates self on therapeutic interventions; can become bored or complacent
Relapses into drug or alcohol use	Feels angry, personally betrayed; withdraws from other clients; doubts own abilities
Asks personal questions about staff qualifications or prior drug or alcohol abuse	Reveals personal information, resents the intrusion, and may regret divulging information
Is silent or divulges minimal information	Tries harder, doubts own therapeutic ability, is angered by client's resistance
Tries to "bend" or ignore milieu and group rules	May permit program rule infractions; may feel pressured, angry, or passive-aggressive
Insists that no one can help him or her	Feels pressure to be the one who can help; may feel angry and inept or helpless

Adapted from Imhoff, J. E. (1991). Countertransference issues in alcoholism and drug addiction. *Psychiatric Annals. 21*(5), 292–306.

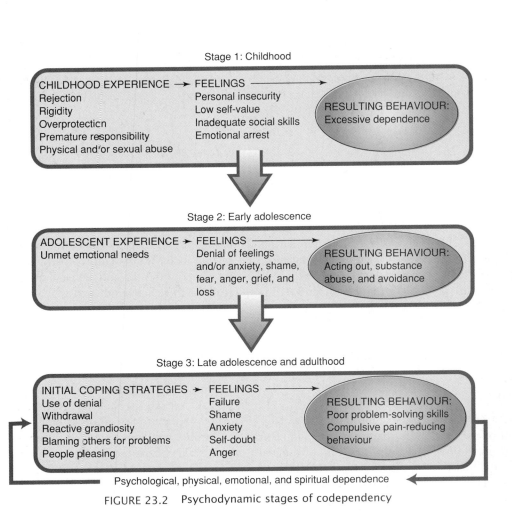

FIGURE 23.2 Psychodynamic stages of codependency

HIV and Substance Use

Intravenous drug users are at high risk for HIV infection because they often share hypodermic needles, syringes, and paraphernalia used in injecting drugs and may not use safe sex practices. Drug-dependent individuals are also likely to engage in risky sexual encounters to obtain money or drugs. Infected intravenous drug users can transmit HIV to their sexual partners, and pregnant intravenous drug users or pregnant women who are sexual partners of intravenous drug users can transmit the virus to the fetus during the neonatal period and the infant during breast-feeding. Other individuals who abuse drugs and alcohol are also often at high risk for sexual transmission of HIV because they may fail to use adequate precautions and preventive methods while intoxicated.

The dual diagnosis of chemical dependency and HIV infection requires extremely careful assessment and intervention planning. Continued alcohol and drug use can interfere with the medical treatment of AIDS; for example, alcohol, marijuana, cocaine, and amphetamines are immunosuppressants that further impair the seriously compromised immune system of a client with HIV. Addicts infected with HIV may have difficulty adhering to medication schedules, and some would not benefit from antiviral medications because of this. Other complicating factors include the financial, social, and emotional stressors experienced by addicts and people with alcoholism who must also cope with the devastating diagnosis of HIV disease.

These clients often experience intense feelings that trying to overcome substance dependence is pointless because they still have to cope with the pain and suffering of a life-threatening illness and may express desires to "die high" (Faltz, 1993). Clients may have mental disorders related to their HIV status, such as adjustment disorder, depression, mania and dementia, and medication-related disorders, in addition to their substance use disorders (U.S. DHHS, 2000).

Addiction treatment programs play an important role in providing care for clients with HIV disease, substance dependence, and concurrent mental health problems (Government of Canada, 1998). Because the issues facing these clients are so complex, planning treatment and setting treatment priorities are essential. Remember that addiction treatment is nearly always necessary for the client to follow with other HIV-related health and mental health interventions. Thus, at the initial diagnosis of HIV infection, substance dependence issues need to be evaluated and addressed (Faltz, 1993).

Harm-Reduction Strategies

The AIDS epidemic has caused addiction treatment professionals to coordinate services with community health and other health care delivery agencies. **Harm reduction**, a community health intervention designed to reduce the harm (consequences) of substance use to the individual, the family, and society, has replaced a moral or criminal approach to drug use and addiction (CCSA, 2005). Contrary to population-based measures aimed at reducing substance consumption and its related risks, harm reduction aims to reduce the risk for adverse consequences arising from substance use without necessarily reducing its use (Single, 2005). It recognizes that the ideal is abstinence but works with the individual regardless of his or her commitment to reduce use. Fischer (2005, p. 13) suggests five general principles of harm reduction:

- Harm reduction focusses on the consequences of substance use, not on the use itself, requiring decisions about which harms to be targeted and in what order based on what we know about client welfare, public health, and the severity of the problem.
- Harm reduction focusses on the pragmatic and effective minimization of use-related harms.
- Meaningful and realistic efforts must be made to actively understand and consider the social and environmental context in which substance use occurs.
- Education, knowledge, and informed decision making by substance users and potential users are key pillars of harm reduction.
- Misinformed or ineffective interventions or policy can be considered sources of substance-related harms, and therefore, must also be targeted for harm reduction interventions.

Interventions for alcohol-related harm reduction include education about the safe use of alcohol, provision of food at bars to reduce the incidence of rapid intoxication, and encouragement of the use of a "designated driver" (Larimer, 1998). Acupuncture has also demonstrated promising effects as a harm reduction strategy for those most severely affected by harmful use of substances. For example, during a 3-month trial among the poorest urban population of Canada, Vancouver's Downtown Eastside (prevalence rate of 30% HIV, 90% hepatitis C), acupuncture resulted in a statistically significant reduction in both the overall use of substances and the intensity of withdrawal symptoms (Janssen, Demorest, & Whynot, 2005).

Pregnancy and Substance Use

Drug and alcohol use during pregnancy can have serious detrimental effects on the course of pregnancy and on the physiologic status of the fetus and newborn. According to the Public Health Agency of Canada (1998), the national rate of fetal alcohol syndrome (FAS; a specific cluster of anomalies associated with the use of alcohol during pregnancy) has been estimated to be 1 to 2 per 1,000 live births, suggesting that each year, more than 350 children are born with FAS. The Canadian Centre on Substance Abuse has estimated the lifetime costs associated with the care of an individual with FAS (extra health care, education, and social services) to be about $1.4 million. Although the severity of problems and complications often depends on the amount of substance abuse during pregnancy, studies show that any amount of substance use during pregnancy puts the newborn at much higher risk for developmental, neurologic, and behavioural problems.

For pregnant women who are substance dependent, social and emotional pressures and concerns associated with their treatment are heightened because treatment affects the well-being of their children. Finkelstein (1993) lists some of the clinical issues facing addicted mothers:

- Feelings of guilt and shame
- Difficulties being a single parent (if applicable)
- Care and responsibility of raising children in early sobriety
- Lack of access to treatment facilities
- Anger and blame from caregivers
- Need for parenting skills training and knowledge of infant care and child development
- Potential for child abuse and neglect
- Lack of medical and other supportive services, such as prenatal care, housing, and child care

Finkelstein suggests that service providers convey hope for the future and assist clients in having realistic expectations for themselves and their children. The nurse should be aware of special social, emotional, and legal issues involving treatment of chemically dependent pregnant women and should be sensitive to their special needs. For example, they may fear that by seeking prenatal care, their drug use will be detected by urine toxicology tests and cause them to lose custody of their children. Marion (1995) suggested a comprehensive approach to treatment in the perinatal period, including prenatal and perinatal care; pharmacologic interventions, such as methadone maintenance programs; life skills training, such as relapse prevention and social skills training; mother–infant development assessment; and early childhood development programs and social work services, if needed.

Interventions and Treatment Modalities

Several treatment modalities are used in most addiction treatment (pharmacologic modalities were discussed earlier), including 12-step–program-focussed, cognitive or psychoeducational, behavioural, group psychotherapy, and individual and family therapy. Discharge planning and relapse prevention are also essential components of successful treatment and are incorporated into most programs. See Table 23-8 and Box 23-8 for different approaches to chemical dependency treatment.

Twelve-Step Programs

Alcoholics Anonymous (AA) was the first 12-step, self-help program. (See Chapter 6 for a list of these steps.) AA is a worldwide fellowship of people with alcoholism who provide support, individually and at meetings, to others who seek help. The program steps

---

BOX 23.8

Principles of Addiction Treatment

Although Canada has developed a number of documents outlining the principles around specific treatments or populations, it has not identified a generic set of principles to encompass all treatment modalities. The United States' National Institute on Drug Abuse in 1999 published a review of the research literature that outlines principles of effective approaches to drug addiction treatment. The summary of these principles follows:

1. No single treatment is appropriate for all individuals.
2. Treatment needs to be readily available.
3. Effective treatment attends to multiple needs of the individual, not just his or her drug use.
4. An individual's treatment and services plan must be assessed continually and modified as necessary to ensure that the plan meets the person's changing needs.
5. Remaining in treatment for an adequate period of time is critical for treatment effectiveness.
6. Counselling (individual and/or group) and other behavioural therapies are critical components of effective treatment for addiction.
7. Medications (eg, methadone, naltrexone) are an important element of treatment for many clients, especially when combined with counselling and other behavioural therapies.
8. Addicted or substance-dependent individuals with coexisting mental disorders should have both disorders treated in an integrated way.
9. Medical detoxification is only the first stage of addiction treatment and by itself does little to change long-term drug use.
10. Treatment does not need to be voluntary to be effective. Note: The evidence supporting this principle is controversial. Canada's Drug Strategy (Health Canada, 2005) recognizes that abstinence is not the only acceptable, realistic, or even primary goal for all substance users (Thomas, 2005) and supports the principles of harm reduction.
11. Possible drug use during treatment must be monitored continuously.
12. Treatment programs should provide assessment for HIV/AIDS, hepatitis B and C, tuberculosis, and other infectious diseases, and counselling to help clients modify or change behaviours that place themselves or others at risk for infection.
13. Recovery from drug addiction can be a long-term process and frequently requires multiple episodes of treatment.

From National Institute on Drug Abuse. (1999). *Principles of drug addiction treatment: A research-based guide* (pp. 1, 3). Rockville, MD: National Institute on Drug Abuse.

Table 23.8   Treatment Approaches to Chemical Dependence

Approach	Psychiatric	Social	Moral	Learning	Disease	12-Step	Dual Diagnosis	Bio-Psychosocial	Multivariant
Conception of etiology	Symptom of underlying emotional problem	Society and environment cause dependence	Person is morally weak—can't say "no"	Abuse is a learned, reinforced behaviour	Probably caused by genetic or biologic factors	Combination of disease concept and "spiritual bankruptry"	Both a primary substance dependence and a mental health disorder	Biologic basis, with social and psychological influences	Many different causes; may be different for each individual
Conception of client	Emotionally disturbed	Victim of circumstance	"Hustler," morally deficient	Has distorted thinking, poor coping skills	Has a chronic progressive disease	Has an allergy and is powerless over substances	Has both mental and substance abuse disorder	Has deficiencies in all three interacting areas	Has multiple issues to be assessed and addressed
Conception of treatment outcome	Emotional conflicts are resolved; there is increased emotional health	Improved social functioning or improved environment	Moral recovery, increased willpower, control, and responsible behaviour	Client learns new ways of thinking and new coping skills	Abstinence, arresting disease progression, and beginning of recovery process	Abstinence, ongoing spiritual recovery	Improvement in both mental health and substance abuse disorders	Improvement in mental and physical health, utilization of social supports	Particular issues for individual addressed, and improvement occurs
Conception of treatment process	Psychotherapy, medication to treat "cause" of substance abuse	Removal of environmental influences and increasing coping responses to it	"Street addict" behaviour and manipulation confronted	Cognitive therapy techniques and coping skills taught	Is treated as a primary disease, reinforces client is an addict and has illness	Use 12 steps, seeking spiritual support, making amends, serving others in need	Concurrent treatment of both disorders	Concurrent treatment of all issues	Treatment strategies are matched with individual client needs
Advantages of approach	Not punitive, treats co-morbidity	Stresses social supports and coping skills	Holds person responsible for actions and making amends	Not punitive, teaches new coping skills	Not punitive, stresses support and education	Widespread success, emphasis is on quality of life and spiritual growth	Treats both mental health disorder and dependency, minimizing relapse potential	Utilizes different modalities; is more inclusive	Treatment matched to individual's needs
Disadvantages of approach	Focus is only on treatment of mental disorder	Blames "ills of society"—the person not responsible for addiction	Punitive, increases low self-esteem and sense of failure	Places emphasis on control of use	Minimizes mental health disorders; discounts return to social use	Self-help group, not a treatment program	Not inclusive enough; does not include social or other issues	Does not match client and specific interventions	Logistical problems can occur in its implementation

include spiritual, cognitive, and behavioural components. Many treatment programs discuss concepts from AA, hold meetings at the treatment facilities, and encourage clients to attend community meetings when appropriate. They also encourage continuing use of AA and other self-help groups as part of an ongoing plan for continued abstinence. Khantzian and Mack (1994) discuss therapeutic elements of Alcoholics Anonymous, pointing out that it does the following:

- Instills hope through seeing that others are not drinking
- Encourages honesty, openness, and a willingness to listen to others
- Emphasizes shared experiences and the development of a friendship network of sober individuals
- Focusses on abstinence and the loss of control over the ability to drink
- Fosters reliance on others, not on isolation and attempts at control of drinking by the use of willpower
- Adds a spiritual dimension that turns away from ego defence mechanisms such as denial and avoidance toward a better quality of life and the capacity to love and help others

Twelve-step programs do not solicit members, engage in political or religious activities, make medical or psychiatric diagnoses, engage in education about addiction to the general population, or provide mental health, vocational, or legal counselling (Nace, 1997). Alternative peer support groups differ from these programs in their approach. Although many have reported benefits from AA-related programs, exactly how effective they are compared with other treatments and how they work have yet to be shown (Brown, & Graves, 2005). For an additional discussion of 12-step programs and mental health clients, see Chapter 31.

Cognitive and Cognitive-Behavioural Interventions and Psychoeducation

Cognitive approaches to addiction hypothesize that if a client can change the way he or she thinks about a situation, both the emotional reaction to it and the behavioural response will change. Psychoeducational materials, groups, and one-on-one interactions with nurses also impart information to reduce knowledge deficits related to alcohol and drug dependence. Cognitive-behavioural therapy (CBT) is a brief treatment that is structured and focussed on immediate problems (Carroll, 1998). It enables clients to examine the thinking process that leads to decisions to use substances, analyze distortions in thinking, and develop rational responses to these distortions. Beck, Wright, Newman, and Liese (1993) developed a cognitive therapeutic approach to substance abuse in response to their model of a continuing use pattern fueled by distorted thinking. There is reasonably good evidence for the effectiveness of a number of CBT interventions in addressing substance use problems (Brown, & Graves, 2005).

Enhancing Coping Skills

Improving coping skills is thought to be one component of preventing relapse into alcohol and drug use. Coping skills include the ability to use thought, emotion, and action effectively to solve interpersonal and intrapersonal problems and to achieve personal goals (Carroll, 1998). Groups in addiction treatment programs that also have a relapse prevention component look at coping skills that are needed when drug and alcohol cravings are triggered. The skills listed in Table 23-9 are often taught as coping strategies for dealing with alcohol and drug cravings (Carroll, 1998). Clients role-play new behaviours and learn from the feedback they receive from other group members. They also increase their sense of competency to use these skills in real-life situations. A lengthier discussion of relapse prevention groups appears in Chapter 31.

Group Therapy and Early Recovery

Isolation and alienation from friends and family are common themes in chemically dependent clients. In addition, thinking that has become distorted is left

Table 23.9 Skills Training Group Topics	
Interpersonal	**Intrapersonal**
Starting conversations	Managing thoughts about alcohol
Giving and receiving compliments	Problem solving
Nonverbal communication	Increasing pleasant activities
Receiving criticism	Relaxation training
Receiving criticism about drinking	Awareness and management of anger
Drink and drug refusal skills	Awareness and management of negative thinking
Refusing requests	Planning for emergencies
Close and intimate relationships	Coping with persistent problems
Enhancing social support networks	

unchallenged without contact with others; thus, change is difficult. When a client enters a group that is working with the goals of continuing recovery, numerous healing advantages can occur. Vanicelli (1989) elaborated the curative elements of a group for people with alcoholism in early recovery first outlined by Yalom and updated in 1995. These groups can accomplish the following:

1. *Reduce the sense of isolation.* Offer a sense of belonging and of being understood.
2. *Instill hope.* Members can see others who are coping and doing well and who have made progress.
3. *Help members learn from watching others.* Members can observe how conflicts are resolved and see successful interactions.
4. *Impart information.* Members learn about group dynamics, how to stay sober, and what works or does not work in various circumstances.
5. *Alter distorted self-concepts.* Members can examine their own behaviour, observe how their behaviour affects others, and give feedback to each other.
6. *Provide a reparative family experience.* Members act and react in groups in ways that are similar to their behaviours in their family of origin. Past behaviours are challenged, and the client has an opportunity to grow and try new behaviours.

Groups in treatment settings focus on immediate goals of maintaining sobriety and not on childhood issues. The emphasis is on using problem-solving and other skills to deal with stressful events that threaten abstinence (Yalom, 1995). This type of support group is also extremely effective in outpatient treatment settings. After a period of successful abstinence, group therapy focusses more on traditional psychotherapy work.

Individual Therapy

Often, individual therapy is helpful, particularly in conjunction with group therapy or family therapy. Kaufman (1994) outlines three phases of long-term individual therapy. The first phase is assessing the problem and its particular emotional and social dynamics, increasing motivation for abstinence, and achieving abstinence. The second phase begins after detoxification and once abstinence is established. It involves maintaining abstinence by using cognitive-behavioural strategies, with the emphasis on immediate issues and their relationship to maintaining abstinence, and encouraging the client to use community self-help support groups. The third phase focusses on establishing intimacy with others and achieving autonomy. Often, issues of childhood trauma are examined during this phase. In addiction treatment settings, counsellors meet with individuals to maintain focus on the goals and objects of their treatment, to review the fears and anxieties that often arise in early recovery, and to devise

new and healthy responses and solutions to stressful and difficult situations (Nagy, 1994).

Family Therapy

Family therapy, a vital part of addiction treatment, can be used in several beneficial ways to initiate change and help the family when the substance-dependent person is unwilling to seek treatment. Behavioural couples therapy for people with alcoholism can improve family functioning, reduce stressors, smooth marital adjustment, and lessen domestic violence and verbal conflict (O'Farrell, 1999). When the substance-dependent person seeks help, family therapy can help stabilize abstinence and relationships. Often, inpatient substance abuse treatment programs have family education and group therapy components that help meet these goals (Laundergan & Williams, 1993). Family therapy can also help to maintain long-term recovery and prevent relapse (O'Farrell, 1999). Families can often unwittingly support addiction by continuing to supply money to the individual, allowing adult children to live at home while continuing their substance use, and "bailing out" individuals from legal and other difficulties that result from substance use. Family therapy can bring these behaviours to light and assist family members to set limits on their further support. Long-term family therapy is often beneficial after the initial stages of detoxification and stabilization. Stanton and Heath (1997) list six stages of marital and family therapy:

1. Defining the problem and negotiating a treatment contract
2. Establishing the context for a chemical-free life
3. Achieving abstinence
4. Managing the crisis and stabilizing the family
5. Reorganizing the family
6. Termination

Goals of family therapy should be realistic and obtainable. Action plans must be specific and organized into manageable increments. Target dates should be realistic so that pressure is minimal, yet there is motivation to act in a timely manner. Planning for the future is very difficult as long as alcohol or drug abuse continues (Box 23-9).

Implementing Nursing Interventions

Because substance-dependent clients differ greatly with respect to severity of the disorder and the biologic, social, and psychological features of their dependence, no one type of treatment program will work for every individual. Often, several approaches can work together, whereas others may be inappropriate. Treatment programs usually combine many different interventions to provide a comprehensive approach based on the individual's needs. Nursing interventions vary depending on the nature of the current problems and their severity. For a client who

Psychoeducation Family Teaching Plan Checklist: Substance Abuse

□ Psychopharmacologic agents, if used (drug action, dosage, frequency, and possible adverse effects)
□ Manifestations of intoxication, overdose, and withdrawal
□ Emergency medical system activation
□ Nutrition
□ Coping strategies
□ Structured planning
□ Safety measures
□ Available treatment programs
□ Family therapy referral
□ Self-help groups and other community resources
□ Follow-up laboratory testing, if indicated

is being detoxified, physical interventions (eg, monitoring vital signs and neurologic functioning) are necessary. When the substance use disorder is secondary to other physical or psychiatric problems, education of client and family may be a priority.

SUMMARY OF KEY POINTS

■ The *DSM-IV-TR* classifies substance use disorders related to the following categories: alcohol, cocaine, amphetamines and other stimulants, cannabis (marijuana), hallucinogens, phencyclidine, opiates, sedative-hypnotics and anxiolytics, inhalants, nicotine, and caffeine.

■ Use is defined as using legal substances within the bounds of socially acceptable circumstances and behaviour that does not pose any harm or risk to the individual or other. Harmful use (abuse), dependence, and addiction are defined as use of substances (legal or illicit) that involves risk to the individual and others and is associated with detrimental or harmful psychological and physiologic effects. Dependence and addiction also include symptoms of tolerance and withdrawal syndromes.

■ Methadone maintenance treatment is a form of treatment for opiate-dependent clients that includes giving a substitute drug, methadone, in lower, controlled dosages to satisfy the individual's intense drug craving and counteract debilitating withdrawal symptoms while the individual simultaneously receives other rehabilitative therapies (individual and group) to overcome addictive behaviours.

■ Opiate intoxication results in sedation, reduced memory and concentration, and euphoria. Withdrawal symptoms are abdominal cramps, runny nose and eyes, diaphoresis, and insomnia.

■ Codependence is a controversial term referring to a maladaptive pattern of coping resulting from prolonged exposure to dysfunctional family dynamics that occur in families of those with active alcohol or drug dependence. Codependence is characterized by boundary distortions, poor relationship and friendship skills, compulsive and obsessive behaviours, inappropriate anger, sexual maladjustment, and resistance to change.

■ A range of effective modalities is used in addiction treatment, and many programs combine several modalities, which can include 12-step programs, social skills groups, psychoeducational groups, cognitive and/or behavioural techniques, group therapy, and individual and family therapies. The research on the effectiveness of each approach varies, and there is no one best treatment method for all people. Evidence-based or best-practice approaches should be the treatments of choice.

■ Fear of acknowledgment (denial) of a substance use disorder is the individual's fear of accepting its diagnosis and can be exhibited by attempts to rationalize the substance use, minimize the harmful results, deflect attention from one's own problem to society's or someone else's, or blame childhood experiences.

■ Nurses should use a nonconfrontational approach when working with clients in fear (denial) of acknowledging their problem. Motivational interviewing approaches are most effective, using empathy and a nonjudgmental approach and helping the client to realize the discrepancy between life goals and engaging in substance use, thus motivating clients to change their self-destructive behaviours and make personal choices regarding treatment goals.

■ Accurate and comprehensive assessment is crucial in planning addiction treatment interventions. Evaluation should consider all substances for pattern of use, including factors of tolerance; withdrawal symptoms; consequences of use; loss of control over amount, frequency, or duration of use; desire or efforts to cease or control use; social, vocational, and recreational activities affected by use; and history of previous addiction treatment. Comprehensive evaluation also includes investigating family and social support systems.

■ Programs and policies should be formulated and delivered with sensitivity to gender, culture, and life stage. In addressing diverse populations, addiction programs should provide staff knowledgeable and responsive to those differences and specialized needs of diverse groups.

■ Substance use disorders have many social and political ramifications. Even the profession of nursing is not immune to substance use disorders among its members.

CRITICAL THINKING CHALLENGES

1 What is your understanding of the etiology of chemical dependence? Based on this understanding, what would be your priorities for client education?

2 Jeff H., a 35-year-old cocaine-dependent client, has entered a rehabilitation program. What goals do you believe would be realistic to achieve by the end of his projected 30-day inpatient stay?

3 You are working in an orthopaedic unit, and Mary L. has been admitted for treatment for a fractured femur. She has been drinking recently and has a blood alcohol level of 0.08%. What further information in the following areas would you need to plan her care?
a. Medical
b. Alcohol and drug use related
c. Other psychosocial issues

4 Medical use of marijuana has been approved in Canada. What is your opinion of this legislation? What are the advantages and disadvantages of this public policy?

5 Normal adolescent behaviour is often similar to that associated with substance abuse. How would you differentiate this normal behaviour from possible substance abuse or dependence?

6 John M. has sought treatment for depression and job stress. He came to your psychiatric assessment unit smelling of alcohol. He believes that he does not have a drinking problem but a job problem. What interventions would you use for possible alcohol abuse or dependence?

7 Sylvia G. has been using heroin intravenously heavily for 2 years. She has come into the hospital with an abscess on her leg. What symptoms would you expect to observe as she experiences withdrawal from opiates? What medications would likely be used to ease these symptoms?

8 After Sylvia G. is free of withdrawal symptoms, she expresses interest in obtaining drug treatment. What are her options? How would you describe them to her?

9 Raymond L. has been treated for hypertension at your clinic. You notice that he complains of peripheral neuropathy and has an unsteady gait. What other medical signs would corroborate alcoholism?

10 What laboratory test results would help confirm a diagnosis of alcoholism?

WEB LINKS

www.ccsa.ca The Canadian Centre on Substance Abuse is a national agency that promotes informed debate on substance abuse; disseminates information on the nature, extent, and consequences of substance abuse; and supports and assists organizations involved in substance abuse treatment, prevention, and educational programming.

www.ccsa.ca/ccendu The Canadian Community Epidemiology Network on Drug Use (CCENDU) is a collaborative project involving federal, provincial, and community agencies, with intersecting interests in drug use, health and legal consequences of use, treatment, and law enforcement.

www.camh.net/about_camh The Centre for Addiction and Mental Health (CAMH) is Canada's leading addiction and mental health teaching hospital.

www.cfdp.ca/sen1841.htm The Canadian Foundation for Drug Policy is a nonprofit organization that recommends effective and humane drug laws and policies in Canada.

www.drugpolicy.org Drug Policy Alliance is the leading organization in the United States working to broaden the public debate on drug policy and to promote realistic alternatives to the war on drugs based on science, compassion, health and human rights.

www.hc-sc.gc.ca/hppb/alcohol-otherdrugs/publications.htm Canada's Drug Strategy Division is the focal point within the federal government for harm reduction, prevention, and health promotion/population health initiatives concerning alcohol and other drugs issues.

www.who.int/dsa/cat98/subs8.htm The World Health Organization website provides access to publications on alcohol and drug abuse.

www.health.org The website of the National Clearinghouse for Alcohol and drug information and PRE-Vline includes a catalog of publications that discuss relevant treatment issues and research findings. It is possible to search several databases using this site.

www.nhic.org The National Health Information Center (NHIC) is consumer focussed and has the ability to conduct searches for health-related topics, including alcoholism and addiction issues.

www.os.dhhs.gov The U.S. Department of Health and Human Services (DHHS) website contains important information links to other relevant websites, including the Substance Abuse and Mental Health Services Administration (SAMHSA).

www.al-anon.org The purpose of Al-Anon is to help families and friends of people with alcoholism recover from the effects of living with the problem drinking of a relative or friend. Similarly, Alateen is the recovery program for young people. The program of recovery is adapted from Alcoholics Anonymous. The only requirement for membership is that there be a problem of alcoholism in a relative or friend.

www.alcoholics-anonymous.org This is the official site for the program of Alcoholics Anonymous. Information about this program and about alcoholism is available.

www.well.com/user/woa Web of Addictions. This site contains fact sheets and in-depth information on special topics, links to resources, and ways to contact various groups and get help with addictions.

www.samhsa.gov The website of the Substance Abuse and Mental Health Services Administration is a federal government site with funding, research, consumer information, and resources.

www.rxlist.com/top200.htm The top 200 prescriptions for 2002 by number of U.S. prescriptions dispensed.

MOVIES

Fix: The Story of an Addicted City: 2002. This NFB documentary focusses on a very controversial issue: Vancouver's efforts to open Canada's first safe injection site for drug users in its Downtown Eastside, one of our nation's poorest neighbourhoods with its highest HIV rate.

VIEWING POINTS: Articulate the arguments for and against safe injection sites. What is your personal position on the issue? Do you find dissent or consensus on the issue among your classmates? Your friends? Your family?

Heroines: The Photographic Obsession of Lincoln Clarkes: 2001. The disturbing world of drug addiction is explored through this NFB documentary. Portraits of addicted women living on the street in Vancouver reveal the harsh reality of their lives. We are confronted by things we may prefer to believe do not occur so close to home.

VIEWING POINTS: What do the lives of the women in this film tell us about addiction? Can you relate to their world? What, as a fellow citizen, do you think about their plight? What, as a nurse, might you offer to them?

The Basketball Diaries: 1995. Loosely based on the memoirs of Jim Carroll, *The Basketball Diaries* follows the experiences of a group of teenage boys as they experiment with drugs. Set in 1960s New York, the film follows Jim (played by Leonardo DiCaprio) and his friends as they play basketball, are expelled from school for using drugs, struggle to survive on the street, and cope with heroin addiction.

VIEWING POINTS: Movies like this one (eg, *Trainspotting*) are sometimes criticized for either glorifying or overly vilifying drug use. What do you think? Do you think they have an influence on adolescent drug use?

REFERENCES

Adams, W. L., Barry, K. L., & Fleming, M. F. (1996). Screening for problem drinking in older primary care patients. *Journal of the American Medical Association, 276*(24), 1964–1967.

Addiction Research Foundation. (1993). *The older adult and alcohol.* Toronto: Addiction Research Foundation

Adlaf, E. M., Paglia, A., & Ivis, F.(1999). Drug use among Ontario students, 1977–1999: Findings from the OSDUS. *CAMH Research Document No. 5.* Toronto: Centre for Addiction and Mental Health, 1999.

Alcoholics Anonymous World Services, Inc. (1976). *Alcoholics anonymous.* New York: Author.

American Psychiatric Association (APA). (2000). *The diagnostic and statistical manual of mental disorders* (4th ed., Text revision). Washington, DC: Author.

Anthenelli, R. M., & Schuckit, M. A. (1997). Genetics. In J. H. Lowinson, P. Ruiz, R. B. Millman, & J. G. Langrod (Eds.), *Substance abuse: A comprehensive textbook* (3rd ed., pp. 41–50). Baltimore: Williams & Wilkins.

Ballesteros, J., Gonzalez-Pinto, A., Querajeta, I., & Cerino, J. C. (2004). Brief interventions for hazardous drinking delivered in primary care and equally effective in men and women. *Addiction, 99*(1), 3–4.

Beck, A. A., Wright, F. D., Newman, C. F., & Liese, B. S. (1993). *Cognitive therapy of substance abuse.* New York: Guilford Press.

Bergob, M. (1994). Drug abuse among senior Canadians. *Canadian Social Trends, Summer,* 25–29.

Blow, F. C., Walton, M. A., Barry, K. L., Coyne, J. C., Mudd, S. A., & Copeland, L. A. (2000). The relationship between alcohol problems and health functioning of older adults in primary care settings. *Journal of the American Geriatrics Society, 48*(7), 769–774.

Brady, K. T., Myrick, H., & Malcolm, R. (1999). Sedative-hypnotic and anxiolytic agents. Specific drugs of abuse: Pharmacological and clinical aspects. In B. S. McCrady & E. E. Epstein (Eds.), *Addictions: A comprehensive guide book* (pp. 98–102). New York: Oxford University Press.

Brehm, N. M., & Khantzian, E. J. (1997). Psychodynamics. In J. H. Lowinson, P. Ruiz, R. B. Millman, & J. G. Langrod (Eds.), *Substance abuse: A comprehensive textbook* (3rd ed., pp. 90–100). Baltimore: Williams & Wilkins.

Brown, T., & Graves, G. (2005). Availability and use of evidence-based treatment (pp. 23–29) In *Substance abuse in Canada: Current challenges and choices.* Ottawa: Canadian Centre on Substance Abuse.

Canadian Centre on Substance Abuse. (1999a). *Canadian profile.* Ottawa: Author. Available at: http://www.ccsa.ca.

Canadian Centre on Substance Abuse. (1999b). *Workplace overview.* Ottawa: Author. Available at: http://www.ccsa.ca.

Canadian Centre on Substance Abuse. (2000). *Straight facts about drugs and drug abuse.* Ottawa: Author. Available at: http://www.ccsa.ca.

Canadian Centre on Substance Abuse. (2004). *Canadian addiction survey: A national survey of Canadian's use of alcohol and other drugs. Prevalence use and related harms.* Ottawa: Author.

Canadian Centre on Substance Abuse. (2005). *Substance abuse in Canada: Current challenges and choices 2005.* Ottawa: Author.

Canadian Community Health Survey (CCHS). *Mental health and well-being.* Ottawa: Statistics Canada. Available at: http://www.statcan.ca.

Canadian Institutes of Health Research. (2005). *North America's first clinical trial of prescribed heroin begins today.* News and Media Resources, Press Releases. February 2005. Available at: http://www.cihr-irsc.gc.ca.

Carroll, K. M. (1998). *A cognitive-behavioral approach: Treating cocaine addiction* (pp. 8–14). Rockville, MD: National Institute on Drug Abuse.

Caulker-Burnett, I. (1994). Primary care screening for substance abuse. *Nurse Practitioner, 19*(6), 42, 44–48.

Centre for Addiction and Mental Health. (2005). *Information about concurrent disorders.* Updated January 14, 2005.

Chassin, L., Pillow, D. R., Curran, P. J., et al. (1993). Relation of parental alcoholism to early adolescent substance abuse: A test of three mediating mechanisms. *Journal of Abnormal Psychology, 102,* 3–19.

Coambs, R. B., & McAndrews, M. P. (1994). The effects of psychoactive substances on workplace performance. In S. Macdonald & P. Roman (Eds.), *Drug testing in the workplace: Research advances in alcohol and drug problems* (Vol. 2, pp. 77–96). New York: Plenum Press.

DeLima, M. S., deOlivera Soceres, B. G., Reisser, A. A., & Farrell, M. (2002). Pharmacological treatment of cocaine dependence: A systematic review. *Addiction, 97*(8), 931–949.

Dewa, C., Lesage, A., Goering, P., Caveen, M. (2004). Nature and prevalence of mental illness in the workplace. *Health Papers, 5(2), Special Issue*.

Dufour, M., & Fuller, R. K. (1995). All in the elderly. *Annual Review of Medicine, 46*, 123–132.

Dunst, C. J., Trivette, C. M., & Deal, A. G. (1994). *Supporting and strengthening families: Methods, strategies and practices.* Cambridge, MA: Brookline Books.

Faltz, B., contributing author. (1993). *Women and HIV: Train the trainer program.* San Francisco: California Nurses Association.

Fingerhood, M. (2000). Substance abuse in older people. *Journal of the American Geriatric Society, 48(8)*, 985–995.

Finkelstein, N. (1993). Treatment programming for alcohol and drug-dependent pregnant women. *International Journal of Addictions, 28(13)*, 1275–1309.

Fischer, B. (2005). Harm reduction. (pp. 11–15) In *Substance abuse in Canada: Current challenges and choices.* Ottawa: Canadian Centre on Substance Abuse.

Fleming, M. F., Manwell, L. B., Barry, K. L., Adams, W., & Stauffacher, E. A. (1999). Brief physician advice for alcohol problems in older adults: A randomized community-based trial. *Journal of Family Practice, 48*, 378–384.

Fu, Q., Heath, A., Bucholz, K. K., Nelson, E., Goldberg, J., Lyons, M. J., True, W. R., Jacob, T., Tsuang, M. T., & Eisen, S. A. (2002). Shared genetic risk of major depression, alcohol dependence, and marijuana dependence: Contribution of antisocial personality disorder in men. *Archives of General Psychiatry, 59(12)*, 1125–1132.

Gardner, E. L. (1997). Brain reward mechanisms. In J. H. Lowinson, P. Ruiz, R. B. Millman, & J. G. Langrod (Eds.) *Substance abuse: A comprehensive textbook* (2nd ed., pp. 51–85). Baltimore: Williams & Wilkins.

Goldstein, R. Z., & Volkow, N. (2002). Drug addiction and its underlying neurobiological basics: Evidence for the involvement of the frontal cortex. *American Journal of Psychiatry, 159(10)*, 1642–1652.

Gomberg, E. S. (1999). Women. In B. S. McCrady & E. E. Epstein (Eds.), *Addictions: A comprehensive guide* (pp. 527–541). New York: Oxford University Press.

Goodwin, D. W. (1979). Alcoholism and heredity. *Archives of General Psychiatry, 36(1)*, 57–61.

Gottlieb, L. N., & Rowat, K. (1987). The McGill model of nursing: A practice-derived model. *Advances in Nursing Science, 9*, 51–61.

Government of Canada. (1998). *Canada's drug strategy.* Ottawa: Interdepartmental Working Group on Substance Abuse, Minister of Public Works and Government Services Canada. Cat. H39-440/1998E. Available at: http://www.hc-sc.gc.ca.

Grimley, D., Prochaska, J. O., Velicer, W. F., Blais, L. M., & DiClemente, C. C. (1994). The transtheoretical model of change. In T. M. Brinthaupt & R. P. Lipka (Eds.), *Changing the self: Philosophies, techniques, and experiences* (pp. 201–227). State University of New York Press.

Hawkins, J. D., Catalano, R. F., & Miller, J. Y. (1992). Risk and protective factors for alcohol and other drug problems in adolescence and early adulthood: Implications for substance abuse prevention. *Psychological Bulletin, 112*, 64–105.

Health Canada. (1996). *Exploring the links between substance use and mental health: Section I. A discussion paper. Section II. A round table.* Canada's Drug Strategy. Cat. No. H39-360/1-1996E. Ottawa: Author.

Health Canada. (1999a). *A second diagnostic on the health of First Nations and Inuit people in Canada: November, 1999.* Ottawa: Author.

Health Canada. (1999b). *Literature review: Evaluation strategies in Aboriginal substance abuse programs. A discussion.* First Nations and Inuit Health Branch (FNIHB), Ottawa: Author.

Health Canada. (2000) *Straight facts about drugs and abuse.* Cat. No. H39-65/2000E. Ottawa: Author.

Health Canada. (2001a). *Best practices: Treatment and Rehabilitation for women with substance use disorders.* Cat. No. H49-153/2001E. Ottawa: Author.

Health Canada. (2001b). *Preventing substance use problems among young people: A compendium of best practices.* Cat. No. H39-580/2001E. Ottawa: Author.

Health Canada. (2002a). *Best practices: Concurrent mental health and substance abuse disorders.* H39-599/2001-2E. Ottawa: Author. Available at: http://www.hc-sc.gc.ca.

Health Canada. (2002b). Sharing the learning: The health transition fund. Synthesis series. Mental Health. Health Canada. Cat. H13-6/2002-8. Ottawa: Author.

Health Canada. (2002c). *A report on mental illnesses in Canada.* Cat. 0-662-32817-5. Ottawa: Author.

Health Canada. (2003a). *Medical marijuana.* Ottawa: Author. Available at: http://www.hc-sc.gc.ca.

Health Canada. (2003b). *Best practices: Treatment and rehabilitation for seniors with substance use problems.* Cat. H46-2/03-295E. Ottawa: Author. Available at: http://www.hc-sc.gc.ca.

Health Canada. (2004). *Canadian tobacco use monitoring survey (CTUMS): Summary of results for the first half of 2004 (February to June).* Ottawa: Health Canada. Retrieved July 19, 2005, from http://www.hc-sc.gc.ca.

Hesselbrock, M. N., Hesselbrock, V. M., & Epstein, E. E. (1999). Theories of alcohol and other drug use disorders. In B. S. McCrady & E. E. Epstein (Eds.), *Addictions: A comprehensive guide* (pp. 50–71). New York: Oxford University Press.

Hughes, J., Hanscom, S., & Broom, B. (2001). *Nursing role report. The substance use practice competencies guideline: Part of the interprofessional faculty training plan on substance use project.* Ottawa: Drug Strategy Division of Health Canada.

Imhoff, J. E. (1991). Countertransference issues in alcoholism and drug addiction. *Psychiatric Annals, 21(5)*, 292–306.

Isaacson, J. H., & Schorling, J. B. (1999). Screening for alcohol problems in primary care. *Medical Clinics of North America, 83(6)*, 1547–1563.

Janssen, P. A., Demorest, L. C., & Whynot, E. M. (2005). Acupuncture for substance abuse treatment in the downtown eastside of Vancouver. *Journal of Urban Health, 82(2)*, 285–295.

Johnston, L. D., O'Malley, P., & Bachman, J. G. (2000). *Monitoring the future: National survey results on adolescent drug use. Overview of key findings, 1999.* Rockville, MD: U.S. Department of Health and Human Services, 2000.

Kaufman, E. (1994). *Psychotherapy of addicted persons.* New York: Guilford Press.

Khantzian, E. J., & Mack, J. E. (1994). How AA works and why it's important for clinicians to understand. *Journal of Substance Abuse Treatment, 11*, 77–92.

Kirby, M., & Keon, W. (2004). *Report 3. Mental health, mental illness and addiction: Issues and options for Canada.* Interim Report on the Standing Senate Committee on Social Affairs, Science and Technology. Ottawa: The Senate.

Kitchens, J. A. (1991). *Understanding and treating codependence.* Englewood Cliffs, NJ: Prentice-Hall.

Kristenson, H. (1995). How to get the best out of Antabuse. *New England Journal of Medicine, 338(9)*, 26.

Larimer, M. E. (1998). Harm reduction for alcohol problems: Expanding access to and acceptability of prevention and treatment services. In G. A. Marlatt (Ed.), *Harm reduction: Pragmatic strategies for managing high-risk behaviors* (pp. 69–121). New York: Guilford Press.

Laundergan, J. C., & Williams, T. (1993). The Hazelden residential family program: A combined systems and disease model approach. In T. J. O'Farrell (Ed.), *Treating alcohol problems: Marital and family interventions* (pp. 145–169). New York: Guilford Press.

Ludwig, M. A., Marecki, M., Wooldridge, P. J., & Sherman, L. M. (1996). Neonatal nurses' knowledge of and attitudes toward caring for cocaine exposed infants and their mothers. *Journal of Perinatal and Neonatal Nursing, 9(4)*, 81–95.

MacKay, R. C., Hughes, J. R., & Carver, E. J. (1990). *Empathy in the helping relationship.* New York: Springer Publishing.

Marion, I. J. (1995). *Pregnant substance abusing women* (pp. 2–11). Rockville, MD: U.S. Department of Health and Human Services.

Markey, B. T., & Stone, J. B. (1997). An alcohol and drug education program for nurses. *AORN Journal, 66*(5), 845–853.

Martin, J. K., Kraft, J. M., & Roman, P. M. (1994). Extent and impact of alcohol and drug use problems in the workplace: A review of the empirical evidence. In S. Macdonald & P. Roman (Eds.), *Drug testing in the workplace: Research advances in alcohol and drug problems* (Vol. 2, pp. 3–31). New York: Plenum Press.

McCaul, M. E., Wand, G. S., Eissenberg, T., Rohde, C. A., & Cheskin L. J. (2000). Naltrexone alters subjective and psychomotor responses to alcohol in heavy drinking subjects. *Neuropsychopharmacology, 22*(5), 480–492.

McNicholas, L. (2002/2003, Winter). Buprenorphine gains FDA approval. *Sudden Impact: Newsletter of the Quality Enhancement Research Initiative, Substance Abuse Module, 1*(1).

Miller, N. S., & Gold, M. S. (1994). A neurochemical basis for alcohol and other drug addiction. *Journal of Psychoactive Drugs, 25*(2), 121–126.

Miller, N. S., Gold, M. S., & Smith D. E. (Eds.). (1997). *Manual of therapeutics for addictions* (pp. 23–152). New York: Wiley-Liss.

Miller, W. R. (1995). Increasing motivation for change. In R. K. Hester & W. R. Miller (Eds.), *Handbook of alcoholism treatment approaches: Effective alternatives* (2nd ed., pp. 89–104). Boston: Allyn & Brown.

Miller, W. R., & Rollnick, S. (1991). *Motivational interviewing: Preparing people to change addictive behavior.* New York: Guilford Press.

Miller, W. R., & Sanchez, V. C. (1994). Motivating young adults for treatment and lifestyle change. In G. Howard & P. E. Nathan (Eds.), *Alcohol use and misuse by young adults.* Notre Dame, IN: University of Notre Dame Press.

Moak, D. H., & Anton, R. F. (1999). Alcohol. Specific drugs of abuse: Pharmacological and clinical aspects. In B. S. McCrady & E. E. Epstein (Eds.), *Comprehensive guidebook of addictions* (p. 78). New York: Oxford University Press.

Moffett, L. A. (1999). *Reality confrontation.* Unpublished manuscript.

Nace, E. P. (1997). Alcoholics Anonymous. In J. H. Lowinson, P. Ruiz, R. B. Millman, & J. G. Langrod (Eds.), *Substance abuse: A comprehensive textbook* (3rd ed., pp. 383–390). Baltimore: Williams & Wilkins.

Nagy, P. D. (1994). *Intensive outpatient treatment for alcohol and other drug abuse* (p. 21). Rockville, MD: U.S. Department of Health and Human Services.

National Institute on Alcohol Abuse and Alcoholism (NIAAA). (2002). Alcohol and minorities: An update. *Alcohol Alert, 55.* Available at: http:// www.niaaa.nih.902.

National Institute on Drug Abuse (NIDA). (1997). *Research report series: Heroin abuse and addiction* (pp. 1–8). Rockville, MD: Author.

National Institute on Drug Abuse (NIDA). (1999). *Principles of drug addiction treatment: A research-based guide* (pp. 1–3). Rockville, MD: Author.

National Institute on Drug Abuse (NIDA), National Institutes of Health. (2000). Marijuana 13551. Available at: http://www.drugabuse.gov.

National Native Addictions Partnership Foundation (NNADAP). (2000). *NNADAP Renewal Framework: For implementing the strategic recommendations of the 1998, General review of the National Native Alcohol and Drug Abuse Program.* Draft working paper, prepared for the Framework Sub-committee of the NNADAP. December 2000.

National Native Addictions Partnership Foundation's Treatment Activity Reporting System. (TARS). Database for health-related information on Aboriginal Canadians.

National Population Survey. Statistics Canada. Ottawa. Collects cross-sectional as well as longitudinal data designed to enhance the understanding of the processes affecting health.

Nemes, S., Rao, P. A., Zeiler, C., Munly, K., Holtz, K. D., & Hoffman, J. (2004). Computerized screening of substance abuse problems in a primary care setting: Older vs. younger adults. *American Journal of Drug and Alcohol Abuse, 30*(3), 627–642.

O'Connor, P. G., & Schottenfeld, R. S. (1998). Departments of Internal Medicine and Psychiatry Medical Progress: Patients with alcohol problems. *New England Journal of Medicine, 338*(9), 592–602.

O'Farrell, J. (1999). Alcoholism treatment and the family: Do family and individual treatments for alcoholic adults have preventative effects for children? *Journal of Studies on Alcohol, 13,* 125–129.

Pandina, R., & Hendren, R. (1999). Other drugs of abuse: Inhalants, designer drugs, and steroids. Specific drugs of abuse: Pharmacological and clinical aspects. In B. S. McCrady & E. E. Epstein (Eds.), *Addictions: A comprehensive guide book* (p. 173). New York: Oxford University Press.

Peele, S. (1985). What treatment for addiction can do and what it can't; what treatment for addiction should do and what it shouldn't. *Journal of Substance Abuse Treatment, 2,* 225–228.

Public Health Agency of Canada. (1998). *Alcohol and pregnancy.* The Canadian Perinatal Surveillance System. Last updated 2003. Available at: http://www.fas-saf.com.

Rosenthal, R. N., & Westreich, L. (1999). Treatment of persons with dual diagnoses of substance use disorder and other psychological problems. In B. S. McCrady & E. E. Epstein (Eds.), *Addictions: A comprehensive guide* (pp. 439–476). New York: Oxford University Press.

Royal Canadian Mounted Police. (2003). *Drug situation in Canada.* Available at: http://www.rcmp.ca.

SAMHSA. (2000). *National household survey on drug abuse.* Office of Applied Studies. Retrieved June 2003, from http://www.samhsa.gov.

Schuckit, M. (1999). New findings in the genetics of alcoholism. *Journal of the American Medical Association, 28*(20), 1875–1876.

Schuckit, M., Goodwin, D., & Winokur, D. (1972). A study of alcoholism in half-siblings. *American Journal of Psychiatry, 128,* 1132–1136.

Segal, B. M., & Stewart, J. C. (1996). Substance use and abuse in adolescence: An overview. *Child Psychiatry and Human Development, 26,* 193–210.

Selwyn, P. A., & Merino, F. L. (1997). Medical complications and treatment. In J. H. Lowinson, P. Ruiz, R. B. Millman, & J. G. Langrod (Eds.), *Substance abuse: A comprehensive textbook* (3rd ed., pp. 597–619). Baltimore: Williams & Wilkins.

Single, E. (2005). New directions in alcohol policy. (pp. 5–9) In *Substance abuse in Canada: Current challenges and choices.* Ottawa: Canadian Centre on Substance Abuse.

Single, E., Robson, L., & Scott, K. (1997). *Morbidity and mortality related to alcohol, tobacco, and illicit drug use among indigenous people in Canada.* Ottawa: Canadian Centre on Substance Abuse.

Single, E., Robson, L., Xie, X., & Rehm, J. (1996). *The costs of substance abuse in Canada.* Ottawa: Canadian Centre for Substance Abuse.

Slade, J. (1999). Nicotine. Specific drugs of abuse: Pharmacological and clinical aspects. In B. S. McCrady & E. E. Epstein (Eds.), *Comprehensive guidebook of addictions* (pp. 163–166). New York: Oxford University Press.

Smith, J. W. (1995). Medical manifestations of alcoholism in the elderly. *International Journal of Addications.* 30(13–14):1749–1798.

Somers, J. Goldner, E., Waraich, P., & Hsu, L. (2004). Prevalence studies of substance-related disorders: A systematic review of the literature. *Canadian Journal of Psychiatry, 49,* 373–384.

Stanton, M. D., & Heath, A. W. (1997). Family and marital therapy. In J. H. Lowinson, P. Ruiz, R. B. Millman, & J. G. Langrod (Eds.), *Substance abuse: A comprehensive textbook* (3rd ed., pp. 448–453). Baltimore: Williams & Wilkins.

Statistics Canada. (1999). Illicit drug use. In *1999 Statistical report on the health of Canadians* (pp. 184–187). Ottawa: Author.

Statistics Canada. (2002). *Statistical snapshots of Canada's seniors.* Available at: http://www.hc.sc.ga.

Statistics Canada. (2003). *2001 Census: Analysis series. Aboriginal peoples of Canada: A demographic profile.* Ottawa: Minister of Industry.

Statistics Canada. (2004). *Health reports: How healthy are Canadians?* Ottawa: Author. Available at: http://www.hc-sc.gc.ca.

Stephens, R. S. (1999). Cannabis and hallucinogens. Specific drugs of abuse: Pharmacological and clinical aspects. In B. S. McCrady & E. E. Epstein (Eds.), *Comprehensive guidebook of addictions* (pp. 122–129). New York: Oxford University Press.

Stewart, K. B., Richards, A. B. (2000). Recognizing and managing your patient's alcohol abuse. Nursing, 30(2):56–59.

Thomas, G. (2005). *Addiction and treatment centres in Canada: An environmental scan*. Ottawa: Canadian Centre on Substance Abuse. June 2005.

Tyas, S. L., & Rush, B. R. (1994). Trends in the characteristics of clients of alcohol/drug treatment services in Ontario. *Canadian Journal of Public Health, 85*(1), 13–16.

U.S. Department of Health and Human Services. (DHHS). (1997). *Alcohol and health* (pp. 1–31). Rockville, MD: Substance Abuse and Mental Health Administration.

U.S. Department of Health and Human Services (DHHS). (1999). *Enhancing motivation for change in substance abuse treatment*. Washington, DC: Author.

U.S. Department of Health and Human Services (DHHS). (2000). *Substance abuse treatment for persons with HIV/AIDS* (pp. 70–71). Washington, DC: Author.

U.S. Department of Health and Human Services (DHHS). (2001). *National household survey on drug abuse: Highlights 2000*. Rockville, MD: Substance Abuse and Mental Health Administration.

Vanicelli, M. (1989). *Removing the roadblocks: Group psychotherapy with substance abusers and family members*. New York: Guilford Press.

Vanyukov, M. M. (1999). Association between a functional polymorphism at the DRD2 gene and the liability to substance abuse. *American Journal of Medical Genetics*, 88(4):446–447.

Wallace, J. (1990). The new disease model of alcoholism. *Western Journal of Medicine, 152*, 501–505.

Weaver, M. F., & Schnoll, S. H. (1999). Stimulants: Amphetamine and cocaine. Specific drugs of abuse: Pharmacological and clinical aspects. In B. S. McCrady & E. E. Epstein (Eds.), *Comprehensive guidebook of addictions* (p. 115). New York: Oxford University Press.

Wennerstrom, P. A., & Rooda, L. A. (1996). Attitudes and perceptions of nursing students toward chemically impaired nurses: Implications for nursing education. *Journal of Nursing Education, 35*(5), 237–239.

Whitfield, C. W. (1997). Co-dependence, addictions, and related disorders. In J. H. Lowinson, P. Ruiz, R. B. Millman, & J. G. Langrod (Eds.), *Substance abuse: A comprehensive textbook* (3rd ed., pp. 672–683). Baltimore: Williams & Wilkins.

Yalom, I. (1995). *The theory and practice of group psychotherapy*. New York: Basic Books.

Zickler, P. (2001, October). Buprenorphine taken three times per week is as effective as daily doses in treating heroin addiction. *NIDA Notes, 16*(4).

For challenges, please refer to the **CD-ROM** in this book.

CHAPTER 24

Personality and Impulse-Control Disorders

Barbara J. Limandri, Mary Ann Boyd, and
Stephen VanSlyke

LEARNING OBJECTIVES

After studying this chapter, you will be able to:

- Identify the common features of personality disorders.
- Distinguish between the concepts of personality and personality disorder.
- Analyze the prevailing biologic, psychological, and social theories explaining the development of personality disorders.
- Discuss the epidemiology of each personality disorder.
- Distinguish among the three clusters of personality disorders.
- Formulate nursing diagnoses and plan interventions for clients with specific personality disorders.
- Compare the psychoanalytic explanation of the borderline personality disorder with biosocial theory.
- Apply the nursing process to individuals with a diagnosis of borderline personality disorder.
- Analyze special concerns within the nurse–client relationship common to treating those with personality disorders.
- Compare and contrast the impulse-control disorders.

KEY TERMS

adaptive inflexibility ▪ affective instability ▪ attachment ▪ cognitive schema ▪ communication triad ▪ dialectical behaviour therapy (DBT) ▪ dichotomous thinking ▪ dissociation ▪ emotional dysregulation ▪ emotional vulnerability ▪ emotions ▪ identity diffusion ▪ impulsivity ▪ inhibited grieving ▪ invalidating environment ▪ kleptomania ▪ parasuicidal behaviour ▪ projective identification ▪ psychopathy ▪ pyromania ▪ self-identity ▪ separation-individuation ▪ skills groups ▪ temperament ▪ tenuous stability ▪ thought stopping ▪ trichotillomania ▪ vicious circles of behaviour

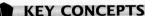 KEY CONCEPTS

personality ▪ personality disorder ▪ personality traits

The concept of personality seems deceivingly simple but is very complex. Historically, the term *personality* was derived from the Greek *persona*, the theatrical mask used by dramatic players. Originally, the term had the connotation of a projected pretense or allusion. With time, the connotation changed from being an external surface representation to the internal traits of the individual.

> **KEY CONCEPT Personality** is a complex pattern of characteristics, largely outside the person's awareness, that compose the individual's distinctive pattern of perceiving, feeling, thinking, coping, and behaving. The personality emerges from a complicated interaction of biologic dispositions, psychological experiences, and environmental situations.

Today, personality is conceptualized as a complex pattern of psychological characteristics that are not easily altered and that are largely outside the person's awareness. These characteristics or traits include the individual's specific style of perceiving, thinking, and feeling about self, others, and the environment. These styles or traits are similar across many different social or personal situations and are expressed in almost every facet of functioning. Intrinsic and pervasive, they emerge from a complicated interaction of biologic dispositions, psychological experiences, and environmental situations that ultimately make up the individual's distinctive personality (Millon & Davis, 1999).

IN A LIFE

Ferdinand Waldo Demara (1921–1982)
The Great Impostor

Public Persona
Ferdinand Waldo Demara spent much of his adult life using forged, stolen, or nonexistent credentials to gain employment in numerous and varied vocations. He became most famous for his masquerade as a commissioned Surgeon-Lieutenant in the Royal Canadian Navy in 1951, having stolen the identity of the Canadian physician Dr. Joseph Cyr. Demara was apparently competent in his role as a physician, relying on medical texts and a medical assistant. Demara had similar success in other branches of the military, as a psychologist in a college, as a prison warden, and as a well-respected school teacher.

Personal Realities
Demara's life was patterned by the establishment of personal connections with individuals (often in the context a religious order), theft of this person's identity, and subsequent employment using these false credentials. Once caught, he would disappear, only to reappear claiming a new identity. It was a sense of emptiness and boredom that would kindle Demara's dreams and his need to act as an impostor to fulfill his seemingly well-intentioned passions.

Source: Crichton, R. (1959). *The great impostor.* New York: Random House.

Personality Disorders

No sharp division exists between normal and abnormal personality functioning. Instead, personalities are viewed on a continuum from normal at one end to abnormal at the other. Many of the same processes involved in the development of a "normal" personality are responsible for the development of a personality disorder.

> **KEY CONCEPT A personality disorder** is an enduring pattern of inner experience and behaviour that deviates markedly from the expectations of the individual's culture, is pervasive and inflexible, has an onset in adolescence or early adulthood, is stable with time, and leads to distress or impairment (American Psychiatric Association [APA], 2000, p. 685).

Personality disorders are classified on Axis II of the *Diagnostic and Statistical Manual of Mental Disorders*, 4th edition, text revision (*DSM-IV-TR*) multiaxial system for diagnoses, separate from the other mental disorders presented thus far, which are classified under Axis I (APA, 2000). Separate classification under Axis II was intended to focus attention on manifestations of behavioural patterns that might be overlooked in light of the more pronounced disorders of Axis I; it does not imply difference in pathogenesis or treatment interventions. Frequently, an Axis II diagnosis coexists with an Axis I diagnosis, in which case the Axis II diagnosis may serve as the background through which the person experiences the other diagnosis. For example, a person who has a dependent personality disorder might also have symptoms of generalized anxiety disorder when faced with demands to function autonomously.

Ten personality disorders are recognized as psychiatric diagnoses and are organized into three clusters based on the dimensions of *odd-eccentric, dramatic-emotional*, and *anxious-fearful* behaviours or symptoms. Cluster A consists of the disorders that most broadly characterize odd and eccentric misfit disorders, including paranoid personality disorder, schizoid personality disorder, and schizotypal personality disorder.

People with cluster B disorders show great impulsivity (acting without considering the consequences of the act or alternate actions) and emotionality; these disorders consist of antisocial personality disorder (APD), borderline personality disorder (BPD), histrionic personality disorder, and narcissistic personality disorder. Dramatic and erratic behaviour best characterizes people with cluster B disorders. Cluster C disorders feature a predominant sense of anxiety and fearfulness and include avoidant personality disorder, dependent personality disorder, and obsessive-compulsive personality disorder.

BPD is highlighted in this chapter because it is severely incapacitating and difficult to treat. APD is also emphasized. Symptoms associated with both of these disorders often provoke negative reactions on the part of the clinician, which interferes with the clinician's ability to provide effective care. Impulse-control disorders are summarized at the end of the chapter. These disorders commonly coexist with other mental disorders.

PERSONALITY DISORDER VERSUS PERSONALITY TRAITS

To receive a diagnosis of a personality disorder, an individual must demonstrate the criteria behaviours persistently and to such an extent that they impair the ability to function socially and occupationally. In some people, the underlying feelings and behaviours may be intermittent and interfere interpersonally without obvious impairment. Instead of having a personality disorder, the individual is said to have traits of the disorder, which also can be noted on Axis II without a formal diagnosis.

> ⬢ **KEY CONCEPT Personality traits** are prominent aspects of personality that are exhibited in a wide range of important social and personal contexts (APA, 2000, p. 770).

Students learning about personality disorders and traits for the first time probably will question whether these personality patterns are truly mental disorders. These questions are shared by much of the general public. Even within the psychiatric community, there is much debate regarding the status of personality disorders. Students may also feel frustrated in caring for individuals with these disorders or traits because sometimes problems may seem to be patterns of behaviours over which the individual could gain control, and because the client may seem otherwise emotionally healthy. Unfortunately, that is not the case. These patterns of thinking and behaviour are not easily changed, and these individuals need a great amount of help and understanding from mental health providers. Changing lifelong personality patterns is difficult and requires much understanding and support.

COMMON FEATURES AND DIAGNOSTIC CRITERIA

The personality disorder diagnosis is based on manifestation of abnormal, inflexible behaviour patterns of long duration, traced to adolescence or early adulthood. These behaviours are pervasive across a broad range of personal and social situations and cause significant distress or impairment to social or occupational functioning. These abnormal behaviour patterns must deviate markedly from expectations of the individual's culture and must manifest in two or more of the following

areas: cognition, or ways of perceiving and interpreting self, other people, and events; affectivity, or the range, intensity, lability, and appropriateness of emotional responses; interpersonal functioning; and impulse control. For immigrants who may be having difficulty learning new acceptable social and cultural behaviour patterns and adjusting to a new culture, the diagnosis of a personality disorder may be delayed beyond this difficult adjustment period.

Maladaptive Cognitive Schema

Cognitive schemas are patterns of thoughts that determine how a person interprets events. Each person's cognitive schemas screen, code, and evaluate incoming stimuli. In personality disorders, maladaptive cognitive schemas cause misinterpretation of other people's actions or reactions and of events that result in dysfunctional ways of responding. For example, if a person thinks that no one can be trusted, an innocent, friendly gesture can be interpreted as a suspicious behaviour, provoking a hostile response, instead of a reciprocal friendly greeting.

Affectivity and Emotional Instability

Emotions are psychophysiologic reactions that define a person's mood and can be categorized as negative (anger, fright, anxiety, guilt, shame, sadness, envy, jealousy, and disgust), positive (happiness, pride, relief, and love), and neutral (hope, compassion, empathy, sympathy, and contentment). Emotions can affect one's ability to learn and function by affecting one's memory and how one accesses and stores information. Emotional arousal, particularly increased negative emotional arousal characteristic of people with personality disorders, can decrease one's ability to remember new information and accurately perceive the environment (Herpertz, Kunnert, Schwenger, & Sass, 1999).

Impaired Self-Identity and Interpersonal Functioning

Self-identity is central to the normal development of one's personality. Self-identity includes an integration of social and occupational roles and affiliations, self-attributed personality traits, attitudes about gender roles, beliefs about sexuality and intimacy, long-term goals, political ideology, and religious beliefs. Without an adequately formed identity, an individual's goal-directed behaviour is impaired, and interpersonal relationships are disrupted. Each individual's abilities, limitations, and goals are shaped by one's identity. In personality disorders, self-identity is often disturbed or absent.

Impulsivity and Destructive Behaviour

People with personality disorders often come to the attention of the mental health clinician because their impulsive behaviour results in negative consequences to others or themselves. They seem unable to consider the consequences of their actions before acting on their impulses. For example, an individual may feel rage toward another and lack skills to resist the impulse to attack that person physically, even though this action may be punished.

SEVERITY OF DISORDER

Three generally agreed-on essential and interdependent criteria are used for determining the severity of personality pathology: tenuous stability, adaptive inflexibility, and tendency to become trapped in rigid and inflexible patterns of behaviour that are self-defeating.

Tenuous Stability

Tenuous stability refers to fragile personality patterns that lack resiliency under subjective stress. These individuals may have exaggerated emotional reactions to stressful situations and cannot cope emotionally with normal stressful situations. They do not easily learn coping skills and may be overwhelmed when new difficulties arise.

Adaptive Inflexibility

Adaptive inflexibility describes rigidity in interactions with others, achievement of goals, and coping with stress. In the normal course of daily living, people learn when to take the initiative and modify environmental factors, as well as when to adapt to the situation. They learn to be flexible in interactions with other people and their environment. Socially appropriate reactions that are proportional to the situation are the norm. Personalities become pathologic when individuals cannot adapt effectively to new circumstances and, instead, begin arranging their lives to avoid stressful situations. Their view of the world and expectations of people within it are inflexible. Consequently, there are no opportunities to learn and practice new coping skills.

The tendency to become trapped in rigid and inflexible patterns of behaviour creates **vicious circles of behaviour** that are self-defeating. These individuals become so rigid and inflexible in their interactions and role functioning that they generate and perpetuate dilemmas, provoke new predicaments, and set into motion self-defeating sequences with others. They restrict opportunities for new learning, misconstrue benign events, and provoke reactions in others that reac-

tivate earlier problems (Millon & Davis, 1999). For example, a normal reaction of feeling angry at receiving a parking ticket usually subsides, and the person decides either to pay the fine or to appeal the case in court. The person with a personality disorder may get angry about receiving the ticket, but the anger controls his actions. For example, he may lash out verbally at the police officer who gave the ticket and get another citation, or when appearing in court, may scream at the judge in the courtroom and end up receiving a more severe sentence such as having to serve time in jail. What begins as a normal stressful daily life event becomes a series of disastrous interpersonal conflicts and ends in a tragic situation for the person with the personality disorder. Modulating emotions and behaviour requires psychoneurologic resources and learned coping skills. The individual with a normal reaction of anger may count to 10 before responding to the ticket or commiserate with a companion. However, the person with a personality disorder lacks cognitive modulation of the emotion and may intimidate others with an irrational angry outburst.

Cluster A Disorders: Odd-Eccentric

PARANOID PERSONALITY DISORDER: SUSPICIOUS PATTERN

The most prominent features of paranoid personality disorder are mistrust of others and the desire to avoid relationships in which one is not in control or loses power. These individuals are suspicious, guarded, and hostile. They are consistently mistrustful of others' motives, even relatives and close friends. Actions of others are often misinterpreted as deception, deprecation, and betrayal, especially regarding fidelity or trustworthiness of a spouse or friend (Millon & Davis, 1999). Minor innocuous incidents are often misinterpreted as having sinister or hidden meaning, and suspicions are magnified into major distortions of reality. People with paranoid personalities are unforgiving and hold grudges; their typical emotional responses are anger and hostility. They distance themselves from others and are outwardly argumentative and abrasive; internally, they feel powerlessness, fearful, and vulnerable (Bodner & Mikulincer, 1998). Other hallmark features of paranoid personality disorder are persistent ideas of self-importance and the tendency to be rigid and controlled. These people are blind to their own unattractive behaviours and characteristics; they often are hypercritical and attribute these traits to others. Their outward demeanour often seems cold, sullen, and humourless. They want to appear controlled and objective, yet often they react emotionally, displaying signs of nervousness, anger, envy, and jealousy. Orderly by nature, they are hypervigilant to any environmental changes that may loosen their control on the world. Because people with this disorder are extremely sensitive about appearing "strange" or "bizarre," they will not seek mental health care until they decompensate into a psychosis (Table 24-1).

Epidemiology

Canadian prevalence data are lacking for paranoid personality disorder as well as for other types of personality disorders (Health Canada, 2002). In the United States, the prevalence of paranoid personality disorder is reported to be 0.5% to 2.5% in the general population. In inpatient settings, 10% to 30% of clients have this disorder, and in outpatient settings, 2% to 10% have the disorder (APA, 2000). Axis I disorders, such as generalized anxiety disorder, mood disorders, and schizophrenia, can coexist with paranoid personality disorder, but minor Axis I symptoms usually are not seen. Other Axis II disorders can also coexist, such as narcissistic, avoidant, and obsessive-compulsive personality disorders (Millon & Davis, 1999).

Table 24.1	Summary of Diagnostic Characteristics of Cluster A Disorders: Diagnostic Criteria and Target Symptoms

Paranoid Personality Disorder 301.0	▪ Pervasive distrust and suspiciousness of others interpreted as malevolent (often with little or no justification or evidence to support it)
	      Assumption of exploitation, harm, or deception; feelings that others are plotting against him or her with possible sudden attacks (associated with feelings of deep or irreversible injury) at any time for no reason
	      Preoccupation with doubts of loyalty or untrustworthiness of friends and associates; deviation from doubts viewed as support for assumptions
	      Reluctance to confide in others or become close in fear that information will be used against him or her
	      Interpretation of hidden meanings into remarks or events, believing them to be demeaning and threatening
	      Holding of grudges with unwillingness to forgive; minor intrusions arouse major hostility, persisting for long periods of time
	      Quick to react and counterattack to perceived insults—possible pathologic jealousy with recurrent suspiciousness about fidelity of spouse or sexual partner
	 ▪ Not occurring exclusively during course of another psychiatric disorder; not a direct physiologic effect of a general medical condition

Schizoid Personality Disorder 301.20	▪ Pervasive pattern of detachment from social relating
	 ▪ Restricted range for emotional expression
	      Lacking desire for intimacy
	      Indifference to opportunities for close relationships
	      Little satisfaction from being part of family or social group
	      Preference for alone time rather than being with others; choosing solitary activities or hobbies
	      Little if any interest in having sexual experiences with others
	      Reduced pleasure from sensory, bodily, or interpersonal experiences
	      No close friends or relatives
	      Indifference to approval or criticism from others
	      Emotional coldness, detachment, or flattened activity
	 ▪ Not occurring exclusively during course of another psychiatric disorder; not a direct physiologic effect of a general medical condition

Schizotypal Personality Disorder 301.22	▪ Pervasive pattern of social and interpersonal deficits evidenced by acute discomfort and reduced capacity for close relationships and cognitive and perceptual distortions and eccentric behaviour
	      Ideas of reference
	      Odd beliefs or magical thinking influencing behaviour, such as superstitions, and preoccupation with paranormal phenomena, special powers
	      Perceptual alterations
	      Odd thinking and speech
	      Suspiciousness or paranoid ideation
	      Stiff, inappropriate, or constricted interactions
	      Odd or eccentric behaviour or appearance
	      Few close friends or confidants (other than first-degree relative)
	      Anxiety in social situation, especially unfamiliar ones; no decrease in anxiety with increasing familiarity
	 ▪ Not occurring exclusively during course of another psychiatric disorder

Etiology

The etiologic factors of paranoid personality disorder are unclear. Experts speculate that there may be a genetic predisposition for an irregular maturation. An underlying excess in limbic and sympathetic system reactivity or a neurochemical acceleration of synaptic transmission may exist. These dysfunctions can give rise to the hypersensitivity, cognitive autism, and social isolation that characterize these clients. As children, these individuals tend to be active and intrusive, difficult to manage, hyperactive, and irritable, and have frequent temper outbursts.

Nursing Management

Nurses are most likely to see these clients for other health problems but will formulate nursing diagnoses based on the client's underlying suspiciousness. Assessment of these individuals will reveal disturbed or illogical thoughts that demonstrate misinterpretation of environmental stimuli. For example, a man was convinced that his wife was having an affair with the neighbour because his wife and the neighbour left their homes for work at the same time each morning. Although the man's beliefs were illogical, he never once considered that he was wrong. He frequently followed them but never caught them together. He continued to believe they were having an affair. The nursing diagnosis of Disturbed Thought Processes is usually supported by the assessment data.

Because of their inability to develop relationships, these individuals are often socially isolated and lack social support systems. Yet, the nursing diagnosis of Social Isolation is not appropriate for the person with paranoid personality disorder because the person does not meet the defining characteristics of feelings of aloneness, rejection, desire for contact with people, and insecurity in social situations.

Nursing interventions based on the establishment of a nurse–client relationship are difficult to implement because of the person's mistrust. If a trusting relationship is established, the nurse helps the individual identify problematic areas, such as getting along with others or keeping a job. Through therapeutic techniques such as acceptance, confrontation, and reflection, the nurse and client examine a problematic area to gain another view of the situation. Changing thought patterns takes time. Client outcomes are evaluated in terms of small changes in thinking and behaviour.

Because paranoid personality disorder has extreme anxiety at its root, there is likely to be disruption in the dopaminergic tracts between the limbic and cortical areas (Cloninger, Bayon, & Svrakic, 1998). Therefore, serotonin-dopamine antagonists such as risperidone (Risperdal), olanzapine (Zyprexa), or quetiapine (Seroquel) may be prescribed. The nurse needs to explain how these drugs work to elicit adherence.

SCHIZOID PERSONALITY DISORDER: ASOCIAL PATTERN

People with schizoid personality disorder are expressively impassive and interpersonally unengaged (Millon & Davis, 1999). They tend to be unable to experience the joyful and pleasurable aspects of life. They are introverted and reclusive, and clinically appear distant, aloof, apathetic, and emotionally detached. They have difficulties making friends, seem uninterested in social activities, and appear to gain little satisfaction in personal relationships. In fact, they appear to be incapable of forming social relationships. Interests are directed at objects, things, and abstractions. As children, they engage primarily in solitary activities, such as stamp collecting, computer games, electronic equipment, or academic pursuits such as mathematics or engineering. In addition, there seems to be a cognitive deficit characterized by obscure thought processes, particularly about social matters. Communication with others is confused and lacks focus. These individuals reveal minimum introspection and self-awareness, and interpersonal experiences are described in a very mechanical way (see Table 24-1).

Epidemiology

Schizoid personality disorder is rarely diagnosed in clinical settings (Lyons, 1995). It is estimated that the prevalence of schizoid disorder ranges from 0% to 8%, with a median prevalence of 1.7% (Torgersen, Kringlen, & Cramer, 2001). The most prevalent comorbid disorder is avoidant personality disorder, which occurs in 5% of the cases. Dependent and obsessive-compulsive disorders may coexist with schizoid personality disorder (Torgersen et al., 2001).

Etiology

The etiologic processes are speculative. There may be defects in either the limbic or reticular regions of the brain that may result in the development of the schizoid pattern (Millon & Davis, 1999). The defects of this personality may stem from an adrenergic–cholinergic imbalance in which the parasympathetic division of the autonomic nervous system is functionally dominant. Excesses or deficiencies in acetylcholine and norepinephrine may result in the proliferation and scattering of neural impulses that may be responsible for the cognitive "slippage" or affective deficits.

Nursing Management

Impaired Social Interactions and Chronic Low Self-Esteem are typical diagnoses of individuals with schizoid personality disorder. Major treatment goals are to enhance the experience of pleasure, prevent social isolation, and increase emotional responsiveness to others. Because these individuals often lack customary social skills, social skills training is useful in enhancing their ability to relate in interpersonal situations. The primary focus is to increase the person's ability to feel pleasure. The nurse balances interventions between encouraging enough social activity that prevents the individual from retreating to a fantasy world and too much social activity that becomes intolerable.

The nurse may find working with these individuals unrewarding and become frustrated, feel helpless, or feel bored during the interactions. It is difficult to establish a therapeutic relationship with these individuals because they tend to shy away from interactions. Evaluation of outcomes should be in terms of increasing the client's feelings of satisfaction with solitary activities.

SCHIZOTYPAL PERSONALITY DISORDER: ECCENTRIC PATTERN

People with the schizotypal personality disorder are characterized by a pattern of social and interpersonal deficits. They are void of any close friends other than first-degree relatives. They have odd beliefs about their world that are inconsistent with their cultural norms. Ideas of reference (incorrect interpretations of events as having special, personal meaning) are often present, as are unusual perceptual delusions and odd, circumstantial, and metaphorical thinking and speech. Their mood is constricted or inappropriate, and they have excessive social anxieties of a paranoid character that do not diminish with familiarity. Their appearance and behaviour are characterized as odd, eccentric, or peculiar. They usually exhibit an avoidant behaviour pattern (see Table 24-1).

If these individuals do become psychotic, they seem totally disoriented and confused. Many will exhibit posturing, grimacing, inappropriate giggling, and peculiar mannerisms. Speech tends to ramble. Fantasy, hallucinations, and bizarre, fragmented delusions may be present. Regressive acts such as soiling and wetting the bed may occur. These individuals may consume food in an infantile or ravenous manner. Symptoms mirror but fall short of features that would justify the diagnosis of schizophrenia. The person's tendency is to remain socially isolated, dependent on family members or institutions. These individuals avoid social interaction that can keep them functional, and well-intentioned relatives or institutional staff will protect them, reinforcing their dependency. People with this disorder are particularly prone to experiencing disorganized schizophrenia.

Epidemiology

The prevalence of schizotypal personality disorder is estimated to range from 0.6% to 5.1%, with a median rate of about 3% of the nonclinical population. In a clinical sample of psychiatric clients, the prevalence ranged from 2.0% to 64%, with a median prevalence of 17.5% (Torgersen et al., 2001). This wide variation in prevalence rates may reflect the controversy surrounding the classification of schizotypal disorder as a separate personality disorder, instead of a component of schizophrenia.

Etiology

The etiology of schizotypal personality disorder is unknown. The neurodevelopmental explanation posits that schizotypy can be explained by insults, such as oxygen deprivation, to the nervous system at critical developmental periods. There is speculation that this disorder is part of a continuum of schizophrenia-related disorders and is really closely related to chronic schizophrenia (Matta et al., 2000). When the genetics of personality disorders are considered, there is evidence of a link between schizotypal personality disorder and schizophrenia (Matta et al., 2000). Additional research is needed to determine whether this disorder is a milder form of schizophrenia.

People with schizotypal personality disorder have widespread cognitive deficits involving the left hemisphere more than the right and impaired cholinergic responsivity. Therefore, they have difficulty with short-term memory and verbal learning (Cadenhead, Perry, Shafer, & Braff, 1999; Voglmaier et al., 2000). They also exhibit visual, perceptual, and working memory deficits (Farmer et al., 2000).

Nursing Management

Depending on the amount of decompensation (deterioration of functioning and exacerbation of symptoms), the assessment of a client with a schizotypal personality disorder can generate a range of nursing diagnoses. If a person has severe symptoms, such as delusional thinking or perceptual disturbances, the nursing diagnoses are similar to those for a person with schizophrenia (see Chapter 17). If symptoms are mild, the typical nursing diagnoses include Social Isolation, Ineffective Coping, Low Self-esteem, and Impaired Social Interactions.

People with schizotypal personality disorder need help in increasing their sense of self-worth and recognizing their positive attributes. They can benefit from interventions such as social skills training and environmental management that increases their psychosocial functioning. Their odd, eccentric thoughts and behaviours alienate them from others. Reinforcing socially appropriate dress and behaviour can improve their overall appearance and ability to relate in the environment. Because they have a hard time generalizing from one situation to another, attention to cognitive skills is important (Waldeck & Miller, 2000).

Continuum of Care

People with cluster A personality disorders are rarely seen in mental health treatment because they seldom admit to mental health problems. They can improve their quality of life through psychotherapy, but their suspiciousness, lack of trust, or impaired social interactions make it difficult to establish a therapeutic relationship. They do not usually seek treatment unless more serious symptoms appear, such as depression or anxiety. Medications are not generally used unless there is coexisting anxiety or depression. Even individuals with schizotypal personality disorder have a relatively stable course. Few actually experience schizophrenia or another psychotic disorder (APA, 2000). They too seek health care for other problems, and come to the attention of mental health professionals when their odd behaviour interferes with their daily activities. At these times, brief interventions are needed, such as self-care assistance, reality orientation, and role enhancement (McCloskey & Bulechek, 2000).

Nursing care is often provided in a home or primary care setting, with the personality disorder being secondary to the purpose of the care. This means that nurses are focussing on other aspects of client care and

may miss the underlying psychiatric disorder. A psychiatric nursing consult may be needed for these individuals to help identify the disorder.

Cluster B Disorders: Dramatic-Emotional
BORDERLINE PERSONALITY DISORDER: UNSTABLE PATTERN
Clinical Course of Disorder

In 1938, the term *borderline* was first used to refer to a group of disorders that did not quite fit the definition of either neurosis or psychosis (Stern, 1938). The term evolved from the psychoanalytic conceptualization of the disorder as a dysfunctional personality structure. In 1980, BPD was formally recognized as a distinct disorder in the *DSM-III*. In the *DSM-IV-TR*, BPD is defined as "a pervasive pattern of instability of interpersonal relationships, self-image, and affects, and marked impulsivity that begins by early adulthood and is present in a variety of contexts" (APA, 2000, p. 706). Table 24-2 outlines the diagnostic characteristics of BPD.

People with BPD have problems in regulating their moods, developing a sense of self, maintaining interpersonal relationships, maintaining reality-based cognitive processes, and avoiding impulsive or destructive behaviour. They appear more competent than they actually are and often set unrealistically high expectations for themselves. When these expectations are not met, they experience intense shame, self-hate, and self-directed anger. Their lives are like soap operas—one crisis after another. Some of the crises are caused by the individual's

Table 24.2	Key Diagnostic Characteristics of Borderline Personality Disorder 301.83	

Diagnostic Criteria and Target Symptoms	Associated Findings

• Pervasive pattern of unstable interpersonal relationships, self-image, and affects
   Frantic efforts to avoid real or imagined abandonment
   Pattern of unstable and intense interpersonal relationships (alternating between extremes of idealization and devaluation)
   Identity disturbance (markedly and persistently unstable self-image or sense of self)
   Impulsivity in at least two areas that are potentially self-damaging (spending, sex, substance abuse, reckless driving, or binge eating)
   Recurrent suicidal behaviour, gestures, or threats; or self-mutilating behaviour
   Affective instability due to a marked reactivity of mood (intense episodes lasting a few hours and only rarely more than a few days)
   Chronic feelings of emptiness
   Inappropriate, intense anger or difficulty controlling anger
   Transient, stress-related paranoid ideation or severe dissociative symptoms
• Beginning by early adulthood and presenting in a variety of contexts
	Associated Behavioural Findings
	• Pattern of undermining self at the moment a goal is to be realized
	• Possible psychotic-like symptoms during times of stress
	• Recurrent job losses, interrupted education, and broken marriages
	• History of physical and sexual abuse, neglect, hostile conflict, and early parental loss or separation

dysfunctional lifestyle or inadequate social milieu, but many are caused by fate—the death of a spouse or a diagnosis of an illness. They react emotionally with minimal coping skills. The intensity of their dysregulation often frightens themselves and others. Friends, family members, and coworkers limit their contact with the person, which furthers their sense of aloneness, abandonment, and self-hatred. It also diminishes opportunities for learning self-corrective measures.

Affective Instability

Affective instability (rapid and extreme shift in mood) is a core characteristic of BPD and is evidenced by erratic emotional responses to situations and intense sensitivity to criticism or perceived slights. For example, a person may greet a casual acquaintance with intense affection, yet later be aloof with the same acquaintance. Friends describe individuals with BPD as moody, irresponsible, or intense. These individuals fail to recognize their own emotional responses, thoughts, beliefs, and behaviours. Clinically, when a stressful situation is encountered, these individuals react with shifts in emotions. They seem to have limited ability to develop emotional buffers to stressful situations. Regulating anger, anxiety, and sadness is particularly problematic (Stein, 1996).

Identity Disturbances

Identity diffusion occurs when a person lacks aspects of personal identity or when personal identity is poorly developed (Erikson, 1968). Four factors of identity are most commonly disturbed: role absorption (narrowly defining self within a single role), painful incoherence (distressed sense of internal disharmony), inconsistency (lack of coherence in thoughts, feelings, and actions), and lack of commitment (Wilkinson-Ryan & Westen, 2000). Other factors of the personality identity (religious ideology, moral value systems, sexual attitudes) appear to be less important in identity diffusion. Clinically, these clients appear to have no sense of their own identity and direction; this becomes a source of great distress to these individuals and is often manifested by chronic feelings of emptiness and boredom. Not surprisingly, adolescent immaturity is a predictor of cluster B disorders (Bernstein, Borchardt, & Perwien, 1996). It is not unusual for people with BPD to direct their actions in accord with the wishes of other people. For example, one woman with BPD describes herself: "I am a singer because my mother wanted me to be. I live in the city because my manager thought that I should. I become whatever anyone tells me to be. Whenever someone recommends a song, I wonder why I didn't think of that. My boyfriend tells me what to wear."

Unstable Interpersonal Relationships

People with BPD have an extreme fear of abandonment as well as a history of unstable, insecure attachments (Sack, Sperling, Fagen, & Foelsch, 1996). This abandonment stems from ambivalent early childhood attachment. Consequently, these individuals are intolerant of being alone, as evidenced by clinging behaviour and attention seeking (Gunderson, 1996). Most never experienced a consistently secure, nurturing relationship and are constantly seeking reassurance and validation. In an attempt to meet their interpersonal needs, they idealize others and establish intense relationships that violate others' interpersonal boundaries, which leads to rejection. When these relationships do not live up to their expectations, they devalue the person. Continually disappointed in relationships, these individuals, who already are intensely emotional and have a poor sense of self, feel estranged from others and feel inadequate in the face of perceived social standards (Miller, 1994). Intense shame and self-hate follow. These feelings often result in self-injurious behaviours, such as cutting the wrist, self-inflicted burns, or head banging.

In social situations, people with BPD use elaborate strategies to structure interactions. That is, they restrict their relationships to ones in which they feel in control. They distance themselves from groups when feeling anxious (which is most of the time) and rarely use their social support system. Even if they are married or have a supportive extended family, they are reluctant to share their feelings. They do not want to burden anyone; they fear rejection and also assume that people are tired of hearing them repeat the same issues (Miller, 1994).

A controversial area of BPD is separating early childhood abuse and trauma from pathologic development. In fact, people with confirmed childhood abuse and neglect histories showed a fourfold likelihood of having a personality disorder (Johnson, Cohen, Brown, Smailes, & Bernstein, 1999). Although trauma and abuse do not seem to cause BPD, they may sufficiently disturb identity and affect regulation to contribute to disordered personality development (Sansone, Wiederman, & Sansone, 1998; Zanarini et al., 1997).

Cognitive Dysfunctions

The thinking of people with BPD is dichotomous. Cognitively, they evaluate experiences, people, and objects in terms of mutually exclusive categories (eg, good or bad, success or failure, trustworthy or deceitful), which informs extreme interpretations of events that would normally be viewed as including both positive and negative aspects. There are also times when their thinking becomes disorganized. Irrelevant, bizarre notions and vague or scattered thought connections are sometimes present, as well as delusions and hallucinations.

Another cognitive dysfunction common in BPD is dissociation, which is defined as splitting or separating closely connected behaviours, thoughts, or feelings (Leichsenring, 1999). Dissociation can be conceptualized as lying on a continuum from minor dissociations of daily life, such as daydreaming, to a breakdown in the usually integrated functions of consciousness, memory, perception of self or the environment, and sensory-motor behaviour. For example, in driving familiar roads, people often get lost in their thoughts or dissociate and suddenly do not remember what happened during that part of the trip. Environmental stimuli are ignored, and there are changes in the perception of reality. The individual is physically present but mentally in another place. Dissociation serves a useful purpose; in the case of driving a familiar road, dissociation alleviates the boredom of driving. It is also a coping strategy for avoiding disturbing events. In dissociating, the person does not have to be aware of or remember traumatic events. There is a strong correlation between dissociation and self-injurious behaviour (Golynkina & Ryle, 1999; Zanarini, Ruser, Frankenburg, & Hennen, 2000).

Dysfunctional Behaviours

Impaired Problem Solving. In BPD, there is often failure to engage in active problem solving. Instead, problem solving is attempted by soliciting help from others in a helpless, hopeless manner (Linehan, 1993a). Suggestions are rarely taken.

Impulsivity. Impulsivity is also characteristic of people with BPD. Because impulse-driven people have difficulty delaying gratification or thinking through the consequences before acting on their feelings, their actions are often unpredictable. Essentially, they act in the moment and clean up the mess afterward. Gambling, spending money irresponsibly, binge eating, engaging in unsafe sex, and abusing substances are typical of these individuals. They can also be physically or verbally aggressive. Job losses, interrupted education, and unsuccessful relationships are common.

Self-Injurious Behaviours. The turmoil and unsuccessful interpersonal relationships and social experiences associated with BPD may lead the person to undermine himself or herself when a goal is about to be reached. The most serious consequences are a suicide attempt or **parasuicidal behaviour** (deliberate self-injury with an intent to harm oneself). For example, in a study of a burn unit from 1980 to 1991, a total of 31 individuals were admitted with self-inflicted burns. Sixteen of the clients had inflicted nonlethal injuries and the other 15 lethal injuries (Tuohig et al., 1995). The prevalence of self-injurious behaviour is estimated to be 43% to 67% of people with BPD (Soloff, Lis, Kelly, Cornelius & Ulrich, 2004). Self-injurious behaviour can

be compulsive, episodic, or repetitive and is more likely to occur when the individual with BPD is depressed; has highly unstable interpersonal relationships, especially problems with intimacy and sociability; and is paranoid, hypervigilant (alert, watchful), and resentful (Yeomans, Hull, & Clarkin, 1994). Some well-known self-injurious behaviours follow:

- *Compulsive self-injurious behaviours* occur many times daily and are repetitive and ritualistic. For example, hair-pulling, which can be a separate disorder (**trichotillomania**) or a behaviour of other personality disorders, involves pulling out hair, especially from the scalp, eyebrows, and eyelashes. Hair is plucked, examined, and sometimes eaten. Hair-pulling sessions may take several hours (Favazza, 1996). Most hair pullers do not seek help unless the symptoms are severe, and then they usually consult dermatologists or family practitioners.

- *Episodic self-injurious behaviours* occur every so often. These are especially common in people with BPD and develop into habitual coping behavioural patterns during periods when stress (progressive tension manifested by feelings of anger, depression, or anxiety) rises to an intolerable level. The individual reports being numb or empty and ends this dissociated state with self-injurious behaviour that elicits feeling. In cutting wrists, arms, or other body parts with sharp objects such as razor blades, glass, or knives, one half to two thirds of people with BPD with self-injurious behaviours experience little or no associated pain (Links, Heslegrave, & van Reekum, 1998); rather, endogenous endorphins (opioids) are released, which dampen pain perception and activate the brain's pleasure centre. In addition, tension is relieved and a sense of calmness or even pleasure may follow. These feelings are believed to be reinforcing, and the person learns to relieve stress and anxiety by self-mutilation. The individuals harm themselves to feel better, get rapid relief from distressing thoughts and emotions, and gain a sense of control.

- *Repetitive self-mutilation* occurs when occasional self-injury turns into an overwhelming preoccupation. These people develop an identity as a "cutter" or "burner" and describe themselves as being addicted to their self-harm. In an interpretive phenomenologic study of people with BPD, Nehls (1999) described the emotional conflict these individuals experience when their perceived efforts to comfort themselves are interpreted by others as manipulation, resulting in their being denied care. Sometimes, clients and nurses determine risk for suicide by whether the intended outcome of a parasuicidal episode is death or injury. The underlying assumption is that those who attempt to kill themselves are at higher risk than those who self-injure.

In reality, there should be no distinction between self-damaging behaviours and suicide attempts. All self-injurious behaviour should be considered potentially life threatening and taken seriously.

BORDERLINE PERSONALITY DISORDER IN SPECIAL POPULATIONS

Many children and adolescents show symptoms similar to those of BPD, such as moodiness, self-destruction, impulsiveness, lack of temper control, and rejection sensitivity. If a family member has BPD, the adolescent should be carefully assessed for this disorder. Because symptoms of BPD begin in adolescence, it makes sense that some of the children and adolescents would meet the criteria for BPD, even though it is not diagnosed before young adulthood. More likely, there are personality traits, such as impulsivity and mood instability, in many adolescents that should be recognized and treated whether or not BPD actually develops.

Epidemiology

The estimated prevalence of BPD in the general population ranges from 0.4% to 2.0%, with a median rate of 1.6%. In clinical populations, BPD is the most frequently diagnosed personality disorder; its prevalence ranges from 11% to 70%, with a median of 31%. The average prevalence among outpatients is 8% to 27%, and among inpatients, 15% to 51% (Lyons, 1995; Widiger & Weissman, 1991). More than three fourths (77%) of the individuals with diagnoses of BPD are young women (mean age, mid-20s) (Lyons, 1995). One explanation for this is that it is more socially acceptable for women than men to seek help from the health care system. Another reason is that childhood sexual abuse, which more commonly affects girls, is one of the strongest risk factors for BPD. Others think that gender bias in diagnosing may have a role.

Ample clinical reports show the coexistence of personality disorders with Axis I disorders, but epidemiologic research is scant. BPD is associated with mood, substance abuse, eating, dissociative, and anxiety disorders (Comtois, Cowley, Dunner, & Roy-Byrne, 1999; Grilo et al., 1996; Oldham et al., 1995).

Risk Factors

Various studies show that physical and sexual abuse appear to be significant risk factors for BPD (Johnson et al., 1999; Laporte & Guttman, 1996; Sansone et al., 1998). Other studies cite parental loss and separation (Zweig-Frank, Paris, & Guzder, 1994a, 1994b). Clearly, more studies are needed to identify risk factors for the development of BPD.

Etiology

What causes BPD remains largely unknown. Little evidence supports a biologic cause. Theories of psychological and social causes are more prolific.

Biologic Theories

There is no consensus regarding a biologic etiology of BPD, and no studies to date show a genetic component. The underlying assumption is that personality disorders develop within the context of the normal personality. Some argue that personality and Axis I disorders actually exist on a continuum and that personality traits and mood episodes are derived from the same underlying neurotransmitter dysfunctions and genetic constitution. These genetically determined traits become the organizing principle for the entire personality. Magnetic resonance imaging studies of 21 female clients with both BPD and post-traumatic stress disorder, compared with a matched healthy control sample, showed that women with BPD had a 16% smaller amygdala than did the healthy control subjects (Driessen et al., 2000). These findings are consistent with neurologic effects of prolonged exposure to cortisol.

Biologic abnormalities are associated with three BPD characteristics: affective instability; transient psychotic episodes; and impulsive, aggressive, and suicidal behaviour. Impulsivity and emotional instability are unusually intense in these individuals, and these traits are known to be inheritable. Associated brain dysfunction occurs in the limbic system and frontal lobe and increases the behaviours of impulsiveness, parasuicide, and mood disturbance. A decrease in serotonin activity and an increase in alpha$_2$-noradrenergic receptor sites may be related to the irritability and impulsiveness common in people with this disorder (Coccaro, Kavoussi, Hauger, Cooper, & Ferris, 1998; Oquendo & Mann, 2000).

It has also been hypothesized that an increase in dopamine may be responsible for transient psychotic states. These dysfunctions could be caused by a number of events, including trauma, epilepsy, and attention deficit hyperactivity disorder (ADHD) (Greene & Ugarriza, 1995; van Reekum, 1993). People with BPD manifest psychotic-like symptoms, including paranoid thinking, dissociation, depersonalization, and derealization. These symptoms seem to be associated with intense anxiety. There is some evidence that these symptoms are associated with excessive dopaminergic activity (Skodol et al., 2002).

Psychological Theories

Psychoanalytic Theories. The psychoanalytic views of BPD focus on two important psychoanalytic concepts: separation-individuation and projective identification. A person with BPD has not achieved the normal and healthy developmental stage of **separation-individuation**, during which a child develops a sense of self, a permanent sense of significant others (object constancy), and integration of seeing both bad and good components of self (Mahler, Pine, & Bergman, 1975). Those with BPD lack the ability to separate from the primary caregiver and develop a separate and distinct personality or self-identity. Psychoanalytic theory suggests that these separation difficulties occur because the primary caregivers' behaviours have been inconsistent or insensitive to the needs of the child. The child develops ambivalent feelings regarding interpersonal relationships and therefore has no basis for establishing trusting and secure relationships in the future. Children experience feelings of intense fear and anger in separating themselves from others. This problem continues into adulthood, and

they continue to experience difficulties in maintaining personal boundaries and in interpersonal interactions and relationships. Often, these individuals falsely attribute to others their own unacceptable feelings, impulses, or thoughts, termed **projective identification**. Projective identification is believed to play an important role in the development of BPD and is a defence mechanism by which people with BPD protect their fragile self-image. For example, when overwhelmed by anxiety or anger at being disregarded by another, they defend against the intensity of these feelings by unconsciously blaming others for what happens to them. They project their feelings onto a significant other with the unconscious hope that the other knows how to deal with it. Projective identification becomes a defensive way of interacting with the world, which leads to more rejection.

Table 24.3 | Maladaptive Schemas

Domain	Schemas With Definitions

I. Disconnection & rejection	1. Abandonment/instability
	   mportant people will not be there
	2. Mistrust/abuse
	   Other people will use client for own selfish end
	3. Emotional deprivation
	   Emotional connection will not be fulfilled
	4. Defectiveness/scheme
	   One is flawed, bad, or worthless
	5. Social isolation/alienation
	   Being different from or not fitting in

II. Impaired autonomy & performance	1. Dependence/incompetence
	   Belief that one is unable to function on one's own
	2. Vulnerability to harm and illness
	   Fear that disaster is about to strike
	3. Enmeshment/undeveloped self
	   Excessive emotional involvement at expense of normal social development
	4. Failure
	   Belief that one has failed

III. Impaired limits	1. Entitlement/grandiosity
	   Belief that one is superior to other; entitled to special rights
	2. Insufficient self-control/self-discipline
	   Difficulty or refusal to exercise sufficient self-control

IV. Other directedness	1. Subjugation
	   Excessive surrendering of control to others because of feeling coerced
	2. Self-sacrifice
	   Excessive focus on voluntarily meeting the needs of others at the expense of one's own gratification
	3. Approval-seeking/recognition-seeking
	   Excessive emphasis on gaining approval, recognition, or attention

V. Overvigilance & inhibition	1. Negativity/pessimism
	   Lifelong focus on negative aspects of life
	2. Emotional inhibition
	   Excessive inhibition of spontaneous action, feeling, or communication
	3. Unrelenting standard/hypercriticalness
	   Belief one must meet very high standard, perfectionistic, rigid
	4. Punitiveness
	   Belief people should be harshly punished

Young, J. E. (2003). *Cognitive therapy for personality disorders: A schema-focused approach*, Sarasota. FL. Professional Resource Press.

Maladaptive Cognitive Processes. Cognitive schemas are important in understanding BPD (and antisocial personality disorder as well). Individuals with personality disorders develop maladaptive schemas leading them to misinterpret environmental stimuli continuously, which in turn leads to rigid and inflexible behaviour patterns in response to new situations and people. Because those with BPD have been conditioned to anticipate rejection and disappointment in the past, they become entrenched in a pattern of fear and anxiety regarding encountering new people or situations. They have fears that disaster is going to strike any minute. Early in life, individuals with BPD and other personality disorders develop maladaptive schemas or dysfunctional ways of interpreting people and events. Table 24-3 explains 18 major maladaptive schemas at work in those with personality disorders. The work of cognitive therapists is to challenge these distortions in thinking patterns and replace them with realistic ones.

Social Theories: Biosocial Theories

The biosocial learning theory was developed by Theodore Millon, who viewed BPD as a distinct disorder that develops as a result of both biologic and psychological factors (Millon & Davis, 1999). Although he believed one's personality was biologically determined, he believed that a child's interaction with the environment and learning and experience could greatly affect biologic predisposition. He argued that each individual possesses a biologically based pattern of sensitivities and behavioural dispositions that shapes his or her experiences, including active-passive behaviour or tendency to take initiative versus reacting to events; sensitivity to pleasure or pain; and sensitivity behaviour to self and others. Millon believed that BPD is a particular cycloid personality pattern representing a moderately dysfunctional dependent or ambivalent orientation, often expressed in intense endogenous moods, described as patterns of recurring dejection and apathy interspersed with spells of anger, anxiety, or euphoria.

A further elaboration of Millon's multidimensional model incorporates biologic explanations into the behaviour. Cloninger and colleagues (1998) described personality disorder behaviours based on temperament and character dimensions derived from a factor analysis design. Cluster A disorders are associated with low-reward dependence and social attachment mediated by norepinephrine and serotonin. Cluster B disorders are associated with high novelty seeking mediated by dopamine. Novelty-seeking behaviour includes exhilaration, exploration, impulsivity, extravagance, and irritability. Cluster C disorders are associated with high harm avoidance mediated by gamma-aminobutyric acid (GABA) and serotonin.

The current biosocial theory of BPD proposed by Marsha Linehan and colleagues at the University of Washington is similar to Millon's theory, with a focus on the interaction of both biologic and social learning influences. Her primary focus is on the particular behavioural patterns observed in BPD, including emotional vulnerability, self-invalidation, unrelenting crises, inhibited grieving, active passivity, and apparent competence (Linehan, 1993a) (Box 24-1).

This biosocial viewpoint presents BPD as a multifaceted problem, a combination of a person's innate **emotional vulnerability** and his or her inability to control that emotion in social interactions (**emotional dysregulation**) and the environment (Linehan, 1993a). The emotional dysregulation and aggressive impulsivity entail both social learning and biologic regulation. Much of the neurobiologic research is directed at neurotransmitter functions involving serotonin, norepinephrine, dopamine, acetylcholine, GABA, and vasopressin (Coccaro et al., 1998; Silk, 2000). In fact,

---

BOX 24.1

Behavioural Patterns in Borderline Personality Disorder

1. *Emotional vulnerability.* Person experiences a pattern of pervasive difficulties in regulating negative emotions, including high sensitivity to negative emotional stimuli, high emotional intensity, and slow return to emotional baseline.
2. *Self-invalidation.* Person fails to recognize one's own emotional responses, thoughts, beliefs, and behaviours and sets unrealistically high standards and expectations for self. May include intense shame, self-hate, and self-directed anger. Person has no personal awareness and tends to blame social environment for unrealistic expectations and demands.
3. *Unrelenting crises.* Person experiences pattern of frequent, stressful, negative environmental events, disruptions, and roadblocks—some caused by the individual's dysfunctional lifestyle, others by an inadequate social milieu, and many by fate or chance.
4. *Inhibited grieving.* Person tries to inhibit and over-control negative emotional responses, especially those associated with grief and loss, including sadness, anger, guilt, shame, anxiety, and panic.
5. *Active passivity.* Person fails to engage actively in solving of own life problems but will actively seek problem solving from others in the environment; learned helplessness, hopelessness.
6. *Apparent competence.* Tendency for the individual to appear deceptively more competent than he or she actually is; usually due to failure of competencies to generalize across expected moods, situations, and time, and failure to display adequate nonverbal cues of emotional distress.

From Linehan, M. (1993). *Cognitive-behavioral treatment of borderline personality disorder* (p. 10). New York: Guilford Press.

restoring balance in these systems permits more consistent neural firing between the limbic system and the frontal and prefrontal cortex. When these pathways are functional, the person has greater capacity to think about his or her emotions and modulate behaviour more responsibly.

The biosocial viewpoint supports the notion that the ability to control one's emotion is in part a learning process, learned from one's private experiences and encounters with the social environment. BPD is believed to develop when these emotionally vulnerable individuals interact with an **invalidating environment**, a social situation that negates the individual's private emotional responses and communication. In other words, when the person's core emotional responses and communications are continuously dismissed, trivialized, devalued, punished, and discredited (invalidated) by others whom the person respects or values, the person receives confused messages about expressing his or her own feelings (Fig. 24-1).

A minor example of invalidating environment or response follows: The parents of Emily, a 4-year-old girl, tell her that the family is going to grandmother's house for a family meal. The child responds, "I am not going to Gramma's. I hate Stevie (cousin)." The parents reply, "You don't hate Stevie. He is a wonderful child.

He is your cousin, and only a spoiled, selfish little girl would say such a thing." The parents have devalued Emily's feelings and discredited her comments, thereby invalidating her feelings and sense of personal worth.

The most severe form of invalidation occurs in situations of child sexual abuse. Often, the abusing adult has told the child that this is a "special secret" between them, that the child should feel guilty if he or she tells anyone, and that telling someone would end their trust and special relationship. The child experiences feelings of fear, pain, and sadness, yet this trusted adult continuously dismisses the child's true feelings and tells the child what he or she should feel. Children often learn to endure sexual abuse for years, suppressing their true feelings. In disclosing the secret to a nonoffending adult, the child risks not being believed or attended to, and possible punishment.

In reality, all children, not just those who are emotionally vulnerable, learn to trust their own feelings and learn when and how to express them by interacting with their environments, including parents, family, friends, and social situations. If they constantly meet with an invalidating environment, they cannot learn to trust their own feelings—when to be angry, sad, or happy—or how to regulate their emotions. They become emotionally dysregulated. This emotional dysregulation leads to further difficulties in identity disturbances, interpersonal relationships, and the development of impulsive, parasuicidal behaviour.

Interdisciplinary Treatment

BPD is a very complex disorder that requires the whole mental health care team. The symptoms of the disorder usually require a variety of medications, including mood stabilizers, antidepressants, and anxiolytics; careful medication monitoring is necessary. Psychotherapy is needed to help the individual manage the dysfunctional moods, impulsive behaviour, and self-injurious behaviours. Specially trained therapists who are comfortable with the many demands of these clients are needed. These therapists represent a variety of mental health disciplines, including psychology, social work, and advanced practice nursing. This is a lifelong disorder requiring ongoing treatment as the individual copes with multiple interpersonal crises.

Dialectical Behaviour Therapy

Dialectical behaviour therapy (DBT), developed by Linehan, is an important biosocial approach to treatment that combines numerous cognitive and behaviour therapy strategies. For DBT to be effective, the therapists and coaches must work with clients as partners and be willing to focus on many interconnected behaviours (eg, parasuicidal and substance abuse) and not a single

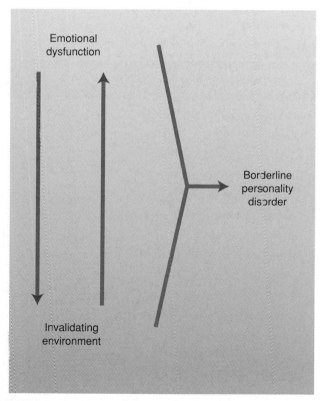

FIGURE 24.1   Biosocial theory of borderline personality disorder. (Courtesy of Marsha M. Linehan, Ph.D., Department of Psychology, Box 351525, University of Washington, Seattle, WA 98195. © 1993 by Marsha M. Linehan.)

diagnosis. It requires clients to understand their disorder by actively participating in formulating treatment goals by collecting data about their own behaviour, identifying treatment targets in individual therapy, and working with the therapists in changing these target behaviours. The core treatment procedures include problem solving, exposure techniques (gradual exposure to cues that set off aversive emotions), skill training, contingency management (reinforcement of positive behaviour), and cognitive modification. **Skills groups** are an integral part of DBT and are taught in group settings in which members practice emotional regulation, interpersonal effectiveness, distress tolerance, and core mindfulness skills.

Emotion regulation skills are taught to manage intense, labile moods and involve helping the client label and analyze the context of the emotion and develop strategies to reduce emotional vulnerability. Teaching individuals to observe and describe emotions without judging them or blocking them helps clients experience emotions without stimulating secondary feelings that cause more distress. For example, describing the emotion of anger without judging it as being "bad" can eliminate feelings of guilt that lead to self-injury.

Interpersonal effectiveness skills include the development of assertiveness and problem-solving skills within an interpersonal context. Clients are given strategies to meet his or her goals in a particular situation, while at the same time maintaining relationships with others and the person's self-respect.

Mindfulness skills are the psychological and behavioural versions of meditation skills usually taught in Eastern spiritual practice and are used to help the person improve observation, description, and participation skills by learning to focus the mind and awareness on the current moment's activity in a nonjudgmental and effective manner.

Distress tolerance skills involve helping the individual tolerate and accept distress as a part of normal life. Self-management skills focus on helping clients learn how to control, manage, or change behaviour, thoughts, or emotional responses to events (Linehan, 1993a; van den Bosch, Verheul, Schippers, & van den Brink, 2002).

The DBT model has been the most researched of any single treatment strategy and consistently demonstrates clinical effectiveness. When used on an inpatient basis, it requires total staff commitment and reinforcement and has shown significant improvement in depression, anxiety, and dissociation symptoms and a highly significant decrease in parasuicidal behaviour (Bohus et al., 2000). DBT is more often incorporated into a long-term outpatient treatment approach because the greatest effectiveness occurs when skills are reinforced over time and practiced in a variety of daily living settings (Bateman & Fonagy, 1999). Members of the treatment team must maintain a positive approach and assume a

skills-coaching role with clients. Probably the most significant interference in treatment with people with BPD is a pessimistic and oppositional attitude of health care professionals (Horsfall, 1999; Nehls, 1998, 1999).

Family Response to Disorder

Individuals with BPD are typically part of a chaotic family system, but they usually add to the chaos. Their family often feels captive to these individuals. Family members are afraid to disagree with them or refuse to meet their multiple needs, fearing that self-destructive behaviour will follow. During the course of the disorder, family members often get "burned out" and withdraw from the individual, only adding to the person's fear of abandonment.

NURSING MANAGEMENT: HUMAN RESPONSE TO DISORDER

People with BPD are unstable in a variety of areas, including mood, interpersonal relationships, self-esteem, and self-identity, and they often exhibit behavioural and cognitive dysregulation. These manifest in a number of ways, the most prominent of which are listed in Box 24-2. These people may have problems in daily living—maintaining intimate relationships, keeping a job, and living within the law (Box 24-3).

BOX 24.2

Response Patterns of Persons With Borderline Personality Disorder

Affective (mood) dysregulation

Mood lability

Problems with anger

Interpersonal dysregulation

Chaotic relationships

Fears of abandonment

Self-dysregulation

Identity disturbance or difficulties with sense of self

Sense of emptiness

Behavioural dysregulation

Parasuicidal behaviour or threats

Impulsive behaviour

Cognitive dysregulation

Dissociative responses

Paranoid ideation

Courtesy of M. Linehan, Department of Psychology, Box 351525, University of Washington, Seattle, WA 98195-1525, 1993.

BOX 24.3

Clinical Vignette: Borderline Personality Disorder

JS is a 22-year-old single woman who was recently fired from her job as a data entry clerk. She is living with her mother and stepfather, who brought her to the emergency room after finding her crouched in a foetal position in the bathroom, her wrists bleeding. She seemed to be in a daze. This is her first psychiatric admission, although her mother and stepfather have suspected that she has "needed help" for a long time. In high school, she received brief treatment for a potential eating disorder. She remains very thin but is able to eat at least one meal per day. During periods of stress, she will go for days without eating. JS is the second of three children. Her parents divorced when she was 3 years old. She has not seen her father since he left. Although she has pleasant memories of her father, her mother has told her that he beat JS and her sisters when he was drinking. When JS was 6 years old, her older sister died following an automobile accident. JS was in the car but was uninjured. As a child, JS was seen as a potential singing star. Her natural musical talent attracted her teachers' support, who encouraged her to develop her talent. She received singing lessons and entered state-wide competitions in high school. Although she enjoyed the attention, she was never really comfortable in the limelight and felt "guilty" about having a talent that she sometimes resented. She was able to make friends but found that she was unable to keep them. They described her as "too intense" and emotional.

She had one boyfriend in high school, but she was very uncomfortable with any physical closeness. After ending the relationship with the boyfriend, she concentrated on dieting to have a "perfect body." When her dieting attracted her parents' attention, she vowed to eat just enough to keep them "off her back about it." She spent much of her leisure time with her grandmother. She attended college briefly but was unable to concentrate. It was during college and after her grandmother's death that JS began cutting her wrists during periods of stress. It seemed to calm her.

After leaving college, JS returned home. She had several jobs and short-lived friendships. She was usually fired from her job because of "moodiness," and it would take her several months before she would again find another. She would spend days in her room listening to music. Her recent episode followed being fired from work and spending 3 days in her bedroom.

What Do You Think?
- How would you describe JS's mood?
- Are JS's losses (father, sister) really severe enough to affect her ability to relate to others now? Do the losses seem to relate to the self-injury?
- What behaviours indicate that there are problems with self-esteem and self-identity?

They may enter the mental health system early (young adulthood or before), but because of their chaotic lifestyle, they do not receive consistent treatment. They drop in and out of treatment as it suits their mood and usually do not remain with one clinician for long-term treatment. People with BPD usually seek help from health care workers because of consequences of their numerous life crises, medical conditions, or other psychiatric disorders (eg, depression), or for physical treatment of self-injury. Thus, other problems usually may need attention before the client's underlying personality disorder can be addressed. Sometimes, the nurse will not know that the person has BPD. However, during an assessment, it becomes clear that these individuals let things bother them more than do others or have an inflexible view of the world. They also seem to have great difficulty changing behaviour, no matter the consequences. Because they see the world differently from the average person, they have difficulty in successfully relating to other people and living a satisfying life.

Biologic Domain

Biologic Assessment

People with BPD are usually able to maintain personal hygiene and physical functioning. Because of the comorbidity of BPD and eating disorders and substance abuse, a nutritional assessment may be needed. The assessment should also include the use of caffeinated beverages, such as coffee, tea, soft drinks, and alcohol. With individuals who engage in binging or purging, assessment should include examining the teeth for pitting and discoloration, as well as the hands and fingers for redness and calluses caused by inducing vomiting. The client should be queried about physiologic responses of emotion. Sleep patterns also should be assessed because sleep alterations may suggest coexisting depression or mania.

Physical Indicators of Self-Injurious Behaviours. Clients with BPD should be assessed for self-injurious behaviour or suicide attempts. It is important to ask the individual about specific self-abusive behaviours, such as cutting, scratching, or overdosing. He or she may wear long sleeves to hide injury on the arms. Specifically asking about thoughts of hurting oneself when experiencing a major upset provides an opportunity for prevention and for coaching the client toward alternative self-soothing measures.

Pharmacologic Assessment. Clients with BPD may be taking several medications. For example, one person may be taking a small dose of an antipsychotic and a mood stabilizer. Another may be taking a selective serotonin reuptake inhibitor (SSRI) and an anxiolytic. Initially, individuals may be reluctant to disclose all the medications they are taking because, for many, there has been a period of trial and error. They are fearful of having medication taken away from them. Development of rapport with special attention to a nonjudgmental approach is especially important when eliciting current medication practices. The effectiveness of the medication in relieving the target symptom needs to be determined. Use of alcohol and street drugs should be carefully assessed to determine drug interactions.

Nursing Diagnoses for the Biologic Domain

Nursing diagnoses focussing on the biologic domain include Disturbed Sleep Pattern, Imbalanced Nutrition, Self-Mutilation or Risk for Self-Mutilation, and Ineffective Therapeutic Regimen Management.

Interventions for the Biologic Domain

The interventions for the biologic domain may address a whole spectrum of problems. Usually, the individuals are managing hydration, self-care, and pain well. This section focuses on those areas most likely to be problematic.

Sleep Enhancement. Facilitation of regular sleep–wake cycles may be needed because of disturbed sleep patterns. Conservative approaches should be exhausted before recommending medication. Establishing a regular bedtime routine, monitoring bedtime snacks and drinks, and avoiding foods and drinks that interfere with sleep should be tried. If relaxation exercises are used, they should be adapted to the tolerance of the individual. Moderate exercises (eg, brisk walking) 3 to 4 hours before bedtime activates both serotonin and endorphins, thereby enhancing calmness and a sense of well-being before bedtime. For individuals who have difficulty falling asleep and experience interrupted sleep, it helps to establish some basic sleeping routines. The bedroom should be reserved for only two activities: sleeping and sex. Therefore, the client should remove the television, computer, and exercise equipment from the bedroom. If the individual is not asleep within 15 minutes, he or she should get out of bed and go to another room to read, watch television, or listen to soft music. The client should return to bed when sleepy. If the person is not asleep in 15 minutes, the same process should be repeated.

Special consideration must be made for individuals who have been physically and sexually abused and who may be unable to put themselves in a vulnerable position (such as lying down in a room with other people or closing their eyes). These clients may need additional safeguards to help them sleep, such as a night light or repositioning of furniture to afford easy exit.

Nutritional Balance. The nutritional status of the person with BPD can quickly become a priority, particularly if the individual has coexisting eating disorders or substance abuse. Eating is often a response to stress, and clients can quickly become overweight. This is especially a problem when the individual has also been taking medications that can promote weight gain, such as antipsychotics, antidepressants, or mood stabilizers. Helping the client to learn the basics of nutrition, make reasonable choices, and develop other coping strategies are useful interventions. If individuals are engaging in purging or severe dieting practices, teaching them about the dangers of both of these practices is important (see Chapter 22). Referral to an eating disorders specialist may be needed.

Prevention and Treatment of Self-Injury. Clients with BPD are usually admitted to the inpatient setting because of threats of self-injury. Observing for antecedents of self-injurious behaviour and intervening before an episode is an important safety intervention. Clients can learn to identify situations leading to self-destructive behaviour and develop preventive strategies. Because individuals with BPD are impulsive and may respond to stress by harming themselves, observation of the person's interactions and assessment of the mood, level of distress, and agitation are important indicators of impending self-injury.

Remembering that self-injury is an effort to self-soothe by activating endogenous endorphins, the nurse can assist the individual to find more productive and enduring ways to find comfort. Linehan (1993b) suggests using the Self-Soothing Exercise and focusing on each of the five senses:

- Vision (eg, go outside and look at the stars or flowers or autumn leaves)
- Hearing (eg, listen to beautiful or invigorating music or the sounds of nature)
- Smell (eg, light a scented candle, boil a cinnamon stick in water)
- Taste (eg, drink a soothing, warm, nonalcoholic beverage)
- Touch (eg, take a hot bubble bath, pet your dog or cat, get a massage)

For clients who injure themselves repeatedly to experience emotional release after the injury, medication that blocks the endogenous opioids system or reward system may help control the behaviour. Preliminary studies show that naltrexone (ReVia) has reduced the incidence of self-injurious behaviour. It has been used to treat dissociative symptoms with some success (Bohus et al., 1999), as have low doses of serotonin-dopamine antagonists, such as clozapine, olanzapine, and risperidone (McDougle, Kresch, & Posey, 2000).

Pharmacologic Interventions. Less medication is better for people with BPD. No specific drug is available for the treatment of BPD. Individuals should take medications only for target symptoms for a short time (eg, an antidepressant for a bout with depression) because they may be taking many medications, particularly if they have a comorbid disorder, such as a mood disorder or substance abuse. Pharmacotherapy is used to control emotional dysregulation, impulsive aggression, cognitive disturbances, and anxiety as an adjunct to psychotherapy.

CONTROLLING EMOTIONAL DYSREGULATION. Target symptoms of emotional dysregulation include instability of mood, marked shifts from or to depression, stress-related and transient mood crashes, rejection sensitivity, and inappropriate and intense outbursts of anger. In some cases, monamine oxidase inhibitors are used to treat depression, but consensus practice guidelines recommend these as third-line choices (APA, 2001).

Because decreased central serotonin neurotransmission has been implicated in the emotional dysregulation and impulsive-aggressive behaviours, the SSRIs have been tried, with some efficacy. Improvement in depressed mood and lability, rejection sensitivity, impulsive behaviour, self-injury, psychosis, and hostility have been shown with fluoxetine (Prozac) in BPD. SSRIs and serotonin-norepinephrine reuptake inhibitors have been most extensively studied and used clinically to treat depression, aggression, and emotional dysregulation. Sertraline (Zoloft), paroxetine (Paxil), and citalopram (Celexa) are most often used, and venlafaxine (Effexor) and mirtazapine (Remeron) have been similarly effective, especially with attentional disturbance and agitation symptoms (Stahl, 2000).

REDUCING IMPULSIVITY. Impulsivity, anger outbursts, and mood lability may be treated effectively with the newer GABA-ergic anticonvulsants such as lamotrigine (Lamictal), gabapentin (Neurontin), and topiramate (Topamax) (Coccaro, 1998; Pinto & Akiskal, 1998). These appear to act by regulating neural firing in the mesolimbic area. Carbamazepine (Tegretol) and lithium have also been used, but these have a less favourable side-effect profile. Divalproex is still the most frequently used drug for impulsivity and aggression (Hollander et al., 2003; Kavoussi & Coccaro, 1998).

MANAGING TRANSIENT PSYCHOTIC EPISODES. Antipsychotic medications may be useful when the client demonstrates thought disorganization, misinterpretation of reality, and high levels of emotional instability. Low doses of antipsychotics are most often used (Soloff, 2000).

DECREASING ANXIETY. If an individual is experiencing anxiety, a nonbenzodiazepine such as buspirone (BuSpar) may be used (Box 24-4). Buspirone appears to be an ideal antianxiety drug. Unlike the benzodiazepines, it does not have the sedation, ataxia, tolerance, and withdrawal effects and does not lead to abuse. However, buspirone takes longer to act than do the benzodiazepines. If a client has been taking benzodiazepines for years, buspirone may not lead to much improvement. When switching from a benzodiazepine to buspirone, the withdrawal symptoms may be unpleasant (or even dangerous), and buspirone will not have any effect on the distress. Because buspirone is a serotonin (5-HT1A) agonist, its use with an SSRI enhances the benefits of both drugs to reduce anxiety and depression symptoms (Stahl, 2000) but exposes the client to serotonin syndrome risk.

More often, people with BPD find buspirone ineffective if their type of anxiety is intense and accompanied by agitation and aggression. Because this anxiety seems to be mediated by serotonergic connections in the prefrontal cortex and anterior cingulum, SSRIs at

BOX 24.4

Drug Profile: Buspirone (Buspar)

DRUG CLASS: antianxiety agent
RECEPTOR AFFINITY: Binds to serotonin receptors and acts as an agonist to 5-HT$_{1B}$. Clinical significance unclear. Exact mechanism of action unknown.
INDICATIONS: Management of anxiety disorders or short-term relief of symptoms of anxiety.
ROUTES AND DOSAGE: Available in 10-mg tablets.
Adults: Initially, 15 mg/d (5 mg tid). Increased by 5 mg/d at intervals of 2–3 d to achieve optimal therapeutic response. Not to exceed 60 mg/d.
Children: Safety and efficacy under 18 years of age not established.
HALF-LIFE (PEAK EFFECT): 3–11 h (40–90 min).
SELECT ADVERSE REACTIONS: Dizziness, headache, nervousness, insomnia, light-headedness, nausea, dry mouth, vomiting, gastric distress, diarrhea, tachycardia, and palpitations.
WARNING: Contraindicated in clients with hypersensitivity to buspirone, marked liver or renal impairment and during lactation. Alcohol and other CNS depressants can cause increased sedation. Decreased effects seen if given with fluoxetine.
SPECIFIC CLIENT/FAMILY EDUCATION:
- Take drug exactly as prescribed; may take with foods or meals if gastrointestinal upset occurs.
- Avoid alcohol and other CNS depressants.
- Notify prescriber before taking any over-the-counter or prescription medications.
- Avoid driving or performing hazardous activities that require alertness and concentration.
- Use ice chips or sugarless candies to alleviate dry mouth.
- Notify prescriber of any abnormal involuntary movements of facial or neck muscles, abnormal posture, or yellowing of skin or eyes.
- Continue medical follow-up and do not abruptly discontinue use.

higher doses than those used for depression are more effective (Best, Williams, & Coccaro, 2002; Gurvits, Koenigsberg, & Siever, 2000).

MONITORING AND ADMINISTERING MEDICATIONS. In inpatient settings, it is relatively easy to control medications; in other settings, clients must be aware that it is their responsibility to take their medication and monitor the number and type of drugs being taken. Individuals who rely on medication to help them deal with stress or those who are periodically suicidal are at high risk for abuse of medications. Those who have unusual side effects are also at high risk for nonadherence. The nurse determines whether the individual is actually taking medication, whether the medication is being taken as prescribed, the effect on target symptoms, and the use of any over-the-counter drugs, such as antihistamines or sleeping pills.

However, the client cannot rely just on the medication. Assuming responsibility for taking the medication regularly, understanding the effects of the medication, and augmenting the medication with other strategies is the most effective approach. The nurse helps the individual assume this responsibility and provides guidance that supports self-efficacy and competence. It is also important for the nurse to emphasize that the medications provide the physiologic balance, but it is the client's effort and skills that provide the social and behavioural balance. By stressing this, the individual does not overinvest in the medication and feels more confident of her or his own skills.

SIDE-EFFECT MONITORING AND MANAGEMENT. Individuals with BPD appear to be sensitive to many of the medications, and they often dose the medication according to their understanding of the side effects. Listen carefully to the person's description of the side effects. Any unusual side effects should be accurately documented and reported to the prescriber.

Teaching Points

Clients should be educated about the medications and their interactions with other drugs and substances. Interventions include teaching individuals about the medication and how and where it acts in the brain and body, helping establish a routine for taking prescribed medication, reporting side effects, and facilitating the development of positive coping strategies to deal with daily stresses, rather than relying on medications. Eliciting the client's partnership in care improves adherence and thereby outcomes.

Psychological Domain

Psychological Assessment

People with BPD have usually experienced significant losses in their lives that shape their view of the world.

They experience **inhibited grieving**, "a pattern of repetitive, significant trauma and loss, together with an inability to fully experience and personally integrate or resolve these events" (Linehan, 1993a, p. 89). They have unresolved grief that can last for years and avoid situations that evoke those feelings of separation and loss. During the assessment, the nurse can identify the losses (real or perceived) and explore the client's experience during these losses, paying particular attention to whether the individual has reached resolution. History of physical or sexual abuse and early separation from significant caregivers may provide important clues to the severity of the disturbances.

Mood fluctuations are common and can be assessed by any number of the depression and anxiety screening scales, or by asking the following questions:

- What things or events bother you and make you feel happy, sad, angry?
- Do these things or events trouble you more than they trouble other people?
- Do friends and family tell you that you are moody?
- Do you get angry easily?
- Do you have trouble with your temper?
- Do you think you were born with these feelings, or did something happen to make you feel this way?

Appearance and activity level generally reflect the person's mood and psychomotor activity. Many of those with BPD have been physically or sexually abused and thus should be assessed for depression. A dishevelled appearance can reflect depression or an agitated state. When feeling good, these individuals can be very engaging; they tend to be dramatic in their style of dress and attract attention, such as by wearing an unusual hairstyle or heavy makeup. Because physical appearance reflects identity, clients may experiment with their appearance and seek affirmation and acceptance from others. Body piercing, tattoos, and other adornments provide a mechanism to define self.

Impulsivity. Impulsivity can be identified by asking the client if he or she does things impulsively or on the spur of the moment. Have there been times when you were hurt by your actions or were sorry later that you acted in the way you did? Direct questions about gambling, choices in sexual partners, sexual activities, fights, arguments, arrests, and alcohol drinking habits can also help in identifying areas of impulsive behaviour.

From a neurophysiologic perspective, impulsively acting before thinking seems to be mediated by rapid nerve firing in the mesolimbic area. This activates psychomotor responses before pathways reach the prefrontal cortex (Best, Williams & Coccaro, 2002). Teaching the client strategies to slow down automatic responses (eg, deep breathing, counting to 10) allows time to think before acting.

Cognitive Disturbances. The mental status examination of those with BPD usually reveals normal thought processes that are not disorganized or confused, except during periods of stress. Those with BPD usually exhibit **dichotomous thinking**, or a tendency to view things as absolute—either black or white, good or bad—with no perception of compromise. Dichotomous thinking can be assessed by asking clients how they view other people. Evidence of dichotomous thinking is indicated with responses of "good" or "bad," "wonderful" or "terrible."

Dissociation and Transient Psychotic Episodes. There may be periods of dissociation and transient psychotic episodes. Dissociation can be assessed by asking if there is ever a time when the person does not remember events or has the feeling of being separate from his or her body. Some individuals refer to this as "spacing out." By asking specific information about how often, how long, and when dissociation first was used, the nurse can get an idea of how important dissociation is as a coping skill. It is important to ask the person what is happening in the environment when dissociation occurs. Frequent dissociation indicates a highly habitual coping mechanism that will be difficult to change. Because transient psychotic states occur, it is also important to elicit data regarding the presence of hallucinations or delusions, their frequency and circumstances.

Risk Assessment: Suicide or Self-Injury. It is critical that individuals with BPD be assessed for suicidal and self-damaging behaviour, including alcohol and drug abuse. (Suicide assessment is discussed in Chapter 37.) An assessment should include direct questions, asking if the person thinks about or engages in self-injurious behaviours. If so, the nurse should continue to explore the behaviours: what is done, how it is done, its frequency, and the circumstances surrounding the self-injurious behaviour. It is helpful to explain briefly to the client that sometimes people cut, scratch, or pick at themselves as a way of bringing some relief and comfort. Although the behaviour brings temporary relief, it also places the person at risk for infection. Approaching the assessment in this way conveys a sense of understanding and is more likely to invite the individual to disclose honestly.

Nursing Diagnoses for the Psychological Domain

One of the first diagnoses to consider is Risk for Self-Mutilation because protection of the individual from self-injury is always a priority. If cognitive changes are present (dissociation and transient psychosis), two other diagnoses may be appropriate: Disturbed Thought Process and Ineffective Coping. The Disturbed Thought Process diagnosis is used if dissociative and psychotic episodes actually interfere with daily living. For example, a secretary could not complete processing letters because she was unable to differentiate whether the

voices on the dictating machine were being transmitted by the machine or by her hallucinations. The nurse helped her learn to differentiate the hallucinations from dictation. The client learned to take her headset off, take a deep breath, and listen to her external environment. When she recognized "the voice" as her partner criticizing her, she was able to use her cognitive reframing strategies to refocus on reality.

If the individual copes with stressful situations by dissociating or hallucinating, the diagnosis Ineffective Coping is used. The outcome in this instance would be the substitution of positive coping skills for the dissociations or hallucinations.

Other nursing diagnoses that are typically supported by assessment data include Personal Identity Disturbance, Anxiety, Grieving, Low Self-Esteem, Powerlessness, Post-trauma Response, Defensive Coping, and Spiritual Distress. The identification of outcomes depends on the nursing diagnoses (Fig. 24-2).

Interventions for the Psychological Domain

The challenge of working with people with BPD is engaging the individual in a therapeutic relationship that will survive its emotional ups and downs. The client needs to understand that the nurse is there to coach her or him to develop self-modulation skills. A relationship based on mutual respect and consistency is crucial for helping the person with those skills. Self-awareness skills, along with access to supervision, are needed by the nurse. Because individuals with BPD are frequently hospitalized, even nurses in acute care settings have an opportunity to develop a long-term relationship (Fig. 24-3).

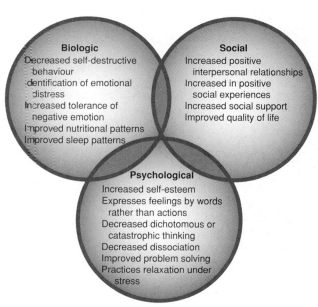

FIGURE 24.2   Biopsychosocial outcomes for individuals with borderline personality disorder.

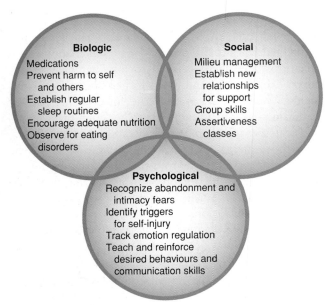

FIGURE 24.3 Biopsychosocial interventions for individuals with borderline personality disorder.

Generalist psychiatric–mental health nurses do not function as the client's primary therapists, but they do need to establish a therapeutic relationship that strengthens the client's coping skills and self-esteem and supports individual psychotherapy. The therapeutic relationship helps the client to experience a model of healthy interac-

tion with consistency, limit-setting, caring, and respect for others (both self-respect and respect for the person). Individuals who have low self-esteem need help in recognizing genuine respect from others and reciprocating with respect for others. In the therapeutic relationship, the nurse models self-respect by observing personal limits, being assertive, and clearly communicating expectations. Consistency is critical in building self-esteem.

ABANDONMENT AND INTIMACY FEARS. A key to helping individuals with BPD is recognizing their fears of both abandonment and intimacy. Informing the client of the length of the relationship as much as possible allows the individual to engage in and prepare for termination with the least pain of abandonment. If the client's hospitalization is time limited, the nurse overtly acknowledges the limit and reminds the person with each contact how many sessions remain (Box 24-5).

In day treatment and outpatient settings, the duration of treatment may be indeterminate, but the nurse may not be available that entire time. The termination process cannot be casual; this would stimulate abandonment fears. However, some clients end prematurely when the nurse informs them of the impending end as a way to leave before being rejected. Anticipating premature closure, the nurse explores with the individual anticipated feelings, including the wish to run away. After careful planning, the nurse anticipates, in advance, the client's feelings, discusses how to cope with them,

---

BOX 24.5

Therapeutic Dialogue: Borderline Personality Disorder

Ineffective Approach

Client: Hey, you know what? You are my favorite nurse. That night nurse sure doesn't understand me the way you do.

Nurse: Oh, I'm glad you are comfortable with me. Which night nurse?

Client: You know, Sue.

Nurse: Did you have problems with her?

Client: She is terrible. She sleeps all night or she is on the telephone.

Nurse: Oh, that doesn't sound very professional to me. Anything else?

Client: Yeah, she said that you didn't know what you were doing. She said that you couldn't nurse your way out of a paper bag (smiling).

Nurse: She did, did she. (Getting angry.) She should talk.

Client: Well, I gotta go to group. Where will you be? I feel so much better if I know where you are. I don't know how I can possibly be discharged tomorrow.

Effective Approach

Client: Hey, you know what? You are my favorite nurse. That night nurse sure doesn't understand me the way you do.

Nurse: I really like you, Sara. Tomorrow you will be discharged, and I'm glad that you will be able to return home.

(Nurse avoided responding to "favorite nurse" statement. Redirected interaction to impending discharge.)

Client: That night nurse slept all night.

Nurse: What was your night like? (Redirecting the interaction to Sara's experience.)

Client: It was terrible. Couldn't sleep all night. I'm not sure that I'm ready to go home.

Nurse: Oh, so you are not quite sure about discharge? (Reflection.)

Client: I get so, so lonely. Then, I want to hurt myself.

Nurse: Lonely feelings have started that chain of events that led to cutting, haven't they? (Validation.)

Client: Yes, I'm very scared. I haven't cut myself for 1 week now.

Nurse: Do you have a plan for dealing with your lonely feelings when they occur?

Client: I'm supposed to start thinking about something that is pleasant—like spring flowers in the meadow.

Nurse: Does that work for you?

Client: Yes, sometimes.

Critical Thinking Questions

- How did the nurse in the first scenario get side-tracked?
- How was the nurse in the second scenario able to keep the client focussed on herself and her impending discharge?

reviews the progress the individual has made, and summarizes what the person has learned from the relationship that can be generalized to future encounters.

Establishing Personal Boundaries and Limitations.

Personal boundaries are highly context specific; for example, stroking the hair of a stranger on the bus would be inappropriate, but stroking the hair and face of one's intimate partner while sitting together would be appropriate. Our personal physical space needs (boundaries) are distinct from behavioural and emotional limits we have. These concepts apply both to the client and the nurse. Furthermore, limits may be temporary (eg, "I can't talk with you right now, but after the change of shift, I can be available for 30 minutes").

Testing limits is a natural way of identifying where the boundaries are and how strong they are. Therefore, it is necessary to state clearly the enduring limits (eg, the written rules or contract) and the consequences of violating them. The limits must then be consistently maintained. Clarifying limits requires making explicit what is usually implicit. Despite the clinical setting (eg, hospital, day treatment setting, outpatient clinic), the nurse must clearly state the day, time, and duration of each contact with the client and remain consistent in those expectations. This may mean having a standing appointment in day treatment or mental health clinic or noting the time during each shift that the nurse will talk individually with the hospitalized client. The nurse should refrain from offering personal information, which is frequently confusing to the person with BPD. At times, the person may present in a somewhat arrogant and entitled way. It is important for the nurse to recognize such a presentation as reflective of internal confusion and dissonance. Responding in a very neutral manner avoids confrontation and a power struggle, which might also unwittingly reinforce the client's internal sense of inferiority.

Some additional strategies for establishing the boundaries of the relationship include the following:

- Documenting in the client chart the agreed-on appointment expectations
- Sharing the treatment plan with the client
- Confronting violations of the agreement in a nonpunitive way
- Discussing the purpose of limits in the therapeutic relationship and applicability to other relationships

When individuals violate boundaries, it is important to respond right away but without taking the behaviour personally. For example, if a client is flirtatious, simply say something like, "X, I feel uncomfortable with your overly friendly behaviour. It seems out of place since we have a professional relationship. That would be more fitting for an intimate relationship that we will never have."

Management of Dissociative States.

The desired outcome for someone who dissociates is to reduce or eliminate the dissociative experiences. The natural tendency is to want to "fix it." Unfortunately, there are limited medications for dissociation, but because the SSRIs, dopamine antagonists, and serotonin-dopamine antagonists affect other target symptoms, the dissociative experiences decrease. Because dissociation occurs during periods of stress, the best approach is to help the individual develop other strategies to deal with stress.

The nurse can teach the client how to identify when he or she is dissociating and then to use some grounding strategies in the moment. Basic to grounding is planting both feet firmly on the floor or ground, then taking a deep abdominal breath to the count of 4, holding it to the count of 4, exhaling to the count of 4, and then holding it to the count of 4. This is called the four-square method of breathing. The benefit of this approach is to bring about a deep, slow breath that activates the calming mechanisms of the parasympathetic system.

After the grounding exercise, the client uses one or more senses to make contact with the environment, such as touching the fabric of a nearby chair or listening to the traffic noise. As the client improves in self-esteem and ability to relate to others, the frequency of dissociation should decrease.

Behavioural Interventions.

The goal of behavioural interventions is to replace dysfunctional behaviours with positive ones. The nurse has an important role in helping individuals control emotions and behaviours by acknowledging and validating desired behaviours and ignoring or confronting undesired behaviours. Clients often test the nurse for a response, and nurses must decide how to respond to particular behaviours. This can be tricky because even negative responses can be viewed as positive reinforcement for the client. In some instances, if the behaviour is irritating but not harmful or demeaning, it is best to ignore rather than focus on it. However, grossly inappropriate and disrespectful behaviours require confrontation. If a client throws a glass of water on an assistant because the client is angry at the treatment team for refusing to increase her hospital privileges, an appropriate intervention would include confronting the individual with her behaviour and issuing the consequences, such as losing her privileges and apologizing to the assistant.

However, this incident can be used to help the individual understand why such behaviour is inappropriate and how it can be changed. The nurse should explore with the client what happened, what events led up to the behaviour, what were the consequences, and what feelings were aroused. Advanced practice nurses or other therapists will explore the origins of the client's behaviours and responses, but the generalist nurse needs to help the person explore ways to change behaviours involved in the current situation. The laboriousness of this analytical process may be a sufficient incentive for the client to abandon the dysfunctional behaviour.

Emotional Regulation.

A major goal of cognitive therapeutic interventions is emotional regulation—

recognizing and controlling the expression of feelings. Clients often fail even to recognize their feelings; instead, they respond quickly without thinking about the consequences. Remember, the time needed for taking action is shorter than the time needed for thinking before acting. Pausing makes up for the momentary lag between the limbic and autonomic response and the prefrontal response.

The nurse can help the client identify feelings and gain control over expressions such as anger, disappointment, or frustration. The goal is for individuals to tolerate their feelings without feeling compelled to act out those feelings on another person or on themselves.

A helpful technique for managing feelings is known as the **communication triad**. The triad provides a specific syntax and order for clients to identify and express their feelings and seek relief. The "sentence" consists of three parts:

- An "I" statement to identify the prevailing feeling
- A nonjudgmental statement of the emotional trigger
- What the individual would like differently or what would restore comfort to the situation

The nurse must emphasize with clients that they begin with the "I" statement and the identification of feelings, although many want to begin with the condition. If the person begins with the condition, the statement becomes accusatory and likely to evoke defensiveness (eg, "When you interrupt me, I get mad."). Beginning with "I" allows the client to identify and express the feeling first and take full ownership. For example, the individual who is angry with another client in the group might say, "Joe, I feel angry ("I" statement with ownership of feeling) when you interrupt me (the trigger or conditions of the emotion), and I would like you to apologize and try not to do that with me (what the individual wants and the remedy)." This simple skill is easy to teach, is easy to reinforce and to encourage others to reinforce, and is a surprisingly effective way of moderating the emotional tone.

Another element of emotional regulation is learning to delay gratification. When clients want something that is not immediately available, the nurse can teach individuals to distract themselves, find alternate ways of meeting the need, and think about what would happen if they have to wait to meet the need.

The practice of **thought stopping** might also help the person to control the inappropriate expression of feelings. In thought stopping, the client identifies what feelings and thoughts exist together. For example, when the person is ruminating about a perceived hurt, the individual might say, "Stop that" (referring to the ruminative thought) and engage in a distracting activity. Three activities associated with thought stopping are effective:

- Taking a quick deep breath when the behaviour is noted (this also stimulates relaxation)

- Visualizing a stop sign or saying "stop" when possible (this allows the person to hear externally and internally)
- Deliberately replacing the undesired behaviour with a positive alternative (eg, instead of ruminating about an angry situation, thinking about a neutral or positive self-affirmation). The sequencing and combining of the steps puts the person back in control.

Challenging Dysfunctional Thinking. The nurse can often challenge the individual's dysfunctional ways of thinking and challenge the person to think about the event in a different way. When a client engages in catastrophic thinking, the nurse can challenge by asking, "What is the worst that could happen?" and "How likely would that be to occur?" Or, in dichotomous thinking, when the client fixates on one extreme perception or alternates between the extremes only, the nurse can ask the person to think about any examples of exceptions to the extreme. The point of the challenge is not to debate or argue with the individual, but to provide different perspectives to consider. Encouraging clients to keep journals of real interactions to process with the nurse or therapist is another effective way of testing the reality of their thinking and anticipations, affording more choices and flexibility (Box 24-6).

In problem solving, the nurse might encourage the individual to debate both sides of the problem and then search for common ground. Practicing communication and negotiation skills through role playing helps the client make mistakes and correct them without harm to her or his self-esteem. The nurse also encourages clients

---

BOX 24.6

Challenging Dysfunctional Thinking

Ms. S had worked for the same company for 20 years with a good job record. Following an accident, she made some minor mistakes in her work that she quickly corrected. She informed her company's nurse that her work was "really slipping" and that she was fearful of her coworkers' disapproval and getting fired from her job. The nurse asked her to keep a journal of coworkers' comments for the next week. At the next visit, the following dialogue occurred:

Nurse: I noticed that you received several compliments on your work. Even a close friend of your boss expressed appreciation for your work.

Ms. S: It was a light week at work. I really don't believe they meant what they said.

Nurse: I can see how you can believe that one or two comments are not genuine, but how do you account for four and five good reports on your work?

Ms. S: Well, I don't know.

Nurse: It looks like your beliefs are not supported by your journal entries. Now, what makes you think that your boss wants to fire you after 20 years of service?

BOX 24.7

Thought Distortions and Corrective Statements

Thought Distortion	Corrective Statement
Catastrophizing	
"This is the most awful thing that has ever happened to me"	"This is a sad thing, but not the most awful."
"If I fail this course, my life is over."	"If you fail the course, you can take the course again. You can change your major."
Dichotomizing	
"No one ever listens to me."	"Your husband listened to you last night when you told him . . ."
"I never get what I want."	"You didn't get the promotion this year, but you did get a merit raise."
"I can't understand why everyone is so kind at first, then always dumps me when I need them the most."	"It is hard to remember those kind things and times when your friends have stayed with you when you needed them."
Self-Attribution Errors	
"If I had just found the right thing to say, she wouldn't have left me."	"There is not a single right thing to say; and she left you because she chose to."
"If I had not made him mad, he wouldn't have hit me."	"He has a lot of choices in how to respond, and he chose hitting. You are responsible for your feelings and actions."

to use these skills in their everyday lives and report back on the results, asking individuals how they feel applying the skills and how doing so affects their self-perceptions. Success, even partial success, builds a sense of competence and self-esteem (Box 24-7).

Management of Transient Psychotic Episodes. During psychotic episodes with auditory hallucinations, the client should be protected from harming self or others. In an inpatient setting, the client should be monitored closely and a determination made as to whether the voices are telling the person to engage in self-harm (command hallucinations). The client may be observed more closely and begin taking antipsychotic medication. In the community setting, the nurse should help the client develop a plan for managing the voices. For example, if the voices return, the individual contacts the clinic and returns for evaluation. There may be a friend or relative who should be contacted or a case manager who can help the person get the necessary protection if it is needed. In some instances, hearing the voices is a prelude to self-injury. Another person can help the individual resist the voices. Once other aspects of the disorder are managed, the episodes of psychosis decrease or disappear.

Teaching and practicing distress tolerance skills help the individual have power over the voices and control intense emotions. When not experiencing hallucinations, the client can practice deep abdominal breathing, which calms the autonomic nervous system. Using brainstorming techniques, the individual identifies early internal cues of rising distress while the nurse writes them on an index card for the client to refer to later. Next, the nurse teaches some skills for tolerating painful feelings or events. To help the client remember, suggest the mnemonic "Wise Mind ACCEPTS" with the following actions:

- **A**ctivities to distract from stress
- **C**ontributing to others, such as volunteering or visiting a sick neighbour
- **C**omparing yourself to people less fortunate than you
- **E**motions that are opposite to what you are experiencing
- **P**ushing away from the situation for awhile
- **T**houghts other than those you are currently experiencing
- **S**ensations that are intense, such as holding ice in your hand (Linehan, 1993b, pp. 165–166)

Client Education

Client education within the context of a therapeutic relationship is one of the most important, empowering interventions for the generalist psychiatric–mental health nurse to use. Teaching individuals skills to resist parasuicidal urges, improve emotional regulation, enhance interpersonal relationships, tolerate stress, and enhance overall quality of life provides the foundation for long-term behavioural changes. These skills can be taught in any treatment setting as a part of the overall facility program (see Box 24-8). If nurses are practicing in a facility where DBT is the treatment model, they can be trained in DBT and can serve as group skills leaders.

Social Domain

Social Assessment

Some individuals with BPD can function very well except during periods when symptoms erupt. They

Psychoeducation Checklist: Borderline Personality Disorder

When caring for the client with borderline personality disorder, be sure to include the following topic areas in the teaching plan:
- ☐ Management of medication, if used, including drug action, dosage, frequency, and possible adverse effects
- ☐ Regular sleep routines
- ☐ Nutrition
- ☐ Safety measures
- ☐ Functional versus dysfunctional behaviours
- ☐ Cognitive strategies (distraction, communication skills, thought-stopping)
- ☐ Structure and limit setting
- ☐ Social relationships
- ☐ Community resources

hold jobs, are active in communities, and can perform well. During periods of stress, symptoms often appear. On the other hand, some individuals with severe BPD function poorly; they are always in a crisis, which they have often created.

Social Support Systems. Identification of social supports, such as family, friends, and religious organizations, is the purpose in assessing resources. Knowing how the person obtains social support is important in understanding the quality of interpersonal relationships. For example, some individuals consider their "best friends" nurses, physicians, and other health care personnel. Because this is a false friendship (ie, not reciprocal), it inevitably leads to frustration and disappointment. However, helping the individual find ways to meet other people and encouraging the client's efforts are more realistic.

Interpersonal Skills. Assessment of the person's ability to relate to others is important because interpersonal problems are linked to dissociation and self-injurious behaviour. Information about friendships, frequency of contact, and intimate relationships will provide data about the person's ability to relate to others. Clients with BPD often are sexually active and may have numerous sexual partners. Their need for closeness clouds their judgment about sexual partners, and it is not unusual to find these individuals in abusive, destructive relationships with people with antisocial personality disorder. During assessment, nurses should use their own self-awareness skills to examine their personal response to the client. How the nurse responds to the individual can often be a clue to how others perceive and respond to this person. For example, if the nurse feels irritated or impatient during the interview, that is a sign that others respond to this person in the same way; on the other hand, if the nurse feels empathy or closeness, chances are this individual can evoke these same feelings in others.

Self-Esteem and Coping Skills. Coping with stressful situations is one of the major problems for people with BPD. Assessment of their coping skills and their ability to deal with stressful situations is important. Because the individual's self-esteem is usually very low, assessment of self-esteem can be done with a self-esteem assessment tool or by interviewing the client and analyzing the assessment data for evidence of personal self-worth and confidence. Self-esteem is highly related to identifying with health care workers. Clients with BPD perceive their families and friends as being weary of their numerous crises and their seeming unwillingness to break the vicious self-destructive cycle. Feeling rejected by their natural support system, these individuals create one within the health system. During periods of crisis or affective instability, especially during the late evening, early morning, or on weekends, they call or visit various psychiatric units, asking to speak to specific personnel who formerly cared for them. They even know different nurses' scheduled days off and make the rounds to several hospitals and clinics. Sometimes they bring gifts to nurses or call them at home. Because their newly created social support system cannot provide the support that is needed, the person continues to feel rejected. One of the goals of the treatment is to help the individual establish a natural support network.

Family Assessment

Family members may or may not be involved with the client. These individuals are often estranged from their families. In other instances, they are dependent on them, which is also a source of stress. Childhood abuse is common in these families, and the perpetrator may be a family member. Ideally, family members are interviewed for their perspectives on the client's problem. Assessment of any mental disorder in the client's family and of the current level of functioning is useful in understanding the client and identifying potential resources for support.

Nursing Diagnoses for the Social Domain

Defensive Coping, Chronic Low Self-Esteem, and Impaired Social Interaction are nursing diagnoses that address the social problems faced by clients with BPD.

Interventions for the Social Domain: Modifying Coping Behaviours

Environmental management becomes critical in caring for a person with BPD. Because the unit can be structured to represent a microcosm of the individual's community, clients have an opportunity to identify relationship problems, boundary violations, and stressful situations. When these situations occur, the nurse can help the individual cope by finding alternative explanations for the situation and practicing new skills. Individual sessions help the client try out some skills, such as putting feelings into words without actions. Role playing may help individuals experience different degrees of effectively relating feelings without the burden of hurting someone they care about. Day treatment and group settings are excellent places for clients to learn more effective feeling management and to practice these techniques with each other. The group helps members develop empathy and diffuses attachment to any one person or therapist.

Building Social Skills and Self-Esteem.
In the hospital, the nurse can use groups to discuss feelings and ways to cope with them. Women with BPD benefit from assertiveness classes and women's health issues classes. Many of the women are involved in abusive relationships and lack the ability to resolve these relationships because of their extreme anxiety regarding separating from those they love and their extreme need to feel connected. These women verbalize desires to leave, but they do not have the strength and self-confidence needed to leave. Exposing them to a different style of interaction as well as validation from other people increases their self-esteem and ability to separate from negative influences.

Exploring Social Supports.
Dependency on family members is a problem for many people with BPD. In some families, a client's positive progress may be met with negative responses, and individuals in these situations need help in maintaining a separate identity while staying connected to family members for social support. Family support groups sometimes help. Usually, the nurse helps the person explore new relationships that can provide additional social contacts.

Teaching Effective Ways to Communicate.
An important area of client education is teaching communication skills. Clients lack interpersonal skill in relating because they often had inadequate modeling and few opportunities to practice. The goals of relationship skill development are to identify problematic behaviour that interferes with relationships and to use appropriate behaviours in improving relationships. The starting point is with communication. The nurse teaches the individual basic communication approaches, such as making "I" statements, paraphrasing what the other party says before responding, checking the accuracy of perceptions with others, compromising and seeking common ground, listening actively, and offering and accepting reactions. Besides modelling the behaviours, the nurse guides clients in practicing a variety of communication approaches for common situations. When role playing, the nurse needs to discuss not only what the skills are and how to perform them, but also the feelings clients have before, during, and after the role play.

In day treatment and outpatient settings, the nurse can give the client homework, such as keeping a journal, applying role-playing skills to actual situations, and observing behaviours in others. In the hospital, the individual can experience the same process, and the nurse is available to offer immediate feedback. Whatever the setting, or even the specific problems addressed, the nurse must keep in mind and remind the client that change occurs slowly. Thus, working on the problems occurs gradually, with severity of symptoms as the guide to deciding how fast and how much change to expect.

EVALUATION AND OUTCOMES

Evaluation and outcomes vary depending on the severity of the disorder, the presence of comorbid disorders, and the availability of resources. For a client with severe symptoms or continual self-injury, keeping the individual safe and alive may be a realistic outcome. Helping the person resist parasuicidal urges may take years. In contrast, individuals who rarely need hospitalization and have adequate resources can expect to recover from the self-destructive impulses and learn positive interaction skills that promote a qualitative lifestyle. Most clients fall somewhere in between, with periods of symptom exacerbation and remission. In these individuals, increasing the symptom-free time may be the best indicator of outcomes.

CONTINUUM OF CARE

Treatment of BPD involves long-term therapy. Hospitalization is sometimes necessary during acute episodes involving parasuicidal behaviour, but once this behaviour is controlled, clients are discharged. It is important for these individuals to continue with treatment in the outpatient or day treatment setting. They often appear more competent and in control than they are, and nurses must not be deceived by these outward appearances. They need continued follow-up and long-term therapy, including individual therapy, psychoeducation, and positive role models (see Nursing Care Plan 24-1).

Antisocial Personality Disorder: Aggrandizing Pattern
CLINICAL COURSE OF DISORDER

In the *DSM-IV-TR*, antisocial personality disorder (APD) is defined as "a pervasive pattern of disregard for, and violation of, the rights of others that begins in childhood or early adolescence and continues into adulthood" (APA, 2000, p. 701).

NURSING CARE PLAN 24.1

Client With Borderline Personality Disorder

YJ, a 28-year-old, single woman, was brought to the emergency department of a hospital by police officers after finding her in a Burger Chef with superficial self-inflicted lacerations on both forearms. She pleaded with the police not to take her to the hospital. The police report noted that she fluctuated between intense crying and pleading to fighting physically and using foul language. By the time she arrived in the emergency department, however, she was calm, cooperative, pleasant, and charming. When asked why she cut herself, YJ reported she wasn't sure but added that her therapist was leaving today for a 4-week trip to Europe. YJ specifically asked the staff not to call her therapist because "she will be angry with me."

After the emergency physician examined YJ, the advanced practice mental health nurse assessed her developmental and psychiatric history and a summary of recent events, before she reached a provisional diagnosis of borderline personality disorder with a primary nursing diagnosis of risk for self-mutilation related to abandonment anticipation. YJ had several previous self-destructive episodes with minor injuries, only one requiring sutures, and two hospitalizations. She lives with her boyfriend, who is cur-

rently on a business trip, and works part time at a bookstore. Her invalid mother lives with her younger sister. There are no other relatives. YJ's father died traumatically in an automobile accident when she was 3 years old. YJ was in the car when it crashed; she received minor injuries.

Because YJ refused to agree not to harm herself, the nurse admitted YJ to the psychiatric unit with suicide precautions. Once on the unit, YJ was assessed by a staff nurse as having a basically normal mental status examination except that her mood was very tearful at times but charming and joking at other times. She said, "Don't mind me, I cry at the drop of a hat sometimes." Toward the middle of the interview she said, "I feel safer here than I ever felt before. It must be you. Are you sure you're just a staff nurse?" YJ agreed to contract for safety just for today, but added, "Are you going to be my nurse tomorrow? I feel safest with you." When the nurse had completed her assessment, she showed YJ around the unit. As the nurse left her in the day room, YJ said, "My therapist doesn't understand me very well. I don't care if she is going out of town. After 4 years, she hasn't helped. If I had you as a therapist, I wouldn't be here now."

SETTING: INPATIENT PSYCHIATRIC UNIT IN A GENERAL HOSPITAL

Baseline Assessment: YJ, a 28-year-old woman, came into the emergency department with superficial self-inflicted wounds on both forearms. There was a marked discrepancy in her behaviour at the scene of the incident reported by emergency medical technicians from her presentation in the emergency department and now on the inpatient unit. She was admitted this time because she refused to agree not to harm herself further if released. She is angry and sad that her therapist is leaving for 4 weeks for a vacation and doesn't know how she will cope while the therapist is gone. She fears the therapist will not return.

Psychiatric Diagnosis	Medications
Axis I: Adjustment disorder with depressed mood Axis II: Borderline personality disorder Axis III: Superficial wounds to both forearms Axis IV: Social support (inadequate social support) Axis V: GAF current = 60; GAF past year = 75	Sertraline (Zoloft) 150 mg qd for anxiety and depression

NURSING DIAGNOSIS 1: SELF-MUTILATION

Defining Characteristics	Related Factors
Cuts and scratches on body Self-inflicted wounds	Fears of abandonment secondary to therapist's vacation Inability to handle stress

Outcomes

Initial	Discharge
1. Remain safe and not harm herself. 2. Identify feelings before and after cutting herself. 3. Agree not to harm herself over the next 24 h.	4. Identify ways of dealing with self-harming impulses if they return. 5. Verbalize alternate thinking with more realistic base. 6. Identify community resources to provide structure and support while therapist is gone.

(continued)

NURSING CARE PLAN 24.1 (Continued)

INTERVENTIONS

Interventions	Rationale	Ongoing Assessment
Monitor client for changes in mood or behaviour that might lead to self-injurious behaviour.	Close observation establishes safety and protection of client from self-harm and impulsive behaviours.	Document according to facility policy. Continue to observe for mood and behaviour changes.
Discuss with client need for close observation and rationale to keep her safe.	Explanation to client for purpose of nursing interventions helps her cooperate with the nursing activity.	Assess her response to increasing level of observation.
Administer medication as prescribed and evaluate medication effectiveness in reducing depression, anxiety, and cognitive disorganization	Allows for adjustment of medication dosage based on target behaviours and outcomes.	Observe for side effects.
After 6–8 h, present written agreement to not harm herself.	Permits client time to return to more thoughtful ways of responding rather than her previous reactive response. Also permits her to save face and avoid embarrassment of a losing power struggle if presented much earlier.	Observe for her willingness to agree to not harm herself.
Communicate information about client's risk to other nursing staff.	The close observation should be continued throughout all shifts until patient agrees to resist self-harm urges.	Review documentation of close observation for all shifts.

EVALUATION

Outcomes	Revised Outcomes	Interventions
Remained safe without further harming self. Identified fears of abandonment before cutting herself and relief of anxiety afterward.	Use hotlines or call friends if fears to harm self return.	Give client hotline number and ask her to record friend's numbers in an accessible place.
She identified friends to call when fears return and hotlines to use if necessary.		
Agreed to not harm herself over the next 3 d.	Does not harm self for 3 d.	Remind her to call someone if urges return.
Enrolled in a day hospital program for 4 wk.	Attend day hospital program.	Follow-up on enrolment.

NURSING DIAGNOSIS 2: RISK FOR LONELINESS

Defining Characteristics	Related Factors
Social isolation	Fear of abandonment secondary to therapist's impending vacation

OUTCOMES

Initial	Discharge
1. Discuss being lonely.	3. Identify strategies to deal with loneliness while therapist is away.
2. Identify previous ways of coping with loneliness.	

INTERVENTIONS

Interventions	Rationale	Ongoing Assessment
Develop a therapeutic relationship	People with BPD are able to examine loneliness within the structure of a therapeutic relationship.	Assess her ability to relate and nurse's response to the relationship.
Discuss past experience with therapist being gone with emphasis on how she was able to survive it.	She has survived therapist's absences before. By identifying the strategies she used, she can build on those strengths.	Assess her ability to assume any responsibility for "living through it." This will become a strength.
Acknowledge that it is normal to feel angry when therapist is gone, but there are other strategies that may help the person deal with the loneliness besides cutting.	Acknowledging feelings is important. Helping client focus on the possibility of other strategies for dealing with the anger helps her regain a sense of control over her behaviour.	Assess whether she is willing to acknowledge that there are other behavioural strategies of handling anger.

NURSING CARE PLAN 24.1 (Continued)

INTERVENTIONS

Intervention	Rationale	Ongoing Assessment
Begin immediate disposition planning with focus on day hospitalization or day treatment for skills training and management of loneliness.	While client is in hospital, she is out of stressful environment in which she can learn more effective behaviours and use the therapy. Moving out of the hospital and back into outpatient therapy decreases possibility of regression and lost learning (Linehan, 1993a and 1993b).	Assess her willingness to learn new skills within a day treatment setting.
Teach her about stress management techniques. Assign her to anger management group while she is in the hospital.	Learning about ways of dealing with feelings and stressful situations helps the client with BPD choose positive strategies rather than self-destructive ones.	Monitor whether she actually attends the groups. She should be encouraged to attend.

EVALUATION

Outcomes	Revised Outcomes	Interventions
YJ was able to verbalize her anger about her therapist leaving and fears of abandonment. The last two times her therapist went on vacation, the client became self injurious and was hospitalized for 2 wk.	None	
YJ was willing to be discharged the next day if she could attend day treatment while her therapist was gone.	Identify other strategies of dealing with therapist vacations besides cutting.	Attend stress management, communication, and self-comforting classes.

McCloskey, J., & Bulechek, G. (2002). Iowa Intervention Report. *Nursing interventions classification* (NIC) (3rd ed., p. 182). St. Louis: Mosby–Year Book.

The term **psychopathy**, which originated in Germany in the late 19th century, initially referred to all personality disorders (Dolan, 1994) but has gradually become equated with only APD. People with this disorder are behaviourally impulsive and interpersonally irresponsible. They fail to adapt to the ethical and social standards of the community. They act hastily and spontaneously, are short-sighted, and fail to plan ahead or consider alternatives. They lack a sense of personal obligation to fulfill social and financial responsibilities, including those involved with being a spouse, a parent, an employee, a friend, or member of the community. Disdainful of traditional values, they fail to conform to social norms and values. They enjoy a sense of freedom and relish being unencumbered and unconfined by people, places, or responsibilities. They can be interpersonally engaging, which is often mistaken for a genuine sense of concern for other people. In reality, they lack empathy, are unable to express human compassion, and tend to be insensitive, callous, and contemptuous of others. Easily irritated, they often become aggressive, disregarding the safety of themselves or others. They lack remorse for transgressions. No matter what the consequences, they are rarely able to delay gratification (APA, 2000).

These individuals have faith only in themselves and are secure only when they are independent from those whom they fear will harm or humiliate them. Their need for independence is based on their mistrust of others, rather than an inherent belief in their own self-worth. They are driven by a need to prove their superiority and see themselves as the centre of the universe. Some of these individuals openly and flagrantly violate laws, ending up in jail. But most people with APD never come in conflict with the law and, instead, find a niche in society, such as in business, the military, or politics, that rewards their competitive, tough behaviour (Millon & Davis, 1999). The most common social problems statistically associated with APD include substance abuse (Bucholz, Heath, & Madden, 2000; Lejoyeux et al., 2000), sexual assault and other criminal behaviour (Gotz, Johnstone, & Ratcliffe, 1999; Hare, 1999; Smallbone & Dadds, 2000), and family violence (Hanson, Cadsky, Harris, & Lalond, 1997) (Table 24-4). This disorder has a chronic course, but the antisocial behaviours tend to diminish later in life, particularly after the age of 40 years (APA, 2000).

Epidemiology and Risk Factors

The prevalence in nonclinical studies ranges from 2% to 3% of the population, with a median value of approximately 2% (Moran, 1999). In prison populations, the prevalence of APD rises to 60%.

Table 24.4	Key Diagnostic Characteristics of Antisocial Personality Disorder 301.7	

Diagnostic Criteria and Target Symptoms	Associated Findings

• Pervasive pattern of disregard for and violation of the rights of others
   Failure to conform to social norms with respect to lawful behaviours (repeatedly performing acts that are grounds for arrest)
   Deceitfulness (repeated lying, use of aliases, or conning others for personal profit or pleasure)
   Impulsivity or failure to plan ahead
   Irritability and aggressiveness (repeated physical fights or assaults)
   Reckless disregard for safety of self or others
   Consistent irresponsibility (repeated failure to sustain consistent work behaviour or honour financial obligations)
   Lack of remorse (being indifferent to or rationalizing having hurt, mistreated, or stolen from another)
• Occurring since 15 years of age
• At least 18 years of age
• Evidence of conduct disorder with onset before 15 years of age
• Not exclusive during the course of schizophrenia or manic episode
	Associated Behavioural Findings
	• Lacking empathy
	• Callous, cynical and contemptuous of the feelings, rights, and suffering of others
	• Inflated and arrogant self-appraisal
	• Excessively opinionated, self-assured or cocky
	• Glib, superficial charm; impressive verbal ability
	• Irresponsible and exploitative in sexual relationships; history of multiple sexual partners and lack of a sustained monogamous relationship
	• Possible dysphoria, including complaints of tension, inability to tolerate boredom, and depressed mood

Age of Onset

To be diagnosed with APD, the individual must have exhibited one or more childhood behavioural characteristics of conduct disorder and ADHD, such as aggression to people or animals, destruction of property, deceitfulness or theft, or serious violation of rules. This requirement of exhibiting antisocial behaviour before 15 years of age is based on older studies of adults with APD (Barry et al., 2000; Faraone, Biederman, Mennin, & Russell, 1998; Myers, Stewart, & Brown, 1998).

Gender

Men receive diagnoses of APD more frequently than do women (Eley, Lichtenstein, & Stevenson, 1999; Marcus, 1999). The best estimate for lifetime prevalence of APD from the Epidemiological Catchment Area (ECA) data is 7.3% for men and 1% for women (Robins, Tipp, & Przybeck, 1991). The cause of this discrepancy between men and women has received considerable speculation. It is generally believed that APD is underdiagnosed in women or manifested differently in men than in women, who usually receive diagnoses of somatization (see Chapter 21) or histrionic disorders (discussed later in this chapter). Some think that males have early-onset and adolescent-onset disorder, whereas females primarily have an adolescent-onset disorder (Silverthorn & Frick, 1999), contributing to less severe symptoms and deficits. Similarly, APD development in females entails more affect dysregulation, resulting in a

competing diagnosis of BPD, even though they meet the overall criteria for APD (Zlotnick, 1999) (Box 24-9).

Cultural and Ethnic Differences

People with APD or psychopathic personalities are found in many cultures, including industrialized and nonindustrialized societies. In an analysis of the Inuit of Northwest Alaska, individuals who break the rules when they are known are called *kunlangeta*, meaning "his mind knows what to do but he does not do it" (Murphy, 1976, p. 1026). This term is used for someone who repeatedly lies, cheats, and steals. He is described as someone who does not go hunting and, when the other men are out of the village, takes sexual advantage of the women. In another culture in rural southwest Nigeria, the Yorubas use the word *arankan* to mean a "person who always goes his own way regardless of others, who is uncooperative, full of malice and bullheaded" (Murphy, p. 1026). In both cultures, the healers and shamans do not consider these people treatable.

The number of people within a culture who actually have APD appears to depend on whether the society is individualistic, where competitiveness and independence are encouraged and temporary relationships the norm, or collectivistic, such as in China, where group loyalties and responsibilities are more important than self-expression (Cooke, 1996). Cultural distribution variation may have more to do with economic conditions, legal structures, social tolerance, and co-occurring conditions than specific diagnostic factors. Poverty and

Clinical Vignette: Antisocial Personality Disorder: Male Versus Female

Stasia (female) and Jackson (male) are fraternal twins, 22 years old, who received diagnoses of antisocial personality disorder. The following are their clinical profiles.

Jackson

Jackson's juvenile probation officer explained that Jackson came from a very violent family and neighbourhood and described the situation by saying, "If gangs hadn't gotten him, his father would have." His lawyer described him as "a likeable guy, but I wouldn't turn my back on him."

Jackson is currently in prison for the third time. Although his juvenile records begin at age 9 and include minor assault and property damage charges, his burglary conviction is his first adult crime. His school teachers thought Jackson was very bright but that he had significant difficulty with peers and authority figures. He fought regularly, was described as a bully, and seemed always to be scamming. At age 16, Jackson dropped out of school and joined a gang.

Stasia

Stasia was recently hospitalized for the sixth time when one of her male friends beat her. She has been working as a prostitute for 5 years. Her physical examination noted not only multiple bruises but also tattoos that cover 50% of

her body. In addition, she has piercings of her tongue, ears, brow, lips, and nipples. She is emotionally volatile, manipulative, and angry. Stasia has many acquaintances and sexual partners, but none are truly intimate. She has periods when she uses drugs regularly.

Stasia and Jackson's mother was jailed when the twins were 18 months old and didn't return until they were 6 years old. They were raised mostly by their paternal grandmother, who hated their mother and reminded Stasia frequently of how much she looked like her mother. Their father, when present, was violent toward Jackson and sexually abused Stasia.

What Do You Think?

- How might gender influence the development of symptoms?
- How might culture influence early recognition of problems and provision of early intervention to prevent future serious mental disorders?
- What are some possible outcomes in this situation?
- How does this case demonstrate the interaction between socialization, biology, and culture?

academic failure were significantly related to delinquency in boys (Pagani, Boulerice, Vitaro, & Tremblay, 1999), and gang entry was seen as a developmental step in boys with conduct disorder (Lahey, Gordon, Loeber, Stouthamer-Loeber, & Farrington, 1999).

Comorbidity

APD is strongly associated with alcohol and drug abuse. Substance-related disorders are common (Lejoyeux et al., 2000; Waldman & Slutske, 2000). The association between substance abuse and APD is stronger in women than in men. It is rare for APD to be the only disorder present. In the ECA study, fewer than 10% of clients with APD had no other diagnoses. In the ECA data, men with active APD were three times more likely to abuse alcohol and five times more likely to abuse drugs than were those without APD. Women with APD were 13 times more likely to use alcohol and 12 times more likely to use drugs (Robins et al., 1991). Other disorders that typically occur with APD include ADHD (Schubiner et al., 2000), depression, and schizophrenia (Nolan, Volavka, Mohr, & Czobor, 1999).

Etiology

Biologic Theories

There appears to be a genetic component in APD, which is five times more common in first-degree biologic relatives of men with the disorder than among the general population. There is a nearly 10 times greater

risk to women who are first-degree biologic relatives. Pooled data of 229 pairs of identical twins from seven twin studies conducted in North America, Japan, Norway, Germany, and Denmark showed a concordance rate of 51.5% for APD, whereas data from 316 fraternal twins yielded a corresponding rate of 23.1% (Gottesman & Goldsmith, 1994).

The biochemical basis of antisocial disorder is not clearly understood. However, some curious biologic markers have been identified. Gotz and colleagues (1999) found significantly higher antisocial behaviour in adolescent and adult men with XYY sex chromosome abnormality than in control subjects. Another study found higher concentration of serum testosterone and sex hormone–binding globulin in incarcerated men who met the criteria for APD (Stalenheim, von Knorring, & Wide, 1998). Serotonin deficiency (Dolan, 1994) and low dopamine levels have also been implicated in APD. In a study of 21 hospitalized boys ages 8 to 16 years who had diagnoses of conduct disorder, oppositional deviant disorder, and ADHD, low levels of dopamine activity were found in those who had been abused or neglected before the age of 3 years (Galvin et al., 1991). These researchers suggested that low levels of dopamine may reflect an attachment disruption that occurs at critical times in the lives of abused and neglected boys. This disruption causes the child to be biologically vulnerable, resulting in low levels of dopamine and less effective regulation of the noradrenergic system when activated by stressors. In addition, researchers consistently find dysregulation in catecholamines with changed activity of the dopaminergic pathways in the frontal cortex (Soderstrom et al., 2003). The limbic-prefrontal cortex (Veit et al., 2002) and dorsolateral prefrontal cortex (Dolan & Park, 2002) are specifically implicated, accounting for poor judgment, emotional distance, aggression, and impulsivity (Kiehl et al., 2001).

Psychological Theories

Learning, social behaviour, empathy, emotional awareness, and regulation are all directly influenced by the nature of the relationship between the caregiver and child. One of the leading explanations of APD is that these individuals had unsatisfactory attachments in early relationships that led to antisocial behaviour in later life. Normal relationships begin with **attachment** that can be defined as:

> Behaviour that results in a person's attaining or retaining proximity to some other differentiated and preferred individual. During the course of healthy development, attachment behaviour leads to the development of affectional bonds or attachments, initially between child and parent and later between adult and adult. The forms of behaviour and the bonds to which they lead are present and active throughout the life cycle. (Bowlby, 1980, p. 39)

An attachment relationship between the child and caregiver depends on the response of both parties. The sense of security in any relationship depends on the quality of the responsiveness experienced with the attachment figure (Smallbone & Dadds, 2000). If the parental figures are overanxious or avoidant, the child does not develop a sense of security with others and instead experiences self as an island (Reti et al., 2002). Secure attachments facilitate a balance between connection to another and the ability to go out into the world autonomously. In a secure attachment, a child feels safe, loved, and valued, but also develops the self-confidence to interact with the rest of the world. Experiences in successive relationships interact with prior experiences to determine an individual's trust in others.

Insecure attachments are formed as a result of faulty interaction between the caregiver and the child and are expressed in relationships as ambivalence, avoidance, or disorganization (Ainsworth, 1989). In APD, a failure to make or sustain stable attachments in early childhood can lead to avoidance of future attachments. Studies have found several childhood situations to be risk factors for developing dysfunctional attachments, such as parental abandonment or neglect, loss of parent or primary caregiver, and physical or sexual abuse. However, evidence supports the theory that ability to foster secure emotional attachments may be a learned parenting skill and that parents who lacked secure attachment relationships in their own childhood may lack the ability to form secure attachment relationships with their own children (Box 24-10).

BOX 24.10   RESEARCH FOR BEST PRACTICE

Antisocial Personality Traits in Children

THE QUESTIONS: At what age can one identify children with high levels of antisocial behaviour? What other factors are associated with these behavioural deficits? What is the prevalence of antisocial behaviour in Canadian children?

METHODS: This research analyzed data from the National Longitudinal Survey of Children and Youth, a nationally representative sample of Canadian children. The analysis included data for children aged 2 to 11 (n = 22,831). A cluster analysis was conducted on standardized reports of behavioural measures including aggression, hyperactivity, prosocial behaviour, emotional disorder/anxiety, and (for those aged 4 to 11) misconduct. Three levels of severity for the antisocial behaviours were identified. The clusters were compared with a number of covariates (structural, family, school, community, and health).

FINDINGS: Even by age 2, antisocial traits were demonstrated in a pattern consistent with the older children and in association with disadvantages in the covariates. The findings suggest that between 5% and 8%, or just over $1/4$ million, Canadian children between the ages of 2 and 11 years demonstrate the most severe level of antisocial behaviour.

IMPLICATIONS FOR NURSING PRACTICE: This study supports the complexity and interactions among the social determinants of health and calls for nurses to make use of assessments and interventions that support the population health approach (eg, family/parenting support, improved neighbourhood safety and cohesion, accessible health care, academic support).

Wade, T., Pevalin, D., & Brannigan, A. (1999). The clustering of severe behavioural, health and educational deficits in Canadian children: Preliminary evidence from the National Longitudinal Survey of Children and Youth. *Canadian Journal of Public Health*, *90*(4), 253–259.

Children are born with a particular **temperament**, a recognizable and distinctive pattern of behaviour that is evident during the first few months of life. Some infants are more relaxed or calm and sleep a lot, whereas others are extremely alert, startled by the slightest noise, cry more, and sleep less. Scientists believe temperament is neurobiologically determined, and many believe that it is central to understanding personality disorders. Children seem to be born with certain temperaments that remain fairly stable throughout development.

Temperament consists of the interaction of two behavioural dimensions—activity and adaptability. Activity patterns in individuals vary along a spectrum, from active or intense children, whose actions display decisiveness and vigour as they continuously relate to their environment, to passive children, who are more cautious and slow to relate to their environment (a wait-and-see pattern of behaviour). Adaptability includes a spectrum, with the extreme at one end being the child who is regular in biologic functions such as eating or sleeping, has a positive approach to new stimuli, and maintains a high degree of flexibility in response to changing conditions. At the other end of the adaptability dimension are children who display irregularity in biologic functions, withdrawal reactions to new stimuli, and minimal flexibility in response to change.

Some studies indicate that extreme temperaments make one vulnerable to antisocial behaviour patterns. A difficult temperament is characterized by withdrawal from novel stimuli, low adaptability, and intense emotional reactions. Four key behaviours are present in a difficult temperament: aggression, inattention, hyperactivity, and impulsivity. There is a strong relationship between difficult temperament and problem behaviours such as those of ADHD, oppositional behaviour, and conduct disorder (Dowson, Sussams, Grounds, & Taylor, 2001; Herpertz et al., 2001; Hill, 2002, 2003; Langbehn & Cadoret, 2001).

Hyperactivity alone is not related to the development of antisocial personality in adults, whereas hyperactivity occurring with aggression and the other behaviours listed is related to APD (Barry et al., 2000; Giancola, 2000; Schubiner et al., 2000). Temperament and problem behaviours are generally consistent throughout a lifetime. There is a strong relationship between conduct disorder in childhood and antisocial behaviour in adulthood with substance abuse (Myers et al., 1998). In a longitudinal study of 961 children whose temperament related to the development of psychiatric problems in childhood, the children with a difficult temperament were more likely to receive diagnoses of APD in adulthood, be a recidivistic offender, and be convicted of a violent offence (Grann, Lanstrom, Tengstrom, & Kullgren, 1999; Hare, 1999).

Social Theories

In many cases, individuals with APD come from chaotic families in which alcoholism and violence are the norm. Individuals who have been victims of abuse or neglect, live in a foster home, or had several primary caregivers are more likely to experience antisocial behaviours, especially aggression (Andrews, Foster, Capaldi, & Hop, 2000; Kim, Hetherington, & Reiss, 1999; Pagani et al., 1999). However, it is difficult to separate the influence of social factors on the development of the disorder because the symptoms of APD are social manifestations—unemployment, divorces and separations, and violence.

Interdisciplinary Treatment of Disorder

People with APD rarely seek mental health care because of the disorder itself, but rather for treatment of depression, substance abuse, or uncontrolled anger or for forensic evaluation (Black, Baumgard, & Bell, 1995). Clients who are admitted through the courts often have a comorbid diagnosis of APD. Treatment is difficult and involves helping the individual alter his or her cognitive schema. The overall treatment goals are to develop empathy for other people and situations and to live within the norms of society.

Priority Care Issues

Although they can be interpersonally charming, these individuals can become verbally and physically abusive if their expectations are not met. Protection of other clients and staff from manipulative and sometimes abusive behaviour is a priority.

Family Response to Disorder

If there are family members, they have probably been abused, mistreated, or intimidated by these individuals. For example, one client sold his mother's possessions while she was at work. Another would abuse his wife after drinking. However, family members may be fiercely loyal to the person and blame themselves for his or her shortcomings.

NURSING MANAGEMENT: HUMAN RESPONSE TO DISORDER

Biologic Domain

Biologic Assessment

Antisocial personality disorder does not significantly impair the biologic dimension unless there are coexisting substance abuse or other Axis I disorders. Because substance abuse is a major problem with this population, the physical effects of chronic use of addictive substances must be considered.

Nursing Diagnoses for the Biologic Domain

A common nursing diagnosis in APD is Dysfunctional Family Processes, Alcoholism.

Interventions for Biologic Domain

In instances in which there are coexisting disorders, the personality disorder may actually interfere with interventions aimed at improving physical functioning. For example, a client with schizophrenia and APD may not develop enough trust within a relationship to examine his or her delusional thoughts or other aspects of dysfunction, such as alcohol or drug abuse.

Psychological Domain

Psychological Assessment

Many individuals with APD are committed to health care agencies by the court system. Assessment generally involves using basic psychological assessment tools to evaluate aberrant behaviours.

Nursing Diagnoses for the Psychological Domain

Because so many individuals with APD have dysfunctional thinking patterns, a common nursing diagnosis is Disturbed Thought Processes and Risk for Other Directed Violence.

Interventions for the Psychological Domain

Therapeutic relationships are difficult to establish because these individuals do not attach to others and are often unable to use the relationship to change behaviour. After the first few meetings with these clients, the nurse may feel that the relationship has a good start, but in reality, a superficial alliance is usually formed. Additional sessions reveal the lack of client commitment to the relationship. These individuals begin to revisit topics discussed in sessions or lose interest in trying to work on problems. By using self-awareness skills and accessing supervision regularly, the nurse can identify blocks in the development of a therapeutic relationship (or lack of) and his or her response to the relationship. The goal of the therapeutic relationship is to identify dysfunctional thinking patterns and develop new problem-solving behaviours.

Self-responsibility facilitation (encouraging a person to assume more responsibility for personal behaviour) is useful with clients with APD (McCloskey & Bulechek, 2000). The nursing activities that are particularly helpful include holding the client responsible for his or her behaviour, monitoring the extent that self-responsibility is assumed, and discussing the consequences of not dealing with responsibilities. The nurse needs to refrain from arguing or bargaining about the unit rules, such as time for meals, use of the television room, and smoking. Instead, positive feedback is given to the individual for accepting additional responsibility or changing behaviour.

Self-awareness enhancement (exploring and understanding personal thoughts, feelings, motivation, and behaviours) is another nursing intervention that is important in helping these individuals develop a sense of understanding about relating peacefully to the rest of the world (McCloskey & Bulechek, 2000). Encouraging clients to recognize and discuss thoughts and feelings helps the nurse understand how the person views the world. The nurse can then use many of the same communication techniques discussed in the section on BPD.

Teaching Points

Client education efforts have to be creative and thought provoking. In teaching a person with APD, a direct approach is best, but the nurse must avoid "lecturing," which the individual will resent. In teaching the client about positive health care practices, impulse control, and anger management, the best approach is to engage the individual in a discussion about the issue and then direct the topic to the major teaching points. These clients often take great delight in arguing or showing how the rules of life do not apply to them. A sense of humour is important, as are clear teaching goals and avoiding being sidetracked (Box 24-11).

Social Domain

Social Assessment

The nursing assessment usually focuses on other problems in addition to the response to the personality disorder. In fact, eliciting data may be difficult because of the basic mistrust individuals with APD have toward authority figures. Clients may not give an accurate history or may embellish aspects to project themselves in a more positive light. Often, they deny any criminal activity, even if they are admitted in police custody. Key areas of assessment are determining the quality of relationships, impulsivity, and the extent of aggression. These individuals do not assume responsibility for their own actions and often blame others for their misfortune. Their disregard for others is manifested in their interactions. For example, one individual with human immunodeficiency virus was engaging in unprotected sex with several different women because he wanted to "have fun as long as I can." He was completely unconcerned about

---

BOX 24.11

Psychoeducation Checklist: Antisocial Personality Disorder

When caring for the client with antisocial personality disorder, be sure to include the following topic areas in the teaching plan:
- ☐ Positive health care practices, including substance abuse control
- ☐ Effective communication and interaction skills
- ☐ Impulse control
- ☐ Anger management
- ☐ Group experience to help develop self-awareness and impact of behaviour on others
- ☐ Analyzing an issue from the other person's viewpoint
- ☐ Maintenance of employment
- ☐ Interpersonal relationships and social interactions

the possibility of transmitting the virus. These individuals often make good first impressions. Self-awareness is especially important for the nurse because of the initial charming quality of many of these individuals. Once these clients realize that the nurse cannot be used or manipulated, they lose interest in the nurse and revert to their normal, egocentric behaviours.

Nursing Diagnoses for the Social Domain

Nursing diagnoses for clients with APD are related to their interpersonal detachment, lack of awareness of others, avoidance of feelings, impulsiveness, and discrepancy between their perception of themselves and others' perception of them. Typical diagnoses are Ineffective Role Performance (unemployment), Ineffective Individual Coping, Impaired Communication, Impaired Social Interactions, Low Self-Esteem, and Risk for Violence. Outcomes should be short term and relevant to a specific problem. For example, if a person has been chronically unemployed, a reasonable short-term outcome would be to set up job interviews, rather than obtain a job.

Interventions for the Social Domain

These clients have a long-standing history of difficulty in interpersonal relationships. In an inpatient unit, interventions can be more intense and focus on helping the individual develop positive interaction skills and experience a consistent environment. For example, the focus of nursing interventions may be the client's continual disregard of the rights of others. On one unit, a client continually placed orders for pizzas in the name of another person on the unit. This individual had limited intelligence and was genuinely afraid of the person with APD. The victimized person always paid for the pizza and gave it to the other client. When the nursing staff realized what was happening, they confronted the client with APD about the behaviour and revoked his unit privileges.

Group interventions are more effective than individual modalities because other individuals on the unit and staff can validate or challenge the client's view of a situation (Messina, Wish, & Nemes, 1999). Problem-solving groups that focus on identifying a problem and developing a variety of alternative solutions are particularly helpful because client self-responsibility is reinforced when fellow clients remind each other of the better alternatives. Clients are likely to confront each other with dysfunctional schemas or thinking patterns. Teaching individuals with APD the same communication techniques as those with BPD will also encourage self-responsibility. These clients often attend groups that focus on the development of empathy.

Milieu interventions, such as providing a structured environment with rules that are consistently applied to clients who are responsible for their own behaviour, are important. While living in close proximity to others, the individual with APD will demonstrate dysfunctional social patterns that can be identified and targeted for correction. For example, these clients often violate ward rules, such as no smoking or limitations on the number of visitors, and may bring contraband, such as illegal drugs, to the unit.

Aggressive behaviour is often a problem for these individuals and their family members. Like clients with BPD, people with APD tend to be impulsive. Instead of self-injury, these individuals are more likely to strike out at those who are perceived to be interfering with their immediate gratification. Anger control assistance (helping to express anger in an adaptive, nonviolent manner) becomes a priority intervention. Because the expression of anger and aggression develops during a lifetime, these individuals can benefit from anger management techniques.

Social support for these individuals is often minimal, just as it is for individuals with BPD, but the reasons are different. These individuals have often taken advantage of friends and relatives who, in turn, no longer trust them. Helping the client build a new support system once new skills are learned is usually the only option. For these individuals to develop friends and re-engage family members, they must learn to interact in new ways, develop empathy, and risk an attachment. For many, this never truly becomes a reality.

Family Patterns

Family members of clients with APD usually need help in establishing boundaries. Because there is a long-term pattern of interaction in which family members are responsible for the client's antisocial behaviour, these patterns need to be interrupted. Families need help in recognizing the client's responsibility for his or her actions.

EVALUATION AND OUTCOMES

The outcomes of interventions for individuals with APD need to be evaluated in terms of management of specific problems, such as maintaining employment or developing a meaningful interpersonal relationship. The nurse will most likely see these clients for other health care problems, so that adherence to treatment recommendations and development of health care practices (eg, reduce smoking and alcohol consumption) can also be factored into the evaluation of outcomes.

CONTINUUM OF CARE

People with APD rarely seek mental health care. In one study, only 14.5% of those with a diagnosis of APD had ever discussed any of its symptoms with a physician. Only 4% had visited a mental health provider during the last 6 months (Robins et al., 1991). Nurses will most likely see these individuals in medical-surgical settings for comorbid conditions. Consistency in interventions is necessary in treating the client throughout the continuum of care.

HISTRIONIC PERSONALITY DISORDER: GREGARIOUS PATTERN

"Attention seeking" and "emotional" describe people with histrionic personality disorders. These individuals are lively and dramatic and draw attention to themselves by their enthusiasm, dress, and apparent openness. They are the "life of the party" and, on the surface, seem interested in others. Their insatiable need for attention and approval quickly becomes obvious. These needs are inflexible and persistent, even after others attempt to meet them. They are moody and

often experience a sense of helplessness when others are disinterested in them. They are sexually seductive in their attempts to gain attention and often are uncomfortable within a single relationship. They are highly suggestible and have a tendency to change opinions often. Their appearance is provocative and their speech dramatic. They express strong opinions without supporting facts. Loyalty and fidelity are lacking (APA, 2000) (Table 24-5).

Gender influences the manifestations of this disorder. Women dress seductively, may express dependency on selected men, and may "play" a submissive role. Men may dress in a very masculine manner and seek attention by bragging about athletic skills or successes in the job. Individuals with this disorder have difficulty achieving any true intimacy in interpersonal relationships. They seem to possess an innate sensitivity to the moods and thoughts of those they wish to please. This hyperalertness enables them to manoeuvre quickly to gain their attention. Then, they attempt to control relationships

---

Table 24.5	Key Diagnostic Characteristics of Histrionic and Narcissistic Personality Disorders 301.50	

Diagnostic Criteria and Target Symptoms for Histrionic Disorders

- Pervasive and excessive emotionality and attention-seeking behaviour
  - Feelings of being uncomfortable and unappreciated when not the centre of attention (lively and dramatic in drawing attention to self)
  - Inappropriately sexually seductive or provocative
  - Shallow and rapidly shifting emotional expression
  - Use of physical appearance to draw attention to self
  - Impressionistic and vague style of speech
  - Exaggerated expression of emotion, theatricality, and self-dramatization
  - Highly suggestible
  - Viewing of relationships as more intimate than they really are

Diagnostic Criteria and Target Symptoms for Narcissistic Disorders

- Pervasive pattern of grandiosity; need for admiration; lack of empathy
  - Grandiose sense of self-importance
  - Preoccupation with fantasies of unlimited success, power of vigilance, beauty, or ideal love
  - Belief of own superiority, specialness, and uniqueness; association with individuals of higher or special status
  - Need for excessive admiration and constant attention
  - Sense of entitlement (unreasonable expectation of highly favourable treatment)
  - Exploitation and taking advantage of others
  - Lack of empathy; difficulty recognizing desires, experiences, and feelings of others
  - Envious of others; feeling that others are envious of him or her
  - Arrogant, haughty behaviour or attitudes

Associated Findings
Associated Behavioural Findings

- Difficulty achieving emotional intimacy in romantic and sexual relationships
- Use of emotional manipulation and seductiveness coupled with marked dependency
- Impaired relationships with same-sex friends
- Constant demanding of attention, leading to alienation of friends
- Craving novelty, excitement, and stimulation; easily bored with routines
- Difficulty in situations involving delayed gratification
- Increased risk for suicidal gestures and threats for attention

Associated Findings
Associated Behavioural Findings

- Sensitive to injury from criticism or deficit
- Criticism causes inward feelings of humiliation, degradation, hollowness, and emptiness
- Social withdrawal
- Impaired interpersonal relationships
- Impaired performance because of intolerance to criticism
- Unwilling to take risk in competitive situation when defeat is possible

by their seductiveness at one level but become extremely dependent on their friends at another level. Their demand for constant attention quickly alienates their friends. They become depressed when they are not the centre of attention.

Epidemiology

The prevalence of histrionic personality disorder is estimated at 2% to 3% of the general population. In mental health settings, the prevalence rate is reported to be 10% to 15% (APA, 2000). A higher rate of this disorder among separated and divorced subjects than among married subjects has been found (Nestadt et al., 1990). This disorder co-occurs with borderline, dependent, and antisocial personality disorders. It also exists with anxiety disorders, substance abuse, and mood disorders (Millon & Davis, 1999). Men with histrionic disorders are more likely to also have substance abuse problems, and women are more likely to experience depressive episodes, suicide attempts, and two or more unexplained medical symptoms (Nestadt et al., 1990).

Etiology

There is a need for research in determining the etiologic factors of histrionic personality disorder. There is speculation that this disorder has a biologic component and that heredity may play a role, but that the biologic influence is less than in some of the previously discussed personality disorders. In infancy and early childhood, these individuals are extremely alert and emotionally responsive. The tendencies for sensory alertness may be traced to responses of the limbic and reticular systems. They demonstrate a high degree of dependence on others and a type of dissociation in which they have reduced awareness of their behaviour in relation to others (Bornstein, 1998). It is believed these highly alert and responsive infants seek more gratification from external stimulation during their first few months of life. Depending on the responsiveness of caregivers to them, they develop behaviour patterns in response to their caregivers. It is believed that these children experience brief, highly charged, and irregular reinforcement from multiple caregivers (parents, siblings, grandparents, foster parents) who are unable to provide consistent experiences.

Parental behaviour and role modeling are also believed to contribute to the development of histrionic personality disorder. Many of the women with this disorder reported that they are just like their mother, who is emotionally labile, bored with the routines of home life, flirtatious with men, and clever in dealing with people. It is believed that through role modeling, these children learn and mimic the behaviours observed in caregivers or adults (Sigmund, Barnett, & Mundt, 1998).

Nursing Management

The ultimate treatment goal for individuals with histrionic personality disorder is to correct the tendency to fulfill all their needs by focussing on others to the exclusion of themselves. When these individuals seek mental health care, they have usually experienced a period of social disapproval or deprivation. Their hope is that the mental health providers will help fulfill their needs. Specific goals are needed to protect the person from becoming dependent on a mental health system. In the nursing assessment, the nurse focuses on the quality of the individual's interpersonal relationships. It is common that the person is dissatisfied with his or her partner, and sexual relations may be nonexistent.

During the assessment, the client will make statements that indicate low self-esteem. Because these individuals believe that they are incapable of handling life's demands and have been waiting for a truly competent person to take care of them, they have not developed a positive self-concept or adequate problem-solving abilities.

Nursing diagnoses that are usually generated include Chronic Low Self-Esteem, Ineffective Individual Coping, and Ineffective Sexual Patterns. Outcomes focus on helping the individual develop autonomy, a positive self-concept, and mature problem-solving skills.

A variety of interventions support the outcomes. A nurse–client relationship that allows the client to explore positive personality characteristics and develop independent decision-making skills forms the basis of the interventions. Reinforcing personal strengths, conveying confidence in the person's ability to handle situations, and examining negative perceptions of self can be done within the therapeutic relationship. Encouraging the client to act autonomously can also improve the individual's sense of self-worth (McCloskey & Bulechek, 2000). Attending assertiveness groups can help increase the individual's self-confidence and improve self-esteem.

NARCISSISTIC PERSONALITY DISORDER: EGOTISTIC PATTERN

People with a narcissistic personality disorder are grandiose, have an inexhaustible need for admiration, and lack empathy. Beginning in childhood, these individuals believe that they are superior, special, or unique and that others should recognize them in this way (APA, 2000). They are often preoccupied with fantasies of unlimited success, power, beauty, or ideal love. They overvalue their personal worth, direct their affections toward themselves, and expect others to hold them in high esteem. They define the world through their own self-centred view. People with narcissistic personality disorder are benignly arrogant and feel themselves above the conventions of their cultural group. They believe they are entitled to be served and that it is their inalienable right to receive special considerations. These individuals are often successful in their jobs but may alienate their significant others, who grow tired of their narcissism (see Table 24-5). Clinically, those with narcissistic personality disorder show overlapping characteristics of BPD.

Epidemiology

The prevalence of narcissistic personality disorder in the general population is estimated to be less than 1%. In the mental health clinical population, the prevalence ranges from 2% to 16% (APA, 2000). In nonclinical samples, the prevalence rate ranges from 0.0% to 0.4% (Lyons, 1995). Narcissistic personality disorder is found more frequently in men than in women (Millon & Davis, 1999). It also commonly occurs in only children and among first-born boys in cultural groups in which males have special privileges. This disorder can coexist with other Axis II disorders, such as antisocial, histrionic, and paranoid disorders and Axis I disorders of mood, anxiety, and substance abuse.

Etiology

There is little evidence of any biologic factors that contribute to the development of this disorder. One notion about its development is that it is the result of parents' overvaluation and overindulgence of a child. These children are overly pampered and indulged, with every whim catered to. They learn to view themselves as special beings and to expect special treatment and subservience from others. They do not learn how to cooperate, share, or consider others' desires and interests. An alternate explanation is that the child never truly separated emotionally from his or her primary caregiver and therefore cannot envision functioning independently. The underlying basis of the outward aggrandizement is one of profound self-hatred and inferiority (Bushman & Baumeister, 1998). To avoid feeling this self-hatred, the person develops a defensive need for power over others (Joubert, 1998; Paulhus, 1998).

Nursing Management

The nurse usually encounters narcissists in medical settings and in psychiatric settings with a coexisting psychiatric disorder. They are difficult clients who are often snobbish, condescending, and patronizing in their attitudes. It is unlikely that these individuals are motivated to develop sensitivity to others and socially cooperative attitudes and behaviours. Nurses need to use their self-awareness skills in interacting with these clients. The nursing process focuses on the coexisting responses to other health care problems.

CONTINUUM OF CARE

Clients with histrionic and narcissistic personality disorders do not seek mental health care unless they have a coexisting medical or mental disorder. They are likely to be treated within the community for most of their lives, with the exception of short hospitalizations for nonpsychiatric problems.

Cluster C Disorders: Anxious-Fearful

AVOIDANT PERSONALITY DISORDER: WITHDRAWN PATTERN

Avoidant personality disorder is characterized by avoiding social situations in which there is interpersonal contact with others. This avoidance is purposeful and deliberate because of fears of criticism and feelings of inadequacy. These individuals are extremely sensitive to negative comments and disapproval. They engage in interpersonal relationships only when they receive unconditional approval. The behaviour becomes problematic when they restrict their social activities and work opportunities because of their extreme fear of rejection. They appear timid, shy, and hesitant. In childhood, they are shy, but instead of growing out of the shyness, it becomes worse in adulthood. They distance themselves from activities that involve personal contact with others. They perceive themselves as socially inept, inadequate, and inferior, which in turn justifies their isolation and rejection by others. They rely on fantasy for gratification of needs, confidence, and conflict resolution. These individuals withdraw into their fantasies as a means of dealing with frustration and anger. They also have underlying feelings of tension, sadness, and anger that vacillate between desire for affection, fear of rebuff, embarrassment, and numbness of feeling (APA, 2000; Millon & Davis, 1999) (Table 24-6).

Epidemiology

The prevalence estimates in nonclinical samples range from 0.0% to 1.3%, with a median value of about 1.1% (Lyons, 1995). Lifetime prevalence of avoidant personality disorder was estimated at 3.6% (Faravelli et al., 2000). Avoidant personality disorder has been reported in about 10% of outpatients in mental health clinics. The problem with examining the epidemiology of avoidant personality disorder is its potential overlap with the Axis I disorder, generalized social phobia. Several studies found that a significant portion of the clients with diagnoses of social phobia also met criteria for avoidant personality disorder. Social phobia was found to be more pervasive and characterized by a higher level of interpersonal sensitivity (Perugi et al.,

Table 24.6	Key Diagnostic Characteristics of Cluster C Disorders

Diagnostic Criteria and Target Symptoms

Avoidant Personality Disorder 301.82	• Pervasive pattern of social inhibition with feelings of inadequacy and hypersensitivity to negative evaluation Avoidance of activities involving significant personal contact because of fear of criticism, disapproval, or rejection Lack of willingness for involvement unless certainty of being liked Restraint within intimate relationships for fear of shame or ridicule Preoccupation with criticism or rejection in social situations Inhibition in new interpersonal situations Viewing self as socially inept, personally unappealing, or inferior Unusual reluctance to take personal risks or engage in new activities
Dependent Personality Disorder 301.6	• Pervasive and excessive need for being taken care of, resulting in submission and clinging with fears of separation Advice and reassurance needed from others for decision making Responsibility for major areas of life assumed by others Difficulty expressing disagreement with others for fear of loss of support or approval Difficulty initiating things by self Excessive methods used to obtain support and nurturance from others Uncomfortable and helpless when alone Urgent seeking of another relationship if previous one ends Unrealistic preoccupation with fears of having to take care of self
Obsessive-Compulsive Personality Disorder 301.4	• Pervasive pattern of preoccupation with orderliness, perfectionism, mental and interpersonal control at the expense of flexibility, openness, and efficiency Major point of activity lost because of preoccupation Task completion interfered with because of perfectionism Excessive devotion to work and productivity, excluding friends and leisure Overly conscientious, scrupulous, and inflexible about morality, ethics, or values Difficulty discarding worn-out or worthless objects Reluctance to delegate tasks or work with others Miserly spending attitude Rigidity and stubbornness

1999). However, avoidant personality disorder involves greater overall psychopathology (Boone et al., 1999). Not surprisingly, social phobia frequently co-occurs with avoidant personality disorder (Moutier & Stein, 1999). Clients with avoidant personality disorder differ from those with generalized social phobia only in the severity of the anxiety symptoms (less than those with social phobia) and in the depressive symptomatology.

Etiology

Experts speculate that individuals with avoidant personality disorder experience aversive stimuli more intensely and more frequently than do others because they may possess an overabundance of neurons in the aversive centre of the limbic system (Millon & Davis, 1999). A general biologic vulnerability may be inherited and interact with environmental factors. The evidence for this biologic influence is the impact of pharmacotherapies on these individuals. When taking medications (benzodiazepines, beta-blockers, and monoamine oxidase inhibitors), symptoms are reduced, but they

resume once medication is stopped (Mattick & Newman, 1991).

Research indicates that those with avoidant personality disorder demonstrate significantly less curiosity and novelty seeking than do healthy control subjects. The research postulated that those with avoidant personality disorder had a more tenuous early attachment (Johnston, 1999). In adulthood, they maintain an ambivalent connection with others, wishing deeply for close, enduring relationships but fearing rejection and loss.

Nursing Management

Assessment of these individuals reveals a lack of social contacts, a fear of being criticized, and evidence of chronic low self-esteem. The nursing diagnoses Chronic Low Self-Esteem, Social Isolation, and Ineffective Coping can be used. The establishment of a therapeutic relationship is necessary to be able to help these individuals meet their treatment outcomes. The development of the nurse–client relationship is a slow process and requires an extreme amount of patience on the part of the nurse.

These individuals have not had positive interpersonal relationships and need time to be able to trust that the nurse will not criticize and demean them. Interventions should focus on refraining from any negative criticism, assisting the client to identify positive responses from others, exploring previous achievements of success, and exploring reasons for self-criticism. The person's social dimension should be examined for activities that increase self-esteem and interventions focussed on increasing these self-esteem–enhancing activities. Social skills training may help reduce symptoms.

DEPENDENT PERSONALITY DISORDER: SUBMISSIVE PATTERN

People with dependent personality disorder cling to others in a desperate attempt to keep them close. Their need to be taken care of is so great that it leads to doing anything to maintain the closeness, including total submission and disregard for self.

Decision making is difficult or nil. They adapt their behaviour to please those to whom they are attached. They lean on others to guide their lives. They ingratiate themselves to others and denigrate themselves and their accomplishments. Their self-esteem is determined by others. Behaviourally, they withdraw from adult responsibilities by acting helpless and seeking nurturance from others. In interpersonal relationships, they need excessive advice and reassurance. They are compliant, conciliatory, and placating. They rarely disagree with others and are easily persuaded. Friends describe them as gullible. They are warm, tender, and noncompetitive. They timidly avoid social tension and interpersonal conflicts (APA, 2000) (see Table 24-6). Dependent personality disorder bears a great deal of resemblance to histrionic personality disorder. People with dependent personality disorder demonstrate high levels of self-attributed dependency needs, whereas those with histrionic personality disorder have greater implicit dependency and will even argue against needing others (Bornstein, 1998).

Epidemiology

Dependent personality disorder is one of the most frequently reported disorders in mental health clinics (APA, 2000). The prevalence in nonclinical samples ranges from 1.5% to 5.1%, with a median value of about 1.8% (Lyons, 1995). In clinical samples, the prevalence of this disorder ranges from 2% to 55%, with a median of 20% (Widiger, 1991). The diagnosis is made more frequently in women than in men. This gender difference may represent a sex bias by clinicians because when standardized instruments are used, men and women receive diagnoses at equal rates. This disorder often coexists with other personality disorders, including borderline, avoidant, histrionic, and schizotypal disorders (Lyons, 1995).

Etiology

It is likely that there is a biologic predisposition to develop the dependency attachments of this disorder. However, no research studies support a biologic hypothesis. Dependent personality disorder most often is explained as a result of parents' genuine affection, extreme attachment, and overprotection. Children then learn to rely on others to meet basic needs and do not learn the necessary skills for autonomous behaviour.

Nursing Management

Nurses can determine the extent of dependency by assessment of self-worth, interpersonal relationships, and social behaviour. They should determine whether there is currently someone on whom the person relies (parent, spouse) or if there has been a separation from a significant relationship by death or divorce.

Nursing diagnoses that are usually generated from the assessment data are Ineffective Individual Coping, Low Self-Esteem, Impaired Social Interaction, and Impaired Home Maintenance Management. Home management skills may be a problem if the client does not have the useful skills and now has to make decisions related to finances, shopping, cooking, and cleaning. The challenge of caring for these individuals is to help them recognize their dependent patterns, motivate them to want to change, and teach them adult skills that have not been developed, such as balancing a checkbook, planning a weekly menu, and paying bills. Occasionally, if a client is extremely fatigued, lethargic, or anxious and the disorder interferes with efforts at developing more independence, antidepressants or antianxiety agents may be used.

These individuals readily engage in a nurse–client relationship and initially will look to the nurse to make all decisions. The nurse can support these individuals to make their own decisions by resisting the urge to tell them what to do. Ideally, these clients are in individual psychotherapy and working toward long-term personality changes. The nurse can encourage clients to stay in therapy and to practice the new skills that are being learned. Assertiveness training is helpful.

OBSESSIVE-COMPULSIVE PERSONALITY DISORDER: CONFORMING PATTERN

Obsessive-compulsive disorder (OCD) stands out in Axis II because it bears close resemblance to obsessive-compulsive anxiety disorder (Axis I). A distinguishing difference is that those with the anxiety disorder tend to use obsessive thoughts and compulsions when anxious but less so when anxiety decreases. With OCD, the person does not demonstrate obsessions and compulsions as much as an overall rigidity, perfectionism, and control. Individuals with this disorder attempt to maintain control by careful attention to rules, trivial details, procedures, and lists (APA, 2000). These people are not fun. They may be completely devoted to work, which typically has a rigid character, such as maintaining financial records or tracking inventory. They are uncomfortable with unstructured leisure time, especially vacations. Leisure activities are likely to be formalized (season tickets to sports, organized tour groups). Hobbies are approached seriously.

Behaviourally, individuals with OCD are perfectionists, maintaining a regulated, highly structured, strictly organized life. A need to control others and situations is common in personal and in work life. They are prone to repetition and have difficulty making decisions and completing tasks because they become so involved in the details. They can be overly conscientious about morality and ethics and value polite, formal, and correct interpersonal relationships. They also tend to be rigid, stubborn, and indecisive and are unable to accept new ideas and customs. Their mood is tense and joyless. Warm feelings are restrained, and they tightly control the expression of emotions (APA, 2000) (see Table 24-6).

Epidemiology

The prevalence of obsessive-compulsive personality disorder is 1% in the general population and 3% to 10% in individuals receiving treatment in mental health clinics (APA, 2000). This disorder is associated with higher education, employment, and marriage. Subjects with the disorder had a higher income than did those without the disorder. This disorder is associated with a greater risk for generalized anxiety disorder and simple phobia and lowered risk for alcohol abuse (Nestadt et al., 1990).

Etiology

As with some of the other personality disorders, there is little evidence for a biologic formulation. The basis of the compulsive patterns that characterize obsessive-compulsive personality disorder is parental overcontrol and overprotection that is consistently restrictive and sets distinct limits on the child's behaviour. Parents teach these children a deep sense of responsibility to others and to feel guilty when these responsibilities are not met. Play is viewed as shameful, sinful, and irresponsible, leading to dire consequences. They are encouraged to resist the natural inclinations toward play and impulse gratification, and parents try to impose guilt on the child to control behaviour.

Nursing Management

These individuals seek mental health care when they have attacks of anxiety, spells of immobilization, sexual impotence, and excessive fatigue. To change the compulsive pattern, psychotherapy is needed. There may be short-term pharmacologic intervention with an antidepressant or anxiolytic as an adjunct.

The nursing assessment focuses on the client's physical symptoms (sleep, eating, sexual), interpersonal relationships, and social problems. Typical nursing diagnoses include Anxiety, Risk for Loneliness, Decisional Conflict, Sexual Dysfunction, Disturbed Sleep Pattern, and Impaired Social Interactions. People with OCD realize that they can improve their quality of life, but they will find it extremely anxiety provoking to make the necessary changes. A supportive nurse–client relationship based on acceptance of the individual's need for order and rigidity will help the person have enough confidence to try new behaviours. Examining the person's belief that underlies the dysfunctional behaviours can set the stage for challenging the childhood thinking. Because the compulsive pattern was established in childhood, it will take a long time to modify the behaviour.

CONTINUUM OF CARE

Long-term therapy is ideal for clients with avoidant personality disorder because it takes time to make the changes. Mental health nurses may see these individuals for other health problems. Encouraging the person to continue with therapy and contacting the therapist when necessary are important in maintaining continuity of care. These individuals are typically hospitalized only for a coexisting disorder.

People with dependent and obsessive-compulsive personality disorders are treated primarily in the community. If there is a coexisting disorder or the person experiences periods of depression, hospitalization may be useful for a short period of time.

Impulse-Control Disorders

This group of mental disorders has as an essential feature: irresistible impulsivity. These disorders are not part of other disorders but often coexist with them. The following impulse-control disorders have been identified:

- Intermittent explosive disorder
- Kleptomania
- Pyromania
- Pathologic gambling
- Trichotillomania

These disorders are characterized by an inability to resist an impulse or temptation to complete an activity that is considered harmful to self or others, an increase in tension before the individual commits the act, and excitement or gratification at the time the act is committed. The release of tension is perceived as pleasurable, but remorse and regret usually follow the act (Gallop, McCay, & Esplen, 1992) (Table 24-7).

INTERMITTENT EXPLOSIVE DISORDER

Episodes of aggressiveness that result in assault or destruction of property characterize people with intermittent explosive disorder. The severity of aggressiveness is out of proportion to the provocation. The episodes can have serious psychosocial consequences, including job loss, interpersonal relationship problems, school expulsion, divorce, automobile crashes, or imprisonment. This diagnosis is given only after all other disorders with aggressive components (delirium, dementia, head injury, BPD, APD, substance abuse) have been excluded. Little is known about this rare disorder. It is more common in men than in women (APA, 2000).

The treatment of this disorder is multifaceted. Psychopharmacologic agents are sometimes used as an adjunct to psychotherapeutic, behavioural, and social

---

Table 24.7	Summary of Diagnostic Characteristics for Impulse-Control Disorders

Diagnostic Criteria and Target Symptoms

Kleptomania 312.32	• Recurrent failure to resist impulse to steal object that is not needed • Increased tension before theft • Pleasure, gratification, or relief at time of theft • Theft not related to anger or vengeance; not in response to delusion or hallucination • Not better accounted for by another psychiatric disorder

Pyromania 312.23	• Multiple episodes of deliberate and purposeful fire setting
	• Tension or affective arousal before act
	• Fascination with, interest in, curiosity about, or attraction to fires
	    Regular fire watchers
	    False alarm setters
	    Pleasure with institution, equipment, and personnel associated with fires
	• Pleasure gratification or tension relief with fire starting, watching its effects or participating in aftermath
	• Not done for monetary gain; expression of ideology, anger, or vengeance; concealing criminal activity; improving living conditions; or as a response to hallucination or delusion
	• Not better accounted for by another psychiatric disorder

Pathologic gambling 312.31	• Persistent and recurrent maladaptive gambling behaviour
	• Disruption of personal, family, or vocational pursuits
	    Preoccupation with gambling
	    Increased amounts of money needed to achieve excitement
	    Unsuccessful efforts to stop, cut back, or control
	    Restlessness and irritability with attempts to control or cut back
	    Means of escape from problems or mood
	    Chasing of losses; attempts to get even
	    Lying to family and others to conceal involvement
	    Commission of illegal acts to finance behaviour
	    Significant relationships, job, or opportunities jeopardized or lost
	    Reliance on others for relief of poor financial situation
	• Not better accounted for by manic episode

Trichotillomania 312.39	• Recurrent pulling of one's hair with subsequent hair loss
	    Brief episodes throughout day or sustained periods of hours
	    Increased during stress and relaxation periods
	• Increased tension immediately before act and with attempts to resist urge
	• Gratification, pleasure, or relief with act
	• Not better accounted for by another psychiatric disorder; not the effect of a general medical condition
	• Significant distress and impairment of functioning

Intermittent explosive episode 312.34	• Discrete episodes of failing to resist aggressive impulses resulting in serious assaultive acts or property destruction • Degree of aggressiveness grossly out of proportion to provocation or stressor • Not better accounted for by another psychiatric disorder; not a direct physiologic effect of a substance or general medical condition

interventions. GABA-ergic mood stabilizers have been used. Anxiolytics are used for obsessive clients who experience tension states and explosive outbursts. Medication alone is insufficient.

KLEPTOMANIA

In **kleptomania**, individuals cannot resist the urge to steal, and they independently steal items that they could easily afford. These items are not particularly useful or wanted. The underlying issue is the act of stealing. The term *kleptomania* was first used in 1838 to describe the behaviour of several kings who stole worthless objects (Goldman, 1992). These individuals experience an increase in tension and then pleasure and relief at the time of the theft. It is a rare condition that occurs in fewer than 5% of shoplifters (APA, 2000). There is little information about this disorder, but it is believed to last for years, despite numerous convictions for shoplifting. It appears to be more common in women. About 81% of reported cases of kleptomania involve women (Goldman, 1991) (see Table 24-7).

Some shoplifting appears to be related to anxiety and stress, in that it serves to relieve symptoms. In a few instances, brain damage has been associated with kleptomania. Depression is the most common symptom identified in a compulsive shoplifter.

Kleptomania is difficult to detect and treat. There are few accounts of treatment. It appears that behaviour therapy is frequently used. Antidepressant medication that helps relieve the depression has been successful in some cases. More investigation is needed (Schatzberg, 2000).

PYROMANIA

Irresistible impulses to start fires characterize **pyromania**. These individuals are aroused before setting a fire and are fascinated with fires. They are attracted to fires, often becoming regular "fire watchers" or even firefighters. These arsonists, people who intentionally set fires or make an effort at fire setting, are not motivated by aggression, anger, suicidal ideation, or political ideology. They may make advanced preparation for the fire. Little is known about this disorder. Most fire setting is not done by people with this disorder. This disorder occurs infrequently, mostly in men (APA, 2000) (see Table 24-7).

Low serotonin and norepinephrine levels are associated with arson (Virkkunen et al., 1989). Little is known about treatment, and as with the other impulse-control disorders, no one approach is uniformly effective. A treatment plan should reflect the special needs of the individual (Soltys, 1992). Education, parenting training, behaviour contracting with token reinforcement, problem-solving skills training, and relaxation exercises may all be used in the management of the individual's responses.

PATHOLOGIC GAMBLING

Social gambling becomes pathologic when it becomes recurrent and disrupts personal, family, or vocational pursuits. These individuals are preoccupied with gambling and experience an aroused, euphoric state during the actual betting. They are drawn to the games and begin making bigger and bigger bets. Characteristically, they relentlessly chase their losses in an attempt to win them back. They are unable to control their gaming and may lie to family, friends, and employers to hide their gambling. These individuals are highly competitive, energetic, restless, and easily bored. The prevalence is estimated at 1% to 3% of the population (APA, 2000); another study found a 3.9% lifetime prevalence (Shaffer, Hall, & Vander Bilt, 1999). Of those individuals in treatment for pathologic gambling, 20% have reported attempting suicide (see Table 24-7).

Over the past two decades, there has been a considerable expansion in legalized gambling in Canada as local and provincial governments have sought to stimulate economic development through tourism and the entertainment sector and to develop new revenue possibilities. The introduction of new technologies, including video lottery terminals (VLTs) and internet-based gambling, has also been a factor in the expansion (Korn, 2001).

It has been challenging for researchers to establish links between the expansion of legalized gambling and trends with problematic or pathologic gambling (Hargreave & Csiernik, 2003). Shaffer and Hall (2001) have studied prevalence rates for pathologic gambling in United States and Canada. Although they find similar rates in both countries, they do suggest that segments of the population may develop problem patterns for different reasons and that the psychosocial profile of gamblers may differ between the countries. The uncertainty surrounding the impact of legalized gambling continues to fuel debate in the media where the balance between risk and benefit is challenged. What is known is that pathologic gambling is associated with depression, suicide attempts, alcohol and drug abuse, family violence, unemployment, and crime (Chacko, Palmer, Corey and Butler, 2003; King, 1999). Other comorbid disorders include ADHD, Tourette syndrome, and personality disorders, especially obsessive-compulsive, avoidant, schizoid, paranoid, and antisocial (Black & Moyer, 1998; Crockford & el-Guebaly, 1998).

This disorder is conceptualized as similar to alcohol and other substances of dependence (Hall et al., 2000; Slutskey, 2000). When substances are used in conjunction with gambling, they cause a deterioration in play and accelerate the progression of the gambling disorder. The disorder has four phases: winning, losing, desperation, and hopelessness. Pathologic gambling can be treated by psychotherapists experienced in this disorder; for many,

Gamblers Anonymous is sufficient (Petry & Armentano, 1999).

Pathologic gamblers feel omnipotent in their ability to win back what was lost. This omnipotence serves as self-deception that leads to denial. Care of these clients involves confronting their omnipotent beliefs. These individuals quickly irritate staff by their self-assurance and overbearing attitude. Staff education about the disorder is important. Family involvement is also crucial. Families often have been dealing with the individual in a dysfunctional manner. Relapse prevention involves learning about specific cues that trigger the gambling behaviour (Selzer, 1992).

With the rise in pathologic gambling and its social consequences, there have been greater efforts to identify supportive pharmacotherapy. Because the underlying mechanisms are anxiety and impulsivity, first-line drugs are SSRIs. These have been moderately effective (Hollander et al., 2000), especially when combined with cognitive-behavioural approaches (Oakley-Browne, Adams, & Mobberly, 2000).

TRICHOTILLOMANIA

Trichotillomania is chronic, self-destructive hair pulling that results in noticeable hair loss, usually in the crown, occipital, or parietal areas, although sometimes of the eyebrows and eyelashes. The individual has an increase in tension immediately before pulling out the hair or when attempting to resist the behaviour. After the hair is pulled, the person feels a sense of relief. Some would classify this disorder as one of self-mutilation. It becomes a problem when there is a significant distress or impairment in other areas of function. A hair-pulling session can last several hours, and the individual may ritualistically eat the hairs or discard them. Hair ingestion may result in the development of a hair ball, which can lead to anorexia, stomach pain, anaemia, obstruction, and peritonitis. Other medical complications include infection at the hair-pulling site. Hair pulling is done alone, and usually clients deny it. Instead of pain, these persons experience pleasure and tension release (APA, 2000; Warmbrodt, Hardy, & Chrisman, 1996) (see Table 24-7).

The onset of trichotillomania occurs among children before the age of 5 years and in adolescence. For the young child, distraction or redirection may successfully eliminate the behaviour. The behaviour in adolescents may begin a chronic course that may last well into adulthood. This disorder is poorly understood. Its prevalence is estimated at 2% to 4% of the population. The cause is unknown (APA, 2000). SSRIs, such as clomipramine and fluoxetine, have shown some success in diminishing the hair-pulling behaviour, as have dopamine antagonists, such as haloperidol (van Ameringen, Mancini, Oakman, & Farvolden, 1999), and opioid antagonists (Kim, 1998).

The assessment includes a review of current problems, developmental history (especially school conflicts, learning difficulties), family history, social history, identification of support systems, previous psychiatric treatment, and health history. Hair-pulling history and pattern are also solicited to determine the duration and severity of the disorders. The typical nursing diagnoses include Self-Mutilation, Low Self-Esteem, Hopelessness, Impaired Skin Integrity, and Ineffective Denial. Within the therapeutic relationship, a cognitive-behavioural approach can be used to help the client to identify when hair pulling occurs, the precipitating events, and the details of the episode. Teaching about the disorder will help individuals understand that they are not alone and that others have also suffered with this problem. The goal of treatment is to help the client learn to substitute positive behaviours for the hair-pulling behaviour through self-monitoring of events that precipitate the episodes.

CONTINUUM OF CARE

Impulse-control disorders require long-term treatment, usually in an outpatient setting. Hospitalization is rare, except when there are comorbid psychiatric or medical disorders.

SUMMARY OF KEY POINTS

- Personality is a complex pattern of characteristics, largely outside of the person's awareness, that compose the individual's distinctive pattern of perceiving, feeling, thinking, coping, and behaving. The personality emerges from a complicated interaction of biologic dispositions, psychological experiences, and environmental situations.
- Personality disorder is an enduring pattern of inner experience and behaviour that deviates markedly from the expectations of the individual's culture, is pervasive and inflexible, has an onset in adolescence or early adulthood, is stable over time, and leads to distress or impairment.
- The severity of personality disorder can be determined by the characteristics of tenuous stability, adaptive inflexibility, and vicious circles of rigid and inflexible behaviour that result in serious interpersonal problems and social dysfunction.
- In the *DSM-IV-TR*, personality disorders are on Axis II and are organized around three clusters or dimensions: cluster A, odd-eccentric disorders; cluster B, dramatic-emotional disorders; and cluster C, anxious-fearful disorders. Any of the personality disorders can coexist with Axis I disorders.
- People with cluster A personality disorders whose odd, eccentric behaviours often alienate them from

others can benefit from interventions such as social skills training, environmental management, and cognitive skill building. Changing patterns of thinking and behaving are difficult and take time; thus, client outcomes must be evaluated in terms of small changes in thinking and behaviour.

◾ In cluster A, paranoid personality disorder is characterized by a suspicious pattern, schizoid personality disorder by an asocial pattern, and schizotypal personality disorder by an eccentric pattern.

◾ People with borderline personality disorder (cluster B) have difficulties regulating emotion and have extreme fears of abandonment, leading to dysfunctional relationships; they often engage in self-injury.

◾ Antisocial personality disorder (cluster B), often synonymous with psychopathy, includes people who have no regard for and refuse to conform to social rules.

◾ Individuals with cluster B personality disorders often have difficulties with emotional regulation or being able to recognize and control the expression of their feelings, such as anger, disappointment, and frustration. The nurse can help these clients identify feelings and gain control over their feelings and actions by teaching communication skills and techniques, thought-stopping techniques, distraction, or problem-solving techniques.

◾ Cluster C personality disorders are characterized by anxieties and fears and include avoidant, dependent, and obsessive-compulsive disorders. The obsessive-compulsive personality disorder differs from the obsessive-compulsive anxiety disorder because the individual demonstrates an overall rigidity, perfectionism, and need for control.

◾ For many people with personality disorders, maintaining a therapeutic nurse–client relationship can be one of the most helpful interventions. Through this therapeutic relationship, the individual experiences a model of healthy interaction, establishing trust, consistency, caring, boundaries, and limitations that help to build the client's self-esteem and respect for self and others. In some personality disorders, nurses will find it more difficult to engage the individual in a true therapeutic relationship because of the person's avoidance of interpersonal and emotional attachment (ie, antisocial personality disorder or paranoid personality disorder).

◾ Individuals with personality disorders are rarely treated in an inpatient facility, except during periods of destructive behaviour or self-injury. Treatment is delivered in the community and over time. Continuity of care is important in helping the individual change lifelong personality patterns.

◾ Although not classified as personality disorders, the impulse-control disorders share one of the primary characteristics of impulsivity, which leads to inappropriate social behaviours that are considered harmful to self or others and that give the individual excitement or gratification at the time the act is committed.

CRITICAL THINKING CHALLENGES

1 Compare and contrast the three common features of personality disorders: tenuous stability, adaptive inflexibility, and vicious circles of behaviour.
2 Define the concepts, *personality* and *personality disorder*. When does a normal personality become a personality disorder?
3 Karen, a 36-year-old woman receiving inpatient care, was admitted for depression; she also has a diagnosis of borderline personality disorder. After a telephone argument with her husband, she approaches the nurse's station with her wrist dripping with blood from cutting. What nursing diagnosis best fits this behaviour? What interventions should the nurse use with the client once the self-injury is treated?
4 A 22-year-old man with borderline personality disorder is being discharged from the mental health unit after a severe suicide attempt. As his primary psychiatric nurse, you have been able to establish a therapeutic relationship with him but are now terminating the relationship. He asks you to meet with him "for just a few sessions" after his discharge because his therapist will be on vacation. What are the issues underlying this request? What should you do? Explain and justify.
5 Compare the psychoanalytic explanation of the development of borderline personality disorder with Linehan's biosocial theory.
6 Compare the characteristics, epidemiology, and etiologic theories of antisocial and borderline personality disorders.
7 Discuss the differences between histrionic and borderline personality disorders.
8 Compare and contrast antisocial and narcissistic personality disorders.
9 Define and summarize the three personality disorders of cluster A. Compare the following among the three disorders:
   a Defining characteristics
   b Epidemiology
   c Biologic, psychological, and social theories
   d Key nursing assessment data
   e Nursing diagnoses and outcomes
   f Specific issues related to a therapeutic relationship
   g Interventions
10 Define and summarize the three personality disorders of cluster C. Compare the following among the three disorders:

a Defining characteristics
b Epidemiology
c Biologic, psychological, and social theories
d Key nursing assessment data
e Nursing diagnoses and outcomes
f Specific issues related to a therapeutic relationship
g Interventions

11 Define and summarize the impulse-control disorders. Compare the following among the three disorders:

a Defining characteristics
b Epidemiology
c Biologic, psychological, and social theories
d Key nursing assessment data
e Nursing diagnoses and outcomes
f Interventions

WEB LINKS

www.mhsanctuary.com/borderline A website for consumers, the Borderline Personality Sanctuary offers a chat room and books.

www.palace.net/~llama/psych/bpd.html This site provides an overview of theories on borderline personality disorder.

www.bpdcentral.com This website of Borderline Personality Disorder Central provides consumer and professional information and resources.

www.borderlineresearch.org The Borderline Research Organization is a research foundation that supports research on borderline personality disorder.

www.mentalhealth.com Internet Mental Health is a website for mental health disorders.

www.responsiblegambling.org/index.cfm The Responsible Gambling Council (RGC) is a non-profit, Ontario-based organization that helps individuals and communities address gambling in a healthy and responsible way.

MOVIES

Fatal Attraction: 1987. This award-winning film portrays the relationship between a married attorney, Dan Gallagher (played by Michael Douglas), and Alex Forest, a single woman (played by Glenn Close). Their one-night affair turns into a nightmare for the attorney and his family as Alex becomes increasingly possessive and aggressive, demonstrating behaviours characteristic of borderline personality disorder: anger, impulsivity, emotional lability, fear of rejection and abandonment, vacillation between adulation and disgust, and self-mutilation.

VIEWING POINTS: Identify the behaviours of Alex that are characteristics of borderline personality disorder. Identify the feelings that are generated by the movie. With which characters do you identify? For which characters do you feel sympathy? If Alex had been admitted to your hospital, what would be your first priority?

REFERENCES

Ainsworth, M. (1989). Attachments beyond infancy. *American Psychologist, 44*(4), 709–716.

American Psychiatric Association. (2000). *Diagnostic and statistical manual of mental disorders* (4th ed., Text revision). Washington, DC: Author.

American Psychiatric Association. (2001). *Practice guidelines for the treatment of patients with borderline personality disorder.* Washington, DC: American Psychiatric Press.

Andrews, J. A., Foster, S. L., Capaldi, D., & Hop, H. (2000). Adolescent and family predictors of physical aggression, communication, and satisfaction in young adult couples: A prospective analysis. *Journal of Consulting Clinical Psychology, 68*(2), 195–208.

Barry, C. T., Frick, P. J., DeShazo, T. M., McCoy, M. G., Ellis, M., & Loney, B. R. (2000). The importance of callous-unemotional traits for extending the concept of psychopathy to children. *Journal of Abnormal Psychology, 109*(2), 335–340.

Bateman, A., & Fonagy, P. (1999). Effectiveness of partial hospitalization in the treatment of borderline personality disorder: A randomized controlled trial. *American Journal of Psychiatry, 156*(10), 1563–1569.

Bernstein, G. A., Borchardt, C. M., & Perwien, A. R. (1996). Anxiety disorders in children and adolescents: A review of the past 10 years. *Journal of the American Academy of Child & Adolescent Psychiatry, 35*(9), 1110–1119.

Best, M., Williams, J. M., & Coccaro, E. F. (2002). Evidence for a dysfunctional prefrontal circuit in patients with an impulsive aggressive disorder. *Processes of the National Academy of Science, 11*(12), 8448–8853.

Black, D., Baumgard, C., & Bell, S. (1995a). The long-term outcome of antisocial personality disorder compared with depression, schizophrenia, and surgical conditions. *Bulletin of the American Academy of Psychiatry and Law, 23*(1), 43–52.

Black, D. W., Baumgard, C. H., & Bell, S. E. (1995b). A 16- to 45-year follow-up of 71 men with antisocial personality disorder. *Comprehensive Psychiatry, 36*(2), 130–140.

Black, D. W., & Moyer, T. (1998). Clinical features and psychiatric comorbidity of subjects with pathological gambling behavior. *Psychiatric Services, 49*(11), 1434–1439.

Bodner, E., & Mikulincer, M. (1998). Learned helplessness and the occurrence of depressive-like and paranoid-like responses: The role of attentional focus. *Journal of Personality & Social Psychology, 74*(4), 1010–1023.

Bohus, M., Haaf, B., Stiglmayr, C., Pohl, U., Bohme, R., & Linehan, M. (2000). Evaluation of inpatient dialectical-behavioral therapy for borderline personality disorder—a prospective study. *Behavior Research and Therapy, 38*(9), 875–887.

Bohus, M. F., Landwehrmeyer, G. B., Stiglmayr, C. E., Limberger, M. F., Bohme, R., & Schmahl, C. G. (1999). Naltrexone in the treatment of dissociative symptoms in patients with borderline personality disorder: An open-label trial. *Journal of Clinical Psychiatry, 60*(9), 598–603.

Boone, M. L., McNeil, D. W., Masia, C. L., Turk, C. L., Carter, L. E., Ries, B. J., & Lewin, M. R. (1999). Multimodal comparisons of social phobia subtypes and avoidant personality disorder. *Journal of Anxiety Disorders, 13*(3), 271–292.

Bornstein, R. F. (1998). Implicit and self-attributed dependency needs in dependent and histrionic personality disorders. *Journal of Personality Assessment, 71*(1), 1–14.

Bowlby, J. (1980). *Loss: Sadness and depression*. New York: Basic Books.

Bucholz, K. K., Heath, A. C., & Madden, P. A. (2000). Transitions in drinking adolescent females: Evidence from the Missouri adolescent female twin study. *Alcohol Clinical Experimental Research, 24*(6), 914–923.

Bushman, B. J., & Baumeister, R. F. (1998). Threatened egotism, narcissism, self-esteem, and direct and displaced aggression: Does self-love or self-hate lead to violence? *Journal of Personality Social Psychology, 75*(1), 219–229.

Cadenhead, K. S., Perry, W., Shafer, K., & Braff, D. L. (1999). Cognitive functions in schizotypal personality disorder. *Schizophrenia Research, 37*(2), 123–132.

Chacko, J., Palmer, M., Gorey, K., & Butler, N. (2003). Social work with problem gamblers: A key informant survey of service needs. In R. Csiernik & W. Rowe (Eds.), *Responding to the oppression of addiction: Canadian social work perspectives* (pp. 335–343). Toronto: Canadian Scholars'.

Cloninger, C., Bayon, C., & Svrakic, D. (1998). Measurement of temperment and character in mood disorders: A model of fundamental states as personality types. *Journal of Affective Disorders, 51*(1), 21–32.

Coccaro, E. F. (1998). Clinical outcome of psychopharmacologic treatment of borderline and schizotypal personality disordered subjects. *Journal Clinical Psychiatry, 59*(Suppl 1), 30–35.

Coccaro, E. F., Kavoussi, R. J., Hauger, R. L., Cooper, T. B., & Ferris, C. F. (1998). Cerebrospinal fluid vasopressin levels: Correlates with aggression and serotonin function in personality-disordered subjects. *Archives of General Psychiatry. 55*(8), 708–714.

Comtois, K. A., Cowley, D. S., Dunner. D. L., & Roy-Byrne, P. P. (1999). Relationship between borderline personality disorder and Axis I diagnosis in severity of depression and anxiety. *Journal of Clinical Psychiatry, 60*(11), 752–758.

Constantino, J. (1996). Intergenerational aspects of the development of aggression: A preliminary report. *Journal of Developmental and Behavioral Pediatrics, 17*(3), 176–182.

Cooke, D. (1996). Psychopathic personality in different culture: What do we know? What do we need to find out? *Journal of Personality Disorders, 10*(1), 23–40.

Crichton, R. (1959). *The great impostor*. New York: Random House.

Crockford, D. N., & el-Guebaly, M. (1998). Psychiatric comorbidity in pathological gambling: A critical review. *Canadian Journal of Psychiatry, 43*(1), 43–50.

Dolan, M. (1994). Psychopathy: A neurobiological perspective. *British Journal of Psychiatry, 165*(2), 151–159.

Dolan, M., & Park, I. (2002). The neuropsychology of antisocial personality disorder. *Psychological Medicine, 32*(3), 417–427.

Dowson, J. H., Sussams, P., Grounds, A. T., & Taylor, J. C. (2001). Associations of past conduct disorder with personality disorders in "non-psychotic" psychiatric inpatients. *European Psychiatry: The Journal of the Association of European Psychiatrists, 16*(1), 49–56.

Driessen, M., Herrmann, J., Stahl, K., Zwaan, M., Meier, S., Hill, A., Osterheider, M., & Petersen, D. (2000). Magnetic resonance imaging volumes of the hippocampus and the amygdala in women with borderline personality disorder and early traumatization. *Archives of General Psychiatry, 57*(12), 1115–1122.

Eley, T. C., Lichtenstein, P., & Stevenson, J. (1999). Sex differences in the etiology of aggressive and nonaggressive antisocial behavior: Results from two twin studies. *Child Development, 70*(1), 155–168.

Erikson, E. (1968). *Identity: Youth and crisis*. New York: Norton.

Faraone, S. V., Biederman, J., Mennin, D., & Russell, R. (1998). Bipolar and antisocial disorders among relatives of ADHD children: Parsing familial subtypes of illness. *American Journal of Medical Genetics, 81*(1), 108–116.

Faravelli, C., Zucchi, T., Viviani, B., Salmoria, R., Perone, A., Paionni, A., Scarpato, A., Vigliaturo, D., Rosi, S., D'adamo, D., Bartolozzi, D., Cecchi, C., & Abrardi, L. (2000). Epidemiology of social phobia: A clinical approach. *European Psychiatry, 15*(1), 17–24.

Farmer, C. M., O'Donnell, B. F., Niznikiewicz, M. A., Voglmaier, M. M., McCarley, R. W., & Shenton, M. E. (2000). Visual perception and working memory in schizotypal personality disorder. *American Journal of Psychiatry, 157*(5), 781–788.

Favazza, A. (1996). *Bodies under siege: Self-mutilation and body modification in culture and psychiatry*. Baltimore: Johns Hopkins University Press.

Gallop, R., McCay, E., & Esplen, J. (1992). The conceptualization of impulsivity for psychiatric nursing practice. *Archives of Psychiatric Nursing, 6*(6), 366–373.

Galvin, M., Shekhar, A., Simon, J., Stilwell, B., Ten Eyck, R., Laite, G., Karwisch, G., & Blix, S.. (1991). Low dopamine-beta-hydroxylase: A biological sequela of abuse and neglect? *Psychiatry Research, 39*(1), 1–11.

Giancola, P. R. (2000). Temperament and antisocial behavior in preadolescent boys with or without a family history of a substance use disorder. *Psychological Addictive Behaviors, 14*(1), 56–68.

Goldman, M. (1991). Kleptomania: Making sense of the nonsensical. *American Journal of Psychiatry, 148*(8), 986–999.

Goldman, M. (1992). Kleptomania: An overview. *Psychiatric Annals, 22*(2), 68–71.

Golynkina, K., & Ryle, A. (1999). The identification and characteristics of the partially dissociated states of patients with borderline personality disorder. *British Journal of Medicine & Psychology, 72*(Pt 4), 429–445.

Gottesman, I., & Goldsmith, H. (1994). Developmental psychopathology of antisocial behavior: Inserting genes into its ontogenesis and epigenesis. In C. Nelson (Ed.), *Threats to optimal development: Integrating biological, social, and psychological risk factors* (Vol. 27, pp. 69–104). Hillsdale, NJ: Erlbaum.

Gotz, M. J., Johnstone, E. C., & Ratcliffe, S. G. (1999). Criminality and antisocial behavior in unselected men with sex chromosome abnormalities. *Psychological Medicine, 29*(4), 953–962.

Grann, M., Lanstrom, N., Tengstrom, A., & Kullgren, G. (1999). Psychopathy (PCL-R) predicts violent recidivism among criminal offenders with personality disorders in Sweden. *Law & Human Behavior, 23*(2), 205–217.

Greene, H., & Ugarriza, D. (1995). The "stably unstable" borderline personality disorder: History, theory, and nursing intervention. *Journal of Psychosocial Nursing, 33*(12), 26–30.

Grilo, C., Becker, D., Fehon, D., Walker, M. L., Edell, W. S., & McGlashan, T. H. (1996). Gender differences in personality disorders in psychiatrically hospitalized adolescents. *American Journal of Psychiatry, 153*(8), 1089–1091.

Gunderson, J. G. (1996). The borderline patient's intolerance of aloneness: Insecure attachments and therapist availability. *American Journal of Psychiatry, 153*(6), 752–758.

Gurvits, I. G., Koenigsberg, H. W., & Siever, I. J. (2000). Neurotransmitter dysfunction in patients with borderline personality disorder. *Psychiatric Clinics of North America, 23*(1), 27–40.

Hall, G. W., Carriero, N. J., Takushi, R. Y., Montoya, I. D., Preston, K. L., & Gorelick, D. A. (2000). Pathological gambling among cocaine-dependent outpatients. *American Journal of Psychiatry, 157*(7), 1127–1133.

Hanson, R. K., Cadsky, O., Harris, A., & Lalond, C. (1997). Correlates of battering among 997 men: Family history, adjustment, and attitudinal difference. *Violence and Victims, 12*(3), 191–208.

Hare, R. D. (1999). Psychopathy as a risk factor for violence. *Psychiatric Quarterly, 70*(3), 181–197.

Hargreave, C., & Csiernik, R. (2003). An examination of gambling and problem gambling in Canada. In R. Csiernik & W. Rowe (Eds.), *Responding to the oppression of addiction: Canadian social work perspectives* (pp. 313–333). Toronto: Canadian Scholars'.

Health Canada (2002). A report on mental illness in Canada. Retrieved August 1, 2005, from http://secure.cihi.ca/cihiweb/dispPage.jsp?cw_page=reports_mental_illness_e.

Herpertz, S. C., Kunnert, H. J., Schwenger, U. B., & Sass, H. (1999). Affective responsiveness in borderline personality disorder: A psychophysiological approach. *American Journal of Psychiatry, 156*(10), 1550–1556.

Herpertz, S. C., Wenning, B., Mueller, B., Qunaibi, M., Sass, H., & Herpertz-Dahlmann, B. (2001). Psychophysiological responses in ADHD boys with and without conduct disorder: Implications for adult antisocial behavior. *Journal of the American Academy of Child & Adolescent Psychiatry, 40*(10), 1222–1230.

Hill, J. (2002). Biological, psychological and social processes in the conduct disorders. *Journal of Child Psychology & Psychiatry & Allied Disciplines, 43*(1), 133–164.

Hill, J. (2003). Early identification of individuals at risk for antisocial personality disorder. *British Journal of Psychiatry-Supplementum, 44*, S11–S14.

Hollander, E., DeCaria, C. M., Finkell, J. N., Begaz, R., Wong, C. M., & Carwight, C. (2000). A randomized double-blind fluvoxamine/placebo crossover trial in pathologic gambling. *Biological Psychiatry, 47*(9), 813–817.

Hollander, E., Tracy, K. A., Swann, A. C., Coccaro, E. F., McElroy, S. L., Wozniak, P., Sommerville, K. W., & Nemeroff, C. B. (2003). Divalproex in the treatment of impulsive aggression: Efficacy in cluster B personality disorders. *Neuropsychopharmacology, 28*(6), 1186–1197.

Horsfall, J. (1999). Towards understanding some complex borderline behaviours. *Journal of Psychiatric Mental Health Nursing, 6*(5), 425–432.

Johnson, J. G., Cohen, P., Brown, J., Smailes, E. M., & Bernstein, D. P. (1999). Childhood maltreatment increases risk for personality disorders during early adulthood. *Archives of General Psychiatry, 56*(7), 607–608.

Johnston, M. A. (1999). Influences of adult attachment in exploration. *Psychological Reports, 84*(1), 31–34.

Joubert, C. E. (1998). Narcissism, need for power, and social interest. *Psychological Report, 82*(2), 701–702.

Kavoussi, R. J., & Coccaro, E. F. (1998). Divalproex sodium for impulsive aggressive behavior in patients with personality disorder. *Journal of Clinical Psychiatry, 59*(12), 676–680.

Kiehl, K. A., Smith, A. M., Hare, R. D., Mendrek, A., Forster, B. B., Brink, J., & Liddle, P. F. (2001). Limbic abnormalities in affective processing by criminal psychopaths as revealed by functional magnetic resonance imaging. *Biological Psychiatry, 50*(9), 677–684.

Kim, J. E., Hetherington, E. M., & Reiss, D. (1999). Associations among family relationships, antisocial peers, and adolescents' externalizing behaviors: Gender and family type differences. *Child Development, 70*(5), 1209–1230.

Kim, S. W. (1998). Opioid antagonists in the treatment of impulse-control disorders. *Journal of Clinical Psychiatry, 59*(4), 159–164.

King, A. (1999). *Diary of a powerful addiction.* Tyndall, MB: Crown.

Korn, D. A. (2001). Research as a foundation for action on gambling. *Canadian Journal of Public Health, 92*(3), 165–166.

Lahey, B. B., Gordon, R. A., Loeber, R., Stouthamer-Loeber, M., & Farrington, D. P. (1999). Boys who join gangs: A prospective study of predictors of first gang entry. *Journal of Abnormal Child Psychology, 27*(4), 261–276.

Langbehn, D. R., & Cadoret, R. J. (2001). The adult antisocial syndrome with and without antecedent conduct disorder: Comparisons from an adoption study. *Comprehensive Psychiatry, 42*(4), 272–282.

Laporte, L., & Guttman, H. (1996). Traumatic childhood experiences as risk factors for borderline and other personality disorders. *Journal of Personality Disorders, 10*(3), 247–259.

Leichsenring, F. (1999). Splitting: An empirical study. *Bulletin Menninger Clinic, 63*(4), 520–537.

Lejoyeux, M., Boulenguiez, S., Fichelle, A., McLoughlin, M., Claudon, M., & Ades, J. (2000). Alcohol dependence among patients admitted to psychiatric emergency services. *General Hospital Psychiatry, 22*(3), 206–212.

Linehan, M. (1993a). *Cognitive-behavioral treatment of borderline personality disorder.* New York: Guilford.

Linehan, M. (1993b). *Skills training manual for treating borderline personality disorder.* New York: Guilford.

Links, P. S., Heslegrave, R., & van Reekum R. (1998). Prospective follow-up study of borderline personality disorder: Prognosis, prediction of outcome, and Axis II comorbidity. *Canadian Journal of Psychiatry, 43*(3), 265–270.

Lyons, M. (1995). Epidemiology of personality disorders. In M. Tsuang, M. Tohen, & G. Zahner (Eds.), *Textbook in psychiatric epidemiology.* New York: Wiley-Liss.

Mahler, M., Pine, F., & Bergman, A. (1975). *The psychological birth of human infant: Symbiosis and individuation.* New York: Basic Books.

Marcus, R. F. (1999). A gender-linked exploratory factor analysis of antisocial behavior in young adolescents. *Adolescence, 34*(133), 33–46.

Matta, I., Sham, P. C., Gilvarry, C. M., Jones, P. B., Lewis, S. W., & Murray, R. M. (2000). Childhood schizotypy and positive symptoms in schizophrenic patients predict schizotypy in relatives. *Schizophrenia Research, 44*(2), 129–136.

Mattick, R., & Newman, C. (1991). Social phobia and avoidant personality disorder. *International Review of Psychiatry, 3*(2), 163–173.

McCloskey, J., & Bulechek, G. (2000). *Iowa Intervention Report. Nursing interventions classification* (NIC) (3rd ed.). St. Louis: Mosby–Year Book.

McDougle, C. J., Kresch, L. E., & Posey, D. J. (2000). Repetitive thoughts and behavior in pervasive developmental disorders: Treatment with serotonin reuptake inhibitors. *Journal of Autism & Development Disorders, 30*(5), 427–435.

Messina, N. P., Wish, E. D., & Nemes, S. (1999). Therapeutic community treatment for substance abusers with antisocial personality disorder. *Journal of Substance Abuse Treatment, 17*(1–2), 121–128.

Miller, S. (1994). Borderline personality disorder from a patient's perspective. *Hospital and Community Psychiatry, 45*(12), 1215–1219.

Millon, T., & Davis, R. (1999). *Personality disorders in modern life.* New York: John Wiley & Sons.

Moran, P. (1999). The epidemiology of antisocial personality disorder. *Social Psychiatry & Psychiatric Epidemiology, 34*(5), 231–242.

Moutier, C. Y., & Stein, M. B. (1999). The history, epidemiology, and differential diagnosis of social anxiety disorder. *Journal of Clinical Psychiatry, 60*(Suppl 9), 4–8.

Murphy, J. (1976). Psychiatric labeling in cross-cultural perspective: Similar kinds of disturbed behavior appear to be labeled abnormal in diverse cultures. *Science, 191*(4231), 1019–1028.

Myers, M. G., Stewart, D. G., & Brown, S. A. (1998). Progression from conduct disorder to antisocial personality disorder following treatment for adolescent substance abuse. *American Journal of Psychiatry, 155*(4), 479–485.

Nehls, N. (1998). Borderline personality disorder: Gender stereotypes, stigma and limited system of care. *Issues in Mental Health Nursing, 19*(2), 97–112.

Nehls, N. (1999). Borderline personality disorder: The voice of patients. *Research in Nursing & Health, 22*(4), 285–293.

Nestadt, G., Romanoski, A., Chahal, R., Merchant, A., Folstein, M., Gruenberg, E., & McHugh, P. (1990). An epidemiological study of histrionic personality disorder. *Psychological Medicine, 20*(2), 413–422.

Nolan, K. A., Volavka, J., Mohr, P., & Czobor, P. (1999). Psychopathy and violent behavior among patients with schizophrenia or schizoaffective disorder. *Psychiatric Services, 50*(6), 787–792.

Oakley-Browne, M. A., Adams, P., & Mobberly, P. M. (2000). Interventions for pathological gambling. *Cochrane Database System Review, 2*, CD001521.

Oldham, J., Skodol, A., Kellman, H., Hyler, S. E., Doidge, N., Rosnick, L., & Gallaher, P. E. (1995). Comorbidity of Axis I and Axis II disorders. *American Journal of Psychiatry, 152*(4), 571–578.

Oquendo, J. A., & Mann, J. J. (2000). The biology of impulsivity and suicidality. *Psychiatric Clinics of North America, 23*(1), 11–25.

Pagani, L., Boulerice, B., Vitaro, F., & Tremblay, R. E. (1999). Effects of poverty on academic failure and delinquency in boys: A change and process model approach. *Journal of Child Psychology & Psychiatry, 40*(8), 119–120.

Paulhus, D. L. (1998). Interpersonal and intrapsychic adaptiveness of trait self-enhancement: A mixed blessing? *Journal of Personality and Social Psychology, 74*(5), 1197.

Perugi, G., Nassini, S., Socci, C., Lenzi, M., Toni, C., Simonini, E., & Akiskal, H. S. (1999). Avoidant personality in social phobia and panic-agoraphobia disorder: A comparison. *Journal of Affective Disorders, 54*(3), 277–282.

Petry, N. M., & Armentano, C. (1999). Prevalence, assessment, and treatment of pathological gambling: A review. *Psychiatric Services, 50*(8), 1021–1027.

Pinto, O. C., & Akiskal, H. S. (1998). Lamotrigine as a promising approach to borderline personality: An open case series without concurrent DSM-IV major mood disorder. *Journal of Affective Disorder, 51*(3), 333–343.

Reti, I. M., Samuels, J. F., Eaton, W. W., Bienvenu, O. J. III, Costa, P. T., Jr., & Nestadt, G. (2002). Adult antisocial personality traits are associated with experiences of low parental care and maternal overprotection. *Acta Psychiatrica Scandinavica, 106*(2), 126–133.

Robins, L., Tipp, J., & Przybeck, T. (1991). Antisocial personality. In L. N. Robins & D. Reiger (Eds.), *Psychiatric disorders in America: The epidemiological catchment area study* (pp. 258–291). New York: Free Press.

Sack, A., Sperling, M., Fagen, G., & Foelsch, P. (1996). Attachment style, history, and behavioral contrasts for a borderline and normal sample. *Journal of Personality Disorders, 10*(1), 88–102.

Sansone, R. A., Wiederman, M. W., & Sansone, L. A. (1998). Borderline personality symptomatology, experience of multiple types of trauma, and health care utilization among women in a primary care setting. *Journal of Clinical Psychiatry, 59*(3), 108–111.

Schatzberg, A. F. (2000). New indications of antidepressants. *Journal of Clinical Psychiatry, 61*(Suppl 11), 9–17.

Schubiner, H., Tzelepis, A., Milberger, S., Lockhart, N., Kruger, M., Kelley, B. J., & Schoener, E. P. (2000). Prevalence of attention-deficit/hyperactivity disorder and conduct disorder among substance abusers. *Journal of Clinical Psychiatry, 61*(4), 244–251.

Selzer, J. (1992). Borderline omnipotence in pathological gambling. *Archives of Psychiatric Nursing, 6*(4), 215–218.

Shaffer, H. J., & Hall, M. N. (2001). Updating and refining prevalence estimates of disordered gambling behaviour in the United States and Canada. *Canadian Journal of Public Health, 92*(3), 168–172.

Shaffer, H. J., Hall, M. N., & Vander Bilt, J. (1999). Estimating the prevalence of disordered gambling behavior in the United States and Canada: A research synthesis. *American Journal of Public Health, 89*(9), 1369–1376.

Sigmund, D., Barnett, W., & Mundt, C. (1998). The hysterical personality disorder: A phenomenological approach. *Psychopathology, 31*(6), 318–330.

Silk, K. R. (2000). Borderline personality disorder. Overview of biologic factors. *Psychiatric Clinical North America, 23*(1), 61–75.

Silverthorn, P., & Frick, P. J. (1999). Developmental pathways to antisocial behavior: The delayed-onset pathway in girls. *Developmental Psychopathology, 11*(1), 101–126.

Skodol, A. E., Siever, L. J., Livesley, W. J., Gunderson, J. G., Pfohl, B., & Widiger, T. A. (2002). The borderline diagnosis II: Biology, genetics, and clinical course. *Biological Psychiatry, 51*, 951–963.

Slutske, W., Eisen, S., True, W., Lyons, M., Goldberg, J., & Tsuang, M. (2000). Common genetic vulnerability for pathological gambling and alcohol dependence in men. *Archives of General Psychiatry, 57*(7), 666–673.

Smallbone, S. W., & Dadds, M. R. (2000). Attachment and coercive sexual behavior. *Sex Abuse, 12*(1), 3–15.

Soderstrom, H., Blennow, K., Sjodin, A. K., & Forsman, A. (2003). New evidence for an association between the CSF HVA: 5-HIAA ratio and psychopathic traits. *Journal of Neurology, Neurosurgery & Psychiatry, 74*(7), 918–921.

Soderstrom, H., Hultin, L., Tullberg, M., Wikkelso, C., Ekholm, S., & Forsman, A. (2002). Reduced frontotemporal perfusion in psychopathic personality. *Psychiatry Research, 114*(2), 81–94.

Soloff, P. H. (2000). Psychopharmacology of borderline personality disorder. *Psychiatric Clinics of North America, 23*(1), 169–192.

Soloff, P., Lis, J., Kelly, T., Cornelius, J., & Ulrich, R. (2004). Risk factors for suicidal behavior in borderline personality disorder. *American Journal of Psychiatry, 151*(9), 1316–1323.

Soloff, P. H., Lis, J. A., Kelly, T., Cornelius, J., & Ulrich, R. (1994). Risk factors for suicidal behavior in borderline personality disorder. *American Journal of Psychiatry, 151*(9), 1316–1323.

Soltys, S. (1992). Pyromania and firesetting behaviors. *Psychiatric Annals, 22*(2), 79–83.

Stahl, S. (2000). *Essential psychopharmacology* (2nd ed.). Cambridge: Cambridge University Press.

Stalenheim, E. G., von Knorring, L., & Wide, L. (1998). Serum levels of thyroid hormones as biological markers in a Swedish forensic psychiatric population. *Biological Psychiatry, 43*(10), 755–761.

Stein, K. (1996). Affect instability in adults with a borderline personality disorder. *Archives of Psychiatric Nursing, 10*(1), 32–40.

Stern, A. (1938). A psychoanalytic investigation and therapy in the borderline group of neuroses. *Psychoanalytic Quarterly, 7*, 467–489.

Stravynski, A., Belisle, M., Marcouiller, M., Lavallee, Y. J., and Elie, R. (1994). The treatment of avoidant personality disorder by social skills training in the clinic or in real-life setting. *Canadian Journal of Psychiatry, 39*(8), 377–383.

Torgersen, S., Kringlen, E., & Cramer, V. (2001). The prevalence of personality disorders in a community sample. *Archives of General Psychiatry, 58*(6), 590–596.

Tuohig, G., Saffle, J., Sullivan, J., Morris, S. and Lento, S. (1995). Self-inflicted patient burns: Suicide versus mutilation. *Journal of Burn Care and Rehabilitation, 16*(4), 429–436.

van Ameringen, M., Mancini, C., Oakman, J. M., & Farvolden, P. (1999). The potential role of haloperidol in the treatment of trichotillomania. *Journal of Affective Disorders, 56*(2–3), 219–226.

van den Bosch, L. M., Verheul, R., Schippers, G. M., & van den Brink, W. (2002). Dialectical behavior therapy of borderline patients with and without substance use problems: Implementation and long-term effects. *Addictive Behaviors, 27*(6), 911–923.

van Reekum, R. (1993). Acquired and developmental brain dysfunction in borderline personality disorder. *Canadian Journal of Psychiatry, 38*(1), 54–58.

Veit, R., Flor, H., Erb, M., Hermann, C., Lotze, M., Grodd, W., & Birbaumer, N. (2002). Brain circuits in emotional learning in antisocial behavior and social phobia in humans. *Neuroscience Letters, 328*(3), 233–236.

Virkkunen, M., Dejong, J., Bartko, J., Goodwin, F. K., and Linnoila, M. (1989). Relationship of psychobiological variables to recidivism in violent offenders and impulsive fire setters. *Archives of General Psychiatry, 46*(7), 600–603.

Voglmaier, M. M., Seidman, L. J., Niznikiewicz, M. A., Dickey, C. C., Shenton, M. E., & McCarley, R. W. (2000). Verbal and nonverbal neuropsychological test performance in subjects with schizotypal personality disorder. *American Journal of Psychiatry, 157*(5), 787–793.

Wade, T., Pevalin, D., & Brannigan, A. (1999). The clustering of severe behavioural, health and educational deficits in Canadian children: Preliminary evidence from the National Longitudinal Survey of Children and Youth. *Canadian Journal of Public Health, 90*(4), 253–259.

Waldeck, T. L., & Miller, L. S. (2000). Social skills deficits in schizotypal personality disorder. *Psychiatry Research, 93*(3), 237–246.

Waldman, I. D., & Slutske, W. S. (2000). Antisocial behavior and alcoholism: A behavioral genetic perspective on comorbidity. *Clinical Psychological Review, 20*(2), 255–287.

Warmbrodt, L., Hardy, E., & Chrisman, S. (1996). Understanding trichotillomania. *Journal of Psychosocial Nursing, 34*(12), 11–15.

Widiger, T. (1991). *DSM-IV* reviews of the personality disorders: Introduction to special series. *Journal of Personality Disorders, 5*(2), 122–134.

Widiger, T., & Weissman, M. (1991). Epidemiology of borderline personality disorder. *Hospital & Community Psychiatry, 42*(10), 1015–1021.

Wilkinson-Ryan, T., & Westen, D. (2000). Identity disturbance in borderline personality disorder: An empirical investigation. *American Journal of Psychiatry, 157*(4), 528–541.

Yeomans, F., Hull, J., & Clarkin, J. (1994). Risk factors for self-damaging acts in a borderline population. *Journal of Personality Disorders, 8*(1), 10–16.

Young, J. E. (1999). Cognitive therapy for personality disorders: A schema-focused approach (3rd ed.). Sarasota, FL: Professional Resource Press.

Young, J. E., Klosko, J. S., Weisharr, M. (2003). *Schema Therapy: A practitioner's guide.* New York: Guilford.

Zanarini, M. C., Ruser, T., Frankenburg, F. R., & Hennen, J. (2000). The dissociative experiences of borderline patients. *Comprehensive Psychiatry, 41*(3), 223–227.

Zanarini, M. C., Williams, A. A., Lewis, R. E., Reich, R. B., Vera, S. C., Marino, M. F., Levin, A., Yong, L., & Frankenburg, F. R. (1997). Reported pathological childhood experiences associated with the development of borderline personality disorder. *American Journal of Psychiatry, 154*(8), 1101–1106.

Zlotnick, C. (1999). Antisocial personality disorder, affect dysregulation and childhood abuse among incarcerated women. *Journal of Personality Disorders, 13*(1), 90–95.

Zweig-Frank, F., Paris, J., & Guzder, J. (1994a). Dissociation in female patients with borderline and non-borderline personality disorders. *Journal of Personality Disorders, 8*(3), 203–209.

Zweig-Frank, F., Paris, J., & Guzder, J. (1994b). Psychological risk factors for dissociation and self-mutilation in female patients with borderline personality disorder. *Canadian Journal of Psychiatry, 39*(5), 259–264.

For challenges, please refer to the **CD-ROM** in this book.

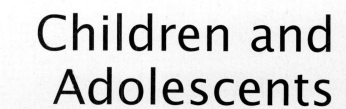

UNIT V

Children and Adolescents

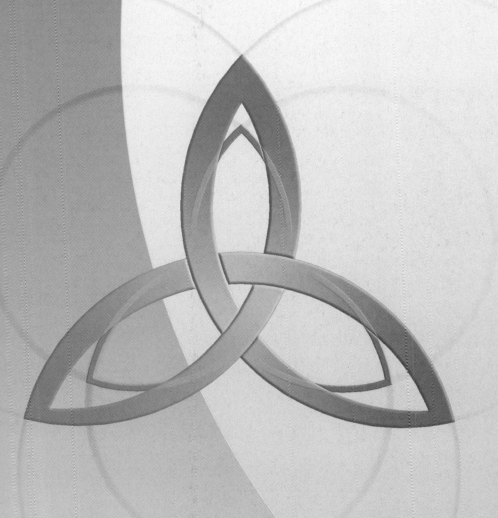

CHAPTER 25

Mental Health Assessment of Children and Adolescents

Vanya Hamrin, Catherine Gray Deering,
Lawrence Scahill, and Jean Robinson Hughes

LEARNING OBJECTIVES

After studying this chapter, you will be able to:

- Define the assessment process for children and adolescents.
- Discuss techniques of data collection used with children and adolescents.
- Discuss the synthesis of biopsychosocial assessment data for children and adolescents.
- Delineate important biopsychosocial areas of assessment for children and adolescents.

◆ KEY TERMS

- assortative mating ▪ attachment ▪ attachment disorganization ▪ developmental delays
- egocentrism ▪ maturation ▪ temperament

◆ KEY CONCEPT

- maturation

The mental health assessment of children and adolescents is challenging. At any given time, 14% of children aged 4 to 17 years (more than 800,000 in Canada) experience mental disorders that cause significant distress and impairment at home, at school, and in the community (Waddell, McEwan, Shepherd, Offord, & Hua, 2005). Yet, fewer than 25% of these children receive specialized treatment services. There are a number of reasons for this situation. First, mental health services are woefully inadequate in many regions of Canada and often are limited to urban areas (eg, Breton, Plante, & St-Georges, 2005). Second, evidence from large studies using national survey data shows that differences in government policies and health care system characteristics cause variances in service use (Sturm, Ringel, & Andreyeva, 2003). Third, some children do not get help when those who serve as gatekeepers to treatment (parents, teachers, and physicians) either fear the stigma that children will carry with mental illness (Jellnick, Patel, & Froehle, 2003) or fail to recognize mental illness as a childhood problem or the impact of early emotional experience on a child's capacity to develop relationships and to learn (Carter, Briggs-Gowan, & Davis, 2004). Given the evidence that the largest determinants of service provision to youth are provider assessment of mental health problems and provider knowledge of service resources (Stiffman, Hadley-Ives, Dore, Polgar, Horvath, Striley, & Elze, 2000), it is crucial that health professionals be knowledgeable and proficient in these areas.

The assessment of children and adolescents is a specialized process that considers their unique problems and responses within the context of their development. The *Standards of Psychiatric and Mental Health Nursing Practice* (3rd ed.) (Canadian Federation of Mental Health Nurses [CFMHN], 2005) serves as a guide for this process. These standards argue that effective diagnosis and monitoring are dependent on a client-centred approach, one that incorporates both theory and an understanding of the meaning of the health or illness experience from the perspective of the client. The nurse acknowledges clients as valued and respected partners throughout the decision-making process and supports them in drawing on their own assets and resources for self-care and mental health promotion. The nurse also incorporates knowledge of family dynamics as well as knowledge of cultural values and beliefs about families in the assessment. The assessment of children and adolescents generally follows the same format as that for adults (see Chapter 10), but there are significant differences. Children think in more concrete terms; thus, the nurse needs to ask more specific and fewer open-ended questions than would typically be asked of adults. The nurse should use simple phrasing because children have a narrower vocabulary than do adults. Examples include saying "sad" instead of "depressed" or "nervous" instead of "anxious." The nurse needs to corroborate information that children offer with more sources (eg, parents, teachers) than they would for adults. The nurse may want to use artistic and play media (eg, puppets, family drawings) to engage children and evaluate their perceptions, inner worlds, fine motor skills, and intellectual functions. Children have a less specific sense of time and a less developed memory than do adults. When children are asked about a sequence of events or specific times when events occurred, they may not be able to provide accurate information.

Mental health assessment involves much more than completing assessment tools and considers far more than the individual. A conceptual framework used as a guide can assist in planning the goals of the assessment, as well as identify the factors, types of information and sources, and the elements within the environment to be considered. A framework that is bio-ecological (Bronfenbrenner, 1986), transactional (Sameroff & Chandler, 1975), and developmental in nature reinforces the importance of placing information about the child's social-emotional functioning and psychopathologic symptoms within the context of the child's cognitive and developmental functioning, family relationships, cultural values and beliefs, and broader family and community risk factors (Carter et al., 2004).

The Canadian Mental Health Association's Framework for Support (Trainor, Pomeroy, Pape, 2004) clusters such knowledge in three resource bases: the Person Resource Base, the Knowledge Resource Base, and the Community Resource Base. By focussing on the **Person Resource Base**, the nurse acknowledges that the child is far more than a repository of illness and symptoms and that positive change builds on existing strengths. Hence, when approaching assessment, the nurse considers children's understanding of their mental health problem/illness as well as their self-esteem, sense of belonging (within their family and community), and sense of purpose and meaning in the world. The nurse also assesses children's skills and capacities (sense of personal control, confidence, resilience, hope) to confront illness. By focussing on the **Knowledge Resource Base**, the nurse takes into consideration not only medical-clinical and social science knowledge but also experiential (first-hand experience) and traditional knowledge (cultural ways). The nurse's assessment considers how children experience mental illness and how the family and community (public attitudes and conventional wisdom) accept it. A critical analysis of such information assists the nurse in building a rich understanding of children and guards against drawing inaccurate assumptions. It can also identify inaccuracies and misconceptions that may be held within the family or community about mental illness. By focussing on the **Community Resource Base**, the nurse gains an understanding of the many factors and social determinants (housing, education, income, meaningful work) that affect the everyday life of children (pp. 8–10). The Community Resource Base also acknowledges the importance of both formal services (mental health services, generic community services) and the network of natural supports (family and friends, self-help and consumer organizations) available to promote mental health and recovery. Equally important, it recognizes the person (child or youth) as having the power (age-appropriate) to make choices about resources to use, if any, and to participate fully in decision making.

The Framework for Support helps the nurse focus assessment on outcomes and, in particular, on those outcomes that play a critical role in recovery from mental illness. Specifically, it assesses whether a child has access to the social determinants of good mental health (housing, school, family, friends, a sense of purpose), feels good and has a sense of personal control, and has various personal resources in place and ways to connect with the formal service system if needed. Finally, the Framework assesses how the individual's age (child or youth) and life circumstances (eg, break-up or death in a family, being dropped from sport team) have challenged the child.

A comprehensive evaluation includes a biopsychosocial history, mental status examination, additional testing (eg, cognitive or neuropsychological)—if necessary, records of the child's school performance and medical-physical history, and information from other agencies that may be providing services (eg, department of child and family services [DCF], juvenile court). The nurse may use various assessment tools, including the Child Attention Profile (CAP) and the Devereux Childhood Assessment (DECA), the Behaviour Assessment System for Children (BASC), the Child Behaviour Checklist (CBCL), or the Children's Depression Inventory (CDI).

CRNE Note

Whenever assessing children or adolescents, developmental level will frame the assessment and implementation of the management plan.

DATA COLLECTION IN THE CLINICAL INTERVIEW

The clinical interview is the primary assessment tool used in child and adolescent psychiatry. A unique set of skills is necessary for interviewing children and adolescents. How the nurse obtains mental health information depends on the developmental level of each child, specifically considering the child's language and cogni-

tive, social, and emotional skills. For example, the nurse should simplify questions for young children or children with developmental delays (eg, mental retardation, Asperger's syndrome, pervasive developmental disorder) so that these children can understand and respond appropriately.

The assessment interview may be the initial contact between the child and parent or guardian and the nurse. The first step is to establish a helping relationship, and the second is to assess the interactions between the child and parent. It is important to understand that children cannot be considered apart from their caregivers and the context in which they live. However, defining the caregiving context is sometimes a challenge (Carter et al., 2004). The nurse needs to identify the child's primary *caregivers*, the patterns of current caregiving relationships (eg, how often the child goes to other caregivers), and the history of these relationships (eg, multiple transitions, abrupt losses) (p. 114). The nurse should also explore the family's definition of *family* and identify those included in the family constellation—both biologic and psychological relationships (eg, friends, neighbours) (pp. 114–115).

Treatment Alliance: The Helping Relationship

The nurse can establish rapport by greeting the child or adolescent in a friendly, polite, open manner and putting him or her at ease. Speaking clearly and at a normal volume and using friendly, reassuring tones are essential measures. The nurse can establish a helping relationship by recognizing the child's individuality and showing respect and concern for that child. The nurse should demonstrate sensitivity, objectivity, and confidentiality. The child will be more forthcoming if he or she believes that the nurse is listening carefully and is interested in what he or she has to say.

Child and Parent Observation

Because the child's primary environment is most often with the parent, child–parent interactions provide important data about the child–parent attachment and parenting practices. The nurse's observations focus on both the child alone and the child within the family. The nurse can actually make some of these observations while the family is in the waiting area, noting behaviours identified in Barnard's Parent–Child Interaction Model (1994):

- Sensitivity/clarity/responsiveness to cues—
  - How the child and parent get each other's attention
  - How parent and child interact with and talk to each other (clarity of cues)
  - How frequently each initiates conversation and how promptly each responds

- How the child and parent separate
- Whether the parent and child play together
- How responsive the parent is to the child's attention-seeking initiatives
- How the parent and child show affection to each other
- How attached the parent and child appear
- Response to distress
  - Whether the parent starts/stops/notes the distress/ changes activity
  - How the parent consoles the child
  - How the parent disciplines the child (clear directive voice, yells, hits)
- Social-emotional growth fostering
  - Use of talking/smiling/laughing/singing/touching (praising or criticising)
- Cognitive growth fostering
  - Parent talks about/describes objects/ideas using developmentally appropriate and stimulating language
  - Parent provides child with/points out objects of interest
  - Parent encourages and/or allows the child to explore

Interview Techniques

To get an accurate picture of the child, the nurse should interview the child and parent individually for some part of the session because each can provide unique meaningful information. Research has shown that during times when parent and child are interviewed separately in a structured interview about the child's psychopathology, they rarely agree on the presence of diagnostic criteria, regardless of the diagnostic type (Jensen et al., 1999). Generally, children provide better information about internalizing symptoms (eg, mood, sleep, suicide ideation), and parents provide better information about externalizing symptoms (eg, behaviour disturbances, oppositionality, relationship with parents).

Discussion With the Child

After talking with the parent and child together, the nurse should ask to speak with the child alone for awhile. Young children may fear separating from their parents. The nurse can reassure children by showing them where the waiting area is and telling them, "Mommy and Daddy are going to be waiting right here for you. You and I are going to be in a room close by. But if you get scared, we can come back out here to check on them." Introducing a toy or game or giving the child a transitional object to hold may help. For example, young children often like holding the family car or house keys, knowing that their parents cannot go anywhere without them. Remember that observing how the child separates from the parent is part of the data needed to complete the assessment.

Adolescents may act indifferent or even hostile when the nurse asks to speak with them alone. Teens tend to be sceptical that adults can really understand their experience, suspicious that they will be blamed for their problems, and fearful that their thoughts and feelings are abnormal. The nurse should be patient with adolescents and show empathy for their concerns through comments such as, "I can see that you're pretty angry about being here. There might be a way that I can help . . . But in order to help, I need to know from *you* what is going on that is making you so angry. I want to assure you that I am not here to judge or blame. I can also promise you that if you tell me anything that I think needs to be shared with your parents, then I will tell you first." If the child is particularly silent, the nurse might comment, "You've been pretty quiet during the last few minutes . . . I'm not sure if that means you're having trouble expressing yourself . . . That can be really frustrating. If that is the case, then, maybe if you just start talking, we can try to find some words together to express your ideas. . . . On the other hand, you may be wondering if it is safe to tell me what you're thinking. It can be really frightening to trust a stranger with your most private thoughts. . . . You may be wondering whether I really meant what I said about confidentiality/ keeping things private . . . or about not judging you. . . . I guess the dilemma/problem is whether it is safer to keep holding on to those tormenting thoughts and feelings or taking a chance that someone might be able to help."

To begin the initial assessment of a child, the nurse introduces himself or herself and explains briefly what they will be doing together. For children younger than 11 years of age, the nurse should explain that he or she helps worried or upset children by talking, playing, and together with his or her parents, thinking of ways to make things better. The nurse should then ask about the child's understanding of why he or she is there. This question often helps to identify children's misconceptions (eg, believing the nurse is going to give them an injection, thinking that they have done something bad) that could create barriers to working with them. When conducting the child interview, the nurse will need to get several releases of information from the child's guardian to obtain corroborating reports, such as the child's physical assessment from the paediatrician or paediatric nurse practitioner; the school's report about the child's academic (report card) and behavioural performance (interactions with peers and adults); and records of diagnosis and treatment from any previous psychiatric provider. Youth are often very sensitive when reports are requested from school. They worry about repercussions if they have had prior difficulties (eg, disciplinary problems). It is important that the nurse explain how these reports will be used, whether the school will be involved in the development of treatment plans, and how the youth and family will participate.

The nurse must adapt communication to the child's age level (Box 25-1). The challenge is to avoid using overly complex vocabulary or talking down to children. Young children often express themselves more easily in the context of play than through adult-like conversation. For example, a child may re-enact a conversation that he had with a sibling or parent using puppets. Children respond well to third-person conversation prompts, such as "Some kids don't like being compared to their brothers and sisters," or "I know a kid who was so sad when he lost his dog that he thought he would never be happy again."

Early in the interview, the goal is to explain the nurse's purpose, elicit any concerns the child may have about what is happening, and establish rapport with the child by engaging in unthreatening discussion. Many adults rarely ask children about things that truly interest them, but expect children to respond readily to adult conversation. The nurse can establish a high degree of credibility simply by taking note of and asking about things that are obviously important to children (eg, a sport that they participate in, a rock group displayed on a shirt, a toy they have brought with them). However, children have an uncanny natural "radar" for dishonest adult behaviour. Attempts to establish rapport work only when the nurse is genuinely interested in the child's life.

Discussion With the Parents

After meeting alone with the child, the nurse should discuss with the child that she or he would now like to talk with the parents alone, just as she or he did with the child. The nurse should be careful to reiterate that she or he wants to help and will not judge anyone in the family. The nurse should ensure that the child has a safe place to wait and age-appropriate activities. When the nurse meets with the parents, she or he should review the expectations and provide similar reassurance around confidentiality, building trust, and being nonjudgmental as that provided the child. The nurse would then proceed to ask parents to describe their view of the problem. When alone, parents often feel more comfortable discussing their children in depth and sharing their frustrations. Parents need this opportunity to speak freely, without being constrained by concern for the child's feelings. Although children often have a pretty good sense about their parents' reactions, it may not be constructive for them to hear the full force of the parents' complaints and feelings, such as their sense of helplessness, anger, or disappointment. Parents sometimes feel guilty and need permission to express their negative feelings without feeling judged. This session is the nurse's opportunity to enlist the help of parents as partners in understanding and addressing the child's problem. This time is also good for filling in any gaps in the history and clarifying the data obtained from the interview with the child.

Parents need the chance to describe the presenting problem in their own words. The nurse can encourage them by asking general questions, such as, "It is not easy for parents to recognize that childhood is sometimes unhappy and that their child needs help. A child's emotions and behaviour can be pretty confusing, even frightening, and most parents hope that, with time, the problems will disappear on their own. Sadly, that is sometimes not the case, and if left unattended over time, the problems can worsen. It takes great courage to seek help, and you took a big step in coming here today. I hope that by working together with your child, we will find some ways of assisting. I am interested in *your* story. Tell me what brings *you* here *today*." The nurse should then reflect his or her understanding of the problem, showing empathy and respect for both parent and child.

BOX 25.1

Strategies for Interviewing Children

- Use a simple vocabulary and short sentences tailored to the child's developmental and cognitive levels.
- Be sure that the child understands the questions and that you do not lead the child to give a particular response. Presenting polar opposite choices (never . . . or all the time), or scaled questions (1–10), is helpful. For example, "Some people feel angry all the time, some only feel angry at certain times, and others don't seem to feel angry at all. On a scale of 1 to 10, where 1 means never and 10 means all the time, how often do you feel angry?" If the child chooses a number greater than 1, she can be asked to describe times when she is angry.
- Select the questions for your interview on an individual basis, using judgment and discretion and considering the child's age and developmental level.
- Be sure that the manner and tone of your voice do not reveal any personal biases.
- Speak slowly and quietly, and try to allow the interview to unfold, using the child's verbalizations and behaviour as guides.
- Use simple terms (eg, "sad" for "depressed") in exploring affective reactions, and ask the child to give examples of how he or she behaves or how other people behave when emotionally aroused.
- Assume an accepting and neutral attitude toward the child's communications.
- Learn about children's current interests by looking at Saturday morning television programs, talking with parents, visiting toy stores, looking at children's books, and visiting day care centres and schools to observe children in their natural habitat (Sattler, 1998).

Asking any other family members about their view of the problem is always a good idea to clarify discrepancies, obtain additional data, and communicate awareness that different family members experience the same problem in different ways.

Building Rapport

To reduce anxiety about the evaluation, the nurse must develop rapport with the family members. Establishing rapport can be facilitated by maintaining appropriate eye contact; speaking slowly, clearly, and calmly with friendliness and acceptance; using a warm and expressive tone; reacting to communications objectively; showing interest in what families are saying; and making the interview a joint undertaking (Sattler, 1998). Suggestions for building rapport with children and adolescents are also addressed in each of the developmental sections that follow. Building rapport, which is often challenging, is fundamental to any mental health assessment of children and youth. The developmental transitions throughout childhood and adolescence are rapid, and there are few guidelines about how information from many sectors should be integrated, how impairment levels should be determined, or how assessing function that may be specific to context (relational or cultural) or caregiver (eg, parents, relatives, day care staff, school teacher) can be achieved practically (Carter et al., 2004). The information in Box 25-2 can serve as a guide to asking specific questions during a comprehensive assessment of the child. The Community Resource Base of the Framework for Support (Trainor, Pomeroy, & Pape, 2004) provides a useful guide for identifying a range of stakeholders from the child's daily living activities (eg, parent, school, day care, recreation, arts) as well as services (formal or informal) that might be consulted (with family permission) for related information about the various contexts in which the child interacts. These stakeholders can provide complementary information (formal or informal) about how the child is functioning in critical developmental domains (language and literacy, physical, cognitive, social, and emotional). They also provide an understanding of how the child is treated within, and copes with, various peer environments involving diverse cultures (eg, ethnic, socioeconomic, language) and activities (eg, scholastic, recreational, artistic). This information can assist the nurse in formulating a well-balanced and integrated mental health assessment (strengths and limitations from multiple contexts) of the child.

Children's Rating Scales

There are a number of instruments available for conducting biopsychosocial assessments. They vary according to age and target areas of interest as well as purpose.

Observational assessment and parent-report questionnaires are generally used for screening, whereas in-depth surveys and interviews help formulate diagnoses of psychopathology. Evidence shows that **screening** for early problems is both feasible and effective in improving rates of referral for mental health services (Murphy, Ichinose, Hicks, Kingdon, Crist-Whitzel, Jordan, Fieldman, & Jellnick, 1996). Screening can be administered in stages starting with short screens of groups of children (eg, in clinics, day care, school) followed by more in-depth screens involving parents and observations of those identified to be at elevated risk. Most effective screening methods involve brief standardized measures that are easy to administer, score, and interpret (Carter et al., 2004). The Ages and Stages Questionnaire-Social-Emotional Version (Squires, Bricker, & Twombly, 2002) is a promising parent-report screen for measuring social-emotional and behavioural problems and competencies from birth to 5 years. It is important to remember, however, that screening measures have proved most effective in evaluating the level of risk for children with socioemotional problems within a population (eg, a community, school) and are less effective in identifying with certainty an individual at risk (Costello, Egger, & Angold, 2005). This means that the nurse should not rely on one source of evidence but, instead, use multiple sources of data to understand a child's emotional well-being.

The Behaviour Assessment System for Children (BASC), developed by Reynolds and Kamphouse (1998), is a tool to measure behaviours and emotions in children ages 2 to 18 years. The scales include a teacher rating scale, parent rating scale, and 180-item self-report of personality. The scale evaluates several dimensions, including attitude toward school, attitude toward teachers, sensation seeking, atypicality, locus of control, somatization, social stress, anxiety, depression, sense of inadequacy, relations with parents, interpersonal relations, self-esteem, and self-reliance. The Child Behaviour Checklist (CBCL) developed by Achenbach and Edelbrock (1983) is a 113-item, self-report tool to identify forms of psychopathology and competencies that occur in children ages 4 to 16 years. This instrument provides scores on internalizing and externalizing behaviours.

Several scales are useful for diagnosing specific problems in children and adolescents. The Children's Depression Inventory (CDI) developed by March (1997) is a 27-item self-rated symptom orientation scale for children ages 7 to 17 years that is useful for diagnosing physical symptoms, harm avoidance, social anxiety, and separation or panic disorder. The paediatric anxiety rating scale (PARS) developed by the RUPP Anxiety Study Group (2001) is a clinician-administered, 50-item semi-structured interview to assess severity of anxiety in children ages 6 to 17 years.

BOX 25.2

Semi-Structured Interview With School-Aged Children

This guide identifies a range of areas and sample questions that can be addressed during an interview with a school-aged or adolescent child. The nurse should note that children generally prefer to be engaged in a conversation, rather than peppered with questions. The interview should be tailored in a way that is comfortable and relevant for the child. Although some direct questions are inevitable, open-ended questions are preferable (Hill & O'Brien, 1999). Similarly, phrasing questions to get at what a child is thinking (eg, "I can see you are trying to tell me something" or "tell me more") is preferable to asking "why" questions that tend to put people on the defensive (Plutchilk, 2000). Finally, trying to match the child's emotional state (unless hostile) helps people feel understood (Forgatch & Patterson, 1989). The interview can begin with a simple greeting, such as the following: "Hi, I am (your name and title). You must be Tom Brown. Come in."

For All School-Aged Children

PRESENTING CONCERN
Thank you for coming to talk with me today. To begin, it would help me if I knew what, if anything, you have been told about why you are here or what will go on today.... Can you tell me *your* story of how you came to be here today (if necessary, probe with specific questions below)? Let the child take the lead and explore issues as he or she raises them. If the child raises a problem, explore it in detail.

DEMOGRAPHIC INFORMATION
I'd like to know you better. Could you tell me about yourself?

Probes
1. How old are you?
2. When is your birthday?
3. Where do you live? (address)
4. And your telephone number is ... ?

SCHOOL
Tell me about your school.

Probes
5. Which school do you go to? Is it close to your home? How do you get there each day?
6. Where do you go after school (home, sitter, etc.) ... and who is there (parent/relative, sitter, no one)?
7. What do most kids think about your school? ... What is it like for you?
8. What grade are you in? What do most kids think about it? ... What is it like for you?
9. What subjects do you like the best? ... Like least?
10. What subjects give you the least trouble? ... Most trouble?
11. How well do you do in school—about the same as, better than, or not as well as other kids in your class?
12. On the whole, would you say that you are doing better or worse than last year?
13. What activities do you participate in at school?
14. How well do you get along with your classmates?
15. How well do you get along with your teachers?
16. Tell me how you spend a usual day at school.

HOME AND FAMILY
To help me understand your family, can you name each of the people who live with you ... and then other important

family members who live somewhere else ... and I'll put them into a picture ... Now using the picture, tell me a little about your family.

(A **genogram** [pronounced: *jen-uh-gram*] [Wright & Leahey, 2005] provides a useful diagram of family relationships. It resembles a family tree but includes additional relationships among individuals. It permits the nurse and the child to quickly see patterns in family history. It maps relationships and traits that may otherwise be missed and includes basic information about number of families, number of children in each family, birth order, and deaths. Some genograms include information on disorders running in the family such as alcoholism, depression, diseases, alliances, and living situations. Older children can provide additional information (eg, about separation/divorce, death) for understanding family dynamics.)

Probes
17. Tell me a little about each of them.
    - Who makes you happy and who makes you sad/angry/worried? Explain.
    - Do you have a favourite photo of you and your family? Tell me about it ... and why you like it.
18. What does your father do during the day—does he work? (other activities at home/with friends)?
19. What does your mother do during the day—does she work? (other activities at home/with friends)?
20. Tell me what your home is like.
21. Tell me about your room at home.
22. What chores do you do at home?
23. How do you get along with your father?
24. What does he do that you like? ... Don't like?
25. How do you get along with your mother?
26. What does she do that you like? ... Don't like?
27. (Where relevant) Some brothers and sisters get along well, whereas others don't get along at all ... How do you get along with your brothers and sisters?
28. What do (does) they (he/she) do that you like? ... That you don't like?
29. Who handles the discipline at home?
30. Tell me about how they (he/she) handle (handles) it.
    - When you do something good, what happens and who is involved?
    - When you get in trouble, what happens and who is involved?
    - If you want to do something different from the rest of your family, would that be okay? Explain ... Who would support you?
    - If you need help, what would you do? Would someone support you? Explain.
    - Are there other relatives who are important to you? Tell me about who they are and how they connect with you (if not already discussed with the genogram).
    - Would you say that your family is like most other families in your school/neighbourhood or different? Explain. Does that make it easy or difficult for you/your family ... and in what ways and in what types of situations? This question gets at culture (ethnicity, socio-economic status, language, beliefs/values, etc.) in a broad way.

(continued)

BOX 25.2 (continued)

INTERESTS
Now let's talk about the things you like to do?

Probes
31. What hobbies and interests do you have?
32. What do you do in the afternoons/evenings after school?
33. Tell me what you usually do on Saturdays and Sundays.
    ■ What do you do on special holidays? Tell me about the best holiday you ever had.
    ■ When you are having fun, what are you doing, who are you with? Tell me about a time when you were really having a good time.

Friends
Tell me about your friends.

Probes
34. What do you like to do with your friends?
    ■ Any best friends?
    ■ If you needed help, could you count on them to support you? Give an example.
    ■ If you wanted to do something different from them, would that be okay?

MOODS AND FEELINGS
Probes
35. Everybody feels happy at times. What things make you feel happiest?
36. What are you most likely to get sad about?
37. What do you do when you are sad?
38. Everybody gets angry at times. What things make you angriest?
39. What do you do when you are angry?

FEARS AND WORRIES
Probes
40. All children get scared sometimes about some things. What things make you feel scared?
41. What do you do when you are scared? ... What takes away the fear?
    ■ How successful are your efforts?
42. Tell me what you worry about ... What takes away the worry?
    ■ How successful are your efforts?
43. Any other things?

SELF-CONCERNS
Probes
44. What do you like best about yourself? ... Anything else?
45. What do you like least about yourself? ... Anything else?
46. Tell me about the best thing that ever happened to you.
47. Tell me about the worst thing that ever happened to you.
    ■ What did you do about this situation?
    ■ How successful were your efforts?
    ■ Overall, how much would you say you believe in yourself?

SOMATIC CONCERNS
Probes
48. Do you ever get headaches?

49. (If yes) Tell me about them. (How often? What do you usually do?)
50. Do you get stomachaches?
51. (If yes) Tell me about them. (How often? What do you usually do?)
52. Do you get any other kinds of body pains?
53. (If yes) Tell me about them.
    ■ What do you do to ease these problems?
    ■ How successful are your efforts?

THOUGHT DISORDER
Probes
54. Do you ever hear things that seem funny or unusual?
55. (If yes) Tell me about them. (How often? How do you feel about them? What do you usually do?)
56. Do you ever see things that seem funny or unreal?
57. (If yes) Tell me about them. (How often? How do you feel about them? What do you usually do?)

HELP-SEEKING
Probes
58. Tell me about a time when you have needed help. What did you do? Who did you ask for help? What kind of help did you get? How did things work out?
59. Have you ever gone to see a counsellor before? Explain. Did it help?

MEMORIES AND FANTASY
Probes
60. What is the first thing you can remember from the time when you were a very little baby?
61. Tell me about your dreams.
62. Which dreams come back again?
63. Who are your favourite television characters?
64. Tell me about them.
65. What animals do you like best?
66. Tell me about these animals.
67. What animals do you like least?
68. Tell me about these animals.
69. What is your happiest memory?
70. What is your saddest memory?
71. If you could change places with anyone in the whole world, who would it be?
72. Tell me about that.
73. If you could go anywhere you wanted to right now, where would you go?
74. Tell me about that.
75. If you could have three wishes, what would they be?
76. What things do you think you might need to take with you if you were to go to the moon and stay there for 6 months?

ASPIRATIONS
77. What do you plan on doing when you become an adult?
78. What things will help you be successful? Is there anything standing in the way of you being successful?
    ■ How hopeful are you that you might be successful? [suggestion–using a visual analogue with a series of faces on a line (sad face–to–very happy face) ask child to choose the face that best describes their hopefulness]
79. If you could do anything you wanted when you become an adult, what would it be?

BOX 25.2 (continued)

CONCLUDING QUESTIONS

80. Do you have anything else that you would like to tell me about yourself?
81. Do you have any questions that you would like to ask me?
    - What are you hoping will happen as a result of our talking today?

For Adolescents

These questions can be inserted after number 57 (the help-seeking section).

SEXUAL RELATIONS

Adolescence is a very confusing time emotionally. Our bodies change as we begin to look more like adults. Our relationships also change. While our sexual relationships are new and exciting, they can also be puzzling, frustrating or even frightening.

1. Do you have any romantic feelings or relationship(s) with guys or girls? Do you feel comfortable talking about them? With girls/guys/ or both?
2. What makes you feel good about it/them?
3. What makes you feel not so good about them?
4. Do you have any special girlfriend (boyfriend)?
5. (If yes) Tell me about her (him).
   Most people have lots of questions about their sexual relationships and yet are not sure whom to trust to talk openly ...
6. What kind of sexual concerns do you have?
7. (If present) Tell me about them.

8. (If applicable) What do you think might be helpful to do about your concerns? (getting information, talking to someone, getting a check-up/some medication)
9. Are you interested in getting help? Would you like me to help you make the right connections?

DRUG AND ALCOHOL USE

10. Do your parents/sister/brothers drink?
11. (If yes) Tell me about their drinking. (How much, how frequently, and where?)
12. Do your friends drink alcohol?
13. (If yes) Tell me about their drinking.
14. Do you drink alcohol?
15. (If yes) Tell me about your drinking.
16. Do your parents use drugs?
17. (If yes) Tell me about the drugs they use. (How much, how frequently, and for what reasons?)
18. Do your friends use drugs?
19. (If yes) Tell me about the drugs they use.
20. Do you use drugs?
21. (If yes) Tell me about the drugs you use. (Sattler, 1998)
22. Are you worried about the way your parents/siblings/friends use alcohol or drugs?
23. Are you worried about the way you use alcohol/drugs?
24. (If yes) Are you interested in getting help?
25. (If applicable) What do you think might be helpful to do regarding your concerns?

The SNAP-IV developed by Swanson (1983) is a 90-item teacher and parent rating scale containing items from the Conners' questionnaire for measuring inattention and overactivity; it is useful for diagnosing attention deficit hyperactivity disorder (ADHD—inattentive and impulsive types) and oppositional defiant disorder. The Children's Yale-Brown Obsessive Compulsive Scale developed by Goodman and colleagues (1989) is a 19-item scale that can help diagnose childhood obsessive-compulsive disorder in children ages 6 to 17 years of age.

Assessments performed for **diagnostic** purposes often require trained administrators and interpreters and are more time consuming and rigorous to administer than screens. However, evidence shows that they are very useful because they highlight both positive and negative aspects of the child and identify delays, evaluate the relative degree of impairment associated with extant problem behaviours, and facilitate the design of interventions that capitalize on children's strengths (Carter et al., 2004).

Preschool-Aged Children

When interviewing preschool-aged children, the nurse should understand that these children may have difficulty putting feelings into words and provide assistance

(eg, "When I see your face all wrinkled up, it tells me that you are mixed up—confused"). The nurse should also understand that young children think in very concrete terms. For example, when talking to a young boy (3 to 6 years) about the death of his father, the nurse needs to recognize that, although children can acknowledge physical death, they consider it as temporary or gradual and not fully separate from life. The young boy may believe that his father continues to live (in the ground where he was buried) and ask questions about his activities (eg, how is Dad eating, going to the toilet, breathing, playing?) (National Cancer Institute, 2005). The child may also believe that something the child thought or did actually caused the father's illness and subsequent death. In response to death, children younger than 5 years will often exhibit disturbances in eating, sleeping, and bladder or bowel control that may result in a parent's seeking help (Grollman, 1990). The nurse should keep language simple and tailored to the child's developmental level. Any discussion about death should include proper words (eg, cancer, died, death) and avoid euphemisms (eg, "he passed away," "he is sleeping," "we lost him") because they can confuse children and lead to misinterpretations (Wass & Corr, 1984).

The nurse can achieve rapport with preschool-aged children by joining their world of play. Play is an activity by which the child transforms an experience from real life into a symbolic, nonliteral representation. Play encourages verbalizations, promotes manual strength, teaches rules and problem-solving, and helps children master control over their environment (Moore-Taylor, Menarchek-Fetkovich, & Day, 2000). With children younger than 5 years of age, the nurse may conduct the assessment in a playroom. Useful materials are paper, pencils, crayons, paints, paint brushes, easels, clay, blocks, balls, dolls, doll houses, puppets, animals, dress-up clothes, and a water supply. The nurse must inform preschool-aged children about any rules for the play. For example, the nurse must tell the child that the nurse must ensure safety, so that there will be no hitting in the playroom.

When observing the child in a free play setting, the nurse should pay attention to initiation of play, energy level, manipulative actions, tempo, body movements, tone, integration, creativity, products, age appropriateness, and attitudes toward adults. In addition, themes of play, expression of emotions, and temperament are important to observe. The nurse must allow children to direct and initiate these themes. When evaluating the young child's peer relationships through play therapy in a play group or school setting, observe play settings and themes, initiation of play, response to peer initiations of play, integration of affect and action during play, resolution of conflicts, responses to suggestions of others during play, and the ability to engage in role taking and role reversals (Howes & Matheson, 1992).

The nurse's roles are to be a good listener; to use appropriate vocabulary; to tolerate a child's anxious, angry, or sad behaviour; and to use reflective comments about the child's play. Through play, the nurse can assess the child's sensory-motor skills, cognitive style, adaptability, language functioning, emotional and behavioural responsiveness, social level, moral development, coping styles, problem-solving techniques, and approaches to perceiving and interpreting the surrounding world. For example, when assessing a child's problem-solving skills, the nurse might say to a preschooler, "I can see that you've noticed the tent in the corner and would like to check it out. Yes, the tent does look interesting … but I can also see that you have a problem … the tent looks a little scary to you … and you do not want to check it out alone. Hmmm … can you think of someone who you would like to take with you? … [then, in response to child's answer] … You say 'Mr. Bear … because he protects you'… Oh, then Mr. Bear is a great choice. You chose a friend who would be sure to keep you safe…. You made a good decision."

In any assessment, the nurse should be careful to assess both strengths and limitations and then build on the strengths to address the child's problem areas. For example, the nurse might engage a preschooler with the comment, "Sara, you are a great story teller; I wonder if

---

BOX 25.3

Lidz Assessment Tool

Child's Name: _____ Birth Date: _____ Age: ____

Assessor: _____ Date of Assessment: _____

Describe typical play style/sequence.

Describe range of levels of play from lowest to highest level with age estimates and within contexts of independent/facilitated, familiar/unfamiliar, single/multiple toys.

Describe language and evidence of self-talk and internalized speech.

Describe interpersonal interactions with assessor and facilitator (if not assessor).

Describe content of any play themes.

What held the child's attention the longest? (For how long?) And what were the child's toy/play preferences?

Describe the child's affective state during play.

Implications of above for intervention:

From Lidz, C. S. (2003). *Early childhood assessment.* Hoboken, NJ: Wiley & Sons, Inc. Copyright 2003, John Wiley & Sons. Used with permission.

---

you could tell me a story about this doll, Jane, who is afraid at day care just like you."

Lidz (2003) developed a tool that the clinician can use to assess preschoolers' play (Box 25-3). Analyzing children's perceptions of fairy tales can provide the clinician with clues to culture, problems, solutions, and elements of mental functioning (LeBuffe & Naglieri, 1999; Trad, 1989).

Drawings are also used in child assessment to illuminate the child's intellect, creative talents, neuropsychological deficits, body image difficulties, and perceptions of family life (Fig. 25-1). Types of drawings used in child assessments are free drawings; self-portraits; the kinetic family drawing; tree, person, house drawing; and a picture of someone of the opposite sex (Cepeda, 2000). The Devereux Early Childhood Assessment (DECA) (LeBuffe & Naglieri, 2003) screening instrument measures protective factors of attachment, self-control, and initiative in children 2 to 5 years of age. The DECA tool is used in the preschool classroom setting with the goal of promoting positive resilience in children.

School-Aged Children

Unlike preschool-aged children, school-aged (5 to 11 years) children can use more constructs, provide longer

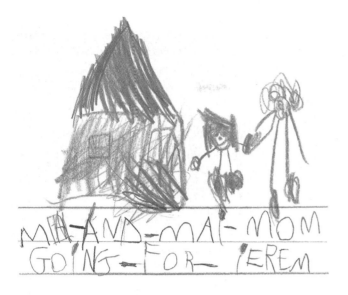

FIGURE 25.1   Me and my mom going for ice cream. Drawing and writing by a 5-year-old girl.

descriptions and make better inferences of others, and acquire more complete conceptions of various social roles. Children in middle school are more capable of verbal exchange and can tolerate limited periods of direct questioning (Box 25-4). The nurse can establish rapport with school-aged children by using competitive board games, such as checkers and playing cards. A therapeutic game helpful in assessing the child's perceptions, cognition, and emotions and in establishing rapport between clinician and child is the thinking–feeling–doing game. In this game, the clinician and child take turns drawing cards that pose hypothetical situations and ask what a person might think, feel, or do in such scenarios. For example, one card might say, "A boy has something on his mind that he is afraid to tell his father. What is he scared to talk about?" Another might read, "A girl heard her parents fighting. What were they fighting about? What was the girl thinking while she listened to her parents?"

Adolescents

Adolescents have an increased command of language concepts and have developed the capacity for abstract and formal operations thinking. Their social world is also more complex. Some early adolescents tend to assume that their subjective experiences are real and congruent with objective reality, which can lead to egocentrism (Shave & Shave, 1989). Egocentrism is a preoccupation with one's own appearance, behaviour, thoughts, and feelings. For example, a preteen may think that he caused his parents to divorce because he fought with his father the day before the parents announced their decision to separate. Because teenagers have a heightened sense of self-consciousness, they may be preoccupied during the interview with applying makeup or other self-grooming tasks.

During early adolescence, cognitive changes include increased self-consciousness, fear of being shamed, and demands for privacy and secrecy. An adolescent's willingness to talk to a nurse will depend partly on his or her perception of the degree of rapport between them. The nurse's ability to communicate respect, cooperation, honesty, and genuineness is important. Rejection by the adolescent, even outright hostility, during the first few interactions is not uncommon, especially if the teen is having behaviour problems at home, at school, or in the community. The nurse should be patient and avoid jumping to conclusions. Hostility or defiance may be a test of how much the teen can trust the nurse, a defence against anxiety, or a transference phenomenon (see Chapter 7).

Adolescents are likely to be defensive in front of their parents and concerned with confidentiality. At the start of the interview, the nurse should clearly convey to the adolescent what information will and will not be shared with parents. Adolescents generally prefer a straightforward, candid approach to the interview because they often distrust those in authority. Making a commitment to adolescents that they do not have to discuss anything that they are not ready to reveal is important, so that they will feel in control while they gradually build trust.

BIOPSYCHOSOCIAL PSYCHIATRIC NURSING ASSESSMENT OF CHILDREN AND ADOLESCENTS

As discussed, the comprehensive assessment of the child or adolescent includes interviews with the child and parents, child alone, and parents alone. After completing these components, the nurse should bring the child and parents back together to summarize his or her view of their concerns and to ask for feedback regarding whether these perceptions agree with theirs. The nurse must give the family a chance to share additional information and ask questions. Then, the nurse should thank them for their willingness to talk and give them some idea of the next steps. Use of an assessment tool is helpful in organizing data for mental health planning and intervention. The nurse should also ask for feedback on the suggested next steps of both child and parents and discuss any areas of disagreement to find a plan with which all can live.

When interviewing both child and parents, the nurse's directly asking the child as many questions as possible is generally the best way to get accurate, first-hand information and to reinforce interest in the child's viewpoint. Asking the child questions about the history of the current problem, previous psychiatric experiences (both

BOX 25.4

Biopsychosocial Psychiatric Nursing Assessment of Children and Adolescents

1. Identifying information

Name
Sex
Date of birth
Age
Birth order
Grade
Ethnic background
Religious preference
List of others living in household

2. Major reason for seeking help

Description of presenting problems or symptoms
When did the problems (symptoms) start?
Describe both the child's and the parent's perspective.

3. Psychiatric history

Previous mental health contacts (inpatient and outpatient)
Other mental health problems or psychiatric diagnosis (besides those described currently)
Previous medications and compliance
Family history of depression, substance abuse, psychosis, etc., and treatment

4. Current and past health status

Medical problems
Current medications
Surgery and hospitalizations
Allergies
Diet and eating habits
Sleeping habits
Height and weight
Hearing and vision
Menstrual history
Immunizations
If sexually active, birth control method used
Date of last physical examination
Paediatrician or nurse practitioner's name and telephone number

5. Medications

Prescription (dosage, side effects)
Over-the-counter drugs

6. Neurologic history

Right handed, left handed, or ambidextrous
Headaches, dizziness, fainting
Seizures
Unusual movement (tics, tremors)
Hyperactivity
Episodes of weakness or paralysis
Slurred speech, pronunciation problems
Fine motor skills (eating with utensils, using crayon or pencil, fastening buttons and zippers, tying shoes)
Gross motor skills and coordination (walking, running, hopping)

7. Responses to mental health problems

What makes problems (symptoms) worse or better?
Feelings about those experiences (what helped and did not help)
What interventions have been tried so far?
Major losses or changes in past year
Fears, including punishment

8. Mental status examination

Appearance, gait, posture, dress, nutrition, gestures
Motor/motility
Interaction with nurse, eye contact
Psychosis, hallucinations, delusions
Mood, affect, anxiety
Speech (clarity, speed, volume), language (articulation, tone, modulation, coherence).
Writing/reading (comprehension), content
Thought patterns (organization, thought content)
Intellectual ability, judgment, insight, general knowledge, orientation to date, time, person
Activity level, stereotypes, mannerisms, obsessions or compulsions, attention, phobia

9. Developmental assessment

Mother's pregnancy, delivery
Child's Apgar score, whether preterm or fullterm, weight at birth
Physical maturation
Psychosocial
Language
Developmental milestones: walking, talking, toileting

10. Attachment, temperament/significant behaviour patterns

Attachment
Concentration, distractability
Eating and sleeping patterns
Ability to adjust to new situations and changes in routine
Usual mood and fluctuations
Excitability
Ability to wait, tendency to interrupt
Responses to discipline
Lying, stealing, fighting, cruelty to animals, fire-setting

11. Self-concept

Beliefs about self
Body image
Self-esteem
Personal identity

12. Risk assessment

History of suicidal thoughts, previous attempts
Suicide ideation, plan, lethality of plan, accessibility of plan
History of violent, aggressive behaviour
Homicidal ideation

13. Family relationships

Relationship with parents
Deaths/losses
Family strengths and conflicts (nature and content)
Nurturing and disciplinary methods
Quality of sibling relationship
Sleeping arrangements
Who does the child relate to or trust in the family?
Relationships with extended family

14. School and peer adjustment

Learning difficulties and strengths
Behaviour problems and strengths at school
School attendance
Relationship with teachers

BOX 25.4 (continued)

Special classes
Best friend
Relationships with peers
Dating
Drug and alcohol use
Participation in sports, clubs, other activities
After-school routine

15. Community resources

Professionals or agencies working with child or family
Day care resources

16. Functional status

Global Assessment of Functioning (GAF) scale

17. Stresses and coping behaviours

Psychosocial stresses
Coping behaviours (strengths)

18. Summary of significant data

---

good and bad), family psychiatric history, medical problems, developmental history (to get an idea of what the child has been told), school adjustment, peer relationships, and family functioning is particularly important. If necessary, the nurse can ask some or all of these same questions of the parents to get consensus or another opinion about the matter, attain supplemental information, or both. Keep in mind that developmental research shows moderate to low correlation between parent and child reports of family behaviour. It is helpful to discuss openly with the family the fact that different perspectives exist and to note that the nurse's role is not to judge or side with one view, but rather to understand the different perspectives and how they might be affecting the family.

Biologic Domain

Nurses should include a thorough history of psychiatric and medical problems in any comprehensive assessment. A physical assessment is necessary to rule out any medical problems that could be mistaken for psychiatric symptoms (eg, weight loss resulting from diabetes, not depression; drug-induced psychosis). Pharmacologic assessment should include prescription and over-the-counter (OTC) medications. Nurses should ask about any allergies to food, medications, or environmental triggers.

Genetic Vulnerability

The line between nature and nurture is not always clear. Characteristics that appear to be inborn may influence parents and teachers to respond differently toward different children, thus creating problems in the family environment. A phenomenon called assortative mating, the tendency for individuals to select mates who are similar in genetically linked traits such as intelligence and personality style, may contribute to the genetic transmission of psychiatric disorders. Research increasingly shows that major psychiatric disorders (eg,

depression, anxiety disorder, schizophrenia, bipolar disorder, substance abuse) run in families. Thus, having a parent or sibling with a psychiatric disorder usually indicates increased risk for the same or another closely related disorder in a child or adolescent. In addition, many childhood psychiatric disorders, such as autism, developmental learning disorders, some language disorders (eg, dyslexia), ADHD, Tourette's syndrome, enuresis (bed wetting) and other trisomy disorders (eg, Down syndrome) appear to be genetically transmitted (American Psychiatric Association, 2000; Health Canada, 2002; Rutter, Silberg, O'Connor, & Simonoff, 1999; State, Lombroso, Pauls, & Leckman, 2000). Certain disorders (eg, ADHD, enuresis, stuttering) are more common in boys than in girls.

Neurologic Examination

A full neurologic evaluation is beyond the scope of practice for a baccalaureate-level or master's-level nurse without specific neuropsychiatric training. However, a screening of neurologic soft signs can help establish a database that will clarify the need for further neurologic consultation. The nurse should ask the child directly the brief neurologic screening questions suggested in Box 25-4 and also should note any soft signs of neurologic dysfunction, such as slurred speech, unusual movements (eg, tics, tremors), hyperactivity, and coordination problems. The nurse can ask young children to hop on one foot, skip, or walk from toe to heel to assess their gross motor coordination and to draw with a crayon or pencil or to play pick-up sticks or jacks to assess their fine motor coordination.

Psychological Domain

Children can usually identify and discuss what improves or worsens their problems. The assessment may be the first time that someone has asked the child to explain his or her view of the problem. It is also a perfect opportunity to discuss any life changes or losses (eg, death of grandparents or pets, parental divorce) and fears, especially of punishment.

Mental Status Examination

The mental status examination of children combines observation and direct questioning. The nurse should note the child's general appearance, including size, cleanliness, dress, masculinity or femininity, and level of attractiveness. Although it perhaps should not be so, social-psychological research shows that the appearance and attractiveness of both children and adults strongly influence their social relationships (Eagly, et al., 1991). The nurse also should note the child's nonverbal behaviour, including posture, tone of voice, eye contact, and mannerisms. How active is the child? Does he or she seem to have difficulty focussing on the interview, sitting still, refraining from impulsive behaviour, and listening without interrupting (possible signs of ADHD)? Does the child seem underactive, lethargic, distant, or hopeless (possible signs of depression)?

The nurse should observe the child's sentence structure and vocabulary for a general sense of his or her intellectual functioning. Does the child seem able to form a relationship with the nurse, or does the child seem distant, uninterested, or in his or her own world? Speech patterns, such as rate (overly fast or slow), clarity, and volume, and any speech dysfluencies (eg, stuttering, halting) are important in screening for mood disorders (eg, depression, mania), language disorders, psychotic processes, and anxiety disorders (see Ch. 20).

Asking children general questions about their everyday lives and observing the content and process of their play (eg, ability to focus on an activity, play themes, boundaries between themselves and others) helps to reveal the level of organization and content of their thinking. The nurse should also note the level of speech organization. Young children normally shift subjects rather abruptly, but adolescents should continue with one train of thought before moving to another. The nurse should note any morbid or eccentric thoughts, violent fantasies, and self-deprecating statements that could reflect a poor self-concept. Assessment of preteens and adolescents should address substance use and sexual activity because responses may provide useful information about high-risk behaviour or harmful substance use. In addition, the nurse should inquire about any obsessions or compulsions (eg, worries about germs, severe hand washing).

Developmental Assessment

Children respond to life's stresses in different ways and in accord with their developmental level. Knowing the difference between normal child development and psychopathology is crucial in helping parents view their children's behaviour realistically and respond appropri-

ately. The key areas for assessment include maturation, psychosocial development, and language.

Maturation

Healthy development of the brain and nervous system during childhood and adolescence provides the foundation for successful functioning throughout life. Such development, called **maturation**, unfolds through sequential and orderly growth processes. These processes are biologically and genetically based but depend on constant interactions with a stimulating and nurturing environment.

> **KEY CONCEPT maturation** is the process of completing a state of development; a ripening.

If trauma or neglect impairs the process of normal biologic maturation, **developmental delays** and disorders that may not be fully reversible can result. For example, babies born with fetal alcohol syndrome experience permanent brain damage, often resulting in mental retardation (Roebuck, Mattson, & Riley, 1999). A pregnant woman's use of crack cocaine deprives the fetus of nutrients and oxygen, leading to developmental delays, deformities, and behaviour disorders (eg, impulsivity, withdrawal, hyperactivity). The nurse can assess for developmental delays by asking questions from specific sections of the mental status examination:

- *Intellectual functioning*: Evaluate the child's creativity, spontaneity, ability to count money and tell time, academic performance, memory, attention, frustration tolerance, and organization.
- *Gross motor functioning*: Ask child to hop on one foot, throw a ball, walk up and down hall, and run.
- *Fine motor functioning*: Ask the child to draw a picture or pick up sticks.
- *Cognition*: The nurse can evaluate the child's general level of cognition by assessing the child's vocabulary, level of comprehension, drawing ability, and responsiveness to questions. Testing, such as the Wechsler Intelligence Scale for Children (WISC-III), provides measures of intelligence quotient (IQ). A psychologist usually performs such tests. The nurse can request cognitive testing if he or she has concerns about developmental delays or learning disabilities.
- *Thinking and perception*: Evaluate level of consciousness; orientation to date, time, and person; thought content; thought process; and judgment.
- *Social interactions and play*: Assess the child's organization, creativity, drawing capacity, and ability to follow rules. Children experiencing developmental delays may remain engaged solely in parallel play, instead of moving to reciprocal play. They may consistently play with toys designed for younger children, draw crude body pictures, or display

receptive (understanding) or expressive (communicative) language problems

Psychosocial Development

Assessment of psychosocial development is very important for children with mental health problems. Various theoretical models are available from which to choose; the most commonly used model is Erikson's stages of development. When considering this model, the nurse should examine the child's gender and cultural background for appropriateness. The nurse also may use the Baker Miller's model for girls (see Chapter 7).

Language

At birth, infants can emit sounds of all languages. Maturation of language skills begins with babbling, or the utterance of simple, spontaneous sounds. By the end of the first year, children can make one-word statements, usually naming objects or people in the environment. By age 2 years, they should speak in short, telegraphic sentences consisting of a verb and noun (eg, "want cookie"). Between ages 2 and 4 years, vocabulary and sentence structure develop rapidly. In fact, the preschooler's ability to produce language often surpasses motor development, sometimes causing temporary stuttering when the child's mind literally works faster than the mouth.

Language development depends on the complex interaction of physical maturation of the nerves, development of head and neck musculature, hearing abilities, cognitive abilities, exposure to language, educational stimulation, and emotional well-being. Social needs create a natural inclination toward communication, but the child needs reinforcement to develop correct pronunciation, vocabulary, and grammar.

Before a diagnosis of a communication disorder (ie, impairment in language expression, comprehension, or both) can be made, the child must be tested to rule out hearing, visual, or other neurologic problems. Brain damage, especially to the left hemisphere (dominant for language in most individuals), can seriously impair the development of communication abilities in children. Any child who has experienced brain damage from anoxia at birth, congenital trauma, head injury, infection, tumour, or drug exposure should be closely monitored for signs of a communication disorder. Before the age of 5 years, the brain has amazing plasticity, and sometimes other intact areas of the brain can take over functions of damaged areas, especially with immediate speech therapy. Genetically based disorders such as autism cause language delays that are sometimes permanent and severe. Children with language delays need particular encouragement to communicate properly because they tend to compensate by using nonverbal signals (Tanguay, 2000).

The nurse must recognize normal variations in child development and assess lags in the development of vocabulary and sentence structure during the critical preschool years. Delays in this area can seriously affect other areas, such as cognitive, educational, and social development. Many children who receive psychiatric treatment have speech and language disorders that are sometimes undetected, either leading to or compounding their emotional problems. Cantwell and Baker (1991) studied 600 consecutive child referrals to an urban community clinic for speech and language disorders and found the psychiatric prevalence was 50% for any diagnosis, 26% for behaviour disorders, and 20% for emotional disorders. The most common individual psychiatric diagnoses were ADHD (19%), oppositional defiant disorder (7%), and anxiety disorders (10%). Beitchman and colleagues (1996) found that children with receptive language disorders also had a high prevalence of ADHD (59%).

Attachment: The Caregiving Context

Current thinking among researchers and clinicians who assess early emerging social-emotional and behavioural problems holds that children must be evaluated in relation to their primary caregivers (Carter et al., 2004). Although parents usually serve as the primary caregivers, in today's world, other family members (biologically or psychologically related), babysitters, day care, and club activity staff, to name a few, often play a significant role in the development of child attachment and should be assessed. In addition, recognizing that children respond differently in different situations, the routine environments in which the child interacts need to be evaluated. Finally, the contexts of culture (values, beliefs, and practices), race, and ethnicity need to be considered (Garcia-Coll & Magnuson, 2000). For meaningful assessments, nurses need to be culturally competent, as suggested in the *Standards of Mental Health Nursing Practice* (CFMHN, 2005). Studies of **attachment** show that the quality of the emotional bond between the infant and parental or caregiver figures provides the groundwork for future relationships. The need to touch and be close to a parental figure appears biologically driven and has been demonstrated in classic studies of monkeys who bonded with a terry cloth surrogate mother (Harlow, Harlow, & Suomi, 1971). A secure attachment is based on the caretaker's consistent, appropriate response to the infant's attachment behaviours (eg, crying, clinging, calling, following, protesting). Children who have developed a secure attachment protest when their parents leave them (beginning at about age 6 to 8 months), seek comfort from their parents in unfamiliar situations, and playfully explore the environment in the parent's presence. When parents are unresponsive to a child's attachment behaviours, the child may develop an insecure attachment, evidenced by clinging and lack of exploratory play when the parent is present, intense protest when the parent leaves, and indifference or even hostility (Thompson, 2002) when the parent returns (Ainsworth, 1989).

Secure attachments in early childhood produce cooperative, harmonious parent–child relationships, in which the child is responsive to the parents' socialization efforts and likely to adopt the parents' viewpoints, values, and goals. Securely attached young children also socialize competently, are popular with well-acquainted peers during the preschool years, and have warm relationships with important adults in their lives. Securely attached children see themselves and others constructively and have relatively sophisticated emotional and moral understanding (Thompson, 2002).

Although the importance of the parent's responsiveness is unquestionable in determining the development of a secure attachment, the process works both ways. Some babies seem to encourage attachment naturally with their parents by responding positively to holding, cuddling, and comforting behaviours. Others, such as those with developmental delays or autistic disorders, may respond less readily and even reject parental attempts at connecting. The interrelatedness of child behaviour and the parenting context is not only reciprocal but also extends over time (Sameroff, 2000). The goodness of fit of the caregiving relationship is, at least in part, dependent on infant temperament, parental perceptions, and the parenting style used, which either lessens or heightens the risk for later psychopathology (Seifer, 2000).

Attachment Theories

Bowlby's early studies (1969) of maternal deprivation formed the initial framework for attachment theory, based on the notion that the infant tends to bond to one primary parental figure, usually the mother. Although this pattern is common, recent studies show that although children make multiple attachments to parents and other caregivers, the high-quality, intense bonds remain essential for healthy development. Contemporary nursing theories, such as Barnard's parent–child interaction model (1994), have stressed the importance of the interaction between the child's spontaneous behaviour and biologic rhythms and the mother's ability to respond to cues that signal distress (Baker et al., 1994). The model provides the foundation for the development of several scales measuring dimensions of attachment. These standardized, observational assessment scales use routine parent–child interaction activities involving feeding (NCAFS scale—76 items, birth to 1 year) and teaching (NCATS scale—73 items, birth to 3 years) to assess a dyad's strengths and limitations during the early years. Areas assessed include contingency (reciprocal communication patterns between caregiver and child), positioning (caregiver's sensitivity to child developmental stage

and needs), verbalness (ability to stimulate language development), sensitivity (psychological availability and responsivity to the child), affect (positive or negative quality of communication patterns), and attention regulation (engaging and disengaging behaviours). Such measures can provide informed assessments to nurses in a variety of settings, such as postpartum hospital care, the home (eg, public health newborn visits), or primary care settings (eg, mental health nurse in community health centre). Doyle, Markiewicz, Brendgen, Lieberman, and Voss (2000) studied 216 parents' attachment style and marital adjustment and found that mothers having an anxious attachment style uniquely predicted that children's attachment to both mother and father would be insecure. Child–mother attachment was associated uniquely with perceived global self-worth and physical appearance for both younger and older children, whereas child–father attachment was associated uniquely with child-perceived school competence and, only for older children, with global self-worth. Although most attachment research has been done with mothers, the father's role in child development has become better understood through research done during the past two decades. Economic support of the family constitutes a major role in which fathers contribute to the rearing and emotional health of their children (Lamb, 1997). Fathers' emotional support tends to enhance the quality of mother–child relationships and facilitates positive adjustment by children, whereas when fathers are unsupportive and marital conflict is high, children suffer (Cummings & O'Reilly, 1997).

Fathers play an important role in children's play, which affects the quality of the child's attachment. Playful interactions involving emotional arousal provide an especially good opportunity to learn how to get along with peers, with fathers' modelling and reinforcing turn taking, affect regulation, and acceptable ways of competing, as well as the sports skills that facilitate acceptance into peer groups. Fathers are also important as role models who assist in their sons' identity formation and serve as models of gender-appropriate behaviour, particularly around aggressive behaviour (DeKlyen, Speltz, & Greenberg, 1998). Biller and Lopez-Kimpton's (1997) review of the literature found that children who have active, committed, and involved fathers generally perform better cognitively, academically, athletically, and socially than do children who do not benefit from such involvement. All these data support the importance of including the father in the mental health assessment of his child, whereas traditionally, the clinician has had contact only with the mother.

Disrupted Attachments

Disrupted attachments resulting from deficits in infant attachment behaviours, lack of responsiveness by caregivers to the child's cues, or both may lead to reactive attachment disorder, feeding disorder, failure to thrive, or anxiety disorder. A reactive attachment disorder is a state in which a child younger than 5 years of age fails to initiate or respond appropriately to social interaction and the caregiver subsequently disregards the child's physical and emotional needs. O'Connor and Rutter (2000) studied 163 adopted children with early severe deprivation at 4 years of age and again at 6 years of age. Longitudinal findings showed that attachment disorder behaviours were correlated with attention and conduct problems. Solomon and George (1999) reviewed the research on a new classification of attachment disorder titled attachment disorganization. **Attachment disorganization** is a consequence of extreme insecurity that results from feared or actual separation from the attached figure. Disorganized infants appear to be unable to maintain the strategic adjustments in attachment behaviour, represented by organized avoidant or ambivalent attachment strategies, with the result that an alteration in both behavioural and physiologic behaviour occurs. Frightening and frightened caregivers can contribute to disorganized attachment in infants. Preschoolers with disorganized attachment manifest behaviours of fear, contradictory behaviour, or disorientation or disassociation in the caregivers' presence.

Temperament and Behaviour

Temperament is a person's characteristic intensity, activity level, threshold of responsiveness, rhythmicity, adaptability, energy expenditure, and mood. According to research findings, temperamental differences can be observed early in life, suggesting that they are at least partly biologically determined, and patterns of temperament can be correlated with emotional and behavioural problems (Kagan et al., 1999). One basic aspect of temperament, the tendency to approach or avoid unfamiliar events, appears moderately stable over time and has been associated with distinct, apparently genetically based, physiologic profiles in 2-year-old children (Caspi & Silva, 1995; Schwartz, Snidman, & Kagan, 1999; Snidman, Kagan, Riordan, & Shannon, 1995). When looking at the cerebral asymmetry of the brain in children with inhibited compared with uninhibited temperaments, Davidson (1994) found that inhibited children in the third year of life showed greater electroencephalographic activation on the right frontal area under resting conditions.

The classic New York Longitudinal Study (Thomas, Chess, & Birch, 1968) identified three main patterns of temperament seen in infancy that often extend into childhood and later life:

- **Easy temperament**, characterized by a positive mood, regular patterns of eating and sleeping, positive approach to new situations, and low emotional intensity

- **Difficult temperament**, characterized by irregular sleep and eating patterns, negative response to new stimuli, slow adaptation, negative mood, and high emotional intensity
- **Slow-to-warm-up temperament**, characterized by a negative, mildly emotional response to new situations that is expressed with intensity and initially slow adaptation but evolves into a positive response

On the positive side, an easy temperament can serve as a protective factor against the development of psychopathology. Children with easy temperaments can adapt to change without intense emotional reactions. Difficult temperament places children at high risk for adjustment problems, such as with adjustment to school or bonding with parents.

Temperament has a major influence on the chances that a child may experience psychological problems; however, temperament is not unchangeable, and environmental influences can change or modify a child's emotional style. Kerr and coauthors (1964) found that temperament remained stable from childhood to adulthood only in those children who were extremely inhibited or uninhibited.

The concept of temperament provides an excellent example of the interaction between biologic–genetic and environmental factors in producing child psychopathology. Although a child may be born with a particular temperament, longitudinal studies show that the temperament itself is less influential than the "goodness of fit" (Chess & Thomas, 2002) between the child's temperament and the reactions of parents and significant others. Difficult children in particular may evoke negative reactions in parents and teachers, thereby creating environments that exacerbate their biologically based behaviour problems, initiating a vicious cycle. Vanden Boom and Hoeksma (1994) found that infants with difficult temperaments received less sensitive caring than did other children, and parents of 2-year-old children with difficult temperaments often resorted to angry, punitive discipline.

Most research in temperament has focussed on the child with a difficult temperament. Studies show that the difficult temperament is correlated with the development of child psychopathology, but only if such temperament persists beyond 3 years of age. Furthermore, the effects of a difficult temperament are more significant in psychiatric populations than in nonpsychiatric populations (Tubman, Lerner, Lerner, & Von Eye, 1992). Extremely difficult temperament shows an association with the development of oppositional and conduct disorders as well as ADHD (Dulcan & Martini, 1999; McClowry, 1995). McClowry developed a school-age temperament inventory (SATI) for parental report of children 8 to 11 years old. Four empirically derived dimensions were proposed: task persistence, negative reactivity, approach/withdrawal, and energy.

BOX 25.5

Social-Emotional Observation Worksheet

Name of child: _____ Date of birth: _____ Age: _____

Name of observer: _____ Discipline or job title: _____ Date of assessment: _____

On the following pages, note specific behaviours that document the child's abilities in the social-emotional categories. Qualitative comments should also be made. The format provided here follows that of the Observation Guidelines for Social-Emotional Development in Transdisciplinary Play-Based Assessment. It may be helpful to refer to the guidelines while completing this form.

1. Temperament
   A. Activity level
      1. Motor activity:
      2. Specific times that are particularly active
         a. Beginning, middle, or end:
         b. During specific activities:
   B. Adaptability
      1. Initial response to stimuli
         a. Persons:
         b. Situations:
         c. Toys:
      2. Demonstration of interest or withdrawal (*circle one*):
         a. Smiling, verbalizing, touching
         b. Crying, ignoring or moving away, seeking security
      3. Adjustment time:
      4. Adjustment time after initially shy or fearful response (*circle one*):
         a. Self-initiation   b. Adult as base of security   c. Resists; stays uninvolved
   C. Reactivity
      1. Intensity of stimuli for discernible response:
      2. Type of stimulation needed to interest child (*circle those that apply*):
         a. Visual, vocal, tactile, combination
         b. Object, social
      3. Level of affect and energy:
      4. Common response mode:
      5. Response to frustration:

From Linder, T. W. (1993). *Transdisciplinary play-based assessment: A functional approach to working with young children* (Revised ed.). Baltimore: Paul H. Brookes Publishing Co., Inc. Copyright © 1993 by Paul H. Brookes Publishing Co., Inc. Used with permission.

The nurses working with parents of young children need to understand temperament so that they can educate families about this concept, particularly because many parents of children with difficult temperaments blame themselves for their children's behaviour. Parents may compare the child with a difficult temperament to children with easier temperaments and wonder what they have done wrong or attribute negative motives to the child. The nurse can help parents accept biologically based differences in their children and learn to adapt their behaviour to each child's needs to improve "fit." Linder (1993) developed a worksheet to assist the clinician in evaluating the child's temperament during play that is divided into measures of activity level, adaptability, and reactivity (Box 25-5).

Self-Concept

For young children, eliciting their view of themselves and the world through projective techniques is helpful. For example, the nurse should ask them what they would

wish for if they had three wishes. Answers can be revealing. An inability to wish for anything beyond a nice meal or place to live may reflect hopelessness, whereas wishes to conquer the world or put one's teacher in jail may indicate feelings of grandiosity. Another technique is to tell a story and ask the child to make up an ending for it. For example, a baby bird fell out of a nest—what happened to it? ... or, a little girl went to the mall with her mother but got lost—what happened to her? The nurse may design stories to elicit particular fears or concerns that he or she suspects may be relevant for the individual child.

Drawings also provide an excellent window into the child's internal world (Fig. 25-2). Asking the child to draw a picture of a person can provide data about the child's self-concept, sexual identity, body image, and developmental level. By age 3 years, children should be able to draw some facial features and limbs, but their drawings may have an "x-ray" quality, in which clothing is transparent and the body can be seen underneath. Older children should produce more sophisticated

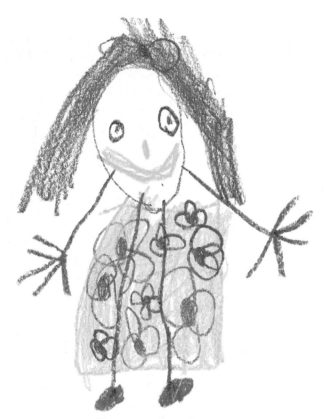

FIGURE 25.2 Self-portrait of a girl, age 5.

drawings, unless they are resistant to the task. After the child has finished the drawing, the nurse can ask what the person in the drawing is thinking and feeling, using this device to assess the child's mental processes. For example, one adolescent with school phobia drew a person fully dressed, in great detail, but with no feet. When asked about the drawing, he said that the boy could not go anywhere because his mother was afraid to let him leave home.

Other ways to assess children's self-concepts include asking them what they want to do when they grow up, what their best subjects are in school, what things they are really good at, and how well-liked they are at school. Before concluding the individual interview with a child, the nurse should always ask whether the child has any other information to share and whether he or she has any questions.

Risk Assessment

The nurse must ask the child about any suicidal or violent thoughts. The best way to assess these areas is to ask straightforward questions, such as, "Have you ever thought about hurting yourself? Have you ever thought about hurting someone else? Have you ever acted on these thoughts? Have you thought about how you would do it? What did you think would happen if you hurt yourself? Have you ever done anything to hurt yourself before?" Contrary to popular belief, talking about suicide with someone who can help can provide great relief to a child or youth. Further, no age should be exempt from assessment because even young children attempt suicide, and they are capable of violent acts toward other children, adults, and animals. When a child shares the intent to commit a suicidal or violent act, the nurse must remind him or her that the nurse will have to discuss this concern with the parent to keep the child and others safe. It is helpful to ask the child if he or she wants anything in particular said to the parent and if he or she wants to be present when the nurse talks with the parents. Although painful, such conversations can serve as an abrupt halt to the charade of happiness that the child may feel forced to portray to the outside world, and often opens honest dialogue within a family in which none has occurred for some time. Alternatively, the conversation can sometimes give words to what the family has long been fearing but lacks the skills or courage to break the silence. The nurse provides a safe environment for the family to begin to face the issues.

Substance use disorders across the life span account for more deaths, illness, and disabilities than any other preventable health condition. Screening for potential use and abuse of substances is becoming a priority in mental health assessment of adolescents. An interview guide has been adapted from questions on substance use developed by Adlaf (Adlaf & Zdanowicz, 1999) to serve as a useful screen for identifying substance use problems in youth. Given that many younger children engage in substance use (see Chapter 23), the nurse should also consider assessing younger children as well (Box 25-6).

Social Domain

Family Relationship

Children depend on adults to create a safe, nurturing, and appropriate environment to support their development. The nurse should assess the quality of the home in terms of its ability to provide appropriate physical space (living space, sleeping arrangements, safety, cleanliness), child care arrangements (age-appropriate supervision), and stimulation (activities or resources), either through a home visit or by discussing these issues with the family. The Home Observation for Measurement of the Environment (HOME) scale (Caldwell & Bradley, 1984) is a widely used, standardized measure to assess the quality of the home environment for fostering child development at any age according to cognitive, social, and emotional growth. It is a 45-item binary (yes/no) scale and best administered in the home through parent interview and observation. The scale addresses six areas: emotional and verbal responsivity of caregiver, avoidance of restriction and punishment, organization of the environment, provision of appropriate play

BOX 25.6

Practice Note 0.1: An Interview Protocol for Reviewing Chemical Use in Youths

As with other topics, questions about substance use are interactive—the answers given determine, to some extent, the subsequent questions. The questions can be used for investigating use of tobacco, alcohol, and drugs.

Tobacco

- Many youth smoke, do you?
- Do you ever feel you should smoke less?
- Do you wish you could smoke less than you do now?
- Have others bothered you by complaining about your smoking?
- Have you felt bad or guilty because of your smoking?
- Have you thought you had a problem because of your smoking?
- Have you ever had a medical problem as a result of your smoking?
- Have you been in hospital because of your smoking?
- Have you gone to anyone for help for a smoking problem?
- How many of your friends smoke occasionally/regularly?
- How many of your family smoke occasionally/regularly?

Alcohol

- Many youth drink, do you?
- Are you always able to stop drinking when you want?
- Have you felt you should drink less?
- Have others bothered you by complaining about your drinking?
- Have you felt bad or guilty because of your drinking?
- Have you been arrested or warned by police because of your drinking?
- Have you ever had "blackouts" or "flashbacks" due to your drinking?
- Have you drunk in the early morning or drunk to get rid of a hangover?
- Have you ever had any medical problem as a result of your drinking?
- Have you been in hospital because of your drinking?
- Have you gone to anyone for help for a drinking problem?
- How many of your friends drink occasionally/regularly?
- How many of your family drink occasionally/regularly?

Drugs

- Many youth use drugs, do you?
- Do you ever feel concerned about your drug use?
- Are you always able to stop using drugs when you want?
- Have you been arrested or warned by police because of your drug use?
- Have you ever had "blackouts" or "flashbacks" due to your drug use?
- Do you wish you could use fewer drugs than you do now?
- Have you ever had any medical problems as a result of your drug use?
- Have you gone to anyone for help for a drug problem?
- Have you ever seen a doctor or been in the hospital because of your drug use?
- How many of your friends use drugs occasionally/regularly?
- How many of your family use drugs occasionally/regularly?

Adapted from Adlaf, E. M., & Zdanowicz, Y. M. (1999). A cluster-analytic study of substance problems and mental health among street youths. American Journal of Drug and Alcohol Abuse, 25(4), 639–660.

material, caretaker involvement with child, and opportunities for variety in daily stimulation.

When gathering a family history, a genogram and timeline are also useful tools to map family members according to birth order and medical and psychiatric histories; family roles, norms, boundaries, strengths, and subgroups; birth dates, deaths, and relationships; stage in the family cycle; and critical events. To understand fully the family's values, goals, and beliefs, the nurse must consider the family's ethnic, cultural, and economic background throughout the assessment (Carter & McGoldrick, 1999). A comprehensive family assessment should be considered (see Chapter 15).

School and Peer Adjustment

The child's adjustment to school is also significant. Often, children are referred for a mental health assessment as a result of changes in behaviour at school. Falling grades, loss of interest in normal activities, decreased concentration, or withdrawal from or aggression toward peers may indicate that the child is experiencing emotional problems. It is very important that the nurse obtain signed permission from the parents to talk to the child's teacher for his or her observations of the child. The nurse may want to observe the child in school, if feasible, to see how the child functions there. The parent can request a treatment planning conference in which the teacher, parent, and nurse discuss the child's school performance and plan ways to promote the child's emotional, cognitive, and social functioning in school. For older children, and in particular youth, the nurse should include the child, if even for only a portion of the meeting. It is critically important that children feel that they are consulted and have an opportunity to participate in the planning processes. Although such involvement is not always comfortable or even desired by all parties, it provides formal recognition of each participant involved in the change process. Suggestions emanating from such panning sessions may range from having the child tested (eg, for learning disabilities) to designing strategies for addressing predictable situations that routinely dissolve into chaos, in which rewards result for each party (eg, extra computer time for the child, quiet time for the parent) for improved functioning.

Community

Assessing the child's economic status, access (psychologically, geographically, economically) to health and other services, housing and home environment, exposure to environmental toxins (eg, lead), neighbourhood safety, and exposure to violence is important in understanding the social context of children and families. Such assessment is also important given the evidence from large, longitudinal population-based studies that have demonstrated the links between social disadvantage (socioeconomic, residential stability, community efficacy and willingness to help neighbours) and mental illness in children (Xue, Levanthal, Brooks-Gunn, Earls, 2005) and adults (Fryers, Melzer, Jenkins, Brugha, 2005).

Children and adolescents function better if they are linked to community supports, such as churches, recreational programs, park district programming, and after-school programming. A number of voluntary organizations such as the YWCA or Big Brothers and Big Sisters offer mentoring relationship programs for children in communities. Before making a commitment, a family should visit the organization and talk with staff to ensure that the programs are well organized and monitored by trained staff. The mentor may perform a wide range of services, from taking a child to community events, helping with homework, or talking about how the child can achieve his or her dreams and goals. Some towns offer community-based juvenile justice programs to rehabilitate children who have had an altercation with the legal system. Juvenile justice programs provide support, such as individual and family counselling and prosocial recreational activities; teach children how to make positive choices about spending free time; and closely monitor their behaviours.

Functional Status

Functional status can be evaluated in children and adolescents using such scales as the Global Assessment of Functioning (GAF) scale, which tallies behaviours related to school, peers, activity level, mood, speech, family relationships, behavioural problems, self-care skills, and self-concept. The GAF scale ranges from 0 to 100; the lower the score, the higher the level of impairment, indicated by psychiatric symptoms and level of general functioning. For example, a score of 30 may indicate that the child is severely homicidal or suicidal and has made previous attempts; that hallucinations or delusions influence the child's behaviour; or that the child has serious impairment in communication or judgment. Moderate impairment scores usually fall in the range of 51 to 69. Indications of moderate impairment include difficulty in one area, such as school phobia, that hinders school attendance or performance, while the child is functioning well within other areas, such as with family and peers. Children in this category are not homicidal or suicidal and usually respond well to outpatient interventions. A score of 70 to 100 usually indicates that the child is functioning well in relation to school, peers, family, and community. The GAF is always measured at the initial assessment so that treatment can be evaluated over time in terms of symptom improvement.

Stresses and Coping Behaviours

Biologic, behavioural, and personality predispositions, family, and community environment may affect a child's ability to cope with stressful life events. Stressful experiences for children include the death of a loved person or pet, parental divorce, violence, physical illness (especially chronic illness), mental illness, social isolation, racial discrimination, neglect, and physical and sexual abuse. The Difficult Life Circumstances (DLC) scale (Barnard, 1989) is a 28-item self-report measure, administered in interview format to a parent, to identify the existence of chronic family problems in a variety of activities of daily life (eg, partner in jail, financial problems, partner or child abuse).

Evaluation of Child Abuse

Thousands of Canadian children suffer maltreatment (intentional physical or emotional abuse, neglect, or sexual exploitation) each year as the result of their parents' action or inaction (Trocmé, McPhee, & Tam, 1995; Wolfe, 1998). The 2003 Canadian Incidence Study of Reported Child Abuse and Neglect (Trocmé, Fallon, 2005) revealed an incidence rate of 21.71 substantiated investigations per 1,000 children in 2003. The three most common categories of substantiated maltreatment comprised neglect (30%), exposure to domestic violence (28%), and physical abuse (24%). Emotional maltreatment accounted for another 15% of cases, whereas sexual abuse cases represented only 3% of all substantiated investigations. Most cases (52%) involved children living in two-parent families, and most referrals (75%) came from professionals (police and school).

The effects of family-engendered maltreatment can result in a lifetime of debilitating biopsychosocial-related problems. A maltreated child may have difficulty managing emotions (Campbell, 1995), communicating effectively (Browne & Sagi, 1988), developing satisfying relationships with others (Crittenden, 1996), and learning in productive ways (Aber, Allen, Carlson, & Cicchetti, 1990; Doherty, 1997). Consequently, there is increasing awareness among Canadian policy makers (Canadian Council on Social Development, 1997; Edwards, 1999; King & Coles, 1992; Steinhauer, 1998; Wolfe, 1998) of the need for child maltreatment policy to concentrate more on ways of building child competence, resilience, and health potential (ie, autonomous self-regulation) (Wolfe, 1998) than simply on issues of protection and deviance.

Although the cause of child abuse is not absolutely clear, best thinking suggests that an ecological model better captures the influencing factors of child abuse and neglect because it understands the child within the context of the family and the larger community (Wachtel, 1999). Such a model uses a broad multifactorial approach for assessment. Such assessment takes into consideration the child's current developmental level and understands that compromises to his or her early development may continue in various ways through all the developmental stages that follow. It is child centred (child welfare is critical), family focussed (most child abuse occurs within the family), has a community context (forms a key part of the child's environment), and is culturally sensitive (the nurse must be culturally competent). It also involves gathering information from a number of stakeholders and ensures that information is gathered in a coordinated way to maximize the integrity of the data collection.

Although a number of assessment tools exist, three general areas should be addressed in any assessment (English, 1996):

1. Are the child's immediate circumstances unsafe? Does the child have to be taken into care or removed to a safe place?
2. For current cases, what is the assessed risk of repeat abuse? What are the issues that merit intervention on a priority basis?
3. For ongoing cases, to what extent are interventions working? What is the current situation of the child, the family, and any substitute care arrangement?

There are several special considerations in interviewing an abused child. First, the nurse must establish a safe and supportive environment in which to conduct the evaluation. Second, the nurse needs to understand the forensic implications of assessment, so that the interview format will be acceptable for disclosure in a court hearing. The Canadian Psychiatric Association (1992) offers practice guidelines for evaluating children who may have been abused. The *Standards of Psychiatric and Mental Health Nursing Practice* (CFMHN, 2005) also identifies a nurse's role in assessing clients for risk of victim violence and abuse. The American Academy of Child and Adolescent Psychiatry (1997) offers practice guidelines for evaluating children who may have been abused. If the child reports abuse, the nurse has a legal responsibility to report the abuse to the child protection agencies. The nurse must use the same language and vocabulary that the child uses to describe the abuse, or anatomical terms, and ask nonleading questions. Nursing professionals who regularly interview children who have been abused may have special training in the use of anatomically correct dolls to obtain information about the abuse.

In the case of family-perpetrated child abuse, the nurse should consider very carefully whether the report will be made *with* or *without* the knowledge of the child's family. The nurse should consider factors such as whether she or he has developed a relationship with the family, the degree of imminent risk to the child, and whether she or he is likely to continue working with the family. The reality is that maltreatment is a complex phenomenon, and families tend to stay connected with services for long periods. Finding ways to build a positive working relationship with families becomes a crucial, yet challenging, goal for nurses. When nurses are open, honest, and direct, families know what to expect. If nurses have an established working relationship with families, they can often share their specific observations about parenting practices and the need to involve child protection services. Nurses might also invite the family to make the call themselves with the nurse's support. For example, the nurse might say, "I know that you love your child but your actions are causing harm ... I don't think your child is safe ... He needs help... I need to call child protection services to get some help for your family. I know this is scary for you ... but you could take an important step in the right direction by making the first call and asking for help for your child and you. I would be happy to support you while you make that call right now ... before I make my call."

Evaluation of Childhood Sexual Abuse

The use of anatomically correct dolls is beneficial because it does not overstimulate or distress the child, assists in identifying and naming specific body parts, increases verbal productivity during the examination, helps to prompt memory, and is useful with immature, language-impaired,

BOX 25.7

Assessing Possible Sexual Abuse of a Child

1. Have you ever been touched on any part of your body?
2. Have you ever touched a part on anybody else's body?
3. Have you ever been hurt on any part of your body?
4. Have you ever hurt a part on anybody else's body?
5. Has anyone done something you didn't like to your body?
6. Have you ever been asked to do something you didn't like to someone else's body?
7. Has anyone put anything on or in any part of your body?
8. Have you ever been without your clothes?
9. Has anyone else asked you to take off your clothes?
10. Have you seen anyone else without clothes?
11. Has anyone asked you not to tell something about your body?
12. Has anyone said that something bad might happen to you or to someone else if you told some secret about your body?
13. Has anyone ever kissed you?
14. Has anyone ever kissed you when you didn't want them to?
15. Has anyone ever taken your picture?
16. Has anyone ever taken your picture without your clothes on?

From White, S. (2000). Using anatomically detailed dolls in interviewing preschoolers. In K. Gitlin-Weiner, A. Sandgrund, & C. Schaefer (Eds.), *Play diagnosis and assessment* (2nd ed., pp. 210–227). New York: Wiley & Sons, Inc. Used with permission.

or cognitively delayed children (Cepeda, 2000). White (2000) provides a detailed chapter on the use of these dolls in interviewing preschoolers. Some questions that may be asked in forensic evaluation of a child for sexual abuse are presented in Box 25-7.

Risk and Protective Factors

The number of stressful events that a child experiences, the supports that the child has in place, and the child's developmental stage may also influence his or her ability to cope with stressors. Werner (1989) performed a longitudinal study of 500 Hawaiian youths considered to be at high risk for mental health problems because they were born into poverty, homelessness, or families whose parents had little education or were alcoholic, mentally ill, or headed by a single parent. Other risk factors included low birth weight, difficult temperament, mental retardation, childhood trauma, exposure to racism, poor schools, and community and domestic violence. One third of the children born at risk did not experience mental health problems by age 18 years. Protective factors that were identified in these children were:

- Individual attributes, such as resilience, problem-solving skills, sense of self-efficacy, accurate processing of interpersonal cues, positive social orientation, and activity level
- A supportive family environment, including attachment with adults in the family, low family conflict, and supportive relationships
- Environmental supports, including those that reinforce and support coping efforts and recognize and reward competence.

Doll's and Lyon's (1998) review of the literature about resilience found that children who show resilience in the face of adversity typically have good intellectual functioning, positive and easygoing temperament, positive social orientation, strong self-efficacy, achievement orientation with high expectations, positive self-concept, faith, high rate of involvement in productive activities, close affective relationship with at least one caregiver, effective parenting, access to positive extrafamilial models, and strong connections with prosocial institutions. Similarly, Steinhausen's (2006) longitudinal study of the determinants and processes of mental disorders in adolescence identified that self-esteem, active coping, parental warmth, and peer acceptance, in different combinations, acted as protective factors against internalizing and externalizing mental disorders.

SUMMARY OF KEY POINTS

- Mental health assessment of children and adolescents includes evaluating the child's biologic, psychological, and social factors.
- Assessment of children and adolescents differs from assessment of adults in that the nurse must consider the child's developmental level, specifically addressing the child's language, cognitive, social, and emotional skills. Establishing a treatment alliance and building rapport are essential to obtaining a good mental health history.
- The mental status examination includes observations and questions about the child's appearance, speech, language, vocabulary, orientation, knowledge base (including reading, writing, and math skills), attention level, activity level, memory, social skills, peer relationships, relationship to interviewer, mood, affect, suicidal or homicidal tendencies, thinking (presence or absence of hallucinations or delusions), substance use, and behaviours.
- Assessment of the child and caregiver together provides important information regarding child–parent attachment and parenting practices.
- The three main types of temperament include the easy temperament, difficult temperament, and slow-to-warm-up temperament. Temperament can be evaluated by assessing the child's sleep and eating habits, mood, emotional intensity, and responses to new stimuli.

■ A child's self-concept can be evaluated using tools such as play, stories, asking three wishes, and asking the child to draw a picture of himself or herself.

■ If a child reveals suicidal ideation in the interview, the nurse must determine whether the child has a plan, let the parent know the child is suicidal, and make a plan to keep the child safe, including consideration of inpatient hospitalization.

■ If a child reports to the nurse neglect or physical or sexual abuse, the nurse must by law report the child's disclosure to Child Protection Services.

■ Protective factors that promote resiliency in children are active coping and the ability to problem solve, a sense of self-efficacy, self-esteem, accurate processing of social cues, supportive family environment, peer acceptance, and environmental supports that promote coping efforts and recognize and reward competence.

CRITICAL THINKING CHALLENGES

1 An adolescent is hostile and refuses to talk in an interview. How would you respond?

2 What are some strategies for building rapport with children?

3 A child reports that he is suicidal. What would be your next question? What measures would you take next?

4 What are some techniques and media for obtaining information about a child's inner world, such as self-concept, sexual identity, body image, and developmental level?

5 Explain why it may be detrimental to interview a child in front of his or her parent. Why may it be detrimental to interview a parent in front of his or her child? Why is it useful, in most cases, to ensure that both parent and child are also interviewed together?

6 Why is obtaining the mental health histories of parents relevant to the child's mental health assessment?

7 What are useful tools in obtaining a family history from the child and parent?

8 Anatomically correct dolls are used in what specific type of child assessment?

9 Describe five characteristics of the resilient child.

WEB LINKS

www.cfc-efc.ca This website of Child and Family Canada is a unique Canadian public education representing 50 Canadian nonprofit organizations. This easy-to-navigate website provides quality, credible resources on children and families.

www.cich.ca The Canadian Institute of Child Health (CICH) is the only national charitable organization dedicated solely to improving the health of children and youth in Canada. It has three main functions: monitoring children's health; educating professionals, caregivers, and policy makers; and advocating for legislation and policies that improve child health.

www.nncc.org The website of the **National Network for Child Care** gives detailed accounts of expected developmental milestones from birth through adulthood and links to numerous articles on child development and parenting.

www.aacap.org The website of the American Academy of Child and Adolescent Psychiatry provides an exhaustive list of links to short articles on many mental health issues and is geared toward families and consumers.

www.phac-aspc.gc.ca/ncfv-cnivf/familyviolence National Clearing House for Family Violence. Public Health Agency of Canada. The NCFV is Canada's resource centre for information on violence within relationships of kinship, intimacy, dependency or trust.

REFERENCES

Aber, J. L., Allen, J. P., Carlson, V., & Cicchetti, D. (1989). The effects of maltreatment on development during early childhood: Recent studies and their theoretical, clinical, and policy implications. In D. Cicchetti & V. Carlson (Eds.), *Child maltreatment: Theory and research on the causes and consequences of child abuse and neglect* (pp. 570–619). New York: Cambridge University Press.

Achenbach, T. M., & Edelbrock, C. (1983). *The Child Behavior Checklist: Manual for the child behavior checklist and revised child behavior profile*. Burlington, VT: Queen City Printers.

Adlaf, E. M., & Zdanowicz, Y. M. (1999). A cluster-analytic study of substance problems and mental health among street youths. *American Journal of Drug and Alcohol Abuse, 25*(4), 639–660.

Ainsworth, M. D. S. (1989). Attachments beyond infancy. *American Psychologist, 44*, 709–716.

American Academy of Child and Adolescent Psychiatry. (1997). Practice parameters for the forensic evaluation of children and adolescents who may have been physically or sexually abused. *Journal of the American Academy of Child and Adolescent Psychiatry, 36*(10 Suppl), 37S–56S.

American Nurses Association. (2000). *Statement on psychiatric–mental health clinical practice and standards of psychiatric–mental health clinical nursing practice*. Washington, DC: American Nurses Publishing.

American Psychiatric Association. (2000). *Diagnostic and statistical manual of mental health disorders* (4th ed., Text revision). Washington, DC: Author.

Armbruster, P. (2002). The administration of school-based mental health services. *Child and Adolescent Psychiatric Clinics of North America, 11*(1), 23–41.

Ayliffe, L., Lagace, C., & Muldoon, P. (2005). The use of a mental health triage assessment tool in a busy Canadian tertiary care children's hospital. *Journal of Emergency Nursing, 31*(2), 161–165.

Baker J. K., Borchers, D. A., Cochran, D. T., et al. (1994). Parent–child interaction model (of Kathryn Barnard). In A. Marriner-Tomey (Ed.), *Nursing theorists and their work*. St. Louis: Mosby.

Barnard, K. E. (1994). The Barnard model. In G. Sumner, & A. Spitz, *NCAST caregiver/parent–child interaction feeding manual* (pp. 6–14). Seattle: NCAST Publications, University of Washington, School of Nursing.

Barnard, K. B. (1989). *Difficult life circumstances manual*. Seattle: NCAST Publications, University of Washington, School of Nursing.

Beitchman, J. H., Cohen, N. J., Konstantareas, M. M., & Tannock, R. (Eds.). (1996). *Language, learning, and behavior disorders: Developmental, biological, and clinical perspectives.* New York: Cambridge University Press.

Biller, H., & Lopez-Kimpton, J. (1997). The father and the school-aged child. In M. Lamb (Ed.), *The role of the father in child development* (3rd ed., pp. 143–161). New York: Wiley & Sons.

Blais, R., Breton, J. J., Fournier, M., St-Georges, M., & Berthiaume, C. (2003). Are mental health services for children distributed according to needs? *Canadian Journal of Psychiatry, 48*(3), 176–186.

Blyth, D. A., & Leffert, N. (1995). Communities as contexts for adolescent development: An empirical analysis. *Journal of Adolescent Research, 10*(1), 64–87.

Bowlby, J. (1969). *Attachment* (Vol. 1 of *Attachment and loss*). New York: Basic Books.

Breton, J. J., Plante, M. A., & St-Georges, M. (2005). Challenges facing child psychiatry in Quebec at the dawn of the 21st century. *Canadian Journal of Psychiatry, 50*(4), 203–212.

Bricker, D., & Squires, J. (1999). The effectiveness of screening at-risk infants: Infant Monitoring Questionnaire. *Topics in Early Special Education, 3*, 67–85.

Bronfenbrenner, U. (1986). Ecology of the family as a context for human development: Research perspectives. *Developmental Psychology, 22*, 723–742.

Browne, K., & Saqi, S. (1988). Approaches to screening for child abuse and neglect. In K. Browne, C. Davies, & P. Stratton (Eds.), *Early prediction and prevention of child abuse* (pp. 57–85). Toronto: John Wiley & Sons.

Caldwell, B., & Bradley, R. (1984). *Home observation for measurement of the environment.* Little Rock, AK: University of Little Rock at Arkansas.

Campbell, S. (1995). Behaviour problems in pre-school children: A review of recent research. *Journal of Child Psychiatry, 36*, 113–149.

Canadian Council on Social Development. (1997). Safer communities: A social strategy for crime prevention in Canada. *Canadian Journal of Criminology, 31*, 359–401.

Canadian Federation of Mental Health Nurses. (2005). *The standards of psychiatric and mental health nursing practice* (3rd ed.). http://www.cfmhn.org/standards.html.

Canadian Psychiatric Association. (1992). *Guidelines for the evaluation and management of family violence.* http://www.epa-apc.org/publications/position-papers/violence.asp

Cantwell, D. P., & Baker, L. (1991). *Psychiatric and developmental disorders in children with communication disorders.* Washington, DC: American Psychiatric Press.

Carter, A. S., Briggs-Gowan, M. J., & Davis, N. O. (2004). Assessment of young children's social-emotional development and psychopathology: Recent advances and recommendations for practice. *Journal of Child Psychology and Psychiatry, 45*(1), 109–134.

Carter, B., & McGoldrick, M. (1999). *The expanded family life cycle: Individual, family, and social perspectives* (3rd ed.). Needham Heights, MA: Allyn & Bacon.

Caspi, A., & Silva, P. A. (1995). Temperamental qualities at age 3 predict personality traits in young adulthood: Longitudinal evidence from a birth cohort. *Child Development, 66*, 486–498.

Cepeda, C. (2000). *The concise guide to the psychiatric interview of children and adolescents.* Washington, DC: American Psychiatric Press.

Chess, S., & Thomas, A. (2002). Temperament and its clinical applications. In M. Lewis (Ed.), *Child and adolescent psychiatry: A comprehensive textbook* (3rd ed.). Philadelphia: Lippincott, Williams & Wilkins.

Costello, E. J., Egger, H., & Angold, A. (2005). Ten-year research update review: The epidemiology of child and adolescent psychiatric disorders. I. Methods and public health burden. *Journal of American Academy of Child and Adolescent Psychiatry, 44*(10), 972–986.

Costello, E. J., Keeler, G. P., & Angold, A. (2001). Poverty, race/ethnicity, and psychiatric disorder: A study of rural children. *American Journal of Public Health, 91*(9), 1494–1498.

Crittenden, P. M. (1996). Research on maltreating families: Implications for intervention. In J. Briere, L. Berliner, A. Bulkey, C. Jenny, & T. Reid (Eds.), *The APSAC handbook on child maltreatment* (pp. 158–174). Thousand Oaks, CA: Sage.

Cummings, E. M., & O'Reilly, A. (1997). Fathers in family context: Effects of marital quality on child adjustment. In M. Lamb (Ed.), *The role of the father in child development* (3rd ed.). New York: Wiley.

Davidson, R. J. (1994). Asymmetric brain function, affective style, and psychopathology. *Developmental Psychopathology, 6*, 741–758.

DeKlyen, M., Speltz, M., & Greenberg, M. (1998). Fathering and early onset conduct problems: Positive and negative parenting, father–son attachment, and the marital context. *Child and Family Psychology Review, 1*, 3–21.

Doherty, G. (1997). *Zero to six: The basis for school readiness.* Ottawa, Canada: Human Resources Development Canada, Applied Research Branch, Strategic Policy.

Doll, B., & Lyon, M. A. (1998). Risk and resilience: Implications for delivery of educational and mental health services in the schools. *School Psychology Review, 27*(3), 348–363.

Doyle, A., Markiewicz, D., Brendgen, M., Lieberman, M., & Voss, K. (2000). Child attachment security and self-concept: Associations with mother and father attachment style and marital quality. *Merrill-Palmer Quarterly, 46*(3), 514–539.

Dulcan, M., & Martini, D. R. (1999). *Child and adolescent psychiatry.* Washington, DC: American Psychiatric Press.

Eagly, A. H., Ashmore, R. D., Makhijani, M. G., & Kennedy, L. (1991). What is beautiful is good, but . . . : A meta-analytic review of research on physical attractiveness stereotype. *Psychological Bulletin, 110*, 109–128.

Edwards, P. (1999). *Fostering knowledge development on the health and well-being of children in Canada: A division paper.* Prepared for Health Canada and the Interim National Expert Advisory Committee for the Centres of Excellence for Children's Well-being.

Egger, H. L., Ascher, B. H., & Angold, A. (1999). *Pre-school Age Psychiatric Assessment: Version 1.1 (unpublished interview schedule).* Center for Developmental Epidemiology, Department of Psychiatry and Behavioral Sciences, Duke University Medical Center.

English, D. T. (1996). The promise and reality of risk assessment: protecting children. Ottawa, ON: Public Health Agency of Canada. Retrieved November 21, 2005, from http://www.phac-aspc.gc.ca/ncfv-cnivf/familyviolence/html/ nfntsptprevention_e.html.

Ezpeleta, L., Keeler, G., Erkanli, A., Costello, E. J., & Angold, A. (2001). Epidemiology of psychiatric disability in childhood and adolescence. *Journal of Child Psychology and Psychiatry, 42*(7), 901–914.

Forgatch, M., & Patterson, G. (1989). *Parents and adolescents: Living together (Part 2: Family problem-solving).* Eugene, OR: Castalia Publishing Company.

Fryers, T., Melzer, D., Jenkins, R., & Brugha T. (2005, Sept. 5). The distribution of the common mental disorders: Social inequalities in Europe. *Clinical Practice in Epidemiology and Mental Health, 1*, 14.

Garcia-Coll, C., & Magnuson, K. (2000). Cultural differences as sources of developmental vulnerabilities and resources. In J. P. Shonkoff & S. J. Meisels (Eds.), *Handbook of early education intervention* (2nd ed., pp. 94–114). New York: Cambridge University Press.

Global Assessment of Functioning (GAF). (1994). *American Psychiatric Association. Diagnostic and statistical manual of mental disorders* (4th ed., Text revision). Washington, DC: American Psychiatric Association.

Goodman, W. K., Price, L. H., Rasmussen, S. A., Mazure, J. C., Fleischmann, R. L., Hill, C. L., Heninger, G. R., & Charney, D. S. (1989). The Children's Yale-Brown Obsessive Compulsive Scale (CYBOCS). I. Development, use, and reliability. *Archives of General Psychiatry, 46*, 1006–1011.

Grollman, E. A. (1990). *Talking about death: A dialogue between parent and child* (3rd ed.). Boston: Beacon Press.

Harlow, H. F., Harlow, M. K., & Suomi, S. J. (1971). From thought to therapy: Lessons from a private laboratory. *American Scientist, 59*(5), 538–549.

Health Canada. (2002). *A report on mental illness in Canada.* Cat. 0-662-32817-5. Ottawa: Author.

Hill, C. E., & O'Brien, K. M. (1999). *Helping skills: Facilitating exploration, insight and action.* Washington, DC: American Psychological Association.

Horwitz, S. M., Hoagwood, K., Stiffman, A. R., Summerfeld, T., Weisz, J. R., Costello, E. J., Rost, K., Bean, D. L., Cottler, L., Leaf, P. J., Roper, M., & Norquist, G. (2001). Reliability of the services assessment for children and adolescents. *Psychiatry Services, 52*(8), 1088–1094.

House, A. (2002). *The first session with children and adolescents: Conducting a comprehensive mental health evaluation.* New York: Guilford Press.

Howes, C., & Matheson, C. (1992). Sequences in the development of competent play with peers: Social and social pretend play. *Developmental Psychology, 28*(5), 961–974.

Jellnick, M., Patel, B. P., & Froehle, M. C. (2003). Bright futures in practice: Mental health (Vol. 1, practice guide and Vol. 2, tool kit). *Journal of the American Academy of Child and Adolescent Psychiatry, 1–2,* 507–508.

Jensen, P., Rubio-Stipac, M., Carnio, G., et al. (1999). Parents and child contributions to diagnosis of mental disorder: Are both informants always necessary? *Journal of the American Academy of Child and Adolescent Psychiatry, 38*(12), 1569–1579.

John, L. H., Offord, D. R., Boyle, M. H., & Racine, Y. A. (1995). Factors predicting use of mental health and social services by children 6–16 years old: Findings from the Ontario Child Health Study. *American Journal of Orthopsychiatry, 65*(1), 76–86.

Kagan, J. (1999). The concept of behavioral inhibition. In L. Schmidt & J. Schulkin (Eds.), *Extreme fear, shyness, and social phobia: Origins, biological mechanisms, and clinical outcomes. Series in affective science.* New York: Oxford University Press.

Kaufman, J., & Cicchetti, D. (1989). Effects of maltreatment on school-aged children's socioemotional development: Assessment in a day-camp setting. *Developmental Psychology, 25,* 516–524.

Kerr WA, Mcgehee EM. (1964). Creative temperament as related to aspects of strategy and intelligence. *Journal of Social Psychology. 62*:211–216.

King, A., & Coles, B. (1992). *The health of Canada's youth.* Ottawa, Canada: Health and Welfare Canada.

Kovacs, M. (1982). *Children's depression inventory.* North Tonawanda, NY: Multi-Health Systems.

Lamb, M. E. (Ed.). (1997). *The role of the father in child development* (3rd ed.). New York: Wiley & Sons.

Le Buffe, P. A., & Naglievi, J. (1999). *Devereux early childhood assessment. The Devereux Foundation.* Lewisville, NC: Kaplan Press.

LeBuffe, P. A., & Naglieri, J. A. (2003). *The Devereux early childhood assessment clinical form (DECA).* Lewisville, NC: Kaplan Press.

Lee, K. A., & Ward, T. M. (2005). Critical components of a sleep assessment for clinical practice settings. *Issues of Mental Health Nursing, 26*(7), 739–750.

Lewis, M. (1996). Psychiatric assessment of infants, children and adolescents. In M. Lewis (Ed.), *Child and adolescent psychiatry: A comprehensive textbook* (2nd ed.). Baltimore: Williams & Wilkins.

Lidz, C. S. (2003). *Early childhood assessment.* Hoboken, NJ: Wiley & Sons.

Linder, T. W. (1993). *Transdisciplinary play-based assessment: A functional approach to working with young children* (Revised ed.). Baltimore: Paul H. Brookes Publishing.

MacMillan, H. L. (2000). Canadian Task Force on Preventive Health Care. Preventive health care, 2000 update: Prevention of child maltreatment. *Canadian Medical Association Journal, 163*(11), 1451–1458.

March, J. (1997). *Multidimensional anxiety scale for children.* North Tonawanda, NY: Multi-Health Systems.

McClowry, S. G. (1995). The development of the School-Age Temperament Inventory. *Merrill-Palmer Quarterly, 41*(3), 271–285.

Moore-Taylor, K. M., Menarchek-Fetkovich, M., & Day, C. (2000). In K. Gitlin-Weiner, A. Sandgrund, & C. Scafer (Eds.), *The play history, interview play diagnosis and assessment* (2nd ed.) New York: Wiley.

Murphy, J. M., Ichinose, C., Hicks, R. C., Kingdon, D., Crist-Whitzel, J., Jordan, P., Fieldman, G., & Jellnick, MS. (1996). Utility of the pediatric symptom checklist as a psychosocial screen to meet the federal Early and Periodic Screening, Diagnosis, and Treatment (EPSDT) standards: A pilot study. *Journal of Pediatrics, 129,* 864–869.

National Cancer Institute, US National Institutes of Health. (2005). Supportive care around bereavement. Retrieved November 7, 2005, from http://www.cancer.gov/cancertopics/pdq/supportive-care/bereavement/HealthProfessional/page8#Section_83.

O'Connor, T., & Rutter, M. (2000). Attachment disorder behavior following early severe deprivation: Extension and longitudinal follow-up. *Journal of the American Academy of Child and Adolescent Psychiatry, 39*(6), 709–712.

Olfson, M., Gameroff, M. J., Marcus, S. C., Greenberg, T., & Shaffer, D. (2005). Emergency treatment of young people following deliberate self-harm. *Archives of General Psychiatry, 62*(10), 1122–1128.

Plutchik, R. (2000). *Emotions in the practice of psychotherapy.* Washington, DC: American Psychological Association.

Reynolds, C. R., & Kamphouse, R. W. (1998). *Behavior assessment system for children (BASC).* Circle Pines, MN: American Guidance Service.

Roebuck, T. M., Mattson, S. N., & Riley, E. P. (1999). Behavioural and psychosocial profiles of alcohol-exposed children. *Alcoholism: Clinical and Experimental Research, 23*(6), 1070–1076.

Research Unit on Pediatric Psychopharmacology (RUPP) Anxiety Study Group (2002), The pediatric anxiety rating scale (PARS): development and psychometric properties. *Journal of the American Academy of Child and Adolescent Psychiatry* 41:1061–1069.

Rutter, M., Silberg, J., O'Connor, T., & Simonoff, E. (1999). Genetics and child psychiatry. I. Advances in qualitative and molecular genetics. *Journal of Psychological Psychiatry, 40,* 3–18.

Sameroff, A., & Chandler, M. (1975). Transactional models in early social relations. *Human Development, 18,* 65–79.

Sameroff, A. J. (2000). Dialectical processes in developmental psychopathology. In A. J. Sameroff, M. L. Lewis, & S. M. Miller (Eds.), *Handbook of developmental psychopathology* (2nd ed., pp. 23–40). New York: Kluwer Academic.

Sattler, J. (1998). *Clinical and forensic interviewing of children and families.* San Diego: Jerome Sattler Publisher.

Schwartz, C., Snidman, N., & Kagan, J. (1999). Adolescent social anxiety as an outcome of inhibited temperament in childhood. *Journal of the American Academy of Child and Adolescent Psychiatry, 38*(8), 1008–1015.

Seifer, R. (2000). Temperament and goodness of fit: Implications for developmental psychopathology. In A. J. Sameroff, M. L. Lewis, & S. M. Miller (Eds.), *Handbook of developmental psychopathology* (pp. 257–276). New York: Kluwer Academic.

Shave, D., & Shave, B. (1989). *Early adolescence and search for self: A developmental perspective.* New York: Praeger Publishers.

Sheldon, C. T., Aubry, T. D., Arboleda-Florez, J., Wasylenki, D., & Goering, P. N. (2005, Dec. 7). CMHEI Working Group. Social disadvantage, mental illness and predictors of legal involvement. *International Journal of Law and Psychiatry.*

Smith, D. H., & Hadorn, D. C. (2002). Steering Committee of the Western Canada Waiting List Project. Lining up for children's mental health services: A tool for prioritizing waiting lists. *Journal of American Academy of Child and Adolescent Psychiatry, 41*(4), 367–376; discussion, 376–377.

Snidman, N., Kagan, J., Riordan, L., & Shannon, D. C. (1995). Cardiac function and behavioural reactivity. *Psychopathology, 32,* 199–207.

Solomon, J., & George, C. (1999). *Attachment disorganization.* New York: Guilford Press.

Squires, J., Bricker, D., & Twombly, E. (2002). *The ASQ: SE user's guide.* Baltimore: Paul H. Brookes Publishing.

State, M., Lombroso, P., Pauls, D., & Leckman, J. (2000). The genetics of childhood psychiatric disorders: A decade of progress. *Journal of the American Academy of Child and Adolescent Psychiatry, 39*(8), 946–962.

Steinhausen HC. (2006). Developmental psychopathology in adolescence: findings from a Swiss study--the NAPE Lecture 2005. *Acta Psychiatr Scand.* 113(1):6–12.

Steinhauer, P. D. (1998). *Developing resiliency in children from disadvantaged populations.* Ottawa: Health Canada.

Stiffman, A. R., Hadley-Ives, E., Dore, P., Polgar, M., Horvath, V. E., Striley, C., & Elze, D. (2000). Youths' access to mental health services: The role of providers' training, resource connectivity, and assessment of need. *Mental Health Services Research, 2*(3), 141–154.

Sturm, R., Ringel, J. S., & Andreyeva, T. (2003). Geographic disparities in children's mental health care. *Pediatrics, 112*(4), e308.

Swanson, J. M. (1983). *The SNAP-IV.* Irvine, CA: University of California, Irvine.

Swartz, H. A., Shear, M. K., Wren, F. J., Greene, C. G., Sales E., Sullivan, B. K., & Ludewig, D. P. (2005) Depression and anxiety among mothers who bring their children to a pediatric mental health clinic. *Psychiatric Services, 56*(9), 1077–1083.

Tanguay, P. (2000). Pervasive developmental disorders: A 10-year review. *Journal of the American Academy of Child and Adolescent Psychiatry, 39,* 1079–1095.

Teplin, L. A., Abram, K. M., McClelland, G. M., Washburn, J. J., & Pikus, A. K. (2005). Detecting mental disorder in juvenile detainees: Who receives services. *American Journal of Public Health, 95*(10), 1773–1780.

Thomas, A., Chess, S., & Birch, H. G. (1968). *Temperament and behavior disorders in childhood.* New York: New York University Press.

Thompson, R. (2002). Attachment theory and research. In: M. Lewis (Ed.), *Child and adolescent psychiatry: A comprehensive textbook* (3rd ed.). Philadelphia: Lippincott, Williams & Wilkins.

Trad, P. (1989). *The pre-school child assessment, diagnosis and treatment.* New York: Wiley.

Trainor, J., Pomeroy, E. & Pape, B. (2004). *A framework for support.* (3rd ed.). Toronto: Canadian Mental Health Association.

Trocmé, N., Fallon, B., MacLaurin B., Daciuk, J., Felstiner, C. Black, T., et al. (2005) *Canadian incidence study of reported child abuse and neglect 2003: Major findings.* Ottawa: Minister of Public Works and Government Services Canada.

Trocmé, N., McPhee, D., & Tam, K. K. (1995). Child abuse and neglect in Ontario: Incidence and characteristics. *Child Welfare, 74,* 563–586.

Tubman, J. G., Lerner, R. M., Lerner, J. V., & Von Eye, A. (1992). Temperament and adjustment in young adulthood: A 15-year longitudinal analysis. *American Journal of Orthopsychiatry, 62,* 564–574.

Vanden Boom, D. C., & Hoeksma, J. B. (1994). The effect of infant irritability on mother–infant interaction: A growth curve analysis. *Developmental Psychology, 30,* 581–590.

Wachtel, A. (1999). *"State of the art" in child abuse prevention.* Prepared for the Family Violence Prevention Unit, Health Canada. Cat. H72-21/151-1997E. Ottawa: Minister of Public Works and Government Services Canada, National Clearing House on Family Violence.

Waddell, C., McEwan, K., Shepherd, C. A., Offord, D. R., & Hua, J. M.. (2005). A public health strategy to improve the mental health of Canadian children. *Canadian Journal of Psychiatry, 50*(4), 226–233.

Wass, H., & Corr, C. A. (1984). *Childhood and death.* Washington, DC: Hemisphere Publishing.

Werner, E. E. (1989). High-risk children in young adulthood: A longitudinal study from birth to 32 years. *American Journal of Orthopsychiatry, 59,* 72–81.

White, S. (2000). Using anatomically detailed dolls in interviewing pre-schoolers. In K. Gitlin-Weiner, A. Sandgrund, & C. Schaefer (Eds.), *Play diagnosis and assessment* (2nd ed., pp. 210–227). New York: Wiley & Sons.

Windle, M., Grunbaum, J. A., Elliott, M., Tortolero, S. R., Berry, S., Gilliland, J., Kanouse, D. E., Parcel, G. S., Wallander, J., Kelder, S., Collins, J., Kolbe, L., & Schuster, M. (2004). Healthy passages: A multilevel, multimethod longitudinal study of adolescent health. *American Journal of Preventive Medicine, 27*(2), 164–172.

Wolfe, D. A. (1998). *Prevention of child abuse and neglect.* Ottawa: Health Canada.

Wren, F. J., Scholle, S. H., Heo, J., & Comer, D. M. (2003). Pediatric mood and anxiety syndromes in primary care: Who gets identified? *International Journal of Psychiatry Medicine, 33*(1), 1–16.

Wright, L. M., & Leahey, M. (2005). The three most common errors in family nursing: How to avoid or sidestep. *Journal of Family Nursing, 11*(2), 90–101.

Xue, Y., Leventhal, T., Brooks-Gunn, J., & Earls, F. J. (2005). Neighborhood residence and mental health problems of 5- to 11-year-olds. *Archives of General Psychiatry, 62*(5), 554–563.

26

Mental Health Promotion With Children and Adolescents

Catherine Gray Deering, Lawrence Scahill, Jean Robinson Hughes, Nazilla Khanlou, and Freida Chavez

LEARNING OBJECTIVES

After reading this chapter, the student will be able to:

- Describe protective factors in the mental health promotion of children and adolescents.
- Identify risk factors for the development of psychopathology in childhood and adolescence.
- Analyze the role of the nurse in mental health promotion with children and families.

KEY TERMS

- attachment ▪ bibliotherapy ▪ child abuse and neglect ▪ developmental delay ▪ early intervention programs ▪ family preservation ▪ fetal alcohol syndrome ▪ formal operations ▪ normalization ▪ protective factor ▪ psychoeducational programs ▪ resilience ▪ risk factor ▪ social skills training

◆ KEY CONCEPTS

- grief in childhood ▪ invincibility fable

Children and adolescents respond to the stresses of life in different ways according to their developmental levels. This chapter examines the importance of childhood and adolescent mental health, identifies core prevention strategies, discusses the effects of common childhood stressors, identifies stressors that create risk for psychopathology, and provides guidelines for mental health promotion and risk reduction. Nurses are in a key position to identify and intervene with children and adolescents at risk for psychopathology by virtue of their close contact with families in health care settings and their roles as educators. Knowing the difference between normal child development and psychopathology is crucial in helping parents to view their children's behaviour realistically and to respond appropriately.

CHILDHOOD AND ADOLESCENT MENTAL HEALTH

According to the goals of Canada's National Children's Agenda (Federal/Provincial/Territorial Council on Social Policy Renewal, 2000), children's needs include physical and emotional health, safety and security, success at learning, and social engagement and responsibility. Supportive social networks and positive childhood and adolescent experiences maximize the mental health of children and adolescents. Children are more likely to be mentally healthy if they have normal physical and psychosocial development, an easy temperament (adaptable, low intensity, positive mood), and secure **attachment** at an early age. These three areas are considered in the mental health assessment of children (see Chapter 25). **Developmental delays** not only slow the child's progress but also can interfere with the development of positive self-esteem. Children with an easy temperament can adapt to change without intense emotional reactions. A secure attachment helps the child test the world without fear of rejection. Parents, in particular, play a critical role in preventing adverse outcomes in their children and, if needed, can be assisted to learn ways of being optimally responsive to their children. Families transmit and interpret values to their children, and teach them how to make connections with, and get along in, the larger world—particularly during the early years of life (Schor & the American Academy of Paediatrics Task Force on the Family, 2003).

CRNE Note

Attachment and temperament are key concepts in the behaviour of children and adolescents in any health care setting. Consider how you would apply these concepts to the care of any paediatric patient.

COMMON CHILDHOOD STRESSORS

Stress is an inevitable part of life and may originate in any one area, or several common areas, including the following:
- ➤ the community
- • violence, poverty, lack of safety and supports, inadequate housing
- ➤ home/family environment
- • family disorganization/conflict/transience/breakup, lack of supplies/resources
- ➤ parent–child interaction
- • parent: insensitive/rejecting parenting responses, angry/harsh discipline, frightened behaviour, failure to protect
- • child: lack of eye contact, controlling of parent
- ➤ parent
- • lack of knowledge and skills, negative attributions of the child, unresolved loss/trauma, developmental delay, undereducated, history of parenting difficulties, high stress, developmental stage of parent, chronic health problems, substance abuse
- ➤ child
- • difficult temperament, birth difficulties (prematurity, developmental delay, failure to thrive), extreme sensitivity to sensory experiences, suspected abuse/neglect, loss of a significant caregiver, withdrawal, extreme activity level, aggressive behaviour and emotional dysregulation/reactivity, substance abuse (Infant Mental Health Promotion, 2005, p. 2)

Regardless of the origin, stress usually causes conflict and difficulty with family relationships. These responses to stress can disrupt parenting as well as the interactions between parent and child, and can lead to short-term or lasting poor outcomes. The earlier these events begin and the longer that the disruption lasts, the worse the outcomes for children (Schor et al., 2003).

Loss: Death and Grief

It is important for nurses to recognize that death and grief are universally experienced by children and therefore are the most common stresses encountered. It is of paramount importance for nurses to understand that children do not respond the same way as adults. The most common losses experienced are death of a grandparent, parental divorce, death of a pet, and loss of friends through moving or changing schools. Learning to mourn losses can lead to a renewed appreciation of the precious value of life and close relationships. Vast research shows that both children and adults who experience major losses are at risk for mental health problems, particularly if the natural grieving process is impeded. The grieving process differs somewhat between children and adults (Table 26-1).

Table 26.1	Grieving in Childhood, Adolescence, and Adulthood	
Children	**Adolescents**	**Adults**
▪ View death as reversible: do not understand that death is permanent until about age 7 years	▪ Understand that death is permanent but may flirt with death (eg, reckless driving, unprotected sex) due to omnipotent feelings	▪ Understand that death is permanent: may struggle with spiritual beliefs about death
▪ Experiment with ideas about death by killing bugs, staging funerals, acting out death in play	▪ May be fascinated by death, enjoy morbid books and movies, listen to rock music about death and suicide	▪ May try not to think about death, depending on cultural background
▪ Mourn through activities (eg, mock funerals, playing with things owned by the loved one); may not cry	▪ Mourn by talking about the loss, crying, and reflecting on it, sometimes becoming dramatic (eg, overidentifying with the lost person, developing poetic or romantic ideas about death)	▪ Mourn through talking about the loss, crying, reviewing memories, and thinking privately about it
▪ May not discuss the loss openly, but express grief through regression, somatic complaints, behaviour problems, or withdrawal	▪ Often withdraw when mourning or seek comfort through peer groups; may feel parents do not understand their feelings	▪ Usually discuss loss openly, depending on level of support available; may feel there is a "time limit" on how long it is socially acceptable to grieve
▪ Need repeated explanations to fully understand the loss; it may be helpful to read children's books that explain death	▪ Need permission to grieve openly because they may believe they should act strong or take care of the adults involved; need acceptance of their sometimes extreme reactions	▪ Need friends, family, and other supportive people to listen and allow them to mourn for however long it takes; need opportunities to review their feelings and memories

KEY CONCEPT Grief in childhood differs from grief in adulthood. Children tend to grieve in stages. They begin without understanding the full effects of the loss and experience some numbness or dulling of emotional pain. This stage progresses to a greater acceptance of the reality of the loss, which leads to more intense psychological pain. Finally, they undergo a reorganization of identity to incorporate the loved person, which may involve engaging in new activities and interests (Van Epps, Opie, & Goodwin, 1997).

Children's responses to loss reflect their developmental level. As early as age 3 years, children have some concept of death. For example, the death of a goldfish provides an opportunity for the child to grasp the idea that the fish will never swim again. However, not until about age 7 years can most children understand the permanence of death. Before this age, they may verbalize that someone has "died" but in the next sentence ask when the dead person will be "coming back." Even adolescents sometimes flirt with death by driving dangerously or engaging in other risky behaviours, as if they believe they are immune to death. This phenomenon is known as the invincibility fable because adolescents view themselves in an egocentric way, as unique and invulnerable to the consequences experienced by others.

KEY CONCEPT Invincibility fable is an aspect of egocentric thinking in adolescence that causes teens to view themselves as immune to dangerous situations, such as unprotected sex, fast driving, and drug abuse.

If the concept of death is difficult for adults to grasp, they should be particularly sensitive to the child's struggle to understand and cope with it. Most children closely watch their parents' response to grief and loss and use fantasy to fill the gaps in their understanding. In many cases, family members take turns grieving, with children sensing that their parents are so overwhelmed by their own emotional pain that they cannot bear the children's grief, with adults taking turns being strong for each other.

Loss and Preschool-Aged Children

The preschool-aged child may react more to the parents' distress about a death than to the death itself. Young children who depend totally on their parents may be frightened when they see their parents upset. Anything the parent can do to alleviate the child's anxiety, such as reassuring him or her that the parent will be okay and continuing the child's normal routine (eg, normal bedtimes, snacks, play times) will help the child to feel secure. Because preschool-aged children have limited ability to verbalize their feelings, they may need to express them through fantasy play and activities, such as mock funerals. Books that explain death, such as *Charlotte's Web* by E. B. White, may also be helpful. Parents should take care not to use euphemisms that could fuel misconceptions of death, such as "He went to sleep" or "Jesus took him." Young children may interpret these messages literally and fear going to sleep (because they

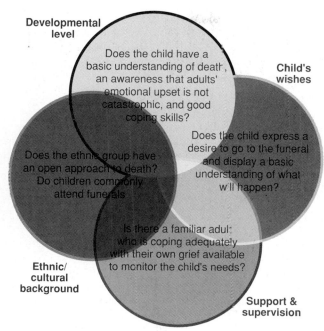

FIGURE 26.1   Factors that influence whether a child should attend a funeral.

might die) or focus their natural, grief-related anger on the irrational idea that the person deliberately has not returned. The best approach is to explain honestly that the person has died and is not coming back, elicit the child's understanding and questions about what has happened, and then repeat this process continually as the child gradually begins to grasp the reality of the situation. The decision of whether to take a small child to a funeral may be particularly complex. Figure 26-1 enumerates some factors to consider.

Loss and School-Aged Children

School-aged children understand the permanence of death more clearly than do preschoolers, but they may be unable to express their feelings in a grown-up way. Children in this age group may express their grief through somatic complaints; finding comfort in behaviours engaged in during earlier developmental stages, also know as regression; behaviour problems; withdrawal; and even hostility toward parents. They may think that others expect them to cry and react with immediate emotional intensity to the death; when they do not react this way, they feel guilty.

Loss and Adolescents

Adolescents who are in Piaget's stage of formal operations can better understand death as an abstract concept. **Formal operations** is the period of cognitive development characterized by the ability to use abstract reasoning to conceptualize and solve problems. Because ado-

lescents tend to be idealistic and to think in extremes, they may even have poetic or romantic notions about death. Many teenagers become fascinated with morbid rock music, movies, and books. Although they may be able to express their thoughts and feelings about death more clearly than younger children, they often are reluctant to do so for fear of being viewed as childish. Some adolescents assume a parental role in the family after a death, denying their own needs. School settings may be particularly helpful in providing group and individual support for grieving adolescents, particularly as a preventive intervention (Van Epps et al., 1997).

Separation and Divorce

According to the Child Support Team of the Department of Justice (2000), separation and divorce are realities for a good number of children in Canada—223 families per 100,000 in 1997, about half the rate reported for the United States. Trends show that divorce now occurs earlier in a child's life, and although joint custody is becoming more common (13%), mothers retain sole custody of the children in about 79% of the cases. In addition, about 40% of the children rarely or never have contact with the other parent after the family breaks up. Although many families adapt to separation and divorce without long-term negative effects for the children, research points out that youth often show at least temporary difficulties dealing with this common stressor in our society (Pruett, Williams, Insabella, & Little, 2003). Parental separation and divorce create changes in the family structure, usually resulting in a substantial reduction in the contact that children have with one of their parents. The child's response to divorce is similar to the response to death. In some ways, divorce may be harder for the child to understand because the noncustodial parent is gone but still alive, and the parents have made a conscious choice to separate. Research shows that children of divorce are at increased risk for emotional, behavioural, and academic problems. However, the response to the loss that divorce imposes varies depending on the child's temperament, the parents' interventions, and the level of stress, change, and conflict surrounding the divorce (Hetherington & Kelly, 2002). Recent studies indicate that a major change in socioeconomic status, that is, moving from dual-earner status to single-parent family status, may account for much of the variation in levels of distress among divorcing families (Jeynes, 2002; Sun & Li, 2002). In fact, single mothers (31%) represent the largest group of families living in poverty in Canada (Child Support Team, 2000). In addition, Statistics Canada (2004) shows that in 1999, 20% of the single-parent mothers who worked full-time lived in poverty.

The first 2 or 3 years after the couple's breakup tend to be the most difficult. Typical childhood reactions include confusion, guilt, depression, regression, somatic symptoms, acting-out behaviours (eg, stealing, disobedience), fantasies that the parents will reunite, fear of losing the custodial parent, and alignment with one parent against the other. After an initial adjustment period, children usually accept the reality of the situation and begin coping adaptively. Most divorced parents eventually remarry to new partners, which often imposes another period of coping difficulties for the children. Children with stepparents and stepsiblings are at renewed risk for emotional and behavioural problems as they struggle to cope with the new relationships (Reifman, Villa, Amans, Rethinam, & Telesca, 2001).

Protective factors against emotional problems in children of divorce and remarriage include a structured home and school environment with reasonable and consistent limit setting and a warm, supportive relationship with stepparents (Hetherington & Kelly, 2002). Helpful interventions for children of divorce include education regarding children's reactions; promotion of regular and predictable visitation; reduction of conflict between the parents through counselling, mediation, and clear visitation policies; continuance of usual routines; and family counselling to facilitate adjustment after remarriage (Table 26-2). Some evidence shows that it is not the divorce itself but rather the continuing conflict between the parents that is most damaging to the child. Parents manage divorce better if they can remember that children naturally idealize and identify with both parents and need to view both of them positively. Therefore, it is helpful for parents to reinforce each other's good qualities and focus on evidence of their former partner's love and respect for the child.

Sibling Relationships

Until recently, the role of siblings in a child's development was underemphasized. A growing body of research shows that sibling relationships significantly influence personality development. Moreover, research shows that positive sibling relationships can be protective factors against the development of psychopathology (Fig. 26-2), particularly in troubled families in which the parents are emotionally unavailable (Brody, 1998). Thus, nurses should emphasize that whatever parents can do to minimize sibling rivalry and maximize cooperative behaviour among their children will benefit their children's social and emotional development throughout life.

Sibling rivalry begins with the birth of the second child. Often, this event is traumatic for the first child who, up until then, was the sole focus of the parents' attention. The older sibling usually reacts with anger and may reveal not-so-subtle fantasies of getting rid of the new sibling (eg, "I dreamed that the new baby

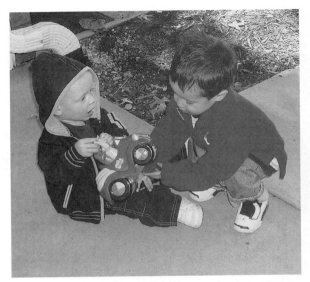

FIGURE 26.2   Play is the work of preschoolers. Here two preschoolers are problem-solving (negotiating) how to take turns with a toy.

died"). Parents should recognize that these reactions are natural and allow the child to express feelings, both positive and negative, about the baby while reassuring the child that he or she has a very special place in the family. Allowing the older child opportunities to care for the baby and reinforcing any nurturing or affectionate behaviour will promote positive bonding.

Some sibling rivalry is natural and inevitable, even into adulthood. However, intense rivalry and conflict between siblings correlate with behaviour problems in children (Moser & Jacob, 2002). One factor that can exacerbate this problem is differential treatment of children. Although it is natural and appropriate for parents to use different methods to manage children with different personalities, parents must be sensitive to their children's perceptions of their behaviour and emphasize each child's strengths. Helping each child to develop a separate identity based on unique talents and interests can minimize rivalry and perceptions of favouritism.

Children with emotionally disturbed siblings are at increased risk for mental health problems. Nurses should be alert to behaviour problems and include siblings in family interventions (Sharpe & Rossiter, 2002).

Physical Illness

Many children experience a major physical illness or injury at some point during development. The experience of hospitalization and intrusive medical procedures is at least acutely traumatic for most children. The likelihood of lasting psychological problems resulting from physical illness depends on the child's developmental level and previous coping mechanisms, the family's level of functioning before and after the illness,

Table 26.2 Play Therapy With a 4-Year-Old Whose Parents Are Divorcing

Child Statement	Nurse Response	Analysis and Rationale
(Child smashes two cars together and makes loud, crashing sound.)	That's a loud crash. They really hit hard.	Child may be experiencing anger and frustration nonverbally through play. Nurse attempts to establish rapport with child by relating at child's level, using age-appropriate vocabulary.
Crrrash!	I know a boy who gets so mad sometimes that he feels like smashing something.	Child is engrossed in fantasy play, typical of preschoolers. Children often use toys as symbols of human figures. Nurse uses indirect method of eliciting child's feelings because preschoolers often do not express feelings directly. Reference to another child's anger helps to normalize this child's feelings.
Yeah!	Sounds like you feel angry too sometimes . . . the same way the other boy feels	Child is beginning to relate to nurse and sense her empathy. Nurse reflects the child's feelings to facilitate further communication
Yeah, when my mom and dad fight.	It's tough to listen to parents fighting. Sometimes it's scary. You wonder what's going to happen.	Child is experiencing frustration and helplessness related to family conflict. Nurse expresses empathy and attempts to articulate child's feelings because preschool children have a limited ability to identify and label feelings.
My mom and dad are getting a divorce.	That's too bad. Children often feel mixed up when their parents get divorced. What's going to happen when they get the divorce?	Child has basic awareness of the reality of parents' divorce, but may not understand this concept. Nurse expresses empathy and attempts to assess the child's level of understanding of the divorce.
Dad's not going to live in our house.	Oh, I guess you'll miss having him there all the time. It would be nice if you all could live together, but I guess that's not going to happen.	Preschool child focusses on the effects the divorce will have on him (egocentrism). Child seems to have a clear understanding of the consequences of the divorce. Nurse articulates the child's perspective and reinforces the reality of the divorce to avoid fueling child's possible denial and reconciliation fantasies.
(Silently moves cars across the floor.)	What do you think is the reason your parents decided to get a divorce?	Child expresses sadness nonverbally. Nurse further attempts to assess the child's understanding of the circumstances surrounding the divorce.
Because I did it.	What do you mean—you did it?	Child provides clue that he may be feeling responsible. Nurse uses clarification to fully assess child's understanding.
I made them mad cause I left my bike in the driveway and Dad ran over it.	How? Do you think that's why they're getting the divorce?	Child uses egocentric thinking to draw conclusion that his actions caused the divorce. Nurse continues to clarify the child's thinking. The goal is to elicit the child's perceptions so that misperceptions can be corrected.
Yeah, they had a big fight.	They may have been upset about the bike, but I don't think that's why they're getting a divorce.	The nurse goes on to explain why parents get divorced and to provide opportunities for the child to ask questions.
Why?	Because parents get divorced when they're upset with *each other*—when they can't get along—not when they're upset with their children.	

and the nature and severity of the illness. As with any major stressor, the perception of the event (ie. meaning of the illness) will influence the family's ability to cope.

Common childhood reactions to physical illness include loss of developmental gains (eg, in toilet training, social maturity, autonomous behaviour), sleep and feeding difficulties, behaviour problems (negativism, withdrawal), somatic complaints that mask attempts at emotional expression (eg, headaches, stomachaches), and depression. Infants and children younger than school age are particularly vulnerable to separation anxiety during illness and may regress to earlier levels of anxiety about strangers, becoming fearful of health care providers. Young children often have magical thinking about the illness, and their tendency to process information in concrete terms may lead to misperceptions about the illness and treatment procedures (eg, dye = die; stretcher = stretch her) (Deering & Cody, 2002). Adolescents may be concerned about body image and maintaining their sense of independence and control.

Nurses must remember that parents are the primary resource to the child and the experts who know the child's needs and reactions. Thus, nurses must maintain a collaborative approach in working with parents of physically ill children. If the child is a sick infant, nurses should take care to allow the normal attachment process between parents and the infant to unfold, despite health care professionals' efforts to assume some parenting functions. Parents who view their children as physically and emotionally fragile will feel disempowered in decision making and limit setting and may develop helpless or overprotective styles of dealing with their children.

Many parents react with guilt to their child's illness or injury, especially if the illness is genetically based or partially the result of their own behaviour (eg, drug or alcohol abuse during pregnancy). Parents may project their guilt onto each other or health care professionals, lashing out in anger and blame. Nurses should view this behaviour as part of the grieving process and help parents to move forward in caring for their children and regaining competence. Teaching parents how to care for their children's medical problems and reinforcing their successes in doing so will help. For example, rather than reacting to what may appear to be an abdication of parenting responsibilities, nurses can, instead, use empathy to acknowledge the parent's feelings and discuss ways to help the parent regain a sense of control with comments, such as,

> It's pretty confusing to know how best to respond to your child's behaviour. Before receiving her diagnosis, you felt comfortable setting reasonable limits on her behaviour, but now your fear and guilt prevent you from taking action because you know how sick she is . . . . It may seem odd, but children actually feel safer and more secure when their parents set some reasonable limits on their behaviour . . . . Can we talk about some of the limits that you might feel most comfortable setting for your daughter to help her feel safe and secure while she is so ill?

Chronic physical illness in childhood presents a unique set of challenges. Although studies show that most children with chronic illnesses and their families are remarkably resilient and adjust to the stressors and regimens involved in their care (LeBlanc, Goldsmith, & Patel, 2003), research shows that children with chronic health conditions are three to four times more likely to experience psychiatric symptoms than are their healthy peers (Lewis & Vitulano, 2003). Conditions that affect the central nervous system (CNS) (eg, infections, metabolic diseases, CNS malformations, brain and spinal

cord trauma) are particularly likely to result in psychiatric difficulties. Nurses who understand pathophysiologic processes are in a unique position to assess the interaction between biologic and psychological factors that contribute to mental health problems in chronically ill children (eg, lethargy from high blood sugar levels or respiratory problems; mood swings from steroid use). Inactivity and lack of sensory stimulation from hospitalization or bed rest may contribute to neurologic deficits and developmental delays. The major challenge for a chronically ill child is to remain active despite the limitations of the illness and to become fully integrated into school and social activities. Children who view themselves as different or defective will experience low self-esteem and be more at risk for depression, anxiety, and behaviour problems. Studies show that parental perceptions of the child's vulnerability predict greater adjustment problems, even after controlling for age and disease severity (Anthony, Gil, & Schanberg, 2003). Educating parents about these facts and helping them to foster maximum independence within the limitations of the child's health problem is the key. For example, nurses might comment,

> Having kidney disease is certainly no fun . . . and it would be wonderful if wrapping your son in a cocoon would ensure that he came to no harm. Unfortunately, there is no such way of protecting him completely . . . . But we know that children seem to manage better with their illness when their parents believe that they have possibilities. Even with all the limitations, what are the best things your son has going for him?

Adolescent Risk-Taking Behaviours

Adolescence is a time of growing independence and, consequently, experimentation. Emotional extremes prevail. To adolescents, the world seems great one day and terrible the next; people are either for them or against them. Adolescents are struggling to consolidate their abilities to control their impulses and react to the many "crises" that may seem trivial to adults but are very important to teens. Biologic changes (eg, onset of puberty, height and weight changes, hormonal changes), psychological changes (increased ability for abstract thinking), and social changes (dating, driving, increased autonomy) are all significant. The primary developmental task of identity formation leads teenagers to test different roles and struggle to find a peer group that fits their unfolding self-image.

Adolescence is a time of experimentation, increasing risk for poor sexual health, smoking, substance use, and psychological distress (Lerner & Galambos, 1998; Walker & Townsend, 1999). Pregnancy occurs in approximately 4% of Canadian females aged 15 to 19 years annually (Dryburgh, 2000), and sexually transmitted diseases (STDs) are most common among younger Canadians (Health Canada, 2000). Some adolescents engage in truancy or criminal behaviours and running away from home. Although most youths eventually become more conventional in their behaviour, some develop harmful behaviour patterns and addictions that endanger their mental and physical health. Adolescents whose psychiatric problems have already developed are particularly vulnerable to engaging in risky behaviours because they have limited coping skills, may attempt to self-medicate their symptoms, and may feel increased pressure to fit in with other teens. Moreover, research shows that risky behaviours tend to be interrelated (Eggert, Thompson, Randell, & Pike, 2002).

Research shows that enhanced life skills and supportive school and family environments can mediate the effect of stressful life events (Burns, Andrews, & Szabo, 2002). Programs that enhance the school environment are associated with improved behaviour and well-being. Interventions that teach cognitive skills are associated with a reduction in one of the most prevalent mental health problems affecting adolescents, depression (Puskar, Sereika, & Tusaie-Mumford, 2003). Current evidence suggests that for an intervention to be sustainable, it must encompass multiple components across several levels, including the classroom, curriculum, whole school, and school–community boundaries. Several approaches to mental health promotion with adolescents are recommended. First, intervening at the peer group level through education programs, alternative recreation activities, and peer counselling is most successful. Adolescents are sceptical of authority figures and tend to take cues from one another. Nurses working with teenagers find it helpful to use a discussion approach that encourages questioning and argument, as opposed to talking down to or "talking at" teenagers (Deering & Cody, 2002).

Second, research has shown that training in values clarification, decision making, problem solving, social skills, and assertiveness helps give adolescents the skills to cope with situations in which they are pressured by their peers (Botvin, 2000). Social psychological research shows that if just one person can find the strength to express an unpopular viewpoint in a group and decline to participate in a destructive activity, others will quickly follow. It takes enormous courage, as well as concrete knowledge and practice with assertiveness, to speak up in these situations.

A third type of intervention is a program that uses team efforts by teachers, parents, community leaders, and teen role models. These programs help at-risk youth by building self-esteem, setting positive examples, and working to involve the youth in community activities. It is important to note that teaching interpersonal skills, including cognitive and problem-solving skills, should be coupled with the promotion of positive school and family environments to prevent mental health problems in young people, notably depression (Burns, Andrews, & Szabo, 2002). Approaches that have not proved effective include more education and information about dangerous activities without behaviour training and programs that provide inadequate training and support for the professionals implementing them.

PROTECTIVE FACTORS AGAINST CHILDHOOD PATHOLOGY

Protective factors include individual, family, and community characteristics that alleviate the impact of risk factors by interacting together to foster resilience in children (Waddell, McEwan, Sheperd, Offord, & Hua, 2005). In the child, these protective factors include learning abilities, social skills, a sense of competence, positive beliefs about one's purpose in the larger world, and long-term support from at least on adult (Werner & Smith, 1992). In the community, protective factors include positive and cohesive families, schools, and neighbourhoods (Box 26-1) (Schoor, 1997).

BOX 26.1 RESEARCH FOR BEST PRACTICE

Khanlou, N., & Crawford, C. (2006). Post-migratory experiences of newcomer female youth: Self-esteem and identity development. *Journal of Immigrant and Minority Health*, 8(1), in press. The study was supported by a research contract from Status of Women Canada's Policy Research Fund.

THE QUESTION: This study explored the postmigratory experiences of newcomer female youth attending secondary school within a multicultural context. The impact of the resettlement process on the self-esteem and identity of newcomer females was considered.

METHODS: Focus groups were held with 10 newcomer female youth, in Toronto. Data were also collected through focus groups or in-depth interviews with school educators, parents, and school and community health centre workers. Also, the Current Self-Esteem (CSE) instrument was used to examine the global self-esteem of youth and the influences on their self-esteem.

FINDINGS: Participants' average age was 17 years; average age at time of immigration to Canada was 13.9 years. The mean for CSE scores was 7.9, indicating that respondents felt, in general, good about themselves. Among the influences on youth's self-esteem were those related to Self, School, Relationships, Achievements, and Lifestyle. The emerging subthemes of the Self-Concept theme, arising from the qualitative data, consisted of Dynamic Self, Silenced Self, Cultural Identity, Female Role Models, and Future Aspirations.

IMPLICATIONS FOR NURSING PRACTICE: This study is an example of a community-based mental health promotion study. The researchers concluded that, in multicultural and post migration societies, context-specific strategies in mental health promotion are needed for youth. Their published report (Khanlou, Beiser, Cole, et al., 2002) provides policy recommendations for health, social services, and educational systems and for resettlement services.

RISK FACTORS FOR CHILDHOOD PSYCHOPATHOLOGY

Poverty and Homelessness

An estimated 14.9% of children in Canada live in poverty (UNICEF, 2005), and 9% of these children had lived in poverty for more than 5 years (Campaign 2000). Forty percent of people of Aboriginal descent, 40% of immigrants, and 34% of visible minority groups also live in poverty in Canada. The effects of poverty on child development and family functioning are numerous and pervasive. Lack of proper nutrition and access to prenatal and mother–infant care place children from poor families at risk for physical and mental health problems. Children from poor rural areas often lack access to educational and other resources. Urban children living in ghetto areas are vulnerable to violent crime, crowded living conditions, and drug-infested neighbourhoods (Leventhal & Brooks-Gunn, 2000). Although crime, drug abuse, gang activity, and teenage pregnancy are seen in adolescents from all socioeconomic backgrounds, children living in poverty may be more vulnerable to these problems because they may view their options as limited. Thus, they may have an increased need to maintain a tough image and struggle more for a sense of control over their environment. The obstacles inherent in overcoming the effects of poverty can seem insurmountable to young people.

A major focus of preventive nursing interventions for disadvantaged families involves simply forming an alliance that conveys respect and willingness to work as an advocate to help patients gain access to resources. In terms of Maslow's need hierarchy, families living in poverty may be more focussed on survival needs (eg, food, shelter) than self-actualization needs (eg, insight-oriented psychotherapy for themselves or their children). Unless the nurse can work as a partner with the family and address the issues most pressing for the family with an active, problem-solving approach, other types of intervention may be fruitless. At the same time, it is inappropriate to assume that poor families will be resistant to or unable to benefit from psychotherapy or other mental health interventions.

Contrary to popular opinion, homelessness is a very complex phenomenon, and the homeless are not a homogenous population. Canada has a growing number of homeless women, children, youth, families, new immigrants, people with mental illness, ethnic minorities, and Aboriginal people (Begin, Casavant, Chenier, & Dupuis, 1999). Homelessness among children and teens may result from a variety of events, including loss of shelter for the entire family, running away, being thrown out of one's home (Barak, 1992), or, in the case of youth, being abandoned by the social service system. Although there is no accurate understanding of the numbers of homeless people in Canada, emergency shelters alone accounted for on average 6,500 homeless in Toronto per night in 1997 (Begin et al., 1999).

Research reveals an increased risk for physical health problems (eg, nutrition deficiencies, infections, chronic illnesses), mental health problems (particularly developmental delays in language, fine or gross motor coordination, and social development; depression; anxiety; disruptive behaviour disorders), and educational underachievement in homeless youth. Many homeless youth have been physically or sexually abused, leading to elevated rates of externalizing disorders for boys and internalizing disorders for girls (Cance et al., 2000). Evidence suggests that at least 50% of homeless youth suffer from serious mental health and drug addiction problems (Adlaf & Zdanowicz, 1999) and are now more likely to be homeless than adults (Ringwalt, Greene, Robertson, & McPheeters, 1998). For adolescents, running away from abusive conditions at home often thrusts them onto the street and into environments where staying alive and developing self-reliance are a daily struggle (Rew, 2003). The living conditions of many shelters place children at risk for lead poisoning and communicable diseases and make the regular sleep, feeding, play, and bathing patterns important for normal development nearly impossible. Nurses working with homeless families need to be aware of the effects of this lifestyle on children because they have a limited ability to speak for themselves and because their needs are often overlooked. Studies show that the demands of parenting often overwhelm parents in homeless shelters. The unstable nature of their living conditions limits the ability of these parents to nurture their children (Gorzka, 1999).

Typically, runaway youth have experienced extreme stress in the course of their lives even before they run away, with most fleeing temporary living arrangements (eg, foster homes, friends, relatives) (Warren, Gary, & Moorhead, 1997). Thus, their runaway experience serves only to compound an already chronic history of trauma and disruption. The key is to prevent the conditions that preceded the runaway behaviour. Unfortunately, much of the response to homelessness has resulted in greater social control measures (eg, rendering panhandling illegal, excluding the homeless from the community) rather than strategies to address the underlying causes (Begin, et al., 1999). Street nurses are often one of the few resources available to marginalized populations who face a variety of barriers to accessing traditional health care services. such as mental health problems, criminal involvement, lack of transportation, lack of ability to pay for prescriptions, lack of specialized or knowledgeable providers, and provider discrimination (Self & Peters, 2005). Street services are effective because they are delivered wherever the person feels comfortable: a school, a drop-in centre, a mall, a youth centre, or simply the street.

Child Abuse and Neglect

Thousands of Canadian children suffer maltreatment (intentional physical or emotional abuse, neglect, or sexual exploitation) each year as the result of their parents' action or inaction (Wolfe, 1998). A recent study (Trocme et al., 2001) confirmed close to half (45%) of the 135,573 child maltreatment investigations in 1998. Child abuse may affect every aspect of a child's life and may have varying consequences depending on its form, duration, severity, and child's gender (Maguire, Mann, Sibert, & Kemp, 2005; Trocme, et al., 2001). The effects may appear immediately or surface only in adolescence or adulthood and may differ according to the nature of the response to the abuse and whether the abuse was disclosed or reported. In some cases, the consequences are fatal (Canadian Centre for Justice Statistics, 2001). Maltreated children often have difficulty managing emotions (Campbell, 1995), communicating effectively (Browne & Sagi, 1988), developing satisfying relationships with others (Crittenden, 1996), and learning in productive ways (Doherty, 1997). Early recognition and reduction of risk factors are the keys to preventing **child abuse and neglect** (Box 26-2).

Risk factors for child abuse and neglect include high levels of family stress, drug or alcohol abuse, a stepparent or parental boyfriend or girlfriend who is unstable or unloving toward the child, and lack of social support for the parents. In addition, young children (particularly those younger than 3 years) and children with a history of prematurity, medical problems, and severe emotional problems are at high risk because they place great demands on the parents. Abuse has a well-known intergenerational pattern, such that children who are abused and neglected are more likely to repeat this behaviour when they become parents (Helfer, Kemper, & Kongman, 1997). However, intergenerational abuse

is not a foregone conclusion. Evidence shows that among abused and nonabused children, having a strong commitment to school, having parents and peers who disapprove of antisocial behaviour, and being involved in a religious community lowered the rates of lifetime violence, delinquency, and status offences (Herrenkohl, Tajima, Whitney, & Huang, 2005).

Table 26-3 lists types of abuse in children. Research clearly documents that child abuse is a risk factor for later psychopathology, especially depression and substance abuse (Putnam, 2003). Nurses should be aware that they are legally mandated to report any reasonable suspicion of abuse and neglect to the appropriate provincial and child protection systems. Mandated reporting laws are designed to allow the provinces and child protection systems to investigate the possibility of abuse, provide protection to children, and link families with the support and services that they need to reduce the risk for further abuse. Nurses are ethically and legally responsible for reporting abuse. The decision to report abuse sometimes poses an ethical dilemma for nurses as they try to balance the need to maintain the family's trust against the need to protect the child. This decision is further complicated by the knowledge that, if temporary out-of-home placement is necessary, the quality of the placement may not be optimum, and the child and family may suffer in the process of the separation.

Experts recommend that nurses report abuse in the presence of the parents, preferably with the parent initiating the telephone call, and that the professional should explain the reporting as necessary to provide safety for the child and to obtain services for the family. If the parents cannot be present when the report is made, the nurse should, at minimum, notify the family that the report was made and explain why to minimize damaging the professional relationship. A major protective factor against psychopathology stemming from abuse and neglect is the

---

BOX 26.2 RESEARCH FOR BEST PRACTICE

The Impact of a Proven Parenting Program on a High-Risk Population

Hughes, J. R, Gottlieb, L. N. (2004). The effects of the Webster-Stratton parenting program on maltreating families: Fostering strengths. *Child Abuse and Neglect, 28*, 1081–1097.

THE QUESTION: This study examined the effects of the nurse-developed, research tested, Webster-Stratton parenting program on the parenting skills of maltreating mothers and on the autonomy of their children (3–8 years of age).

METHODS: Twenty-six maltreating families were randomly assigned to one of two conditions: the 16-hour weekly intervention group or the 4-month wait list control group. Preintervention and postintervention independent assessments included a 2-hour home visit involving videotaped mother–child interactions during two prescribed (structured and unstructured), 10-minute play activities.

FINDINGS: Compared with the control group, treatment mothers demonstrated significant improvement in involvement and marginally significant improvement in autonomy–support. Treatment group children showed no significant improvement in autonomy when compared with control group children.

CONCLUSIONS AND IMPLICATIONS FOR NURSING PRACTICE: This parenting program proved effective with maltreating parents. The lack of demonstrated effect on children may reflect the need for a larger and more sustained treatment dose and/or the need to include parent–child interaction opportunities in the program. This study shows that conventional promotion programs may need additional supports to be effective with high-risk populations.

Table 26.3 Types and Rates of Abuse in Canada

Type	Description	Rate
Neglect	Is often chronic and usually involves repeated incidents of failing to provide what a child needs for his or her physical, psychological, or emotional development and well-being.	3.66 confirmed cases per 1,000 children
Physical abuse	May consist of just one incident or happen repeatedly. It involves deliberately using force against a child in such a way that the child is either injured or is at risk for being injured. Injuries may include bruises, lacerations, burns, fractures caused by another person or object (eg, belt, cords, cigarette). *Note:* Many injuries do not represent child abuse; therefore, when abuse is suspected, bruising must be assessed in the context of medical, social, and developmental history, the explanation given, and the patterns of nonabusive bruising (Maguire, Mann, Sibert, & Kemp, 2005)	2.25 confirmed cases per 1,000 children
Emotional abuse	Involves harming a child's sense of self. It includes acts (or omissions) that result in, or place a child at risk for, serious behavioural, cognitive, emotional, or mental health problems.	2.20 confirmed cases of per 1,000 children
Sexual abuse and exploitation	Involves using a child for sexual purposes resulting in physical wounds such as bruises or bleeding of the genitals or rectum, sexually transmitted infections, sore throat, enuresis/encopresis, pregnancy, foreign objects in the vagina or rectum. The child may also display sophisticated knowledge/behaviour/preoccupation with sexual activity, withdrawal, hypervigilance, or sleep difficulties.	0.86 confirmed cases per 1,000 children

From Trocme, N., MacLaurin, B., Fallon, B., et al. (2001). Canadian incidence study of reported child abuse and neglect. Ottawa: Minister of Public Works and Government Services Canada.

establishment of a supportive relationship with at least one adult, who can provide empathy, consistency, and possibly, a corrective experience (eg, a foster parent or other family member) for the child (Taussig, 2002).

Preventing child abuse and neglect occurs with any intervention that supports the parents with physical, financial, mental health, and medical resources that will reduce stress within the family system. Early intervention and family support programs are considered the cornerstones of preventive efforts. Nurses working with abused children should resist the temptation to view the child as the only victim. Remembering that most abusive parents were abused themselves as children and, therefore, may have limited coping mechanisms or little access to positive parental role models will help the nurse maintain empathy toward the parents. Once agencies intervene to establish the child's safety, a family systems approach that is supportive of the whole family unit is most effective.

Child and Family Services

The tendency to blame parents and view out-of-home placement as a refuge for children has sharply declined

IN A LIFE

Charleen Touchette (1954–)

Public Persona
Charleen Touchette is a celebrated artist, writer, and activist. Her book, *It Stops With Me: Memoirs of a Canuck Girl*, is her own rich story of hope and self-discovery that is grounded in her French Canadian and Aboriginal heritage. The artwork and text of the book tell of her healing from childhood abuse and her determination that abuse would no longer be a family legacy: "[C]'est fini. No more. It stops with me" (Touchette, 2004, p. 245).

Personal Realities
As a child, Charleen's family life was shaped by anger, alcohol abuse, and physical violence. She writes, "At eight, I wrote a letter to my future grown-up self. *Never forget how it feels to be a little kid with a crazy mean daddy*" (p. 19). She left her birthplace, a French Canadian community in Rhode Island, US, at 17 and began a journey that took her to the world of art, Aboriginal culture, marriage, and motherhood. Today, she shares what she learned about healing in her books and painting.

in recent years. This change in attitudes results from public awareness of the deficiencies in the foster care system, greater support for parents' rights, and increased knowledge of the biologic basis for many of the disorders of parents and children that lead to out-of-home placement. **Family preservation** involves efforts made by professionals to preserve the family unit by preventing the removal of children from their homes by providing support and education to secure the attachment between children and parents. Today children are removed from their homes only as a last resort. Family support services are designed to assist families with access to resources and education regarding childrearing, to monitor and facilitate the development of the bond between child and caregiver, and to increase the caregiver's confidence in his or her abilities (MacLeod & Nelson, 2000).

However, despite recent trends toward family preservation, an increasing number of children are placed in foster homes, group homes, or residential treatment centres—in many cases for months to years. Factors leading to the increased number of children in out-of-home placement include increased willingness of the public and professionals to report child abuse and neglect, the epidemic proportions of substance abuse and cases of AIDS, and the increasing number of families living in poverty, which may lead to abuse, neglect, and homelessness. In 2003, 76,183 children and youth in Canada were under the protection of Child and Family Services across the country. Infants who are abandoned by drug-abusing parents and children with HIV whose parents are sick or deceased need permanent out-of-home placements, which are often difficult to find.

The adjustment to an out-of-home placement can be viewed through the conceptual framework of Bowlby's stages of coping with parental separation. According to Bowlby (1960), the child initially responds to separation from parents with protest (crying, kicking, screaming, pleading, and attempting to elicit the parent's return). The child then moves to a state of despair (listlessness, apathy, and withdrawal, which lead to some acceptance of caregiving by others, but a reluctance to reattach fully). Finally, the child experiences detachment if the child and new parent cannot manage to form an emotional bond. Because children often experience multiple placements, the potential for a disrupted attachment may be great by the time the child faces the prospect of a permanent family. After repeatedly undergoing separation and mourning, the child learns that rejection is inevitable and may automatically maintain distance from a new caregiver.

Typical coping styles seen in children exposed to multiple placements include detachment, diffuse rage, chronic depression, antisocial behaviour, low self-esteem, and chronic dependency or exaggerated demands for nurturing and support. Sometimes these symptoms develop into attachment disorders that can be difficult to treat (O'Connor, Bredenkamp, & Rutter, 1999). It takes a very committed and resilient parent to continue caring for a child who does not reinforce attempts at caregiving and who exhibits these kinds of significant emotional and behaviour problems.

Parent With Mental Illness

Children who grow up with a depressed parent, the most common form of mental illness among adults (approximately 8% of the adult population) (Health Canada, 2002) are themselves at increased risk for mental illness—both in childhood and in later life (Health Canada & Canadian Mental Health Association, 1999). These children are also more likely to be at sociodemographic disadvantage—they are more likely to be living with a single mother and living on low income (Federal/Provincial/Territorial Advisory Committee on Population Health, 1999). Infants whose mothers experience postpartum depression (approximately 10%) or are otherwise troubled are at most risk for losing the opportunity to establish a secure attachment (Federal/Provincial/Territorial Advisory Committee on Population Health, 1999). Many children know that something is wrong when a parent has a mental illness but may not be able to identify the problem specifically (Health Canada & Canadian Mental Health Association, 1999). They feel alone, left out, distanced, and powerless to participate in decisions. They report feeling angry, sad, and guilty that somehow they are to blame for their parent's illness. They also worry that they will, in turn, become ill and fear the stigma that surrounds mental illness. Fortunately, the likelihood or severity of these problems can be reduced or eliminated when families have the knowledge and support they need. Children need information, their questions answered, opportunity to talk about how they feel, and routine childhood experiences. As with other family stressors, it is important to keep children informed, in manageable ways and doses, and at times that the children determine (Health Canada & Canadian Mental Health Association, 1999, p. 13). Nurses can helps parents get started by modelling.

Mommy isn't feeling well. She feels sad, it's because of an illness and it's not her fault. It is a sad time for all of us but I'm here to talk with you about it when you need to.

Children need hope that depression is treatable and that their mother will get better. They also need to be reassured that their parents love them—no matter what the challenge involves . . . or how long it takes (Health Canada & Canadian Mental Health Association, 1999). Children also need supportive relationships outside the home with someone (eg, a teacher, coach, neighbour) who can provide a listening ear, extra support, and a measure of respite for the family. Children need to know that their routine in life will continue, including the fun times, and that their relationship with both parents is valued by the parents. Evidence shows that when children and their families are given information about the affected parent's mental illness, they show improved knowledge and long-standing positive effects in how they problem solve (a resilient-related quality) around parental illness (Beardslee, Gladstone, Wright, & Cooper, 2003).

Parent With a Substance Abuse Problem

A number of Canadian children live in homes (in urban or rural communities) with a parent who is dependent on alcohol (2.6% of adults: men 3.9%, women 1.3%) or illicit drugs (0.8% of adults: men 1.1%, women 0.5%) (Statistics Canada, 2004). Many of the parents with an alcohol or illicit substance dependence are also suffering or have suffered from depression, which acts as both a *precursor* and an *outcome* of heavy substance use, and are more likely to be living on a low income and have a relatively low education level (Statistics Canada, 2004). Children whose parents are dependent on alcohol live in an unpredictable family environment, coping with stress that may disrupt their ability to perform in school and lead to other emotional problems (Casa-Gil & Navarro-Guzman, 2002). Many individuals with alcoholism become polysubstance abusers, addicted to other drugs as well. The codependency movement, which emphasizes the effects of addiction on family members, and groups such as Adult Children of Alcoholics (ACOA) and Al-Anon have brought increasing attention to the effects of parental substance abuse on child development. Any review of this topic must examine the role of biologic-genetic mechanisms and environmental mechanisms in creating increased risk for psychological problems among children of those who abuse substances.

Biologic factors affecting children of those who abuse substances include **fetal alcohol syndrome**, nutritional deficits stemming from neglect, and neuropsychiatric dysfunction related to overstimulation or understimulation (Kaemingk & Paquette, 1999). Genetic factors are at least partly responsible for the well-documented increased risk for substance abuse among those who abuse substances. Recent studies are beginning to link a family history of anxiety disorders and alcoholism with genetically transmitted anxiety disorders, which may be a precursor to alcohol abuse. The precise mechanism of family transmission of alcoholism remains unknown. Recent studies suggest that children of those who abuse substances may inherit a predisposition to a nonspecific form of biologic dysregulation that may be expressed phenotypically, either as alcoholism or some other psy-

chiatric disorder (eg, hyperactivity, conduct disorder, depression), depending on the individual's developmental history.

Children of those who abuse substances are at high risk for both substance abuse and behaviour disorders (Mylant, Ide, Cuevas, & Meehan, 2002). Moreover, some evidence shows that other factors related to addiction, such as family stress, violence, divorce, dysfunction, and other concurrent parental psychiatric disorders (eg, depression, anxiety), are as important as the alcoholism itself in increasing this risk (Ritter, Stewart, Bernet, Coe, & Brown, 2002). The experience of growing up in a substance-abusing family is marked by unpredictability, fear, and helplessness because of the cyclic nature of addictive patterns.

The literature on children of parents who are alcoholic has described several typical roles that children assume, including the "hero" (overly responsible children who may ignore their own needs to take care of parents and other children), "scapegoat" (problem children who divert attention away from the parent with alcoholism), "mascot" (family clowns who relieve tension and mask feelings through joking), and "lost child" (children who suffer in silence but may exhibit difficulties at school or in later life) (Veronie & Freuhstorfer, 2001). These roles, combined with the enabling behaviours of other family members who attempt to cover up and minimize the effects of the addiction, may become so rigid and effective in masking the problem that children of substance abusers may not come to the attention of mental health professionals until after the parent stops drinking and family roles are disrupted.

Even for children who do not experience significant psychopathology, the experience of growing up in a substance-abusing family can lead to a poor self-concept when children feel responsible for their parents' behaviour, become isolated, and learn to mistrust their own perceptions because the family denies the reality of the addiction. Despite the well-documented risk for children in substance-abusing families, there is no uniform pattern of outcomes, and many children demonstrate resilience (Harter, 2000). **Resilience** is the phenomenon by which some children at risk for psychopathology—because of genetic or experiential circumstances—attain good mental health, maintain hope, and achieve healthy outcomes (Masten, 2001). Again, individual protective factors and preventive interventions are paramount.

MENTAL ILLNESS AMONG CHILDREN AND ADOLESCENTS

Fourteen percent of children aged 4 to 17 years experience mental health disorders (more than 50% have at least two concurrent disorders) that cause significant distress and impairment at home, school, and in the community (Federal/Provincial/Territorial Advisory Committee on Population Health, 1999; Waddell et al., 2005). Suicide is the second leading cause of death among youth (24%) (Health Canada, 2002), and the rates are two to seven times higher among Aboriginal populations (Federal/Provincial/Territorial Advisory Committee on Population Health, 2000). Sadly, fewer than 25% of the children with a mental disorder receive treatment, and youth rate professionals as the last resource, behind peers and parents, for seeking assistance regarding depression, drugs, and alcohol (Federal/Provincial/Territorial Advisory Committee on Population Health, 2000). Fortunately, there is growing recognition of these service challenges (Canadian Paediatric Society, 1999) and a growing interest in understanding better which approaches are most effective in preventing mental illness during the early years (Goldner, 2002).

INTERVENTION APPROACHES

Mental health promotion with children, adolescents, and their families encompasses the full range of preventive efforts discussed in Chapter 2. Current thinking argues that a mix of psychological and social determinants affect health overall and mental health in particular (Health Canada, 2002, p. 23).

> At the *individual level*, such factors as secure attachment, good parenting, friendship and social support, meaningful employment and social roles, adequate income,

physical activity, and internal locus of control will strengthen mental health and, indirectly, reduce the impact or incidence of some mental health problems.

> At a *system level*, strategies that create supportive environments, strengthen community action, develop personal skills, and orient health services can help to ensure that the population has some control over the psychological and social determinants of mental health.

The overall philosophy of nursing is to advocate for the least restrictive type of intervention possible. This means focussing on interventions that allow maximal autonomy for the child and family, that keep the family unit intact, if possible, and that provide the appropriate level of care to meet the needs of the child and family. A continuum of modalities of care is available to children and families.

Professional nursing emphasizes an interdisciplinary approach in which the nurse acts as collaborator, coordinator, case manager, and advocate to establish linkages with physicians and nurse practitioners, teachers, speech and language specialists, social workers, and other professionals to develop and implement a comprehensive biopsychosocial plan of intervention (Box 26-3). A view of parents as partners should be foremost. In the past, parents were viewed as the culprits in creating children's mental health problems and were treated as patients themselves. Recent insights into the biologic and genetic origins of psychiatric disorders have contributed to a shift from blaming parents to seeking their collaboration in treatment. Promotion and prevention

---

BOX 26.3

Clinical Vignette: Preventive Interventions With an Adolescent in Crisis

Ben and Rita were just transferred to a second foster home after being removed from their mother's care when she relapsed on cocaine and left them unattended. The plan is for the two children to return to their mother's home after she completes a 30-day drug treatment program. Ben, a high school freshman, is in the school nurse's office asking for aspirin for another headache.

The nurse notices that Ben's nose looks inflamed, he is sniffling, and he seems more "hyper" than usual. In a concerned tone of voice, she asks him if he's been using cocaine and he snaps back, "Just because my mother's a coke head doesn't give you the right to suspect me!" When the nurse gently says, "Tell me about what's happening with your mother; I had no idea," Ben responds less defensively and explains the situation about the foster home and his mother's drug problem. He says that if it weren't for Rita, his younger sister, he would have run away by now. His foster parents are "making him" go to school, but he's going to drop out as soon as he returns to live with his mother. The only thing that he likes about school is playing basketball, and the basketball coach, who is his gym teacher, wants him on the team.

After a lengthy talk with Ben, the nurse finishes the assessment interview and concludes that he is at risk for

drug abuse, running away, and dropping out of school. He is also showing symptoms of depression, which he may be attempting to medicate with cocaine. Protective factors for Ben include his strong attachment to his sister, his ability and willingness to express his thoughts and feelings, his interest in basketball, and a positive relationship with the basketball coach.

The nurse develops a plan with Ben to attend the weekly drug and alcohol discussion group at the school, so that he can talk with other teens from substance-abusing families and learn coping skills to prevent addiction. The nurse contacts the basketball coach, who agrees to find a student mentor who can shoot hoops with Ben and help him come up with a plan to stay in school, maybe find a part-time job, and join the basketball team. Ben agrees to check in regularly with the nurse to report how the plan is working and revise it if needed. The nurse feels optimistic that with support from his peers, coach, mentor, and herself, Ben can overcome what is probably a genetically based risk for depression and addiction. Ben shows signs of resilience. He is motivated to "keep his act together for Rita," capable of forming positive attachments, and willing to seek help when he knows where to find it.

programs incorporate a range of techniques to provide reassurance and education, skill training, or direct intervention. The programs may use face-to-face techniques (eg, home visits, educational groups), literature (eg, pamphlets, books), phone (eg, crisis lines) or electronic mechanisms (eg, Internet, telehealth).

Psychoeducational programs are a particularly effective form of mental health intervention. These programs are designed to teach parents and children basic coping skills for dealing with various stressors. Among other techniques, they use the process of **normalization** (ie, teaching families what are normal behaviours and expected responses) and provide families with information about normal child development and expected reactions to various stressors so that they will feel less isolated, know what to expect, and put their reactions into perspective. For example, if families learn that anger is a natural part of grieving, they will be less likely to view it as abnormal and more likely to accept and cope with it constructively. Parallel curricula can be established, with concurrent psychoeducational groups for adults and children. Most foster care agencies now provide a program of education and training for prospective foster parents to help them know what to expect and how to help the child adjust to placement.

Social skills training is one psychoeducational approach that has been useful with youth who have low self-esteem, aggressive behaviour, or a high risk for substance abuse (Cavell, Ennett, & Meehan, 2001). Social skills training involves instruction, feedback, support, and practice with learning behaviours that help children to interact more effectively with peers and adults. When combined with assertiveness training, social skills training can be particularly helpful in providing children with coping skills to resist engaging in addictive or antisocial behaviours and to prevent social withdrawal under stress. Social skills training may be particularly helpful for children who are bullies or who are rejected by their peers (Fopma-Loy, 2000).

Bibliotherapy involves the use of books and other reading materials to help individuals cope with various life stressors. It is a particularly potent form of intervention because it empowers families to learn and develop coping mechanisms on their own. A wide variety of books are available to help children understand issues such as death, divorce, chronic illness, stepfamilies, adoption, and birth of a sibling. In addition, many mental health organizations such as the Canadian Mental Health Association, public health agencies, and Health Canada have pamphlets or website information designed for parents, or children and youth about various physical and psychological problems. In addition to providing concrete information and advice, these reading materials help to reduce anxiety by pointing out common reactions to the various stressors so that families do not feel alone.

Support groups are available for just about every kind of stressor that a family can experience, including substance abuse, death, divorce, and coping with a chronic illness. Both parents and children in groups can experience Yalom's (1985) healing effects of group therapy, including group cohesiveness, universality (awareness of the normalcy and commonality of one's reactions), catharsis, hope, and altruism (being able to help others).

Finally, **early intervention programs**, possibly the most important form of primary prevention available to children and families, offer regular home visits, support, education, and concrete services to those in need. Research supports the effectiveness of these programs, which may be the key to preventing the placement of children outside the home (Gimpel & Holland, 2003; Tomlin & Viehweg, 2003). The assumption underlying these programs is that parents are the most consistent and important figures in children's lives, and they should be afforded the opportunity to define their own needs and priorities. With support and education, parents will be empowered to respond more effectively to their children.

Canada has made several recent investments in early intervention to promote healthy child development by enhancing such programs as paid parental leave (now 1 year), child care, family resource centres, and early learning (Waddell et al., 2005). A number of jurisdictions have introduced promotion and prevention programs aimed at high-risk families (low-income, lone parents) around the birth of a newborn (eg, Better Beginnings, Brighter Futures in Ontario; Healthy Beginnings in Nova Scotia). Many of these programs involve nurse home visitation. There is growing evidence that *intensive* postpartum support (more than antenatal support) provided by a health professional prevents postpartum depression (Dennis, 2005) and that early interventions are effective in preventing child maltreatment among *first time* disadvantaged mothers (MacMillan & Canadian Task Force on Preventive Health Care, 2000). Other population-based early intervention initiatives are aimed at older children in socioeconomically disadvantaged communities. These universal programs are directed toward the child (eg, classroom enrichment, quality child care), parent (eg, home visiting, parent help/information/crisis phone lines, parent–child play groups), and neighbourhood (information that engages families and connects them to community supports), with an emphasis on providing intensive services to children directly. They have demonstrated improvements in children's emotional problems, behavioural problems, social skills, and a decreased need for special education during the early years (ages 4 to 8 years) (Peters, Petrunka, & Arnold, 2003).

Current thinking around prevention and promotion programs designed for adolescent mental health argues that offerings should support and educate youth (eg, through peer mentoring in community organizations and schools); enhance self-help and self-responsibility, coping skills, self-esteem, and skill development in ways that foster mental health; and teach youth when and how to seek assistance for problems (Federal/Provincial/Territorial Advisory Committee on Population Health, 2000). Particular emphasis has been given to ways of creating healthy images related to gender, body image, and empowerment.

Historically, nurses have been underused in school-based mental health efforts, although schools are good locations for other early intervention programs because they are physically near the families they serve and are less intimidating than mental health centres. Programs can be targeted for very young children before symptoms have time to develop. Studies show that by fourth grade, a large number of young children already use some kind of substance (eg, inhalants, which are toxic); therefore, prevention efforts may be crucial in the early grades (Finke et al., 2002). In numerous schools throughout Canada, Youth Health Centres have become familiar resources.

The number of promotion and early intervention mental health services provided through electronic mechanisms (eg, Internet, telehealth) is growing. Targeted support groups are increasingly available through the Internet. Dedicated websites providing both universal mental health information and confidential intervention services by e-mail are also available through some school systems. Similar services around specific mental health issues are also being tested with high-risk populations. Telehealth, which involves telephone and video support to rural and remote Canada, is increasingly offered both to practitioners and children or their parents (Urness, Hailey, Delday, Callanan. & Orlik, 2004). The full capacity of these approaches is largely unknown, and contrary to professional fears, the users are generally more than satisfied with the services (Williams, May, & Esmail, 2001). Some users even prefer the anonymity of the electronic mechanisms. Nurses are playing instrumental roles in many of these initiatives, both as direct service providers and as on-site support services (Elford, 1998).

Although a number of children's mental health promotion and prevention programs have proven effective on their own, not well understood is the effect of programs that include an array of comprehensive health care services, parent education, and support on the mental health of children and youth (Breton, 1999; Peters et al., 2003). Best thinking to date suggests that the most effective strategies for reducing the burden of suffering from child psychiatric disorders are those that consist of a number of concurrent steps (Offord, Kraemer, Kazdin, Jensen, & Harrington, 1998). First, effective universal programs should be in place. Targeted programs should follow for those not helped sufficiently by the universal programs. Finally, for those unaffected by the targeted programs, clinical services should be available. To be effective, prevention programs need to start early, continue long-term, and involve multiple domains in a child's life (Offord & Bennett, 2002).

In conclusion, undertaking interventions to promote the mental health of children and adolescents is time and effort well spent. Many adult mental health problems can be prevented, coped with more effectively, or at least reduced in their scope and severity through focussed intervention with children and families. Children lack the power and voice to fight for their own needs, making them one of the most vulnerable groups in society. By virtue of their close interaction with families, nurses are in a key position to identify the mental health needs of children and intervene, particularly in times of crisis. The feeling that comes from making a difference can be fulfilling and long-lasting.

NEW DIRECTIONS IN COMMUNITY-BASED MENTAL HEALTH PROMOTION

Mental health promotion with children and youth can occur at individual, familial, community, and global levels. There is growing recognition that multiple factors affect mental well-being, that mental health does not equate to a lack of mental illness and is also affected by the social determinants of mental well-being, and that health promotion efforts need to span across systems (Khanlou, 2003; Khanlou, Beiser, Cole, Friere, Hyman, & Kilbride, 2002). Mental health promotion initiatives need to be individualized to the circumstances of the youth we work with (including their familial and social resources), must be sensitive to context (eg, rural setting or urban multicultural setting), and must incorporate the latest empirical and theoretical developments (see Box 26-1). Among children and youth, in addition to the health and social services systems, the education system can be among the sites where mental health promotion initiatives take place.

SUMMARY OF KEY POINTS

▢ Nurses working with children and adolescents are in a key position to identify risk and protective factors for psychopathology and to intervene to reduce risk.

▢ Nurses who are aware of normal developmental processes can educate parents about their children's behaviours, help them better understand their children's reactions to stress, and decide when intervention may be warranted.

▢ If the process of normal biologic maturation in childhood is disrupted through trauma or neglect, developmental delays and disorders can occur, some of which may have irreversible effects.

▢ From early infancy, children exhibit different kinds of temperaments that are at least partially biologically determined.

▢ Studies of attachment show that the quality of the emotional bond between the child and parental figure is an important determinant of the success of later relationships.

■ Research shows that children who experience major losses, such as death or divorce, are at risk for developing mental health problems.

■ Sibling relationships have significant effects on personality development. Positive sibling relationships can be protective factors against the development of mental health problems.

■ Medical problems in childhood and adolescence may cause psychological problems when illness leads to behaviours common to an earlier developmental stage (regression) or lack of full participation in family, school, and social activities.

■ Striving for identity and independence may lead adolescents to participate in high-risk activities (eg, drug use, unprotected sex, smoking, delinquent behaviours) that may lead to mental health problems.

■ Poverty, homelessness, abuse, neglect, and parental alcoholism all create conditions that undermine a child's ability to make normal developmental gains and contribute to vulnerability for various emotional and behavioural problems.

■ Children who experience disrupted attachments because of out-of-home placements may have difficulty forming close relationships with their new parents and trusting others.

■ Family support services and early intervention programs are designed to prevent removal of the child from the family as a result of abuse or neglect and to maintain a strong, nurturing family system.

■ Psychoeducational approaches, such as training opportunities, group experiences, and bibliotherapy, provide children and families with the information and skills to promote their own mental health.

CRITICAL THINKING CHALLENGES

1 Analyze a case of a family that is grieving a loss and compare the parents' and children's reactions. Include an evaluation of how each child's reactions differ, depending on his or her developmental level.

2 Watch a movie or read a book that provides a child's view of death, divorce, or some other loss and consider how adults may be insensitive to the child's reactions.

3 Examine your own developmental history and pinpoint periods when stressful life events might have increased risk for emotional problems for you or other family members. What protective factors in your own personality and coping skills and in the environment around you helped you to maintain your good mental health?

4 What aspects of life are more stressful for children than for adults (ie, how is it different to experience life as a child)?

5 Examine how your own social and cultural background may either facilitate or create barriers to your ability to interact with families from other ethnic groups or those who are poor or homeless.

6 Allow yourself to reflect on how your own judgmental attitudes might interfere with your ability to communicate effectively with families who have abused or neglected their children.

7 Why is the process of normalization of feelings such a powerful intervention with children and families? What kinds of mental health issues, developmental processes, or both would benefit from teaching related to normal reactions? How can nurses incorporate this kind of intervention into their practice roles?

8 How can nurses expand their roles to have maximal effects on primary, secondary, and tertiary mental health intervention with children and families?

WEB LINKS

www.socialunion.gc.ca The Centres of Excellence for Children's Well-Being website provides the latest information on issues concerning the National Children's Agenda in Canada.

www.cfc-efc.ca The website of the Child and Family Canada, representing about 50 not-for-profit organizations, provides public education on children and families.

www.hc-sc.gc.ca The Health Canada Mental Health Promotion website provides extensive publications, including information on capacity building in youth mental health promotion as well as youth projects.

www.canadiancrc.com This website of the Canadian Children's Right's Council includes the 2005 article, "Homeless Children and Youths in Canada."

www.phac-aspc.gc.ca This is the website of the Public Health Agency of Canada. At this site information and resources on child health can be found. The National Clearinghouse on Family Violence, Canada's resources centre for information on violence within relationships, can be found here.

MOVIES

My Girl: 1991. This story lovingly portrays a young girl coping with her mother's death. It provides a thoughtful general analysis of death because the family runs a funeral parlour.

VIEWING POINTS: How is the depiction of the child's grieving process in this film typical of childhood mourning? What aspects of it appear to be uniquely influenced by her family and the circumstances? How could the adults in the film have been more sensitive to the child's fears and anxieties about death?

To Kill a Mockingbird: 1962. The narrator of this beautiful film is a young girl growing up in the southern United States. The story illustrates several important factors that can influence a child's development, including single-parent families, cultural factors, the effects of abuse and alcoholism, and the child's attempt to reconcile good and evil forces in the world.

VIEWING POINTS: How effective is this single-parent family in coping with life stresses and developmental changes? What aspects of the family's functioning appear particularly strong? Compare Scout and Jem's upbringing to that of the young woman from the family with alcoholism. In what ways does this young girl appear to be at risk for developing mental health problems?

The Breakfast Club: 1985. This funny, poignant portrayal of adolescence is told through the eyes of several teens from different backgrounds brought together when they are assigned to all-day Saturday detention. It illustrates the heightened sense of drama that typifies adolescence, identity concerns, and peer relationship struggles.

VIEWING POINTS: Which of these adolescents do you consider to be most at risk for having mental health problems? State the reasons for your choice. What are some factors that appear to be contributing to the risk-taking and acting-out behaviours among these adolescents?

What's Eating Gilbert Grape?: 1997. Johnny Depp plays Gilbert, a frustrated young man who struggles to be free from emotional stagnation, his sleepy Iowa town, and his 500-pound reclusive mother. This story highlights complex family dynamics and revolves around Gilbert's relationship with his mentally handicapped brother, played by Leonardo Di Caprio.

Significance: Family interaction centres on food and the impact of the mother's obesity on the rest of the family.

VIEWING POINTS: Observe the interaction of the family during meal times. How has the mother's disability affected the family? How would you provide nursing care to this very complex family?

REFERENCES

Adlaf, E. M., & Zdanowicz, Y. M. (1999). A cluster-analytic study of substance problems and mental health among street youths. *American Journal of Drug and Alcohol Abuse, 25*(4), 639–660.

Anthony, K. K., Gil, K. M., & Schanberg, L. E. (2003). Parental perceptions of child vulnerability in children with chronic illness. *Journal of Pediatric Psychology, 28*(3), 185–190.

Barak, G. (1992). *A social history of homelessness in contemporary America.* New York: Praeger.

Beardslee, W. R., Gladstone T. R., Wright, E. J., & Cooper, A. B. (2003) A family-based approach to the prevention of depressive symptoms in children at risk: Evidence of parental and child change. *Paediatrics, 112*(2), e119–131.

Begin, P., Casavant, L., Chenier, N. M., & Dupuis, J. (1999). *Homelessness.* Ottawa: Library of Parliament, Parliamentary Research Branch.

Botvin, G. J. (2000). Preventing drug abuse in schools: Social and competence enhancement approaches targeting individual-level etiologic factors. *Addictive Behaviors, 25*(6), 887–897.

Bowlby, J. (1960). Grief and mourning in infancy and early childhood. *Psychoanalytic Study of the Child, 15,* 9–52.

Breton JJ. (1999). Complementary development of prevention and mental health promotion programs for Canadian children based on contemporary scientific paradigms. *Canadian Journal of Psychiatry.* 44(3):227–234.

Brody, G. H. (1998). Sibling relationship quality: Its causes and consequences. *Annual Review of Psychology, 49,* 1–24.

Browne, K., & Saqi, S. (1988). Approaches to screening for child abuse and neglect. In K. Browne, C. Davies, & P. Stratton (Eds.), *Early prediction and prevention of child abuse* (pp. 57–85). Toronto: John Wiley & Sons.

Burns, J. M., Andrews, G., & Szabo, M. (2002). Depression in young people: What causes it and can we prevent it? *Medical Journal of Australia, 177*(Suppl), S93–96.

Campaign 2000. *One million too many: Implementing solutions to child poverty in Canada. 2004 Report Card on Child Poverty.* Available at: http://www.campaign2000.ca.

Campbell, S. (1995). Behaviour problems in preschool children: A review of recent research. *Journal of Child Psychiatry, 36,* 113–149.

Canadian Centre for Justice Statistics. (2001). *Family violence in Canada: A statistical profile.* Cat. No. 85-224-XPE. Ottawa: Statistics Canada.

Cance, A. M., Paradise, M., Ginzler, J. A., Embry, L., Morgan, C. J., Lohr, Y., & Theofelis, J. (2000). The characteristics and mental health of homeless adolescents: Age and gender differences. *Journal of Emotional & Behavior Disorders, 8*(4), 230–239.

Casa-Gil, M. J., & Navarro-Guzman, J. I. (2002). School characteristics among children of alcoholic parents. *Psychological Reports, 90*(1), 341–348.

Cavell, T., Ennett, S. T., & Meehan, B. T. (2001). Preventing alcohol and substance abuse. In J. N. Hughes, A. M. LaGreca, & J. C. Conoley (Eds.), *Handbook of psychological services for children and adolescents* (pp. 133–160). Oxford: Oxford University Press.

Child Support Team. (2000). *Selected statistics on Canadian families and family law* (2nd ed.). Ottawa: Department of Justice Canada.

Crittenden, P. M. (1996). Research on maltreating families: Implications for intervention. In J. Briere, L. Berliner, A. Bulkey, C. Jenny, & T. Reid (Eds.), *The APSAC handbook on child maltreatment* (pp. 158–174). Thousand Oaks, CA: Sage.

Deering, C. G., & Cody, D. J. (2002). Communicating effectively with children and adolescents. *American Journal of Nursing, 102* (3), 34–42.

Dennis, C. L. (2005). Psychosocial and psychological interventions for prevention of postnatal depression: Systematic review. *British Medical Journal, 331*(7507), 15–24.

Doherty, G. (1997). *Zero to six: The basis for school readiness.* Hull, Quebec: Applied Research Branch, Human Resources Development Canada.

Dryburgh, H. (2000). Teenage pregnancy. *Health Reports, 12,* 9–19.

Eggert, L. L., Thompson, E. A., Randell, B. P., & Pike, K. (2002). Preliminary effects of brief school-based prevention approaches for reducing youth suicide: Risk behaviors, depression, and drug involvement. *Journal of Child and Adolescent Psychiatric Nursing, 15*(2), 48–64.

Elford, R. (1998). Telemedicine activities at memorial University of Newfoundland: A historical review, 1975–1997. *Telemedicine Journal, 4*(3), 207–224.

Farris-Manning, C., & Zandstra, M. (2003). *Children in care in Canada.* Ottawa: Child Welfare League of Canada. Available at: http://www.nationalchildrensalliance.com.

Federal/Provincial/Territorial Advisory Committee on Population Health (1999). *Toward a healthy future: Second report on healthy Canadians*. Cat. N(o): H39-468/1999E. Ottawa: Author.

Federal/Provincial/Territorial Advisory Committee on Population Health. (2000). *The opportunity of adolescence: The health sector contribution*. Cat. N(o): H39-548/200E. Ottawa: Author.

Federal/Provincial/Territorial Council on Social Policy Renewal. (2000). *Public report: Dialogue on the national children's agenda—Developing a shared vision*. Ottawa: Author.

Finke, L., Williams, J., Ritter, M., Kemper, D., Kersey, S., Nightenhauser, J., Autry, K., Going, C., Wulfman, G., & Hail, A. (2002). Survival against drugs: Education for school-age children. *Journal of Child and Adolescent Psychiatric Nursing, 15*(4), 163–169.

Fopma-Loy, J. (2000). Peer rejection and neglect of latency age children: Pathways and group psychotherapy model. *Journal of Child and Adolescent Psychiatric Nursing, 13*, 29–38.

Goldner, E. (2002). *Sharing the learning: The health transition fund-synthesis series. Mental Health*. Cat. N(o): H13-6/2002-8. Ottawa: Health Canada.

Gorzka, P. (1999). Homeless parents' perceptions of parenting stress. *Journal of Child and Adolescent Psychiatric Nursing, 12*, 7–16.

Guruge, S., & Khanlou, N. (2004). Intersectionalities of influence: Researching health of immigrant and refugee women. *Canadian Journal of Nursing Research, 36*(3), 32–47.

Harter, S. (2000). Psychosocial adjustment of adult children of alcoholics: A review of recent empirical literature. *Clinical Psychology Review, 20*(3), 311–337.

Health Canada. (1998). *The consequences of child maltreatment: A reference guide for health practitioners*. Ottawa: Author.

Health Canada & Canadian Mental Health Association. (1999). *All together now: How families are affected by depression and manic depression*. Cat. N(o): H39-461/1999E. Ottawa: Author.

Health Canada. (2000). 1998/1999 Canadian sexually transmitted disease surveillance report. Centre for Infectious Disease Prevention. *Canada Communicable Disease Report (CCDR), 26S6*, 1–46. Available at: http://www.phac-aspc.gc.ca.

Health Canada. (2002). *A report on mental illness in Canada*. Cat. N(o): 0-662-32817-5. Ottawa: Author.

Helfer, M. E., Kemper, S., & Kongman, R. D. (1997). *The battered child*. Chicago: University of Chicago Press.

Herrenkohl, T. I., Tajima, E. A., Whitney, S. D., & Huang, B. (2005). Protection against antisocial behavior in children exposed to physically abusive discipline. *Journal of Adolescent Health, 36*(6), 457–465.

Hetherington, E. M., & Kelly, J. (2002). *For better or for worse: Divorce reconsidered*. New York: WW Norton.

Hughes, J. R., & Gottlieb, L. N. (2004). The effects of the Webster-Stratton parenting program on maltreating families: fostering strengths. *Child Abuse and Neglect, 28*, 1081–1097.

Infant Mental Health Promotion. (2005). *Core prevention and intervention for the early years*. Toronto: The Hospital for Sick Children.

Jeynes, W. (2002). *Divorce, family structure, and the academic success of children*. New York: Haworth Press.

Kaemingk, K., & Paquette, A. (1999). Effects of prenatal alcohol exposure on neuropsychological functioning. *Developmental Neuropsychology, 15*, 111–140.

Khanlou, N. (2003). Mental health promotion education in multicultural settings. *Nursing Education Today, 23*, 96–103.

Khanlou, N., Beiser, M., Cole, E., Freire, M., Hyman, I., & Kilbride, K. M. (2002). *Mental health promotion among newcomer female youth: Post-migration experiences and self-esteem*. Ottawa: Status of Women Canada (English and French versions). Available at: http://dsp-psd.communication.gc.ca.

Khanlou, N., & Crawford, C. (2006). Post-migratory experiences of newcomer female youth: Self-esteem and identity development. *Journal of Immigrant and Minority Health, 81*(1), 45–56.

Khanlou, N., & Peter, E. (2005). Participatory action research: Considerations for ethical review. *Social Science & Medicine, 60*, 2333–2340.

LeBlanc L. A., Goldsmith, T., & Patel, D. R. (2003). Behavioral aspects of chronic illness in children and adolescents. *Pediatric Clinics of North America, 50*(4), 859–878.

Lerner, R. M., & Galambos, N. L. (1998). Adolescent development: Challenges and opportunities for research, programs and policies. *Annual Review Psychology 49*, 413–436.

Leventhal, T., & Brooks-Gunn, J. (2000). The neighborhoods they live in: The effects of neighborhood residence on child and adolescent outcomes. *Psychological Bulletin, 126*, 309–337.

Lewis, M., & Vitulano, L. A. (2003). Biopsychosocial issues and risk factors in the family when the child has a chronic illness. *Child & Adolescent Psychiatric Clinics of North America, 12*(3), 389–399.

MacLeod, J., & Nelson, G. (2000). Programs for the promotion of family wellness and the prevention of child maltreatment: A meta-analytic review. *Child Abuse & Neglect, 24*(9), 1127–1149.

MacMillan, H. L., & Canadian Task Force on Preventive Health Care. (2000). Preventive health care, 2000 update: Prevention of child maltreatment. *Canadian Medical Association Journal, 163*(11), 1451–1458.

MacMillan, H. L., Thomas, B. H., Jamieson, E., Walsh, C. A., Boyle, M. H., Shannon, H. S., & Gafni, A. (2005). Effectiveness of home visitation by public-health nurses in prevention of the recurrence of child physical abuse and neglect: A randomised controlled trial. *Lancet, 365*(9473), 1786–1793.

Maguire, S., Mann, M. K., Sibert, J., & Kemp, A. (2005). Are there patterns of bruising in childhood which are diagnostic or suggestive of abuse? A systematic review. *Archives of Diseases in Childhood, 90*(2), 182–186.

Masten, A. S. (2001). Ordinary magic: Resilience processes in development. *American Psychologist, 56*(3), 227–238.

Menke, E. M. (1998). The mental health of homeless school-age children. *Journal of Child and Adolescent Psychiatric Nursing, 11*, 87–98.

Moser, R. P., & Jacob, T. (2002). Parental and sibling effects in adolescent outcomes. *Psychological Reports, 91*(2), 463–479.

Murray, S. K., Baker, A. W., & Lewin, L. (2002). Screening families with young children for child maltreatment potential. *Pediatric Nursing, 26*, 47–54.

Mylant, M. L., Ide, B., Cuevas, E., & Meehan, M. (2002). Adolescent children of alcoholics: Vulnerable or resilient? *Journal of the American Psychiatric Nurses Association, 8*(2), 57–64.

National Children's Agenda. (2005). *Public dialogue on the National Children's Agenda: Developing a shared vision*. Retrieved July 7, 2005, from http://socialunion.gc.ca/nca/June21-2000/english/sharedvision_e.html.

O'Connor, T. G., Bredenkamp, D., & Rutter, M. (1999). Attachment disturbances and disorders in children exposed to early severe deprivation. *Infant Mental Health Journal, 20*(1), 10–29.

Offord, D. R., & Bennett, K. J. (2002). Prevention. In: M. Rutter, & E. Taylor (Eds.), *Child and adolescent psychiatry* (4th ed.). Oxford, UK: Blackwell Science.

Offord, D. R., Kraemer, H. C., Kazdin, A. E., Jensen, P. S., & Harrington, R. (1998). Lowering the burden of suffering from child psychiatric disorder: Trade-offs among clinical, targeted, and universal interventions. *Journal of the American Academy of Child and Adolescent Psychiatry, 37*(7), 686–694.

Peters, R., Petrunka, K., & Arnold, R. (2003). The better Beginnings, Brighter Futures Project: A universal, comprehensive, community-based prevention approach for primary school children and their families. *Journal of Clinical Child and Adolescent Psychology, 32*, 215–227

Pruett, M. K., Williams, T. Y., Insabella, G., & Little, T. D. (2003). Family and legal indicators of child adjustment to divorce among families with young children. *Journal of Family Psychology, 17*(2), 169–180.

Puskar, K. R., Sereika, S., & Tusaie-Mumford, K. (2003). Effect of the Teaching Kids to Cope (TKC) Program on outcomes of depression and coping among rural adolescents. *Journal of Child and Adolescent Psychiatric Nursing, 16*(2), 71–80.

Putnam, F. W. (2003). Ten-year research update review: Child sexual abuse. *Journal of the American Academy of Child & Adolescent Psychiatry, 42*(3), 269–278.

Raphael, S. (2001). A national action agenda for children's mental health. *Journal of Child and Adolescent Psychiatric Nursing, 14*(4), 193–198.

Reifman, A., Villa, L. C., Amans, J. A., Rethinam, V., & Telesca, T. Y. (2001). Children of divorce in the 1990's: A meta-analysis. *Journal of Divorce and Remarriage, 35*(1–2), 27–36.

Rew, L. (2003). A theory of taking care of oneself grounded in experiences of homeless youth. *Nursing Research, 52*(4), 234–241.

Ringwalt, C. L., Greene, J. M., Robertson, M., & McPheeters, M. (1998). The prevalence of homelessness among adolescents in the United States. *American Journal of Public Health, 88*(9), 1325–1329.

Ritter, J., Stewart, M., Bernet, C., Coe, M., & Brown, S. A. (2002). Effects of childhood exposure to familial alcoholism and family violence on adolescent substance use, conduct problems, and self-esteem. *Journal of Traumatic Stress, 15*(2), 113–122.

Schoor, L. B. (1997). *Common purpose: Strengthening families and neighborhoods to rebuild America.* New York: Doubleday.

Schor, E. L., & the American Academy of Pediatrics Task Force on the Family. (2003). Family pediatrics: Report of the task force on the Family. *Pediatrics, 111*(6 Pt 2), 1541–1571.

Self, B., & Peters, H. (2005). *Canadian Nurse, 101*(1):20–24. Street outreach with no streets

Sharpe, D., & Rossiter, L. (2002). Siblings of children with a chronic illness: A meta-analysis. *Journal of Pediatric Psychology, 27*(8), 699–710.

Slomkowski, C., Rende, R., Conger, K. J., Simons, R. L., & Conger, R. D. (2001). Sisters, brothers, and delinquency: Evaluating social influence during early and middle adolescence. *Child Development, 72*(1), 271–283.

Statistics Canada. (2004). *Health reports: How healthy are Canadians? 2004 Annual Report. Supplement to Vol. 15.* Cat. N(o): 82-003-S1E. Ottawa: Author.

Sun, U., & Li, Y. (2002). Children's well-being during parents' marital disruption process: A pooled time-series analysis. *Journal of Marriage and the Family, 64*(2), 472–488.

Taussig, H. N. (2002). Risk behaviors in maltreated youth placed in foster care: A longitudinal study of protective and vulnerability factors. *Child Abuse & Neglect, 26* (11), 1179–1199.

Tomlin, A. M., & Viehweg, S. A. (2003). Infant mental health: Making a difference. *Professional Psychology: Research and Practice, 34*(6), 617–625.

Trocme, N., MacLaurin, B., Fallon, B., Daciuk, J., Billingsley, D., Tourigny, M., Mayer, M., Wright, J., Barter, K., Burford, G.,

Hornick, J., Sullivan, R., & McKenzie, B. (2001). *Canadian incidence study of reported child abuse and neglect.* Ottawa: Minister of Public Works and Government Services Canada.

Trocme, N., McPhee, D., & Tam, K. K. (1995). Child abuse and neglect in Ontario: Incidence and characteristics. *Child Welfare, 74*, 563–586.

UNICEF. (2005). Child poverty in rich countries, 2005. Innocenti Report Card No.6. Florence, Italy: UNICEF Innocenti Research Centre. Available at: http://www.unicef.org/irc.

Urness, D., Hailey, D., Delday, L., Callanan, T., & Orlik, H. (2004). The status of telepsychiatry services in Canada: A national survey. *Journal of Telemedicine and Telecare. 10*(3), 160–164.

U.S. Department of Commerce News. (2003, September 26). Available at: http://www.census.gov.

Van Epps, J., Opie, N. D., & Goodwin, T. (1997). Themes in the bereavement experience of inner city adolescents. *Journal of Child and Adolescent Psychiatric Nursing, 10*, 25–36.

Veronie, L., & Freuhstorfer, D. B. (2001). Gender, birth order and family role identification among children of alcoholics. *Current Psychology: Developmental, Learning, Personality, Social, 20*(1), 53–67.

Waddell, C., McEwan, K., Shepherd, C. A., Offord, D. R., & Hua, J. M. (2005). A public health strategy to improve the mental health of Canadian children. *Canadian Journal of Psychiatry, 50*(4), 226–233.

Walker, Z. A. K., & Townsend, J. (1999). The role of general practice in promoting teenage health: A review of the literature. *Family Practice, 16*, 164–172.

Warren, J. K., Gary, F. A., & Moorhead, M. S. (1997). Runaway youths in a Southern community: Four critical areas of inquiry. *Journal of Child and Adolescent Psychiatric Nursing, 10*(2), 26–35.

Werner, E. E., & Smith, R. S. (1992). *Overcoming the odds: High risk children from birth to adulthood.* Ithaca, NY: Cornell University Press.

Williams, T. L., May, C. R., & Esmail, A. (2001). Limitations of patient satisfaction studies in telehealthcare: A systematic review of the literature. *Telemedicine Journal and E-Health, 7*(4), 293–316.

Wolfe, D. A. (1998). *Prevention of child abuse and neglect.* Ottawa: Health Canada.

Yalom, I. D. (1985). *The theory and practice of group psychotherapy* (2nd ed.). New York: Basic Books.

Zenah, C. H., Larrieu, J. A., Heller, S. S., Valliere, J., Hinshaw-Fuselier, S., Aoki, Y., & Drilling, M. (2001). Evaluation of a preventive intervention for maltreated infants and toddlers in foster care. *Journal of the American Academy of Child & Adolescent Psychiatry, 40*(2), 214–221.

For challenges, please refer to the **CD-ROM** in this book.

Psychiatric Disorders Diagnosed in Children and Adolescents

Lawrence Scahill, Vanya Hamrin,
Catherine Gray Deering, and Julia Noel

LEARNING OBJECTIVES

After studying this chapter, you will be able to:

- Identify the disorders usually first diagnosed in infancy, childhood, or adolescence, according to the *Diagnostic and Statistical Manual of Mental Disorders,* 4th edition, Text revision *(DSM-IV-TR).*
- Identify the biopsychosocial dimensions of the developmental disorders of childhood.
- Discuss the nursing care of children with pervasive developmental disorders.
- Compare the disruptive behaviour disorders: attention deficit hyperactivity disorder, oppositional defiant disorder, and conduct disorder.
- Relate the assessment data of children with attention deficit hyperactivity disorder to the development of nursing diagnoses, interventions, and evaluation of outcomes.
- Identify the steps involved in fundamental behaviour modification interventions, such as "time out," for children.
- Discuss the epidemiology, etiology, psychopharmacologic interventions, and nursing care of children with disorders of mood and anxiety.
- Discuss the epidemiology, etiology, psychopharmacologic interventions, and nursing care of children with tic disorders.
- Discuss behavioural intervention strategies for the treatment of encopresis.

KEY TERMS

ascertainment bias ▪ autism ▪ communication disorders ▪ concordant ▪ dyslexia ▪ encopresis ▪ enuresis ▪ externalizing disorders ▪ internalizing disorders ▪ learning disorder ▪ mental retardation ▪ phonologic processing ▪ school phobia ▪ stereotypic behaviour

⬠ KEY CONCEPTS

attention ▪ autistic disorder ▪ developmental delay ▪ hyperactivity ▪ impulsiveness ▪ pervasive developmental disorders ▪ tics

The understanding of child psychiatric disorders has benefited from advances in several related fields, including developmental biology, neuroanatomy, psychopharmacology, genetics, and epidemiology. Before the introduction of the third edition of the American Psychiatric Association's (APA's) *Diagnostic and Statistical Manual of Mental Disorders (DSM-III)* in 1980, clinicians based their diagnostic decisions on subjective impressions, rather than on clearly defined diagnostic criteria. Because the clinician's theoretic orientation directly influenced these subjective impressions, psychiatric diagnoses were notoriously unreliable.

The aims of any diagnostic system are to (1) foster communication between clinicians, (2) provide insight concerning etiology, and (3) predict long-term outcomes. Thus, a reliable method for making psychiatric diagnoses is necessary for ongoing research efforts concerning the etiology and outcome of childhood disorders. Because they are categorical in nature without clear categorical boundaries, current psychiatric diagnoses for children and adolescents provide only limited explanations of a condition's etiology or outcomes. However, the clear diagnostic criteria and the multiaxial system introduced by *DSM-III* facilitate communication among clinicians. This chapter uses criteria from the current *Diagnostic and Statistical Manual of Mental Disorders) (DSM-IV-TR;* APA, 2000) in defining childhood disorders. The *DSM-IV-TR* contains 10 categories of disorders, as listed in Table 27-1. Despite their limitations, the *DSM-III* and *DSM-IV-TR* represent major steps forward in defining psychiatric disorders of childhood.

Child psychopathology can be classified according to several broad categories: developmental disorders, disruptive behaviour disorders, mood and anxiety disorders, tic disorders, and psychotic disorders. The prevalence of child psychiatric disorders varies across these categories. For example, child schizophrenia is rare, whereas attention deficit hyperactivity disorder (ADHD) is relatively common. In cited estimates of prevalence for psychiatric disorders of childhood, the numbers usually include adolescents; however, it should be noted that some of these disorders vary with age. For example, depression is more common in adolescents than in younger children. Gender ratio may also vary with some disorders according to age. For example, depression is probably more common in boys in children younger than 12 years of age but is more common in girls during adolescence.

In Canada, at any given time, approximately 14% of children aged 4 to 17 years (more than 800,000) experience mental disorders that cause significant distress and impairment at home, at school, and in the community— fewer than 25% of these children receive specialized treatment (Waddell, McEwan, Shepherd, Offord, & Hua, 2005). This discrepancy appears to be the result of

limited access to treatment facilities, either because of financial constraints or because appropriate mental health services for children are simply unavailable. Psychiatric problems are less easily diagnosed in children than they are in adults. One factor contributing to this difference is that sometimes the symptoms of disorders are difficult to distinguish from the turbulence of normal growth and development. For example, a 4-year-old child who has an invisible imaginary friend is normal; however, an adolescent with an invisible friend might be experiencing a hallucination. The certainty of current estimates for the frequency of the various psychiatric disorders is also inconsistent, partly because of changing definitions of these disorders.

This chapter presents an overview of the childhood disorders that the psychiatric–mental health nurse may encounter and discusses the nursing care of children with these problems. Because it is beyond the scope of this text to present all child psychiatric disorders, this chapter focuses on developmental disorders, excluding mental retardation/intellectual disability, disruptive behaviour, mood and anxiety, and tic disorders. It highlights in detail ADHD. It also briefly describes childhood schizophrenia and elimination disorders.

CRNE Note

All of the psychiatric disorders of childhood and adolescence should be viewed within the context of growth and development models. Safety and self-esteem are priority considerations.

Developmental Disorders of Childhood

Under the primary influences of genes and environment, development may be said to proceed along several pathways, such as attention, cognition, language, affect, and social and moral behaviour. The developmental disorders of childhood include several conditions that are etiologically unrelated; however, their common feature is a significant delay in one or more lines of development. Some of these developmental pathways and developmental delays are closely interwoven. For example, a language delay can interfere with a child's social development and contribute to behaviour problems (Paul, 2002). The *DSM-IV-TR* classifies developmental disorders in several categories, including mental retardation/intellectual disability, pervasive developmental disorders, and specific developmental disorders. It places mental retardation/intellectual disability, on Axis II and records pervasive developmental disorders and specific developmental disorders on Axis I. This is a change from the *DSM-III*, which could be a

Table 27.1	Disorders Usually First Diagnosed in Infancy, Childhood, or Adolescence

Disorder	Characteristics
Mental Retardation/Intellectual Disability Mild Moderate Severe Profound Severity unspecified	Significantly below-average intellectual functioning (IQ about 70 or below) with onset before age 18 years and concurrent impairments in adaptive functioning
Learning Disorders Reading disorder Mathematics disorder Disorder of written expression Learning disorders not otherwise specified	Academic functioning substantially below that expected given the person's chronologic age, measured intelligence, and age-appropriate education
Motor Skills Disorders Developmental coordination disorder	Motor coordination substantially below that expected given the person's chronologic age and measured intelligence
Communication Disorders Expressive language disorder Mixed receptive–expressive language disorder Phonologic disorder Stuttering Communication disorder not otherwise specified	Significant delay or deviance in speech or language
Pervasive Developmental Disorders Autistic disorder Asperger's disorder Pervasive developmental disorder not otherwise specified Rett's disorder Childhood disintegrative disorder	Severe deficits in multiple areas of development; these include impairment in reciprocal social interaction, impairment in communication, and the presence of stereotyped behaviour, restricted interests, and activities
Attention Deficit and Disruptive Behaviour Disorders Predominantly inattentive type Predominantly hyperactive–impulsive type Combined type Conduct disorder Oppositional defiant disorder	Prominent symptoms of inattention and/or hyperactivity–impulsivity A pattern of behaviour that violates the basic rights of others or major age-appropriate societal norms or rules A pattern of negativistic hostile, and defiant behaviour
Feeding and Eating Disorders of Infancy or Early Childhood Pica Rumination disorder Feeding disorder of infancy or early childhood	Persistent disturbances in feeding and eating
Tic Disorders Tourette disorder Chronic motor or vocal tic disorder Transient tic disorder Tic disorder not otherwise specified	Vocal or motor tics
Elimination Disorders Encopresis Enuresis	Repeated passage of feces into inappropriate places Repeated voiding of urine into inappropriate places
Other Disorders of Infancy, Childhood, or Adolescence Separation anxiety disorder Selective mutism Reactive attachment disorder of infancy or early childhood Stereotypic movement disorder	Developmentally inappropriate and excessive anxiety concerning separation from home or those to whom the child is attached A consistent failure to speak in specific social situations despite speaking in other situations Markedly disturbed and developmentally inappropriate social relatedness that occurs in most contexts and is associated with physical and/or emotional neglect Repetitive, seemingly driven, and nonfunctional motor behaviour that markedly interferes with normal activities and at times may result in bodily injury

Data from American Psychiatric Association. (2000). *Diagnostic and statistical manual of mental disorders* (4th ed., Text revision, pp. 39–41). Washington, DC: Author.

source of confusion when reading child psychiatric literature or past medical records.

PERVASIVE DEVELOPMENTAL DISORDERS

Children with pervasive developmental disorders (PDDs) may or may not have an intellectual disability, but they commonly show an uneven pattern of intellectual strengths and weaknesses. Children with PDDs may show a lifelong pattern of being rigid in style, intolerant of change, and prone to behavioural outbursts in response to environmental demands or changes in routine (Box 27-1).

> **KEY CONCEPT Developmental delay** means that the child's development is outside the norm, including delayed socialization, communication, peculiar mannerisms, and idiosyncratic interests.

> **KEY CONCEPT Pervasive developmental disorders** are a group of syndromes marked by severe developmental delays in several areas that cannot be attributed to an intellectual disability.

Types

The *DSM-IV-TR* includes several categories of PDDs, but it is beyond the scope of this chapter to review all of them (Koenig & Scahill, 2001). This section focuses on autistic disorder and Asperger's disorder.

Autistic Disorder

Autistic disorder, or autism, has been a subject of considerable interest and research effort since its original description more than 50 years ago, when Leo Kanner

BOX 27.1

History and Hallmarks of Childhood and Adolescent Disorders

- Maternal age and health status during pregnancy
- Exposure to medication, alcohol, or other substances during pregnancy
- Course of pregnancy, labor, and delivery
- Infant's health at birth
- Eating, sleeping, and growth in first year
- Health status in first year
- Interest in others in first 2 years
- Motor development
- Mastery of bowel and bladder control
- Speech and language development
- Activity level
- Response to separation (eg, school entry)
- Regulation of mood and anxiety
- Medical history in early childhood
- Social development
- Interests

(1943) described the profound isolation of these children and their extreme desire for sameness. Two features distinguish autism from other PDDs: early age of onset (before age 30 months) and severe disturbance in social relatedness. These children appear aloof and indifferent to others and often seem to prefer inanimate objects.

The impairment in communication is severe and affects both verbal and nonverbal communication (APA, 2000). Children with autism manifest delayed and deviant language development, as evidenced by *echolalia* (repetition of words or phrases spoken by others) and a tendency to be extremely concrete in interpretation of language. Pronoun reversals and abnormal intonation are also common. Other common features of autism categorized as **stereotypic behaviour** include repetitive rocking, hand flapping, and an extraordinary insistence on sameness. The child may also engage in self-injurious behaviour, such as hitting, head banging, or biting. For some children, their unusual interests may evolve into fascination with specific objects, such as fans or air conditioners, or a particular topic, such as Prime Ministers of Canada.

> **KEY CONCEPT Autistic disorder** is marked impairment of development in social interaction and communication with a restrictive repertoire of activity and interest.

Epidemiology and Etiology

As currently defined, autism affects between 2 and 20 people per 10,000 in the general population (Chakrabarti & Fombonne, 2001). It occurs in boys more often than girls, with the ratio ranging from 2:1 to 5:1. However, when girls are affected, they tend to be more severely impaired and have poorer outcomes (Volkmar, Klin, & Paul, 2004). About half of children with autism are intellectually disabled, and about 25% have seizure disorders. Recent claims that the prevalence of autism is increasing are confounded by improved diagnosis in lower functioning (eg, low IQ) and higher functioning children.

Numerous theories suggest various causes for autism, including genetics, perinatal insult, and impaired parent–child interactions (Volkmar et al., 2004). It was fashionable in the 1950s and 1960s to believe that the "indifference" of professional parents was a contributing cause of autism. This explanation is no longer seriously considered and almost certainly reflected an **ascertainment bias** (a bias that occurs when the method of identifying cases creates a sample that differs from the population it purports to represent) because professional families were more likely to use the services of major medical centres. It also represents a failure to recognize that the child's disability may have contributed to disturbed parent–child interactions, rather than being an effect of these interactions.

Low IQ and autism recur at a higher-than-expected rate in the siblings of children with autism, and monozygotic twins are more likely to be **concordant** (mutually affected) than are dizygotic twins, suggesting that genetic factors play a role in the disorder. Other proposed causes include perinatal complications, such as exposure to infectious agents or medications during gestation; prematurity; and gestational bleeding. The findings of minor physical anomalies in these children have led to a hypothesis of a first-trimester insult, but controlled studies fail to support a prominent role for perinatal complications in autism (Bolton et al., 1997). Biochemical studies have shown increased platelet serotonin levels, excessive dopaminergic activity, and alteration of endogenous opioids (Novotny, Evers, Barboza, Rawitt, & Hollander, 2003). Despite the substantial body of evidence pointing to a neurobiologic basis, the specific cause remains unknown and may result from multiple factors. Structural and functional imaging studies provide intriguing leads for future inquiry (Courchesne et al., 2003; Schultz et al., 2000; see Fig. 27-1).

Psychopharmacologic Interventions

No medication has proved effective at changing the core social and language deficits of autism. However, numerous psychiatric medications have been used to treat the associated behavioural difficulties in PDDs (see McDougle & Posey, 2003, for a detailed review). Medications can reduce the frequency and intensity of behavioural disturbances, including hyperactivity, agitation, mood instability, aggression, self-injury, and stereotypic behaviour. Haloperidol has demonstrated efficacy in reducing hyperactivity, stereotypic behaviour, and emotional lability (McDougle & Posey, 2003).

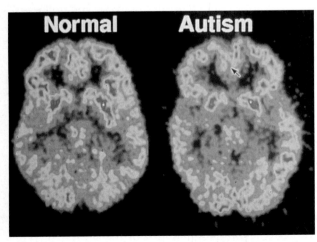

FIGURE 27.1 The client with autism (*right*) may have decreased metabolic rates in the cingulate gyrus and other associated areas; however, wide heterogeneity in brain metabolic patterns is seen in clients with autism. (Courtesy of Monte S. Buchsbaum, MD, The Mount Sinai Medical Centre and School of Medicine, New York, NY.)

Despite these reported benefits, haloperidol is associated with a range of side effects. Findings from a review of 224 children with autism treated with haloperidol showed that 12.5% had either tardive dyskinesia (n = 5) or withdrawal dyskinesias (n = 23) (Campbell et al., 1997). Given these findings, drug holidays every 6 to 12 months are often recommended to observe the child's continued need for medication. The less potent antipsychotics, such as chlorpromazine, tend to cause excessive sedation without clinical improvement.

Preliminary reports on the efficacy of the newer atypical antipsychotics in treating autism show promise (see Koenig & Scahill, 2001; McDougle & Posey, 2003). A multisite placebo-controlled study showed that risperidone (Risperdal) was safe and effective for reducing aggression, tantrums, and self-injury in children with autism (Research Units on Paediatric Psychopharmacology [RUPP] Autism Network, 2002). Long-term results are pending.

Methylphenidate (Ritalin) may reduce target symptoms of inattention, impulsivity, and overactivity in children and adolescents with PDD (Handen, Johnson, & Lubetsky, 2000). A multisite placebo-controlled study of methylphenidate in PDD is currently underway and will provide important new information on efficacy and safety in this population.

Several controlled studies of the opioid antagonist naltrexone have found modest improvements in activity level reported, but this was not supported in a recent study. The selective serotonin reuptake inhibitors (SSRIs) may be helpful in managing compulsive behaviour, withdrawal, and irritability, but they have not been well studied in children with PDD (McDougle & Posey, 2003). Lithium has been reported to reduce manifestations of mood disturbances in individuals with autism. There is also an open study showing that buspirone may reduce agitation and explosive outbursts in some individuals (Buitelaar, van der Gaag, & van der Hoeven, 1998), but these findings have not been replicated.

Continuum of Care

Autism is a chronic disorder usually requiring long-term care at various levels of intensity. Treatment consists of designing academic, interpersonal, and social experiences that support the child's development. Children with autism, even those who are severely affected, may be able to live at home and attend a special school for children with autism that uses behavioural modification. Other outpatient services may include family counselling, home care, and medication. As the child moves toward adulthood, living at home may become more difficult, given the appropriate need for greater independence. The level of structure required depends primarily on IQ and adaptive functioning.

Asperger's Disorder

Although Asperger's disorder was also described about 50 years ago, it was not included in *DSM-III* or *DSM-III-R*. It has been incorporated into *DSM-IV-TR* and is defined as severe and sustained impairment in social interaction and restricted, repetitive patterns of behaviour, interests, and activities (APA, 2000). Children with Asperger's disorder have profound social deficits marked by inappropriate initiation of social interactions, inability to respond to usual social cues, and a tendency to be concrete in their interpretation of language. They also display stereotypic behaviours, such as rocking and hand flapping, and highly restricted areas of interest, such as train schedules, fans, air conditioners, dogs, or British royalty. Signs of developmental delay may not be apparent until preschool or school age, when social deficits become evident (Box 27-2). The differences in intelligence, language development, and age of clear onset suggest that Asperger's is distinguishable from autism. However, it may not be differentiated from autism in the literature (Volkmar et al., 2004).

Asperger's disorder is defined by severe and sustained impairment in social interaction and restricted, repetitive patterns of behaviour, interests, and activities not associated with intellectual disability. Communication deficits are less severe than in autism.

Epidemiology and Etiology

The prevalence of this disorder is difficult to determine because of shifts in its definition and lack of population data on the newly established diagnostic criteria. The current estimate is in the range of 1 to 3 per 10,000. Asperger's disorder appears to be more common in boys. Although no genetic marker has been identified, the disorder often runs in families, with high recurrence in fathers (Volkmar et al., 2004; Volkmar, Klin, Schultz, Rubin, & Bronen, 2000).

Psychopharmacologic Interventions

Psychopharmacologic management is targeted to specific manifestations, such as compulsive behaviour, or comorbid conditions, such as depression. Although no medication studies have been conducted on children with carefully diagnosed Asperger's, approaches to the treatment of depression and anxiety disorders would be the same as those used in typically developing young children.

Continuing Care

Asperger's disorder has been recognized only recently. As with autism, the family needs help in supporting the child's development and in managing symptoms.

BOX 27.2

Clinical Vignette: Frank (Asperger's Disorder)

A paediatrician refers Frank, age 5 years 6 months, for an evaluation because of Frank's unusual preoccupation with ceiling fans and lawn sprinklers. According to his mother, Frank became interested in ceiling fans at age 3 years when he began drawing them, tearing pictures of them out of magazines, and engaging others in discussions about them. In the months before the evaluation, Frank also became fascinated by lawn sprinklers. These preoccupations so dominated Frank's interactions with others that he was practically incapable of discussing any other topics. He remained on the periphery of his kindergarten class and had few friends. Although he tried to make friends, his approaches were inept, and he had trouble reading others.

Frank was the product of a full-term uncomplicated pregnancy, labor, and delivery to his then 25-year-old mother. It was her first pregnancy, and both parents eagerly anticipated Frank's birth. As an infant, Frank was healthy but seemed to cry a lot and was difficult to comfort, causing his mother to feel inadequate and depleted. His motor development was also delayed, and at age 3 years, nonfamily members had difficulty understanding his speech. His articulation, however, was within normal limits at the time of consultation. Frank received regular paediatric care and had no history of serious illness or injury. There was no family history of intellectual disability or psychiatric illness; results of genetic testing for chromosomal abnormality were negative.

In addition to his unusual preoccupations and social deficits, Frank resisted any change in his routine, was easily frustrated, and was prone to temper tantrums. His parents sharply disagreed about the nature of and appropriate response to his problems.

What Do You Think?

1. What effect do you think Frank's preoccupation may have on his family and their relationships?
2. What kind of teaching program would you develop if you were the nurse assigned to this family?

NURSING MANAGEMENT: HUMAN RESPONSE TO DISORDER

Biologic Domain

Assessment

The assessment of children with PDD is a complex endeavour (Koenig & Scahill, 2001). Biologic assessment should include a review of physical health and neurologic status, giving particular attention to coordination, childhood illnesses, injuries, and hospitalizations. The nurse should assess sleep, appetite, and activity patterns because they may be disturbed in these children. Lack of adequate sleep can increase irritability. Comorbid seizure disorders are common in autism, and depression is often seen concurrently with Asperger's. Thus, the nurse should consider these conditions in the assessment.

Youngsters with additional psychiatric disorders or seizures may be receiving multiple medications and require the care of several clinicians. Therefore, the assessment should include a careful review of current medications and treating clinicians.

Nursing Diagnoses for the Biologic Domain

Assessment data generate a variety of potential nursing diagnoses, including Self-Care Deficits, Impaired Verbal Communication, Disturbed Sensory Perceptions, Delayed Growth and Development, and Disturbed Sleep Pattern. Treatment outcomes need to be individualized to the child, family, and social environment.

Interventions for the Biologic Domain

In teaching self-care skills, the nurse needs to consider the child's current adaptive skills and language limitations. Developing a list of activities for the child to post in his or her bedroom may be effective for some children. Drawings or symbols may be useful for nonverbal children. Physical safety is an important concern for children who are cognitively delayed and may have impaired judgment.

As noted earlier, children with PDD may be treated with multiple medications in novel combinations (Martin, Van Hoof, Stubbe, Sherwin, & Scahill, 2003). In some cases, these unusual combinations are the result of careful management; in other cases, the combinations are the result of clinical mismanagement, perhaps because of poor coordination among treating prescribers. Consequently, the nurse should carefully review the target symptoms for each drug treatment with the parents. This review includes possible drug interactions that are especially important for this clinical population.

Psychological Domain

Assessment

Critical elements to evaluate include intellectual ability, communication skills, and adaptive functioning. Direct behavioural observation is critical to evaluate the child's ability to relate to others, to verify the selection of age-appropriate activities, and to watch for stereotypic behaviours. Children with PDD often need specific behavioural interventions to reduce the frequency of inappropriate or aggressive behaviour. These interventions follow from a careful evaluation of the circumstances that precede or accompany the behaviour and the usual consequences of the behaviour (Volkmar et al., 2004). For example, a child may exhibit angry outbursts in response to routine transitions. If the tantrum is dramatic, the consequence may be that the transition does not take place. By structuring the environment and using visual cues to signal the end of one activity and the start of another, it may be possible to reduce the number and intensity of responses to transitions.

Nursing Diagnoses for the Psychological Domain

Assessment data generate a variety of potential nursing diagnoses, including Anxiety and Disturbed Thought Processes. Because of the long-term nature of these disorders, outcomes may change with time.

Interventions for the Psychological Domain

Managing the repetitive behaviours of these children will depend on the specific behaviour and its effects on others or the environment. If the behaviour, such as rocking, has no negative effects, ignoring it may be the best approach. If the behaviour, such as head banging, is unacceptable, redirecting the child and using positive reinforcement are recommended. In some cases, especially in severely delayed children, these strategies may not work, and environmental alterations and perhaps protective headgear are needed.

Social Domain

Assessment

The nursing assessment is an ongoing process in which attention is given to establishing a positive relationship with the child and the family. The assessment should include a review of the child's capacity for self-care and maladaptive behaviours (Koenig & Scahill, 2001). Self-injury and aggression are sometimes present, and children may need to be protected from hurting themselves and others. Inquiry should also include the presence of perseverative behaviours and preoccupation with restricted interests. These odd behaviours may not necessarily cause a problem, but they often interfere with the child's relationships.

Another important domain to consider in the nursing assessment is the effects of the child's developmental delays on the family. Having a child with PDD is bound to influence family interaction, and responding to the child's needs may adversely affect family functioning. For example, sleep disruption in family members who care for these children may increase family stress.

Nursing Diagnoses for the Social Domain

Assessment data generate a variety of potential nursing diagnoses, including Social Isolation. The family may be grieving the loss of the normal child they had expected and are trying to cope with the multitude of problems inherent in raising a child with a disability. Because of the long-term nature of these disorders, the aims of treatment may change with time. However, throughout childhood, the focus should be on the development of age-appropriate adaptive and social skills.

Interventions for the Social Domain

Planning interventions for youngsters with severe developmental problems considers the child, family, and community supports, such as schools, rehabilitation centres, mental health centres, or group homes. First and foremost, the various clinicians involved in the child's treatment should collaborate with the family toward the same general goals. As the number of clinicians and educators involved increases, the chance of fragmentation in treatment planning also increases. The nurse can serve as a case coordinator.

Promoting Interaction

Structuring interventions for social isolation should fit the child's cognitive, linguistic, and developmental levels. Interventions fostering nonverbal social interactions may be more useful than those based on speech. For higher functioning children, activities such as getting the mail, passing out snacks, or taking turns in the context of simple games can engage the child in social activities without requiring the use of their limited language skills. Structuring social interactions so that the child has to share a task with another, such as carrying a load of books, may help to boost confidence in relating to others.

Ensuring Predictability and Safety

When children with PDD are hospitalized, milieu management—a consistent, structured environment with predictable routines for activities, mealtimes, and bedtimes—is necessary for successful treatment. Changes in routine may provoke disorganization in the child with PDD, leading to emotional disequilibrium and explosive behaviour. The safety of the inpatient unit offers an opportunity to try behavioural strategies, such as rewards for managing transitions. Health care professionals can pass on successful strategies to parents or primary caretakers.

Managing Behaviour

Because children with PDD have difficulty relating to others, they should spend most of their time within the therapeutic environment of the unit. These children can learn social and communication skills, such as taking turns in conversation and warning the listener before changing the subject in the context of milieu. If a child requires isolation for control of aggressive or assaultive behaviour, a brief "time out" followed by prompt re-entry into unit activities is optimum.

Autism and related disorders are chronic conditions that call for extraordinary patience and determination. Unfortunately, lack of integration of medical, psychiatric, social, and educational services can add to the family's burden. Parents may manifest denial, grief, guilt, and anger at various points as they adjust to their child's disability. The nurse can offer parents the opportunity to express their frustrations and disappointments and can be alert for indications that parents are in need of additional assistance, such as parent support groups or respite care.

Residential care may be necessary in some cases. After making the decision to place a child into a residential facility, family members may experience guilt, loss, and a sense of failure concerning their inability to care for the child at home.

Supporting Family

Family interventions include support, education, counselling, and referral to self-help groups. Whenever possible, the nurse provides education to help parents determine appropriate expectations for their child with PDD and to meet the child's special needs. The following are examples of potentially useful nursing interventions focusing on the family:

- Interpreting the treatment plan for parents and child
- Modeling appropriate behaviour modification techniques
- Including the parents as cotherapists for the implementation of the care plan
- Assisting the family in identifying and resolving their sense of loss related to the diagnosis
- Coordinating support systems for parents, siblings, and family members
- Maintaining interdisciplinary collaboration

EVALUATION AND TREATMENT OUTCOMES

Evaluation of client and family outcomes is an ongoing process. Short-term outcomes might consist of discrete behavioural improvements, such as reducing self-injurious behaviour by 50%. The long-term goal is for the client to achieve the highest level of functioning. The prognosis depends on the severity of the impairments, the interventions available, and the cognitive ability of the child. The use of standardized rating scales before and after treatment can improve the precision of outcome measurement (Arnold et al., 2000; RUPP Autism Network, 2002).

SPECIFIC DEVELOPMENTAL DISORDERS

In contrast to intellectual disability and PDD, specific developmental disorders are characterized by a narrower range of deficits. These more discrete delays can occur in various developmental domains. However, some children have more than one specific developmental disorder, and some of these disorders may have a common etiology (Paul, 2002; Shaywitz, 2003).

Types

Specific developmental disorders are generally classified as learning, communication, and motor skills disorders. This section focuses primarily on learning and communication disorders.

Learning Disorders

Learning disorders (also called *learning disabilities*) are typically classified as verbal (reading and spelling) or nonverbal (mathematics). This distinction between verbal and nonverbal learning disorders comes from documented differences in their nature and etiology (Shaywitz, 2003).

Generally, learning disorders are defined as a discrepancy between actual achievement and expected achievement based on the person's age and intellectual ability. The definition varies depending on the source and state statute.

Reading disability, also called *dyslexia*, has been recognized for more than 100 years. It is defined as a significantly lower score for mental age on standardized tests in reading that is not the result of low intelligence or inadequate schooling. This relatively common problem affects about 5% of school-aged children, with some studies reporting higher prevalence. In clinical samples, dyslexia affects boys more often than girls; however, a large community-based sample of children with reading disorders found no gender difference. This discrepancy suggests that the observed difference in clinic samples may be related to biases in seeking treatment, rather than a true gender difference (Shaywitz, 2003).

Although it is clear that no single cause will provide a sufficient explanation for reading disability, the underlying problem appears to be a deficit in **phonologic processing**, which involves the discrimination and interpretation of speech sounds. A disturbance in the development of the left hemisphere is believed to cause this deficit. Both genetic and environmental factors have been implicated in the etiology of reading disability. Data from family studies show that reading disability is familial and that shared environmental factors alone cannot explain the high rate of recurrence in affected families. Additional evidence from twin studies indicates that specific weaknesses in phonologic processing are more likely to be observed in monozygotic twins than in dizygotic twins (Willcutt, Pennington, & DeFries, 2000).

Less is known about the prevalence of nonverbal learning disorder (mathematics disorder), with estimates of occurrence ranging from 0.1% to 1.0% of school-aged children, and no apparent difference between boys and girls. Mathematics disorder (which is manifested by significant delay in learning mathematics) appears to be a right-hemisphere disorder. Right-hemisphere dysfunction and math problems have been shown in fragile X syndrome and Turner's syndrome, both of which are genetic syndromes. Other reports from clinical populations have shown that acquired problems, such as early-onset seizure disorders, can produce right hemisphere dysfunction and mathematic disability.

Communication Disorders

Communication disorders involve speech or language impairments. *Speech* refers to the motor aspects of speaking; *language* consists of higher-order aspects of formulating and comprehending verbal communication. A large community survey of 5-year-old children in Canada found a combined prevalence of 19% for speech and language disorders (Beitchman, Nair, Clegg, & Patel, 1986), suggesting they are fairly common in young school-aged children. However, available evidence also suggests that many communication deficits appearing at this age do resolve (Toppelberg & Shapiro, 2000). Nonetheless, speech and language disorders are also associated with psychiatric disability (Tomblin, Zhang, Buckwalter, & Catts, 2000). As with reading disability, there are undoubtedly multiple causes of speech or language handicap.

A delay in speech or language development can adversely affect the child's socialization and education. For example, peers may rebuff or tease a child with an articulation defect or stutter, contributing to withdrawal and a negative self-image. The resulting isolation could limit opportunities to negotiate rules, take turns, and learn cooperation. These same tasks could also be difficult for children with language delay. Moreover, language appears to play a role in the regulation of behaviour and impulses. Not surprisingly, impaired language appears to be a risk factor for ADHD (Shaywitz, 2003; Toppelberg & Shapiro, 2000). Children with language delays may also be at greater risk for reading disability, which may share the same underlying phonologic defect (Tomblin et al., 2000; Willcutt et al., 2000).

NURSING MANAGEMENT: HUMAN RESPONSE TO DISORDER

Nursing assessment of children with a known specific developmental disorder includes (1) evidence of interference in daily life, (2) determination of the youngster's ability (and limitations) to communicate during the interview, (3) assessment of the child's perception about his or her disability, (4) observation for impaired learning and communication, and (5) past and current interventions for the learning or communication deficit, with data gathered through direct interview of the child and significant others such as parents. Several nursing diagnoses can be generated from these data, such as Impaired Verbal Communication and Social Isolation. For the child with learning disabilities, nurses can focus on building self-confidence and helping the family connect with guidance and educational resources that support the child's development into adulthood. For the child with communication disorders, the interventions focus on fostering social and communication skills and making referrals for specific speech or language therapy. Modeling appropriate communication in spontaneous situations with the child can be a useful intervention for some children. The following is an overview of nursing interventions for the child with specific developmental difficulties:

- Introduce strategies for increasing communication skills (eg, initiating conversation, taking turns in conversation, facing the listener).
- Identify and develop specific intervention strategies for problems secondary to learning communication disorders, such as low self-esteem (Tomblin et al., 2000).
- Provide parental support for coping with the disorder.
- Maintain interdisciplinary medical, psychiatric, dental, speech therapy, and educational collaboration.
- Refer to a learning or speech specialist for evaluation and assistance (Toppelberg & Shapiro, 2000).

CONTINUUM OF CARE

Children with learning disabilities obviously require careful psychoeducational and cognitive testing to identify their strengths and deficits. School or clinical psychologists usually perform this type of specialized testing. When a learning disability has been identified, families may need help in advocating for the required services.

The same is true for children with communication disorders, although the services requested may be different. Speech pathologists conduct the diagnostic assessment of speech and language disorder. Nurses may be involved with formal screening for communication disorders (Tomblin et al., 2000). Services such as speech therapy (directed at the motor aspects of speaking) or social skills groups (directed at the social and interpersonal aspects of language) may be available in some school districts and can be obtained if a speech or language disorder has been identified. For some children with communication disorders, the services offered by the school may be insufficient. In such cases, the nurse can help the family locate resources that can provide these needed services.

Disruptive Behaviour Disorders

The disruptive behaviour disorders, which include ADHD, oppositional defiant disorder, and conduct disorder, are a group of syndromes marked by significant problems of conduct. Because these disorders are characterized by "acting out" behaviours, they are sometimes referred to as **externalizing disorders**. In contrast, disorders of mood (eg, anxiety, depression) are classified as **internalizing disorders** because the symptoms tend to be within the child.

The disruptive behaviour disorders are more common in boys and are associated with lower socioeconomic status, urban living (Scahill et al., 1999), learning disabilities (Shaywitz, 2003; Tomblin et al., 2000), and language delay (Toppelberg & Shapiro, 2000). These disorders are relatively common in school-aged children and are frequently presenting complaints in child psychiatric treatment settings.

ATTENTION DEFICIT HYPERACTIVITY DISORDER

ADHD is a common disorder in school-aged children. It is almost certainly a heterogeneous disorder with multiple etiologies. The relatively high frequency of ADHD and associated behaviour problems virtually guarantees that nurses will meet these children in all paediatric treatment settings.

Clinical Course and Diagnostic Criteria

Attention deficit hyperactivity disorder is a persistent pattern of inattention, hyperactivity, and impulsiveness that is pervasive and inappropriate for developmental level (APA, 2000).

Parents and teachers describe children with ADHD as restless, always on the go, highly distractible, unable to wait their turn, heedless, and frequently disruptive. Indeed, it is often disruptive behaviour that brings these children into treatment. The historical debate concerning the nature of ADHD is reflected in the labels used to describe it: organic brain syndrome, hyperkinetic impulse disorder, minimal brain dysfunction, hyperkinetic reaction of childhood, hyperkinesis, attention deficit disorder, and most recently, in *DSM-IV-TR*, attention deficit hyperactivity disorder. This long list of terms also implies the various theories regarding the cause and the presumed site of the primary defect. The *DSM-IV-TR* represents yet another formulation of

Table 27.2	**Key Diagnostic Characteristics of Attention Deficit Hyperactivity Disorder** **314.10: Attention deficit hyperactivity disorder, combined type** **314.00: Attention deficit hyperactivity disorder, predominantly** **inattentive type** **314.01: Attention deficit hyperactivity disorder, predominantly** **hyperactive–impulsive type** **314.9: Attention deficit hyperactivity disorder, not otherwise specified**	DSM IV

Diagnostic Criteria and Target Symptoms	Associated Features

• Symptoms of inattention (at least six)
  Lacks close attention to details; makes careless
    mistakes in activities
  Has difficulty sustaining attention
  Appears to not listen when spoken to directly
  Has difficulty following-through on instructions; fails
    to finish work or activities
  Has difficulty organizing tasks and activities
  Has difficulty with tasks requiring sustained mental
    effort; commonly avoids, dislikes, or is reluctant to
    engage in them
  Loses items necessary for tasks
  Is easily distracted by outside stimuli
  Is often forgetful in daily activities
• Symptoms of hyperactivity-impulsivity (at least six):
  Hyperactivity
    Fidgets or squirms
    Gets up when expectation is to remain seated
    Excessively runs about or climbs inappropriately
    Has difficulty with quiet leisure activities
    Often appears "on the go" or "driven by a motor"
    Talks excessively
  Impulsivity
    Blurts out answers before question completion
    Has difficulty awaiting turn
    Is interruptive or intrusive or others
• Symptoms are maladaptive and inconsistent with
  developmental level, persisting for at least 6 months
• Some symptoms present before age 7 years
• Evidence of significant impairment in social, academic,
  or occupational functioning
• Not exclusive during other psychiatric disorder; not
  better accounted for by another mental disorder
	• Low frustration tolerance
	• Temper outbursts
	• Bossiness, stubbornness
	• Excessive and frequent insistence for requests to be met
	• Mood lability
	• Demoralization
	• Dysphoria
	• Rejection by peers
	• Low self-regard
	• Resentment and antagonism within family
	• Reduced vocational achievement

ADHD by defining ADHD as predominantly hyperactive type, predominantly inattentive type, or combined type (Table 27-2). Despite the historical shifts in terminology and the various proposals regarding the etiology of ADHD, the accumulated consensus during the past several decades is that three core symptoms define the disorder: inattention, impulsiveness, and hyperactivity.

Attention is a complex mental process that involves the ability to concentrate on one activity to the exclusion of others, as well as the ability to sustain focus. Children with ADHD are easily distracted and lack persistence in the performance of age-appropriate tasks, reflecting an inability to filter stimuli, sustain attention, or both. The inability to screen stimuli leaves the child unable to identify salient stimuli. The child may then treat all incoming stimuli with equal regard and respond to multiple incoming stimuli. Alternatively, it

has been argued that the distractibility seen in ADHD is the result of stimulus-seeking behaviour. Given the heterogeneity of ADHD, either of these models may be true for subgroups of affected children.

Both clinical observation and laboratory studies support the conclusion that children with ADHD are prone to impulsive, risk-taking behaviour (Barkley, 1998).

KEY CONCEPT Attention is a complex process that involves the ability to concentrate on one activity to the exclusion of others and the ability to sustain that focus.

A fundamental question that some have raised is whether impulsiveness is truly separate from distractibility or hyperactivity. Alternatively, some have argued that children with ADHD have an impaired capacity to learn through reinforcement, which predisposes them to impulsive behaviour. Indirect support for this view comes from studies showing that animals with lesions of the frontal lobe are less able to make use of reinforcement without additional external structure and greater rewards (Barkley, 1998). In behavioural terms, children with ADHD often fail to consider the consequences of their actions, exercise poor judgment, and tend to have more than the usual lumps, bumps, and bruises because of their risk-taking behaviour. They often require a high degree of structure and supervision.

> ⬟ **KEY CONCEPT Impulsiveness** is the tendency to act on urges, notions, or desires without adequately considering the consequences.

Although hyperactivity is a characteristic often associated with ADHD, controversy is long-standing about whether attention deficit can occur without overactivity. The decision by *DSM-IV-TR* to define ADHD as predominately hyperactive, predominately inattentive, or combined offers a compromise in the debate regarding attention deficit disorder with or without hyperactivity. Even those who argue in favour of attention deficit disorder without hyperactivity acknowledge that it is probably much less common than attention deficit disorder with hyperactivity.

In many cases, it is the hyperactivity that prompts the search for treatment. Parents typically report that the child's hyperactivity was manifest early in life and evident in most situations. However, the child's overactivity may be more noticeable in the classroom because it is poorly tolerated there (Barkley, 1998).

> ⬟ **KEY CONCEPT Hyperactivity** is excessive motor activity, as evidenced by restlessness, inability to remain seated, and high levels of physical motion and verbal output.

Epidemiology and Risk Factors

Although prevalence estimates vary depending on the diagnostic criteria used, the sources of data, and the sampling procedure, ADHD is a common psychiatric disorder of childhood. The current estimate in school-aged children is about 6%, with a range of 2% to 14%. Boys are affected three to eight times more often than are girls (for a review, see Scahill & Schwab-Stone, 2000). Longitudinal studies that followed groups of children with ADHD into adulthood have shown that 30% to 40% continued to have problems with impulsiveness and inattention, although hyperactivity was less evident (Weiss & Weiss, 2002). Older adolescents and young adults with a history of ADHD were more likely to have multiple arrests, arrests for more serious offenses, and more car accidents than were individuals

Temple Grandin, Ph.D. (1949–)
Scientist and a Person With Autism

Public Persona
Dr. Temple Grandin is a gifted scientist and world-renowned expert on cattle. Her book, *Thinking in Pictures and Other Reports of My Life With Autism* (1996), is an astonishing revelation of the profoundly different way in which a person with autism conceives and experiences the world. Her story shows the extraordinary way in which she uses her visual thinking ability to develop her field of animal science. It gives us a view of her world and helps us understand the reason she identifies with Data, the android in *Star Trek*.

Personal Realities
As a child, Temple experienced life as chaotic, full of engulfing sensations of sound, smell, and touch. She would scream, rock, or spin continually and shut the world out by fixing for hours on one object. At first thought to be deaf when she did not learn to speak, she was taken to a neurologist and labeled "brain-damaged." Although she gained a sense of language and speech, connecting with others was affected by her inability to understand them or them, her. She dreamed of a magic machine that could give her safe "hugging." Her mother's dedication to her and the guidance of a gifted science teacher enabled her to create a life as a scientist.

in the control group (Weiss & Weiss, 2002). Clearly, a substantial percentage of children do not "grow out of" ADHD. These findings bolster the connection between ADHD and "antisocial" behaviour (see Chapter 24).

Etiologic Factors

Despite more than a half century of investigation, the etiology of ADHD remains unclear (Weiss & Weiss, 2002). Numerous environmental exposures, including perinatal insult, head injury, psychosocial disadvantage, lead poisoning, and diet (eg, food allergies or sensitivity to food additives) have been proposed as potential causes. Although these hypotheses may explain some cases, none of these exposures alone is likely to account for a significant portion of children with ADHD (Weiss & Weiss, 2002). The claim that food additives or allergies cause ADHD has very limited data to support it (Weiss & Weiss, 2002).

Biologic Factors

Although the etiology of ADHD is uncertain, persuasive evidence from several lines of research has shown that the frontal lobe and functional connections with specific subcortical structures are dysregulated in clients with ADHD. For example, structural magnetic resonance imaging (MRI) studies of 57 boys with ADHD compared with those of 55 control subjects showed reduced volumes of the right dorsolateral frontal region and of selected regions of the basal ganglia (Castellanos et al., 1996). Using single-photon emission computed tomography (SPECT) to measure brain activity, Lou, Henriksen, and Bruhn (1990) found reduced blood flow in these same subcortical regions (caudate and putamen) of individuals with ADHD compared with those of control subjects. Additional evidence linking ADHD to dysfunction of the frontal lobe comes from a positron emission tomography (PET) study of adults who had a personal history of ADHD and were parents of children with ADHD. This study found hypoperfusion (decreased metabolic activity) in the frontal lobe of the adults with a history of ADHD compared with the control group (Zametkin et al., 1990). These investigators used similar techniques to evaluate frontal lobe functioning in a group of adolescents with ADHD. Although the findings were in the same direction, the difference between control subjects and the adolescents with ADHD was not statistically significant (Zametkin et al., 1993). More recently, Vaidya and colleagues (1998) showed differences in frontal-subcortical function during an attentional task. The difference between control subjects and subjects with ADHD was reduced when the subjects with ADHD received methylphenidate.

Genetic factors have also been implicated in the etiology of ADHD, and they clearly play a fundamental role for at least a subgroup of children. Several twin studies have shown that, although identical twins are not fully concordant for ADHD, they are far more likely to be mutually affected than are dizygotic twins (Levy et al., 1997). In this large twin study, investigators examined the concordance of ADHD symptoms in a large community sample of monozygotic and dizygotic twins across a wide range of symptoms, from none to severe (Levy et al., 1997). In that study, roughly 82% of the monozygotic (MZ) twin pairs were mutually affected (concordant), compared with 38% in the dizygotic (DZ) twins. Moreover, the MZ twin pairs showed greater similarity on a parent rating of ADHD symptoms across the entire range (from no symptoms) when compared with the DZ twin pairs. These findings suggest that ADHD can be viewed as one or more heritable traits (eg, attention and impulsiveness) on a continuum from mild to severe. Family genetic studies also support a prominent role for genetics in the etiology of ADHD. In the largest family study to date, Biederman and colleagues (1992) showed that ADHD is roughly six times more likely to affect biologic relatives of children with ADHD than biologic relatives of paediatric control subjects.

Psychological and Social Factors

Although genetic endowment clearly plays a fundamental role in the etiology of ADHD, environmental factors are also important. Psychosocial influences (family stress and marital discord) are associated with ADHD, but the direction of causality is difficult to determine (Scahill et al., 1999; Szatmari, Boyle, & Offord, 1989). Other psychosocial correlates that have been observed in large community samples (Scahill et al., 1999; Szatmari et al., 1989) and clinical samples (Biederman et al., 1995) are poverty, overcrowded living conditions, and family dysfunction.

NURSING MANAGEMENT: HUMAN RESPONSE TO DISORDER

Biologic Domain

The nursing assessment for the biologic domain may be initiated either before or after the diagnosis of ADHD is made. In the school setting, the teacher may suspect ADHD and consult the school nurse. The nurse in collaboration with the teacher will collect assessment data similar to that collected by the nurse in a psychiatric facility.

Assessment

In the school setting, the primary focus of the assessment is the impact of ADHD on classroom behaviour and school performance. In the hospital, the nurse tries to determine the contribution of ADHD to the acute psychiatric problem. In both cases, the nurse collects assessment data through direct interview, observation of the child and parent, and teacher ratings. Because children with ADHD may have difficulty sitting through long sessions, interviews are typically brief. Parents and teachers are extremely important sources for assessment data. To this end, the nurse can make use of several standardized instruments (Box 27-3).

As with other psychiatric disorders with onset in childhood, the nursing assessment of children with ADHD begins with identification and exploration of the presenting problem. This typically entails a review of the child's developmental course, the onset and pattern of the current symptoms, factors that have worsened or improved the child's problems, and prior treatment or self-initiated efforts to remedy the situation. The association of ADHD and communication disorders suggests a need for careful consideration of language development and current language functioning. Medical history is also essential, consisting of perinatal course, childhood illnesses, hospital admissions, injuries, seizures, tics, physical growth, general health status, and timing of the child's last physical examination. Family history is also an important part of assessment data.

BOX 27.3

Standardized Tools for ADHD Diagnosis

The Conners Parent Questionnaire is a 48-item scale that a parent completes about his or her child. Each item is a statement that the parent rates on a 4-point scale from 0 (not at all) to 3 (very much). The Conners Teacher Questionnaire is a 28-item questionnaire that the child's teacher completes according to the same 4-point scale as the Parent Questionnaire. Both questionnaires have been standardized by age and gender for a mean of 50 and a standard deviation of 10 (Conners, 1989; Goyette et al., 1978).

The ADHD Rating Scale is a recently developed measure that asks parents or teachers to respond directly to 18 items in the *DSM-IV-TR* criteria (see Barkley, 1998, for a description of this scale). A similar scale called the SNAP-IV is available on-line for free at www.adhd.net. The SNAP-IV was used as the primary outcome measure in the MTA Cooperative Group Study (1999).

The Child Behaviour Checklist (CBCL) is a 118-item questionnaire that a parent completes. In addition to the 118 questions about specific behaviours and psychiatric symptoms, the CBCL also includes questions concerning the child's competence in social and academic spheres as well as age-appropriate activities. Normative data are available allowing the conversion of raw scores to standard scores for age and gender. There is also a teacher version of this scale.

*Note that the diagnosis of ADHD is not made on the basis of questionnaires alone. Data from these rating scales augment the information gathered through interview and observation. These questionnaires can be especially useful before and after initiating a treatment plan to measure change.

Behaviour of these children is characteristically very active and can often be observed in the office. They cannot sit still. They fidget. Even in sleep, they may be more active than normal children. Thus, a careful assessment of eating, sleeping, and activity patterns is essential. Assessing daily food intake, typical diet, and frequency of eating will help identify any nutrition problems. Caffeinated products can contribute to hyperactivity. Sleep is often disturbed for children with ADHD and consequently the family. A detailed sleep assessment can provide points for interventions and help the interpretation of drug effects.

Nursing Diagnoses for the Biologic Domain

Depending on the severity of the responses, family situation, and school environment, several nursing diagnoses could be generated from the assessment data, including Self-Care Deficit, Risk for Imbalanced Nutrition, Risk for Injury, and Disturbed Sleep Pattern. The outcomes should be individualized to the child.

Interventions for the Biologic Domain

The planning of nursing interventions must be done within the context of the family, treatment setting, and school environment. With the parents, clinical team members, and school personnel, the nurse participates in designing a plan of care that fits the child's and family's needs. Medication can help the hyperactivity, impulsiveness, and inattention; therefore, teaching the parent, child, and school personnel about the importance of the medication in ADHD and the potential side effects is a place to begin. Explaining to the child that the medication improves concentration and the ability to sit still can help strengthen client motivation.

Several medications may be used in the treatment of ADHD, although the stimulants are by far the most common (Table 27-3). Commonly used stimulants include methylphenidate, D-amphetamine, and D-, L-amphetamine. Although each of these medications has demonstrated efficacy in controlled studies, methylphenidate has received considerably more research effort and is typically the first medication tried in the treatment of ADHD (MTA Cooperative Group, 1999). Another psychostimulant, pemoline, has fallen out of use because of concerns about liver toxicity. It should be noted that the stimulants are not effective in all cases; thus, alternatives to the stimulants may be prescribed for children who do not experience response to the stimulants or develop tics when taking them (Biederman & the ADHD Study Group, 2002; Scahill, Chappell, et al., 2001).

Methylphenidate is a short-acting medication that peaks in about 90 minutes to 2 hours and has a total duration of action of about 4 hours. Thus, parents or teachers often describe a return of overactivity and distractibility as

Table 27.3   Stimulant Medications Used in Treating ADHD

Medication	Total Daily Dosage*	Common Side Effects
Methylphenidate	10–60 mg in two or three divided doses	Loss of appetite, insomnia, rebound activation, increase in tics or compulsive behaviour, psychotic reaction
D-Amphetamine	5–40 mg in two divided doses	Similar to methylphenidate
D, L-Amphetamine	5–40 mg in two divided doses	Similar to methylphenidate

*Dosage ranges are similar for long-acting products Concerta, Metadiate, and Adderall.

BOX 27.4

Drug Profile: Methylphenidate (Ritalin)

DRUG CLASS: CNS stimulant

RECEPTOR AFFINITY: The mechanisms of effect are not completely clear. At low doses, it provides mild cortical stimulation similar to that of amphetamines. This stimulation results from methylphenidate's ability to promote release and interfere with the reuptake of dopamine in the synaptic cleft. Main sites appear to be the cerebral cortex, striatum, and pons.

INDICATIONS: Treatment of narcolepsy, attention deficit disorders, and hyperkinetic syndrome; unlabeled uses for treatment of depression in elderly patients and patients with cancer or stroke.

ROUTES AND DOSAGE: Available in 5- to 10-mg immediate-release tablets and 20-mg sustained-release tablets (Ritalin-SR). Newer long-acting preparations such as Concerta and Metadate, in various dose strengths, are also available.

Adult Dosage: Must be individualized; range from 10 to 60 mg/d orally in divided doses bid to tid, preferably 15 to 30 min before meals. If insomnia is a problem, drug should be administered before 6 PM.

Child Dosage: The immediate release formulation can be started at 5 mg twice or three times daily on a 4-hour schedule with weekly increases depending on response. Starting doses of the long-acting preparations are equivalent to the total tid dose (eg, 5 tid of short-acting would translate into 18 mg of Concerta). Usually given on a tid schedule, with the last dose being roughly half that of the first and second dose. Daily dosage of > 60 mg not recommended. Discontinue after 1 month if no improvement.

PEAK EFFECT: 1 h; *half-life:* 3–4 h for the immediate-release preparations.

SELECT ADVERSE REACTIONS: Nervousness, insomnia, dizziness, headache, dyskinesias (including tics), toxic psychosis, anorexia, nausea, abdominal pain, increased pulse and blood pressure, palpitations, tolerance, psychological dependence.

WARNING: The drug is discontinued periodically to assess the client's condition. Contraindications include marked anxiety, tension and agitation, glaucoma, severe depression, and obsessive-compulsive symptoms. Use cautiously in clients with a personal or family history of tic disorders, seizure disorders, hypertension, drug dependence, alcoholism, or emotional instability.

SPECIFIC CLIENT/FAMILY EDUCATION

- Do not chew or crush sustained-release tablets—they must be swallowed whole.
- Take the drug exactly as prescribed; if insomnia is a problem, time and dose may need adjustment. The drug is rarely taken after 5 PM.
- Avoid alcohol and OTC products, including decongestants, cold remedies, and cough syrups—these could accentuate side effects of the stimulant.
- Keep appointments for follow-up, including evaluations for monitoring the child's growth and use of parent and teacher ratings to monitor benefit.
- Note that the prescriber may discontinue the drug periodically to confirm effectiveness of therapy.

---

the first dose of medication wears off. This "rebound effect" can often be managed by moving the second dose of the day slightly closer to the first dose. Similar phenomena may be observed with the amphetamines, although the rebound typically occurs later because the duration of action is slightly longer than that for methylphenidate (see Box 27-4). To obviate the need for redosing during the day, several new long-acting formulations of methylphenidate and amphetamine compounds have been developed (Ford, Greenhill, & Posner, 2003).

Psychological Domain

Assessment

Hyperactivity, impulsivity, and inattention are typically pervasive problems that are evident both at school and at home. Discipline is frequently an issue because parents may have difficulty controlling their child's behaviour, which is disruptive and occasionally destructive.

Nursing Diagnoses for the Psychological Domain

Assessment of the psychological domain may generate several diagnoses, including Anxiety and Defensive Coping. The outcomes should be individualized to the child.

Interventions for the Psychological Domain

As a complement to medication, behavioural programs based on rewards for positive behaviour, such as waiting turns and following directions, can foster new social skills. Interventions may also include specific cognitive behavioural techniques in which the child learns to "stop, look, and listen" before doing. These approaches have been refined, and several useful treatment manuals are available (Barkley, 1997). In general, these manuals emphasize problem solving and development of prosocial behaviour. Interactions with children can be guided by the following:

- Set clear limits with clear consequences. Use few words and simplify instructions.
- Establish and maintain a predictable environment with clear rules and regular routines for eating, sleeping, and playing.
- Promote attention by maintaining a calm environment with few stimuli. These children cannot filter extraneous stimuli and react to all stimuli equally.
- Establish eye contact before giving directions; ask the child to repeat what was heard.
- Encourage the child to do homework in a quiet place, outside of a traffic pattern.
- Assist the child to work on one assignment at a time (reward with a break after each completion).

Social Domain

Assessment

Dysfunctional interactions can develop within the family. Reviewing the problem behaviours and the situations in which they occur is a way to identify negative interaction patterns. These children are often behind in their work at school because of poor organization, off-task behaviour, and impulsive responses. They can exhaust their parents, aggravate teachers, and annoy siblings with their intrusive and disruptive behaviour. Because ADHD often occurs in the context of psychosocial adversity, it is important to review the family situation, including parenting style, stability of household membership, consistency of rules and routines, and life events, such as divorce, moves, deaths, and job loss. Identification of these factors can be useful in shaping a care plan that builds on potential strengths and mitigates the effects of environmental factors that may perpetuate the child's disruptive behaviour. Data regarding school performance, behaviour at home, and comorbid psychiatric disorders are essential for developing school interventions and behaviour plans and establishing the baseline severity for medication.

Nursing Diagnoses for the Social Domain

Depending on the severity of the child's responses, family situation, and school environment, several nursing diagnoses could be generated from the assessment data, including Impaired Social Interaction, Ineffective Role Performance, and Compromised Family Coping. Short-term outcomes, such as decreasing the number of classroom ejections within a 2-week period, may be useful for one child, whereas reducing the frequency and amplitude of angry outbursts at home may be relevant to another child.

Interventions for the Social Domain

Family treatment is nearly always a component of cognitive behavioural treatment approaches with the child. This may involve parent training that focuses on principles of behaviour management, such as appropriate limit setting and use of reward systems, as well as revising expectations about the child's behaviour. School programming often involves increasing structure in the child's school day to offset the child's tendency to act without forethought and to be easily distracted by extraneous stimuli. Specific remediation is required for the child with comorbid deficits in learning or language. Some children may require small, self-contained classrooms.

EVALUATION AND TREATMENT OUTCOMES

Children may not notice any effects after taking medication, but people in their environment do. Often, within 1 to 2 weeks of initiating therapy, children with ADHD become more attentive, less impulsive, and less active. Parents and teachers are often the first to notice improvement. Useful tools for tracking changes in behaviour are the Parent and Teacher Conners Questionnaires (Conners, 1989), the ADHD Rating Scale (Barkley, 1998), and the SNAP-IV (MTA Cooperative Group, 1999). With time, academic achievement also may improve (Fig. 27-2).

CONTINUUM OF CARE

Treatment of ADHD typically is conducted in community clinic settings. Optimal treatment is multimodal (includes several types of interventions), encompassing four main areas: individual treatment for the child, family treatment, school accommodations, and medication. The Multi-modal Treatment of ADHD Study (MTA Cooperative Group, 1999) showed that well-managed medication is the most important intervention for the core symptoms of ADHD. Parent training and social skills training also help diminish disruptive and defiant behaviour. See Nursing Care Plan 27-1.

OPPOSITIONAL DEFIANT DISORDER AND CONDUCT DISORDER

Oppositional defiant disorder is characterized by a persistent pattern of disobedience, argumentativeness, angry outbursts, low tolerance for frustration, and tendency to blame others for misfortunes, large and small. Conduct disorder is characterized by serious violations of social norms, including aggressive behaviour, destruction of property, and cruelty to animals. Children with oppositional defiant disorder have trouble making friends and often find themselves in conflict

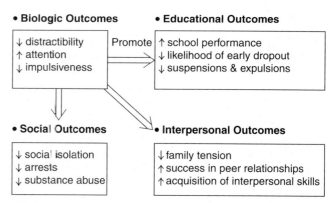

FIGURE 27.2   Long-term outcomes of optimal treatment for clients with attention deficit hyperactivity disorder.

NURSING CARE PLAN 27.1

Attention Deficit Hyperactivity Disorder

Jamie, age 6 years, comes to the mental health clinic with his mother Lillian because of motor restlessness, distractibility, and disruptive behaviour in the classroom. According to Lillian, Jamie had a reasonably good year in kindergarten, but early in the first grade, the teacher began to report disruptive behaviour. On reflection, Lillian recalls that kindergarten was a half-day program with more activity. By contrast, Jamie is expected to sit in his seat and pay attention for longer periods in first grade.

Jamie's medical history is unremarkable. Lillian's pregnancy with Jamie was her first and unplanned. Although there were no complications during the pregnancy, the period was marked by significant marital discord, culminating in divorce before Jamie's first birthday. Jamie was born by cesarean section after a long, unproductive labor. He was healthy at birth and grew normally, with no devel-

opmental delays. Despite genuine interest in other children, his intrusive style and inability to wait his turn resulted in frequent conflicts with them. The family history is positive for substance abuse in his father. In addition, Lillian reports that her ex-husband was disruptive in school, had trouble concentrating, and was highly impulsive. These problems have continued into adulthood.

During the two evaluation sessions, Jamie is active but cooperative. His speech is fluent and normal in tone and tempo, but somewhat loud. His discourse is coherent, but at times he makes rather abrupt changes in conversation without warning his listeners. Psychological testing done at the school revealed average to above-average intelligence. Parent and teacher questionnaires concurred that Jamie was overactive, impulsive, inattentive, and quarrelsome, but not defiant.

SETTING: MENTAL HEALTH CENTRE—CHILD & ADOLESCENT SERVICES

Baseline Assessment: Jamie is a 6-year-old boy with prominent hyperactivity and disruptive behaviour. He lives with Lillian, his single mother. These problems interfere with his interpersonal relationships and academic progress. Lillian is discouraged and feels unable to manage Jamie's behaviour.

Associated Psychiatric Diagnosis	*Medications*

Axis I: Attention deficit hyperactivity disorder
Axis II: None
Axis III: None
Axis IV: Problems with primary support (mother is exhausted)
Educational problems (failing in school)
Economic problems (mother in entry-level
  job with no health insurance)
Axis V: GAF = 52
	Methylphenidate 5 mg at breakfast and lunch (ie, at
	  8 AM and 12 noon), then adding 5 mg at 4 PM. The
	  likely dose would be 7.5 mg at 8 AM & 12 noon &
	  5 mg at 7 PM.

NURSING DIAGNOSIS 1: IMPAIRED SOCIAL INTERACTION

Defining Characteristics	*Related Factors*

Cannot establish and maintain developmentally
  appropriate social relationships
Has interpersonal difficulties at school
Is not well accepted by peers
Is easily distracted
Interrupts others
Cannot wait his turn in games
Speaks out of turn in the classroom
	Impulsive behaviour
	Overactive
	Inattentive
	Risk-taking behaviour (tried to climb out the window to
	  get away from Lillian)
	Failure to recognize effects of his behaviour on others.

Outcomes

Initial	*Discharge*
1. Decrease hyperactivity and disruptive behaviour. 2. Improve attention and decrease distractibility. 3. Decrease frequency of acting without forethought.	4. Improve capacity to identify alternative responses in conflicts with peers. 5. Improve capacity to interpret behaviour of age-mates.

Interventions

Intervention	*Rationale*	*Ongoing Assessment*
Educate mother and teach about ADHD and use of stimulant medication.	Better understanding helps to ensure adherence; also parents and teachers often miscast children with ADHD as "troublemakers."	Determine extent to which parent or teacher "blames" Jamie for his problems.
Monitor adherence to medication schedule.	Uneven compliance may contribute to failed trial of medication.	Administer parent and teacher questionnaires; inquire about behaviour across entire day.

NURSING CARE PLAN 27.1 (Continued)

Interventions

Intervention	Rationale	Ongoing Assessment
Ensure that medication is both effective and well tolerated.	Stimulants can affect appetite and sleep and can cause "behavioural rebound" (Barkley, 1998).	Administer parent and teacher questionnaires; check height and weight; ask about sleep and appetite.

Evaluation

Outcomes	Revised Outcomes	Interventions
Jamie shows decreased hyperactivity and less disruption in the classroom.	Improve ability to identify disruptive classroom behaviour.	Initiate point system to reward appropriate behaviour.
Jamie shows improved attention and decreased distractibility.	Improve school performance.	Move to front of classroom as an aid to attention.
Mother and teacher attest to Jamie's decreased impulsive behaviour.	Increase Jamie's capacity to recognize effects of his behaviour on others.	Encourage participation in structured activities.
Jamie identifies alternative responses such as walking away until it is his turn.	Increase frequency of acting on these alternative approaches.	Inquire about social skills group at school, if available.
Jamie improves interpretation of motives and behaviours of others.	Improve acceptance by peers.	Encourage participation in community activities.

NURSING DIAGNOSIS 2: INEFFECTIVE COPING (LILLIAN)

Defining Characteristics	Related Factors
Verbalizes discouragement and inability to handle situation with Jamie	Chronicity of ADHD More than average childrearing problems

Outcomes

Initial	Discharge
1. Verbalize frustration at trying to raise a child with ADHD alone. 2. Identify positive methods of interacting and disciplining Jamie that will support the parent–child relationship as well as meet Jamie's development needs.	3. Identify coping patterns that decrease the sense of frustration and increase parental competence. 4. Initiate a collaborative relationship with teacher. 5. Identify sources of support in the community and begin to access these resources.

Interventions

Intervention	Rationale	Ongoing Assessment
Assess mother's discouragement and feelings about parenting, identifying specific problem areas.	Helping the mother verbalize her feelings and identify problem areas helps in formulating problem-solving strategies.	Assess the severity of the problems with which she is living.
Refer mother to community health centre for free parenting class.	Parent training based on clear directives and rewards can be effective for decreasing impulsive and disruptive behaviour.	Monitor mother's level of confidence and perceived change in Jamie's behaviour.
Refer mother to self-help organization.	Parent groups such as Children and Adults With Attention Deficit Disorder (CHAAD) can be sources of support and information.	Determine whether contact was made and whether it was helpful.
Make contact with school to enhance collaboration with mother.	Assess effectiveness of medication and other interventions, need feedback from teachers.	Determine whether mother has been able to contact teacher.

Evaluation

Outcomes	Revised Outcomes	Interventions
After four sessions, Lillian expresses her frustrations, but she has begun to identify different ways of relating to Jamie and his developmental needs.	None	None
Through attending the parenting class and joining a support group, Lillian begins to change her coping patterns, decrease her frustrations, and increase parental competence.	Complete parenting class; attend at least two support group meetings each month.	If necessary, refer for additional parent counselling.
Lillian initiates a collaborative relationship with Jamie's teacher	Lillian and teacher mutually develop and implement behaviour plans for home and school.	Have mother observe in the classroom; have mother visit highly structured classroom.

BOX 27.5

Clinical Vignette: Leon (Conduct Disorder)

Leon, a 14-year-old boy, was admitted to the child psychiatric inpatient service from the emergency department after a fight with his mother. His mother reported that she and Leon had argued earlier in the evening and that he stormed out of the house screaming and vowing he would never return. Several hours later, Leon came back, yelling and demanding entry into the apartment. Leon's father was working. While his mother was getting up to open the door, Leon continued to yell and scream, waking the neighbours. This led to further arguing between Leon and his mother. Before long, the police were called, and Leon was taken to the emergency department.

The admission interview revealed that Leon had run away on several occasions and had even stayed away overnight. Although he strongly denied drug use, he had gotten drunk on several occasions. He had also been in several fights, the latest of which resulted in an expulsion from school. Three months before admission he was caught trying to steal a CD from a music store. More recently, he boasted that he and his friends had snatched a purse at an outdoor concert and had broken into a car to steal its contents. Leon's school performance has been declining; he was truant on several occasions and will probably have to repeat ninth grade.

Leon was born in Cape Breton, N.S. and is the oldest of three children. His family moved to Toronto shortly after his birth. His father is employed as a janitor and is illiterate. His mother works as a secretary and has recently completed BA in English. There is much marital discord at home. Leon has received no treatment except for consulation with the school social worker.

What Do You Think?

1. When conducting a nursing assessment, what would you want to learn about Leon's school performance?
2. What information could you provide Leon's parents about pharmacotherapy? About behaviour management?
3. How would you present the material so it meets the learning needs of both parents?

with adults. This disorder is distinguishable from conduct disorder, which is characterized by more serious violations of social norms. Youngsters with conduct disorder often lie to achieve short-term ends, may be truant from school, may run away from home, and may engage in petty larceny or even mugging (Box 27-5).

The prevalence of conduct disorder is greater in boys and ranges from 6% to 16%, compared with a range of 2% to 9% in girls. Conduct disorder is one of the most frequently diagnosed disorders in children in mental health facilities. Individuals with conduct disorder are at greater risk for experiencing mood or anxiety disorders and substance-related disorders (APA, 2000). Other common comorbid conditions that may precede conduct disorder include specific developmental delays, such as learning disabilities and language delay, ADHD, and oppositional defiant disorder. Several reports from large community surveys, family studies, and studies of clinical samples confirm the high comorbidity among these disorders (Weiss & Weiss, 2002).

Children with ADHD, a learning disability, or a language deficit may frequently encounter failure and acquire a bitter and hostile attitude. Appropriate treatment focussed on the ADHD or the specific developmental delay may foster more positive interactions and promote success at school. Success in these areas may lead to more positive behaviour in some cases.

The etiology of oppositional defiant disorder and conduct disorder is complex. More attention has been paid to conduct disorder, probably because it is the more serious of the two. Models used to understand antisocial personality disorder (see Chapter 24) and aggressiveness (see Chapter 35) are useful in examining these childhood disorders, which appear to have both genetic and environmental components. For example, the risk for conduct disorder is increased in the offspring of individuals with conduct disorder. However, physical abuse by fathers, whether biologic or adoptive, also increases the risk for conduct disorder (Blackson et al., 1999).

NURSING MANAGEMENT: HUMAN RESPONSE TO DISORDER

Biologic Domain

Assessment

The nurse gathers data from multiple sources and domains, including biologic, psychological (mood, behavioural, cognitions), and social. These adolescents are at high risk for physical injury as a result of fighting and impulsive behaviour. Sexual promiscuity is common, resulting in an increased frequency of pregnancy and sexually transmitted diseases.

Another important aspect of assessment of adolescents presenting with defiance or aggressive behaviour is to rule out comorbid conditions that may partially explain or complicate their lack of behavioural control. These conditions include ADHD, learning disabilities, chemical dependency, depression, bipolar illness, or generalized anxiety. Young people who are chronically depressed may be irritable and easily frustrated. Given the tendency of adolescents to act out their frustration, chronic depression may exacerbate their behaviour. Conduct problems can also elevate the risk for depression because young people who regularly elicit negative attention from parents and teachers and are constantly at odds with their environment may become despondent.

Nursing Diagnoses for the Biologic Domain

Typical nursing diagnoses in the biologic domain are Risk for Other-Directed Violence, Risk for Self-Directed

Violence, and Impaired Verbal Communication. Although the outcomes are individualized for each client, some outcomes for these clients are as follows:

- Maintenance of physical safety in the milieu (or other treatment setting)
- Decreased frequency of verbal and physical aggressive episodes

Interventions for the Biologic Domain

Children with oppositional defiant disorder or conduct disorder who also have specific developmental disorders should be referred to appropriate programs for remediation. If a diagnosis of ADHD or depression emerges from the evaluation, appropriate pharmacotherapy should be considered (see previous discussion of ADHD and after the discussion regarding depression).

Several medications have been used to treat extremely aggressive behaviour, including antipsychotics, such as haloperidol and thioridazine; the anticonvulsant carbamazepine; the α-blocking agent propranolol; and the antimanic medication lithium carbonate. With the exception of haloperidol, most of these medications have limited support for their use in children and adolescents (Werry & Aman, 1998). More recently, several placebo-controlled studies have shown that low-dose risperidone therapy is effective for the treatment of aggression in children across a wide range of diagnostic groups (Aman et al., 2002; RUPP Autism Network, 2002).

Psychological Domain

Assessment

Adolescents with conduct problems are usually brought or coerced into the mental health system by family, school, or the court system because of fighting, truancy, speeding tickets, car accidents, petty crimes, substance abuse, or suicide attempts. These young people may be hostile, sarcastic, defensive, and provocative. At the same time, they may appear calm, outgoing, and engaging. Inconsistencies, distortions, and misrepresentations of the truth are common when interviewing these children, so obtaining a clear history may be difficult. Therefore, instead of asking if an event or behaviour occurred, it may be better to ask when it occurred. A structured interview, such as the Diagnostic Schedule for Children (DISC), or self-reports, such as the Youth Self-Report (Achenbach, 1991), can aid the assessment. These adolescents are adept at changing the subject and diverting discussions from sensitive issues. They often use denial, projection, and externalization of anger as defence mechanisms when asked for self-disclosure. The assessment, which may take several sessions, should be conducted in a nonjudgmental fashion.

Nursing Diagnoses for the Psychological Domain

In the psychological domain, a typical nursing diagnosis is Ineffective Coping. Outcomes are individualized for each client but can include the following:

- Increased personal responsibility for behaviour
- Increased use of problem-solving skills as evidenced by decreased interpersonal conflicts
- Decreased rule violations and conflicts with authority figures

Interventions for the Psychological Domain

In planning interventions for clients with oppositional defiant disorder or conduct disorder, the focus is on problem behaviours. Therapeutic progress may be slow, at least partly because these clients often lack trust in authority figures.

Social Skills Training

The nurse should communicate behavioural expectations clearly and enforce them consistently. Consequences of appropriate and inappropriate actions also should be clear. Specific approaches for improving social and problem-solving skills are fundamental features for school-aged children and adolescents. Insofar as children and adolescents with conduct problems fail to recognize the adverse effects of their verbal and nonverbal behaviour, their deficit can be formulated as an interpersonal problem. Social skills training teaches adolescents with these behaviour disorders to recognize the ways in which their actions affect others. Training involves techniques such as role playing, modeling by the therapist, and giving positive reinforcement to improve interpersonal relationships and enhance social outcomes.

Problem Solving Therapy

In contrast to social skills training, which proposes that problems of conduct are the result of poor interpersonal skills, problem-solving therapy conceptualizes conduct problems as the result of deficiencies in cognitive processes. These processes include assessment of situations, interpretation of events, and expectations of others that are congruent with behaviour. As reviewed in Kazdin & Weisz (2003), these children often misinterpret the intentions of others and may perceive hostility with little or no cause. Problem-solving skills training teaches these children to generate alternative solutions to social situations, to sharpen thinking concerning the consequences of those choices, and to evaluate responses after interpersonal conflicts.

Social Domain

Assessment

High levels of marital conflict, parental substance abuse, and parental antisocial behaviour often mark family history.

Nursing Diagnoses for the Social Domain

In the social domain, nursing diagnoses include Compromised Family Coping and Impaired Social Interaction. Some outcomes for these clients are as follows:

- Increased use of problem-solving skills as evidenced by decreased interpersonal conflicts
- Decreased rule violations and conflicts with authority figures

Interventions for the Social Domain

Parent education for preschool- and school-aged children with disruptive behaviour problems appears to be the most effective psychosocial intervention.

Management Training

Parent training begins with educating parents about disruptive behaviour disorders, focusing particularly on impulsiveness, impaired judgment, and self-control. Children with long-standing problems in these areas often elicit punitive responses and negative attributions about their behaviour from their parents. Ironically, because these parental responses focus on the child's failure, they may contribute to the child's behaviour problems. An important second step is to clarify parental expectations and interpretation of the child's behaviour. Parent management training may be offered to a group of parents or to individuals (Kazdin & Weisz, 2003).

Educating Parents

The aims of education are to provide parents with new ways of understanding their child's behaviour and to promote improved interactions between parent and child. The most commonly presented techniques include the importance of positive reinforcement (praise and tangible rewards) for adaptive behaviour, clear limits for unacceptable behaviour, and use of mild punishment, such as time out (Box 27-6).

Family therapy is directed at assisting the family with altering maladaptive patterns of interaction or improving adjustment to stressors, such as changes in membership or losses. Multisystemic family therapy, which considers the child in the context of multiple family and

BOX 27.6

Time Out

Time Out Procedure

- *Labelling behaviour:* Identify the behaviour that the child is expected to perform or cease. The aim of this statement is to make clear what is required of the child. It typically takes the form of a simple declarative sentence: "Threatening is not acceptable."
- *Warning:* In this step, the child is informed that if he or she does not perform the expected behaviour or stop the unacceptable behaviour, he or she will be given a "time out." "This is a warning: if you continue threatening to hit people, you'll have a time out."
- *Time out:* If the child does not heed the warning, he or she is told to take a time out in simple straightforward terms: "take a time out."
- *Duration:* The usual duration for a time out is 5 minutes for children 5 years of age or older.
- *Location:* The child sits in a designated time-out chair without toys and without talking. The chair should be located away from general activity but within view. A kitchen timer can be used to mark the time, but the clock does not start until the child is sitting quietly in the designated spot.
- *Follow-up:* The child is asked to recount why he or she was given the time out. The explanation need not be detailed, and no further discussion of the matter is required. Indeed, long discourse about the child's behaviour is not helpful and should be avoided.

community systems, has shown promise in the treatment of adolescents with conduct disorder (Henggeler et al., 1999).

EVALUATION AND TREATMENT OUTCOMES

The nurse can review treatment goals and objectives to assess the child's progress with respect to verbal and physical aggression, socially appropriate resolution of conflicts, compliance with rules and expectations, and better management of frustration. As is true for the initial assessment, evaluation of treatment outcomes relies on input from parents, teachers, and other team members.

CONTINUUM OF CARE

Children and adolescents with disorders of conduct may be involved in many different agencies in the community, such as child and family services, school authorities, and the legal system. Mental health services are requested when a child or adolescent's behaviour is out of control or a comorbid disorder is suspected. Helping the youngster and the family negotiate their way through this maze of services may be an essential part of the treatment plan.

Disorders of Mood and Anxiety

ANXIETY DISORDERS

Anxiety is a universal human condition. Indeed, it may well be that common anxiety-provoking stimuli have biologically protective value. For example, a fear of snakes and the dark may have contributed to the survival of early humans through vigilance and avoidance behaviour. Some degree of worry and specific fears is considered normal during the course of childhood (eg, anxiety about strangers in the 1-year-old child). However, when the level of anxiety is excessive and hinders daily functioning, the diagnosis of an anxiety disorder may be appropriate. This section focuses on separation anxiety, a disorder diagnosed in childhood, and obsessive-compulsive disorder (OCD), a disorder that occurs in both adults and children (see Chapter 20).

SEPARATION ANXIETY DISORDER

Some have suggested that separation anxiety disorder is the childhood equivalent of panic disorder in adults. Although many children experience some discomfort on separation from their mothers or major attachment figures, children with separation anxiety disorder suffer great distress when faced with ordinary separations, such as going to school. In most cases, the mother is the focus of the child's concern, but this may not be so, especially if the mother is not the primary caregiver. The child may exhibit extraordinary reluctance or even refusal to separate from the primary caregiver. When asked, most children with separation anxiety disorder will express worry about harm or permanent loss of their major attachment figure. Other children may express worry about their own safety (Table 27-4).

A common manifestation of anxiety is **school phobia**, in which the child refuses to attend school, preferring to stay at home with the primary attachment figure. However, it should be noted that school phobia is a common presenting complaint in child psychiatric clinics and may be part of separation anxiety disorder, general anxiety disorder, social phobia, OCD, depression, or conduct disorder. In rare cases, school phobia can be a side effect of antipsychotic medication (see Scahill, Leckman, Schultz, Katsovich, & Peterson, 2003). The term *school phobia* was coined to distinguish it from truancy—whether it is a phobia in the usual sense is a matter of some debate. When another disorder such as depression is identified, it becomes the focus of treatment. In some cases, the school phobia may resolve when the primary disorder is successfully treated.

Separation anxiety disorder is excessive anxiety on separation from home or major attachment figure before age 18 years. It is manifested by acute distress, frequent nightmares about separation, and reluctance or refusal to separate. It lasts for at least 1 month, and causes clinically significant impairment in social or academic functioning.

Epidemiology and Etiology

The prevalence of separation anxiety disorder is estimated at 4% of school-aged children; thus, it is relatively common. Anxiety disorders run in families, and it

---

Table 27.4 Key Diagnostic Characteristics of Separation Anxiety Disorder 309.21

Diagnostic Criteria and Target Symptoms	Associated Findings

▪ Inappropriate and excessive anxiety about being away from home or primary attachment figure
  Excessive distress when separation occurs or is anticipated
  Persistent, excessive worry about losing or having harm come to attachment figures
  Persistent and excessive worry about an event that might cause separation from attachment figure
  Persistent reluctance or refusal to go to school or somewhere else because of separation anxiety
  Reluctance to be alone without attachment figures at home or without significant adults in other settings
  Persistent reluctance or refusal to go to sleep without being near attachment figure or sleep away from home
  Repeated nightmares about being separated
  Repeated complaints of physical symptoms when separated or when separation from attachment figures is anticipated
▪ Duration of at least 4 weeks
▪ Onset before age 18 years (for early-onset type, onset before age 6 years)
▪ Not exclusively occurring during course of other psychotic disorder; not better accounted for by panic disorder with agoraphobia
	▪ Social withdrawal, apathy
	▪ Difficulty concentrating
	▪ Fears of other situations, such as animals, monsters, accidents, and plane travel
	▪ Concerns about death and dying
	▪ School refusal and subsequent academic difficulties
	▪ Anger or lashing out with prospect of separation
	▪ Unusual perceptual experiences when alone
	▪ Demanding and needing constant attention and reassurance
	▪ Somatic complaints
	▪ Depressed mood
	▪ Other recurring worries that do not involve attachment figure

appears that both environmental and genetic factors affect the risk for separation anxiety disorder. For example, it may emerge after a move, change to a new school, or death of a family member or pet. By contrast, recent evidence suggests that traits such as shyness and behavioural inhibition (reluctance in new situations) are inherited (Koda, Charney, & Pine, 2003; Schwartz, Snidman, & Kagan, 1999). Furthermore, not only are children with an enduring "inhibited" temperament at greater risk for anxiety disorders themselves, but their immediate family members are also at greater risk for anxiety disorders compared with a psychiatric control group. Others have argued in favour of environmental determinants of separation anxiety, contending that anxious parents communicate to the child that the world is inhospitable and menacing to keep the child near. Available data suggest that the long-term outcome of childhood disorders is favourable in many cases but may evolve and take other forms in adulthood. For example, separation anxiety in childhood may re-emerge as panic disorder in adults (Koda et al., 2003).

Psychopharmacologic Interventions

The tricyclic antidepressant medication imipramine has been used as an adjunct to behavioural treatment or as a primary therapy for several years (Velosa & Riddle, 2000). However, in the largest controlled study to date, imipramine was no better than a placebo in managing separation anxiety (reviewed in Velosa & Riddle, 2000). In addition, some children display drowsiness and irritability when taking imipramine. Other side effects may include tachycardia, dry mouth, constipation, urinary retention, and dizziness. As a class of medications, the tricyclics can alter cardiac conduction; thus, baseline and follow-up electrocardiograms are recommended (King, Scahill, Lombroso, & Leckman, 2003). A recent multicenter study showed that the SSRI fluvoxamine is effective for reducing separation anxiety (RUPP Anxiety Study Group, 2001). The inconsistent results with the tricyclics and the positive results with fluvoxamine suggest that an SSRI would be a first-line treatment.

NURSING MANAGEMENT: HUMAN RESPONSE TO DISORDER

School phobia is often what prompts the family to seek consultation for the child. The onset of school refusal may be gradual or acute. Because school phobia can be a behavioural manifestation of several different child psychiatric disorders, it requires careful assessment. Issues to consider are whether the parents have been aware that the child is avoiding school (separation versus truancy); what efforts the family has used to return the child to school; the presence of significant subjective distress in the child with anticipation of going to

school; and whether the school refusal occurs in the context of other behavioural, social, or emotional problems. The nurse should also review the purpose and dose of current medications.

The child's developmental history and response to new situations and prior separations provide essential background information for understanding the child's current separation anxiety. The assessment should also include a review of recent life events and the methods the family has used to promote the child's return to school. Finally, the family history with respect to anxiety, panic attacks, or phobias is also informative.

Most clinicians agree that the child should return to school as soon as possible because resistance to attending school invariably mounts the longer the child remains absent. Several therapeutic approaches are used in treating separation anxiety disorder, including individual psychotherapy, behavioural treatment, and pharmacotherapy. Although individual psychotherapy is a common treatment, data to support this approach are sparse. By contrast, evidence suggests that behavioural techniques can be effective in reducing separation anxiety. These techniques include flooding (rapid and forcible return to school) and desensitization in which the child is gradually returned to school (Labellarte & Ginsberg, 2003). To be successful, these techniques require close collaboration with the family and the school and may also include medication (Labellarte & Ginsberg, 2003).

OBSESSIVE-COMPULSIVE DISORDER

Obsessive-compulsive disorder (OCD) is characterized by intrusive thoughts that are difficult to dislodge (obsessions) or ritualized behaviours that the child feels driven to perform (compulsions). Historically, OCD was regarded as a neurosis, and the primary symptoms were viewed as the expression of unresolved sexual and aggressive impulses. Recent evidence from family genetic studies, pharmacologic trials, and neuroimaging studies has dramatically shifted the conceptualization of OCD (see Chapter 20). The notion that OCD is the manifestation of internal conflict concerning sexual and aggressive impulses has given way to a more biologic model (Murphy, Voeller, & Blier, 2003).

Epidemiology and Etiology

Until recently, OCD was considered uncommon in adults and even more rare in children; the multicenter ECA study estimated a 2% to 3% prevalence in the general population for adults. In addition, many of these adults reported that their symptoms began in childhood (Karno, Golding, Sorenson, & Burnam, 1988). A large community sample of high school students found a prevalence of about 2% (Flament et al.,

1988). Thus, OCD is far more prevalent than previously supposed and can be expressed in childhood (Scahill, Kano, et al., 2003).

Family genetic studies indicate that OCD recurs with a greater-than-expected frequency in the families of clients with OCD or Tourette disorder, suggesting an inherited vulnerability in some cases (Murphy et al., 2003). OCD has also been associated with other movement disorders, such as Sydenham's chorea (Murphy et al., 2003). This observation led to speculation that autoimmune mechanisms may underlie some cases of OCD (Morshed et al., 2001; Taylor et al., 2002).

Regardless of etiology, most researchers now conceptualize OCD as a disorder of the basal ganglia (Murphy et al., 2003). Results from neuroimaging studies, which have shown functional abnormalities in the brain circuits connecting the frontal cortex and basal ganglia structures such as the caudate nucleus, strongly support this view (see Murphy et al., 2003 for a review). OCD is accompanied by anxiety disorders in some cases and tic disorders in others (Scahill et al., 2003).

> ⬟ **KEY CONCEPT Obsessions** are unwanted persistent, intrusive thoughts, impulses, or images related to anxiety.

> ⬟ **KEY CONCEPT Compulsions** are unwanted behavioural patterns or acts.

Psychopharmacologic Interventions

Double-blind trials with clomipramine, fluoxetine, fluvoxamine, and sertraline have demonstrated the effectiveness of these agents in reducing symptoms of OCD in children and adolescents (DeVeaugh-Geiss et al., 1992; Geller et al., 2001; March et al., 1998; Riddle et al., 2001). Although the precise mechanism for their positive effects on OCD is not completely clear, these agents block the reuptake of serotonin in the brain. This property appears to be essential to the therapeutic effects of these agents because other antidepressants that do not block the reuptake of serotonin are not effective in treating OCD.

NURSING MANAGEMENT: HUMAN RESPONSE TO DISORDER

Recurrent worries and ritualistic behaviour can occur normally in children at particular stages of development. The first step in the assessment of OCD in children is to distinguish between normal childhood rituals and worries and pathologic rituals and obsessional thoughts (King & Scahill, 2001). Obsessional thoughts are recurrent, nagging, and bothersome. Although children may describe obsessions as occurring "out of the blue," external events may trigger obsessions. For example, a child may fear contamination whenever he or she is in contact with a certain person or object. Likewise, compulsions waste time, cause distress, and interfere with daily living (Box 27-7).

Several measures are now available to assist in the assessment of OCD in children. The Leyton Survey is a 20-item self-report used in both epidemiologic studies and clinical trials; high scores appear to be predictive of a clinical diagnosis of OCD (Flament et al., 1988). The Children's Yale-Brown Obsessive Compulsive Scale (CY-BOCS) is a semistructured interview designed to measure the severity of OCD once the diagnosis has been made. The CY-BOCS is a revision of the original adult instrument, and available evidence suggests that it is a reliable and valid measure of OCD severity in children (Scahill et al., 1997).

BOX 27.7

Clinical Vignette: Kimberly and OCD

Kimberly, an 11-year-old fifth grader, comes for evaluation because her mother and teacher have become increasingly concerned about her repetitive behaviours. In retrospect, Kim's mother recalls first noticing repetitive rituals about 2 years before, but she did not become alarmed about these behaviours until recently when they began to interfere with daily living. At the time of referral, Kim exhibits complicated jumping rituals that involve a specific number of jumps and a particular manner of jumping. She also turns light switches off and on and performs complex movements, such as blinking in patterns and thrusting her arms back and forth a certain number of times. Her mother also reports Kim's near-constant request for reassurance about her own safety. In recent months, her incessant demands for reassurance have been more frequent and elaborate. For example, Kim's mother has to answer three times that everything is all right and then say, "I swear to it."

At the evaluation, Kim expresses fears that some ill fate, such as catastrophic illness or injury, will befall her. This fear is triggered by contact with any individual who seems sick, chance exposures to foul smells or dirt, or minor scrapes or bumps. Once the fear is triggered, she becomes increasingly anxious and consumed with the fear that she will develop an illness and die. Sometimes, her fears are specific, such as cancer or AIDS. Other times, her fears are more ambiguous, as evidenced by statements such as, "something bad will happen" if she doesn't complete the ritual. Kim acknowledges that the ritual is probably not related to the feared event, but she is reluctant to take a chance. If the ritual does not reduce her anxiety, she seeks reassurance from her mother.

Kim's medical history was negative for serious illness or injury; she was born after an uncomplicated pregnancy, labor, and delivery and achieved developmental milestones at appropriate times. Indeed, her mother could recall no unusual problems in the first few years of life except that Kim was typically anxious in new situations. Kim's mother reports a prior history of panic attacks, but the family history is otherwise negative for anxiety disorders, including obsessive-compulsive disorder.

The severity of the child's and family's response to OCD will determine the appropriate nursing diagnoses. When the obsessions and compulsions emerge, these children or adolescents are in distress because of the disturbing and relentless nature of the symptoms. Parents may be pulled into the child's rituals (King & Scahill, 2001). Ineffective Coping, Compromised Family Coping, and Ineffective Role Performance are likely nursing diagnoses.

Treatment goals focus on reducing the obsessions and compulsions and their effects on the child's development. Behaviour modification techniques have demonstrated benefit in reducing the primary symptoms of OCD in adults. However, behaviour therapy has not been well studied in children and adolescents (Piacentini, 1999). Consistently effective OCD treatment techniques include exposure and response prevention (Piacentini, 1999). Exposure consists of gradual confrontation with events or situations that trigger obsessions and cause the urge to ritualize. According to the theory behind behaviour therapy, repeated exposure works because the client learns that the immediate anxiety will subside even if he or she does not complete the ritual. Response prevention complements exposure and consists of instructing the client to delay execution of the ritual. When exposure and response prevention are combined, the client is confronted with a triggering stimulus such as dirt (exposure) but agrees not to do the hand washing for a brief period (response prevention) and tracks the anxiety level during the exercise. Successful cognitive behavioural treatment of children with OCD includes parents, both to include them in the treatment plan and to reduce parental involvement in the ritualized behaviour. For example, the child may demand that the parent participate in a washing and checking ritual (Piacentini, 1999).

MOOD DISORDERS: MAJOR DEPRESSIVE DISORDER

The *DSM-IV-TR* includes several mood disorders, among them major depressive disorder, dysthymic disorder, bipolar I and bipolar II disorders, and cyclothymic disorder. Although these disorders occur in children and adolescents, they are less common in prepubertal children. These disorders are reviewed in detail in Chapter 19. Thus, this section is confined to a brief discussion of major depressive disorder in children and adolescents.

Depression is characterized by profound sadness, loss of interest in usual activities, loss of appetite with weight loss, sleep disturbance, loss of energy, feeling worthless or guilty, and recurrent thoughts of death or suicide. To meet *DSM-IV* criteria, these symptoms must be present on a daily basis and persist for at least 2 weeks (see Chapter 19).

Epidemiology

The prevalence of depression in children and adolescents is estimated at 1% to 5%, with adolescents being at the high end of this range and young children at the low end. Boys appear to be at higher risk for depression until adolescence, when depression becomes more common in girls.

NURSING MANAGEMENT: HUMAN RESPONSE TO DISORDER

The clinical picture of a child with depression may be similar to that of an adult, but children may not spontaneously express feelings of sadness and worthlessness. Thus, clinical experience is helpful when trying to elicit the symptoms of depression from young children. Reports from parents are important sources of information about changes in sleep patterns, appetite, activity level and interests, and emotional stability. In addition, quantitative measures, such as the Children's Depression Rating Scale and the Children's Depression Inventory, can assist in the assessment of childhood depression (Birmaher & Brent, 2003).

Nursing diagnoses for children or adolescents who are depressed are similar to those for adults, including Ineffective Coping, Chronic Low Self-Esteem, Disturbed Thought Processes, Self-Care Deficit, Imbalanced Nutrition, and Disturbed Sleep Pattern.

Treatment goals include improving the depressed mood and restoring sleep, appetite, and self-care. Interventions for responses to major depressive disorder in children and adolescents are also similar to those for adults. The psychiatric nurse develops a therapeutic relationship with the child and provides parent education and support. These children may act out their feelings, rather than discuss them. Thus, behaviour problems may accompany depression. Younger children may respond to the use of art or play therapy as a safe way to encourage expression of painful feelings. Older children and adolescents may also respond positively to board games that have been specifically designed to encourage the expression of emotions. Developing sensitivity to the influence of environmental events on the child is important for the nurse, parents, and teachers (Box 27-8). These children are likely to be treated with an antidepressant medication and may also be undergoing psychotherapy with a mental health specialist. Unfortunately, outcome data concerning the superiority of any psychotherapeutic method are scarce. In addition, there are surprisingly few studies supporting the use of antidepressant medications in children (Birmaher & Brent, 2003). Much more research is needed to confirm the best methods of treating children with major depression.

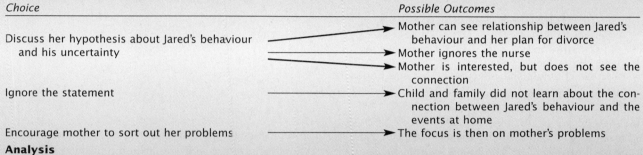

BOX 27.8

Questions, Choices, and Outcomes

Mrs. S has just returned with her son Jared to the child psychiatric inpatient services following an overnight pass. She reports that the visit did not go well due to Jared's anger and defiance. She remarked that this behaviour was distressingly similar to his behaviour before the hospitalization. She expressed additional concern because of the upcoming discharge from the hospital. After saying goodbye to Jared, she pulled the nurse aside and stated that she had decided to file for divorce.

Mrs. S indicated that she had not told her husband or the family therapist. When asked whether Jared knew about her decision, Mrs. S suddenly realized that he may have overheard her discussing the matter with her sister on the telephone during this home visit.

How should the nurse approach this situation?

Choice	Possible Outcomes
Discuss her hypothesis about Jared's behaviour and his uncertainty	Mother can see relationship between Jared's behaviour and her plan for divorce
	Mother ignores the nurse
	Mother is interested, but does not see the connection
Ignore the statement	Child and family did not learn about the connection between Jared's behaviour and the events at home
Encourage mother to sort out her problems	The focus is then on mother's problems

Analysis

The best response is focusing on the possible relationship between Jared's recent behavioural deterioration and his uncertainty of his family's future. If the nurse ignores the statement or focuses on the mother's interpretation of Jared's behaviour, the mother is less likely to appreciate the connection between pending divorce and Jared's behaviour. The nurse should also emphasize the importance of discussing the matter in family therapy.

Tic Disorders and Tourette Disorder

Motor tics are usually quick, jerky movements of the eyes, face, neck, and shoulders, although they may involve other muscle groups as well. Occasionally, tics involve slower, more purposeful, or dystonic movements. Phonic tics typically include repetitive throat clearing, grunting, or other noises, but may also include more complex sounds, such as words, parts of words, and, in a minority of clients, obscenities. Transient tics by definition do not endure over time and appear to be fairly common in school-aged children.

> **KEY CONCEPT Tics** are sudden, rapid, repetitive, stereotyped motor movements or vocalizations.

Tic disorder is a general term encompassing several syndromes that are chiefly characterized by motor tics, phonic tics, or both. The *DSM-IV-TR* includes four tic disorders: Tourette syndrome or disorder, chronic motor or vocal tic disorder, transient tic disorder, and tic disorder not otherwise specified. This section focuses on the most severe tic disorder, Tourette disorder (Table 27-5). Because no diagnostic tests are used for this disorder, the diagnosis is based on the type and duration of tics present (Leckman, Peterson, King, Scahill, & Cohen, 2001). The typical age of onset for tics is about 7 years, and motor tics generally precede phonic tics. Parents often describe the seem-

ing replacement of one tic with another. In addition to this changing repertoire of motor and phonic tics, Tourette disorder exhibits a waxing and waning course. The child can suppress the tics for brief periods. Thus, it is not uncommon to hear from parents that their child has more frequent tics at home than at school. Older children and adults may describe an urge or a physical sensation before having a tic. The general trend is for tic symptoms to decline by early adulthood (Leckman et al., 1998).

Tourette disorder is defined by multiple motor and phonic tics for at least 1 year.

Epidemiology and Etiology

The prevalence of Tourette disorder is estimated to be between 1 and 10 per 1,000 in school-aged children, with boys being affected three to six times more often than girls (Scahill, Tanner, & Dure, 2001). The observation in the 1970s that the potent dopamine blocker haloperidol could reduce tics sparked interest in the biologic mechanisms, with particular focus on central dopaminergic systems.

The precise nature of the underlying pathophysiology is unclear, but the basal ganglia and functionally related cortical areas are presumed to play a central role (Mink, 2001). The basal ganglia, which consist of the caudate, putamen, and globus pallidus, are located at the base of the cortex and play an important role in planning and executing movement. This functional role is accomplished by means of parallel circuits that connect the basal ganglia

Table 27.5	Key Diagnostic Characteristics of Tourette Syndrome 307.23
Diagnostic Criteria and Target Symptoms	**Associated Findings**
<ul><li>Multiple motor tics and one or more vocal tics Sudden rapid recurrent, nonrhythmic, stereotyped motor movements or vocalizations Motor tics typically involving the head and other parts of body Vocal tics typically involving throat clearing, grunting, and occasionally words or parts of words</li><li>Tics occurring many times a day, present for at least 1 year Appear simultaneously or at different periods during the illness No tic-free period of more than 3 consecutive months</li><li>Onset before age 18 years</li><li>Not a direct physiologic effect of a substance or general medical condition</li></ul>	<ul><li>Obsessions and compulsions</li><li>Hyperactivity, distractibility, and impulsivity</li><li>Social discomfort, shame, self-consciousness, and depressed mood</li><li>Impaired social, academic, and occupational functioning</li><li>Possible interference with daily activities if tics are severe</li></ul>

to the cortex and the thalamus. To date, no specific lesions in the basal ganglia have been found in Tourette disorder. Nonetheless, findings from neuroimaging studies are consistent with the presumption that a dysregulation of frontal cortical and basal ganglia circuits underlies Tourette disorder (Peterson et al., 2001).

In the 1980s, data from family genetic studies suggested that Tourette disorder is inherited as a single autosomal dominant gene. However, more recent studies suggest that the inheritance may involve more than a single gene (Tourette Syndrome Association, 1999; Walkup et al., 1996). The range of expression is presumed to be variable and includes Tourette disorder, chronic motor or chronic vocal tics, and OCD. Twin studies have shown that monozygotic twins are far more likely to be concordant for Tourette disorder than are dizygotic twins, further supporting the genetic hypotheses. However, even when monozygotic twins are concordant, the twins may not be equally affected. Thus, although substantial evidence supports a genetic etiology, environmental factors affect the expression of the gene (for a more complete review, see Walkup et al., 1996).

Several neurochemical systems have been implicated in the etiology of Tourette disorder, including dopamine systems, noradrenaline, endogenous opioids, and serotonin. The consistent observation that boys are more likely to be affected than girls has also led to speculation about the potential role of androgens in the pathophysiology of tic disorders. However, treatment strategies based on this theory appear to be ineffective (Peterson, Zhang, Anderson, & Leckman, 1998).

Psychopharmacologic Interventions

Two classes of drugs are commonly used in the treatment of tics: antipsychotics and α-adrenergic receptor agonists. Historically, the most commonly used antipsychotics include haloperidol and pimozide. These potent dopamine blockers are often effective at low doses. Attempts to erad-

icate all tics by increasing the dosages of these antipsychotics almost certainly results in diminishing therapeutic returns and additional side effects. The most frequently encountered side effects include drowsiness, dulled thinking, muscle stiffness, akathisia, increased appetite and weight gain, and acute dystonic reactions. Long-term use carries a small risk for tardive dyskinesia. Recently, the atypical antipsychotics ziprasidone and risperidone have been evaluated for the treatment of tics in children and adolescents (Sallee et al., 2000; Scahill et al., 2003). Both were found to be superior to placebo.

The α₂-adrenergic receptor agonist clonidine (Catapres) has been used in treating Tourette disorder for more than 20 years. Guanfacine (Tenex) is a newer α₂-adrenergic receptor agonist that has only recently been studied in children with Tourette disorder. Both drugs were originally developed as antihypertensive agents, but their regulatory action on the brain's norepinephrine system led researchers to try these medications in clients with Tourette disorder. Results from double-blind, placebo-controlled studies indicate that both are effective in reducing tics (King et al., 2003; Scahill, Chappell, et al., 2001). However, the level of improvement in tic symptoms is generally less than that observed with the antipsychotics. In the study by Scahill, Chappell, and colleagues (2001), guanfacine was also effective in reducing symptoms of ADHD. (For additional discussion of pharmacotherapy in Tourette disorder, see King et al., 2003).

NURSING MANAGEMENT: HUMAN RESPONSE TO DISORDER

Nursing assessment of a child with tics includes a review of the onset, course, and current level of the symptoms. The goals of the assessment are to identify the frequency, intensity, complexity, and interference of the tics and their effects on functioning; determine the child's level of adaptive functioning; identify the child's areas of strength and weakness in general and in school; and identify social supports for the child and family (Leckman et al., 2001). Another important aspect of the assessment is to determine the effects of the tic symptoms on the child and family. Some children and families adjust well; however, others are embarrassed or devastated and tend to withdraw socially. About half of school-aged children with Tourette disorder have ADHD, and a substantial percentage have symptoms of OCD (Leckman et al., 2001). Therefore, in addition to inquiring about tics, the nurse should assess the child's overall development, activity level, and capacity to concentrate and persist with a single task, as well as explore repetitive habits and recurring worries. The completion of a family history of tic disorder may also provide some critical assessment data.

Nursing diagnoses could include Ineffective Coping, Impaired Social Interaction, Anxiety, and Compromised Family Coping. Children with Tourette disorder typically have normal intelligence, although clinical samples may show a higher frequency of learning problems. These learning problems may include subtle problems of organization and planning or more severe problems with reading (Schultz et al., 1998). Handwriting, including both speed and legibility, is another common problem for these youngsters. The use of a computer can obviate difficulties with handwriting in some cases.

The approach to planning nursing interventions depends on the primary source of impairment: tics themselves, OCD symptoms, or the triad of hyperactivity, inattention, and poor impulse control. The nurse can provide counselling and education for the client, education for the parents, and consultation for the school. Most children and their families need some education about Tourette disorder. Individual psychotherapy with a mental health specialist (such as a psychologist or an advanced practice nurse) may be indicated for some children and adolescents with Tourette disorder to deal with maladaptive responses to the chronic condition.

Before evaluation and diagnosis of Tourette disorder, most families struggle with various explanations for the child's tics. Because tics fluctuate in severity with time and may be more prominent in some settings than in others, family members may have difficulty understanding their involuntary nature. Some parents may be convinced that the tics are deliberate and done to secure attention; others may judge that the tics are "nervous habits" indicative of underlying trouble. Such views require reconciliation with the currently accepted view that tics are involuntary. Some parents may conclude that the child is incapable of controlling any behaviour because of Tourette disorder. They may subsequently feel uncertain about setting limits. In these families, delineating the boundaries of Tourette disorder can be helpful (Leckman et al., 2001).

On learning that this disorder is probably genetic, some parents may harbor guilt for having passed it on to their child. The nurse can assist such families by listening to these concerns and providing information about the natural history of Tourette disorder—it is not a progressive condition, tics often diminish in adulthood, and it need not restrict what the child can achieve in life.

Teaching

Teachers, guidance counsellors, and school nurses may need current information about Tourette disorder and related problems. Discussions with school personnel often include issues such as how to deal with tic behaviours that are disruptive in the classroom, how to manage teasing from other children, and how to handle medication side effects. A careful discussion of the boundaries of Tourette disorder and tic symptomatology usually can resolve these matters. Teachers who understand the involuntary nature of tics can often generate creative solutions, such as excusing the child for errands. This maneuver allows the child to step out of the classroom briefly to release a bout of tics, thereby reducing stress. In some situations, a brief presentation about Tourette disorder to the class will reduce teasing and help both teachers and classmates tolerate the tic symptoms (Leckman et al., 2001) (see Box 27-9).

Before initiating these interventions, it is essential to identify the child's needs and to pursue these strategies in collaboration with the family and other clinical team members. If evidence shows that Tourette disorder is hindering academic progress, the nurse can help families negotiate with the school to obtain appropriate services.

Childhood Schizophrenia

Childhood (early-onset) schizophrenia is diagnosed by the same criteria as those used in adults (see Chapter 17). The difficulty in diagnosing a psychiatric disorder in children has led to years of debate and controversy regarding whether childhood schizophrenia differs from the adult type or is merely an early manifestation of the same disorder. For many years, it was believed that autism represented the childhood form of schizophrenia. However, in recent years, autism and childhood schizophrenia have been differentiated (Volkmar et al., 2004). As currently defined, childhood schizophrenia (occurring before the age of 13 years) is rare, with an estimated 2 cases per 100,000 in the population. Other forms of psychosis, falling short of diagnostic criteria for schizophrenia, can occur in children.

Childhood schizophrenia is usually characterized by poorer premorbid functioning than later-onset schizophrenia. Common premorbid difficulties include social, cognitive, linguistic, attentional, motor, and perceptual delays (Volkmar et al., 2004). Taken together, these findings suggest that early-onset schizophrenia is a more severe form of the disorder.

BOX 27.9

Therapeutic Dialogue: Tics and Disruptive Behaviours

Ineffective Approach

Teacher: I see the tics. He jerks his head, makes faces, and flicks his hands.

Nurse: What do you do about them?

Teacher: What can I do? If he isn't disrupting the class, I leave him alone. Even when he is throwing spitballs.

Nurse: Spitballs! He shouldn't be allowed to throw spitballs.

Teacher: Oh, I thought that was a part of his problem.

Nurse: Well, throwing spitballs has nothing to do with tics.

Effective Approach

Teacher: I see the tics. He jerks his head, makes faces, and flicks his hands.

Nurse: He cannot help the tics that you are seeing. Tic disorders can exhibit a wide range of severity, from mild to severe and from simple to complex. Some complex tics may be difficult to distinguish from habits or rituals.

Teacher: What about things like throwing spitballs? When he does things like that, I try to ignore that behaviour.

Nurse: Sounds like you give him the benefit of the doubt. (Validation) However, throwing a spitball is not a tic behaviour.

Teacher: What should I do?

Nurse: How do you usually handle that type of behaviour? (A modification of reflection)

Teacher: I'd ask him to stop and sometimes go into the hall.

Nurse: Disruptive behaviour that is voluntary in a student with a tic disorder should be handled as you would handle any other child.

Critical Thinking Challenge

- Compare the responses of the nurse in these scenarios. What made the difference in the teacher's responsiveness to the nurse?

Nursing care for these children follows an approach similar to that used in treatment of PDDs. Antipsychotic medication is prescribed for symptoms (Kumra, 2000). Increasingly, clinicians are using the newer atypical antipsychotics, such as risperidone, olanzapine, and quetiapine (Kumra, 2000). To varying degrees, these medications have both dopamine-blocking and serotonin-blocking properties. This combined effect is presumed to decrease the risk for neurologic side effects associated with the traditional antipsychotics (see Chapters 9 and 13 for more detailed description of the atypical antipsychotics).

Development of an individualized care plan for children with schizophrenia begins with a nursing assessment to identify functional problems specific to the child. Similarly, the recognition that childhood schizophrenia is a chronic and severe condition should guide the identification of outcomes. Goals should be realistic, and the nurse should pay special attention to the child's support systems. Parent education about the disorder, medications, and long-term management (including use of community resources) is an essential part of the treatment plan. Long-term management also requires monitoring of chronic antipsychotic therapy. Although the newer, atypical antipsychotic medications appear to have a lower risk for neurologic effects, other side effects such as weight gain also warrant careful monitoring (Martin et al., 2000).

Elimination Disorders
ENURESIS

Enuresis usually means involuntary bedwetting, although repeated urination on clothing during waking hours can occur (diurnal enuresis). For nocturnal enuresis, the *DSM-IV-TR* specifies that bedwetting occurs at least twice per week for a duration of 3 months and that the child is at least 5 years of age. Even without treatment, 50% of these children can achieve dryness by age 10 years.

Enuresis is the involuntary excretion of urine after the age at which the child should have attained bladder control.

Epidemiology and Etiology

The prevalence of nocturnal enuresis varies with age and gender, being most common in young boys—an estimated 15% of 5-year-old boys, 7% of boys aged 7 to 9 years, and 1% of 14-year-old boys have nocturnal enuresis (Mikkelsen, 2002; Reiner, 2003). The frequency in girls is about half that of boys in each age group. The etiology of enuresis is unknown, with probably no single cause. Most children with nocturnal enuresis are urologically normal. Some evidence has shown that at least some children with nocturnal enuresis secrete decreased amounts of antidiuretic hormone during sleep, which may play a role in enuresis (Reiner, 2003).

NURSING MANAGEMENT: HUMAN RESPONSE TO DISORDER

The nursing assessment should include the child's developmental history, the onset and course of enuresis, prior treatment, presence of emotional problems, and medical history. The nurse should also explore the family's home environment, family attitudes about the child's enuresis, and the family's medical history. Routine laboratory tests such as urinalysis and a urine culture are used to determine the presence of infection. The nurse should obtain baseline data regarding toileting habits, including daytime incontinence, urinary frequency, and constipation. He or she should refer children with persistent daytime enuresis for consultation with a urologist (Reiner, 2003).

In many cases, limiting fluid intake in the evening and treating constipation (if present) is sufficient to decrease the frequency of bedwetting.

Pharmacologic Interventions

If conservative methods fail, both drug and behavioural treatment have been beneficial for nocturnal enuresis. Imipramine (Tofranil), a tricyclic antidepressant, has shown efficacy in the treatment of enuresis (Reiner, 2003). The nasal spray preparation of desmopressin (DDAVP) has also shown promise, but beneficial effects may not endure (Hamano et al., 2000). DDAVP is a synthetic antidiuretic hormone that actually inhibits the production of urine. One review suggests that DDAVP helps about 25% of children who use it, with minimal risk for adverse effects (Harari & Moulden, 2000). Given its safety margin, DDAVP is preferred to imipramine.

Behavioural Interventions

The most effective nonpharmacologic treatment is the use of a pad and buzzer. In this form of behavioural treatment, the bed is equipped with a pad that sets off a buzzer if the child wets. The buzzer then wakes up the child, thereby reminding the child to void. Bedwetting can often be extinguished with this method in a relatively brief period.

ENCOPRESIS

Encopresis involves soiling clothing with feces or depositing feces in inappropriate places. Additional diagnostic criteria include that the child is older than 4 years, that the soiling occurs at least once per month, and that the soiling is not the result of a medical disorder, such as aganglionic megacolon (Hirschsprung's disease). The most common form of encopresis is fecal impaction accompanied by leakage around the hardened mass of stool. Because of the loss of muscle tone in the lower bowel, the child loses the usual urge to defecate and may not feel the leakage. Surprisingly, the child may not detect the smell of the stool because the olfactory apparatus becomes accustomed to the odor. If left untreated, this problem generally resolves independently by middle adolescence. Nonetheless, the social consequences may be substantial (Mikkelsen, 2002).

Epidemiology and Etiology

As with enuresis, encopresis is more common in boys, and the frequency of the condition declines with age.

The current estimate of prevalence is 1.5% of school-aged children, with boys three to four times more likely to have encopresis than girls (Mikkelsen, 2002).

The reasons for withholding stool and starting the cycle of fecal impaction are unclear but are usually not the result of physical causes. However, as noted, once the fecal impaction occurs, there is a loss of tone in the bowel and leakage.

NURSING MANAGEMENT: HUMAN RESPONSE TO DISORDER

The assessment includes a detailed interview with the child and parent regarding the pattern of the encopresis. A calm, matter-of-fact approach can help to reduce the child's embarrassment. A physical examination is also necessary; thus, collaboration with the child's family physician or consulting paediatrician is essential. The presence of encopresis does not necessarily signal severe emotional or behavioural disturbances, but the nurse should inquire about other psychiatric disorders. The diagnosis of encopresis is presumed given a history of intermittent constipation and soiling. Collaboration with family physician and paediatrician often is helpful to rule out rare medical conditions, such as Hirschsprung's disease.

Teaching

Effective intervention begins with educating the parents and the child about normal bowel function and the self-perpetuating cycle of fecal impaction and leakage of stool around the hardened mass of feces. The short-term goal of this educational effort is to decrease the anger and recrimination that often complicate the picture in these families. Because encopresis often results in a loss of bowel tone, it may help to motivate children by emphasizing the need to strengthen their muscles. In many cases, cleaning out the bowel is necessary before initiating behavioural treatment. The bowel catharsis is usually followed by administration of mineral oil, which is often continued during the bowel retraining program. A high-fiber diet is often recommended.

The behavioural treatment *program* involves daily sitting on the toilet after each meal for a predetermined period (eg, 10 minutes). The child and parents can measure the time with an ordinary kitchen timer, and the parents can encourage the child to read or look at picture books while sitting. They can give the child rewards in the form of stars, stickers, or points for complying with the retraining *program* and add bonuses for successful defecation. The family can tally stickers or points on a calendar, and the child can "cash in" collected points for small prizes (Mikkelsen, 2002; Reiner, 2003). All the disorders discussed in this chapter are summarized in Table 27-6.

Table 27.6   Summary of Diagnostic Characteristics

Disorder	Diagnostic Characteristics

Pervasive Developmental Disorder Not Otherwise Specified	▪ Impairment of reciprocal social interaction
	    Marked impairment in use of nonverbal behaviours
	    Failure to develop appropriate peer relationships
	    Absence of spontaneously seeking to share enjoyment, interest, or achievements (eg, pointing out things of interest)
	    Lack of social or emotional reciprocity (oblivious to others, not noticing another's distress)
	▪ Repetitive and stereotypic behaviour patterns and activities
	    Preoccupation with pattern that is abnormal in intensity or focus
	    Inflexible adherence to nonfunctional routines or rituals
	    Stereotypic, repetitive motor mannerisms
	    Persistent preoccupation with idiosyncratic interests (eg, train schedules, air conditioners)

Autism	▪ As listed above for pervasive developmental disorders
	▪ Severe impairment in communication
	    Delay or total lack of spoken language
	    Impaired ability to initiate or sustain a conversation
	    Use of stereotypic, repetitive, or idiosyncratic language
	    Lack of varied, spontaneous make-believe or social imitative play
	▪ Abnormal social interaction, use of language for social communication, or symbolic or imaginative play before age 3 years
	▪ Not better accounted for by another psychiatric disorder

Asperger's disorder	▪ As listed above for pervasive developmental disorders ▪ Clinically significant impairment in social, occupational, or other areas of functioning ▪ No general delay in language ▪ Less likely to have delay in cognitive development or daily living skills ▪ Overfocus on an area of restricted interest is a prominent feature ▪ Not better accounted for by another pervasive developmental disorder or schizophrenia
Learning Disorders	▪ Discrepancy between academic achievement and intellectual ability
Reading disorders	▪ Reading achievement substantially below that expected for age, intelligence, and education
Mathematics disorders	▪ Mathematic ability substantially below that expected for age, intelligence, and education
Disorders of written expression	▪ Writing skills substantially below that expected for age, intelligence, and education
Communication Disorders	▪ Interference with academic or occupational achievement or social communication

Expressive language disorder	▪ Deficits not explained by retardation or deprivation
	▪ Impairment of expressive language development
	    Limited amount of speech
	    Limited range of vocabulary
	    Vocabulary errors
	    Sentence structure problems
	    Unusual word order
	    Slow rate of language development
	    Difficulty in communication, both verbally and with sign language
	▪ As listed above for communication disorders
	▪ Deficits cannot be explained by pervasive developmental disorder

Mixed receptive–expressive language disorder	▪ Impairment of receptive and expressive language development
	    Markedly limited vocabulary
	    Errors in tense
	    Difficulty recalling words or appropriate-length sentences
	    General difficulty expressing ideas
	    Difficulty understanding words, sentences, or types of words or statements
	    Multiple disabilities such as inability to understand basic vocabulary or simple sentences; deficits in sound discrimination, storage, recall, and sequencing
	▪ As listed above for communication disorders
	▪ Deficits not explained by pervasive developmental disorder

Table 27.6 (Summary of Diagnostic Characteristics (Continued)

Disorder	Diagnostic Characteristics

Phonologic disorder	▪ Failure to use appropriate developmentally expected speech sounds
	    Errors in sound production
	    Substitution of one sound for another
	    Omission of sounds
	▪ As listed above for communication disorders

Stuttering	▪ Disturbed fluency and timing patterns of speech
	    Repetition of sounds and syllables
	    Prolongation of sound
	    Interjections
	    Broken words
	    Filled or unfilled pauses in speech
	    Substitutions of words to avoid problematic sounds
	    Production of words with an excess of physical tension
	    Repetitions of monosyllabic whole word
	▪ As listed above for communication disorders

Disruptive Behaviour Disorders	▪ Significant impairment in social, academic, or occupational functioning ▪ Not accounted for by antisocial personality disorder if older than 18 years

Conduct disorder	▪ Repetitive and persistent behaviour that violates the rights of others or major age-appropriate societal norms
	    Aggression to people and animals
	    Destruction of property
	    Deceitfulness or theft
	    Serious violations of rules
	▪ As listed above for disruptive behaviour disorders

Oppositional defiant disorder	▪ Negativistic, hostile behaviour pattern
	    Loss of temper
	    Frequently argumentative
	    Active defiance or refusal to comply with adult requests or rules
	    Deliberate annoyance of others
	    Blaming of others for own mistakes or misbehaviour
	    Anger and resentment
	    Spitefulness and vindictiveness
	▪ As listed above for disruptive behaviour disorders
	▪ Not exclusive during course of psychotic or mood disorder

Anxiety Disorders Obsessive-compulsive disorders	See Chapter 20.
Mood Disorders Major depressive disorder	See Chapter 19.
Tic Disorders	▪ Single or multiple tics ▪ Onset before age 18 years ▪ Not due to substance (eg, amphetamine) or general medical condition
Chronic motor or vocal tic disorder, 307.22	▪ Motor or vocal tics occurring many times per day nearly every day or intermittently throughout more than 1 year, no tic-free period greater than 3 months ▪ As listed above for tic disorders
Transient tic disorder, 307.21	▪ Motor or vocal tics occurring many times during the day for at least 4 weeks; not longer than 12 consecutive months
Tourette disorder	▪ Motor and phonic tics lasting more than 12 months
Childhood Schizophrenia *Elimination Disorders*	See Chapter 17
Enuresis, 307.6	▪ Repeated voiding into bed or clothes (involuntary or intentional) ▪ Occurring twice a week for at least 3 consecutive months or significant impairment in social, academic, or other area of functioning ▪ At least 5 years of age or developmental equivalent ▪ Not a physiologic effect of a substance or general medical condition
Encopresis	▪ Repeated passage of feces into inappropriate places, such as clothing or floor
307.7 without constipation and overflow incontinence	▪ Occurring at least once a month for at least 3 months ▪ At least 4 years of age or developmental equivalent
787.6 with constipation and overflow incontinence	▪ Not the physiologic effect of a substance or general medical condition except involving constipation

BOX 27.10

Research for Best Practice

QUESTIONS: What are the perceived levels of informal and formal social supports among families of autistic children? What are the coping strategies used by parents of children with autism?

METHODS: The conceptual framework for this study was the Resiliency Model of Family Stress, Adjustment, and Adaptation. The study used a descriptive survey design and a convenience sample. Participants were parents of children with autism (ages 5–13) who were enrolled in selected special education classes. A convenience sample of 72 was identified; however, only 18 families completed and returned the questionnaires. Participants completed a demographic questionnaire, which included questions about concurrent stressors in the family, and two Likert-type scales that examined coping strategies and formal and informal types of social support.

FINDINGS: Significant stressors in addition to a child's autism were reported by 50% of the families. Identified stressors were finances, unemployment, absentee fathers, transportation problems, recent divorce, and concurrent chronic health problems such as diabetes and asthma. Reframing scored highest as a coping strategy for participants. Reframing enabled families to define problems in more positive ways to avoid becoming depressed. Social support ranked second as a coping method for families. There were individual differences in accessing social supports because of difficulties such as inability to speak English, low income, and lack of transportation. Approximately 50% of the parents indicated that they attended or were interested in attending a support group. Eighty-three percent of participants strongly agreed with the statement that having faith in God was a way of coping; however, fewer than half coped by attending church services or sought the advice of a minister, priest, or rabbi. Participants scored high on the Passive Appraisal subscale. This subscale focussed on inactive or passive behaviour that the family might use, such as avoidance responses based on a lack of confidence in their ability to change the situation. Passive behaviours may also be used as a means of coping with stress. Responses regarding formal and informal social support were consistently high for close friends and family members; few, however, relied on neighbours for help or support. Responses for obtaining help when needed and feeling comfortable within the community were variable. The variation may have resulted from differing cultural and socioeconomic levels, as well as differing lengths of time families may have resided in the neighbourhood.

IMPLICATIONS FOR NURSING PRACTICE: This study found that half of the children with autism had coexisting medical conditions. School nurses are the link between educational and medical institutions and are valuable members of the educational intervention team. The school nurse can assist parents or caregivers to examine information and make informed decisions about the child's needs. Understanding parents' preferred coping strategies and their access to informal and formal support systems will assist nurses as they strive to help them meet their own and their families' needs.

From Luther, E. H., Canham, D. L., Young-Cureton, V. (2005). Coping and social supports for parents of children with autism. *Journal of School Nursing, 21*(1), 40–47.

SUMMARY OF KEY POINTS

- Improved methods of assessing and defining psychiatric disorders have enhanced appreciation for the frequency of psychiatric disorders in children and adolescents.
- An estimated 14% of children 4 to 17 years of age (more than 800,000) in Canada experience mental disorders that cause significant distress and impairment at home, at school, and in the community.
- The developmental disorders include intellectual disability, pervasive developmental disorders (PDDs), and specific developmental disorders. Assessment findings should guide nursing management. Specific developmental disorders include communication disorders and learning disorders. These disorders are fairly common in the general population, but they are more common in children with other primary psychiatric disorders.
- Child psychiatric disorders can be divided into externalizing and internalizing disorders. Externalizing disorders include the disruptive behaviour disorders: attention deficit hyperactivity disorder (ADHD), oppositional defiant disorder, and conduct disorder. Internalizing disorders include depression and anxiety disorders.
- ADHD is defined by the presence of inattention, impulsiveness, and in most cases, hyperactivity. As currently defined, ADHD is the most common disorder of childhood. This heterogeneous disorder affects boys more often than girls.
- Effective treatment of ADHD often involves multiple approaches, including medication and parent training.
- Primary features of oppositional defiant disorder include persistent disobedience, argumentativeness, and tantrums.
- Conduct disorder is characterized by lying, truancy, stealing, and fighting.
- Assessment of children with disruptive behaviour problems involves securing data from multiple sources, including the child, parents, and school personnel.
- Standardized rating instruments can assist data collection from multiple informants.
- Separation anxiety and obsessive-compulsive disorder (OCD) are relatively common anxiety disorders in school-aged children. (OCD becomes more common in adolescents.)
- Treatment of separation anxiety and OCD may include medication, behavioural therapy, or a combination of these treatments.
- Major depression in children is believed to be similar to major depression in adults.
- The efficacy of antidepressant medications is less well established in children and adolescents than in adults.

▣ Tourette disorder is a tic disorder characterized by motor and phonic tics. Common comorbid conditions include ADHD and OCD.

▣ Childhood schizophrenia is a rare disorder.

▣ Elimination disorders include encopresis and enuresis. Behavioural therapy approaches are the most effective treatment for these disorders. Medication may also be used.

CRITICAL THINKING CHALLENGES

1 Discuss the distinguishing features of ADHD and conduct disorder.

2 What brain region is believed to play a fundamental role in the pathophysiology of Tourette disorder?

3 Discuss the advantages of using a developmental framework to assess a child or adolescent psychiatric client.

4 Analyze how genetic and environmental factors may interact in the etiology of child psychiatric disorders.

5 Learning disabilities and communication disorders are more common in children with psychiatric disorders than in the general population. How might a learning disability or a communication disorder complicate a psychiatric illness in a school-aged child?

6 Compare and contrast nursing approaches for a child with ADHD with those used for a child with autistic disorder. How are they different? How are they similar?

7 Many children have imaginary playmates. What are the benefits to the child? At what age level is this appropriate? When does it become inappropriate?

8 How would you answer these questions from a parent: "What causes ADHD? Is it my fault?"

WEB LINKS

www.chaddcanada.org This site of the Children and Adults With Attention-Deficit/Hyperactivity Disorder (CHADD) organization provides information and resources on ADHD.

www.tourette.ca This website contains information and resources about Tourette disorder.

www.wpi.edu/~trek/aspergers.html This website describes Asperger's disorder.

www.schizophrenia.ca This website provides links to all the provincial association websites. See "resources & links."

www.autism.org The website of the Centre for Study of Autism contains information and resources about autism and related disorders.

MOVIES

Rain Man: 1988. This classic film stars Dustin Hoffman as Raymond Babbitt, a man who has autism (savant).

Tom Cruise plays his brother Charlie, a self-centered hustler who believes that he has been cheated out of his inheritance. Discovering Raymond in an institution, Charlie abducts Raymond in a last-ditch effort to get his fair share of the family estate. The story evolves around the relationship that develops as the brothers drive across the country.

Dustin Hoffman brilliantly portrays the behaviours and symptoms of high functioning autism, such as the monotone speech, insistence on sameness, and repetitive behaviour.

VIEWING POINTS: Identify and describe Raymond's ritualistic behaviours. Identify the behaviours that depict extreme autistic isolation. Observe Raymond's language patterns and any distinct abnormalities. What happens when Raymond's rituals are interrupted?

REFERENCES

Achenbach, T. (1991). *Manual for the child behavior checklist and behavior profile*. Burlington, VT: University of Vermont.

American Psychiatric Association. (2000). *Diagnostic and statistical manual of mental disorders* (4th ed., Text revision). Washington, DC: Author.

Arnold, L. E., Aman, M. G., Martin, A., Collier-Crespin, A., Vitiello, B., Tierney, E., Asarnow, R., BellBradshaw, F., Freeman, B. J., Gates-Ulanet, P., Klin, A., McCracken, J. T., McDougle, C. J., McGough, J. J., Posey, D. J., Scahill, L., Swiezy, N. B., Ritz, L., & Volkmar, F. (2000). Assessment in multisite randomized clinical trials (RCTs) of clients with autistic disorder. *Journal of Autism Development, 30*, 99–111.

Barkley, R. A. (1997). *Defiant children: A clinician's manual for parent training*. New York: Guilford Press.

Barkley, R. A. (1998). *Attention deficit hyperactivity disorder: A handbook for diagnosis and treatment*. New York: Guilford Press.

Beitchman, J. H., Nair, R., Clegg, M., & Patel, P. G. (1986). Prevalence of speech and language disorders in 5-year-old kindergarten children in the Ottawa-Carleton Region. *Journal of Speech and Hearing Disorders, 51*, 98–110.

Biederman, J., Faraone, S. V., Keenan, K., et al. (1992). Further evidence for family-genetic risk factors attention deficit disorder. *Archives of General Psychiatry, 49*, 728–738.

Biederman, J., Milberger, S., Faraone, S. V., et al. (1995). Family-environment risk factors for attention-deficit hyperactivity disorder. *Archives of General Psychiatry, 52*, 464–470.

Biederman, J., & the ADHD Study Group. (2002). Efficacy of atomoxetine versus placebo in school-age girls with attention-deficit/hyperactivity disorder. *Paediatrics, 110*(6), 75–79.

Birmaher, B., & Brent, D. (2003). Depressive disorders. In A. Martin, L. Scahill, D. S. Charney, & J. F. Leckman (Eds.), *Paediatric psychopharmacology: Principles and practice* (1st ed.; pp. 466–483). New York: Oxford.

Blackson, T. C., Butler, T., Belsky, J., et al. (1999). Individual traits and family contexts predict sons' externalizing behavior and preliminary relative risk ratios for conduct disorder and substance use disorder outcomes. *Drug and Alcohol Dependence, 56*(2), 115–131.

Bolton, P. F., Murphy, M., Macdonald, H., et al. (1997). Obstetric complications in autism: Consequences or causes of the condition? *Journal of the American Academy of Child and Adolescent Psychiatry, 36*(2), 272–281.

Buitelaar, J. K., van der Gaag, R. J., & van der Hoeven, J. (1998). Buspirone in the management of anxiety and irritability in children with pervasive disorders: Results of an open-label study. *Journal of Clinical Psychiatry, 59*(2), 56–59.

Campbell, M., Armenteros, J. L., Malone, R. P., et al. (1997). Neuroleptic-related dyskinesias in autistic children: A prospective, longitudinal study. *Journal of the American Academy of Child and Adolescent Psychiatric Nursing, 36,* 835–843.

Carroll, D. H., Scahill, L., & Phillips, K. (2002). Current concepts in body dysmorphic disorder. *Archives of Psychiatric Nursing, 16,* 72–79.

Carroll, D. H., Shyam, R., & Scahill, L. (2002). Cardiac conduction and antipsychotic medication: A primer on electrocardiograms. *Journal of Child and Adolescent Psychiatric Nursing, 15*(4), 170–177.

Castellanos, F. X., Giedd, J. N., Marsh, W. L., et al. (1996). Quantitative brain magnetic resonance imaging in attention-deficit hyperactivity disorder. *Archives of General Psychiatry, 53*(7), 607–616.

Chakrabarti, S., & Fombonne, E. (2001). Pervasive developmental disorders in preschool children. *Journal of the American Medical Association, 285*(24), 3093–3142.

Conners, C. K. (1989). *Conners' rating scales manual.* North Tonawanda, NY: Multi-Health Systems.

DeVeaugh-Geiss, J., Moroz, G., Biederman, J., et al. (1992). Clomipramine hydrochloride in childhood and adolescent obsessive-compulsive disorder: A multicenter trial. *Journal of American Academy of Child and Adolescent Psychiatry, 31,* 45–49.

Flament, M. F., Whitaker, A., Rapoport, J. L., et al. (1988). Obsessive compulsive disorder in adolescence. *Journal of the American Academy of Child and Adolescent Psychiatry, 27,* 764–771.

Ford, R. E., Greenhill, L. L, & Posner, K. (2003). Stimulants. In A. Martin, L. Scahill, D. S. Charney, & J. F. Leckman (Eds.), *Pediatric psychopharmacology: Principles and practice* (1st ed.; pp. 255–263) New York: Oxford.

Geller, D. A., Hoog, S. L., Heiligenstein, J. H., Ricardi, R. K., Tamura, R., Kluszynski, S., Jacobsen, J. G., & Team TFPOS (2001). Fluoxetine treatment for obsessive-compulsive disorder in children and adolescents: A placebo-controlled clinical trial. *Journal of the American Academy of Child & Adolescent Psychiatry, 40,* 773–779.

Grandin, T. (1996). *Thinking in pictures and other reports from my life with autism.* New York: Vintage Books.

Hamano, S., Yamanishi, T., Igarashi, T., et al. (2000). Functional bladder capacity as predictor of response to desmopressin and retention control training in monosymptomatic nocturnal enuresis. *European Urology, 37*(6), 718–722.

Handen, B. L., Johnson, C. R., & Lubetsky, M. (2000). Efficacy of methylphenidate among children with autism and symptoms of attention-deficit hyperactivity disorder. *Journal of Autism and Developmental Disorder, 30,* 245–255.

Harari, M. D., & Moulden, A. (2000). Nocturnal enuresis: What is happening? *Journal of Pediatrics and Child Health, 36*(1), 78–81.

Henggeler, S. W., Rowland, M. D., Randall, J., Ward, D. M., Pickrel, S. G., Cunningham, P. B., Miller, S. L., Edwards, J., Zealberg, J. J., Hand, L. D., & Santos, A. B. (1999). Home-based multisystemic therapy as an alternative to the hospitalization of youths in psychiatric crisis: Clinical outcomes. *Journal of the American Academy of Child and Adolescent Psychiatry, 38*(11), 1331–1339.

Jensen, P. S., Edelman, A., & Nemeroff, R. (2003). Paediatric psychopharmacoepidemiology: Who is prescribing? And for whom, how and why? In A. Martin, L. Scahill, D. S. Charney, J. F. Leckman (Eds.), *Pediatric psychopharmacology: Principles and practice* (1st ed.; pp. 701–711). New York: Oxford.

Kanner, L. (1943). Autistic disturbances of affective contact. *Nervous Child, 2,* 217–250.

Karno, M., Golding, J. M., Sorenson, S. B., & Burnam, M. A. (1988). The epidemiology of obsessive compulsive disorder in five US communities. *Archives of General Psychiatry, 45,* 1094–1099.

Kazdin, A. E., & Weisz, J. K. (2003). *Evidence-based psychotherapies for children and adolescents.* Guilford: New York.

King, R. A., & Scahill, L. (2001). Emotional and behavioral difficulties associated with Tourette syndrome. *Advances Neurology, 85,* 79–88.

King, R. A., Scahill, L., Lombroso, P. J., & Leckman, J. F. (2003). Tourette's syndrome and other tic disorders. In A. Martin, L. Scahill, D. S. Charney, J. F. Leckman (Eds.), *Pediatric psychopharmacology: Principles and practice* (1st ed.; pp. 526–542). New York: Oxford.

Koda, V. H., Charney, D. S., & Pine, D. S. (2003). In A. Martin, L. Scahill, D. S. Charney, J. F. Leckman (Eds.), *Pediatric psychopharmacology: Principles and practice* (1st ed.; pp. 138–149). New York: Oxford.

Koenig, K., & Scahill, L. (2001). Assessment of children with pervasive developmental disorders. *Journal of Child and Adolescent Psychiatric Nursing, 14,* 159–166.

Kumra, S. (2000). The diagnosis and treatment of children and adolescents with schizophrenia: 'My mind is playing tricks on me.' *Child and Adolescent Psychiatric Clinics of North America, 9*(1), 183–199.

Labellarte, M. J., & Ginsberg, G. S. (2003). Anxiety disorders. In A. Martin, L. Scahill, D. S. Charney, J. F. Leckman (Eds.), *Pediatric psychopharmacology: Principles and practice* (1st ed.; pp. 497–510). New York: Oxford.

Leckman, J. F., Peterson, B. S., King, R. A., Scahill, L., & Cohen, D. J. (2001). Phenomenology of tics and natural history of tic disorders. *Advances Neurology, 85,* 1–14.

Leckman, J. F., Zhang, H., Vitale, A., et al. (1998). Course of tic severity in Tourette syndrome: The first two decades. *Pediatrics, 102,* 14–19.

Levy, F., Hay, D. A., McStephen, M., et al. (1997). Attention-deficit hyperactivity disorder: A category or a continuum? Genetic analysis of a large-scale twin study. *Journal of the American Academy of Child and Adolescent Psychiatry, 36,* 737–744.

Lou, H. C., Henriksen, L., & Bruhn, P. (1990). Focal cerebral dysfunction in developmental learning disabilities. *Lancet, 335,* 8–11.

Luther, E., Canham, D., & Young Curetan, V. (2005). Coping and social support for parents of children with autism. *Journal of School Nursing, 21*(1), 40–47.

March, J. S., Biederman, J., Wolkow, R., et al. (1998). Sertraline in children and adolescents with obsessive-compulsive disorder: A multi-center randomized controlled trial. *Journal of the American Medical Association, 280,* 1752–1755.

Martin, A., Landau, J., Leebens, P., et al. (2000). Risperidone-associated weight gain in children and adolescents: A retrospective chart review. *Journal of Child and Adolescent Psychopharmacology, 10,* 259–268.

Martin, A., Van Hoof, T., Stubbe, D., Sherwin, T., & Scahill, L. (2003). Multiple psychotropic pharmacotherapy in children and adolescents: A study of Connecticut Medicaid managed care recipients. *Psychiatric Services, 54,* 72–77.

McDougle, C. J., & Posey, D. J. (2003). Autistic and other pervasive developmental disorders. In A. Martin, L. Scahill, D. S. Charney, & J. F. Leckman (Eds.), *Pediatric psychopharmacology: Principles and practice* (1st ed.; pp. 563–579). New York: Oxford.

Mikkelsen, E. J. (2002). Modern approaches to enuresis and encopresis. In M. Lewis (Ed.), *Child and adolescent psychiatry: A comprehensive textbook* (3rd ed.; pp. 700–711). Philadelphia: Lippincott Williams & Wilkins.

Mink, J. W. (2001). Neurobiology of basal ganglia circuits in Tourette syndrome: Faulty inhibition of unwanted motor patterns? *Advances in Neurology, 85,* 113–122.

Moss, N. E., & Racusin, G. R. (2002). Psychological assessment of children and adolescents. In M. Lewis (Ed.), *Child and adolescent psychiatry: A comprehensive textbook* (3rd ed.). Philadelphia: Lippincott Williams & Wilkins.

Morshed, S. A., Parveen, S., Leckman, J. F., Mercadante, M. T., Bittencourt Kiss, M. H., Miguel, E. C., Arman, A., Yazgan, Y.,

Fujii, T., Paul, S., Peterson, B. S., Zhang, H., King, R. A., Scahill, L., & Lombroso, P. J. (2001). Antibodies against neural, nuclear, cytoskeletal, and streptococcal epitopes in children and adults with Tourette's syndrome, Sydenham's chorea, and autoimmune disorders [erratum appears in *Biol Psychiatry* 2001(Dec 15);50(12): following 1009]. *Biology Psychiatry, 50*(8), 566–577.

MTA Cooperative Group. (1999). A 14-month randomized clinical trial of treatment strategies for attention-deficit/hyperactivity disorder. *Archives of General Psychiatry, 56,* 1073–1086.

Murphy, T. K., Voeller, K. K. S., & Blier, P. (2003). Neurobiology of obsessive-compulsive disorder. In A. Martin, L. Scahill, D. S. Charney, & J. F. Leckman (Eds.), *Pediatric psychopharmacology: Principles and practice* (1st ed.; pp. 150–163). New York: Oxford.

Novotny, S., Evers, M., Barboza, K., Rawitt, R., & Hollander, E. (2003). Neurobiology of affiliation: Implications for autism spectrum disorders. In A. Martin, L. Scahill, D. S. Charney & J. F. Leckman (Eds.), *Pediatric psychopharmacology: Principles and practice* (1st ed.; pp. 195–209). New York: Oxford.

Paul, R. (2002). Disorders of communication. In M. Lewis (Ed.), *Child and adolescent psychiatry: A comprehensive textbook* (3rd ed.; pp. 612–621). Philadelphia: Lippincott Williams & Wilkins.

Peterson, B. S., Staib, L., Scahill, L., Zhang, H., Anderson, C., Leckman, J. F., Cohen, D. J., Gore, J. C., Albert, J., & Webster, R. (2001). Regional brain and ventricular volumes in Tourette syndrome. *Archives of General Psychiatry, 58,* 427–440.

Peterson, B. S., Zhang, H., Anderson, G. M., & Leckman, J. F. (1998). A double-blind, placebo-controlled, crossover trial of an antiandrogen in the treatment of Tourette's syndrome. *Journal of Clinical Psychopharmacology, 18*(4), 324–331.

Piacentini, J. (1999). Cognitive behavioral therapy of childhood OCD. *Child and Adolescent Psychiatric Clinics of North America, 8*(3), 599–616.

Reiner, W. G. (2003). Elimination disorders: Enuresis and encopresis. In A. Martin, L. Scahill, D. S. Charney, & J. F. Leckman (Eds.), *Pediatric psychopharmacology: Principles and practice* (1st ed.; pp. 686–698). New York: Oxford.

Research Units on Pediatric Psychopharmacology (RUPP) Anxiety Study Group. (2001). Fluvoxamine for the treatment of anxiety disorders in children and adolescents. *New England Journal of Medicine, 344*(17), 1279–1285.

Research Units on Pediatric Psychopharmacology (RUPP) Autism Network. (2002). Risperidone in children with autism and serious behavioral problems. *New England Journal of Medicine, 347,* 314–321.

Riddle, M. A., Reeve, E. A., Yaryura-Tobias, J. A., et al. (2001). Fluvoxamine for children and adolescents with obsessive-compulsive disorder: A controlled multicenter trial. *Journal of American Academy of Child and Adolescent Psychiatry, 40*(2), 222–229.

Sallee, F. R., Kurlan, R., Goetz, C. G., et al. (2000). Ziprasidone treatment of children and adolescents with Tourette's syndrome: A pilot study. *Journal of the American Academy of Child and Adolescent Psychiatry, 39*(3), 292–299.

Scahill, L., Chappell, P. B., Kim, Y. S., et al. (2001). A placebo-controlled study of guanfacine in the treatment of attention deficit hyperactivity disorder and tic disorders. *American Journal of Psychiatry, 158*(7), 1064–1074.

Scahill, L., Kano, Y., King, R. A., Carlson, A., Peller, A., LeBrun, U., Rosario-Campos, M. C., & Leckman, J. F. (2003). Influence of age and tic disorders on obsessive-compulsive disorder in a pediatric sample. *Journal Child Adolescent Psychopharmacology*

Scahill, L., Leckman, J. F., Schultz, R. T., Katsovich, L., & Peterson, B. S. (2003). A placebo-controlled trial of risperidone in Tourette syndrome. *Neurology, 60,* 1130–1135.

Scahill, L., Riddle, M. A., McSwiggan-Hardin, M., et al. (1997). Children's Yale-Brown Obsessive Compulsive Scale: Reliability and validity. *Journal of the American Academy of Child and Adolescent Psychiatry, 36,* 844–852.

Scahill, L., & Schwab-Stone, M. (2000). Epidemiology of attention deficit hyperactivity disorder in school-age children. *Child and Adolescent Psychiatric Clinics of North America, 9*(3), 541–555.

Scahill, L., Schwab-Stone, M., Merikangas, K., Leckman, J., Zhang, H., & Kasl, S. (1999). Psychosocial and clinical correlates of ADHD in a community sample of young school-age children. *Journal of the American Academy of Child and Adolescent Psychiatry, 38,* 976–983.

Scahill, L., Tanner, C., & Dure, L. (2001). Epidemiology of tic disorders and Tourette syndrome: Toward a common definition. *Advances in Neurology, 85,* 261–272.

Schultz, R. T., Carter, A. S., Gladstone, M., et al. (1998). Visual-motor integration functioning in children with Tourette syndrome. *Neuropsychology, 12*(1), 134–145.

Schwartz, C. E., Snidman, N., & Kagan, J. (1999). Adolescent social anxiety as an outcome of inhibited temperament in childhood. *Journal of the American Academy of Child and Adolescent Psychiatry, 38*(8), 1008–1015.

Shaywitz, S. E. (2003). *Overcoming dyslexia* (1st ed.). New York: Knopf.

Sparrow, S. S., Balla, D. A., & Cicchetti, D. V. (1984). *Vineland Adaptive Behavior Scales.* Circle Pines, MN: American Guidance Clinic.

Szatmari, P., Boyle, M., & Offord, D. R. (1989). ADHD and conduct disorder: Degree of diagnostic overlap and differences among correlates. *Journal of the American Academy of Child and Adolescent Psychiatry, 28,* 865–872.

Taylor, J. R., Morshed, S. A., Parveen, S., Mercadante, M. T., Scahill, L., Peterson, B. S., King, R. A., Leckman, J. F. & Lombroso, P. J. (2002). An animal model of Tourette's syndrome. *American Journal of Psychiatry, 159*(4), 657–660.

Tomblin, J. B., Zhang, X., Buckwalter, P., & Catts, H. (2000). The association of reading disability, behavioral disorders, and language impairment among second-grade children. *Journal of Child Psychology and Psychiatry and Allied Disciplines, 41*(4), 473–482.

Toppelberg, C. O., & Shapiro, T. (2000). 10-year update review: Language disorders. *Journal of the American Academy of Child and Adolescent Psychiatry, 39*(2), 143–152.

Tourette Syndrome Association International Consortium for Genetics. (1999). A complete genome screen in sib pairs affected by Gilles de la Tourette syndrome. *American Journal of Human Genetics, 65*(5), 1428–1436.

Tourette Syndrome Study Group. (1999). Short versus longer term pimozide therapy in Tourette's syndrome: A preliminary study. *Neurology, 52,* 874–877.

Vaidya, C. J., Austin, G., Kirkorian, G., et al. (1998). Selective effects of methylphenidate in attention deficit disorder: A functional magnetic resonance study. *Proceedings of the National Academy of Sciences, 95,* 14494–14499.

Velosa, J. F., & Riddle, M. A. (2000). Psychopharmacologic treatment of anxiety disorders in children and adolescents. *Child and Adolescent Psychiatric Clinics of North America, 9*(1), 119–133.

Volkmar, F. R., Klin, A., & Paul, R. (2004). *Handbook of autism and pervasive developmental disorders* (3rd ed.). New York: Wiley.

Volkmar, F. R., Klin, A., Schultz, R. T., Rubin, E., & Bronen, R. (2000). Asperger's disorder. *American Journal of Psychiatry, 157*(2), 262–267.

Waddell, C., McEwan, K., Shepherd, C., Offord, D., & Hua, J. M. (2005). A public health strategy to improve the mental health of Canadian children. *Canadian Journal of Psychiatry, 50*(4), 226–233.

Walkup, J. T., LaBuda, M. C., Singer, H. S., et al. (1996). Family study and segregation analysis of Tourette syndrome: Evidence of a mixed model of inheritance. *American Journal of Human Genetics, 59,* 684–693.

Weiss, M., & Weiss, G. (2002). Attention deficit hyperactivity disorder. In M. Lewis (Ed.), *Child and adolescent psychiatry: A comprehensive textbook* (3rd ed.; pp. 645–670). Philadelphia: Lippincott Williams & Wilkins.

Werry, J. S., & Aman, M. G. (1998). *Practitioner's guide to psychoactive drugs for children and adolescents.* New York: Plenum Press.

Willcutt, E. G., Pennington, B. F., & DeFries, J. C. (2000). Twin study of the etiology of comorbidity between reading disability and attention-deficit/hyperactivity disorder. *American Journal of Medical Genetics, 96*(3), 293–301.

Zametkin, A. J., Liebenauer, L. L., Fitzgerald, G. A., et al. (1993). Brain metabolism in teenagers with attention-deficit hyperactivity disorder. *Archives of General Psychiatry, 50,* 333–340.

Zametkin, A. J., Nordahl, T. E., Gross, M., et al. (1990). Cerebral glucose metabolism in adults with hyperactivity of childhood onset. *New England Journal of Medicine, 323*(20), 1361–1366.

Acknowledgments

This work was supported in part by the following United States Public Health Service grants: Children's Clinical Research Center Grant RR06022; Program Project Grant MH49351 from the National Institute of Mental Health; Program Project Grant HD-03008 from the National Institute of Child Health and Human Development; Research Units on Pediatric Psychopharmacology; contract MH-70009 from the National Institute of Mental Health.

Older Adults

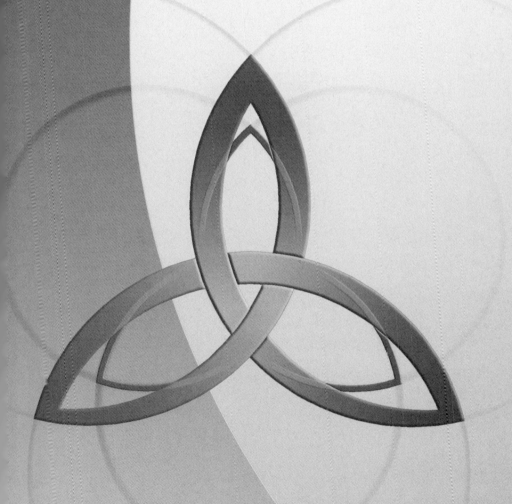

CHAPTER 28

Mental Health Assessment of the Older Adult

Mary Ann Boyd, Mickey Stanley, and Annette M. Lane

LEARNING OBJECTIVES

After studying this chapter, you will be able to:

- Compare changes in normal aging with those associated with mental health problems in older adults.
- Select various techniques in assessing older adults who have mental health problems.
- Delineate important areas of assessment for the biologic domain in completing the geriatric mental health nursing assessment.
- Delineate important areas of assessment for the psychological domain in completing the geriatric mental health nursing assessment.
- Delineate important areas of assessment for the social domain in completing the geriatric mental health nursing assessment.

KEY TERMS

dysphagia ▪ functional activities ▪ insomnia ▪ instrumental activities ▪ polypharmacy ▪ xerostomia

⬟ KEY CONCEPTS

biopsychosocial geriatric mental health nursing assessment ▪ normal aging

In 1920, the average life span in Canada was 60 years (Statistics Canada, 2005). By 1997, this life span increased to approximately 76 years for men and 81 years for women (Health Canada, 2002a). Health care providers will face new and increased challenges as the baby boomers move into the ranks of older adults. By the year 2021, projections are that there will be almost 7 million older adults (65 years of age and older), composing 19% of the Canadian population. The fastest growing segment of the older population is the group 85 years of age and older (Public Health Agency of Canada, 2005a).

Normal aging is associated with some physical decline, such as decreased sensory abilities and decreased pulmonary and immune function, but many important functions do not change. Intellectual function, capacity for change, and productive engagement with life remain stable. Many myths exist about normal aging. Some people believe that "senility" is normal, or that depression or hopelessness is natural for older individuals. If family members believe these myths, they will be less likely to seek treatment for their elders with real problems. Even if family members seek help for their older adults, health care providers may fail to identify depression, or simply attribute symptoms to normal aging (Rabheru, 2004). Approximately 15% to 30% of older adults experience symptoms of mental illness (SAGMHS, 2003). Older adults with mental health problems comprise different population groups. One group consists of those with long-term mental illnesses who have reached the ranks of the older adult population. These individuals usually understand their disorders and treatments. Unfortunately, the changes associated with aging can affect a patient's control of his or her chronic mental illness. Symptoms may reappear, and medications may need to be adjusted. Another group includes individuals who are relatively free of mental health problems until their later years. These individuals, who may already have other health problems, develop late-onset mental disorders, such as depression, schizophrenia, or dementia. For these individuals and their family members, the development of a mental disorder can be very traumatic.

Mental health problems in older adults can be especially complex because of coexisting medical problems and treatments. Many symptoms of somatic disorders mimic or mask psychiatric disorders. For example, fatigue may be related to anaemia, but it also may be symptomatic of depression. In addition, older individuals are more likely to report somatic symptoms, rather than psychological ones, making identification of a mental disorder even more difficult.

The purpose of this chapter is to present a comprehensive geriatric mental health nursing assessment process that serves as the basis of care for older individuals (discussed in Chapters 29 and 30). A mental health assessment is necessary when psychiatric or mental health issues are identified or when patients with mental illnesses reach their later years (usually about age 65 years). The assessment generally follows the same format as described in Chapter 10. However, the overall health care issues for older adults can be very complex, so it follows that certain components of the geriatric mental health nursing assessment are unique. Thus, the geriatric assessment emphasizes some areas that are less critical to the standard adult assessment.

> ⬟ **KEY CONCEPT Normal aging** is associated with some physical decline, such as decreased sensory abilities and decreased pulmonary and immune function, but many important functions do not change.

TECHNIQUES OF DATA COLLECTION

The nurse assesses the older client using an interview format that may take a few sessions to complete. He or she also may rely on self-report standardized tests, such as depression and cognitive functioning tools. A wide variety of physiologic disorders may cause changes in mental status for older adults; thus, results of laboratory tests often are significant. For example, urinalysis can detect a urinary tract infection that has affected a client's cognitive status. Box 28-1 contains a representative listing of common physiologic causes of changes in mental status. In addition, medical records from other health care providers are useful in developing a complete picture of the client's health status.

An important source of client data is family members, who often notice changes that the older individual overlooks or fails to recognize. A client with memory impairment may be unable to give an accurate history. By interviewing family members, the nurse expands the scope of the client assessment. Moreover, the nurse has an opportunity to evaluate the caregivers themselves to determine whether they can care for the older individual adequately and how they are coping with the situation. For example, a husband may be unable to care for his wife but is unwilling to admit it. If the nurse can

---

BOX 28.1

Changes That Affect Mental Status

- Acid–base imbalance
- Dehydration
- Drugs (prescribed and over-the-counter)
- Electrolyte changes
- Hypothyroidism
- Hypothermia and hyperthermia
- Hypoxia
- Infection and sepsis

establish rapport with the husband, the nurse may use the assessment interview as an opportunity to help the husband to examine his wife's care requirements realistically. The nurse may be able to explain to the husband the impact of caregiving on his health. For instance, it is not uncommon for the caregiving spouse to die before his or her spouse with dementia, because of the extreme and prolonged stresses.

BIOPSYCHOSOCIAL GERIATRIC MENTAL HEALTH NURSING ASSESSMENT

> ◆ **KEY CONCEPT** A **biopsychosocial geriatric mental health nursing assessment** is the comprehensive, deliberate, and systematic collection and interpretation of biopsychosocial data that is based on the special needs and problems of older adults to determine current and past health, functional status, and human responses to mental health problems, both actual and potential (Box 28-2).

At the beginning of the assessment, the nurse should determine the client's ability to participate. For example, if a client is using a wheelchair, he or she may have physical limitations that prevent full participation in the assessment. The older client must be able to hear the nurse. For a client with compromised hearing, the nurse must attend to voice projection and volume. Shouting at the older individual is unnecessary. The nurse should remember to lower the pitch of his or her voice because higher-pitched sounds are often lost with presbycusis (loss of hearing sensitivity associated with aging). The nurse should eliminate distracting noises, such as from a television or radio, and ensure that the client's hearing aid is in place and turned on. Facing the client and using distinct enunciation will help lip-reading clients understand what is being said. Sometimes, deafness is mistaken for cognitive dysfunction. If a client's hearing is questionable, the nurse should enlist the help of a speech and language specialist. Generally, the pace of the interview should mirror the older adult's ability to move through the assessment. Usually, the pace will be slower than the nurse uses with younger populations.

Biologic Domain

Collecting and analyzing data for assessment of the biologic domain includes areas similar to those discussed in Chapter 10. The assessment components include present and past health status, physical examination results, physical functioning, and pharmacology review. When focussing on the biologic domain, the nurse pays special attention to the client's general physical appearance as well as any observable manifestations of illness. The nurse should assess how all physical problems affect the client's mental well-being. For example, pain and immobility are physical problems that can negatively affect mental health. Low energy level may be immediately apparent. Women with obvious osteoporosis are experiencing pain most of the time. Men undergoing radiation for prostate cancer worry about sexual functioning and urinary incontinence.

Present and Past Health Status

A review of the older adult's current health status includes examining health records and collecting information from the client and family members. The nurse must identify chronic health problems that could affect mental health care. For example, the client's management of diabetes mellitus could provide clues to the likelihood of complications such as retinopathy or neuropathy, which in turn will affect the individual's ability to follow a mental health treatment regimen. The nurse must document a history of psychiatric treatment.

Physical Examination

The psychiatric nurse reviews the physical examination findings, paying special attention to recent laboratory values, such as urinalysis, white and red blood cell counts, and fasting blood glucose data (see Chapter 9). Results of neurologic tests could indicate compromise of the neuromuscular systems. Many psychiatric medications lower the seizure threshold, making a history of seizures, which can cause behaviour changes, an important assessment component. The nurse should note any evidence of movement disorders, such as tremors, abnormal movements, or shuffling. If a client has been taking conventional antipsychotics, the nurse should consider assessment for symptoms of tardive dyskinesia, using one of the appropriate assessment tools (see Chapter 17 for additional discussion of tardive dyskinesia).

The nurse should take routine vital signs during the assessment. He or she should note any abnormalities in blood pressure (ie, hypertension or hypotension) because many psychiatric medications affect blood pressure. Generally, these medications may cause orthostatic hypotension, which can lead to dizziness, unsteady gait, and falls. A baseline blood pressure is needed for future monitoring of medication side effects. Lying, sitting, and standing blood pressures are especially useful in assessing for orthostatic hypotension.

Physical Functions

The nurse must consider the older client's physical functioning within the context of the normal changes that accompany aging and the presence of any chronic disorders. The nurse should note the client's use of any personal devices, such as canes, walkers, wheelchairs, or

BOX 28.2

Biopsychosocial Geriatric Mental Health Nursing Assessment

I. Major reason for seeking help _____

II. Initial information

   Name _____

   Age _____ Current marital status _____

   Gender _____ Caregiver's name _____

   Living arrangements _____

III. Level of independence:

   High (needs no help) _____

   Moderate (lives independently, but needs some help with instrumental activities) _____

   Low (relies on others for help in meeting functional and instrumental activities) _____

   Physical limitations _____

   Level of education completed _____

	Normal	Treated	Untreated
Physical functions: system review	☐	☐	☐
Activity/exercise	☐	☐	☐
Sleep patterns	☐	☐	☐
Appetite and nutrition	☐	☐	☐
Hydration	☐	☐	☐
Sexuality	☐	☐	☐
Existing physical illnesses	☐	☐	☐

List any chronic illnesses _____

Presence of pain (Use standardized instrument if pain is present.) No _____ Yes _____

Score _____ Treatment of pain _____

Medication (prescription and over-the-counter)	Dosage	Side Effects	Frequency of Side Effects

Significant Laboratory Tests	Values	Normal Range

BOX 28.2

Biopsychosocial Geriatric Mental Health Nursing Assessment (Continued)

IV. Responses to mental health problems

   Major concerns regarding mental health problem _____

   Major loss/change in past year: No _____ Yes _____

   Fear of violence: No _____ Yes _____

   If yes, Type of violence _____

   Strategies for managing problems/disorder _____

V. Mental status examination

   General observation (appearance, psychomotor activity, attitude) _____

   Orientation (time, place, person) _____

   Mood, affect, emotions (Geriatric Depression Scale should be used if evidence of depression)

   Speech (verbal ability, speed, use of words correctly) _____

   Thought processes (hallucinations, delusions, tangential, logic, repetition, rhyming of words, loose connections, disorganized) (*Describe content of hallucinations, delusions.*)

   Cognition and intellectual performance (*Use standardized test scores as well as observations.*)

   Attention and concentration _____

   Abstract reasoning and concentration _____

   Memory (recall, short-term, long-term) _____

   Judgment and insight _____

   (MMSE, CASI scores) _____

VI. Significant behaviours (psychomotor, agitation, aggression, withdrawn) (*Use standardized test if behaviours are problematic.*) _____

   When did problem behaviour begin? Has it gotten worse? _____

VII. Self-concept (beliefs about self—body image, self-esteem, personal identity) _____

VIII. Risk assessment

   Suicide: High _____ Moderate _____ Low _____ Assault/homicide: High _____ Low _____

   Suicide thoughts or ideation: No _____ Yes _____

   Current thoughts of harming self _____ Plan _____

   Means _____

   Means available

   Assault/homicide thoughts: No _____ Yes _____

   What do you do when angry with a stranger? _____

   What do you do when angry with family or partner? _____

   Have you ever hit or pushed anyone? No _____ Yes _____

   Have you ever been arrested for assault? No _____ Yes _____

   Current thoughts of harming others _____

IX. Functional status (*Use standardized test such as FAQ.*) _____

X. Cultural assessment

   Cultural group _____

   Cultural group's view of health and mental illness _____

   By what cultural rules do you try to live? _____

   Special, cultural foods that are important to you _____

(continued)

BOX 28.2

Biopsychosocial Geriatric Mental Health Nursing Assessment (Continued)

XI. Stresses and coping behaviours _____

    Social support _____

    Family members _____

    Which members are important to you? _____

    On whom can you rely? _____

    Community resources _____

XII. Spiritual assessment _____

XIII. Economic status _____

XIV. Legal status _____

XV. Quality of life _____

Summary of significant data that can be used in formulating a nursing diagnosis:

SIGNATURE/TITLE _____ Date _____

---

oxygen, or environmental devices, such as grab bars, shower benches, or hospital beds. Specific areas to consider are nutrition and eating, elimination, and sleep patterns.

Nutrition and Eating

Assessment of the type, amount, and frequency of food eaten is standard in any assessment of the older adult. The nurse should note any unintentional weight loss of more than 4.5 kg. He or she must consider such nutrition changes in light of mental health problems. For example, is a client's weight loss related to an underlying physical problem or to the client's belief that she is being poisoned, which makes her afraid to eat? Or, is the older adult not eating because of an active wish to die?

Eating is often difficult for older adults, who may experience a lack of appetite. The nurse must assess eating and appetite patterns because many psychiatric medications can affect digestion and may impair an already compromised gastrointestinal tract. A common problem of older individuals who live in long-term care facilities is **dysphagia**, or difficulty swallowing. Dysphagia can lead to dehydration, malnutrition, pneumonia, or asphyxiation. People who have been exposed to conventional antipsychotics (eg, haloperidol, chlorpromazine) may have symptoms of tardive dyskinesia, which can make swallowing difficult. Thus, the nurse should evaluate any client who has been exposed to the older psychiatric medications for symptoms of tardive dyskinesia.

Xerostomia, or dry mouth, which is common in older adults, also may impair eating. The nurse should pay particular attention to those who are currently receiving treatment for mental illnesses, particularly with medications that have anticholinergic properties. Dry mouth is also a side effect of many other anticholinergic medications, such as cimetidine, digoxin, and furosemide. Frequent rinsing with a non–alcohol-based mouthwash will help to correct the dry condition. Decreased taste or smell is common among older adults and may reduce the pleasure of eating so that the client may eat less. Making meal times social and relaxing experiences can help the older individual compensate for some of the loss of pleasure associated with decreased taste or smell. Preparing favourite foods will also enhance the quality of meals and meal times.

The nurse also must determine the client's use of alcohol. Alcoholism is a growing problem in the older adult population. It is estimated that 8.9% of older Canadian adults meet the criteria for alcohol abuse, and another 3.7% may abuse alcohol (Thomas & Rockwood, 2001). There is a substantially increased mortality risk for heavy drinkers and slightly reduced risk for lighter drinkers. Limited data suggest a more favourable mortality experience for drinkers of wine than for drinkers of liquor or beer (Klatsky, Friedman, Armstrong, & Kipp, 2003). The use of the CAGE questionnaire may be helpful in this area (see Appendix G).

Elimination

The nurse must assess the client's urinary and bowel functions. Older individuals are more likely to experience constipation because the peristaltic movement of the bowel slows. Medications with anticholinergic properties can cause constipation, leading to fecal impaction. Abuse of laxatives is common among older adults and requires evaluation. Although the addition of fibre is recommended for constipation, such measures may cause bloating and excessive gas production. Older clients are also more likely to experience urinary frequency because the strength of the sphincter muscle decreases. Because many older adults drink fewer fluids to manage urinary incontinence, fluid intake also becomes an important factor in assessing urinary functioning and constipation. The nurse should remember that urinary incontinence is a symptom of a disorder that requires follow-up and treatment.

Sleep

During the normal aging process, sleep patterns change, and clients often sleep less than they did when younger. The nurse must assess any recent changes in sleep patterns and evaluate whether they are related to normal aging or are symptomatic of an underlying disorder. **Insomnia**, the inability to fall or remain asleep throughout the night, can lead to increased risk for depression and regular use of sleep medications. Clients with insomnia report that they cannot sleep at night and do not feel rested in the morning. They often sleep during the day. In a large 3-year study of 10,430 women, 70 to 75 years of age, more than 60% reported difficulty sleeping and 15% reported using sleep medications (Byles, Mishra, Harris, & Nair, 2003). Sleep problems are also often linked to the use of alcohol. If an older individual reports sleep problems, the nurse should ask about his or her use of alcohol, over-the-counter medications, and prescription drugs (Box 28-3).

Pain

Older adults are more likely to experience pain than younger adults because they are at increased risk for chronic illness and may be suffering from the consequences of a lifetime of injuries. For a number of older individuals, pain is a constant companion; for instance, in 1999, 27% of home-dwelling older adults admitted to living with chronic pain (Public Health Agency of Canada, 2005b). The experience of chronic pain often contributes to unexplained behaviour and personality changes. To assess pain, the nurse can use many pain instruments. One of the most popular is the Wong-Baker Faces Pain Rating Scale, initially developed for children but now used for all age groups (Fig. 28-1). This scale is especially useful in communicating with people from different cultures and languages than the nurse's. See Chapter 32 for further discussion of pain.

Assessment of pain is especially critical for those older adults who are cognitively impaired and living in long-term care institutions. One study determined the relationship between cognitive status of older individuals and pain medication orders and administration through a retrospective medication review of residents' charts (Kaasalainen et al., 1998). The pain ratings of 25 registered nurses using a visual analogue scale were correlated with pain medications given to residents on the day of the ratings. Results indicated that the nurses' ratings of residents' pain and administration of pain medications were not significantly related. Residents with cognitive impairment were prescribed significantly fewer scheduled medications and received significantly fewer pain medications (either PRN or scheduled) than did those without cognitive impairment. The researchers theorized that nurses based their medication administration on verbal reports of pain. Because residents with cognitive impairment could not verbalize their pain, they subsequently did not receive pain medication. These results indicate that pain is underrecognized and undertreated in older adults with cognitive impairment.

BOX 28.3   RESEARCH FOR BEST PRACTICE

Alcohol, Drugs, and Key Problems in the Elderly

THE QUESTION: This research study examined the potential for additional health problems resulting from the combination of alcohol and medications in a retrospective sample of community resident elderly people with sleep complaints. Insomnia is a common complaint of older people, and they frequently use alcohol and over-the-counter or prescription medications as sedatives. The potential for adverse drug and alcohol interactions is a serious threat to health and functional status.

METHODS: A retrospective sample of community resident older individuals with sleep complaints was studied. The sample consisted of 19 people ranging in age from 65 to 88 years who reported daily alcohol consumption.

FINDINGS: The most commonly voiced reasons for seeking care were problems related to the central nervous system, including depression, anxiety, and memory loss or forgetfulness. Other problems included urinary incontinence or retention, unexplained falls, bruises, trauma, and pain. Of the 19 people, 18 (95%) were using medications that adversely interact with alcohol, and 16 (84%) of the 19 reported sleep problems, and sleep maintenance was the most common complaint.

IMPLICATIONS FOR NURSING: Nurses should ask clients aged 65 years and older who report insomnia about their use of alcohol, over-the-counter drugs, and prescription drugs. They should carefully assess older individuals for drug and alcohol interactions during the initial health history. Nurses should encourage clients to try nonpharmacologic sleep interventions first.

Tabloski, P. A., & Church, O. M. (1999). Insomnia, alcohol and drug use in community-residing elderly persons. *Journal of Substance Use,* 4(3), 147–154.

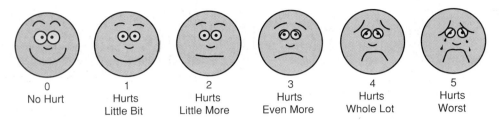

Wong-Baker FACES Pain Rating Scale

Each face represents a person who is happy or sad depending on how much or how little pain he/she has:

0   "a person who is very happy because he/she doesn't hurt at all"
1   "it hurts just a little bit"
2   "it hurts a little more"
3   "it hurts even more"
4   "it hurts a whole lot"
5   "it hurts as much as you can imagine, but you don't have to be crying to feel this bad"

Subject ID #:_____ Date:___/___/___ Visit #_____

Client name: _____

RA:_____

FIGURE 28-1   Wong-Baker FACES Pain Rating Scale.

Pharmacologic Assessment

One of the most important areas of the biologic domain is the pharmacologic assessment. **Polypharmacy**, the concurrent use of several different medications, is common in older individuals. The nurse must ask the client and family to list all medications and times that the client takes them. Asking family members to bring in all the medications the client is taking, including over-the-counter medications, vitamins, and herbal supplements, is a good idea. Because older adults are more sensitive than younger people to medications, the possibility of drug–drug interactions is greater. When considering potential drug interactions, the nurse should ask the older individual about his or her consumption of grapefruit juice, which contains narginin, a compound that inhibits the CYP3A4 enzyme involved in the metabolism of many medications (eg, antidepressants, antiarrhythmics, erythromycin, and several statins).

Psychological Domain

Assessment of the psychological domain provides the nurse with the opportunity to identify limitations, behaviour symptoms, and reactions to illness. The nurse assesses many of the same areas as in other adult assessments, but again, the emphasis may be different. The following discussion focuses on the responses of older adults to mental health problems, mental status examination, behaviour changes, stress and coping patterns, and risk assessments.

Responses to Mental Health Problems

Many older clients are reluctant to admit that they have psychiatric symptoms, particularly if their culture stigmatizes mental illness, and may deny having mental or emotional problems. They may also fear that if they admit to any symptoms, they may be placed outside their home. If clients do not recognize or admit to having psychiatric symptoms, their vulnerability to being taken advantage of or injured increases.

Throughout the assessment, the nurse evaluates the client's verbal reports, obvious symptoms, and family reports. If a client flatly denies any psychiatric symptoms (eg, depression, mood swings, outbursts of anger, memory problems), the nurse should respectfully accept the older adult's answer and avoid arguments or confrontation (Box 28-4). If the client's family members contradict the client's report or symptoms are obvious during the interview, the nurse can approach the issue while planning care. Nurses may need to use conflict resolution strategies in helping families and clients obtain appropriate care despite disagreement about symptoms experienced by the older adults.

Mental Status Examination

The areas of special interest in the mental status examination are mood and affect, thought processes, and cognitive functioning. The nurse should interpret the results in light of any accompanying physical problems, such as chronic pain, or life changes, such as loss of a spouse.

BOX 28.4

Therapeutic Dialogue: Assessment Interview

Tom, 79 years old, is being seen for the first time in a geriatric mental health clinic because of recent changes in his behaviour and his accusations that family members are trying to steal his house and car. He locked his wife out of the house, accusing her of being unfaithful. When Susan, the psychiatric nurse assigned to his case, is conducting the assessment interview, Tom cooperates and is very pleasant until the nurse begins to assess the psychological domain.

Ineffective Approach

Nurse: Have there been times when you have had problems with any members of your family?
Patient: No. (Silence)
Nurse: Have you noticed that lately you have been getting more upset than usual?
Patient: No. Who has been talking to you?
Nurse: Your wife seems to think that you may be getting a little more upset than usual.
Patient: You are just like her. She keeps telling me something is wrong with me. (Getting very agitated)
Nurse: Please, I'm trying to help you. I understand that you locked your wife out of the house last week.
Patient: Leave me alone. (Gets up and leaves)

Effective Approach:

Nurse: How have things been going at home?
Patient: All right.
Nurse: (Silence)
Patient: Well, my wife and I sometimes argue.

Nurse: Oh. Most husbands and wives argue. Any special arguments?
Patient: No. Just the usual. I don't pick up after myself enough. I don't dress right to suit her. But, lately, she's gone a lot.
Nurse: She is gone a lot?
Patient: Yeah! A lot.
Nurse: The way you say that, it sounds like you have some feelings about her being gone.
Patient: You're damned right I do—and you would, too.
Nurse: I'm missing something.
Patient: Well, if you must know, I think she's having an affair with the man next door.
Nurse: Really? That must upset you to think your wife is having an affair.
Patient: I am devastated. I feel so bad.
Nurse: Would you say that you are depressed?
Patient: Well, wouldn't you be? Yes, I'm feeling pretty low.

Critical Thinking Challenge

- How do the very first questions differ in the two interviews?
- What therapeutic techniques did the nurse use in the second interview to avoid the pitfalls the nurse encountered in the first scenario?
- How did the nurse in the second scenario elicit the client's delusion about his wife's affair?
- From the data that the second nurse gathered, how many of the client's problems can be identified?

Mood and Affect

Depression in older adults is common and associated with the following risk factors: loss of spouse, physical illness, education below high school, impaired functional status, and heavy alcohol consumption. In older people, other disorders may mask depression. When symptoms are present, they may be attributed to normal aging or atherosclerosis or other age-related problems. Older clients are less likely to report feeling sad or worthless than are younger patients. As a result, family members and primary care providers often overlook depression in older adults.

Depressive symptoms are much more common than a full-fledged depressive disorder, as characterized by the *Diagnostic and Statistical Manual of Mental Disorders* (APA, 2000). Between 10% to 15% of older adults living in the community experience depressive symptoms (Conn, 2002). Approximately 50% of older adults living in long-term care facilities show signs of depression (Canadian Coalition for Seniors Mental Health, 2003). Research suggests that untreated depression in older adults may result in overuse of health care services, longer hospital stays, decreased treatment compliance, and increased morbidity and mortality (Conn, 2002). The Geriatric Depression Scale (GDS) is a useful screening tool with demonstrated validity and reliability

(Hyer & Blount, 1984). The GDS was designed as a self-administered test, although it also has been used in observer-administered formats. One advantage of the test is its "yes/no" format, which may be easier for older adults than the Hamilton Rating Scale for Depression (HAM-D), which uses a scale from 0 to 4 (see Chapter 19). This tool is easy to administer and provides valuable information about the possibility of depression (Box 28-5). If results are positive, the nurse should refer the client to a psychiatrist or advanced practice nurse for further evaluation.

Among residents in long-term care facilities, the usefulness of the GDS depends on the degree of cognitive impairment. Residents who are mildly impaired may be able to answer yes/no questions; however, moderately to severely impaired older adults will be unable to do the same. The best validated scale for individuals with dementia is the Cornell Scale for Depression in Dementia (CSDD) (Alexopoulos et al., 1998). The CSDD is an interview-administered scale that uses information both from the client and an outside informant.

Anxiety is another important mood for nurses to assess in older adults because it can interfere with normal functioning. In dementia, anxiety is common (Lopez et al., 2003). The Rating Anxiety in Dementia (RAID) scale was developed as a global scale to assess anxiety in

BOX 28.5 RESEARCH FOR BEST PRACTICE

Geriatric Depression Scale (Short Form)

1. Are you basically satisfied with your life?	Yes	No
2. Have you dropped many of your activities and interests?	Yes	No
3. Do you feel that your life is empty?	Yes	No
4. Do you often get bored?	Yes	No
5. Are you in good spirits most of the time?	Yes	No
6. Are you afraid that something bad is going to happen to you?	Yes	No
7. Do you feel happy most of the time?	Yes	No
8. Do you often feel helpless?	Yes	No
9. Do you prefer to stay at home rather than go out and do new things?	Yes	No
10. Do you feel you have more problems with memory than most?	Yes	No
11. Do you think it is wonderful to be alive now?	Yes	No
12. Do you feel pretty worthless the way you are now?	Yes	No
13. Do you feel full of energy?	Yes	No
14. Do you feel that your situation is hopeless?	Yes	No
15. Do you think that most people are better off than you are?	Yes	No

Score: ____/15 One point for "No" to questions 1, 5, 7, 11, 13

One point for "Yes" to other questions

Normal	3 ± 2
Mildly depressed	7 ± 3
Very depressed	12 ± 2

Adapted from Sheikh, J. I., & Yesavage, J. A. (1986). Geriatric Depression Scale (GDS): Recent evidence and development of a shorter version. In T. L. Brink (Ed.), *Clinical gerontology: A guide to assessment and intervention* (pp. 165–173). Binghamton, NY: Haworth Press. © By the Haworth Press, Inc. All rights reserved. Reprinted with permission.

clients with dementia (Shankar, Walker, Frost, & Orrell, 1999). The domains that the RAID scale assesses include worry, apprehension and vigilance, motor tension, autonomic hyperactivity, and phobias and panic attacks.

Thought Processes

Thought processes and content are critical in the assessment of older adults. Can the client express ideas and thoughts logically? Can the client understand questions and follow the conversation of others? If the older adult shows any indication of hallucinations or delusions, the nurse should explore the content of the hallucination or delusion. If the client has a history of mental illness, such as schizophrenia, these symptoms may be familiar to family members, who can validate whether they are old or new problems. If this is the first time the client has experienced these abnormal thought processes, the nurse should further evaluate the content. Suspicious and delusional thoughts that characterize dementia often include some of the following beliefs:

- People are stealing my things.
- This house is not my house.
- My relative is an impostor.

If a client shares any such thoughts, the nurse can complete further assessment by using the Behavioural Pathology in Alzheimer's Disease rating scale (BEHAVE-AD). This 25-item scale is based on caregivers' reports within the previous 2 weeks (Reisberg & Ferris, 1985). The BEHAVE-AD measures thought and behaviour disturbances in seven major categories, with each item scored on a four-point scale of severity (0 to 3), including delusions, hallucinations, activity disturbances, aggressiveness, diurnal rhythm disturbances, mood disturbances, and anxieties and phobias. The BEHAVE-AD also contains a four-point global assessment of the overall magnitude of the behaviour symptoms in terms of disturbance to the caregiver, dangerousness to the client, or both. The reliability of the BEHAVE-AD (0.95 and 0.96; $p < 0.01$) is comparable to that of the Mini-Mental State Examination (Reisberg, Auer, & Monteiro, 1996).

Cognition and Intellectual Performance

Cognitive functioning includes such parameters as orientation, attention, short- and long-term memory, consciousness, and executive functioning. Intellectual functioning, also considered a cognitive measure, is rarely formally assessed with a standardized intelligence test in older adults. Considerable variability among individuals depends on lifestyle and psychosocial factors. Some changes in cognitive capacity accompany aging, but important functions are spared. Normal cognitive changes during aging include a slowing of information processing and memory retrieval. Abnormalities of consciousness, orientation, judgment, speech, or language are not related to age but to underlying neuropathologic changes. Cognitive changes in older adults are associated with delirium or dementia (see Chapter 30) or with schizophrenia (see Chapter 17).

The assessment includes the number of years of education. An inverse relationship between Alzheimer disease and the number of years of education exists. When

BOX 28.6

Cognitive Status: Documentation Versus Standardized Assessments

THE QUESTION: How does standard nursing documentation compare with standard assessment tests in identifying problems of cognitive function in older adults? Although the literature discusses the importance of assessing cognitive status, few studies have explored the concordance of nurses' documentation of cognitive status and standardized assessment.

METHODS: This study examined nurses' documentation of cognitive status in 42 medically hospitalized individuals (mean age, 51.9 years; SD, 10.1 years) using various standardized measures.

FINDINGS: Although the chart review revealed no documentation of impaired cognitive status, it identified impaired performance in 24% to 67% of the cognitive measures.

IMPLICATIONS FOR NURSING: This study suggests nurses are missing cognitive impairment in hospitalized individuals by limiting assessment of orientation. Use of a combination of several brief screening measures, such as the clock-drawing test and the standardized Mini-Mental State Examination (MMSE), would provide timely, effective, and inexpensive assessment of cognitive status (abstract). This article supports the use of standardized instruments in assessing cognitive status.

Souder, E., & O'Sullivan, P. S. (2000). Nursing documentation versus standardized assessment of cognitive status in hospitalized medical patients. *Applying Nursing Research, 13*(1), 29–36.

assessing cognitive functioning, the nurse should use standardized instruments and not rely on observations or chart documentation (Box 28-6) (Souder & O'Sullivan, 2000). Of such instruments, the Mini-Mental State Examination (MMSE), discussed in Chapter 10, is most widely used in screening for cognitive functioning related to dementia. Various studies suggest that an MMSE score below 24 of 30 has a reasonable sensitivity (80% to 90%) and specificity (80%) for discriminating between those with dementia and those without. However, some data suggest that the MMSE may have a built-in bias against those with fewer than 8 years of education or among those who belong to ethnic minority groups (Mulgrew et al., 1999).

Evidence suggests that severe cognitive deterioration may occur in older individuals with schizophrenia. In assessing the cognitive status of this population, the Cognitive Abilities Screening Instrument (CASI) demonstrates greater specificity than does the MMSE (Sherrell, Buckwalter, Bode, & Strozdas, 1999). The CASI is a 25-item instrument test developed as a research instrument and piloted in Japan and the United States (Teng et al., 1994). The total score ranges from 0 (poor) to 100 (good), with a suggested cutoff of 74 for classifying dementia. The CASI provides quantitative assessment of nine domains: attention, concentration, orientation, long-term memory, short-term memory, language, visual construction (copying pentagons), fluency (naming four-legged animals), and abstraction and judgment. Because it determines the level of cognitive impairment, the CASI could be used in establishing individualized care plans.

Behaviour Changes

Behaviour changes in older adults can indicate neuropathologic processes and thus require nursing assessment. If such changes occur, it is most likely that family members will notice them before the client does. Apraxia (inability to execute a voluntary movement despite normal muscle function) is not attributed to age but indicates an underlying disease process, such as Alzheimer disease, Parkinson's disease, or other disorders. Various other behaviour problems are associated with psychiatric disorders in older individuals, including irritability, agitation, apathy, and euphoria. Other behaviours in older adults who are experiencing psychiatric problems include wandering and aggressive behaviours. The BEHAVE-AD identifies these behaviours

The Neuropsychiatric Inventory (NPI) was developed in 1994 to assess behaviour problems associated with dementia. The scale assesses 10 behaviour problems: delusions, hallucinations, dysphoria, anxiety, agitation/aggression, euphoria, inhibition, irritability/lability, apathy, and aberrant motor behaviour (Cummings et al., 1994). This very popular tool is used in many medication clinical trials. There are two versions. The standard version is used when the client is still at home, whereas a different version is used when the client is in a long-term care facility.

Stress and Coping Patterns

Identifying stresses and coping patterns is just as important for older individuals as it is for younger adults. Unique stresses for older clients include living on a fixed income, handling declining health, losing partners and friends, and ultimately confronting death. Coping ability varies, depending on clients' unique circumstances. For example, some older adults respond to stressful events with amazing adaptability, whereas others become depressed and suicidal.

Loss of a spouse is common in late life, especially for women. For instance, in 1998, one million older women were widowed, compared with 208,000 older men (National Advisory Council on Aging, 1998). Bereavement, a natural response to the death of a loved one, includes crying and sorrow, anxiety and agitation, insomnia, and loss of appetite. These symptoms, while overlapping with those of major depression, do not constitute a mental disorder. Only when these symptoms persist for 2 months or longer can a diagnosis of either adjustment disorder or major depressive disorder be made (APA, 2000). Although bereavement is a normal response, the nurse must identify it and develop interventions to help the individual successfully resolve the loss. Bereavement is an important and well-established risk factor for depression. Factors such as previous mental or physical health conditions in the surviving spouse, high levels of caregiver strain before the death of the spouse, and a lack of social support increase the likelihood of depression post bereavement (Schum, Lyness, & King, 2005).

Risk Assessment

Suicide is a major mental health risk for older adults. Men 80 years of age and older have the highest suicide rate of all age groupings (58.4 per 100,000) (Health Canada, 2002b). Most older individuals who commit suicide have visited their family physician within the month of their death (Juurlink, Herrmann, Szalai, Kopp, & Redelmeier, 2004).

When caring for the older client with mental health problems, the nurse always should consider the individual's potential to commit suicide. Depression is the greatest risk factor for suicide. In assessing an older client, the nurse should consider the following characteristics as indications of high risk for committing suicide:

- Depression
- Attempted suicide in the past
- Family history of suicide
- Firearms in the home
- Abuse of alcohol or other substances
- Unusual stress
- Chronic medical condition (eg, cancer, neuromuscular disorders)
- Social isolation

CRNE ALERT

Suicide assessment is a priority for the older adult experiencing mental health problems. It is important to carefully assess recent behaviour changes and loss of support.

Social Domain

Assessment of the social domain includes determining the client's interactions with others in his or her family and community. The nurse targets social support because it is so important to the well-being of older adults, functional status because of the potential physical changes that can affect this area, and social systems, which encompasses all community resources.

Social Support

Remaining active throughout one's life is one of the best predictors of mental health and wellness in an older individual. People obtain their sense of self-worth through their interactions with others in their environment. A sense of "who one is" is closely tied to the roles that a person plays in life. When older adults relinquish such roles because of physical disabilities, become isolated from friends and family, or begin to sense that they are a burden to those around them, rather than contributing members of society, a sense of hopelessness and helplessness often follows.

The role of social support is critical to assess in this age group. Social support is a reciprocal concept, meaning that simply receiving assistance increases the person's sense of being a burden. Those older individuals who also believe that they contribute to the welfare of others are most likely to remain mentally healthy. For this reason, pets are often "life savers" for older adults who live alone. Nothing can be more understanding and accepting of an older adult's behaviour or disabilities than a beloved pet.

The nurse should assess the client's number of formal and informal social contacts. The nurse should ask about the frequency of contacts with others (in person and through telephone calls, letters, and cards) that the older adult has. Determining whether these contacts are actually satisfying and supporting to the patient is essential. If family members are important to the client's well-being, the nurse should complete a more in-depth family assessment (see Chapter 16).

The nurse can use the following questions to focus on social support (Kane, 1995):

- In the past 2 weeks, how often would you say that others let you know that they care about you?
- In the past 2 weeks, how often has someone provided you with help, such as giving you a ride somewhere or helping around the house?
- Do you have any one special person you could call or contact if you needed help? Who?
- In general, other than your children, how many relatives do you feel close to and have contact with at least once a month?

For older clients who are isolated with few social contacts, the nurse can develop interventions to improve social support.

Functional Status

As part of a complete assessment, the nurse will need to assess the older adult's functional status. **Functional**

activities or activities of daily living (ADLs) are the activities necessary for self-care (ie, bathing, toileting, dressing, and transferring). **Instrumental activities** of daily living (IADLs) include those that facilitate or enhance the performance of ADLs (ie, shopping, using the telephone, using transportation). These aspects are critical to consider for any older adult living alone. When possible, the older adult should be observed for his or her ability to complete ADLs, rather than relying on self-report or report of the family. The most common tools used to assess functional status are the Index of Independence in Activities of Daily Living and the Instrumental Activities of Daily Living Scale (Katz & Akpom, 1976). The Functional Activities Questionnaire (FAQ) measures an adult's functional abilities based on information from family members and caregivers. The older person is rated on 10 complex, higher-order activities, such as writing checks, assembling tax records, and driving (Costa et al., 1996).

Social Systems

Community resources are essential to an older adult's ability to maintain mental health and wellness, as well as to his or her ability to remain at home throughout the later years. Senior centres are federally or provincially funded community resources that provide a wide array of services to Canada's older population. They may provide daily balanced meals at a nominal cost. In addition, they provide opportunities for socialization, which is key to combating loneliness and social isolation. Many senior centres provide annual influenza and pneumonia vaccination clinics and education on such topics as fall prevention and recognition and prevention of elder abuse. Additional community resources that are specific to older individuals include geriatric assessment clinics and adult day programs.

During the assessment, the nurse must determine which community resources are available and if the older client uses them. Lack of transportation to and from these community resources may be a barrier to use. Most communities have buses available for older or handicapped individuals. The nurse may need to assist the older adult in accessing this important resource.

One in five older adults in Canada is classified as living in a low-income situation (Public Health Agency of Canada, 2005c). A number of older adults rely on Canada Pension Plan (CPP), Old Age Security (OAS), and Guaranteed Income Supplement (GIS) for their monthly income. For these older individuals, this financial support, although less than adequate in most instances, is their only source of income. The nurse should assess a client's sources of financial support. Sometimes, nurses are uncomfortable asking for financial information, fearing that they are invading the client's privacy. However, such data are important for the nurse to determine whether an older individual's resources adequately meet his or her needs. The source of financial support is also important. For example, a client whose income is adequate and comes from personal resources is more likely to be independent than is a client who depends on family members for income.

The nurse should ask the client about accessible health care facilities, formal supports such as physicians, nurses, and other health care professionals and about the client's ability to pay for medications and health aids. Information about available health care resources beyond standard provincial health care (eg, plans to pay for additional services such as medications or foot care) will alert the nurse to what services the client currently can and cannot access. In urban areas that are likely to have adequate health care resources, cultural and language barriers may prohibit access. People who live in rural areas where health care resources are limited are less likely to enjoy the full range of health care resources than are those in urban areas. For instance, older adults in Canadian rural settings have greater difficulty accessing geriatric mental health services than those in urban sites (Conn, 2003). Even in centres with geriatric mental health services, however, many older adults are reluctant to access services because of lack of awareness of available help, stigma, or cultural issues (Sadavoy, Meier, & Ong, 2004).

Spiritual Assessment

Spiritual needs are basic for all age groups and are requirements for establishing meaning and purpose, love and relatedness, and forgiveness. Spirituality is sometimes expressed through commitment to organized religion and, other times, is expressed differently. Aging is a process that can bring individuals closer to understanding the finite nature of existence and evokes an awareness of their spiritual needs. With advanced age, many people begin to reflect on their successes and failures. During such reflection, many seek out God or a higher being to make sense of the past and establish hope for the future.

The process of spiritual assessment involves active listening, thoughtful observing, and sensitive questioning. The nurse may simply ask if the older adult would find comfort from a visit from a minister or a spiritual leader. Many forms of religion use various rituals that are important to the older individual's daily routine. The nurse should explore and honour these aspects to the extent possible.

Legal Status

A growing trend in Canada and the United States is to view older adults as a special population whose rights deserve increased attention. Instances of elder abuse are far too common. Every nurse must consider himself or herself a patient advocate and be vigilant in recognizing the signs of neglect or abuse, such as unexplained injuries. At times, abuse can take the form of another individual (sometimes an adult child) usurping the rights of the older person. Unless the older person is determined to be incompetent, he or she has the same rights to personal decision making as any other adult, including the right to refuse treatment.

Quality of Life

Sense of quality of life is closely tied to values and beliefs. For many older individuals, quality of life is not reflected in material possessions or physical health. At this stage, quality of life is connected more with contentment over how the person has lived life and the extent to which his or her life has had meaning and purpose. Keeping close personal contacts with friends and family and having the opportunity to share stories of lifetime experiences are essential to maintaining mental health and wellness for older adults. For older individuals, physical illnesses may affect the quality of life more than psychiatric disorders. The assessment of quality of life becomes especially important when assessing a client living in a long-term care facility or isolated in his or her own home. The assessment of quality of life of older adults is similar to that for younger adults (see Chapter 10).

SUMMARY OF KEY POINTS

- Normal aging is associated with some physical decline, but most functions do not change. Intellectual functioning, capacity for change, and productive engagement with life remain stable.
- Mental health assessments are necessary when older clients face psychiatric or mental health issues. The biopsychosocial geriatric mental health nursing assessment examines many sources of data, including self-reports, laboratory test results, and reports from family members.
- The biopsychosocial geriatric mental health nursing assessment is based on the special needs and problems of older individuals. This assessment examines current and past health, functional status, and human responses to mental health problems.
- Assessment of the biologic domain involves collecting data about past and present health status, physical examination findings, physical functions (ie, nutrition and eating, elimination patterns, sleep), pain, and pharmacologic information.
- Assessment of the psychological domain includes the client's responses to mental health problems, mental status examination, behavioural changes, stress and coping patterns, and risk assessment.

- When conducting an assessment, the nurse may find several tools useful. For clients with possible depression, the Geriatric Depression Scale (GDS) may be helpful. For clients with anxiety, nurses can use the Rating Anxiety in Dementia (RAID) scale. In addition to a careful interview, the nurse can use the Behavioural Pathology in Alzheimer's Disease (BEHAVE-AD) scale to determine delusions, hallucinations, activity disturbances, aggressiveness, diurnal rhythm disturbances, mood disturbances, anxieties, or phobias.
- The nurse can conduct cognitive assessments using the Mini-Mental State Examination (MMSE) or the Cognitive Abilities Screening Instrument (CASI).
- Coping with the stresses of aging varies among clients. Determining stresses and coping skills for dealing with stresses is important.
- Social support is critical to clients in this age group and requires assessment.
- Determination of the client's ability to perform functional and instrumental activities of daily living is critical in the assessment of older adults. The Functional Activities Questionnaire (FAQ) measures the functional abilities based on information from others.
- Social systems, spiritual assessment, legal information, and quality of life are components within the social domain that the nurse should consider.

CRITICAL THINKING CHALLENGES

1 The director of your church's senior centre has asked you to be the guest speaker at the monthly meeting of the Retired Active Citizens group. The subject is to be "Maintaining Your Mental Health After Retirement." What key points will you touch on in your presentation? What activities or handouts will you use to highlight your talk?

2 When asking about current illnesses, a client begins telling you her whole life story. What approach would you take to elicit the most important information needed to develop an individualized plan of care for your older client?

3 A caregiver tells you that her mother has become suspicious of the neighbours and other family members. How would you assess this perceptual experience? What other data should you gather from this client?

4 A caregiver brings a bag of medications to the client's assessment interview. What information should you obtain from the caregiver regarding the older individual's use of these medications?

5 A woman brings her father, who has a long history of frequent psychiatric hospitalizations for depression,

to the clinic. The client's wife recently died, and the daughter fears that her father is becoming depressed again. What approach would you use in assessing for changes in mood?

6 Obtain a listing of the social services available in your community. Examine the list for areas of duplication and omission of services needed by an older adult living alone in his or her own home.

WEB LINKS

www.alzheimer.ca   The Alzheimer Society of Canada website includes information about the Society, Alzheimer Disease (AD), how to care for someone with AD, and research updates.

www.canada.gc.ca   The Government of Canada website provides information on government financial plans for older adults (e.g., Canada Pension Plan).

www.ccsmh.ca   The Canadian Coalition for Seniors Mental Health (CCSMH) website explains the mission of this organization and offers resources for education, assessment, and treatment for older adults living with mental illness.

www.cmhc-schl.gc.ca   The Canada Mortgage and Housing Corporation (CMHC) website provides information about how older adults can adapt their homes for increasing disabilities and financial assistance programs for housing for older adults.

MOVIES

On Golden Pond: 1981. In this classic film, Henry Fonda portrays a crotchety, retired professor named Norman Thayer. Norman is angry that he is 80 years old and scared that he may lose his cognitive abilities. His wife, played by Katherine Hepburn, provides support and encouragement in maintaining his independence. The story revolves around Norman's relationship with his estranged daughter (played by Jane Fonda) as they try finally to understand each other during Norman's later years.

VIEWING POINTS: Identify the physical impairments that are obvious throughout the movie. Identify specific memory problems that Norman experiences. Are these problems part of normal aging? If you were Norman Thayer's nurse, what key assessment areas would you explore?

REFERENCES

Alexopoulos, G. S., Abrams, R. C., Young, R. C., et al. (1998). Cornell Scale for Depression in Dementia. *Biological Psychiatry, 23,* 271–284.

American Psychiatric Association (APA). (2000). *Diagnostic and statistical manual of mental disorders* (4th ed., Text revision). Washington, DC: Author.

Byles, J. E., Mishra, G. D., Harris, M. A., & Nair, K. (2003). The problems of sleep for older women: Changes in health outcomes. *Age and Ageing, 32*(2), 123–124.

Canadian Coalition for Seniors Mental Health. (2003). Depression fought in seniors. *Canadian Coalition for Seniors Mental Health, 1*(4), 2.

Conn, D. K. (2003). Oral presentation to the Standing Senate Committee on Social Affairs, Science and Technology. *Bulletin of the Canadian Academy of Geriatric Psychiatry, 10*(3), 5–8.

Conn, D. K. (2002). An overview of common mental disorders among seniors. *National Advisory Council on Aging, Writing in Gerontology, Mental Health and Aging.* Minister of Public Works and Government Services Canada.

Costa, P. T., Williams, R. F., Somerfield, M., et al. (1996). *Recognition and initial assessment of Alzheimer's disease and related dementias.* No. 19, AHCPR Publication No. 97-0703. Rockville, MD: U.S. Department of Health and Human Services, Public Health Service, Agency for Health Care Policy and Research.

Cummings, J. L., Mega, M., Gray, K., et al. (1994). The Neuropsychiatric Inventory: Comprehensive assessment of psychopathology in dementia. *Neurology, 44*(12), 2308–2314.

Health Canada. (2002a). *Canada's aging population.* Minister of Public Works and Government Services Canada.

Health Canada. (2002b). *A report on mental illness in Canada.* Ottawa: Health Canada.

Hyer, L., & Blount, J. (1984). Concurrent and discriminant validities of the geriatric depression scale with older psychiatric inpatients. *Psychological Reports, 54,* 611–616.

Juurlink, D. N., Herrmann, N., Szalai, J. P., Kopp, A., & Redelmeier, D. A. (2004). Medical illness and the risk of suicide in the elderly. *Archives of Internal Medicine, 164*(11), 1179–1184.

Kaasalainen, S., Middleton, J., Knezacek, S., et al. (1998). Pain and cognitive status in the institutionalized elderly: Perceptions and interventions. *Journal of Gerontological Nursing, 24*(8), 24–31, 50–51.

Kane, R. A. (1995). Assessment of social functioning: Recommendations for comprehensive geriatric assessment. In Z. Rubenstein, D. Wieland, & R. Bernabei (Eds.), *Geriatric assessment technology: The state of the art* (pp. 91–110). New York: Springer.

Katz, S., & Akpom, A. (1976). A measure of primary sociobiological functions. *International Journal of Health Science, 6,* 493.

Klatsky, A. L., Friedman, G. D., Armstrong, M. A., & Kipp, H. (2003). Wine, liquor, beer, and mortality. *American Journal of Epidemiology, 158*(6), 585–595.

Lopez, O. L., Becker, J. T., Sweet, R. A., Klunk, W., Kaufer, D. I., Saxton, J., Habeych, M., & Dekosky, S. T. (2003). Psychiatric symptoms vary with the severity of dementia in probable Alzheimer's disease. *Journal of Neuropsychiatry and Clinical Neuroscience, 15*(3), 346–353.

Mulgrew, C., Morgenstern, N., Shetterly, S., et al. (1999). Cognitive functioning and impairment among rural elderly Hispanics and non-Hispanic whites as assessed by the Mini-Mental State Examination. *Journal of Gerontology, 54B*(4), 223–230.

National Advisory Council on Aging. (1998). Bereavement: A life passage. *Newsletter of the National Advisory Council on Aging, 12*(1), 2–8.

Public Health Agency of Canada. (2005a). *A growing population: Statistical snapshot #1.* Statistics Canada. Retrieved July 25, 2005, from http://www.phac.aspc.gc.ca/seniors-aines.

Public Health Agency of Canada. (2005b). *Seniors experiencing chronic pain: Statistical snapshot # 34.* Statistics Canada. Retrieved July 25, 2005, from http://www.phac.aspc.gc.ca/seniors-aines.

Public Health Agency of Canada. (2005c). *Low income across the country: Statistical snapshot #18.* Statistics Canada. Retrieved July 25, 2005, from http://www.phac.aspc.gc.ca/seniors-aines.

Rabheru, K. (2004). Special issues in the management of depression in older patients. *Canadian Journal of Psychiatry, 49*(Suppl 1), 41S–50S.

Reisberg, B., & Ferris, S. (1985). A clinical rating scale for symptoms of psychosis in Alzheimer's disease. *Psychopharmacology Bulletin, 21,* 101–104.

Reisberg, B., Auer, S., & Monteiro, I. (1996). Behavioural Pathology in Alzheimer's Disease (BEHAVE-AD) rating scale. *International Psychogeriatrics, 8*(3), 301–308.

Sadavoy, J., Meier, R., & Ong, A. Y. M. (2004). Barriers to access to mental health services for ethnic seniors: The Toronto study. *Canadian Journal of Psychiatry, 49*(3), 192–199.

SAGMHS (Southern Alberta Geriatric Mental Health Working Group). (2003, Sept.). *Summary Report of the Southern Alberta Geriatric Mental Health Working Group,* 1–12.

Schum, J. L., Lyness, J. M., & King, D. A. (2005). Bereavement in late life: Risk factors for complicated bereavement. *Geriatrics, 60*(4), 18–20, 24.

Shankar, K. K., Walker, M., Frost, D., & Orrell, M. W. (1999). The development of a valid and reliable scale for rating anxiety in dementia (RAID). *Aging & Mental Health, 3*(1), 39–49.

Sheikh, J. I., & Yesavage, J. A. (1986). Geriatric Depression Scale (GDS): Recent evidence and development of a shorter version. In T. L. Brink (Ed.), *Clinical gerontology: A guide to assessment and interventions* (pp. 165–177). Binghamton, NY: Haworth Press.

Sherrell, K., Buckwalter, K., Bode, R., & Strozdas, L. (1999). Use of the Cognitive Abilities Screen Instrument to assess elderly persons with schizophrenia in long-term care settings. *Issues in Mental Health Nursing, 20,* 541–558.

Souder, E., & O'Sullivan, P. S. (2000). Nursing documentation versus standardized assessment of cognitive status in hospitalized medical patients. *Applying Nursing Research, 13*(1), 29–36.

Statistics Canada. (2005). Life expectancy at birth, by sex, by provinces. Retrieved June 06, 2005, from http://www.40.statcan.ca/101/cst01/health26.htm.

Tabloski, P. A., & Church, O. M. (1999). Insomnia, alcohol and drug use in community-residing elderly persons. *Journal of Substance Use, 4*(3), 147–154.

Teng, E., Kazuo Hasegawa, K., Homma, A., et al. (1994). The Cognitive Abilities Screen Instrument (CASI): A practical test for cross-cultural epidemiological studies of dementia. *International Psychogeriatrics, 6*(1), 45–58.

Thomas, V. S., & Rockwood, K. J. (2001). Alcohol abuse, cognitive impairment, and mortality among older people. *Journal of the American Geriatrics Society, 49*(4), 415–420.

For challenges, please refer to the **CD-ROM** in this book.

29

Mental Health Promotion With the Older Adult

Mary Ann Boyd and Sharon Moore

LEARNING OBJECTIVES

After studying this chapter, you will be able to:

- Identify important biopsychosocial factors occurring in late adulthood.
- Identify risk factors related to geriatric psychopathology.
- Analyze the nurse's role in mental health promotion with elders and their families.
- Discuss mental health prevention and promotion interventions that are especially effective with older patients.

KEY TERMS

gerotranscendence middle-old ▪ old-old ▪ self-care ▪ young-old

⬟ KEY CONCEPT

late adulthood

Canada, like many other countries, is experiencing a boom in population growth of seniors. At the turn of the 21st century, nearly 4 million of the 30 million Canadians were older adults. Statistics Canada estimates this number will grow to 5.7 million by the year 2016 and will double to more than 8 million by the year 2031(NACA, 2003; Statistics Canada, 2001, 2003). The National Advisory Council on Aging (NACA) reports that seniors are the fastest growing age group in the country.

Mental health concerns among older adults are a significant problem in Canada. With the increase in aging population, there is a concomitant increase in the number of older persons with psychiatric disorders. The Southern Alberta Geriatric Mental Health Working Group reported 15% to 30% prevalence rates in the community, whereas the Canadian Coalition for Seniors Mental Health reported a 50% to 80% prevalence rate for mental disorders within nursing homes and long-term care settings in Canada. Further, older adults (men, in particular) compose a significant risk group for suicide, with men older than 80 years having the highest rate of suicide in Canada (Conn, 2003). "These disorders can substantially impair functioning and can result in unnecessary hospitalizations and nursing home placement, poorer health outcomes, and increased rates of mortality. For example, older persons who suffer from depression have worse outcomes after medical events such as hip fractures, heart attacks, or cancer, and individuals who are age 75 and older have the highest suicide rate of any age group" (NAMI, 2001, p. 1). It is well documented that, for older persons, it takes less alcohol to exacerbate medical and mental problems, and, in turn, medical and emotional problems may contribute to further alcohol use (Sattar, Petty, & Burke, 2003). It is important for nurses to understand and respond well to the unique needs of this special population.

MENTAL HEALTH OF THE OLDER ADULT

This chapter explains the effect of aging on mental health and identifies risk factors related to geriatric psychopathology.

> ■ **KEY CONCEPT Late adulthood** can be divided into three chronologic groups: **young-old** (ages 65 to 74 years), **middle-old** (ages 75 to 84 years), and **old-old** (age 85 years and older).

People 85 years and older are the most rapidly growing segment of the Canadian population. From 1921 until 1998, the population of oldest old (those over age 85) has increased 20 times. It is estimated that by 2041, the numbers in this age group will jump to 1.6 million (Lindsay & Almay, 1999). The transition from young-old to old-old is more than a series of birthdays; it is a gradual biopsychosocial process that may be viewed as both positive and negative. From a positive perspective, the later years provide time for personal growth and development, providing an opportunity to do all the things that were impossible when work and family responsibilities took precedence. Travelling, visiting friends, and engaging in neglected hobbies enhance quality of life and improve well-being.

In late adulthood, changes in health status can lead to negative outcomes. A loss in physical functioning can lead to a loss in independence, which can result in an unplanned change in residence. Family relationships change, as once-dependent children grow into adulthood and become parents themselves. Friendships change, and losses occur. Many elders retire from meaningful lifelong work and are faced with establishing new meaning in life. To have a sense of meaning and purpose is a critical factor in older persons' mental health and is one of the factors that serves as a protection against suicide and despair in later life (Moore, 1997; Moore, Metcalf, & Schow, 2000).

In all health care settings, communication is an integral factor in nursing care. Communication with older persons requires special attention to verbal interactions and environmental influences. Box 29-1 highlights some of the necessary considerations.

BOX 29.1

Communicating With Older Adults

- Focus the person's attention on the exchange of communication; the older adult may need extra time to begin to process information.
- Face the person when speaking to him or her.
- Minimize distractions in the room, including other people, objects in your hands, noise, and other activities.
- Reduce glare from room lighting by dimming too-bright lights. Conversely, avoid sitting in shadows.
- Speak slowly and clearly. Older adults may depend on lip reading, so ensure that the individual can see you. Speak loudly, but do not shout.
- Use short, simple sentences and be prepared to repeat or revise what you have said.
- Limit the number of topics discussed at one time to prevent information overload.
- Ask one question at a time to minimize confusion. Allow plenty of time for the person to answer and express ideas.
- Frequently summarize the important points of the conversation to improve understanding and comprehension.
- Avoid the urge to finish sentences.
- If the communication exchange is going poorly, postpone it for another time.

Biologic Domain

During the later years, changes in vital biologic structure and processes can occur in a particular organ or tissue or in the whole body. Changes may occur from disuse after the function of the organ has been fulfilled (eg, the uterus or thymus gland) or from disuse associated with insufficient exercise or movement (eg, in neuromusculoskeletal systems). Body fat increases (18% to 36% in men, 33% to 48% in women), total body water decreases (10% to 15%), and muscle mass decreases. Distinguishing whether changes occur because of decreased physical activity, level of motivation, influence of societal expectations, or cumulative effects of disease is difficult.

When changes occur in the organ systems, functional capacity is often decreased. However, many older adults can integrate profound decrements in physical capacity without affecting the ability to function under normal conditions. It is only when functional reserves are needed, such as during an infection, that the absence of these reserves is observed. The following sections highlight significant biologic changes that occur in later adulthood.

Renal Changes

Even without disease, a predictable decline in glomerular filtration and tubular secretion occurs with aging. Renal blood flow decreases by as much as 10% every decade after age 40 years. Renal clearance is estimated to decrease by as much as 35% between the ages of 20 and 90 years. These changes result in decreased renal excretion, which is of particular concern because the kidneys excrete most drugs (Tiao, Semmens, Masarei, & Lawrence-Brown, 2002).

Gastrointestinal Changes

Blood flow in the liver tends to decline with advancing age, decreasing as much as 40% to 50% by the age of 65 years. Reduced cardiac output is the major factor slowing blood flow through the liver. Reduced blood flow decreases the liver's opportunity to metabolize medications; consequently, medications may remain in the blood longer, increasing the risk for toxicity. As a result, fat-soluble drugs become sequestered in fatty tissue, rather than remaining in the circulating plasma. These factors increase the risk for accumulation and drug toxicity (Anantharaju, Feller, & Chedid, 2002).

Neurologic Changes

Nervous system changes that occur with aging include central and peripheral neuronal cell loss; slowed transmission of nerve impulses; slowed reaction time; diminished proprioception, balance, and postural control; poor thermoregulation; and altered sleep patterns. The effects of changes in the nervous system are confounded by changes in other systems, such as the cardiovascular system (eg, decreased arterial elasticity) and respiratory system (eg, diminished response to hypoxia and hypercapnia). Physiologic changes occurring with physical illness may precipitate altered mental status (eg, delirium) or exacerbate symptoms of existing psychiatric illness (eg, depression).

The brain, like most other body organs, undergoes changes with aging. Although brain weight begins to decline after the age of 30 years, visible atrophy is not apparent until about 60 years of age. Brain weight decreases by about 10% from early life to the ninth decade; this change is reflected in enlarged ventricles and widened sulci. Brain atrophy may result from a net loss of neurons (Scahill et al., 2003).

Sensory Changes

All five senses decline with age. This factor is important to remember when assessing psychiatrically ill elderly patients because diminished senses may affect attention and perception, potentially affecting interpretation of standard mental status examinations. Structural changes in the eye include rigidity of the iris, accumulation of yellow substance in the lens, and diminished lens elasticity. These changes result in decreased pupil size, alteration in colour perception, presbyopia, impaired adaptation to darkness, and significant vision impairment in the presence of glare (Bakker, 2003). Auditory changes are noticeable as early as 40 years of age; however, age of onset varies according to lifestyle (eg, previous exposure to occupational noise). Cochlear neurons are lost, resulting in hearing loss that may affect performance on intelligence tests. Several other factors beyond loss of hearing can influence age-related differences in performance on intelligence tests. Research on taste, touch, and smell is sparse, but a uniform dulling of these senses occurs with aging. The rate of decline is highly variable among individuals.

Sexuality

Misinformation and attitudinal barriers continue to plague the study of sexuality in the aging individual. Several generalizations have emerged: older persons retain interest in sex; frequency of sexual activity is less than desired; and increasing problems with sexual performance are associated with increasing age in both men and women. Although several physical changes with aging affect sexual functioning, interest in and enjoyment of sexual activities can continue until one's death. Health, desire to remain sexually active, access to a partner, and a conducive environment contribute to positive sexual functioning.

Physiologic changes in women include decreasing estrogen levels, alterations in the structural integrity of the vagina (eg, decreased blood flow, decreased flexibility, diminished lubrication, and diminished response during orgasm), and decreased breast engorgement during arousal (Wright, 2001). The sexual response continues as in younger women, but with less intensity. Even with chronic illness, many older women remain interested in and satisfied with a variety of sexual activities. Although being older is often associated with decrease in sexual interest in women, sexual attitudes and knowledge are also important predictors of interest, participation, and satisfaction with sexual activity. In reality, sexual activity in aging women often depends on availability of a partner.

Physiologic changes in men include a decline in testosterone production, increased time to achieve erection, less firm erections, decreased urgency for ejaculation, decreased sperm production, and a longer refractory period (ie, the amount of time before the man can achieve another erection) (Wright, 2001). Problems with sexual performance in aging men are usually centred around erectile dysfunction.

In men, frequency and desired frequency for coitus decline as age increases. Men are more likely to be sexually active, but are less satisfied with their level of sexual activity than are women. As with women, partner availability and willingness influence the frequency of sexual activity.

Access to a conducive environment may be hindered if the parent resides with an adult child or in a nursing home. Although nursing home residents may remain interested in maintaining sexual relationships, the attitudes of the staff and physicians constitute an additional barrier for this population beyond those noted previously (Bauer, 1999; Gott & Hinchliff, 2003).

Psychological Domain

Cognitive Function

Changes in cognition are most likely accounted for by structural and functional changes in the brain (Rosenzweig & Barnes, 2003). These alterations are probably highly specific because aspects of cognitive decline are very specific (eg, secondary memory), and many abilities are preserved. Moreover, external factors, including activity levels, socioeconomic status, education, and personality, may modify the development or expression of age-related changes in cognition (see Chapter 28). Normal aging does not impair consciousness. Alertness is required for attention, but the alert patient may not necessarily be able to attend. Attention has two aspects: sustained attention (vigilance) and selective attention (ability to extract relevant from irrelevant information). Numerous studies indicate that elderly people perform well on tests of sustained and selective attention. Earlier findings of poor performance on tests of selective attention have been attributed to lack of control for perceptual difficulties (eg, vision and hearing deficits).

Slower reaction time may affect how quickly the elder responds to questions. Hurrying elders to answer questions may interfere with their ability to provide the correct answer. This has been labelled the *speed-accuracy* shift, by which the older person focusses more on accuracy than on speed in responding. Caution tends to increase, whereas risk-taking behaviour tends to decrease; older adults are more likely to make errors of omission (leave the answer out) than errors of commission (make a guess) (Zimprich, 2002).

Learning

Intelligence and personality are stable across the life span in the absence of disease; however, the learning abilities of older people may be more selective, requiring motivation ("How important is this information?"), meaningful content ("Why do I need to know this?"), and familiarity with the idea or content. Although age causes no differences in the ability to process knowledge to learn a skill, younger people are more likely to employ strategies to learn tasks. Level of education needs to be considered in evaluating responses on mental status examinations because it may represent socioeconomic status and occupation.

Memory

Other than overall intelligence, age-related memory alterations have been more widely studied than any other aspect of cognition. Memory loss is not a normal part of aging. To remember events, humans must first attend to information and process it. Older people may well dismiss information that is not important to them. Memory problems in later life are believed to result from encoding problems, or "getting" the information in the first place. This problem may be related to sensory problems, not paying attention, or a general failure to link the "to be remembered" information to existing knowledge through association or to strengthen the memory through repetition. However, it is important not to confuse decline with deficit. Although a decline in memory ability may be frustrating for the older individual, it does not necessarily hamper his or her ability to function daily. Threats to memory include medications, depression (impairs concentration and attention), poor nutrition, infection, heart and lung disease (lack of oxygen), thyroid problems (can cause symptoms of depression or confusion that mimic memory loss), alcohol use, and sensory loss (interferes with perception).

BOX 29.2   RESEARCH FOR BEST PRACTICE

Practical Application of Gerotranscendence Theory

Wadensten, B., & Carlsson, M. (2003) Theory-driven guidelines for practical care of older people, based on the theory of gerotranscendence. *Journal of Advanced Nursing, 41*(5), 462–470.

THE QUESTION: The developmental process toward gerotranscendence can be obstructed or accelerated by life crises and grief, but elements in the culture can also facilitate or impede the process. Similarly, the caring climate can obstruct or accelerate the process toward gerotranscendence. This study was undertaken to find out what practical guidelines could be devised for use in the care of older people.

METHODS: The method of deriving guidelines from the theory was focus group interviews. The theory of gerotranscendence was used as a foundation for stimulating the discussions in the focus groups, as well as for organizing the proposals that emerged.

FINDINGS: Concrete guidelines at three levels, focussing on the individual, activity, and organization, were derived.

The following guidelines were generated to support older people in their process toward gerotranscendence.
- Accept the possibility that behaviours resembling the signs of gerotranscendence are normal signs of aging.
- Reduce preoccupation with the body.
- Allow alternative definitions of time.
- Allow thoughts and conversations about death.
- Choose topics of conversation that facilitate and further older people's personal growth.
- Accept, create, and introduce new types of "activities."
- Encourage and facilitate quiet and peaceful places and times.

IMPLICATIONS FOR NURSING: These guidelines could support staff in their practical care of older people and could be used as a supplement to enrich current care. The guidelines should be used to promote development toward gerotranscendence.

Development

Late-life adult developmental phenomena have not been well defined (see Chapter 7). Although Erik Erikson identified "integrity versus despair" as a developmental task specific to late adulthood, his wife recently published an extension of his theory that included old age as a ninth stage, **gerotranscendence** (Erikson & Erikson, 1997). Rather than emphasizing decrements in physical capacity for function, gerotranscendence theory provides for continued growth in dimensions such as spirituality and inner strength. The concept of gerotranscendence may be used in establishing health promotion interventions (Box 29-2).

Relationship Strains

As family relationships change, interpersonal relationship strains can develop. Disappointments with lifestyles of adult children and changes in caregiving responsibilities may affect the quality of a long-time family relationship. In some instances, the young-old assume caregiving responsibilities for their old-old relatives. It is also common for grandparents to assume some caregiving responsibilities for their grandchildren. A change in work status of grandparents (the fact that many of them work today) has drastically changed the "face" of grandparenting in Canada.

With Canadians living longer and healthier lives, grandparents are playing a larger part in the lives of their families. A century ago, grandparents could expect to have only 10 years with their grandchildren; that statistic has doubled to 20 years today. As most Canadian women can expect to live to be 82 years of age, many will spend nearly half of their lives as grandmothers. As well, many more Canadians can expect to become great-grandparents than those in the past. (NACA, 2005).

Social Domain

Functional Status

Functional status, the extent to which a person can carry out independently personal care, home management, and social functions in everyday life in a way that has meaning and purpose, often changes during the later years (see Chapter 28). Estimates of the prevalence of functional dependency vary, but, in general, studies show that difficulty in performing activities of daily living (ADLs) increases with advancing age, and that rates of dependency are significantly higher for women than for men, particularly for women who live alone (von Strauss, Aguero-Torres, Kareholt, Winblad, & Fratiglioni, 2003).

Although older women and men have similar paths to life satisfaction, the recent Canadian study conducted by Bourque and colleagues (2005) reported that there are important differences. Men's greater independence allows them to be less dependent on environmental and social factors for life satisfaction; women's greater social embeddedness enables them to be as satisfied as men with life in general, even though their life circumstances may be poorer (p. 43).

Retirement

The average age of retirement decreased from age 66 years in the period 1955 to 1960 to age 63 years in the period 1985 to 1990 (U.S. DHHS, 1999). The transition from a paid work role to a potentially less structured and purposeful pattern of living can lead to alterations in self-concept. Retirement is frequently characterized as a stressful life event that may bring psychological, social, and economic uncertainty. It affects social roles, income, use of health services, and participation in leisure activities. Although these changes are often associated with negative myths and stereotypes, most people do very well in retirement (U.S. DHHS, 1999). Adequate pensions, savings/investments, and social assistance contribute to its success.

Cultural Impact

As the population ages in Canadian society, it is also becoming more culturally diverse. Our North American communities are increasingly a reflection of multiple ethnic histories and values (Hayes-Bautista, Hsu, Perez, & Gamboa, 2002). Before the 1960s, immigrants to Canada were mostly from Europe; since the late 1980s, immigrants are increasingly from Asia, Central and South America, and Africa (Tam, Fletcher, & Chi, 2004). Wide cultural variations exist in family expectations of and responsibilities for the older adult. Some groups, such as Aboriginal and Asian cultures, tend to highly value the experience and wisdom of their elderly, and family members feel a responsibility for their care. Further research is needed to understand and address the relationships between cultural issues related to aging, health, and health care delivery. We do know that treatment and intervention are most effective when patients, families, and the health care team can work together to integrate patients' beliefs and cultural values into the plan of care.

Social Activities

Health conditions may also prevent participation in home maintenance and leisure activities, especially walking, gardening, and active sports. Among serious health conditions in the years after retirement, lung disease and diabetes most seriously affect leisure activities. As age increases, participation decreases. Higher education levels are associated with increased participation in both formal and informal activities (Holmes & Dorfman, 2000).

Community Strains

Older adults can find themselves living in changing or deteriorating neighbourhoods. With decreasing social support, they are often faced with either living in a familiar but increasingly socially isolated environment or moving to an unfamiliar place (U.S. DHHS, 1999). One major problem is housing and the prox-imity of home to social resources, such as church, community centres, shopping, health care, and related social services. Although most elders live in their own homes, relocating to smaller and more protective housing may be welcomed by some and fiercely resisted by others.

Residential Care

Various residential care models are in part a response to the medical model emphasized in most long-term care facilities and the need to develop alternatives to nursing home care. Residential care models include a spectrum of residential living environments, such as foster care homes, family homes, personal care homes, residential care facilities, and assisted living arrangements.

For every person currently in institutional care, an estimated four others who require some form of long-term care are in the community. How and by whom will they be provided care? Approaches to this looming problem include the following:

- Reducing the need for home care by improving the health of older people
- Finding and paying for home care when disability and frailty preclude continued independence
- Ensuring better integration across the total continuum of care and coordination of different care providers who subscribe to a biopsychosocial view of health care that includes both medical and social components

Consumers should question residential providers about all aspects of services, including staff training and staffing patterns, medication supervision, approaches to behaviour management, activities provided, services available (eg, care management, family support, counselling, day care), safety and security issues, provision of personal care with attention to dignity and privacy, health and nutrition concerns, and full disclosure of costs and funding and payment issues, to determine whether the older adult's needs and abilities match the care provided in that facility.

Assisted Living

The assisted living concept has emerged as an important long-term care alternative for the mentally and physically frail. Assisted living provides community-based, residential services for older persons and adults with physical disabilities who need help with ADLs. Assisted living services combine housing, personal services, and light medical or nursing care. Perhaps the most important feature of these assisted living facilities is the orientation toward the older resident that empowers the frail older adult by sharing responsibilities for care and ADLs, enhancing their choices, and managing risks. The need for alternative long-term care strategies for this population is expected to continue, with the growing number of older adults in need of supportive services.

RISK FACTORS FOR GERIATRIC PSYCHOPATHOLOGY

Chronic Illnesses

Although the frequency of acute conditions declines with advancing age, about 90% of older adults have chronic medical conditions that can adversely affect function. Poor physical health is a well-established risk factor for mental disorders. The major chronic conditions experienced by older adults are ischemic heart disease, hypertension, vision impairment, hearing impairment, musculoskeletal impairment, and diabetes (U.S. DHHS, 2001). Chronic illnesses can reduce physiologic capacity and consequently increase functional dependency. In addition, during acute episodes of illness, many elders lose functional ability because they have limited reserves or cannot mobilize reserves to regain their premorbid performance levels.

Polypharmacy

Polypharmacy, the use of several medications, is often associated with chronic illness and long-term drug therapy (see Chapter 28). Those older than 65 years purchase 30% of all prescription drugs and 40% of all over-the-counter drugs (Cohen, 2000). The aging process affects pharmacokinetics (primarily the mechanisms of drug absorption, distribution, metabolism, and excretion) and the strength and number of protein-binding sites. These changes place the older adult at increased risk for adverse drug reactions. In a review of literature, the reported prevalence of older patients using at least one inappropriately prescribed drug ranged from 40%

of nursing home patients to 21.3% of community-dwelling patients (Liu & Christensen, 2002). Serious problems result when coordination of the care delivery and treatment regimen specific to prescribed medications is lacking. These problems are compounded when the patient uses over-the-counter drugs, herbal remedies, and home or folk remedies without considering their potential interaction with prescribed drugs. Nurses can follow the principles delineated in Box 29-3 to improve drug therapy with older adults.

Bereavement and Loss

The older person experiences many losses—friends and family members die, physical health compromises, and social status diminishes. Loss of one's spouse, particularly when the relationship has been long and satisfying, constitutes a major life event. Women are more likely to lose their spouses and tend to be widowed at a younger age than are men. Consequently, women have more time to adjust and develop substitute social relationships to replace the spouse. Conversely, men tend to lose their wives at an older age, have fewer social networks to replace the spouse, and express feelings of loneliness and abandonment. Because of differences in longevity, men and women usually experience life events at different ages.

Gender differences in reactions to loss through death have been reported. One study asked 391 individuals who had lost a spouse, parent, child, other relative, or friend to recall their experiences at the time of the loss. Significantly, more women than men recalled being highly emotional at the time of the loss; the recovery

---

BOX 29.3

Drug Therapy Interventions

- Minimize the number of drugs that the person uses, keeping only those drugs that are essential. One-third of the residents in one long-term care facility received 8 to 16 drugs daily.
- Always consider alternatives among different drug classifications or dosage forms that are more suitable for elderly patients.
- Implement preventive measures to reduce the need for certain medications. Such prevention includes health promotion through proper nutrition, exercise, and stress reduction.
- Most age-dependent pharmacokinetic changes lead to potential accumulation of the drug; therefore, medication dosage should start low and go slow.
- Exercise caution when administering medication with a long half-life or in an older adult with impaired renal or liver function. Under these conditions, the time may be extended between doses.
- Be knowledgeable of each drug's properties, including such factors as half-life, excretion, and adverse effects.

For example, venlafaxine HCl (Effexor), a structurally novel antidepressant that inhibits the reuptake of serotonin and norepinephrine, requires regular monitoring of the patient's blood pressure.

- Assess the patient's clinical history for physical problems that may affect excretion of medications.
- Monitor laboratory values (eg, creatinine clearance) and urinary output in patients receiving medications eliminated by the kidneys.
- Monitor plasma albumin levels in patients receiving drugs that have high binding affinity to protein.
- Regularly monitor the patient's reaction to all medications to ensure a therapeutic response.
- Look for potential drug interactions that may complicate therapy. Antacids lower gastric acidity and may decrease the rate at which other medications are dissolved and absorbed.
- Remind patients to consult with their provider before taking any over-the-counter medications.

period after the loss was longer for women. However, more men than women wished that they could have changed past relationships with their families. One possible explanation for the findings in this study is that a significantly higher percentage of women (38.5%) than men (15.1%) had lost a spouse; whereas, men more often reported the loss of a parent (52.4% for men versus 39.8% for women) (Benedict & Zhang, 1999).

Regardless of gender differences, survivors are at higher risk for depression and face financial issues after the death of a loved one. Health care professionals should work closely with grieving survivors to help the survivors understand that their lives will be displaced for some time. Support sessions on the grief process and financial and employment planning could become a standard part of care.

Poverty

Because retirement and widowhood are common events in late life, older adults can be at higher risk for poverty than other age groups. Two groups of poor older persons include those who have lived in poverty all their lives and those who become impoverished in late life. Poverty may result from inadequate retirement income, illness, discrimination against women in pension plans, and financial exploitation of older individuals. Poverty has significant effects on this population, including higher mortality rates, poorer health, lower health-related quality of life, lower likelihood of participating in health screening programs, and higher likelihood of using the emergency department for acute illness (Fleming, Evans, & Chutka, 2003).

Suicide and the Lack of Social Support

Suicide is a leading cause of preventable death in Canada and worldwide. The Canadian Association for Suicide Prevention (CASP) reports that more than 400,000 Canadians engage in some type of self-harm behaviour every year and that in the past 30 years, many of the 100,000 people who have died by suicide in Canada have been older adults (CASP, 2004). Older adults tend to use more lethal methods than younger persons in their suicide attempts. Firearms are the most common method of suicide for men, although women tend to use self-poisoning or suffocation (Moore, Grek, Heisel & Jackson, 2006). The general population engages in suicidal behaviour approximately 20 times for every death to suicide; older adults, in contrast, may do so fewer than 4 times (Conwell et al., 1998; McIntosh et al., 1994). "The lethality of suicidal behaviour and related likelihood of death among older adults is especially disturbing in light of large estimated increases in the older Canadian population in coming years" (Statistics Canada, 2005, p. 1).

A lack of social support has been linked to the rate of suicide in the elderly (Heisel, 2004; Heisel & Duberstein, 2005), the highest rates being for divorced or widowed men. Risk factors for suicide in older persons include being white, male, widowed or divorced, retired or unemployed, living alone in an urban area, in poor health (including poor mental health) or lonely, and having a history of poor interpersonal relationships (Waern, Rubenowitz, & Wilhelmson, 2003).

PREVENTION OF MENTAL ILLNESS

Preventing Depression and Suicide

Depression is one of the most common mental disorders of the older adult (see Chapter 19). Recognition and early intervention are the keys to avoiding ongoing depressive episodes. Early indications of symptomatology can be identified in primary care settings. Several preventive interventions, such as grief counselling for widows and widowers, self-help groups, and social activities, are helpful. Community-based projects have been effective in significantly reducing suicide rates in older adults (Heisel & Duberstein, 2005).) By assessing and addressing cognitive and social-cognitive vulnerability factors and by focussing on the promotion of life satisfaction, nurses can help not only to prevent suicide but also to assist the older adult in achieving a healthier and more meaningful life (Heisel, 2004). Increasingly, studies are exploring concepts such as meaning and hope and the role that these play in helping older adults live well (Heisel & Duberstein, 2005; Moore, 1997).

Reducing the Stigma of Mental Health Treatment

The stigma of mental illness continues to interfere with the willingness of older adults to seek treatment. Today's older Canadians grew up during a time when institutionalization in asylums, electroconvulsive treatments, and other treatment approaches were regarded with fear. This fear can lead to denial of problems. Nurses can help reduce the stigma through education interventions and facilitation of access to services.

CRNE Note

Safety concerns are a priority. Carefully explore any suicidal ideation and develop a plan for intervention and prevention.

Use of Medications

With the approval of new medications, older adults will be able to treat health problems with pharmacologic agents that were not previously available. Side effects and drug interactions should be carefully monitored to detect untoward symptoms and delirium (see Chapter 30).

Education of older adults and their families regarding a medication regimen is crucial to ensure adherence and to minimize untoward effects. Basic principles regarding neurobiologic changes in normal aging (as previously discussed) should be applied when designing teaching strategies. The nurse must consider the older adult's pace of learning as well as any visual and hearing deficits. Education should include the reason for administering the drug and important side effects of the drug. The nurse should provide instructional aids, large-print labelling, and devices such as medication calendars that encourage adherence to the treatment plan. Patients should be aware that they can reject childproof containers for their medications if they have trouble opening them.

Avoiding Premature Institutionalization

In Canada, as in many countries around the world, health care reform has drastically affected how health care is delivered. Such reform has focussed on a move from institutional care to home care. Research has demonstrated that there is significant potential for home care to support mental health and well-being of seniors in the community (Parent, Anderson, & Huestis, 2002). Supportive community-based services can help to avoid premature institutionalization in seniors.

PROMOTION OF MENTAL HEALTH

Social Support Transitions

Older adults may compensate for loss of family by expanding friendship networks, and employment may become an important method of establishing a network in late life. The elder can be prepared for the transition by receiving information about internal developmental processes, sources of social support, and opportunities for personal growth and role supplementation.

Lifestyle Support

Lifestyle interventions, such as exercise promotion and nutrition counselling, are particularly important in late life because a tendency to slow down and to become more sedentary usually accompanies aging. For many, retirement provides an opportunity to restructure the time that was previously spent working. Developing regular exercise habits can help maintain physical and psychological well-being. Self-help programs generally include components of exercise, nutrition, health screening, and health habits.

Spiritual Support

Humanists suggest that the main purpose of life is to find meaning and that this can be accomplished through creations (or accomplishments), experiences in the world, and attitude toward suffering (Frankl, 1963). In nursing, spirituality is recognized as a basic quality, inherent in all humans. The spiritual perspective includes three critical attributes:

- Connectedness (with other humans, nature, universal forces, or God)
- Beliefs in powers or forces beyond the self, and a faith that affirms life
- A creative energy

The spiritual perspective also can provide a path for the quest for the meaning of life and can organize and guide human values and motivations.

Spirituality can be extremely important to the older adult and can positively affect attitude, particularly as health declines (Lowry & Conco, 2002). Supporting contact with spiritual leaders important to the patient is

IN A LIFE

Verna Splane (1914–) and Dr. Helen Mussallem (1915–):

Outstanding Canadian Nurses Shown at Dr. Mussallem's birthday party, 2005.

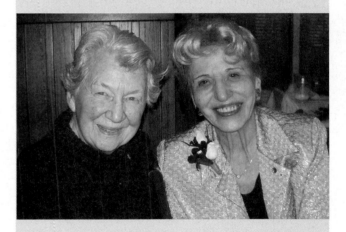

Dr. Helen Mussallem
(*right*) celebrated her 90th birthday in 2005. Currently living in Ottawa, she is a former chairperson of the Board of the Victorian Order of Nurses and continues to serve on 23 boards. Beginning her career in 1937, she has dedicated her life to nursing.
Verna Splane
(*left*) celebrated her 90th birthday in 2004. She was Chief Nursing Officer in National Health and Welfare and worked with the World Health Organization in International Nursing and Public Health. She was also Vice President of the International Council of Nurses (ICN). She continues to meet with nursing students at the University of British Columbia who have an interest in international nursing.

an ongoing mental health promotion intervention. The nurse can also support a patient's spiritual growth by exploring the meanings that a particular life change has for the elder. In late life, existential issues such as experiencing losses, redefining meanings in existence, and living in the present become the standard, replacing the performance and future orientation that characterize earlier adulthood.

Community Services

More emphasis should be placed on community care options, services that provide both sustenance and growth. Examples of supportive services that foster independent community living include information and referral services, transportation and nutrition services, legal and protective services, comprehensive senior centres, homemaker and handyman services, matching of older with younger individuals to share housing, and use of the supports available through churches, community groups, or mental health and other community agencies (eg, area agencies on aging) to maintain elderly individuals in the community for as long as possible. The availability and accessibility of these services vary greatly, and eligibility requirements may exist. A Canadian Mental Health Association project, funded by Population Health in Canada, examined seniors' mental health and home care using mental health promotion principles. A variety of methods grounded in the principle of participation explored the perspectives of seniors, family caregivers, and home care providers. A policy guide was developed as an outcome of the project to provide direction for a holistic model of care, incorporating both medical and psychosocial supports to meet the needs of seniors.

SUMMARY OF KEY POINTS

- Major changes in social roles with aging include retirement, loss of partner, and residence.
- The brain changes with aging; these changes include a decline in weight and reduction in synapses.
- The nervous system has a considerable degree of plasticity and can sustain some structural losses without losing function.
- All five special senses (sight, hearing, touch, taste, and smell) decline with age.
- Intelligence and personality are stable throughout the life span; however, reaction time slows with age.
- The concept of **gerotranscendence** emphasizes continued spiritual growth and development of inner strength rather than decrements in physical capacity in the last stage of life.
- Threats to memory in the older adult include medications, depression, poor nutrition, infection, heart and lung disease, thyroid problems, alcohol use, and sensory loss.

- Polypharmacy is prevalent in older adults, particularly in nursing homes. Ongoing assessment of medication is needed to prevent inappropriate medication administration.
- Older adults are at higher risk for poverty and suicide.
- Although older adults experience many physical changes, they can desire and have the urge to remain sexually active.
- Aging affects pharmacokinetics, including drug absorption, distribution, metabolism, and excretion; aging also affects the strength and number of protein-binding sites.
- Residential care environments ideally emphasize family-oriented care that optimizes existing functional capacities.
- Assisted living is a supportive housing environment that provides routine nursing services within a philosophy of patient empowerment.

CRITICAL THINKING CHALLENGES

1 Compare the three late adulthood chronologic groups in terms of age. Using the recommendations of Box 29-1, interview people representing each of the three chronologic groups about their views of mental health.
2 Highlight normal biologic changes that occur during the aging process.
3 Hypothesize why IQ tests and personality do not change with time.
4 Use the concept of *gerotranscendence* to explain differences between the young-old and the old-old.
5 Identify positive and negative perspectives of retirement.
6 Explain why chronic illnesses, polypharmacy, and poverty are all risk factors for mental health problems in later life.
7 Describe mental health promotion interventions that relate to social support transitions, lifestyle support, and self-care.

WEB LINKS

www.naca-ccnta.ca The National Advisory Council on Aging was created on May 1, 1980, to assist and advise the Minister of Health on all matters related to the aging of the Canadian population and the quality of life of seniors.

www.nami.org This website includes a guide book written for older adults with mental health concerns and their family members and caregivers.

www.ccsmh.ca The Canadian Coalition for Seniors' Mental Health, established in 2002, has as its goal to support collaborative initiatives that will facilitate positive mental health for seniors through innovation and dissemination of best practices.

www.cgna.net The Canadian Gerontological Nurses Association represents nurses who work with and for older adults in a wide variety of settings. Their interests include education, research, and clinical practice. They encourage and support members through research grants, scholarships, conference funding, and certification study sessions.

MOVIES

Emile: 2004. Emile returns to western Canada to receive an honorary degree for his life achievements. Ironically, in this reconnection with his past, he must face things left undone. This movie, part of a trilogy on self-transition, is about searching for one's identity in the latter part of life.

VIEWING POINTS: What were the turning points in Emile's life? Do you believe he would truly choose differently if he could live his life over? Is Emile's experience an example of gerotranscendence or not?

Driving Miss Daisy: 1989. This delightful and beautiful film, starring Jessica Tandy as Daisy Werthan, a cantankerous old woman, and Morgan Freeman as Hoke Colburn, Daisy's chauffeur, examines a relationship between two people who have more in common than just growing old. The film also challenges some of the myths about aging.

VIEWING POINTS: Identify the normal behaviours in the growth and development of the older adult. Observe the verbal and nonverbal communication of Daisy and Hoke. How do they support each other?

REFERENCES

Anantharaju, A., Feller, A., & Chedid, A. (2002). Aging liver: A review. *Gerontology, 48*(6), 343–353.

Bakker, R. (2003). Sensory loss, dementia, and environments. *Generations, 27*(1), 46–51.

Bauer, M. (1999). Their only privacy is between their sheets: Privacy and the sexuality of elderly nursing home residents. *Journal of Gerontological Nursing, 25*(8), 37–41.

Benedict, A., & Zhang, X. (1999). Reactions to loss among men and women: A comparison. *Activities, Adaptation & Aging, 24*(1), 29–38.

Bourque, P., Pushkar, D., Bonneville, L., & Beland, F. (2005). Contextual effects on life satisfaction of older men and women. *Canadian Journal on Aging, 24*(1), 31–44.

Canadian Coalition for Seniors Mental Health. (2003). Depression fought in seniors. *Canadian Coalition for Seniors Mental Health, 1*(4), 2.

Cohen, J. S. (2000). Avoiding adverse reactions: Effective lower-dose drug therapies for older patients. *Geriatrics, 55*(2), 54–64.

Conn, D. (2003). Presentation to the Standing Senate Committee on Social Affairs, Science and Technology. *Bulletin of the Canadian Academy of Geriatric Psychiatry, 10*(3), 5–8.

Conwell, Y., Lyness, J. M., Duberstein, P. R., Cox, C., Seidlitz, L. Caine, E. D. (1998). Physical illness & suicide among elderly

patients in primary care practices. (Abstract). Toronto: American Psychiatric Association.

Erikson, E. H., & Erikson, J. M. (1997). *The lifecycle completed, extended version.* New York: WW Norton.

Fleming, K. C., Evans, J. M., & Chutka, D. S. (2003). A cultural and economic history of old age in America. *Mayo Clinic Proceedings, 78*(7), 914–921.

Frankl, V. (1963). *Man's search for meaning: An introduction to logotherapy.* New York: Pocket Books.

Goodman, C., & Silverstein, M. (2002). Grandmothers raising grandchildren: Family structure and well-being in culturally diverse families. *Gerontologist, 42*(5), 676–689.

Gott, M., & Hinchliff, S. (2003). How important is sex in later life? The views of older people. *Social Science Medicine, 56*(8), 1617–1628.

Hayes-Bautista, D. E., Hsu, P., Perez, A., & Gamboa, C. (2002). The "browning" of the graying of America: Diversity in the elderly population and policy implications. *Generations, 26*(3), 15–24.

Heisel, M. J. (2004). Suicide ideation in the elderly. *Psychiatric Times, XXI*(3).

Heisel, M. J., & Duberstein, P. R. (2005). Suicide prevention in older adults. *Clinical Psychology: Science and Practice, 12*(3), 242–259. Available at: http://psychiatrictimes.com/p040350.html.

Holmes, J. S., & Dorfman, L. T. (2000). The effects of specific health conditions on activities in retirement. *Activities, Adaptation & Aging, 25*(1), 47.

Lindsay, C., & Almay, M. (1999). *A portrait of seniors in Canada.* Ottawa: Statistics Canada.

Liu, G. C., & Christensen, D. B. (2002). The continuing challenge of inappropriate prescribing in the elderly: An update of evidence. *Journal of the American Pharmaceutical Association, 7*(12), 634–638.

Lowry, L. W., & Conco, D. (2002). Exploring the meaning of spirituality with aging adults in Appalachia. *Journal of Holistic Nursing, 20*(4), 388–402.

McIntosh, J. L., Santos, J. F., Hubbard, R. W., & Overholser, J. C. (1994). Elder Suicide Research, Theory & Treatment. Washington, D.C.: American Psychological Association.

Moore, S. L. (1997). A phenomenological study of meaning in life in suicidal older adults. *Archives in Psychiatric Nursing, XI*(1), 29–36.

Moore, S. L., Grek, A., Heisel, M. & Jackson, F. (2006). *Canadian Coalition for Seniors Mental Health: National guidelines initiative. Suicide assessment and prevention.* Toronto: Canadian Coalition for Seniors Mental Health.

Moore, S. L., Metcalf, B., & Schow, E. (2000). Meaning in life: Examining the concept. *Geriatric Nursing, 21*(1), 27–29.

National Advisory Council on Aging. (NACA). (2003). *Interim report card on seniors.* Ottawa: Government of Canada.

NACA. (2005). Grandparenting today. Available at: http://www.naca-ccnta.ca.

NACA. (2003). Interim Report Card: Seniors in Canada. Ottawa: Government of Canada.

NAMI. (2001). Mental illness, healthy aging: A NH guide for older adults and caregivers. Retrieved June 2004, from http://www.nami.org/Content/ContentGroups/Home4/HomePageSpotlight1/Guidebook.pdf.

Parent, K., Anderson, M., & Huestis, L. (2002). *Supporting seniors' mental health through home care: A policy guide.* Toronto: Canadian Mental Health Association.

Public Health Agency of Canada. (2002). A report on mental illnesses in Canada. Ottawa: Author. Retrieved July 25, 2005, from http://www.phac-aspc.gc.ca/publicat/miic-mmac/.

Rosenzweig, E. S., & Barnes, C. A. (2003). Impact of aging on hippocampal function: Plasticity, network dynamics and cognition. *Progress in Neurobiology, 69*(3), 143–179.

Sattar, S. P., Petty, F., & Burke, W. J. (2003). Diagnosis and treatment of alcohol dependence in older alcoholics, *Clinics in Geriatric Medicine, 19,* 743–764.

Scahill, R. I., Frost, C., Jenkins, R., Whitwell, J. L., Rossor, M. N., & Fox, N. C. (2003). A longitudinal study of brain volume changes in normal aging using serial registered magnetic resonance imaging. *Archives of Neurology, 60*(7), 989–994.

Southern Alberta Geriatric Mental Health Working Group (SAGMHS). (2003, September). *Summary report of the Southern Alberta Geriatric Mental Health Working Group.* Calgary, AB: 1–12.

Stanford, E., & Usita, P. M. (2002). Retirement: Who is at risk? *Generations, 26*(2), 45–48.

Statistics Canada. (2005). *Selected highlights from portrait of seniors in Canada.* Available at: http://www.statcan.ca.

Statistics Canada. (2001). Seniors in Canada. Available at: http://www.statcan.ca/bsolc/english/bsolc?catno=85F0033m2001008

Statistics Canada. (2003). Population by sex and age. Available at: http://www40.statcan.ca/l01/cst01/demo31c.htm

Tiao, J. Y., Semmens, J. B., Masarei, J. R., & Lawrence-Brown, M. M. (2002). The effect of age on serum creatinine levels in an aging population: Relevance to vascular surgery. *Cardiovascular Surgery, 10*(5), 445–451.

Tam, E. Y., Fletcher, P. C., & Chi, I. (2004). Cultural and gender diversity in health. *STRIDE, 1.* Retrieved December 18, 2005, from http://www.stridemagazine.com.

U.S. Department of Health & Human Services (DHHS). (1999). The Surgeon General's Report on Mental Health. Washington, D.C.: U.S. Public Health Service.

U.S. Department of Health and Human Services (DHHS). (2001). Older Adults and Mental Health: Issues and Opportunities. Washington, DC: Administration on Aging.

von Strauss, E., Aguero-Torres, H., Kareholt, I., Winblad, B., & Fratiglioni, L. (2003). Women are more disabled in basic activities of daily living than men only in very advanced ages: A study on disability, morbidity, and mortality from the Kungsholmen Project. *Journal of Clinical Epidemiology, 56*(7), 669–677.

Wadensten, B., & Carlsson, M. (2003). Theory-driven guidelines for practical care of older people, based on the theory of gerotranscendence. *Journal of Advanced Nursing, 41*(5), 462–470.

Waern, M., Rubenowitz, E., & Wilhelmson, K. (2003). Predictors of suicide in the old elderly. *Gerontology, 49*(5), 328–334.

World Health Organization. (1999). Facts and figures about suicide. Geneva: Author. Retrieved June 29, 2005, from http://www.who.int/mental_health/media/en/382.pdf.

Wright, L. (2001). Sexuality-reproductive pattern: Normal changes with aging. In M. L. Maas, K. C. Buckwalter, M. D. Hardy, et al. (Eds.), *Nursing care of older adults: Diagnoses, outcomes, and interventions* (pp. 729–732). St. Louis: Mosby.

Zimprich, D. (2002). Cross-sectionally and longitudinally balanced effects of processing speed on intellectual abilities. *Experimental Aging Research, 28,* 231–251.

For challenges, please refer to the **CD-ROM** in this book.

30

Delirium, Dementias, and Related Disorders

Mary Haase

LEARNING OBJECTIVES

After studying this chapter, you will be able to:

- Distinguish the clinical characteristics, onset, and course of delirium and Alzheimer disease.
- Analyze the prevailing biologic, psychological, and social theories that relate to delirium and Alzheimer disease in older adults.
- Integrate biopsychosocial theories into the analysis of human responses to delirium and dementia, with emphasis on the concepts of impaired cognition and memory.
- Discuss various etiologies for cognitive impairment in other patients (other than those with delirium and dementia).
- Formulate nursing diagnoses based on a biopsychosocial assessment of patients with impaired cognitive function.
- Identify expected outcomes for patients with impaired cognition and their evaluation.
- Discuss nursing interventions used for patients with impaired cognition.

KEY TERMS

acetylcholine (ACh) ▪ acetylcholinesterase (AChE) ▪ acetylcholinesterase inhibitor (AChEI) ▪ agnosia ▪ aphasia ▪ apraxia ▪ butyrylcholinesterase (BuChE) ▪ bradykinesia ▪ catastrophic reactions ▪ cortical dementia ▪ disinhibition ▪ disturbance of executive functioning ▪ hyperkinetic delirium ▪ hypokinetic delirium ▪ hypersexuality ▪ hypervocalization ▪ illusions ▪ beta-amyloid plaques ▪ neurofibrillary tangles ▪ subcortical dementia

▪ KEY CONCEPTS

cognition ▪ delirium ▪ dementia ▪ memory

Cognition and memory are important in many psychiatric disorders, but in this chapter, they are the key concepts. Cognition is the ability to think and know. Now the definition is further refined to be understood as a relatively high level of intellectual processing in which perceptions and information are acquired, used, or manipulated.

> ⬟ KEY CONCEPT **Cognition** is based on a system of interrelated abilities, such as perception, reasoning, judgment, intuition, and memory, that allow one to be aware of oneself and one's surroundings. Impairments in these abilities can result in a failure of the afflicted person to recognize that he or she is ill and in need of treatment.

Cognition involves both how reality is perceived and how those perceptions are understood in relation to internal representations of reality previously acquired. In the broadest sense, cognition denotes how the brain processes information. Cognition includes a number of specific functions, such as the acquisition and use of language, the ability to be oriented in time and space, and the ability to learn and solve problems. It includes judgment, reasoning, attention, comprehension, concept formation, planning, and the use of symbols, such as numbers and letters used in mathematics and writing.

Memory, a facet of cognition, refers to the ability to recall or reproduce what has been learned or experienced. It is more than simple storage and retrieval; it is a complex cognitive mental function that includes most areas of the brain, especially the hippocampus, which is believed to be essential to the transfer of some memories from short-term to long-term storage. Defects of memory are an essential feature of many cognitive disorders, particularly dementia.

> ⬟ KEY CONCEPT **Memory** is a facet of cognition concerned with retaining and recalling past experiences, whether they occurred in the physical environment or internally as cognitive events.

The disorders discussed in this chapter—delirium, dementia, and related cognitive disorders—are characterized by deficits in cognition or memory that represent a clear-cut deterioration from a previous level of functioning. Delirium is a disorder of acute cognitive impairment and can be caused by a medical condition (eg, infection) or substance abuse, or it may have multiple etiologies. Dementia is characterized by chronic cognitive impairments and is differentiated by underlying cause, not by symptom patterns, which are often similar. Some dementias are irreversible and progressive, such as Alzheimer type, but not all dementias are irreversible. For example, some organic compounds and

Table 30.1	Selected Compounds and Chemicals That May Produce Dementia
Substance	**Related Symptoms**
Arsenic	Headache
	Drowsiness
	Confusion
Mercury	Tremors
	Extrapyramidal signs
	Upper and lower extremity ataxia
	Depression
	Confusion
Lead	Abdominal cramps
	Anemia
	Peripheral neuropathy
	Encephalopathy (rare)
Manganese	Extrapyramidal symptoms
	Delirium
Aluminum	Myoclonus
	Speech disorders
	Seizure disorders
	Cognitive impairment
Toluene (methyl benzene)	Profound cognitive impairment
	Tremor
	Ataxia
	Loss of vision and hearing

chemicals, such as lead, aluminum, manganese, and toluene (one of the toxins in glue and paint), may produce symptoms of dementia (Table 30-1). Once evaluated and treated, the symptoms of dementia can resolve in many of these disorders (eg, endocrine disorders).

> ⬟ KEY CONCEPT **Delirium** is a disorder of acute cognitive impairment and is caused by a medical condition (eg, infection), substance abuse, or multiple etiologies.

> ⬟ KEY CONCEPT **Dementia** is characterized by chronic cognitive impairments and is differentiated by underlying cause, not by symptom patterns, which are often similar. Dementia can be further classified as cortical or subcortical to denote the location of the underlying pathology.

Cortical dementia results from a disease process that globally afflicts the cortex. **Subcortical dementia** is caused by dysfunction or deterioration of deep grey- or white-matter structures inside the brain and brain stem. Symptoms of subcortical dementia may be more localized and tend to disrupt arousal, attention, and motivation, but they can produce a variety of clinical behavioural manifestations. In this chapter, a type of cortical dementia, Alzheimer disease, is highlighted because it is the most prevalent form of dementia.

Delirium

CLINICAL COURSE OF DISORDER

Delirium is a disturbance in consciousness and a change in cognition that develops over a short time. It is usually reversible if the underlying cause is identified and treated quickly. It is a serious disorder that is associated with high morbidity and mortality.

Emergency!

Individuals who are delirious arrive in the emergency room in a state of confusion and disorientation that developed during a period of a few hours or days. If delirium is not treated in a timely manner, irreversible neurologic damage can occur. About 25% of patients do not survive.

DIAGNOSTIC CRITERIA

Impaired consciousness is the key diagnostic criterion. The patient becomes less aware of his or her environment and loses the ability to focus, sustain, and shift attention. Associated cognitive changes include problems in memory, orientation, and language. The patient may not know where he or she is, may not recognize familiar objects, or may be unable to carry on a conversation. Another important diagnostic indicator is that the problem developed during a short period (compared with dementia, which develops gradually) (American Psychiatric Association [APA], 2000). Table 30-2 presents the

CRNE Note

Delirium can be life-threatening, so identifying potential underlying causes of the symptoms is a priority.

diagnostic criteria of delirium caused by a general medical condition. Delirium is different from dementia, but the presenting symptoms are often similar. Table 30-3 highlights the differences among delirium, dementia, and depression (pseudo-dementia).

DELIRIUM IN SPECIAL POPULATIONS

Children

Delirium can occur in children and may be related to medications (anticholinergic agents) or fever. Children seem to be especially susceptible to this disorder, probably because of their immature brain. However, delirium may be hard to diagnose and may be mistaken for uncooperative behaviour.

Older Adults

Although delirium may occur in any age group, it is most common among the older adults. Nurses must recognize that delirium, dementia, and depression present with overlapping clinical features and may coexist in the older adult (Registered Nurses Association of Ontario [RNAO], 2003).

Table 30.2	Key Diagnostic Characteristics of Delirium Caused by a General Medical Condition 293.0	

Diagnostic Criteria	Associated Findings
Disturbance of consciousness Reduced clarity of awareness Decreased ability to focus, sustain, or shift attention **Developing over a short period of time**—usually hours to days; fluctuating during the course of the day **Cognitive changes** Memory deficit, disorientation, language disturbance Development of perceptual disturbance not better accounted for by a pre-existing, established, or evolving dementia **History, physical examination, or laboratory tests** indicating change as a direct cause of physiologic effects of medical condition	*Associated Behavioural Findings* • Attention wandering • Perseveration • Easily distracted • Recent memory changes • Dysnomia, dysgraphia • Speech is rambling, irrelevant, incoherent • Misinterpretations, illusions, and hallucinations
Etiologies • Substance intoxication delirium • Substance withdrawal delirium • Multiple etiologies (due to more than one medical condition, substance effect, or medication side effect) • Not otherwise specified	*Associated Physical Findings* • Daytime sleepiness • Nighttime agitation • Difficulty falling asleep • Restlessness, hyperactivity, or sluggishness and lethargy • Anxiety, fear, irritability, anger, euphoria, and apathy • Rapid unpredictable shifts from one emotional state to another *Associated Laboratory Findings* • Abnormal electroencephalogram

Table 30.3	Differentiating Delirium, Dementia, and Depression (Pseudo-Dementia)		
Characteristics	**Delirium**	**Dementia**	**Depression (Pseudo-Dementia)**
Onset	Sudden; over hours or days; often at twilight	Insidious; slow; chronic	Coincides with major life event; can be abrupt or gradual
Course	Short; generally worse at night, in darkness, and on wakening	Long; symptoms progressive yet stable over time; often worse at night	Typically worse in the morning; situational fluctuations
Duration	Hours to less than a month	Months to years	At least 2 weeks; can be several months or years
Consciousness	Reduced	Clear	Clear
Orientation	Impaired; fluctuates with severity	May be impaired	Selective disorientation
Memory	Impaired recent and immediate	Impaired recent and remote; tries to hide loss	Selective impairment; complains of memory loss
Awareness	Reduced	Clear	Clear
Alertness	Fluctuates	Generally normal	Normal
Attention	Impaired; fluctuates	Generally normal	Distractible
Thought processes	Disorganized, distorted, and fragmented	Difficulty with abstraction, poverty of thought, and impaired judgment	Intact but themes of hopelessness, helplessness, or self-criticism
"Don't know" answers	Uncommon	Uncommon	Common
Perceptions	Distorted; illusions, delusions, and hallucinations	Generally not impaired	Generally intact; hallucinations and delusions in psychotic depression
Psychomotor activity	Hypo- and/or hyperkinetic	Normal; may have apraxia.	Variable; psychomotor slowing or agitation
Sleep/wake cycle	Days and nights reversed		
Speech	Incoherent, slowed, or speeded	Fragmented	Generally disturbed; early morning wakening and/or initial insomnia
Distinguishing feature	Associated with acute physical illness; fluctuating levels of consciousness	Difficulty finding words Attempts to conceal intellectual deficiencies; insight lacking; memory impairment	Often slowed speech Affect depressed, dysphoric mood, somatic concerns, and/or self-neglect; suicide risk

From Arnold, 2005; Blair, 2000; Forman, Fletcher, Mion, & Trygstad, 2003; Gleason, 2003; and New Zealand Guidelines Group, 1998.

EPIDEMIOLOGY AND RISK FACTORS

Statistics concerning prevalence are based primarily on elderly individuals in acute care settings. Estimated prevalence rates range from 10% to 30% of patients. In nursing homes, the prevalence is much higher, approaching 60% of those older than the age of 75 years. Delirium occurs in as many as 30% of patients hospitalized for cancer and in 30% to 40% of those hospitalized with acquired immunodeficiency syndrome (AIDS). Near death, 80% of patients experience delirium (APA, 2000).

Delirium is particularly common in older postoperative patients. The most powerful risks for developing delirium are present before admission. For example, pre-existing cognitive impairment is one of the greatest risk factors for delirium. Severe illness and age also put patients at higher risk for delirium, and male gender, alcohol abuse, and comorbidities contribute significantly. Risk factors include a fracture, depression, and impaired vision (Schuurmans, Duursma, & Shortridge-Baggett, 2001). One study concluded that patients with

or without dementia had persistant symptoms of delirium up to 12 months after diagnosis. The same study found that a quicker in-hospital recovery is associated with better outcomes (McCusker, Cole, Dendukuri, Han and Belzile, 2003). Patients experiencing mental confusion are also more likely to be victims of falls and fractures. Box 30-1 lists proposed risk factors for delirium, and Box 30-2 presents a vignette of a patient who experienced delirium after using an over-the-counter (OTC) sleeping medication.

ETIOLOGY

The etiology of delirium is complex and usually multifaceted. A lack of generally accepted theories of causation has resulted in considerable variability in the research. Thus, integrating the research and applying it to practice has been difficult. To date, studies focus almost exclusively on biologic causes of delirium, with psychosocial factors viewed as contributing or facilitating. Because environmental and psychosocial factors

BOX 30.1

Risk Factors for Delirium

- Advanced age
- Pre-existing dementia
- Functional dependence
- Pre-existing illness
- Bone fracture
- Infection
- Medications (both number and type)
- Changes in vital signs (including hypotension and hyper- or hypothermia)
- Electrolyte or metabolic imbalance
- Admission to a long-term care institution
- Postcardiotomy
- AIDS
- Pain

have been explored only in small, uncontrolled studies, conclusions cannot be drawn about these factors. For this reason, the following discussion of etiology covers biologic theories of cause.

The most commonly identified causes of delirium, in order of frequency, follow:

- Medications
- Infections (particularly urinary tract and upper respiratory)
- Fluid and electrolyte imbalance; metabolic disturbances
- Hypoxia/ischemia (Schuurmans et al., 2001).

The probability of the syndrome developing increases if certain predisposing factors, such as advanced age, brain damage, or dementia, are also present. Sensory overload or underload, immobilization, sleep deprivation, and psychosocial stress also contribute to delirium.

Because delirium has multiple causes, a wide variety of brain alterations may also be responsible for its development. Major theories of causation follow:

- A general reduction in brain functioning, which can result from a decrease in the supply, uptake, or use of substances for metabolic activity
- Damage of enzyme systems, the blood–brain barrier, or cell membranes
- Reduced brain metabolism resulting in decreased acetylcholine synthesis
- Imbalance of neurotransmitters, such as acetylcholine, norepinephrine, and dopamine
- Increased plasma cortisol level in response to acute stress, which affects attention and information processing
- Involvement of the white matter, especially in the thalamocortical projections (Tune, 2000).

INTERDISCIPLINARY TREATMENT AND PRIORITY CARE ISSUES

Although delirium may be recognized and diagnosed in any health care setting, appropriate intervention requires that the patient be admitted to an acute care setting for rigourous assessment and rapid treatment. The priority in care is identifying the underlying cause of the delirium. Interdisciplinary management of delirium includes two primary aspects: (1) elimination or correction of the underlying cause, and (2) symptomatic and supportive measures (eg, adequate rest, comfort, maintenance of fluid and electrolyte balance, and protection from injury) (House, 2000).

When developing a treatment plan for a patient in whom delirium is suspected, close attention must be paid to correcting any organic or disease-related factors. Initially, life-threatening illnesses, such as cerebral hypoxia,

BOX 30.2

Clinical Vignette: Delirium

Mrs. Campbell, a widowed 72-year-old woman living in her own home, has been having trouble sleeping. Her daughter visits her and suggests that Mrs. Campbell try an over-the-counter sleeping medication. Mrs. Campbell has also been taking antihistamines for allergies and the antidepressant amitriptyline. Three nights later, a neighbour calls the daughter, concerned because she encountered Mrs. Campbell wandering the streets, unable to find her home. When the neighbour approached Mrs. Cambell to help her home, Mrs. Campbell began to scream and strike out at the neighbour.

The daughter visits immediately and discovers that her mother does not know who she is, does not know what time it is, appears disheveled, and is suspicious that people have been in her home stealing the things she cannot find. Mrs. Campbell does not recall taking any medication, but when her daughter investigates she finds that 10 pills

of the new sleeping aid have already been used. Mrs. Campbell is irritable and refuses to go to the hospital, but over the course of a few hours, she appears to calm down, and her daughter is able to take her to see her physician the following morning. After hearing the history, the physician hospitalizes Mrs. Campbell, withholds all medication, and provides intravenous hydration. Within 3 days, Mrs. Campbell is again able to recognize her daughter, and her mental status appears to be greatly improved.

What Do You Think?

- Identify risk factors that may have contributed to Mrs. Campbell experiencing delirium.
- How could the addition of an OTC sleeping medication interact with the antihistamine and antidepressant to be responsible for Mrs. Campbell's delirium?

hypertensive encephalopathy, intracranial hemorrhage, meningitis, severe electrolyte and metabolic imbalances, hypoglycemia, and intoxication, must be ruled out or corrected. If possible, the use of all suspected medications should be stopped and vital signs monitored at least every 2 hours. Because many patients with delirium are seriously ill, excellent nursing care is vital. The plan of care requires close observation of the patient with particular regard to changes in vital signs, behaviour, and mental status. Patients are monitored until the delirium subsides or until discharge. If the delirium still exists at discharge, it is critical that referrals for postdischarge follow-up assessment and care be implemented.

NURSING MANAGEMENT: HUMAN RESPONSE TO DISORDER

By definition, a biologic insult must be present for delirium to occur, but psychological and environmental factors are often involved. Because delirium develops quickly during a matter of hours or days and has been associated with increased mortality, nurses should be particularly vigilant in assessing patients who are at increased risk for this syndrome. If the patient is a child, the assessment process presented in Chapter 25 should be used. If the patient is an elderly person, the assessment in Chapter 28 should serve as a guide. Special efforts should be made to include family members in the nursing process.

CRNE Note

Nurses need to be able to differentiate between the characteristics of dementia and those of delirium. Remember that it is possible for people with dementia to develop delirium, so that if agitation and a sudden change in mental status occur, assess the person for delirium.

Biologic Domain

Biologic Assessment

The onset of symptoms is typically signalled by a rapid or acute change in behaviour. To assess the symptoms, the nurse needs to know what is normal for the individual. Caregivers, family members, or significant others should be interviewed because they can often provide valuable information. Family members may be the only resource for accurate information.

Current and Past Health Status

History should include a description of the onset, duration, range, and intensity of associated symptoms. Chronic physical illness, dementia, depression, or other psychiatric illnesses should be identified. Sorting out historical information may be particularly problematic when delirium accompanies acute illness, recent surgery, or infection.

Physical Examination and Review of Systems

If the patient is cooperative, a physical examination will be conducted in the emergency room. Vital signs are crucial. A review of systems must be conducted in each patient suspected of having delirium or other organic mental disorders. Laboratory data, including a complete blood count, glucose, blood urea nitrogen, creatinine, and electrolyte analyses; liver function and oxygen saturation; as well as fluid balance, signs of constipation, or a recent history of diarrhea should be assessed in an attempt to discover an underlying cause.

Physical Functions

Functional assessment includes physical functional status (activities of daily living), use of sensory aids (eyeglasses and hearing aids), usual activity level and any recent changes, and pain assessment. Because sleep is often disturbed in patients with delirium, sleep patterns must be assessed, including what is typical for the individual and recent changes. Often, the sleep–wake cycle of the patient with delirium becomes reversed, with the individual attempting to sleep during the day and be awake at night. Sleep disturbances are a symptom of delirium, and sleep deprivation may add to the confusion. Restoration of a normal sleep cycle is extremely important.

Pharmacologic Assessment

A substance use history (including alcohol intake and smoking history) should be obtained (see Chapters 23 and 31). In addition, information regarding medication use must be obtained, with particular attention given to new medications or changes in dose of current medications. Table 30-4 lists some of the drugs that can cause an acute change in mental status. Special attention should be given to combinations of these medications because drug interactions can cause delirium.

Information regarding OTC medications should be included in this assessment. OTC medications are often thought of as harmless, but several, such as cold medications, taken in sufficient quantities may produce confusion, especially in older individuals.

Findings from the medication assessment are integrated with findings of the physical assessment, including such things as fluid and electrolyte balance, lack of adequate pain management, or serum drug levels, if available. For example, chronic pain may lead an individual to use more medication for pain relief than has been intended. Careful monitoring of the effectiveness of pain medications may lead to the use of a different medication that is more effective with less potential for misuse. Because many classes of medications have been

Table 30.4	Categories of Drugs That Can Cause "Acute Change in Mental Status"*
Mnemonic: Drug Category	**Examples of Drugs**
A ntiparkinsonian drugs	Trihexyphenidyl, benzatropine, bromocriptine, levadopa, selegiline (deprenyl)
C orticosteroids	Prednisolone
U rinary incontinence drugs	Oxybutinin (Ditropan), flavoxate (Urispas)
T heophylline	Theophylline
E mptying drugs (motility drugs)	Metoclopramide (Reglan), cisapride (Prepulsid)
C ardiovascular drugs (including antihypertensives)	Digoxin, quinidine, methaldopa, reserpine, beta blockers (propanolol—to a less amount), diuretics, ACE inhibitors (captopril, Enalapril), calcium channel antagonists (nifedipine, verapamil, diltiazem)
H $_2$ blockers	Cimetidine (uncommon on its own but increased risk with renal impairment)
A ntimicrobials	Cephalosporins, penicillin, quinolones, others
N SAIDs	Indomethacin, ibuprofen, naproxen, salicylate compounds
G eropsychiatry drugs	1. Tricylic antidepressants (eg, amitriptyline, desipramine – to a lesser extent, imipramine, nortriptyline) 2. SSRIs—safer but watch if hyponatremia present 3. Benzodiazepines (eg, diazepam) 4. Antipsychotics (eg, haloperidol (Haldol), chlorpromazine, risperidone)
E NT drugs	Antihistamines, decongestants, cough syrups in over-the-counter preparations
I nsomnia	Nitrazepam, flurazepam, diazepam, temazepam
N arcotics	Meperdine, pentazocine (risky)
M uscle relaxants	Cyclobenzaprine (Flexeril), methocarbamol (Robaxin)
S eizure drugs	Phenytoin, primidone

* This table notes some examples of possible medications that can contribute to delirium. It is the physiologic status of the older adult and the combination of medications, among other factors, that increase risk. Therefore: "Watch and Beware."
Reprinted from Flaherty, J. H., Commonly prescribed and over-the-counter medications: Causes of confusion *Clinics in Geriatric Medicine, 14*(1), 101–125, copyright (1998), with permission from Elsevier.

associated with delirium, the focus is on changes in the type and number of medications and how medications relate to other findings in the history and physical assessment.

Nursing Diagnoses for the Biologic Domain

The nursing diagnoses typically generated from assessment data are Acute Confusion, Disturbed Thought Processes, or Disturbed Sensory Perception (visual or auditory) (North American Nursing Diagnosis Association [NANDA], 2006). However, an astute nurse will also use nursing diagnoses based on other indicators, such as Hyperthermia, Acute Pain, Risk for Infection, and Disturbed Sleep Pattern.

Interventions for the Biologic Domain

Important interventions for a patient experiencing acute confusional state include providing a safe and therapeutic environment, maintaining fluid and electrolyte balance and adequate nutrition, and preventing aspiration and decubitus ulcers, which are often complications. Other interventions relate to a particular nursing diagnosis focused on individual symptoms and underlying causes, for example, for patients with Disturbed Sleep Patterns, the Sleep Enhancement inter-

vention is appropriate (McCloskey & Bulechek, 2000). Interventions to prevent delirium can reduce length of stay (McCusker, Cole, Dendukuri, & Belzile, 2003).

Safety Interventions

Behaviours exhibited by the delirious patient, such as hallucinations, delusions, illusions, aggression, or agitation (restlessness or excitability), may pose safety problems. The patient must be protected from physical harm by using low beds, guardrails, and careful supervision. The intervention Surveillance: Safety or Fall Prevention may be implemented (McCloskey & Bulechek, 2000) for any patient at risk for falls.

Pharmacologic Interventions

The goal of psychopharmacologic management is treatment of the behaviours associated with delirium, such as symptoms of agitation, inattention, sleep disorder, and psychosis, so that the patient can be more comfortable. The decision to use medications should be based on the specific symptoms. Dosages are usually kept very low, especially with elderly patients. There is no consensus on the use of psychopharmacologic agents to control the symptoms of delirium, and limited studies have been conducted. Use of these medications usually relates to agitation, combativeness, or hallucinations. However, medication should be chosen in light of the potential side effects (particularly anticholinergic effects, hypotension, and respiratory suppression) and in light of making the delirium worse. For most patients with delirium, short-term use of an antipsychotic agent, such as risperidone (Risperdal), is recommended (Schwartz & Masand, 2002). The use of antipsychotic agents in older individuals is discussed in greater detail later in the chapter. Benzodiazepines have also been tried but should be used only when the delirium is related to alcohol withdrawal. In some patients, these medications may further impair cognition because of the sedation, so in some cases, a paradoxic agitation may develop (Gleason, 2003).

Administering and Monitoring Medications

Patients experiencing delirium may resist taking medication because of their confusion. If medication is given, ideally it should be oral.

MONITORING AND MANAGING SIDE EFFECTS. Monitoring drug action and side effects is especially important because the cause of the delirium may not be known, and the patient may inadvertently be affected by the medication. Patients should be monitored for sedation, hypotension, or extrapyramidal symptoms. Although mental status often fluctuates during delirium, it may also be influenced by these medications, and any changes or worsening of mental status after administration of the medication should be reported immediately to the prescriber. Some side effects may also be confused with the symptoms of delirium. For example, akathisia (see Chapter 13) may appear to be agitation or restlessness. The patient's physical condition and concurrent medication regimen may also influence the bioavailability, metabolism, and elimination of these medications. Adequate hydration and nutrition must be maintained. When using antipsychotic medications, closely monitor the patient for symptoms of neuroleptic malignant syndrome (see Chapter 13). The appearance of these symptoms may be missed because many may be confused with those related to delirium.

Finally, the use of antipsychotic agents or other medications for treating symptoms related to delirium should be discontinued as soon as possible. These medications should not be stopped abruptly, but rather should be withdrawn gradually during a period of several days or weeks.

IDENTIFYING DRUG INTERACTIONS. The etiology of delirium is often a drug–drug interaction. OTC sleeping, cold, or allergy medication may be the cause. If medication is the underlying cause, it is important to identify accurately which medications are involved before administering any other drugs. A consultation with a clinical pharmacist may also be helpful.

Teaching Points

To prevent future occurrences, the nurse needs to educate the patient and family about the underlying cause of the delirium. If the delirium is not resolved before discharge, family members need to know how to care for the patient at home.

Psychological Domain

Assessment

Psychological assessment of the individual with delirium focuses on cognitive changes revealed through the mental status examination as well as the resulting behavioural manifestations. Changes in mental status must be monitored frequently for early detection of delirium, especially in older individuals. In addition, other factors, such as stressors and environmental change, may contribute to the symptoms.

Mental Status

Rapid onset of global cognitive impairment that affects multiple aspects of intellectual functioning is the hallmark of delirium. Mental status evaluation reveals several changes:

- Fluctuations in level of consciousness with reduced awareness of the environment
- Difficulty focusing and sustaining or shifting attention
- Severely impaired memory, especially immediate and recent memory

Patients may be disorientated to time and place but rarely to person. Environmental perceptions are often disturbed. The patient may believe shadows in the room are really people. Thought content is often illogical, and speech may be incoherent or inappropriate to the context. Each variation in mental status tends to fluctuate over the course of the day. During the same day, an individual with delirium may appear confused and uncooperative, whereas later, may be lucid and able to follow instructions. Nurses must continually assess the cognitive status of the individual throughout the day so that interventions can be modified accordingly.

Calculations, orientation (especially to time), and recall are most affected in delirium, whereas naming and registration are relatively preserved. Several rating scales are available for use in assessing the cognitive and behavioural fluctuations of delirium (Box 30-3).

Behaviour

Delirious patients exhibit a wide range of behaviours, complicating the process of making a diagnosis and planning interventions. At times the individual may be restless or agitated, and at other times, lethargic and slow to respond. Delirium can be categorized into three types.

- **Hyperkinetic delirium** involves behaviours most commonly recognized as delirium (eg, psychomotor hyperactivity, marked excitability, and a tendency toward hallucinations).

BOX 30.3

Rating Scales for Use With Delirium

The Confusion Assessment Method (CAM)

Inouye, S. K., van Dyck, C. H., Alessi, C. A., et al. (1990). Clarifying confusion: The confusion assessment method. *Annals of Internal Medicine, 113*, 941–948.

Confusion Rating Scale (CRS)

Williams, M. A., Ward, S. E., & Campbell, E. B. (1988). Confusion: Testing versus observation. *Journal of Gerontological Nursing, 14*(1), 25–30.

Delirium Symptom Interview

Levkoff, S., Liptzin, B., Cleary, P., et al. (1991). Review of research instruments and techniques used to detect delirium. *International Psychogeriatrics, 3*, 253–271.

Delirium Rating Scale (DRS)

Trzepacz, P. T., Baker, R. W., & Greenhouse J. (1988). A symptom rating scale for delirium. *Psychiatry Research, 23*, 89–97.

High Sensitivity Cognitive Screen (HSCS)

Faust, D., & Fogel, B. S. (1989). The development and initial validation of a sensitive bedside cognitive screening test. *Journal of Nervous and Mental Disease, 177*, 25–31.

NEECHAM Confusion Scale

Neelon, V. J., Champagne, M. T., McConnell, E., et al. (1992). Use of the NEECHAM Confusion Scale to assess acute confusional states of hospitalized older patients. In S. G. Funk, E. M. Tornquist, M. T. Champagne, & R. A. Wiese (Eds.), *Key aspects of elder care*. New York: Springer.

Visual Analog Scale for Acute Confusion (VASAC)

Cacchione, P. Z. (2002). Assessment. Four acute confusion assessment instruments: Reliability and validity for use in long-term care facilities. *Journal of Gerontological Nursing, 28*(1), 12–19.

- **Hypokinetic delirium** is marked by lethargy, sleepiness, and apathy, and psychomotor activity decreases; this is the "quiet" patient for whom the diagnosis of delirium often is missed.
- **Mixed variant delirium** involves behaviour that fluctuates between the hyperactive and hypoactive states.

Nursing Diagnoses for the Psychological Domain

The nursing diagnosis Acute Confusion is also associated with impaired cognitive functioning. Although the underlying cause of confusion is physiologic, nursing care should focus on the psychological domain, as well as the physical. Other typical nursing diagnoses related to the psychological domain include Disturbed Thought Process, Ineffective Coping, and Disturbed Personal Identity.

Interventions for the Psychological Domain

Staff should have frequent interaction with patients and support them if they are confused or hallucinating. Patients should be encouraged to express their fears and discomforts that result from frightening or disconcerting psychotic experiences. Adequate lighting, easy-to-read calendars and clocks, a reasonable noise level, and frequent verbal orientation may reduce this frightening experience. If the patient wears eyeglasses or uses a hearing aid, these devices should be used. Including familiar personal possessions in the environment may also help. Interventions that may be useful for these individuals are discussed in detail later in the chapter (see the section on dementia).

Social Domain

Assessment

Discussion should be initiated with the family to determine whether the patient's behaviours are new. An assessment of living arrangements may provide information about sensory stimulation or social isolation. Cultural and educational background must be considered when the patient's mental capacity is evaluated. Individuals from certain ethnic backgrounds may not be familiar with the information used in tests of general knowledge (eg, names of prime ministers, geographic knowledge), memory (eg, date of birth in cultures that do not routinely celebrate birthdays), and orientation (eg, sense of placement and location may be conceptualized differently in some cultures) (APA, 2000). Some cultural practices may involve using substances such as elixirs that contain chemicals that may exacerbate delirium. Assessment should address these practices.

Family Roles

Family support for the individual and understanding of the disorder must be assessed. The behaviours exhibited by the person experiencing delirium may be frightening or at least confusing for family members. Some family members may actually contribute to the patient's increased agitation. Assessing family interactions and family members' ability to understand delirium is important. If feasible, family presence may help to calm and reassure the patient.

Nursing Diagnoses for the Social Domain

Several nursing diagnoses associated with the social domain can be generated. Interrupted Family Processes, Ineffective Protection, Ineffective Role Performance, and Risk for Injury are the most typical. Risk for Injury is a high-priority diagnosis because individuals with delirium are more likely to fall or injure themselves during a confused state (Carpenito-Moyet, 2004).

Interventions for the Social Domain

The environment needs to be safe to protect the patient from injury. A predictable, orienting environment will help to re-establish order to the patient's life. That is, a calendar, clocks, and other items may be provided to help orient the patient to time, place, and person. If the patient is agitated, de-escalation techniques should be used (see Chapter 12). Physical restraint should be avoided.

Support from Families

Families can be encouraged to work with staff to reorient the patient and provide a supportive environment. Families need to understand that important decisions requiring the patient's input should be delayed if at all possible until the patient has recovered. Although patients may be able to participate in decision making, they may not remember the decision later; therefore, it is important to have several witnesses present.

EVALUATION AND TREATMENT OUTCOMES

The primary treatment goal is prevention or resolution of the delirious episode with return to previous cognitive status. Outcome measures include

- correction of the underlying physiologic alteration
- resolution of confusion
- family member verbalization of understanding of confusion
- prevention of injury.

Resolution of confusion is the primary goal; however, the nurse makes important contributions to all four of these outcomes. The end result of delirium is either full recovery, incomplete recovery, incomplete recovery with some residual cognitive impairment, or a downward course leading to death.

CONTINUUM OF CARE

The nurse may encounter patients with delirium in a number of treatment settings (eg, home, nursing home, ambulatory care, day treatment, outpatient setting, hospital). Patients usually are admitted to an acute care setting for rapid evaluation and treatment of the underlying etiology. An abrupt change in cognitive status can also occur while the patient is hospitalized for another reason. Delirium often persists beyond discharge from the hospital. Discharge planning should routinely include family education and referrals to community health care providers. If the patient will return to a res-

BOX 30.4

Psychoeducation Checklist: Delirium

When caring for the patient with delirium, be sure to include the caregivers, as appropriate, and address the following topic areas in the teaching plan:

☐ Psychopharmacologic agents, if used, including drug action, dosage, frequency, and possible adverse effects
☐ Underlying cause of delirium
☐ Mental status changes
☐ Safety measures
☐ Hydration and nutrition
☐ Avoidance of restraints
☐ Decision-making guidelines

idential long-term care setting, communication with facility staff about the patient's hospital stay and treatment regimen is crucial. For more information on caring for patients with delirium, see Box 30-4.

Dementia of the Alzheimer Type

CLINICAL COURSE OF DISORDER

Alzheimer disease (AD) is a degenerative, progressive neuropsychiatric disorder that results in cognitive impairment, emotional and behavioural changes, physical and functional decline, and ultimately death. Gradually, the patient's ability to carry out activities of daily living declines, although physical status often remains intact until late in the disease. Primarily a disorder of older individuals, AD has been diagnosed in patients as young as age 35 years.

Two subtypes have been identified: early-onset AD (age 65 years and younger) and late-onset AD (age older than 65 years). Late-onset AD is much more common than early-onset AD, but early-onset AD has a more rapid progression. AD is also routinely conceptualized in terms of three stages: mild, moderate, and severe. Signs and symptoms of AD change as the patient passes from one phase of the illness to another (Fig. 30-1). It is unclear whether all patients with AD pass through a specific sequence of deterioration and whether the staging of a patient at initial assessment has any prognostic implications in terms of speed of decline. Nevertheless, staging is a useful technique for determining the patient's current cognitive status and provides a sound basis for decisions in clinical management.

DIAGNOSTIC CRITERIA

The diagnosis of AD is made on clinical grounds, and verification is confirmed at autopsy by abnormal

Early Stage (2–4 years)	Middle Stage (2–10 years)	Late Stage (1–3 years)
Mild forgetfulness Difficulty processing new information Reduced concentration Communication difficulties Problems with orientation Mood shifts Passive Restless	Deterioration in mental abilities, mood and behaviour Disorientation Personality changes Wandering, pacing Disinhibited Assistance needed for ADL	Mental capacities severely compromised Restricted emotions Increased sleep Incontinent Unable to perform ADL Increasingly nonverbal

FIGURE 30.1   Signs and symptoms of the stages of Alzheimer Disease
Reference: National Advisory Council on Aging (2004).

degenerative structures, neuritic plaques, and neurofibrillary tangles. The essential feature of AD is multiple cognitive deficits, especially memory impairment, and at least one of the following cognitive disturbances: **aphasia** (alterations in language ability), **apraxia** (impaired ability to execute motor activities despite intact motor functioning), **agnosia** (failure to recognize or identify objects despite intact sensory function), or a **disturbance of executive functioning** (ability to think abstractly, plan, initiate, sequence, monitor, and stop complex behaviour).

The cognitive deficits must be sufficiently severe to impair occupational or social functioning and must represent a decline from a previously higher level of functioning (APA, 2000). These symptoms are common to all presentations of dementia, regardless of the underlying pathology. Table 30-5 lists essential symptoms of dementia, along with other possible behavioural and psychological changes that may or may not be present. To make a diagnosis of AD, all other known causes of dementia must be excluded (eg, vascular,

AIDS, Parkinson's disease, and others). Box 30-5 lists 10 warning signs of AD.

Mild Cognitive Impairment

When people experience memory problems but do not meet the diagnostic criteria for dementia, they are thought to have mild cognitive impairment (MCI). In some studies, about 40% of these individuals develop AD within 3 years. Others never develop AD (United States Department of Health and Human Services [U.S. DHHS], 2003).

EPIDEMIOLOGY AND RISK FACTORS

In 1991, 8% of the Canadian population 65 years and older suffered from dementia. It is forecasted that the number of Canadians with dementia will triple between 1991 and 2031, increasing from 253,000 to 778,000. The proportion of the population older than 65 years of age will double during the same time period. The 1991 data show that the probability of suffering from dementia rises with age: 2.4% among those 65 to 74, 11.1% among those 75 to 84, and 34.5% among those 85 and older. The prevalence doubles every 5.1 years after the age of 65 years (Canadian Study of Health and Aging Working Group, 1994; Daziel, 1994; Ebly et al., 1994).

To date, only age, a familial tendency for either AD or Down's syndrome, female gender, head trauma, and low educational level or illiteracy are identified risk factors for AD. Studies evaluating other factors, including impaired immunity, viruses, and environmental toxins (eg, aluminum), are ongoing. Alzheimer type dementia is twice as common in women as in men, but this may be because women tend to live longer than men, and the incidence of AD increases with age.

BOX 30.5

10 Warnings Signs of Alzheimer Disease

To help the public know the warning signs of AD, the Alzheimer Society of Canada lists the following:
1. Memory loss that affects day-to-day function
2. Difficulty performing familiar tasks
3. Problems with language
4. Disorientation of time and place
5. Poor or decreased judgment
6. Problems with abstract thinking
7. Misplacing things
8. Changes in mood and behaviour
9. Changes in personality
10. Loss of initiative
See http://www.alzheimer.ca for more information.

Table 30.5   Key Diagnostic Characteristics for Dementia of the Alzheimer's Type 290

With early onset:
With delirium 290.11
With delusions 290.12
With depressed mood 290.13
Uncomplicated 290.10
With late onset:
With delirium 290.3
With delusions 290.20
With depressed mood 290.21
Uncomplicated 290.0

Diagnostic Criteria

- Development of multiple cognitive deficits
- Involvement of both memory impairment and one or more of the following cognitive disturbances: aphasia, apraxia, agnosia, or disturbance in executive functioning
- Significant impairment in social or occupational functioning resulting from cognitive deficits; significant decline from previous level of functioning
- Cognitive deficits not due to: other CNS conditions causing progressive deficits in memory or cognition; systemic conditions known to cause dementia; substance-induced conditions
- Not occurring exclusively during course of a delirium
- Not better accounted for by another Axis I disorder
    Early onset: age 65 y or less
    Late onset: over age 65 y

Target Symptoms and Associated Findings

- Memory impairment
- Cognitive disturbances

Associated Behavioural Findings
- Spatial disorientation and difficulty with spatial tasks
- Poor judgment and poor insight
- Little or no awareness of memory loss or other cognitive abnormalities
- Unrealistic assessment of abilities; underestimation of risks involved in activities
- Possible suicidal behaviours (usually in early stages when individual is more capable of carrying out a plan of action)
- Possible gait disturbances and falls
- Disinhibited behaviour, such as inappropriate jokes, neglect of personal hygiene, undue familiarity with strangers, or disregard for conventional rules of social conduct
- Delusions, especially ones involving persecution
- Superimposed delirium

Associated Physical Examination Findings
- Few motor or sensory signs (in the first year of illness)
- Myoclonus and gait disorder (later)
- Seizure possible

Associated Laboratory Findings
- Brain atrophy (with computed tomography or magnetic resonance imaging)
- Senile plaques, neurofibrillary tangles, granulovascular degeneration, neuronal loss, astrocytic gliosis, and amyloid angiopathy on microscopic examination

AD can run in families. Compared with the general population, first-degree biologic relatives of individuals with early-onset AD are more likely to experience the disorder. So far, studies point toward genetically related risk factors only in familial AD, which accounts for only a small proportion of cases of AD (less than 5%) (Cummings, 2003). The hypothesis that low educational level may increase the risk for AD remains a matter of controversy. The connection between AD and education is unclear at this time. One theory is that education has a direct biologic effect on the brain, which increases synaptic reserve. Prior head injury leading to unconsciousness may represent a significant risk factor for the later development of AD, perhaps accounting for 5% to 10% of the attributable risk (Guo et al., 2000).

ETIOLOGY

Researchers have yet to identify a definitive cause of AD. In general, the brain appears normal in the early phases of AD, but it undergoes widespread atrophy as the disease advances. Although causation remains in question, new research using a brain scan–based computer program that measures brain metabolism in the hippocampus supports the possibility of screening for early AD (Mosconi et al., 2005).

Dame Iris Murdoch (1919–1999)

Public Persona

Born in Dublin, Ireland, Dame Iris Murdoch became a much loved philosopher and writer, the author of 36 novels, several plays, essays and philosophical works, and a critical study of Jean-Paul Sartre. Over her life, she filled 95 diaries with her aspirations and self-analysis of her own shortcomings. Her book, *The Sea, The Sea* won the Booker Prize in 1978. Iris Murdoch was elected as a fellow to St. Anne's College, Oxford in 1948 and remained a tutor there until 1963.

Personal Realities

Iris Murdoch married John Bayley in 1955. In the mid-1990s, she began to show signs of Alzheimer disease. Her extensive vocabulary became diminished; she had difficulty in answering questions, and there was a noticeable decline in the quality of her last book, *Jackson's Dilemma*. She died of AD in 1995. Her husband's book about her life, an *Elegy for Iris* (1999), was made into a movie, *Iris*, in 2001.

Beta-amyloid Plaques

One piece of the puzzle is partially explained by a leading theory that, in AD, beta-amyloid deposits destroy cholinergic neurons, in a manner similar to cholesterol causing atherosclerosis. It is hypothesized that **beta-amyloid plaques**, dense, mostly insoluble deposits of protein and cellular material outside and around neurons, gradually increase in number and are abnormally distributed throughout the cholinergic system. Plaques are partly made of a protein, beta-amyloid protein, which is a fragment snipped from a larger protein called amyloid precursor protein (APP) and apolipoprotein A (apoA) cores. Neuritic plaque densities are highest in the temporal and occipital lobes, intermediate in the parietal lobes, and lowest in the frontal and limbic cortex. Symptoms such as aphasia and visuospatial abnormalities are attributable to plaque formation (Cummings, 2003). Study continues as investigators examine the process by which APP releases beta-amyloid protein, how the fragments accumulate in the brain, and whether the plaques cause AD or are a by-product.

Neurofibrillary Tangles

Neurofibrillary tangles are made of paired helical filaments of a chemically altered protein, or tau proteins, that disrupt normal intracellular transport and result in cell death. They are initially found in the limbic area and then progress to the cortex. Neurofibrillary tangles contribute to memory disturbance and psychiatric symptoms (Cummings, 2003). It is thought that formation of these neurofibrillary tangles is related to the apolipoprotein E4

(apoE$_4$). Apolipoprotein (apoE) is a normal cholesterol-carrying protein produced by a gene on chromosome 19, which has three forms: apoE$_2$, apoE$_3$, and apoE$_4$. It appears that apoE$_3$ protects against abnormal changes in proteins that lead to neurofibrillary tangles, associated with late-onset dementia, but apoE$_4$ appears to leave these proteins unprotected and increases the patient's risk for AD (Stahl, 2000) (Fig. 30-2).

Cell Death and Neurotransmitters

In patients with AD, neurotransmission is reduced, neurons are lost, and the hippocampal neurons degenerate. Several major neurotransmitters are affected. **Acetylcholine** (ACh) is associated with cognitive functioning, and disruption of cholinergic mechanisms damages memory in animals and humans (see Chapter 9). Cell loss in the nucleus basalis leads to deficits in the synthesis of cortical acetylcholine, but the number of ACh receptors is relatively unchanged. The reduced ACh is related to a decrease in *choline acetyltransferase* (a critical enzyme in the synthesis of ACh), especially in the forebrain. That is, there are fewer enzymes available to synthesize ACh, which leads to a reduction in cholinergic activity. Positron emission tomography (PET) scans, such as those in Figure 30-3, show changes in brain function.

Other neurotransmitters that are affected include norepinephrine and serotonin. Deficiencies in norepinephrine are associated with loss of cells in the locus ceruleus, and neuronal loss in the raphe nuclei leads to a loss of serotoninergic activity (Cummings, 2003).

Genetic Factors

Approximately half of the cases of early-onset AD appear to be transmitted as a pure genetic, autosomal dominant trait caused by mutations in genes on chromosomes 1 and 14 (Rogaeva, 2002; Suh & Checler, 2002). Mutations on chromosome 14 account for most cases of early-onset familial AD (Taddei et al., 2002). Chromosome 21 is also associated with AD because amyloid plaques and neurofibrillary tangles accumulate consistently in older people with Down's syndrome (trisomy 21) who have AD. The role of chromosome 19 in the production of apoE was previously discussed.

Oxidative Stress and Free Radicals

One theory of aging and neurodegeneration is that damage from oxygen free radicals (highly reactive molecules) can build up in neurons over time. This **oxidative stress** can modify or damage cellular molecules, such as proteins, lipids, and nucleic acids. This type of damage has been observed in AD, especially in the late stages when the beta-amyloid plaques and neurofibrillary

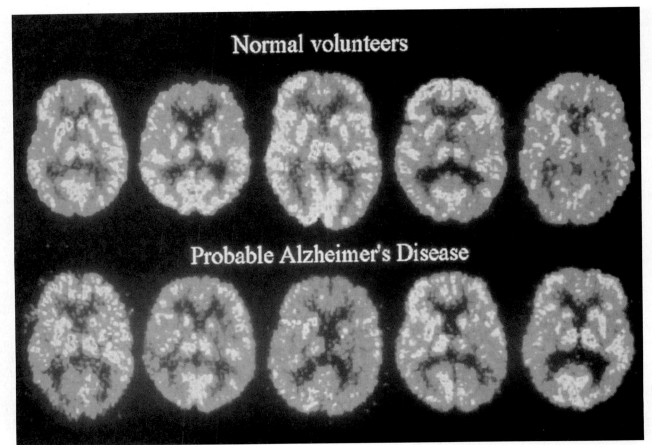

FIGURE 30.2   Series comparison of elderly control subjects (*top row*) and patients with Alzheimer disease (*bottom row*). Although there are some decreases in metabolism associated with age, in most patients with Alzheimer's disease, there are marked decreases in the temporal lobe, an area important in memory functions. (Courtesy of Monte S. Buchsbaum, MD, The Mount Sinai Medical Centre and School of Medicine, New York, NY.)

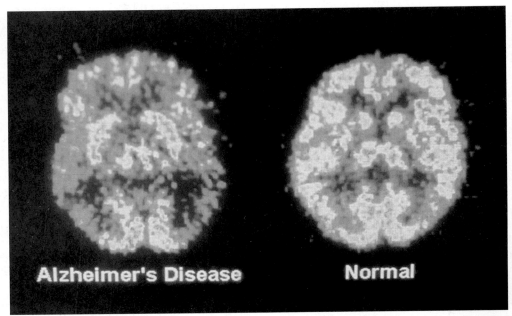

FIGURE 30.3   Metabolic activity in a subject with Alzheimer disease (*left*) and in a control subject (*right*). (Courtesy of Monte S. Buchsbaum, MD, The Mount Sinai Medical Center and School of Medicine, New York, NY.)

tangles are present. However, it is not known whether the oxidative stress causes or results from the process of plaque formation (U.S. DHHS, 2003).

Inflammation

Inflammation in the brain is one of the early hallmarks of AD, but it is unknown whether it is a cause or effect. The use of certain medications, such as nonsteroidal anti-inflammatory drugs and estrogen, may delay the onset of the disorder (Tarkowski, Andreasen, Tarkowski, & Blennow, 2003). Vitamin E and the drug selegiline (Deprenyl) appear to delay important milestones in the course of AD, including severe functional impairments, even as the disease progresses (Sano et al., 1997).

INTERDISCIPLINARY TREATMENT

In designing services and interventions, the interdisciplinary team must keep in mind that AD has a progressively deteriorating clinical course and that the anatomic and neurochemical changes that occur in the brain are accompanied by impairments in cognition, sensorium, affect (facial expression representing mood), behaviour, and psychosocial functioning. The nature and range of services needed by patients and families throughout the illness can vary dramatically at different stages.

Initial assessment of the patient suspected of having dementia has three main objectives: (1) confirmation of the diagnosis, (2) establishment of baseline levels in a number of functional spheres, and (3) establishment of a therapeutic relationship with the patient and family that will continue through subsequent phases of the disease. Treatment efforts currently focus on managing the cognitive symptoms, delaying the cognitive decline (eg, memory loss, confusion, and problems with learning, speech, and reasoning), treating the noncognitive symptoms (eg, psychosis, mood symptoms, agitation), and supporting the caregivers as a means of improving the quality of life for both patients and their caregivers.

PRIORITY CARE ISSUES

The priority of care will change throughout the course of AD. Initially, the priority is delaying cognitive decline and supporting family members. Later, the priority changes to protecting the patient from injury because of lack of judgment. Near the end, the physical needs of the patient are the focus of care.

FAMILY RESPONSE TO DISORDER

Families are the first to be aware of the cognitive problem, often before the patient, who can be unaware of the extent of memory impairment. When finally con-

firmed, the actual diagnosis can be devastating to the family and patient (Werezak & Stewart, 2002). Unlike delirium, a diagnosis of AD means long-term care responsibilities, while the essence of a family member diminishes day by day. Most families keep their relative at home as long as possible to maintain contact and to avoid costly nursing home placement. The two symptoms that often result in nursing home placement are incontinence that cannot be managed and behavioural problems, such as wandering and aggression.

Especially in dementia, the needs of family members should also be considered. Caring for a family member with dementia takes its toll. Caregivers' health is often compromised, and normal family functioning is threatened. Caregiver distress is a major health risk for the family, and "caregiver burnout" is a common cause of institutionalization of patients with dementia.

NURSING MANAGEMENT: HUMAN RESPONSE TO DISORDER

The development and implementation of appropriate, effective, and safe nursing services for the care and support of patients with dementia and their families is a particular challenge because of the complex nature of the illness. Although AD is caused by biologic changes, the psychological and social domains are seriously affected by this disorder. The assessment of the patient with AD should follow the geriatric mental health nursing assessment in Chapter 28.

Biologic Domain

Assessment

The nursing assessment should include a medical history, current medication profile (prescription and OTC medications or home remedies), substance abuse history (including alcohol intake and smoking history), chronic physical or psychiatric illness, and a description of the onset, duration, range, and intensity of symptoms associated with dementia. The onset of symptoms in dementia is typically gradual, with insidious changes in behaviour. To conduct a thorough assessment of the patient with dementia, the nurse needs to know what is typical for the individual; therefore, caregivers, family members, or significant others can be sources of valuable information.

Physical Examination and a Review of Body Systems

A review of body systems must be conducted on each patient suspected of having dementia. Specific biologic assessment parameters for a patient with dementia include vital signs, neurologic status, nutritional status, bladder and bowel function, hygiene (including oral hygiene), skin integrity, rest and activity level, sleep patterns, and fluid and electrolyte balance. The neurologic function of the patient with AD is usually preserved through the early and middle stages of the disease, although seizures, gait disturbances, and tremors may occur at any time. In the later stages of the disease, neurologic signs, such as flexion contractures and primitive reflexes, are prominent features.

Physical Functions

At first, limitations may primarily involve instrumental activities, such as shopping, preparing meals, and performing other household chores. Later in the disease process, basic physical dysfunctions occur, such as incontinence, ataxia, dysphagia, and contractures. Incontinence can be a major source of stress and a considerable burden to family caregivers. Evaluation of the patient's functional abilities includes bathing, dressing, toileting, feeding, nutritional status, physical mobility, sleep patterns, and pain.

Assessment of physical functions includes activities of daily living, recent changes in functional abilities, use of sensory aids (glasses and hearing aids), activity level, and assessment of pain. Eyeglasses and hearing aids may need to be in place before other assessments can be made.

Self-Care

Alterations in the central nervous system (CNS) associated with dementia impair the patient's ability to collect information from the environment, retrieve memories, retain new information, and give meaning to current situations. Therefore, patients with dementia often neglect self-care activities. Periodically, biologic assessment parameters need to be re-evaluated because patients with dementia may neglect activities such as bathing, eating, or skin care.

Sleep–Wake Disturbances

The sleep–wake disturbances that commonly occur in dementia are hypersomnia, insomnia, and reversal of the sleep–wake cycle. These disturbances may be attributable partly to physiologic changes, neurotransmitters, or metabolic changes resulting from a dementia-causing disease or injury, but they are often of environmental or iatrogenic origin. Patients with dementia have frequent daytime napping and nighttime periods of wakefulness, with little rapid eye movement (REM) sleep. Lowered levels of REM sleep are associated with restlessness, irritability, and general sleep impairment (Turner, D'Amato, Chervin, & Blaivas, 2000).

Activity and Exercise

One of the earliest symptoms of AD is withdrawal from normal activities. The patient may just sit staring at a blank wall.

Nutrition

Eating can become a problem for a patient with dementia. As the disease progresses, patients may lose the ability to feed themselves or recognize what is offered as food. The hyperactive patient requires frequent feedings of a high-protein, high-carbohydrate diet in the form of finger foods (which they can carry while on the go). It may be wise to secure a fanny pack around the patient's waist with an assortment of nutritious finger foods appropriate for the patient who can no longer use eating utensils properly. Most patients with dementia prefer to feed themselves with their fingers rather than have someone feed them.

Some patients with dementia are bulimic or hyperoral (eating or chewing almost everything possible and sometimes with an insatiable appetite). In fact, some patients with advanced dementia put inedible objects into their mouths, presumably because they fail to recognize the objects as nonfood items. Other patients with dementia experience anorexia and have no appetite. It is important to monitor patients with altered appetites for hydration and electrolyte imbalances. Maintaining weight and proper hydration status are signs of effective nursing interventions.

Pain

Assessment and documentation of any physical discomfort or pain the patient may be experiencing is a part of any geropsychiatric nursing assessment (see Chapter 10). Although AD is not usually thought of as a physically painful disorder, patients often have other comorbid physical diseases that may be painful. In the early stages of AD, the patient can usually respond to verbal questions regarding pain. Later, it may be difficult to assess objectively the comfort level, especially if the patient cannot communicate. Some patients in the end stage of dementia become hypersensitive to touch.

Pain can be assessed by obtaining vital signs, completing a physical assessment, and using one of the pain assessment scales (see Chapter 10). Sometimes, laboratory tests must be conducted to help identify the source of discomfort. Subtle behavioural changes, such as lethargy, anxiety, or restlessness, or more obvious physical signs, such as pyrexia, tachypnea, or tachycardia, may be the only indications of actual or impending illness. Observing for changes in patterns of nonverbal communication, such as facial expressions, may help the nurse identify indicators of pain. Hypervocalizations (disturbed vocalizations), restlessness, and agitation are other possible signs of pain.

Nursing Diagnoses for the Biologic Domain

The unique and changing needs of these patients present a challenge for nurses in all settings. A multitude of potential nursing diagnoses focusing on the biologic domain can be identified for this population. A sample of common nursing diagnoses include Imbalanced

Nutrition: Less (or More) Than Body Requirements; Feeding Self-Care Deficit; Impaired Swallowing; Bathing/Hygiene Self-Care Deficit; Dressing/Grooming Self-Care Deficit; Toileting Self-Care Deficit; Constipation (or Perceived Constipation); Bowel Incontinence; Impaired Urinary Elimination; Functional Incontinence; Total Incontinence; Deficient Fluid Volume; Risk for Impaired Skin Integrity; Impaired Physical Mobility; Activity Intolerance; Fatigue; Disturbed Sleep Pattern; Pain; Chronic Pain; Ineffective Health Maintenance; and Impaired Home Maintenance.

Interventions for the Biologic Domain

The numerous interventions for the biologic domain vary throughout the course of the disorder. Initially, the patient requires simple directions for self-care activities and initiation of psychopharmacologic treatment. At the end of the disorder, total patient care is required.

Self-Care Interventions

Patients should be encouraged to maintain as much self-care as possible (See Box 30-6). Promotion of self-care supports cognitive functioning and a sense of independence. In the early stages, the nurse should maximize normal perceptual experiences by making sure that the patient and family have appropriate eyeglasses and working hearing aids. If eyeglasses and hearing aids are needed, but not used, patients are more likely to have false perceptual experiences (hallucinations). Ongoing monitoring of self-care is necessary throughout the course of AD. Oral hygiene can be a problem and requires excellent basic nursing care. Aging and many medications reduce salivary flow, which can lead to a painfully dry and cracking oral mucosa. Drugs that have xerostomia (dry mouth) as a side effect and are commonly prescribed for patients with progressive dementia include antidepressant, antispasmodic, antihypertensive, bronchodilator, and some antipsychotic agents. For patients with xerostomia, hard candy or chewing gum may stimulate salivary flow, or modification of the drug regimen may be necessary. Glycerol mouthwash can provide as much relief from xerostomia as artificial saliva.

Nutritional Interventions

Maintenance of nutrition and hydration are essential nursing interventions. The patient's weight, oral intake, and hydration status should be monitored carefully. Patients with dementia should eat well-balanced meals that are appropriate to their activity level and eating abilities, with special attention given to electrolyte balance and fluid intake.

When swallowing is a problem for the patient, thick liquids or semisoft foods are more effective than traditionally prepared foods. If a patient is likely to choke or aspirate food, less liquid (pureed) and more semisolid foods should be included in the diet because liquid flows into the pharyngeal cavity more quickly than does solid food.

The dining environment should be calm and food presentation appealing. If the patient eats only a small portion of food at one meal, reduce the presentation of food in terms of the amount and number of choices. One-dish meals (eg, a casserole) are ideal. If the patient is stressed or upset, it is better to delay feeding because eating, chewing, and swallowing difficulties are accentuated (Schell & Kayser-Jones, 1999).

As dementia progresses, intensive feeding efforts are needed to ensure adequate food and fluid intake. If food intake is low, vitamin and mineral supplements may be indicated. If weight loss cannot be stopped by skillful feeding or dietary adjustments, then enteral or parenteral feedings may be considered. The patient's quality of life is an important issue to consider when the family or other health care proxy must decide whether to use artificial feeding mechanisms. By inserting a feeding tube, the goal of sustaining weight can be met, but patient comfort may be jeopardized, especially if restraints are used to keep the tube in place.

BOX 30.6   RESEARCH FOR BEST PRACTICE

Learning to Live With Early Dementia

THE QUESTION: Few studies address the needs and concerns of dementia patients from their own perspective. To address this gap, research was undertaken to explore and conceptualize the process of learning to live with memory loss in older adults with early-stage dementia.

METHODS: A qualitative grounded theory approach was used to explore the subjective experience of people with early-stage dementia. Theoretical sampling was carried out to obtain six participants who were interviewed twice. Data from the first interviews were coded and analyzed, and a preliminary theory was developed. The second interview, which was less structured, was used to verify and clarify the emerging theory.

FINDINGS: The theory that emerged can best be described as a *continuous process of adjusting to early-stage dementia*. The process consists of five core categories or stages: antecedents, anticipation, appearance, assimilation, and acceptance.

IMPLICATIONS FOR NURSING: The proposed framework offers a base of valuable information to nurses working with people who have early-stage dementia, whereas the core concepts provide a foundation for future research to test the applicability of the model in the larger population of people with dementia.

From Werezak, L., & Stewart, N. (2002). Learning to live with early dementia. *Canadian Journal of Nursing Research, 34*(1), 67–85.

The patient with dementia should be presented food that is easy to chew (soft) and swallow and not too hot or cold. In the later stages of progressive dementia, some patients hoard food in their mouths without actually swallowing it; others swallow too rapidly or fail to chew their food sufficiently before attempting to swallow. The nurse needs to watch for swallowing difficulties that place the patient at risk for aspiration and asphyxiation. Swallowing difficulties may result from changes in esophageal motility and decreased secretion of saliva.

Supporting Bowel and Bladder Function

Urinary or bowel incontinence affects many patients with dementia. During middle phases of the disease, incontinence may be caused by the patient's inability to communicate the need to use the toilet or locate a toilet quickly; undress appropriately to use the toilet; or recognize the sensation of fullness signalling the need to urinate or defecate; or the patient may show apathy with lack of motivation to remain continent.

For the patient who is incontinent because of an inability to locate the toilet, orientation may be helpful. Signs and active training should help to modify disorientation in older people. Displaying pictures or signs on bathroom doors provides visual cues; words should use appropriate terminology.

If the patient cannot recognize the need to void because of impaired sensory perception of fullness, increasing fluid intake can help to fill the bladder sufficiently to give a clear message of the need to urinate. In addition, getting to know the patient's habits and moods can help the nurse to identify signals that indicate a need to void. The patient can then be assisted to reach the bathroom in time. Positioning the patient near the toilet or placing a portable commode nearby may help if the patient cannot reach a toilet quickly. If the patient demonstrates dressing apraxia (cannot undress appropriately), clothing can be modified with easy-to-open fasteners in place of zippers or buttons. For nocturnal incontinence, other strategies may be effective. Limiting the amount of fluid consumed after the evening meal and taking the patient to the toilet just before going to bed or upon awakening during the night should reduce or eliminate nocturia.

Indwelling urinary catheters are contraindicated in patients with dementia because they are generally not well tolerated and because hand restraints are often used to prevent them from removing the catheter. In addition, indwelling urinary catheters foster the development of urinary tract infections and may compromise the patient's dignity and comfort. Urinary incontinence can be managed with the use of disposable, adult-size diapers that must be checked regularly and changed expeditiously when soiled.

Patients with dementia often experience constipation, although they may not be able to tell the nurse about this change. Therefore, subtle signs such as lethargy, reduced appetite, and abdominal distention need to be assessed frequently. Medications, decreased food and liquid intake, lack of motor activity, and decreased intestinal motility contribute to developing constipation. In such cases, the patient's diet should be rich in fiber, including bran or whole grains, vegetables, and fruit. Adequate oral intake (minimum of 1,500 to 2,000 mL/day) helps to prevent constipation. A gentle laxative such as milk of magnesia (1 to 2 tablespoons every other evening) is commonly used to promote bowel elimination. Enemas and harsher chemical cathartics should be avoided because they may increase pain or discomfort. Care must be taken to ensure that the patient does not become dehydrated in the process of treating constipation.

Sleep Interventions

Disturbed sleep cycles are particularly stressful to both family caregivers and nursing staff. Disturbed sleep is difficult to manage from a behavioural perspective, and the patient's overall level of health may suffer because sleep serves a restorative function. Sedative–hypnotic agents may be prescribed for a short time for restlessness or insomnia, but they may also cause a paradoxic reaction of agitation and insomnia (especially in older adults).

Sleep hygiene interventions are appropriate for patients with dementia, although morning and afternoon naps (or rest periods for patients who do not nap) may be the most effective intervention for a patient with altered diurnal rhythms. Morning naps are likely to produce REM sleep patterns and may help patients who are restless from a loss of REM sleep, whereas afternoon naps produce deep sleep and are suitable for restlessness associated with fatigue. Rest periods (in reclining chairs) in the morning and afternoon may help to eliminate late-day confusion (sundowning) and nighttime awakenings.

Activity and Exercise Interventions

Activity and exercise are important nursing interventions for patients with dementia. To promote a feeling of success, any activity or exercise plan must be culturally sensitive and adapted to the patient's functional ability and interests. The activity or exercise must be designed to prevent excess stress (both physical and psychological), which means that it must be individualized for each patient with dementia, based on their relative strengths and deficits. If the program of rest, activity, and exercise is truly individualized, the resultant feelings of value and competency will enhance the patient's morale and self-esteem.

Pain and Comfort Management

Nursing care of noncommunicative patients who have dementia and who also have pain can be challenging. Because of the difficulty in identifying and monitoring the pain, the patients are often undertreated. However, several measures may be used to assess the efficacy of pharmacologic interventions, such as decreased restlessness and agitation. Small doses of oral morphine solution appear to reduce discomfort during routine nursing procedures. The main side effect of morphine is constipation.

Relaxation

Approaching patients in a calm, confident, unhurried manner; maintaining a soothing, quiet environment; avoiding unnecessary noise or chatter around patients and lowering vocal tone and rate when addressing them; maintaining eye contact; and using touch judiciously are likely to promote a sense of security conducive to patient relaxation and comfort. Simple relaxation exercises can be used to reduce stress and should be performed by the patient.

Administering and Monitoring Medications

Because no medication can cure AD, psychopharmacologic interventions have two goals: restoration or maintenance of cognitive function and treatment of related psychiatric and behavioural disturbances that cause discomfort for the individual, interfere with treatment, or worsen the individual's cognitive status. However, medications for AD must used with caution. Doses must be kept extremely low, and individuals should be monitored closely for any side effects or worsening of cognitive status. "Start low and go slow" is the principle guiding the administration of psychopharmacologic agents to older adults.

Often, convincing the patient to take the medication is one of the biggest nursing challenges. Patients may be unwilling, even though they previously agreed to take the drugs. The nurse will need to investigate and hypothesize the reason for the reluctance to take medication. It may be because of difficulty swallowing pills, paranoid ideas, or lack of understanding. The underlying reason for medication refusal will determine the strategy. If the patient has difficulty swallowing, most medications come in concentrate liquid form and can be easily swallowed. Some medications can also be mixed in food. If suspicion or paranoia is the reason, the nurse will need to try to identify the conditions under which the patient feels safe to take the medication, such as in the presence of favorite nurse or relative.

CHOLINESTERASE INHIBITORS. **Acetylcholinesterase** (AChE) is the key enzyme that inactivates the neurotransmitter acetylcholine. AChE is found in high concentrations in the brain and is one of two cholinesterase enzymes capable of breaking down ACh. **Butyrylcholinesterase** (BuChE), a nonspecific cholinesterase, is also found in the brain, but especially in the glial cells. Both AChE and BuChE work in the gastrointestinal tract. If these enzymes are inhibited, the destruction of ACh will be delayed, resulting in an increase in ACh activity. The increase in ACh activity helps maintain cognitive functioning and delay its decline. **Acetylcholinesterase**

inhibitors (AChEIs) are the mainstay of pharmacologic treatment of dementia because they inhibit AChE, resulting in an enhancement of cholinergic activity. Because these medications have been shown to delay the decline in cognitive functioning, but generally do not improve cognitive function once it has declined, it is important that this medication be started as soon as the diagnosis is made. The primary side effect of these medications is gastrointestinal distress—nausea, vomiting, and diarrhea.

Three AChEI drugs have been approved for use in Canada: donepezil (Aricept), rivastigmine (Exelon), and galantamine (Reminyl). Clinical trials have demonstrated that people with mild to moderate AD treated with any of these medications experience modest improvements in cognition, function, behaviour, or global clinical state (Hogen & Patterson, 2002). Doses at the higher end of the recommended ranges are associated with greater benefits, but more side effects. The main side effects are nausea, vomiting, and diarrhoea. These three drugs are only effective in the treatment of mild to moderate AD. A decision is made to discontinue usage when the Mini-Mental Status Examination (MMSE) score is less than 10 or when the person with AD is institutionalized (Hogen & Patterson, 2002).

The cholinesterase inhibitors are oral medications usually taken once or twice a day. If the patient is suspicious or paranoid, the most difficult aspect in administering the drug is convincing the patient to take it. The earlier in the disease process these medications are initiated, the more likely they will delay cognitive decline.

There are no special monitors for these medications. With cholinesterase inhibitors, patients should not be taking any anticholinergic medication.

NMDA ANTAGONISTS. Overstimulation of the N-methyl-D-aspartate (NMDA) receptor by glutamate (excitatory neurotransmitter) is considered to have a role in AD. Approximately 70% of all excitatory synapses in the CNS are stimulated by this neurotransmitter. Dysfunction of glutamatergic neurotransmission is involved in the pathology of dementia. In dementia, it is hypothesized that there is a chronic release of glutamate that causes a permanent increased intracellular calcium concentration that leads to neuronal degeneration. Memantine is an NMDA-receptor antagonist that has been shown to improve cognition and activities of daily living in patients with moderately severe to severe symptoms of dementia, as well as the mild to moderate symptoms (Resiberg et al., 2003). Health Canada has issued a Notice of Compliance with conditions for use of memantine (Ebixa) (Perras, 2005). Memantine can be used in combination with AChEI drugs.

ANTIPSYCHOTIC AGENTS. Antipsychotic agents are often effective in reducing psychosis, agitation, or aggressive behaviours that are common in the moderate to severe stages of AD. With the introduction of the atypical antipsychotic drugs, the use of conventional antipsychotic agents, such as haloperidol, in elderly patients immediately declined. Risperidone, quetiapine, and olanzapine have all been studied in elderly patients. Clozapine is not prescribed as a front-line agent because of its side-effect profile.

Health Canada (2005) issued an advisory that studies have shown that elderly demented patients prescribed atypical antipsychotics had a 1.6 times greater death rate than those taking a placebo. Risperidone (Risperdal), quetiapine (Seroquel), olanzepine (Zyprexa), and clozapine (Clozaril) are not approved for treating behavioural disorders in elderly patients with dementia (Health Canada).

When using atypical antipsychotics in older patients, the dosage should be much lower than in younger adults. These medications can usually be given once a day, except for quetiapine, which has a shorter half-life than the others. It is also important for the nurse to monitor side effects of these medications and recognize that the side effects of the various agents are different (see Chapter 13).

ANTIDEPRESSANT AGENTS AND MOOD STABILIZERS. A depressed mood is common in patients with dementia, and they often experience response to psychotherapeutic intervention alone (individual or group therapy) or in combination with pharmacotherapy. Low doses of the selective serotonin reuptake inhibitors and other newer antidepressive agents should be considered.

ANTIANXIETY MEDICATIONS (SEDATIVE–HYPNOTICS). Antianxiety medications, also known as benzodiazepines, should be used with caution in elderly patients and, if used, should be administered on a short-term basis. An antianxiety medication may be considered in an emergency, but ideally, the patient should try a non-benzodiazepine before being prescribed a benzodiazepine. In elderly people, the benzodiazepines can cause a paradoxic reaction.

OTHER MEDICATIONS. Clinical observations indicate that elderly patients with defects in the cholinergic system are more vulnerable to the effects of anticholinergic drugs that can cause confusion and amnesia. Anticholinergic medications should be avoided in patients with AD if at all possible. See Box 30-7 for examples of medications that are commonly prescribed to older adults, all of which have anticholinergic receptor activity.

Psychological Domain

Psychological Assessment

Personality changes almost always accompany dementia and can take the form of either an accentuation or a marked alteration of a patient's previous lifelong character traits. The neural substrates underlying personality change in AD are not understood, but researchers

---

BOX 30.7

Medications With Anticholinergic Effects*

Captopril (Capoten)
Codeine
Cimetidine (Tagamet)
Digoxin (Lanoxin)
Dipyridamole (Trental)
Furosemide (Lasix)
Isosorbide (Ismotic)
Nifedipine (Procardia)
Prednisolone
Ranitidine (Zantac)
Theophylline (Bronkodyl)
Triamterene (Dyrenium) and hydrochlorothiazide (HCTZ)
Warfarin (Coumadin)

*These medications are commonly prescribed for older adults.

---

have identified two contrasting patterns. One is marked by apathy, lack of spontaneity, and passivity. The other involves growing irritability, sarcasm, self-preoccupation, and intolerance of and lack of concern for others. Assessment of the psychological domain includes sexuality and spirituality.

Cognitive Status

The mental status should always be assessed and can follow the process suggested in Chapter 10, including the use of the MMSE.

Cognitive disturbance is the clinical hallmark of dementia. The intellectual status of the patient is usually assessed by the traditional, neurologically oriented mental status assessment. If cognitive deterioration occurs rapidly, delirium should be suspected. The patient should be quickly evaluated by a physician because delirium calls for immediate attention to diagnose and treat the underlying cause (Box 30-8).

MEMORY. The most dramatic and consistent cognitive impairment is in memory. Patients with dementia appear mildly forgetful and repetitive in conversation. They misplace objects, miss appointments, and forget what they were just doing. They may lose track of a conversation or television story. Initially, they may complain of memory problems, but rapidly in the course of the illness, insight is lost and they become unaware of what is lost. Sometimes, they may confabulate, making what appears to be an appropriate explanation of why the information or object is missing. Eventually, all aspects of memory are impaired, and even long-term memories are affected. During the interview, short-term memory loss is usually readily evident by the patient's inability to recall three or four words given to him or her at the beginning of the assessment. Often, the earliest symptom of AD is the inability to retain new information.

LANGUAGE. Language is also progressively impaired. Individuals with AD may initially have agnosia, difficulty finding a word in a sentence or in naming an

BOX 30.8

Rating Scales for Use With Dementia

Mental Status Questionnaires

Mini-Mental State Examination

Folstein, M. F., Folstein, S. E., & McHugh, P. R. (1975). "Mini mental state" a practical method for grading the cognitive state of patients for the clinician. *Journal of Psychiatric Research, 12,* 189–198. See Chapter 11.

Cognitive Abilities Screening Instrument (CASI)

Teng. E. L., Hasegawa, K., Homma, A., et al. (1994). The Cognitive Abilities Screening Instrument (CASI): A practical test for cross-cultural epidemiological studies of dementia. *International Psychogeriatrics, 6,* 45–58.

Short Portable Mental Status Questionnaire

Pfeiffer, E. (1975). A short portable mental status questionnaire for the assessment of organic brain deficit in elderly patients. *Journal of the American Geriatrics Society, 23,* 433–441.

Combination of Cognitive and Functional Assessment

Brief Cognitive Rating Scale

Reisberg, B., Schneck, M. K., & Ferris, S. H. (1983). The Brief Cognitive Rating Scale (BCRS): Findings in primary degenerative dementia. *Psychopharmacology Bulletin, 19,* 47–50.
Includes five scales: concentration, recent memory, remote memory, orientation, and functioning and self-care.

Alzheimer's Disease Assessment Scale

Rosen, W. G., Mohs, R. C., & Davis, K. L. (1984). A new rating scale for Alzheimer's disease. *American Journal of Psychiatry, 141,* 1356–1364.
Includes 21 items in the cognitive section and 10 items that are noncognitive, such as mood, appetite, delusions, and pacing.

Rating Scales of Activities of Daily Living

Progressive Deterioration Scale (PDS)

DeJong, R., Osterlund, O. W., Roy, G. W. (1989). Measurement of quality-of-life changes in patients with Alzheimer's disease. *Clinical Therapeutics, 11,* 545–554.

Dependence Scale

Stern, Y., Albert, S. M., Sano, M., et al. (1994). Assessing patient dependence in Alzheimer's disease. *Journal of Gerontology, 49,* M216–M222.

Ratings Scales for Relatives

Geriatric Evaluation by Relatives Rating Scale Instrument (GERRI)

Schwartz, G. E. (1983). Development and validation of the Geriatric Evaluation by Relatives Rating Instrument (GERRI). *Psychological Reports, 53,* 478–488.

---

object. They may be able to talk around it, but the loss is noticeable. Later, fluent aphasia develops, comprehension diminishes, and, finally, they become mute and unresponsive to directions or information.

VISUOSPATIAL IMPAIRMENT. Deficits in visuospatial tasks that require sensory and motor coordination develop early, drawing is abnormal, and the ability to write may change. Inaccurate drawings on the MMSE or clock drawings (see Chapter 10) is diagnostic of impairment in this area. Sequencing tasks, such as cooking or other self-care skills, become impaired. The individual becomes unable to complete complex tasks that require calculations, such as balancing a checkbook.

EXECUTIVE FUNCTIONING. Judgment, reasoning, and the ability to problem-solve or make decisions are also impaired later in the disorder, closer to the time of nursing home placement. It is hypothesized that as the disease progresses, the degeneration of neurons is spread diffusely throughout the neocortex.

Psychotic Symptoms

Delusional thought content and hallucinations are common in people with dementia. These psychotic symptoms differ from those of schizophrenia.

SUSPICIOUSNESS, DELUSION, AND ILLUSIONS. During the early and middle stages of dementia, many patients are aware of their cognitive losses and compensate with hyperalertness. In a hyperalert state, one becomes aware of many environmental stimuli that are not readily understood. Suspiciousness is a variant of the hyperalert or hypervigilant state in which stimuli are interpreted as dangerous. **Illusions**, or mistaken perceptions, also occur commonly in patients with dementia. For example, a woman with dementia mistakes her husband for her father. He resembles her father in that he is roughly her father's age when he was last alive. If an illusion becomes a false fixed belief, it is a delusion.

As the disease progresses, delusions develop in 34% to 50% of the people with dementia. These characteristic delusions are different from those discussed in the psychotic disorders. Common delusional beliefs include the following:

- Belief that his or her partner is engaging in marital infidelity
- Belief that other patients or staff are trying to hurt him or her
- Belief that staff or family members are impersonators
- Belief that people are stealing his or her belongings
- Belief that strangers are living in his or her home
- Belief that people on television are real.

HALLUCINATIONS. Hallucinations occur frequently in dementia and are usually visual or tactile (they can also be auditory, gustatory, or olfactory). Visual, rather than auditory, hallucinations are the most common in dementia. A frequent complaint is that children, adults, or strange creatures are entering the house or the patient's room. These hallucinations may not seem unusual to the patient. If possible, the content and form of hallucination should be ascertained because this information may suggest a treatable disorder. For example, an auditory hallucination commanding the patient to commit suicide may be caused by a treatable depression, not dementia. In some cases, hallucinations may be pleasant, such as children being in the room; or they may frightening and uncomfortable.

Mood Changes

Recognition of coexisting (and often treatable) psychiatric disorders in patients with dementia is often ignored. A depressed mood is common and is reported in 40% to 50% of AD cases. A diagnosis of major depression is less common, occurring in 10% to 20% of patients with AD. A number of people with AD experience one or more depressive episodes with symptoms such as psychomotor retardation, anxiety, feelings of guilt and worthlessness, sadness, frequent crying, insomnia, loss of appetite, weight loss, and suicidal rumination. Depressive symptoms are most prevalent in the early stages of dementia, which may be attributed to the patient's awareness of cognitive changes, memory loss, and functional decline. However, dysphoric symptoms can occur at any stage, even in the most disoriented elderly patients. In more advanced stages of dementia, assessment of depression depends more on changes in behaviour than on verbal complaints.

ANXIETY. Symptoms of anxiety develop in a high proportion of geriatric patients with dementia and those without dementia with major depression (Alexopoulos, 1991). Therefore, it is important to assess for depression when signs of anxiety appear. Moderate anxiety is a natural reaction to the fear engendered by gradual deterioration of intellectual function and the realization of impending loss of control over one's life. Failure to complete a task once regarded as simple creates a source of anxiety in the patient with AD. As patients with AD become unsure of their surroundings and the expectations of others, they frequently react with fear and distress. It is thought that anxious behaviour occurs when the patient is pressed to perform beyond his or her ability.

CATASTROPHIC REACTIONS. **Catastrophic reactions** are overreactions or extreme anxiety reactions to everyday situations. Catastrophic responses occur when environmental stressors are allowed to continue or increase beyond the patient's threshold of stress tolerance. Behaviours indicative of catastrophic reactions typically include verbal or physical aggression, violence, agitated or anxious behaviour, emotional outbursts, noisy behaviour, compulsive or repetitive behaviour, agitated night awakening, and other behaviours in which the patient is cognitively or socially inaccessible. Factors that contribute to catastrophic responses in patients with pro-

gressive cognitive decline include fatigue, change in routine (pace or caregiver), demands beyond the patient's ability, overwhelming sensory stimuli, and physical stressors, such as pain or hunger.

Behavioural Responses

APATHY AND WITHDRAWAL. Apathy, the inability or unwillingness to become involved with one's environment, is common in AD, especially in moderate to late stages. Apathy leads to withdrawal from the environment and a gradual loss of empathy for others. The lack of empathy is very difficult for families and friends to understand. In a study comparing the prevalence of symptoms of those with dementia (n = 329) and those with no dementia (n = 629), the most prevalent symptom (27.4%) of those with dementia was apathy (no dementia, 3.1%) (Lyketsos et al., 2000).

RESTLESSNESS, AGITATION, AND AGGRESSION. Restlessness, agitation, and aggression are relatively common in moderate to later stages of dementia (Lyketsos et al., 2000). Restlessness should be further evaluated to determine its underlying cause. If the restlessness occurs during medication change or adjustment, side effects should be suspected.

Agitation and aggressive physical contacts are among the most dangerous behaviour management problems encountered in any setting. They often result in placement of a family member in a nursing home. Careful evaluation of the antecedents leading up to the behaviour enable the nurse to plan nursing care that prevents future occurrences.

ABERRANT MOTOR BEHAVIOUR. Symptoms such as fidgeting, picking at clothing, wringing hands, loud vocalizations, and wandering may all be signs of such underlying conditions as dehydration, medication reaction, pain, or infection (suggesting delirium). One of the most difficult behaviours for which to determine an underlying cause is **hypervocalization,** the screams, curses, moans, groans, and verbal repetitiveness that are common in the later stages of disease in cognitively impaired elderly patients, often occurring during a hospitalization or nursing home placement. In the assessment of these hypervocalizations, it is important to identify when the behaviour is occurring, antecedents of the behaviour, and any related events, such as a family member leaving or a change in stimulation.

DISINHIBITION. One of the most frustrating symptoms of AD is **disinhibition,** acting on thoughts and feelings without exercising appropriate social judgment. In AD, the patient may decide that he or she is more comfortable naked than with clothes. Or the patient may not be able to find his or her clothes and may walk into a room of people without any clothes on. This behaviour is extremely disconcerting to family members and can also lead to nursing home placement.

HYPERSEXUALITY. A closely related symptom is **hypersexuality,** inappropriate and socially unacceptable sexual behaviour. The patient begins talking and behaving in ways that are uncharacteristic of premorbid behaviour. This behaviour is very difficult for family members and nursing home staff.

STRESS AND COPING SKILLS. Patients with dementia seem extremely sensitive to stressful situations and often do not have the coping abilities to deal with the situation. A careful assessment of the triggers that precede stressful situations will help in understanding a provoking event.

Nursing Diagnoses for the Psychological Domain

A multitude of potential nursing diagnoses can be identified for the psychological domain of this population. A sample of common nursing diagnoses includes Impaired Memory; Disturbed Thought Processes; Chronic Confusion; Disturbed Sensory Perception; Impaired Environmental Interpretation Syndrome; Risk for Violence: Self-Directed or Directed at Others; Risk for Loneliness; Risk for Caregiver Role Strain; Ineffective Sexuality Patterns; Ineffective Individual Coping; Hopelessness; and Powerlessness (Carpenito-Moyet, 2004).

Interventions for the Psychological Domain

The therapeutic relationship is the basis for interventions for the patient and family with dementia. Care of the patient entails a long-term relationship needing much support and expert nursing care. Interventions should be delivered within the relationship context (Williams & Tappen, 1999).

Cognitive Impairment

VALIDATION THERAPY. Validation therapy emerged in the 1970s as a method for communicating with patients with AD. It was developed as a contrast to reality therapy, which attempted to provide a here-and-now, factual focus to the interaction. **Validation therapy** focuses on the emotions and subjective reality of the patients. In validation therapy, individuals with cognitive impairment are viewed on one of four stages of a continuum: malorientation, time confusion, repetitive motion, and vegetation. The benefits of validation therapy for patients are reported as restoration of self-worth, less withdrawal from the outside world, communication and interaction with other people, reduction of stress and anxiety, help in resolving unfinished life tasks, and facilitation of independent living for as long as possible. These outcomes are highly desirable, but no substantive research supports its effectiveness (Neal &

Briggs, 2003). Validation therapy is a useful model for nursing care of the patient with dementia. The nurse does not try to reorient the patient, but rather respects the individual's sense of reality.

MEMORY ENHANCEMENT. Interventions for progressive memory impairment should always be a part of the treatment plan. The sooner patients begin taking AChE inhibitors, the slower the cognitive decline. However, pharmacologic agents are only a small part of the intervention picture. The nursing goal is to maintain memory functioning as long as possible. The nurse should make a concerted effort to reinforce short- and long-term memory. For example, reminding patients what they had for breakfast, which activity was just completed, or who their visitors were a few hours ago will reinforce short-term memory. Encouraging patients to tell the stories of their earlier years will help bring long-term memories into focus. In the earlier stages of AD, there is considerable frustration when the patient realizes that he or she has short-term memory loss. In a matter-of-fact manner, the nurse should "fill in the blanks" and then redirect to another activity. Pictures of familiar people, places, and activities are also important tools in memory retrieval. Using scents (perfume, shaving lotions, spices, different foods) to stimulate memory retrieval and asking patients to relate memories are also useful. Formalized reminiscence groups also help patients relive their earlier experiences and support long-term memories.

ORIENTATION INTERVENTIONS. To enhance cognitive functioning, attempts should be made to remind patients of the day, time, and location. However, if the patient begins to argue that he or she is really at home or that it is really 1992, the patient need not be confronted by facts. Any confrontation could easily escalate into an argument. Instead, the nurse should either redirect the patient or focus on the topic at hand (see Box 30-9).

MAINTAINING LANGUAGE. Losing the ability to name an object (agnosia) is frustrating. For example, the patient may describe a flower in terms of color, size, and fragrance but never be able to name it a flower. When this happens, the nurse should immediately say the name of the item. This reinforces cognitive functioning and prevents disruption in the interaction. Referral to speech therapists may also be useful if the language impairment impedes communication.

SUPPORTING VISUOSPATIAL FUNCTIONING. The patient with visuospatial impairments loses the ability to sequence automatic behaviours, such as getting dressed or eating with silverware. For example, patients often put their clothes on backward, inside out, or with undergarments over outer garments. Once dressed, they become confused as to how they arrived at their current state. If this happens, the nurse should begin to place clothes for dressing in a sequence so that the patient can move from one article to the next in the correct

BOX 30.9

Therapeutic Dialogue: The Patient With Dementia of the Alzheimer Type

Lois's daughter has told the home care nurse that on several occasions, Lois has been found cowering and fearful under the kitchen table, saying she was hiding from voices. The nurse also knows that Lois denies having any difficulty with her memory or her ability to care for herself.

Ineffective Approach

Nurse: I'm here to see you about your health problems.
Patient: I have no problems. Why are you here?
Nurse: I'm here to help you.
Patient: I do not need any help. I think there is a mistake.
Nurse: Oh, there is no mistake. Your name is Ms. W, isn't it?
Patient: Yes, but I don't know who you are or why you are here. I'm very tired, please excuse me.
Nurse: OK. I will return another day.

Effective Approach

Nurse: Hello, my name is Susan Miller. I'm the home health nurse and I will be spending some time with you.
Patient: Oh, alright. Come in. Sit here.
Nurse: Thank you.
Patient: There is nothing wrong with me, you know.
Nurse: Are you wondering why I am here? (open-ended statement)
Patient: I know why you are here. My children think that I cannot take care of myself.
Nurse: Is that true? Can you take care of yourself? (restatement)

Patient: Of course I can care for myself. When people get older they slow down. I'm just a little slower now and that upsets my children.
Nurse: You are a little slower? (reflection)
Patient: I sometimes forget things.
Nurse: Such as . . . (open-ended statement)
Patient: Sometimes, I cannot remember a telephone number or a name of a food.
Nurse: Does that cause problems?
Patient: According to my children, it does!
Nurse: What about you? What causes problems for you?
Patient: Sometimes the radio says terrible things to me.
Nurse: That must be frightening. (Acceptance)
Patient: It's terrifying. Then, my daughter looks at me as if I am crazy. Am I?
Nurse: It sounds like your mind is playing tricks on you. Let's see if we can figure out how to control the radio. (Validation)
Patient: Oh, OK. Will you tell my daughter that I am not crazy?
Nurse: Sure, I would be happy to meet with both you and your daughter if you would like. (Acceptance)

Critical Thinking Challenge

- How did the nurse's underlying assumption that the patient would welcome the nurse in the first scenario lead to the nurse's rejection by the patient?
- What communication techniques did the nurse use in the second scenario to open communication and set the stage for the development of a sense of trust?

---

sequence. This same technique can be used in other situations, such as eating, bathing, and toileting.

INTERVENTIONS FOR PSYCHOSIS. Patients who are experiencing psychosis usually are prescribed an antipsychotic agent. Interventions associated with antipsychotic therapy were presented earlier in this chapter.

MANAGING SUSPICIONS, ILLUSIONS, AND DELUSIONS. Patients' suspiciousness and delusional thinking must be addressed to be certain that patients do not endanger themselves or others. Often, delusions are verbalized when patients are placed in a situation they cannot master cognitively. The principle of nonconfrontation is most important in dealing with suspiciousness and delusion formation. No efforts should be made to ease the patient's suspicions directly or to correct delusions. Efforts should be directed at determining the circumstances that trigger suspicion or delusion formation and creating a means of avoiding these situations.

Frequent causes of suspicion are changes in daily routine and strangers. The common accusations that "Someone has entered my room," or "Someone has changed my room," can be managed by asking, "Do you want to see if anything is missing?" Such accusations usually arise when a patient cannot remember what the room looked like or when the room was rearranged or cleaned.

Patients with dementia often hide or misplace their belongings and later complain that the item is missing.

It is helpful if the nurse and other caregivers pay attention to the patient's favorite hiding places and communicate this so that objects can be more easily retrieved. An outburst of delusional accusations after a social outing or other activity may indicate that the activity was too long, the setting was too stimulating, there was too much activity, or the pace was too fast for the patient. All these elements can be modified, or it may be necessary to exclude or significantly diminish the delusional patient's participation in overstimulating activities.

Patients with dementia have delusions that a spouse, child, or other significant person is an impostor. If this situation occurs, it is important to assert in a matter-of-fact manner, "This is your wife Barbara" or "I am your daughter Jenny." More vigorous assertions, such as offering various types of proof, tend to increase puzzlement as to why a person would go so far to impersonate the spouse or child.

When patients experience illusions, the nurse needs to find the source of the illusion and remove it from the environment if possible. For example, if a patient is watching a television program featuring animals and then verbalizes that the animal is in the room, switch the channel and redirect the conversation. Some patients with dementia may no longer recognize the reflection in the mirror as self and become agitated, thinking that a stranger is staring at them. Potentially misleading or disturbing stimuli, such as mirrors or art work, can be easily covered or removed from the environment.

MANAGING HALLUCINATIONS. Reassurance and distraction may be helpful for the hallucinating patient. For example, an 89-year-old patient with AD in a residential care facility would get up each night, walk to the nursing station, and whisper to the nurses, "There's a man in my bed who won't let me sleep. You should patrol this place better!" If the hallucination is not too disturbing for the patient, it can often be dismissed calmly with diversion or distraction. Because this patient did not seem too concerned by the man in her bed, the nurse may gently respond by saying, "I'm sorry you have to put up with so much. Just wait here (or come with me) and I'll make sure your room is ready for you." The nurse should then take the patient back to her room and help her into bed.

Frightening hallucinations and delusions usually require antipsychotic medications to dampen the patient's emotional reactions, but they can also be dealt with by optimizing perceptual cues (cover mirrors or turn off the television) and by encouraging patients to stay physically close to their caregivers. For example, one patient complained to her visiting nurse that she was being poisoned by deadly bugs that crawled up and down her arms and legs while she tried to sleep at night. Antipsychotic medication may help this patient sleep at night, and she would also likely benefit from reassurance and protection. Patients benefit more if nurses give them a specific intervention to help the hallucination, such as applying moisturizing lotion to her legs and arms to repel the bugs at night. The nurse does not have to agree with the patient's hallucination or delusion but should let the patient know that the feelings are justified based on the patient's perception of the threat.

Interventions for Mood Changes

MANAGING DEPRESSION. Psychotherapeutic nursing interventions for depression that accompanies dementia are similar to interventions for any depression. It is important to spend time alone with patients and to personalize their care as a way of communicating the patient's value. Encouraging expression of negative emotions is helpful because patients can talk honestly to a nonjudgmental person about their feelings. Although depressed patients with dementia are likely to be too disorganized to commit suicide, it is wise to remove potentially harmful objects from the environment (Box 30-10).

Do not force depressed patients to interact with others or participate in activities, but encourage activity and exercise. One of the psychogenic aspects of depression is a sense of lowered worth related to the patient's actual decreased competence to work and to deal with the problems of daily living. Therefore, it may be helpful to involve the person in a simple repetitive task or

project (such as folding linens or setting the table), especially one that involves helping someone else. Assist the patient to meet self-care needs while encouraging independence when possible.

MANAGING ANXIETY. Cognitively impaired patients are particularly vulnerable to anxiety. As patients with dementia become more unsure of their surroundings or of what is expected of them, they tend to react with fear and distress. They may feel lost, insecure, and left out. Failure to complete a task once regarded as simple creates anxiety and agitation. Often, they cannot explain the source of their anxiety. The difficulty in developing interventions for the anxious patient with dementia is that the symptoms may also be a sign of underlying illnesses, such as depression, pain, infection, or other physical illnesses.

In many cases, lowering the demands, or perceived demands, on the patient will be conducive to promoting comfort. Although maintaining autonomy in any remaining function is a high priority in nursing care of the patient with dementia, it may decrease the patient's anxiety or stress level to have things done for him or her at certain points along the illness continuum. In addition, being sensitive to the pronounced startle reflexes and potential hypersensitivity to touch also helps reduce stress.

BOX 30.10

Clinical Vignette: A Nurse's Dilemma

It is 8 o'clock and you are working as a nurse on an inpatient general medical unit of a large urban hospital. A 72-year-old man is admitted to your unit with symptoms of disorientation to time and place, and he is intermittently exhibiting signs of agitation. He thinks you are his child, and he falls asleep while you ask him questions about his symptoms. When you ask him to sign a consent form and hand him a pen, he looks at you as if he didn't understand your request.

The patient's wife tells you that he has had trouble with his memory for the past 3 or 4 years but that her husband has been "acting strange for the past 4 days." The patient's wife denies any history of substance abuse or head injury, but states that her husband has been recently diagnosed as having dementia of the Alzheimer's type.

The patient's physician gives a verbal order to restrain the patient "as needed" while writing orders for lab work.

What Do You Think?
- What assessment techniques would you use to determine whether this patient has dementia, delirium, or both?
- What nursing diagnosis would be included in the patient's plan of care?
- What nursing interventions would promote comfort and safety for this patient?
- Is this patient able to give consent?
- What would be the possible outcomes of physically restraining this patient (eg, would restraints be helpful or harmful for the patient)?

The threshold for stress is progressively lowered in AD and other progressive dementias. A healthy person frequently uses cognitive coping strategies when under stress, whereas the person with dementia can no longer use many of these strategies. Effective nursing interventions include simplifying routines, making routines as consistent and predictable as possible, reducing the number of choices the patient must make, identifying areas in which control can be maintained, and creating an environment in which the patient feels safe. With any of the therapeutic interventions discussed, the nurse is reminded that each patient has relative strengths and weaknesses and that sound nursing judgment must be used in each situation.

Commonly used therapeutic approaches may exacerbate anxiety in a patient with dementia. For example, reality orientation is usually an effective intervention for acutely confused patients. Reality orientation is contraindicated in dementia because it is possible that the patient's disoriented behaviour or language has inherent meaning. If the disoriented behaviour or language is continuously neglected or corrected by the nurse, the patient's sense of isolation and anxiety may increase.

Another therapeutic intervention that may (or may not) be contraindicated in patients with dementia is providing the patient with information before a difficult or painful procedure. Anticipatory preparation for non-routine events may produce anxiety because the patient is unable to retain information, use reasoning skills, or make sound judgments. Telling the patient that he or she is scheduled for an upcoming diagnostic test only communicates, on an emotional level, that something distressing is about to happen. A simple explanation immediately before the event may be more helpful.

MANAGING CATASTROPHIC REACTIONS. If a patient reacts catastrophically, the nurse needs to remain calm, minimize environmental distractions (quiet the environment), get the patient's attention, and softly assure the patient that he or she is safe. Give information slowly, clearly, and simply, one step at a time. Let the patient know that you understand the fear or other emotional response, such as anger or anxiety.

As the nurse becomes skilled at identifying antecedents to the patient's catastrophic reactions, it becomes possible to avoid situations that provoke such reactions. Patients with AD respond poorly to change and respond well to structure. Attempts to argue or reason with them only escalate their dysfunctional responses.

Interventions for Behaviour Problems

MANAGING APATHY AND WITHDRAWAL. As the patient withdraws and becomes more apathetic, the nurse is challenged to engage the patient in meaningful activities and interactions. To provide this level of care, the nurse must know the premorbid functioning of the patient. Close contact with family helps give the nurse ideas about meaningful activities.

MANAGING RESTLESSNESS AND WANDERING. Restlessness and wandering are major concerns for caregivers, especially in the community (home) or long-term care setting. The principal means of dealing with restless patients who wander into other patient's rooms or out the door is to have an adequate number of staff (or caregivers, in the home setting) to provide supervision, as well as electronically controlled exits. Wandering behaviour may be interrupted in more cognitively intact patients by distracting them verbally or visually. Colour and structure of the care setting can serve as cues to enable patients to locate their own rooms (Gibson, MacLean, Barrie & Geiger, 2004). Patients who are beyond verbal distraction can be distracted by physically joining them on their walk and then interrupting their course of action and gently redirecting them back to the house or facility. Many times, wandering is a result of a patient's inability to find his own room or may represent other agenda-seeking behaviours.

MANAGING ABERRANT BEHAVIOUR. When patients are picking in the air or wringing hands, simple distraction may work. Hypervocalizations are another story. Direct care staff tend to avoid these patients, which only makes the vocalizations worse. In reality, these vocalizations may have meaning to the patient. The nurse should develop strategies to try to reduce the frequency of vocalizations (Table 30-6).

MANAGING AGITATED BEHAVIOUR. Agitated behaviour is likely to occur when patients are pressed to assist in their own care. A calm, unhurried, and undemanding approach is usually most effective. Attempts at reasoning may only aggravate the situation and increase the patient's resistance to care. If the nurse is unable to determine the source of the patient's anxiety, the patient's restless energy can often be channelled into activities such as walking. Relaxation techniques also can be effective for reducing behavioural problems and anxiety in patients with dementia.

REDUCING DISINHIBITION. Anticipation of disinhibiting behaviour is the key to nursing interventions for this problem. Disinhibition can take many forms, from undressing in a public setting, to touching someone inappropriately, to making cruel, but factual statements. This behaviour can usually be viewed as normal by itself but abnormal within its social context. With keen behavioural assessment of the patient, the nurse should be able to anticipate the likely socially inappropriate behaviour and redirect the patient or change the context of the situation. If the patient starts undressing in the dining room, offering a robe and gently escorting him or her to another part of the room might be all that is needed. If a patient is trying to fondle a staff member or another patient, having the staff member leave the immediate area or redirecting the patient may alleviate the situation.

Table 30.6   Messages, Meanings, and Management Strategies

Possible Underlying Meanings	Related Management Strategies
"*I hurt!*" (eg, from arthritis, fractures, pressure ulcers, degenerative joint disease, cancer)	• Observe for pain behaviours (eg, posture, facial expressions, and gait in conjunction with vocalizations) • Treat suspected pain judiciously with analgesics and nonpharmacologic measures (eg, repositioning. careful manipulation of patient during transfers and personal care, warm/cold packs, massage, relaxation)
"*I'm tired*" (eg, sleep disturbances possibly related to altered sleep–wake cycle with day–night reversal, difficulty falling asleep, frequent night awakenings)	• Increase daytime activity and exercise to minimize daytime napping and promote nighttime sleep • Promote normal sleep patterns and biorhythms by strengthening natural environmental cues (eg, provide light exposure during the day, avoid bright, artificial lights at night), provide large calendars and clocks • Establish a bedtime routine • Reduce night awakenings: avoid excess fluids, diuretics, caffeine at bedtime; minimize loud noises; consolidate nighttime care activities (eg, changing, medications, treatments)
"*I'm lonely*"	• Encourage social interactions between patients and their family, caregivers, and others • Increase time the patient spends in group settings to minimize time in isolation • Provide opportunity to interact with pets
"*I need . .*" (eg, food, a drink, a blanket, to use the toilet, to be turned or repositioned)	• Anticipate needs (eg, assist patient to toilet soon after breakfast when the gastrocolic reflex is likely) • Keep patient comfort and safety in mind during care (eg, minimize body exposure to prevent hypothermia)
"*I'm stressed*" (eg, inability to tolerate sensory overload)	• Promote rest and quiet time • Minimize "white noise" (eg, vacuum cleaner) and background noise (eg, televisions and radios) • Avoid harsh lighting and busy, abstract designs • Limit patient's contacts with other agitated people • Reduce behavioural expectations of patient, minimize choices, promote a stable routine
"*I'm bored*" (eg, lack of sensory stimulation)	• Maximize hearing and visual abilities (eg, keep external auditory canals free from cerumen plugs, ensure glasses and hearing aids are worn, provide reading material of large print, soften lighting to reduce glare) • Play soft, classical music for auditory stimulation • Offer structured diversions (eg, outdoor activities)
"*What are you doing to me?*" (eg, personal boundaries are invaded)	• Avoid startling patients by approaching them from the front • Always speak before touching the patient • Inform patients what you plan to do and why before you do it • Allow for flexibility in patient care
"*I don't feel well*" (eg, a urinary or upper respiratory tract infection, metabolic abnormality, fecal impaction)	• Identify etiology through patient history, examination, possible tests (eg, urinalysis, blood work, chest radiograph, neurologic testing) • Treat underlying causes
"*I'm frustrated—I have no control*" (eg, loss of autonomy)	• When possible, allow patient to make own decisions • Maximize patient involvement during personal care (eg, offer patient a washcloth to assist with bathing) • Treat patients with dignity and respect (eg, dress or change patient in private)
"*I'm lost*" (eg, memory impairment)	• Maintain familiar routines • Label the patient's room, bathroom, drawers, and possessions with large name signs • Promote a sense of belonging through displays of familiar personal items, such as old family pictures
"*I feel strange*" (eg, side effects from medications that may include psychotropics, corticosteroids, β-blockers, nonsteroidal antiinflammatories)	• Minimize overall number of medications; consider nondrug interventions when possible • Begin new medications one at a time; start with low doses, titrate slowly. Suspect drug reaction if patient's behaviour (eg, vocal) changes • Educate caregivers about patient medications
"*I need to be loved!*"	• Provide human contact and purposeful touch • Acknowledge or verify patient's feelings • Encourage alternative, nonverbal ways to express feelings, such as through music, painting, or drawing • Stress a sense of purpose in life; acknowledge achievements; reaffirm that the patient is still needed

From Clavel, D. S. (1999). Vocalizations among cognitively impaired elders. *Geriatric Nursing, 20*, 90–93.

Social Domain

Social Assessment

Dementia interferes with a person's ability to interact socially as much as it disrupts intellectual functioning. The social domain assessment should include those areas explained in Chapter 28, including functional status, social systems, spiritual assessment, legal status, and quality of life (see Chapter 10). The Global Assessment of Functioning scale presented in Chapter 10 also can be used.

The patient's whole social network is affected by dementia, and the primary caregiver of a person with dementia (usually the partner or offspring in a community setting) is often considered a copatient. It is important to assess the family caregiver's ability to use supportive mechanisms to maintain his or her own integrity throughout the disease process.

The extent of the primary caregiver's personal, informal, and formal support systems must also be assessed, as well as personal resources, skills, and stressors. The assessment of the social domain provides objective data on the patient's social circumstances and impressions of the patient's family structure, sociocultural beliefs, attitudes toward health and disease, myths about dementia, patterns of communication, and degree of psychopathology (such as potential for abuse). If the patient still resides in the community, a home visit will prove useful because it gives the nurse information about the patient in the natural environment. From this assessment, the nurse can identify the situational and psychosocial stressors that affect the family and patient and can begin to develop interventions to strengthen coping strategies, including the ability to seek help from appropriate community resources.

Nursing Diagnoses for the Social Domain

Typical nursing diagnosis for the social domain are Deficient Diversional Activity; Impaired Social Interaction; Social Isolation; Risk for Loneliness; Caregiver Role Strain; Ineffective Coping; Hopelessness; and Powerlessness (Carpenito-Moyet, 2004). Outcomes are determined according to nursing diagnoses.

Interventions for the Social Domain

Safety Interventions

One of the primary concerns of the nurse should be patient safety. In the early stages of the illness, safety may not seem to be a prime issue because the individual is cognitively intact. However, early behaviours suggesting dementia are often related to safety, such as the patient getting lost while driving or going the wrong way on the highway. Patients may be prevented from driving even though they can continue to live at home. Determining the ability of a dementia patient to drive is recognized to be a challenge for health care providers (Byszewski et al., Guzman, 2003). Safety continues to be an issue in the home when patients engage in unsupervised cooking, cleaning, or household tasks. Day care centres provide a structured, yet safe, environment for these individuals. Family members should be encouraged to assess continually the abilities of members to live at home safely.

During hospitalizations or nursing home care, the safety issues are different. There are more people with the patient, which presents more opportunity for wandering into unsafe areas. Most geropsychiatric units are locked, and in a dementia unit, there often is an electronic alarm system to alert staff of patients attempting to leave the secured floor. Staff and visitors need to be vigilant for perilous situations.

Environmental Interventions

The need for stimulation can also be an antecedent to catastrophic reactions. The need for stimulation varies from individual to individual and can change, depending on many factors, including cognitive intactness, alertness, emotional state, and physical state. The amount of stimulation received also influences each patient's behaviour. Lack of stimulation or intense stimulation may cause emotional distress and aggression. Generally speaking, the more severe the dementia, the less stimulation can be integrated. The nurse should attempt to determine each patient's optimal level of stimulation at various times of the day. It may be that stimulating environments can be tolerated early in the morning but not in the afternoon when the patient is tired.

Socialization Activities

Overlearned social skills are rarely lost in patients with AD. It is not unusual for the patient with dementia to respond appropriately to a handshake or smile well into the disease process. Even patients who are no longer able to communicate coherently will carry on long discussions with people who are willing to listen and respond (to language that does not make sense). There is a strong risk for social isolation in patients with dementia because of communication difficulties. Reinforcing social remarks and gestures, such as eye contact, smiling, greetings, and farewells, can promote a sense of competency and self-esteem (Box 30-11). Pet therapy and "stuffed animal" therapy can also enhance social interaction in cognitively impaired individuals. It is important to remember that patients with dementia do not lose their ability to laugh and play, and the psychosocial benefits of humor are well known.

The nurse who engages a patient with dementia in an activity is encouraged to (1) avoid confronting the patient

BOX 30.11   RESEARCH FOR BEST PRACTICE

Nurse–Patient Communication in Dementia

THE QUESTIONS: What are the communication strategies used by expert nurses in communication with people diagnosed with advanced dementia? How effective are these strategies in supporting participation in social conversations?

METHOD: This is a descriptive study of interactions in a weekly socialization group composed of eight women with advanced dementia (MMSE 0–19) in a residential facility and led by two researchers. Ten sessions, 30 to 50 minutes in length, were audiotaped and then transcribed. There were no specific agendas for the groups, but the leaders addressed such topics as holidays, the weather, unit activities, and members' well-being. A line-by-line analysis of the first group session by the researchers resulted in two taxonomies that were used to code the other nine transcripts.

FINDINGS: With effective support and prompting, people with advanced dementia were able to engage in social conversations beyond what would be expected given their diagnosis and MMSE scores.

IMPLICATIONS FOR NURSES: Communication strategies should be adapted to the nursing situation at hand. Useful strategies included clarifying (attempting to ensure that the nurse understood the resident), exploring (searching for information about the resident and helping the resident to articulate experience or thoughts), moderating (initiating and maintaining the conversation), validating (recognizing expressed or inferred feelings), and rescuing (suggesting relevance for specific, isolated, or unconnected sentences). The use of socialization groups to enrich conversation with institutionalized individuals with dementia may be a cost-effective way of enhancing quality of life.

From Perry, J., Galloway, S., Bottorff, J. I., & Nixon, S. (2005). Nurse-patient communication in dementia: Improving the odds. *Journal of Gerontological Nursing, 31*(4), 43–52.

with the disability; (2) allow the level of autonomy best tolerated by the patient; (3) simplify activities and directions to the point that they can be mastered (eg, avoid directions such as "use right or left arm" because the patient may be unable to distinguish one from the other); (4) provide adequate structure or directions; and (5) recognize that instructions may not be carried out correctly. It is important to monitor the length of time, crowding, and noise level when the patient participates in a group activity because all these factors may increase the patient's stress level.

Activities that elicit pleasant memories from an earlier time in the patient's life (reminiscence) may produce a soothing effect. Eliciting pleasant memories may be enhanced by gentle stimulation of the patient's senses, for example, viewing and discussing photo albums, looking at personal memorabilia, providing a favorite food item, playing a musical instrument, or listening to music the person preferred in younger years.

It may be useful to incorporate movement or dance along with a singing exercise. If the patient with dementia resists structured exercise, it may be because of a fear of falling or injury, or of demonstrating to others that his or her health is failing. Patients with dementia often forget how to move or how to coordinate their movements in relation to objects. Therefore, exercise should be light and enjoyable. Encourage the patient to take rest periods at intervals throughout the activity in an effort to minimize stress.

Home Visits

The goal of in-home and community-based long-term care services is to maintain patients in a self-determining environment that provides the most home-like atmosphere possible, allows maximum personal choice for care recipients and caregiver, and encourages optimal family caregiving involvement without overwhelming the resources of the family network. All services for patients with dementia and their families must be provided within a context of continuity of care, a concept that mandates access to a variety of health and supportive services over an unpredictable and changing clinical course.

The effectiveness of having nurses make home visits was recently demonstrated. In a randomized study, older residents with psychiatric disorders living in six public housing sites in Baltimore were identified by building staff. Residents in three of the buildings were assigned to receive nursing interventions by visiting nurses, whereas the residents in the other three did not. The interventions included patient counselling and education, liaisons with the patient's social worker, preparation of patient medication with monitoring of adherence and side effects, facilitation of care and support for patient physical health problems, discussion with home care providers about medication, and monitoring of patient vital signs. Each patient was seen an average of five times. At the end of 26 months, patients receiving the interventions were significantly less depressed and had fewer psychiatric symptoms than did those who did not receive the intervention (Rabins et al., 2000).

Community Actions

Nurses working with patients with dementia are especially knowledgeable about all aspect of the illness and care. These nurses are often involved in local organizations, such as the Alzheimer Society of Canada. Issues of care and safety and access to services often require professional expertise and influence.

Family Interventions

Caregivers are faced with extreme pressures. Caregivers are either spouses of the person with AD or children,

BOX 30.12

Psychoeducation Checklist: Tips for Caregivers

When caring for the patient with dementia, be sure to include the caregivers, as appropriate, and address the following topic areas in the teaching plan:
□ Psychopharmacologic agents, if used, including drug action, dosage, frequency, and possible adverse effects
□ Rest and activity
□ Consistency in routines
□ Nutrition and hydration
□ Sleep and comfort measures
□ Protective environment
□ Communication and social interaction
□ Diversional measures
□ Community resources

BOX 30.13 RESEARCH FOR BEST PRACTICE

Helping Families Provide Safe Care

THE QUESTION: Because family members care for 80% of people with Alzheimer disease (AD) and related disorders and often lack adequate support and training for this all-consuming job, research was undertaken to determine the efficacy of a longitudinal, multisite, community-based intervention designed to teach home caregivers to manage behavioural problems in people with AD.

METHODS: A psychoeducational nursing intervention was implemented for 132 caregiver/care recipient dyads. Family members were taught to modify the environment to compensate for the care recipients' cognitive and functional impairment, as well as their decreased tolerance to environmental stimuli. Interventions included lowering the temperature on the hot water heater to prevent inadvertent scalding, installing a toilet seat of contrasting color to facilitate visualization, and removing mirrors to eliminate misinterpretation of environmental stimuli. In addition, caregivers were encouraged to develop activities that would promote the care recipient's past interests and minimize television viewing. The comparison group (105) received routine information and referrals for case management, community-based services.

FINDINGS: These interventions had a positive impact on both the frequency of and response to problem behaviours among spouses who were caregivers.

IMPLICATIONS FOR NURSING: Family interventions are important for the person with dementia. Formally including these interventions on the treatment plan will help ensure the implementation of these strategies within families.

From Gerdner, L. A., Buckwalter, K. C., & Reed, D. (2002). Impact of a psychoeducational intervention on caregiver response to behavioral problems. *Nursing Research, 51*(6), 363–374.

usually a daughter, who also have other responsibilities, such as children and a job. The caregiver often feels isolated, frustrated, and trapped. The potential for patient abuse is significant, especially if agitated and aggressive behaviours are present in the relative. The use of home care nurses has been investigated relative to their impact on the burden and depression of elderly caregivers. The caregivers who used the home care services were significantly less burdened and less depressed than were those who did not use these services (Mignor, 2000). A Canadian nurse, Dorothy Forbes, and her colleagues (2005) are studying the role of home care and other agencies in meeting the needs of people with dementia and their unpaid caregivers, such as family members.

It is important that the nurse recognize the need of the caregivers for support and relief from the 24-hour responsibility. Determining availability of family members or friends to assist with personal care of the patient should be included in the assessment (see Box 30-12). Caregivers should be encouraged to attend support groups and carve out personal time. Educational and training programs may help in understanding the complex nature of the disorder. Community resources, such as day care centres, home care agencies, and other community services, can be an important aspect of nursing care for the patient with dementia. (See Box 30-13.)

EVALUATION AND TREATMENT OUTCOMES

The objectives of nursing interventions are to help the patient with dementia remain as independent as possible and to function at the highest cognitive, physical, emotional, spiritual, and social levels. The maximum level of functional ability can be promoted when nursing care is related to and based on the remaining abilities of the patient. Patients who receive diagnoses of AD or other types of dementia have a wide and varying range of functional abilities. As cognitive decline progresses, there is a tendency for caregivers to perform more and more tasks for the patient. It is essential to assess for strengths and to assist in the maintenance of existing skills. Adaptive and appropriate behaviours continue to some degree in people with dementia, even in the presence of increasing cognitive decline. It is important for nursing interventions to focus on more than the maintenance of optimal physical functional ability; interventions also must focus on meeting psychological, social, and spiritual needs of the patient with dementia.

Nurses can maintain quality of life if they protect a patient's overall well-being by balancing physical, mental, social, and spiritual health. Figure 30-4 illustrates the truly biopsychosocial aspects of the treatment of individuals with dementia by summarizing potential outcomes of nursing care.

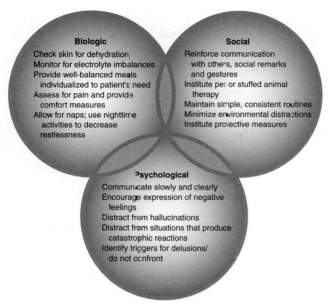

FIGURE 30.4 Biopsychosocial interventions for patients with dementia.

CONTINUUM OF CARE

Community Care

In 1991, approximately 50% of elderly dementia patients lived in the community. The remainder lived in an institution (Canadian Study of Health & Aging Working Group, 1994). In 1991, dementia costs in Canada were $3.9 billion. This is expected to increase to $12 billion by 2031 if no advances are made in prevention or treatment (Ostbye & Crosse, 1994; Dalziel, 1994). Use of community-based services (eg, home health aides, home-delivered meals, adult day care, respite care, caregiver support groups) often extends the amount of time an individual with AD or a related disorder can safely remain in the home. However, the progressive impairment associated with dementia often culminates with placement in a long-term care facility. The nurse working in a physician's office or ambulatory setting may provide ongoing information about management and problem solving. The public health nurse may provide intermittent assessment and ongoing case management. Nurses working in programs designed specifically for patients with dementia, such as adult day care, also practice the role of educator. The nurse who is simply a neighbour or family member is often asked to advise about care of the person with dementia. The complex and interrelated problems often observed in patients with neuropsychiatric disorders will increasingly demand the attention of nurses in all health care settings. Cooperation among health care providers of different disciplines and in various settings is needed to meet the highly individualized needs of patients with neuropsychiatric deficits.

Inpatient-Focused Care

Comprehensive admission assessment, followed by the development of an individualized (and constantly updated) care plan that involves the patient, significant others, and a variety of health care professionals, is the foundation of an effective and efficient postdischarge plan. Attention to all aspects of this process is necessary to ensure that the goal of continuity of care is achieved. The hospital-based nurse may initiate family education and counselling as part of discharge planning. For more information on caring for the patient with dementia, see Nursing Care Plan 30-1.

Nursing Home Care

As the dementia progresses, most patients are placed in a nursing home for care. Nursing care in a nursing home is usually delivered by nurses' aides, who need support and direction. Interestingly, people with dementia require complex nursing care, but the skill level of people caring for these individuals often is minimal. Education and support of the direct caregiver is the focus of most nursing homes.

Other Dementias

Dementia symptoms may occur as a result of a number of disorders and underlying etiologies. The subsequent sections provide a brief description of some of the dementias listed in the *Diagnostic and Statistical Manual of Mental Disorders,* 4th edition, text revision (*DSM-IV-TR*; APA, 2000). In each case, the classic symptoms of dementia (eg, memory impairment with a number of other cognitive deficits) must be present. Nursing interventions for all dementias are similar to those described for individuals with AD.

VASCULAR DEMENTIA

Vascular dementia (also known as *multi-infarct dementia*) is seen in about 20% of patients with dementia, most commonly people between the ages of 60 and 75 years. Slightly more men than women are affected. Vascular dementia results when a series of small strokes damage or destroy brain tissue. These are commonly referred to as "ministrokes" or transient ischemic attacks (TIAs), and several TIAs may occur before the affected individual becomes aware of the symptoms of vascular dementia. Most often, a blood clot or plaques (fatty deposits) block the vessels that supply blood to the brain, causing a stroke. However, a stroke can also occur when a blood vessel bursts in the brain.

The primary causes of strokes include high blood cholesterol levels, diabetes, heart disease, and high blood pressure. Of these, high blood pressure is the

NURSING CARE PLAN 30.1

Patient with Dementia

LW is a 76-year-old widow who lives independently. Recently, her children have noticed that she is becoming more forgetful and seems to have periods of confusion. She has agreed to having someone help her during the day. Her oldest son lives with her and is with her during the evening and night. LW refuses to see a health care provider but did agree to go in for a routine checkup. Her daughter helped her get dressed and took her to the primary health care clinic.

SETTING: PRIMARY HEALTH CARE CLINIC

Baseline Assessment: A well-groomed woman is accompanied by her daughter. LW says there is nothing wrong, but daughter disagrees. A review of body systems reveals poor hearing and vision but is otherwise unremarkable. MMSE score is 19. Daughter reports that LW has become very suspicious of neighbours and has changed her locks several times.

Associated Psychiatric Diagnosis	Medications
Axis I: Probable dementia of the Alzheimer's type Axis II: None Axis III: History of breast cancer, unilateral mastectomy, arthritis Axis IV: Social problems (suspiciousness) GAF = Current 70 Potential 70	Galantamine (Reminyl) 4 mg bid, titrate to 8 mg bid over 4 weeks. Consider risperidone 0.5–1 mg od, if psychotic symptoms occur.

NURSING DIAGNOSIS 1: IMPAIRED MEMORY

Defining Characteristics	Related Factors
Inability to recall information Inability to recall past events Observed instances of forgetfulness Forgets to perform daily activities—grooming	Neurocognitive changes associated with dementia

Outcomes

Initial	Long Term
Maintain or improve current memory	Delay cognitive decline associated with dementia

Interventions

Interventions	Rationale	Ongoing Assessment
Develop memory cues in home. Have clocks and calendars well displayed. Make lists for patients.	Maintaining current level of memory involves providing cues that will help patient recall information.	Contact family members for patient's ability to use memory cues.
Teach patient and family about taking an acetylcholinesterase inhibitor. Review expected effects, side effects, and adverse effects. Develop a titration schedule with family to decrease the appearance of side effects.	Confidence and self-esteem improve when a person looks well groomed.	Monitor response to suggestions.
Observe patient for visuospatial impairment. If present, sequence habitual activities, such as eating, dressing, bathing, etc.	Visuopatial impairment is one of the symptoms of dementia.	Observe for appropriate dress, bathing, eating, etc.

Evaluation

Outcomes	Revised Outcomes	Interventions
LW did have some improvement in memory. Suspiciousness and behavioural symptoms improved.	Continue maintaining memory.	Continue with memory cues and galantamine.

greatest risk factor for vascular dementia. It is essential that anyone who demonstrates symptoms of dementia or who has a history of stroke should have a complete physical examination that includes neurologic and neuropsychological evaluation, diet and medication history, review of recent stressors, and an array of laboratory tests. Damage to the brain in vascular dementia is usually apparent using computed tomography scans or magnetic resonance imaging. At autopsy, multifocal lesions may be found, rather than the more generalized cortical atrophy characteristic of AD.

The behaviour changes that result from vascular dementia are similar to those found in AD, such as memory loss, depression, emotional lability or emotional incontinence (including inappropriate laughing or crying), wandering or getting lost in familiar places, bladder or bowel incontinence, difficulty following instructions, gait changes such as small shuffling steps, and problems handling daily activities such as money management. However, these symptoms usually begin more suddenly, rather than developing slowly, as is the case in AD. Often, the neurologic symptoms associated with a TIA are minimal and may last only a few days, including slight weakness in an extremity, dizziness, or slurred speech. Thus, the clinical progression is often described as intermittent and fluctuating, or of step-like deterioration, with the patient's cognitive and functional status improving or plateauing for a period of time, followed by a rapid decline in function after another series of small strokes. The Hachinski Ischemia Score in Box 30-14 may be helpful in differentiating vascular dementia from AD and in summarizing the symptoms more closely related to vascular dementia.

BOX 30.14

Hachinski Ischemia Score

Abrupt onset	2
Stepwise progression	1
Fluctuating course	2
Nocturnal confusion	1
Relative preservation of personality	1
Depression	1
Somatic complaints	1
Emotional incontinence	1
History of hypertension	1
History of stroke	2
Evidence of associated atherosclerosis	1
Focal neurologic symptoms	2
Focal neurologic signs	2
Alzheimer's disease if scores total	4 or less
Vascular dementias if scores total	7 or more

From Hachinski, V. C. (1983). Differential diagnosis of Alzheimer's dementia: Multi-infarct dementia. In B. Reisberg (Ed.), *Alzheimer's disease* (pp. 188–192). New York: Free Press/Macmillan.

Treatment aims to reduce the primary risk factors for vascular dementia, including hypertension, diabetes, and additional strokes. Interventions that reduce the tendency of the blood to clot and of platelets to aggregate include using medications and lifestyle changes, such as diet, exercise, and smoking cessation to control hypertension, high cholesterol, heart disease, and diabetes. Increasingly, physicians are recommending drugs such as aspirin to help prevent clots from forming in the small blood vessels. Occasionally, surgical procedures such as carotid endarterectomy may be needed to remove blockages in the carotid artery.

DEMENTIA CAUSED BY OTHER GENERAL MEDICAL CONDITIONS

People of any age, race, or gender are at risk for dementia caused by a medical condition known to cause cerebral pathology. Older adults are particularly vulnerable to the development of dementia caused by general medical conditions because so many older people are affected by one or more chronic medical illnesses. Strong relationships have been reported between chronic medical illness and the development of dementia. Of the conditions that cause dementia, about 10% are completely treatable, and about 25% to 30% cease to progress as long as treatment is initiated before irreversible brain damage has occurred. Finally, about 50% to 60% of patients with dementia have a disorder for which no specific medical treatment is available.

Dementia Caused by AIDS

Dementia associated with AIDS has been called AIDS dementia complex (ADC). ADC has been observed in nearly two thirds of all patients with AIDS. AIDS is caused by human immunodeficiency virus 1 (HIV-1), which infects and destroys T lymphocytes as well as the central nervous system (CNS). HIV-1 directly invades the CNS and allows opportunistic infections of the CNS and other organ systems. Although there has been a proportional increase in ADC at AIDS diagnosis, survival after ADC has improved markedly in the era of highly active antiretroviral therapy (HAART) (Dore et al., 2003).

Dementia Caused by Head Trauma

When head trauma occurs in the context of a single injury, the resulting dementia is usually not progressive, but repeated head injury (eg, from the sport of boxing) may lead to a progressive dementia. When the nurse observes progressive decline in intellectual functioning after a single incident of head trauma, the possibility of another superimposed process must be considered. Head injury associated with a prolonged loss of consciousness (days to months) may be followed by delirium, dementia, or a profound alteration in personality.

The degree and type of cognitive impairment or behavioural disturbances demonstrated by a person with head trauma depend on the location and extent of the brain injury (as with other forms of dementia). Repeated head injuries, such as those sustained by young, healthy boxers, may lead to *dementia pugilistica,* or "punch-drunk syndrome." Although the exact mechanism of this disorder is unknown, it appears likely that early damage to neurons and their connections becomes clinically manifest later, when the combination of normal neuronal cell loss and prior damage summate to reach a threshold of impaired cognitive function.

Dementia Caused by Parkinson's Disease

Parkinson's disease is a neurologic syndrome of unknown etiology, which manifests as a disorder of movement, with a slow and progressive course. Clinical manifestations of Parkinson's disease are **bradykinesia** (the slowing of body movements), rigidity, resting tremor, and postural changes. The person's gait is unstable, which results in frequent falls. Parkinson's disease may appear at any time after a person reaches 30 years of age, but the median age of onset is about 70 years of age. A subcortical dementia can be diagnosed in about 20% to 60% of patients with Parkinson's disease (APA, 2000). Although investigators do not know why, there is considerable pathologic overlap between Parkinson's disease and AD. Medical treatment of Parkinson's disease typically is with anticholinergics and dopamine agonists. It is important for nurses to know that in patients with dementia caused by Parkinson's disease, anticholinergic medications are likely to increase cognitive impairment (Katzenschlager, Sampaio, Costa, & Lees, 2003).

Dementia Caused by Huntington's Disease

Huntington's disease is a progressive, genetically transmitted autosomal dominant disorder characterized by choreiform movements and mental abnormalities. The onset is usually between the ages of 30 and 50 years, but onset occurs before 5 years of age in the juvenile form or as late as 85 years of age in the late-onset form. The disease affects men and women equally. A person with Huntington's disease usually lives for 15 to 20 years after diagnosis (APA, 2000). The dementia syndrome of Huntington's disease is characterized by insidious changes in behaviour and personality. Typically, the dementia is frontal, which means that the person demonstrates prominent behavioural problems and disruption of attention.

Dementia Caused by Pick's Disease

Pick's disease is a rare form of dementia that is clinically similar to AD. The etiology of Pick's disease is unknown. Pick's disease particularly affects the frontal and temporal lobes of the brain (APA, 2000). The disorder usually manifests in individuals between the ages of 50 and 60 years, although it can occur among older individuals. Pick's disease is not readily distinguishable from AD until autopsy (APA, 2000), when the distinctive intraneuronal Pick's bodies can be identified microscopically.

Dementia Caused by Creutzfeldt-Jakob Disease

Creutzfeldt-Jakob disease is a rare, rapidly fatal brain disorder. Many of the symptoms seen in Creutzfeldt-Jakob disease are similar to those found in AD and other dementias. However, changes in the brain tissue are different in Creutzfeldt-Jakob disease and are best differentiated by surgical biopsy or on autopsy. Scientists speculate that Creutzfeldt-Jakob disease is caused by infectious agents known as *prions,* which are abnormal proteins that collect in central nervous tissue and cause the nerve cells to die by an, as yet, unknown process.

At present, there is no effective treatment for the disease, and nothing has been found to slow progression of the illness. Because of its rapid clinical course, an important nursing role is assisting family members to understand and come to terms with the illness and to make decisions related to treatment setting and life-sustaining treatments. Creutzfeldt-Jakob disease progresses much more rapidly than most dementias, and death usually occurs within 1 year after onset, although some evidence suggests that extensive changes in the brain may be present before symptoms appear.

Only about 3,000 cases of Creutzfeldt-Jakob disease have been reported worldwide in the past 70 years, resulting in an annual incidence of about 1 per 1 million population. The disease strikes both men and women, most commonly between the ages of 50 and 75 years. Interestingly, there appears to be a genetic component to Creutzfeldt-Jakob disease (Cummings, 2003). Inhabitants of certain rural areas of the world, such as Slovakia and Chile, and Libyan-born Jews living in Israel have a much higher incidence of the disease.

Person-to-person transmission of Creutzfeldt-Jakob disease is rare (but possible), and it can be transmitted from people to animals and between animals. Evidence indicates that the prions can be introduced into the nervous system of healthy patients during medical procedures, such as corneal transplantation, implantation of contaminated electrodes in the brain, and injection of contaminated growth hormones (a few health care workers, probably exposed to the infectious agent through blood and spinal fluids, have experienced the disease). Because of the transmissible nature of Creutzfeldt-Jakob disease, strict criteria for the handling of infected tissues and other contaminated materials have been developed.

A variant type of Creutzfeldt-Jakob disease (vCJD) now exists that is linked to eating beef products from cattle infected with bovine spongiform encephalopathy (BSE). There has been only one case in Canada, and the person affected had been living in the United Kingdom. Nevertheless, the third occurrence of BSE in Canadian cattle was confirmed in January 2005 (Public Health Agency of Canada, 2005).

Substance-Induced Persisting Dementia

If dementia results from the persisting effects of a substance (eg, drugs of abuse, a medication, or exposure to toxins), substance-induced persisting dementia is diagnosed. Other causes of dementia (eg, dementia caused by a general medical condition) must always be considered, even in a person with a dependence on or exposure to a substance. For example, head injuries often result from substance use and may be the underlying cause of the dementia syndrome (APA, 2000).

Drugs of abuse are the most common toxins in young adults, and prescription drugs are the most common toxins in elderly people. In older patients, dementia results from use of long-acting benzodiazepines, barbiturates, meprobamate (Equanil), and a host of other drugs, depending on their dose and the length of time they have been used. Drugs such as flurazepam (Dalmane), with a half-life of more than 120 hours, accumulate rapidly in a person's body. Other drugs accumulate more slowly or require relatively high doses for toxicity to develop. A toxic etiology should be suspected in every patient with a probable diagnosis of dementia. The nurse should inquire about exposure to drugs and toxins (exposure to toxins at work sites, medication use, and recreational drug use) for each patient with dementia, and any substances known to be potentially injurious to the nervous system should be withdrawn if at all possible.

Most of the dementias in this category are related to chronic alcohol abuse. Understanding the cognitive deficits associated with chronic alcohol consumption is complicated. Alcoholic dementia is directly related to the toxic effects of alcohol, although the vitamin deficiencies associated with alcoholism (thiamine and niacin) are also known to be etiologically related to dementia. Individuals with alcoholism also have a high incidence of systemic illnesses that can affect cognition (eg, cirrhosis, cardiomyopathy), and they are susceptible to repeated head injuries, which carry cognitive consequences of their own.

Much of our knowledge about cognitive deficits in individuals with alcoholism comes from the study of patients with Korsakoff's syndrome, which is a profound deficit in the ability to form new memories and is associated with a variable deficit in recall of old memories, despite a clear sensorium. Further careful examination reveals a flattening of drives, unconcern about incapacity, and profound apathy. Nonetheless, Korsakoff's syndrome does not qualify as a dementia; rather, it is considered an amnestic syndrome (or restricted deficit of memory). In alcohol-induced dementia, the cognitive deficits span a wider range of functioning than with Korsakoff's syndrome (see Chapter 23).

Chemicals and organic compounds that impair functioning of the CNS usually have their primary effects on other body systems: the gastrointestinal, renal, hepatic, blood-forming, and peripheral nervous systems. For example, metal poisonings generally produce gastrointestinal symptoms and peripheral neuropathy. Cognitive changes with poisoning tend to be more characteristic of delirium than dementia, with altered levels of consciousness a prominent feature. Table 30-1 lists some of the organic compounds or chemicals that can cause symptoms of dementia; related distinguishing symptoms are also included.

Many adolescents and indigent adults engage in the act of "huffing" because the cost of purchasing spray paint, hair spray, glue, and other aerosol products is relatively inexpensive (compared with illicit street drugs). The nurse is reminded to evaluate people who abuse drugs for signs of cognitive impairment because neural and cognitive symptoms tend to appear before permanent brain damage occurs. It is also important to realize that the patient's cognitive status may not immediately improve after discontinuation of use of the offending agent. The effects of drugs taken for a long period may be long lasting, and improvement may follow discontinuation of drug use only slowly. For example, in dementia associated with chronic alcoholism, cognition may improve only after many months of abstinence.

Amnestic Disorder

Amnestic disorder is characterized by an impairment in memory that is caused either by the direct physiologic effects of a general medical condition or by the persisting effects of a substance (eg, a drug of abuse, a medication, or exposure to a toxin) (APA, 2000). More specifically, amnestic disorder is diagnosed when there is severe memory impairment without other significant cognitive impairments (eg, aphasia, apraxia, agnosia, or disturbances in executive functioning) or impaired consciousness, which would indicate a diagnosis of either delirium or dementia.

The amnestic disorders share a common symptom, memory impairment, but are differentiated by etiology. Amnestic disorders often occur as the result of pathologic processes. Traumatic brain injury, cerebrovascular events, or specific types of neurotoxic exposure (eg, carbon monoxide poisoning) may lead to an acute onset of an amnestic disorder. Other conditions, such as prolonged substance abuse, chronic neurotoxic exposure, or sustained nutritional deficiency (eg, thiamine deficiency), create a more insidious onset. The age of the patient and course of amnestic disorder may vary, depending on the pathologic process causing the disorder.

Amnestic disorder is characterized by an impaired ability to learn new information or an inability to recall previously learned information (short-term recall) or past events (long-term recall), with preservation of immediate recall (immediate-recall deficits are commonly associated with dementia) (APA, 2000). Although short-term and long-term memory are impaired in most patients who have a form of organic brain disease, the occurrence of memory impairment as a relatively circumscribed deficit is rare. Short-term or recent memory is usually more severely impaired than remote memory with an amnestic disorder, and no deficit may be observed when the patient is asked to recall events or dates that have been overlearned. Most patients with deficits in short-term recall are disoriented to place and time; therefore, disorientation is a common sign of amnestic disorder. However, in some forms of amnestic disorder, the patient may remember information from the very remote past better than more recent events (eg, the patient may have a vivid memory of a hospital stay that occurred many years ago, but may have no idea that he or she is currently in the hospital) (APA, 2000).

Amnestic disorders are often preceded by an evolving and variable clinical picture, which includes confusion and disorientation, occasionally with attentional deficits that suggest a delirium (eg, amnestic disorder caused by thiamine deficiency). Confabulation (filling gaps in memory with imaginary events) may be noted during the early stages of amnestic disorder but usually disappears with time. For this reason, it may be important for the nurse to obtain corroborating information from family members or other informants when gathering historical information on the patient. Most patients with a severe amnestic disorder lack insight into their memory deficits and may adamantly deny the presence of memory impairment despite evidence to the contrary. This lack of insight may lead to accusations against others or, in some instances, to agitation. Some individuals may acknowledge that they have memory problems but appear unconcerned. Apathy, lack of initiative, emotional blandness, or other changes in personality are not uncommon with amnestic disorder.

SUMMARY OF KEY POINTS

- Neuropsychiatric disorders, such as delirium and dementia, are characterized clinically by significant deficits in cognition or memory that represent a clear-cut change from a previous level of functioning. In some disorders, the loss of cognitive function is progressive, such as in Alzheimer disease.

- Two major syndromes of cognitive impairment in elderly people are delirium and chronic cognitive impairments, such as dementia. It is important to recognize the differences because the interventions and expected outcomes of the two syndromes are different.

- Delirium is characterized by a disturbance in consciousness and a change in cognition that develops over a short period of time. It requires rapid detection and treatment because in 25% of cases, it is a sign of impending death.

- Usually, delirium is caused by a combination of precipitating factors. The most commonly identified causes are medications, infections (particularly urinary tract and upper respiratory tract infections), fluid and electrolyte imbalance, and metabolic disturbances such as electrolyte imbalance or poor nutrition. Other important predisposing factors include advanced age, brain damage, pre-existing dementia, and biopsychosocial stressors.

- The primary goal of treatment of delirium is prevention or resolution of the acute confusional episode with return to previous cognitive status and interventions focusing on (1) elimination or correction of the underlying cause and (2) symptomatic and safety and supportive measures.

- Dementia is characterized by the gradual onset of decline in cognitive function, especially memory, usually accompanied by changes in behaviour and personality. There are numerous causes of the symptoms of dementia, some of which are reversible, such as hypoxia, carbon monoxide poisoning, and vitamin deficiencies.

- Alzheimer disease (AD) is an example of a progressive, degenerative dementia. Treatment efforts currently focus on reduction of cognitive symptoms (eg, memory loss, confusion, and problems with learning, speech, and reasoning) in attempts to improve the quality of life for both patients and their caregivers.

- No one cause of dementia or AD has been discovered. Research efforts continue to pinpoint a singular identifiable genetic basis while focusing on other implicated etiologies, including neurochemical (ie, decreased acetylcholine believed to play a major role in memory impairment), neuropathologic (ie, degeneration of glutamatergic nerve terminals, head injury causing damage to the blood–brain barrier, defects in the immune system), and even some environmental factors (ie, aluminum and other heavy metals).

◙ Some of the psychosocial stressors known to precipitate delirium and contribute to worsening dementia include sensory overload or underload, immobilization, sleep deprivation, fatigue, pain or hunger, change in routine (pace or caregiver), or demands beyond the patient's ability. Nursing interventions should include reducing the impact of these stressors on patients and educating their families or caregivers.

◙ Educating families and caregivers about what to expect, progressive cognitive decline and behaviour changes, environment safety, and community resources for patients with dementia is essential to ensuring proper care.

◙ Symptoms of dementia may occur as a result of a number of disorders, including vascular and amnestic disorders, head trauma, AIDS, and substance abuse and as a symptom of Parkinson's, Huntington's, Pick's, and Creutzfeldt-Jakob diseases.

CRITICAL THINKING CHALLENGES

1 What factors should the nurse consider in differentiating Alzheimer's disease from vascular dementia?

2 Compare the defining characteristics and related risk factors of acute confusion with those for the NANDA diagnoses of Impaired Thought Processes and Sensory/Perceptual Disturbances. What are the differences and similarities between the recommended nursing interventions for delirium and dementia? What is the theoretic base for these similarities and differences?

3 Describe three ways in which medical disease can disrupt brain functioning, and relate these mechanisms to the neuropsychiatric disorders presented in this chapter.

4 Suggest reasons that older adults are particularly vulnerable to the development of neuropsychiatric disorders.

5 In what ways can culture and education influence mental status test scores?

6 The physical environment is particularly important to the patient with dementia. Every effort should be made to modify the physical environment to compensate for the cognitive and functional impairment associated with AD and related disorders, including safety measures and the avoidance of misleading stimuli. Visualize your last experience in a health care setting (hospital, nursing home, day care program, or home care setting). Identify environmental factors that could be misleading or stress producing to a person with impaired cognition (dementia), and identify ways to modify this environment to alleviate some of the stressors or misleading stimuli.

WEB LINKS

www.alz.org   This Alzheimer's Association website provides information, resources, and consumer and caregiver support.

www.rnao.org/bestpractices   Screening & Selecting Care Strategies for Delerium, Dementia & Depression in Older Adults.

www.pdsg.org.uk   This website of the Pick's Disease Support Group provides information on Pick's disease, Lewy bodies, and other dementias.

www.alzheimer.ca/english/misc/redirect.htm   This site of the Alzheimer's Association of Canada provides information and resources related to the disease.

www.pieces.cabhru.com/prc/videos.htm   A. Tassonyi. Recognizing Delirium in the Elderly.

M O V I E S

Iris: 2001. Based on the book by her husband, John Bayley, this movie (directed by Richard Eyre) tells the story of an influential British woman of letters, Dame Iris Murdoch. Young Iris is played by Kate Winslet, and the older Iris by Dame Judi Dench, in the unfolding of her rich and interesting life. The story reveals the couple's struggle with Iris's Alzheimer disease as her exceptional capabilities are increasingly diminished.

VIEWING POINTS: Consider how the love and friendship of the couple is both strengthened and challenged by AD. Are there any external supports and resources that might have made their situation in living with AD less difficult?

The Notebook: 2004. Every day an elderly man reads to a woman from his faded notebook. They are in a nursing home, and it is their own love story that he is reading. It is a story about how they met, fell in love, and then spent their lives together. Based on a novel by Nicholas Sparks, the movie reveals the fleeting moments of clarity that Noah's story brings to Allie, his wife, who is suffering from dementia. It shows the hope that keeps him trying to reach her.

VIEWING POINTS: Consider what it might be like to hear your own life story and to recognize it only momentarily and vaguely. Can you think of other ways people cope with the loss of a loved one who remains, at least physically, before them?

REFERENCES

Alexopoulos, G. S. (1991). Anxiety and depression in the elderly. In C. Salzman & B. D. Lebowitz (Eds.), *Anxiety in the elderly*. New York: Springer.

American Psychiatric Association. (2000). *Diagnostic and statistical manual of mental disorders* (4th ed., Text revision). Washington, DC: Author.

Arnold, E. (2004). Sorting out the 3 D's: Learn how to sift through overlapping signs and symptoms so you can help improve an older patient's quality of life. *Nursing (2004), 34*(b), 36–42.

Arnold, E. (2005). Sorting out the 3 D's: Delirium, dementia, depression. Learn how to sift through overlapping signs and symptoms so you can help improve an older patient's quality of life. *Holistic Nursing Practice, 19*(3), 99–105.

Benson, S. (1999). Hormone replacement therapy and Alzheimer's disease: An update on the issues. *Health Care Women International, 20*(6), 619–638.

Blair, B. D. (2000). Presentations and recognition of common psychiatric disorders in the elderly. *Clinical Geriatrics, 8*(2), 26, 28–29, 33–34.

Byszewski, A. M., Graham, I. D., Amos, S., et al. (2003). A continuing Medical Education Initiative for Canadian Primary Care Physicians. The Driving and Dementia Tool Kit: A pre and post evaluation of knowledge, confidence gained, and satisfaction. *Journal of the American Geriatrics Society, 51*(10), 1484–1489.

Canadian Study of Health and Aging Working Group. (1994). Canadian Study of Health and Aging. Study methods and prevalence of dementia. *Canadian Medical Association Journal, 150*, 899–913.

Cacchione, P. Z. (2002). Assessment. Four acute confusion assessment instruments: Reliability and validity for use in long-term care facilities. *Journal of Gerontological Nursing, 28*(1), 12–19.

Carpenito-Moyet, L. (2004). *Nursing diagnosis.* Philadelphia: Lippincott Williams & Wilkins.

Clavel, D. S. (1999). Vocalizations among cognitively impaired elders. *Geriatric Nursing, 20*, 90–93.

Cummings, J. L. (2003). *The neuropsychiatry of Alzheimer's disease and related dementias.* London: Martin Dunitz, Ltd.

Dalziel, W. B. (1994). Dementia: No longer the silent epidemic. *Canadian Medical Association Journal, 151*, 1407–1409.

DeJong, R., Osterlund, O. W., Roy, G. W. (1989). Measurement of quality-of-life changes in patients with Alzheimer's disease. *Clinical Therapeutics, 11*, 545–554.

Dore, G. J., McDonald, A., Li, Y., Kaldor, J. M., Brew, B. J., & National HIV Surveillance Committee. (2003). Marked improvement in survival following AIDS dementia complex in the era of highly active antiretroviral therapy. *AIDS, 17*(10), 1539–1545.

Ebly, E. M., Parhad, I. M., Hogan, D. B., & Fung, T. S. (1994). Prevalence and types of dementia in the very old: Results from the Canadian Study of Health and Aging. *Neurology, 44*, 1593–1600.

Faust, D., & Fogel, B. S. (1989). The development and initial validation of a sensitive bedside cognitive screening test. *Journal of Nervous and Mental Disease, 177*, 25–31.

Flaherty, J. H. (1998). Commonly prescribed and over the counter medications: Causes of confusion. *Clinics in Geriatric Medicine, 14*(1), 101–125.

Folstein, M. F., Folstein, S. E., & McHugh, P. R. (1975). Mini-mental state: A practical method for grading the cognitive state of patients for the clinician. *Journal of Psychiatric Research, 12*, 189–198.

Forbes, D. A., Anderson, M., Hawranik, P., Henderson, S., Leipert, B., Markle-Reid, M., Morgan, D., & Parent, K. (2005). The role of homecare in dementia care. Unpublished research proposal.

Forman, M., Fletcher, K., Mion, L., & Trygstad. (2003). Assessing cognitive function. In M. Mezey, T. Fulmer, I. Abraham, & D. Zwicker (Eds.), *Geriatric Nursing Protocols for Best Practice* (2nd ed, pp. 102–103). New York: Springer.

Gerdner, L. A., Buckwalter, K. C., & Reed, D. (2002). Impact of a psychoeducational intervention on caregiver response to behavioural problems. *Nursing Research, 51*(6), 363–374.

Gibson, M., MacLean, J., Barrie, M., & Geiger, J. (2004). Orientation behaviors in residents relocated to a redesigned dementia care unit. *American Journal of Alzheimer's Disease, 19*(1), 45–49.

Gleason, O. C. (2003). Delirium. *American Family Physician, 67*(5), 1027–1034.

Guo, Z., Cupples, L. A., Kurz, A., Auerbach, S. H., Volicer, L., Chui, H., Green, R. C., Sadovnick, A. D., Duara, R., DeCarli, C., Johnson, K., Go, R. C., Growden, J. H., Haines, J. L., Kukull, W. A., & Farrer, L. A. (2000). Head injury and the risk of AD in the MIRAGE study. *Neurology, 54*, 1316–1323.

Hachinski, V. C. (1983). Differential diagnosis of Alzheimer's dementia: Multi-infarct dementia. In B. Reisberg (Ed.), *Alzheimer's disease* (pp. 188–192). New York: Free Press/Macmillan.

Health Canada (2005). Health Canada advises consumers about important safety information on atypical antipsychotic drugs and dementia. Advisory 2005-63. June 13, 2005. Ottawa: Health Canada.

Hogen, D., & Patterson, C. (2002). Treatment of Alzheimer's disease and other dementias: Review and comparison of the cholinesterase inhibitors. *Canadian Journal of Neurological Sciences, 29*(4), 306–314.

House, R. M. (2000). Delirium and agitation. *Current Treatment Options in Neurology, 2*(2), 141–150.

Inouye, S., K., van Dyck, C. H., Alessi, C. A., Balkin, S., Siegal, A. P., & Horwitz, R. I. (1990). Clarifying confusion: The confusion assessment method. *Annals of Internal Medicine, 113*, 941–948.

Katzenschlager, R., Sampaio, C., Costa, J., & Lees, A. (2003). Anticholinergics for symptomatic management of Parkinson's disease. *Cochrane Database of Systematic Reviews, (2),* CD003735.

Levkoff, S., Liptzin, B., Cleary, P., Reilly, C. H., & Evans, D. (1991). Review of research instruments and techniques used to detect delirium. *International Psychogeriatrics, 3*, 253–271.

Lyketsos, C. G., Steinberg, M., Tschanz, J. T., Norton, M. C., Steffan, D. C., & Breither, J. C. (2000). Mental and behavioral disturbances in dementia: Findings from the Cache County Study on memory in aging. *American Journal of Psychiatry, 157*, 707–714.

McCloskey, J. C., & Bulechek, G. M. (2000). *Nursing interventions classification* (NIC). St. Louis: Mosby.

McCusker, J., Cole, M., Dendukuri, N., & Belzile, E. (2003). Does delirium increase hospital stay. *Journal of American Geriatrics Society, 51*(11), 1539–1546.

McCusker, J., Cole, M., Dendukuri, N., Han, L., & Belzile, E. (2003). The course of delirium in older medical inpatients: A prospective study. *Journal of General Internal Medicine, 18*, 696–704.

Mignor, D. (2000). Effectiveness of use of home health nurses to decrease burden and depression of elderly caregivers. *Journal of Psychosocial Nursing & Mental Health Services, 38*(7), 34–41.

Mosconi L., Herholz, K., Prohovnik, I., Nacmias, B., De Cristofaro, M. T., Fayyaz, M., Bracco, L., Sorbi, S., & Pupi, A. (2005). Metabolic interaction between ApoE genotype and onset age in Alzheimer's disease: Implications for brain reserve. *Journal of Neurology, Neurosurgery & Psychiatry, 76*(1), 15–23.

North American Nursing Diagnosis Association (NANDA) (2006). *Nursing diagnoses: Definition and Classification* 2005–2006. Philadelphia, PA: NANDA International.

National Advisory Council on Aging. (2004). The NACA position on Alzheimer disease and related dementias, No. 23. Minister of Public Works and Government Services Canada. Available at: http://www.naca.ca. [on-line].

Neal, M., & Briggs, M. (2003). *Validation therapy for dementia.* Oxford, UK: The Cochrane Library, 2, CD001394.

Neelon, V. J., Champagne, M. T., McConnell, E., et al. (1992). Use of the NEECHAM Confusion Scale to assess acute confusional states of hospitalized older patients. In S. G. Funk, E. M. Tornquist, M. T. Champagne, & R. A. Wiese (Eds.), *Key aspects of older care.* New York: Springer.

New Zealand Guidelines Group. (1998). *Guideline for the support and management of people with dementia.* Auckland, New Zealand: Enigma.

Ostbye, T., & Crosse, E. (1994). Net economic costs of dementia in Canada. *Canadian Medical Association Journal, 151*, 1407–1464

Perras, C. (2005). Memantine for treatment of moderate to severe Alzheimer's disease. *Issues in Emerging Health Technologies, 64*, 1–4.

Perry, J., Galloway, S., Bottorff, J. L., & Nixon, S. (2005). Nurse-patient communication in dementia: Improving the odds. *Journal of Gerontological Nursing, 31*(4), 43–52.

Pfeiffer, E. (1975). A short portable mental status questionnaire for the assessment of organic brain deficit in elderly patients. *Journal of the American Geriatrics Society, 23,* 433–441.

Public Health Agency of Canada. Infectious diseases: CJD/vCJD. Retrieved September 17, 2005, from http://www.phac-aspc.gc.ca.

Rabins, P. V., Black, B. S., Roca, R., German, P., McGuire, M., Robbins, B., Rye, R., & Brant, L. (2000). Effectiveness of a nurse-based outreach program for identifying and treating psychiatric illness in the elderly. *Journal of the American Medical Association, 283,* 2802–2809.

Registered Nurses Association of Ontario. (2003). *Screening for delirium, dementia and depression in older adults.* Toronto, Canada: Author.

Reisberg, B., Doody, R., Stöffler, A., Schmitt, F., Ferris, S., & Jörg Möbius, H. (2003). Memantine in moderate-to-severe Alzheimer's disease. *New England Journal of Medicine, 343*(14), 1333–1334.

Reisberg, B., Schneck, M. K., & Ferris, S. H. (1983). The Brief Cognitive Rating Scale (BCRS): Findings in primary degenerative dementia. *Psychopharmacology Bulletin, 19,* 47.

Rogaeva, E. (2002). The solved and unsolved mysteries of the genetics of early-onset Alzheimer's disease. *Neuromolecular Medicine, 2*(1), 1–10.

Rosen, W. G., Mohs, R. C., & Davis, K. L. (1984). A new rating scale for Alzheimer's disease. *American Journal of Psychiatry, 141,* 1356–1364.

Sano, M., Ernesto, C., Thomas, R. G., Klauber, M., Schafer, K., Grundman, M., Woodbury, P., Growden, J., Cotman, C. W., Pfeiffer, E., Schneider, L. S., & Thal, L. J. (1997). A controlled trial of selegiline, alpha-tocopherol, or both as treatment for Alzheimer's disease. The Alzheimer's Disease Cooperative Study. *New England Journal of Medicine, 336,* 1216–1222.

Schell, E. S., & Kayser-Jones, J. (1999). The effect of role-taking ability on caregiver resident mealtime interaction. *Applied Nursing Research, 12,* 38–44.

Schuurmans, M. J., Duursma, S. A., & Shortridge-Baggett, L. M. (2001). Early recognition of delirium: Review of the literature [Review]. *Journal of Clinical Nursing, 10*(6), 721–729.

Schwartz, G. E. (1983). Development and validation of the Geriatric Evaluation by Relatives Rating Instrument (GERRI). *Psychological Reports, 53,* 478–488.

Schwartz, T. L., & Masand, P. S. (2002). The role of atypical antipsychotics in the treatment of delirium. *Psychosomatics, 43*(3) 171–174.

Stahl, S. M. (2000). *Essential psychopharmacology: Neuroscientific basis and practical applications* (2nd ed.) New York: Cambridge University Press.

Stern, Y., Albert, S. M., Sano, M., et al. (1994). Assessing patient dependence in Alzheimer's disease. *Journal of Gerontology, 49,* M216–M222.

Suh, Y. H., & Checler, F. (2002). Amyloid precursor protein, presenilins, and alpha-synuclein: Molecular pathogenesis and pharmacological applications in Alzheimer's disease. *Pharmacological Reviews, 54*(3), 469–525.

Taddei, K., Fisher, C., Laws, S. M., Martins, G., Paton, A., Clarnette, R. M., Chung, C., Brooks, W. S., Hallmayer, J., Miklossy, J., Relkin, N., St. George-Hyslop, P. H., Gandy, S. E., & Martins, R. N. (2002). Association between presenilin-I Glu318Gly mutation and familial Alzheimer's disease in the Australian population. *Molecular Psychiatry, 7*(7), 776–781.

Tarkowski, E., Andreasen, N., Tarkowski, A., & Blennow, K. (2003). Intrathecal inflammation precedes development of Alzheimer's disease. *Journal of Neurology, Neurosurgery, and Psychiatry, 74*(4), 1200–1205.

Thorpe, L., Middleton, J., Russell, G., & Stewart, N. (2000). Bright light therapy for demented nursing home patients with behavioral disturbance. *American Journal of Alzheimer's Disease, 15*(1), 18–26.

Trzepacz, P. T., Baker, R. W., & Greenhouse, J. (1988). A symptom rating scale for delirium. *Psychiatry Research, 23,* 89–97.

Tune, L. (2000). Delirium. In C. E. Coffey & J. L. Cummings (Eds.), *American Psychiatric Press textbook of geriatric neuropsychiatry* (2nd ed.; pp. 441–462). Washington, DC: American Psychiatric Press.

Turner, R. S., D'Amato, C. J., Chervin, R. D., & Blaivas, M. (2000). The pathology of REM sleep behavior disorder with comorbid LEWY body dementia. *Neurology, 55*(11), 1730–1732.

United States Department of Health and Human Services (U.S. DHHS). (2003). *National Institute on Aging, 2001–2002. Alzheimer's Disease Progress Report.* National Institutes of Health Publication No. 03-533.

Werezak, L., & Stewart, N. (2002). Learning to live with early dementia. *Canadian Journal of Nursing Research, 34*(1), 67–85.

Williams, C., & Tappen, R. (1999). Can we create a therapeutic relationship with nursing home residents in the later stages of Alzheimer's disease? *Journal of Psychosocial Nursing, 37*(3), 28–35.

Williams, M. A., Ward, S. E., & Campbell, E. B. (1988). Confusion: Testing versus observation. *Journal of Gerontological Nursing, 14*(1), 25–30.

For challenges, please refer to the **CD-ROM** in this book.

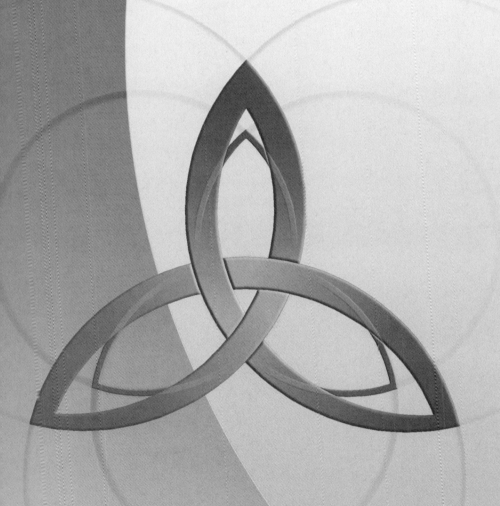

UNIT VII

Care of Special Populations

CHAPTER 31

Issues in Dual Diagnosis

Barbara G. Faltz, Sandra C. Sellin, and
Brad F. Hagen

LEARNING OBJECTIVES

After studying this chapter, you will be able to:

- Define the term *dual disorders.*
- Discuss the epidemiology of dual disorders.
- Describe the cycle of relapse.
- Describe the effects of alcohol and other drugs on mental illness.
- Analyze barriers to the treatment of patients with dual disorders.
- Discuss four etiologies of dual disorders.
- Integrate relapse prevention concepts into the care of a patient with dual disorders.

KEY TERMS

alcohol-induced persisting amnestic disorder ▪ deinstitutionalization ▪ dual disorders
▪ Korsakoff's psychosis ▪ motivational interviewing ▪ substance use ▪ 12-step programs
▪ Wernicke's syndrome

KEY CONCEPT

- relapse cycle

We drank for joy and became miserable;
We drank for exhilaration and became depressed;
We drank for friendship and became enemies;
We drank to diminish our problems and saw
   them multiply.

—Anonymous, from "Positively Negative"

Dual disorders, or the coexistence of a substance use disorder and a mental health disorder, raises many issues for the psychiatric and mental health (PMH) nurse. Other terms that may be used to describe dual disorders include "comorbidity," "concurrent disorders," and "dual diagnosis," although in Canada, the term "dual diagnosis" generally refers to a person with both a mental illness and a developmental disability. Traditionally, substance use and mental health treatment providers have attempted to treat only one aspect of a dual problem. This approach can lead to recurrent relapses into drug or alcohol use or to successive psychiatric hospitalizations. The relapse cycle becomes continuous unless both the mental illness and the substance use disorder are treated.

> **KEY CONCEPT** In the **relapse cycle**, re-emerging psychiatric symptoms lead to ineffective coping strategies, increased anxiety, substance use to avoid painful feelings, adverse consequences, and attempted abstinence, until psychiatric symptoms emerge once more and the cycle repeats itself.

Figure 31-1 shows the relationship between increased psychiatric symptoms and the use of substances as a coping strategy. Without alternative effective coping behaviours, the patient will continue to experience this cycle of relapse and abstinence. The goal of treatment for patients with dual disorders is a comprehensive recovery plan for the complex problems presented—one that offers the patient a way out of what can be a downward spiral of debilitation (Fig. 31-1).

This chapter highlights methods of assessing dual disorders, explores the psychodynamics of their development, and discusses specific mental illnesses and the adverse effects of concurrent substance use. It offers treatment strategies and nursing interventions to address this complex yet common presentation in psychiatric and substance use treatment settings. A complete discussion of related substance use disorders is provided in Chapter 23.

Relationship of Substance Use to Mental Illness

Although it has been prevalent throughout the history of mental illness treatment, the problem of dual disorders has been inadvertently magnified by the community mental health reform movement that began in the 1950s. One major facet of this reform was a rational movement toward **deinstitutionalization** of the mentally ill, which resulted in large numbers of homeless mentally ill people living on the streets (Joseph, 1997). Along with homelessness came the increased use of drugs and alcohol and increased incidence of mental illness (Hwang, 2001).

Chronically mentally ill people are vulnerable to exploitation by others, particularly the more astute and street-wise addicts. It is impossible to make any meaningful distinction between simple recreational use of a substance and actual **substance use** with this population because even small amounts of alcohol or other drugs can be damaging to people who have concurrent psychiatric problems. All substances of abuse exert profound effects on mental states, perception, psychomotor function, cognition, and behaviour. The specific neurochemical and other biologic mechanisms that evoke these psychological features are discussed in Chapter 23. Table 31-1 lists the psychological effects of substances of abuse.

The pattern of alcohol and illicit drug use by the mentally ill varies. Some mentally ill people can use alcohol and drugs recreationally, whereas others experience severe problems from the use of these substances. Individuals can become caught in a "revolving door" of repeated hospitalizations because of the distressing symptoms of mental illness that are exacerbated by substance use. When the presenting symptoms are stabilized and the patient is released, perhaps with new medications or a new discharge plan in place, the patient may fail to follow the therapeutic regimen. The patient may increase use of alcohol or drugs, resulting in an exacerbation of the emotional problem and leading to another episode of hospitalization. This cyclic pattern of mental health or substance use decompensation, hospitalization, stabilization, discharge, and decompensation accounts largely for the difficulty in providing nursing care for patients who have dual disorders.

Manifestations of Dual Disorders

The four possible manifestations of dual disorders and a clinical example describing each follows. For additional information, see Table 31-2.

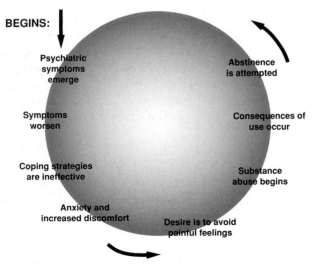

FIGURE 31.1   Relapse cycle.

Table 31.1 Psychological Effects of Substances of Abuse

Substance	Psychological Effects
Alcohol	Organic brain disorders—alcohol amnestic syndrome; dementia Agitation, anxiety disorders, sleep disorders Alaxia, slurred speech Withdrawal symptoms, which may include hallucinations, confusion, illusions, delusions; protracted withdrawal delirium can occur Depression, increased rate of suicide, disinhibition
Cocaine	Anxiety, agitation, hyperactivity, sleep disorders, delusions, paranoia, euphoria, internal sense of interest and excitement Rebound withdrawal symptoms, such as prolonged depression, somnolence, anhedonia
Amphetamines	Similar to cocaine but more prolonged Hyperactivity, agitation, anxiety, increased energy
Hallucinagens (MOMA Ecstacy) and phencyclidine	Hallucinations, delusions, paranoia, confusion Withdrawal can produce severe depression, somnolence Hallucinations, illusions, delusions, perceptual distortions, paranoia, rage, anxiety, agitation, confusion
Marijuana	Acute reactions: panic, anxiety, paranoia, sensory distortions, rare psychotic episodes; patients with schizophrenia use these reactions to distance themselves from painful symptoms and to gain control over symptoms Antimotvational syndrome: apathy, diminished interest in activities and goals, poor job or school performance, memory and cognitive deficits
Opiates	Confusion, somnolence Withdrawal can produce anxiety, irritability, and depression and can trigger suicidal ideation
Sedative-hypnotics	Confusion, slurred speech, ataxia, stupor, sleep disorders, withdrawal delirium, dementia, amnestic disorder, sleep disorders
Volatile solvents	Hallucinations, delusions, hyperactivity, sensory distortions, dementia

Adapted from Beauchamp, J. K., & Olson, K. R. (2000). Drug overdoses and dependence. In R. M. Wachter, L. Goldman, H. Hollander (Eds.), *Hospital medicine*. Philadelphia: Lippincott Williams & Wilkins.

Table 31.2 Assessment and Classification of Dual Disorder Conditions

Assessment Issue	Primary Mental Illness With Substance Use	Substance Use With Psychiatric Sequelae	Dual Primary Disorders	Common Etiology
Are dual syndromes present?	Yes	Yes	Yes	Yes
Which came first?	Mental illness	Substance use	None	None
What is the family history?	Mental illness, if any	Substance use, if any	Mental illness, substance use, or both	Mental illness, substance use, or both, if any
What are the psychosocial factors?	Vulnerable to victimization by peers because of primary mental illness	Often can maintain family and employment during periods of sobriety	Prognosis is less favourable; may often be incarcerated or hospitalized	Common risk factor possible (eg, homelessness)
What is the treatment and response to treatment?	Treatment for mental illness alleviates both syndromes; discharge plan focuses on mental health maintenance	Treatment for substance use alleviates both syndromes; discharge plan focuses on maintenance of sobriety	Treatment for both mental illness and substance use required	Treatment for common risk factor alleviates both mental illness and substance use

Adapted from Lehman, A. F., Myers, C. P., & Corty, E. (1989). Assessment and classification of patients with psychiatric and substance abuse syndromes. *Hospital and Community Psychiatry, 40*(10), 1019–1024.

• *A primary mental illness with subsequent substance use.* In this manifestation, a primary mental illness leads to addictive behaviour when the patient self-medicates to cope with the symptoms of the illness. It includes abuse resulting from impaired judgment, poor impulse control, impaired social skills, and inappropriate coping strategies.

When she was 18 years old, Sylvia G. was raped and held by her assailant for 2 days. She has frequent nightmares, relives the experience almost daily, and is extremely anxious around men whom she does not know. She began drinking heavily after this incident and states that it provides some relief from her anxiety. Drinking also enables her to numb painful feelings. Her alcohol use has had numerous adverse consequences. She was recently fired from her job as a clerk when she was found drinking at her desk. Sylvia has received diagnoses of post-traumatic stress disorder and alcohol dependence.

• *A primary substance use disorder with psychopathologic sequelae.* Psychiatric symptoms are consequences of drug or alcohol intoxication, of withdrawal symptoms (such as severe depression after cessation of prolonged cocaine abuse), or of cognitive impairments related to chronic alcohol or drug use.

Ralph D. has been smoking crack cocaine for 3 years. He has lost his job because of absenteeism. His wife has left him, and he is now homeless. He has attempted suicide three times in moments of despair after cocaine binges. He has been unable to stop using crack and continues to be chronically depressed.

• *Dual primary diagnoses.* Psychiatric and substance use diagnoses interact to exacerbate each other.

Joan K. has a diagnosis of bipolar type II disorder. For many years, she has engaged in heavy drinking, which began in early adolescence. When she is binge drinking, she does not take her medication and experiences manic episodes and deep depressions. She has attempted periods of sobriety, but frequently discontinues use of her medication. She has difficulty controlling impulsive alcohol use.

• *A common etiology.* One common factor causes both disorders. The factor can be (1) genetic; (2) a defect in dopaminergic function that predisposes patients to conditions such as schizophrenia or abuse of dopamine agonists such as amphetamines; or (3) a defect in cholinergic activity that may predispose patients to affective disorders and to substance use affecting cholinergic pathways (Lehman, Myers, & Corty, 1989).

Frank L. received a diagnosis of attention deficit hyperactivity disorder as a child. His parents, both of whom had alcoholism, had a hard time controlling him and would give him alcohol to attempt to "calm him down." Frank continues to have difficulty concentrating, is hyperactive, and has developed numerous medical problems related to his alcohol abuse as an adult.

Epidemiology

It can be difficult to know precisely how many people have a dual or concurrent disorder, although it is

---

BOX 31.1 RESEARCH FOR BEST PRACTICE

Factors Associated With Depression and Alcohol Dependence

THE QUESTIONS: (1) What are the 12-month prevalence of alcohol dependence (AD) among subjects with major depressive episodes (MDEs) and the 12-month prevalence of MDEs among those with AD? (2) What are the associations between demographic and sociodemographic characteristics and comorbid MDE and AD? (3) What are the rates of mental health service use between groups having high and low risk for comorbid conditions?

METHODS: Data were used from the 1996–1997 Canadian National Population Health Survey to calculate the 12-month prevalence of MDEs among participants with AD and of AD among those with MDEs. In addition, the associations between demographic and socioeconomic characteristics and comorbidity were calculated.

FINDINGS: Of participants with MDEs, 8.6% had AD; 19.6% of participants with AD reported having at least 1 MDE in the past 12 months. Being young (aged 12–24 years); being divorced, separated, or widowed; and

having low family income level were positively associated with MDE, AD, and comorbidity. Among participants with comorbid MDE and AD, those who were aged 12 to 24 years were less likely to have used any mental health services in the past 12 months than were others.

IMPLICATIONS FOR NURSING PRACTICE: Because the rate of participants with AD reporting having at least 1 MDE in the past year was quite high (19.6%), nurses working with clients with AD should be sure to screen for the coexistence of depression. In addition, this research study reminds nurses to recognize youth, single marital status, and low family income as factors associated with comorbid depression and AD. Finally, nurses may need to specifically target adolescents and young adults when providing services for depression and alcohol misuse because this age group appears to be less likely to seek and use mental health services.

Wang, J. L., & El-Guebaly, N. (2004). Sociodemographic factors associated with comorbid major depressive episodes and alcohol dependence in the general population. *Canadian Journal of Psychiatry, 49*(1), 37–44.

IN A LIFE

Michael J. Fox (1961–)
Famous Canadian Actor

Public Persona

Michael J. Fox is one of the more famous Canadian-born actors, and he has charmed audiences with his wit, sensitivity, and charisma in such movies and TV series as *Back to the Future, Family Ties, The Secret of My Success,* and *Spin City.* Born the son of a Canadian army officer, Michael J. Fox, like many other Canadian kids, originally wanted to play hockey for a living. He decided to pursue acting instead, however, and moved to Hollywood at the age of 18. An Emmy Award winner, Michael J. Fox first became well known for the hit TV series *Family Ties,* and proceeded to enjoy a successful career involving a number of hit movies and TV series. In 1998, he publicly announced that he was suffering from Parkinson's disease, a condition he had managed to keep hidden from the public for 7 years.

Personal Realities

In his autobiography, *Lucky Man: A Memoir,* Michael J. Fox describes how he was heavily addicted to alcohol in his early celebrity years, an addiction that continued as he struggled with the increasing disability associated with Parkinson's disease. In his memoir, Fox describes his climb up from his periods of depression and addiction, how he has begun to deal with his Parkinson's disease, and the opportunity he now has to help search for a cure for Parkinson's disease and to raise public awareness of the disease.

From: Fox, M. J. (2002). *Lucky man: A memoir.* New York: Hyperion.

generally accepted that people suffering from a mental illness have much higher rates of substance abuse than those without a mental illness. For example, a study cited by the Canadian Mental Health Association (1997) found that approximately one in three people who suffer from a mental illness also have a substance abuse problem. A British Columbia study found an even higher rate, with 55% of mental health service clients also having substance abuse issues with their first episode of mental illness (B.C. Partners for Mental Health and Addictions Information, 2003). Similarly, a high proportion of people experiencing substance abuse problems also face mental health challenges. Ross (1995) found that more than half (55%) of an Ontario sample of people with an alcohol disorder also had a mental health diagnosis during their lifetime. In an earlier Ontario study, Ross, Glaser, and Germanson (1988) found that of people seeking assistance with alcohol and other drug problems at a treatment facility, four fifths (78%) had a lifetime mental disorder, and two thirds (65%) had a current mental disorder.

Given these Canadian and other U.S. studies, there is strong epidemiologic evidence for the widespread coexistence of mental health issues and substance abuse

problems. Therefore, nurses need to incorporate thorough assessment and screening techniques into their care of clients with mental health or substance abuse issues, to ensure that complete and appropriate treatment is provided.

Psychodynamic Model of Dual Disorders

Confusion and professional disagreement exist about the etiology of dual disorders. Differing views of the etiology affect the proposed treatment strategies. Biologic aspects and theories of mental illness have been integrated into each chapter of this text. Chapter 23 examines several different models of substance use etiology. The psychodynamic model is particularly relevant to dual disorders. This section examines this model of chemical dependency and dual disorders.

Current psychodynamic thought views substance use as an attempt by a person to return to homeostasis after experiencing psychological suffering (Brehm & Khantzian, 1997). The person attempts to alleviate or control disturbing feelings such as anxiety, depression, or anger through use of alcohol or drugs. The patient's inability to achieve homeostasis or relief from those feelings without substance use results from "self-regulatory deficiencies" (Brehm & Khantzian, 1997).

Ineffective self-regulation leads to the use of substances to achieve emotional homeostasis. Addicts often do not seek a "high" but rather desire to feel "normal" or comfortable in their lives. The purpose of psychotherapy is to help the patient acquire insight into the reasons for the psychological suffering, increase tolerance and modulation of painful feelings, learn skills to care for and nurture the self, and adopt a reality that is not based on childhood illusions (Brehm & Khantzian, 1997).

Searches have been numerous for an addictive personality or other personality traits associated with substance use. A person's problematic chemical use may also be viewed as a symptom of or a response to family dysfunction. Models that regard alcohol and drug abuse as symptoms of another primary psychiatric or family dysfunctional problem are problematic. If these models offered the only explanation for dual disorders, the logical treatment would be to seek insight into substance-abusing behaviour through psychotherapy. The goal would be to decrease substance use as insight emerges. This model of addiction is helpful in viewing the possible etiologies of dual disorders, but it is narrowly focussed and is only one of many models (see Chapter 23).

Because of the barriers to treatment (described below) and differing views on the etiology of addiction, completing a careful and thorough assessment is essential in mental health, chemical dependency, and medical settings. Comprehensive assessment will help ensure that interventions meet patients' needs. Current research trends in dual disorders are empiric studies to test the validity of cherished treatment beliefs and efficacy studies of treatment approaches.

Barriers to Treatment

High comorbidity rates point to the need for effective treatment of dual disorders. However, patients with dual disorders often face barriers to obtaining proper treatment because of specific cultural, economic, and health-related issues. These include the nature of substance use, countertransference and the position of substance users in society, misunderstandings about and stigmatization of mental illness, and related health issues.

NATURE OF SUBSTANCE USE

Substance users are often unwilling to seek mental health treatment because they may dismiss disturbing emotions as unrelated to their drug or alcohol abuse or to withdrawal symptoms. They may view the disturbing emotions as just a "bad trip," viewing drugs and alcohol as the "cure," rather than the cause of their distress. Conversely, patients who are substance users may seek mental health treatment for problems associated with the consequences of their abuse but may fail to mention their substance use. In addition, they may seek medications to alleviate symptoms that are caused by their abuse, such as anxiety, depression, and insomnia, although effective nonpharmacologic interventions are available. Beeder and Millman (1997) pointed out the dilemma facing these patients. The patient with dual disorder must choose between two equally unsatisfactory options:

1. Take the substance of choice to experience fleeting moments of joy and escape, even though doing so will prompt a decline in overall function and worsen psychiatric symptoms.
2. Accept prescribed treatments, including medications such as neuroleptics or antidepressants, which promote a better level of functioning and a better treatment outcome but are not intoxicating.

COUNTERTRANSFERENCE

PMH professionals in psychiatric treatment programs are often frustrated in their efforts to assist substance using patients. Behaviour often associated with addiction, such as denial of a substance use diagnosis, manipulative behaviour, and noncompliance with health-related protocols, is often regarded as a sign of treatment failure. This type of behaviour can provoke hostility from the staff and can make planning for mental health recovery difficult. Drug-dependent patients may have the additional stigma of being regarded as criminals because they commit illegal acts every time they purchase, use, or distribute illicit drugs. Strong public feelings about alcohol-related motor vehicle crashes, negative experiences with family members or friends with drinking problems, and cultural biases against public intoxication can prejudice interactions with patients who are alcohol dependent.

PMH professionals may have difficulty understanding the compelling nature of drug or alcohol cravings, may not understand differences in drug use patterns and behaviours associated with particular drugs of abuse, and may overdiagnose personality disorders in those who take drugs and commit crimes (Churchill, 2003). Mental health care providers may also be reluctant to endorse the use of 12-step programs, which they may view as nothing more than "prayer meetings," and instead initiate pharmacotherapy prematurely (Beeder & Millman, 1997).

A treatment approach often used in psychodynamic therapies is to seek the underlying cause of the patient's symptoms by uncovering unconscious conflict, and thereby producing heightened anxiety (Wallen & Weiner, 1989). However, if the patient experiences too much anxiety, it may trigger renewed substance use. The relapse may then be mistakenly viewed as a failure on the patient's part, not a result of inappropriate treatment.

MISUNDERSTANDINGS ABOUT AND STIGMATIZATION OF MENTAL ILLNESS

Some professionals who treat substance dependence regard mental illness as outside their area of interest or expertise and may not accept patients with mental health disorders into addiction treatment programs. They may lack a general understanding of the nature of mental illness or fear unpredictable behaviour, recurrent substance use relapses, and the inability of some patients with dual disorders to understand or use 12-step programs. Sometimes, counsellors may view patients as unmotivated by not recognizing possible cognitive impairments. Patients who are recovering from alcoholism and addicts who are employed in treatment programs may also feel uncomfortable working with mentally ill patients, not only because of a lack of knowledge, but also because of denial of the influence of their own personality or psychopathology on their former drug-taking behaviours.

Such common symptoms of mental illness as depression, anxiety, and sleep disturbances are often attributed to substance use or withdrawal (Beeder & Millman, 1997). Thus, underlying or concurrent mental health disorders may remain undiagnosed and untreated. Providers may also misunderstand the second step of the Alcoholics Anonymous (AA) program, which states, "We came to believe that a power greater than ourselves could restore us to sanity," thinking that mental health-related symptoms will abate if a patient "works the program" (Wallen & Weiner, 1989). In addition, confusion exists about the use of psychoactive medication to treat these common psychiatric symptoms.

HEALTH ISSUES

Numerous health hazards are associated with alcohol and drug abuse (see Chapter 23). Patients with dual disorders are more likely than others to use emergency departments for primary health care, waiting until they can no longer ignore physical illness. They are more likely to be unclear about the medical plan they need to follow and to be noncompliant with health care directives. The use of alcohol and illicit substances in addition to medications prescribed for mental illness can lead to drug interactions and may exacerbate side effects of these medications. Homelessness can increase these patients' medical problems (Hwang, 2002), with inadequate nutrition, poor hygiene, and the adverse effects of exposure to the elements adding to their difficulties. Health care providers often become frustrated with patients' noncompliance and with what they see as behaviours that are difficult to manage. Their frustration may negatively affect the way they treat patients with dual disorders. Because of providers' biases against patients with dual disorders, the nature of these patients' behaviour, and confusion about what is the primary and most immediate problem to treat, these patients are often underserved and only partially treated.

Disorder-Specific Assessment and Interventions

It is crucial for patients with dual disorders to receive a thorough assessment of both psychiatric and substance use disorders (Petrakis, Gonzalez, Rosenheck, & Krystal, 2002). An important part of assessment is to delineate the relative contribution of each diagnosis to the severity of the current symptoms presented and to determine treatment priorities accordingly. Because patients with dual disorders often make unreliable historians or distort the reality of their mental health problems and the severity of their substance use, obtaining objective data is especially important. Ideally, one should obtain an objective history of the patient from family, significant others, board and care operators, other health care providers, or anyone familiar enough with the patient to provide an accurate history. Box 31-2 lists

---

BOX 31.2

Methods of Assessment of Dual Disorders

History and physical examination, laboratory tests (eg, liver function tests, complete blood count) to confirm medical indicators related to substance use and also to rule out medical disorders with psychiatric presentations
- Substance use history and severity of consequences, and physical symptoms
- Mental status examination and severity of symptoms (eg, suicidal, homicidal, florid psychosis)

Interview with and assessment of family members, to verify or determine: (1) the accuracy of the patient's self-reported substance use or mental health history; (2) the patient's history of past mental health problems during periods of abstinence; and if possible, (3) the sequence of the diagnoses (ie, what symptoms appeared first)
- Interviews with partner, friends, social worker, and other significant people in the patient's life
- Review of court records, medical records, and previous psychiatric and substance use treatment
- Urine and blood toxicity screens; use of breath analyzer to test blood alcohol level

Revision of initial assessment by observation of the patient in the clinical setting; full assessment of the underlying psychiatric problem may not be possible until there is a long (up to 6 months) period of total abstinence
- Observation of patient for reappearance of psychiatric symptoms after a period of sobriety
- Assessment of patient's motivation to seek treatment, desire to change behaviour, and understanding of diagnoses

---

basic assessment tools and methods used for patients with dual disorders. The following concepts are paramount to diagnosis and assessment of dual disorders (Drake, 2001):

CRNE Note

Patients with both mental illness and substance abuse disorders have responses to both disorders. Prioritizing nursing care will depend upon the immediate issue, but responses to both disorders should be assessed.

- Substance use can cause psychiatric symptoms and mimic psychiatric syndromes.
- Substance use can initiate or exacerbate a psychiatric disorder.
- Substance use can mask psychiatric symptoms and syndromes.
- Withdrawal from alcohol and other drugs can cause psychiatric symptoms and mimic psychiatric syndromes.
- Psychiatric and substance use disorders can coexist.
- Psychiatric behaviours can mimic alcohol and other drug use problems.

PSYCHOTIC ILLNESSES AND SUBSTANCE USE

About half of patients with schizophrenia have a concurrent substance use disorder (Bellack & Gearon, 1998). The diagnosis of schizophrenia can be made only if the symptoms, as described in the *Diagnostic and Statistical Manual of Mental Disorders*, 4th edition, Text revision (*DSM-IV-TR*) (American Psychiatric Association [APA], 2000), last at least 6 months. A diagnosis of schizophrenia can be made accurately only without the added complication of substance use. The patient with a psychotic disorder may have an altered thought process or delusional thinking and may experience auditory hallucinations. He or she may also be cognitively impaired and have poor memory. These patients can have negative symptoms, such as poor motivation and poor hygiene. They often have low self-esteem and poor social skills, and may have a general sense of not belonging to a community. Their sense of self in relation to the world may be altered. These symptoms also can result from intoxication with or withdrawal from substances of abuse (Olson, 2004).

Acute and chronic psychotic disorders may be precipitated in predisposed people by the use of cocaine, amphetamines, marijuana, and the hallucinogens, as well as during severe withdrawal states (Beeder & Millman, 1997). Whereas all people are vulnerable to experiencing psychotic episodes from the use of various drugs, one psychotic episode renders a person more susceptible to subsequent episodes (Olson, 2004). Rosenthal and Westreich (1999) caution that the default diagnosis for patients presenting with substance use disorders and psychotic symptoms should be that these symptoms are related to substance use until proved otherwise.

Assessing the needs of people with schizophrenia who are also chemically dependent is complicated by the changing interaction among psychotic symptoms, the antipsychotic effects of medications, and the side effects of medications. Management and treatment of the psychotic substance user may vary according to the severity of symptoms. Drake (2001) suggested the following is the dual-focus approach for assessment and treatment:

- Initial focus on severity of presenting symptoms, not on diagnosis of one disorder or another
- Acute crisis intervention and crisis management
- Acute, subacute, and long-term stabilization of the patient
- Ongoing diagnostic efforts
- Multiple-contact longitudinal treatment

The emphatic confrontative approach of addressing a patient's denial of his or her problems would not benefit this population (see Chapter 23 for additional discussion of confrontation) and could alienate a patient. A more supportive approach is appropriate, in which relapses are treated as an expected part of the recovery process. Addressing relapse risk is part of treatment planning. Focus on examining behaviour, feelings, and the thinking process that led to the relapse. The nurse must avoid blame and guilt-inducing statements.

Bellack and Gearon (1998) suggest a multifaceted approach for treating the patient with concurrent schizophrenia and substance use. Their treatment approach, behaviour treatment for substance abuse in schizophrenia (BTSAS), consists of four parts:

1. Social skills training to help the patient learn ways to interact in a sober living situation and problem-solving training to review and refine their behaviours
2. Education about the nature of substance use, including triggers and cravings
3. **Motivational interviewing**, which helps the patient clarify personal goals and increases commitment to recovery (see Chapter 23)
4. Education regarding relapse prevention techniques

Another important intervention is to integrate the administration of antipsychotic medication into the chemical dependency treatment plan to reduce the chances of relapse. Relapse is frequently secondary to medication noncompliance, especially if patients experience side effects associated with the use of neuroleptics (Beeder & Millman, 1997).

ANXIETY DISORDERS AND SUBSTANCE USE

The *DSM-IV-TR* (APA, 2000) includes acute distress disorder, generalized anxiety disorder, agoraphobia, obsessive-compulsive disorder, panic disorder, post-traumatic stress disorder (PTSD), social phobia, and other specific phobias as some of the anxiety disorders. Nineteen percent of patients with anxiety disorder have a concurrent alcohol problem, and 28% have a drug problem (Scott, Gilvarry, & Farrell, 1998). PTSD increases the risk for substance use relapse and is associated with poor treatment outcome (Rosenthal & Westreich, 1999). Among patients with substance use disorders, coexisting anxiety disorder is likely (Drake, 2001).

The symptoms of anxiety may result from an anxiety disorder, such as panic attack, and may be secondary to drug or alcohol use, as part of a withdrawal syndrome. Symptoms are so subjectively disturbing that they can lead to drug or alcohol abuse as self-medication for the emotional pain; therefore, they require prompt evaluation and treatment. Pharmacologic treatment of anxiety is difficult because the traditional medications used, the benzodiazepines, are themselves addicting.

Kushner, Sher, and Beitman (1990) helped to clarify the relationship between specific anxiety disorders and substance use. They found that alcohol problems in patients with agoraphobia and social phobia may result from attempts to self-medicate symptoms of anxiety, whereas panic disorder and generalized anxiety disorder may result from pathologic alcohol consumption. Confusion about whether alcohol consumption is a cause or an effect of anxiety can be explained by the ability of alcohol in initial use to reduce anxiety, but that of alcohol abuse for extended periods to increase anxiety (Marx, Hockberger, & Walls, 2002).

Patients with anxiety disorders should also pay particular attention to their physical health. Regular, balanced meals, exercise, and sleep are ways to decrease and manage stress levels. Patients should avoid excessive consumption of caffeine and sugars. If the patient has a fear of crowds, he or she may benefit from gradual desensitization techniques. Ries (1995) suggests the following guidelines for treating anxiety and coexisting substance use disorders:

- Treatment of anxiety can be postponed unless the anxiety interferes with substance use treatment.
- Anxiety symptoms may resolve with abstinence and substance use treatment.
- Affect-liberating therapies should be postponed until the patient is stable.
- Psychotherapy, when required, should be recovery oriented.
- Nonpsychoactive medications are preferred when medication is required.
- Antianxiety treatments such as relaxation techniques can be used with and without medications.
- A healthy diet, aerobic exercise, and avoiding caffeine can reduce anxiety.

MOOD DISORDERS AND SUBSTANCE USE

The term *mood disorder* describes various mood disturbances, including major depressive disorder, dysthymic disorder, bipolar I and bipolar II disorders, and cyclothymic disorder (APA, 2000). Thirty-two percent of patients with a mood disorder have a comorbid substance use disorder, whereas 56% of patients with a bipolar disorder have a comorbid substance use disorder (Regier et al., 1990). Substance use disorders occur concurrently in 13.4% of patients with any affective disorder (Regier et al., 1990). Substance use is more common in patients with a bipolar disorder than in those with any other Axis I diagnosis and

may also contribute to treatment noncompliance and less positive outcomes (Goldberg et al., 1999). Mood disorders may be more prevalent among patients using opiates than among other drug users (Drake, 2001). During the first few months of sobriety, symptoms of depression may persist. Initiation of pharmacologic interventions may be delayed until the diagnosis of underlying depression or other mood disorder can be made.

In 1996, there were 3,941 suicides in Canada, resulting in a national rate of 13 suicides per 100,000 population (Federal, Provincial and Territorial Advisory Committee on Population Health, 1999). In Canada, suicide is the leading cause of death for men aged 25 to 29 and 40 to 44, and for women aged 30 to 34 (Senate Committee on Social Affairs, Science and Technology, 2004). In addition, certain groups experience higher suicide rates than others. For example, Aboriginal adolescents have a suicide rate roughly five to six times greater than that of their non-Aboriginal counterparts (Royal Commission on Aboriginal Peoples, 1996). More than 90% of completed suicides are associated with psychiatric disorders and substance abuse. The most common psychiatric disorders associated with completed suicide are major depression and alcohol abuse. Depression during withdrawal from alcohol, cocaine, opiates, and amphetamines puts patients at severe risk for suicide. A person's presenting behaviours may not have included depression, but depression may develop as the withdrawal syndrome unfolds. Hyperactivity often appears with stimulant use and at times with alcohol abuse. Patients may be treated for hypomania or bipolar disorder when they are in fact hyperactive. Symptoms usually improve as the person maintains abstinence.

As with anxiety disorders, determining whether mood disorders are the cause or the effect of protracted substance use is difficult (Table 31-3). One important assessment is to determine whether drug use relates to mood states. Patients may be attempting to alleviate uncomfortable symptoms, such as depression or agitation, or to enhance a mood state, such as hypomania. Symptoms that persist during periods of abstinence are a clue to the degree that the mood disorder contributes to the presenting symptoms. When possible, the use of medication for mood disorders should be initiated after a period of abstinence (Beeder & Millman, 1997) so

Table 31.3	Drugs That Precipitate or Mimic Mood Disorders	
Mood Disorders	**During Use (Intoxication)**	**After Use (Withdrawal)**
Depression and dysthymia	Alcohol, benzodiazepines, opioids, barbiturates, cannabis, steroids (chronic use), stimulants (chronic use)	Alcohol, benzodiazepines, opioids, barbiturates, cannabis, steroids (chronic use), stimulants (chronic use)
Mania and cyclothymia	Stimulants, alcohol, hallucinogens, inhalants, steroids (chronic and acute use)	Alcohol, benzodiazepines, barbiturates, opiates, steroids (chronic use)

that indications are clear as to whether the alcohol or other drug use was not the sole cause of the symptoms.

Patients with bipolar disorders can benefit from chemical dependency treatment if their medications are stabilized and they can tolerate group treatment approaches, focus on and complete simple goals, and follow simple ground rules in a treatment program. Evans and Sullivan (2001) suggest these guidelines for treatment:

- Limit responses in group sessions (eg, to less than 5 minutes of total group time).
- Limit the length of responses to simple exercises.
- Work with patients to heal interpersonal relationships that may have become impaired as a result of manic episodes.
- Relate patients' substance use and manic episodes to out-of-control behaviour for which ongoing treatment (recovery) plans are needed.

For patients who have depression and a substance use disorder, employing interventions centred on examining cognitive distortions (eg, "I'll never get better, no one likes me, alcohol is my only friend") and cognitive therapy techniques can help improve mood. Use of positive self-talk can be helpful for both the depression and the substance use disorders. Working on unresolved grief can be appropriate. However, assignments that deal with patients' previous actions can evoke guilt, self-blame, and expressions of low self-esteem, thereby increasing depression (Evans & Sullivan, 2001).

ORGANIC MENTAL DISORDERS AND SUBSTANCE USE

Current terminology refers to cognitive impairment and deficits related to substance use as **alcohol-induced persisting amnestic disorder**. **Wernicke's syndrome** is a reversible alcohol-induced amnestic disorder caused by a thiamine-deficient diet. Thiamine is an essential element in producing fatty acids for synthesis and maintaining cerebral myelin. Wernicke's syndrome is marked by diplopia from palsy of the third or fourth cranial nerves, hyperactivity and delirium from stimulation of cortical brain and thalamic lesions, and coma caused by lesions in cranial nerve nuclei and in the mesencephalon and diencephalon of the brain (Goodwin, 1997). Thiamine treatment can reverse this process if initiated rapidly. All the B vitamins are essential for myelination. Deficiencies can lead to the development of lesions in distal peripheral nerves, causing neuropathies.

A second syndrome, which can occur concurrently with Wernicke's, is **Korsakoff's psychosis**. It is characterized by a loss of recent memory and confabulation (or filling in the blanks in memory by making up facts to cover this deficit). The patient with this condition is highly suggestible, has poor judgment, and cannot reason critically. Korsakoff's psychosis often follows Wernicke's encephalopathy and is also associated with prior peripheral neuropathy (Goodwin, 1997). It is treated with thiamine and can often be partially reversed.

Patients with alcohol-induced persisting amnestic disorder usually have histories of many years of heavy alcohol abuse, are generally older than 40 years, can experience sudden onset of symptoms, or may have had symptoms develop during a period of many years (APA, 2000). Impairment can be severe, and once the disorder is established, it can persist indefinitely (APA, 2000). Sedative-hypnotics, anxiolytic agents, and anticonvulsants are also known to cause a persisting amnestic disorder.

Cerebellar degeneration can occur from increased levels of acetaldehyde, a toxic by-product of alcohol metabolism, resulting from years of alcohol abuse. Symptoms are impaired coordination, a broad-based unsteady gait, and fine tremors. Alcohol is directly toxic to the brain, causing atrophy of the frontal cortex and eventually, chronic brain syndrome. Sedative-hypnotic effects of long-term alcohol abuse lead to disturbances in rapid–eye-movement sleep and chronic sleep disorders.

Organic brain disorders resulting from head trauma are more common in substance users than in the general population. This discrepancy is largely attributable to motor vehicle crashes, fights, physical abuse, and other trauma.

COGNITIVE IMPAIRMENT IN EARLY STAGES OF RECOVERY FROM SUBSTANCE USE

Most cognitive impairment in the population of patients seeking alcohol or drug abuse treatment is transitory and resolves within the first month of abstinence. Patients often experience difficulties with disorientation, clouding of consciousness, incoherent thoughts, memory loss, and delirium, which may hinder their ability to learn new concepts (Miller, 1998). In addition to the biologically based etiologies discussed, psychosocial factors can have a negative influence on cognitive ability. Fear of legal or relationship difficulties, depression, grief, and feelings of guilt and shame all may contribute to cognitive impairment (Petrakis et al., 2002). Psychological testing and other methods of assessment are necessary to determine whether the patient's cognitive functioning can improve and whether chemical dependency treatment can be used (Shivani, Goldsmith, & Anthenelli, 2002). The nurse must assess the patient's abilities for self-care, independent living, impulse control, control of assaultiveness, direction taking, and development of new responses to new situations and ideas. The nurse must also evaluate changes in mental status during the past 6 months and examine previous treatment outcomes (Evans & Sullivan, 2001).

Intervention for patients with cognitive or memory impairment must consist of clear, direct, simple messages.

The following points (Evans & Sullivan, 2001) illustrate this approach:

- Use reading material that is relevant to recovery and that can be referred to in short study sessions.
- For patients who have trouble grasping abstract concepts, read first-person accounts of addiction and recovery found in AA and Narcotics Anonymous (NA) literature.
- Concentrate on basic concepts of recovery, such as those in AA slogans, and on patients' need for continuing care after discharge.
- Show films with scenes illustrating relevant family problems or other problems related to substance use. Movies can be more effective than lectures.
- Avoid discussing extraneous issues and avoid theoretic or technical discussions.

PERSONALITY DISORDERS AND SUBSTANCE USE

Personality disorders are frequently diagnosed in alcohol and other drug abusers. Regier and associates (1990) noted that 14.3% of people with an alcohol-related disorder and 17.8% of those with a drug-related disorder had a lifetime prevalence rate of antisocial personality disorder. Conversely, people with an antisocial personality disorder had a lifetime prevalence rate of 83.6% for any substance use disorder. Those with borderline personality disorder had a 28% rate of substance dependence (Thomas, Melchert, & Banker, 1999).

Another study suggested a 40% to 50% concurrent diagnosis of antisocial personality disorder and substance dependence. In addition, the study reported that 90% of patients with antisocial personality disorders who are criminal offenders are substance users (Messina, Wish, & Nemes, 1999). Thomas and colleagues (1999) noted that this population has a higher rate of involuntary hospital admissions, greater resistance to treatment, poor coping skills, poorer interpersonal relationships, and a higher level of impulsivity.

Beeder and Millman (1997) noted that the label *personality disorder* is often incorrectly applied to patients who seek treatment because of legal problems, interpersonal violence, or other difficulties. Chronic drug use can cause personality changes and even psychiatric illness. Alcohol and other drug use in patients with personality disorders are often secondary to these disorders. For example, people with antisocial personality disorder may use alcohol and other drugs to enhance their view of the world as fast-paced and dramatic and may be involved in crime and other sensation-seeking, high-risk behaviour (Ball & McCann, 2001).

Addiction treatment based on tight structure, peer support, and confrontation that addresses the significant destructive behaviour on the part of patients with personality disorders appears to be the most useful approach (Beeder & Millman, 1997). Formally structured groups may improve patients' ability to learn new and more appropriate behaviours and to develop new perceptions that may help them in relating to others. Cognitive therapy approaches may help these patients examine the cognitive distortions that contribute to their substance use.

General Treatment Elements

Patients with dual disorders enter treatment at various stages of recovery. Flexible treatment programs that can meet each patient's needs are the most effective. Regardless of the patient's primary diagnosis or degree of recovery, some common elements exist in the treatment of dual disorders. The following discussion highlights these essential components of treatment.

SETTING PRIORITIES WHEN HOSPITALIZATION IS NECESSARY

Often, patients with dual disorders can be treated effectively in community mental health settings if their symptoms are stable, they are following their treatment plan, they are compliant with use of psychiatric medications, and they remain alcohol and drug free. Dackis & Gold (1997) specified that patients who meet any of the following criteria should be admitted to the hospital for treatment:

- Serious medical needs, such as the need for detoxification
- An exacerbated medical disorder or an illness that prevents abstinence or outpatient treatment
- Suicidal or homicidal ideation, psychotic disorganization, or other serious psychiatric illnesses
- Failed outpatient treatment
- Addiction severity that prevents any significant period of abstinence
- Serious psychosocial problems, such as immediate risk for incarceration, homelessness, or abusive relationships
- Continued abuse of substances during pregnancy

CRISIS STABILIZATION

Setting priorities is essential for hospitalized patients with dual disorders. The first priorities are gathering data from a physical examination and nursing assessments, stabilizing psychiatric symptoms, and treating withdrawal symptoms (Beeder & Millman, 1997) (see Chapter 23). After these issues have been addressed, the patient can enter the rehabilitation phase of treatment for both diagnoses. Rehabilitative therapy is appropriate if the patient (1) can participate in a group process, (2) can focus attention on groups or reading material, (3) does not engage in behaviour that is detrimental to the group process, (4) can listen to and receive feedback from others, and (5) can benefit from the group process.

ENGAGEMENT

Engagement entails establishing a treatment relationship and enhancing motivation to make behaviour changes and a commitment to treatment (Miller, 2000). Patients who are abusing substances may experience repeated cycles of detoxification and relapse. Mentally ill patients may have prolonged cycles of "revolving-door" admissions and persistent medication noncompliance before acknowledging the need to engage in continuous treatment (Kertesz, Horton, Friedmena, & Samet, 2003). Each admission is a "window of opportunity." Relapse does not mean that a treatment intervention, the health care provider, or the patient has failed. Readmission and clear, realistic goals can further the patient's engagement in the treatment process. Effective programs emphasize a combination of empathic, long-term relationship building and the use of leverage and possible confrontation by family, other caregivers, or the legal system.

Engaging patients with dual disorders in treatment presents two main challenges. The first is developing relationships with people who tend to have difficulties in their relationships and with trusting authority figures. The second is patients' lack of motivation and the need to encourage them to enter drug and alcohol treatment programs.

Possible social barriers to patients becoming motivated to seek treatment are homelessness, unemployment, and lack of social support for abstinence. In addition, patients or their therapists may excuse substance use because of the patients' psychiatric symptoms. Patients who deny a problem with substances do not seek treatment because they do not view themselves as needing it. These patients do not fully understand their mental illness or the effect of substance use on their mood or behaviour.

Engagement in treatment is a process that may take many contacts with a patient and requires patience. Patients who struggle with authority and control issues must be convinced that the treatment team members have something to offer and are worth listening to before they will begin to trust them. The engagement process is enhanced if staff can deal with presenting crises concretely (eg, provide help in avoiding legal penalties and obtaining food, housing, entitlements, relief from psychiatric symptoms, vocational opportunities, recreation, and socialization). Harm reduction may be a first step toward a goal of abstinence.

The process of engagement is often characterized by approach–avoidance behaviour by the patient. Intake and assessment procedures may discourage the patient from engagement or be intolerable if they are protracted and begin with asking the patient numerous pointed personal questions. These procedures may have to be adjusted to tailor treatment and accommodate the needs or reactions of the patient with dual disorders.

MEDICATION MANAGEMENT

One essential feature of dual disorder treatment is medication management. Noncompliance with prescribed medications is associated with increased behaviour problems after discharge and is a direct cause of relapse and rehospitalization. Impulsive behaviour in response to transient exacerbations of psychotic symptoms, depressed mood, or anxiety symptoms may lead to relapse. Treating a patient with dual disorders can be as complex as the presenting symptoms. Errors in treatment can include treating temporary psychiatric symptoms resulting from withdrawal as if they were a permanent feature of the individual, withholding needed medication for a psychiatric disorder, or setting arbitrary limits on medication based on a belief that medication for all psychiatric symptoms should be suspended for a time.

Collaboration between the patient's prescriber and other treatment providers is important to minimize the possible misuse of prescription drugs. In addition, caution is essential in prescribing medications that can increase the patient's potential for relapse into abusing the drug of choice (Sullivan, 2001). The patient in recovery is often reluctant to use potentially mind-altering drugs, and the nurse should explore any concerns (Sullivan, 2001). Figure 31-2 presents an algorithm, developed by Sowers and Golden (1999). A cooperative partnership between the health care provider and the patient will help determine which medication is most effective and offers the greatest chance of patient compliance.

The term *abuse* can be applied to the improper use of prescription drugs. Portenoy and Payne (1997) listed the following as clear examples of abuse: (1) prescription forgery; (2) selling of prescription drugs by unauthorized people; (3) acquisition of drugs from nonmedical sources; (4) use of illicit opiates to supplement therapy; (5) unsanctioned drug dose escalation; (6) use of drugs to treat symptoms other than those targeted by the therapy; (7) frequent visits to emergency departments to obtain drugs; (8) contacts with multiple prescribers to obtain drug prescriptions; and (9) drug hoarding.

PATIENT EDUCATION

Patient education is an essential element in treating dual disorders. Topics for group sessions should encourage interaction among patients. Sharing their experiences with their peers, patients can enhance these presentations. Topics should be clear, relevant to the

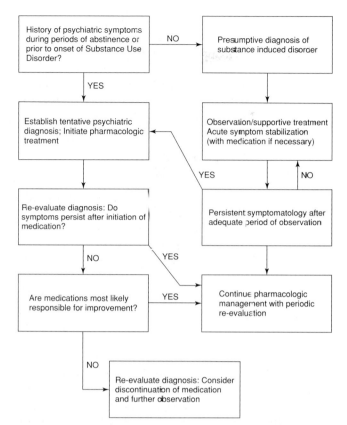

FIGURE 31.2   From Sowers, W., & Golden, S. (1999). Psychotropic medication management in persons with cooccurring psychiatric and substance use disorders. *Journal of Psychoactive Drugs, 31*(1), 59–70. Used with permission.

group members, and illustrated with charts, handouts, or appropriate films. Each lecture or discussion group should be relatively short and not contain too many new or difficult concepts. Reinforcing and reviewing previous discussions can be helpful to remind patients of particularly relevant concepts. Box 31-3 lists some suitable topics for nurse-led discussion groups. Individual patient education can focus on areas of knowledge deficits and reinforce topics discussed in group settings. Group sessions can also assist patients in learning interpersonal skills (eg, assertiveness) and problem-solving skills and in relapse prevention planning.

MUTUAL SELF-HELP GROUPS

Several mutual self-help groups are appropriate for many patients with dual disorders. The most common groups are **12-step programs**, such as AA and NA (see Chapter 23). Zweben (1987) raised the issue of whether a patient who is taking psychotropic medications may participate in a 12-step program. AA published a landmark report by a group of physicians in AA that addressed this issue. In it, the physicians gave guidelines to members for the sensible use of medications and indicated pitfalls that can occur with psychoactive prescription drug use. The report presented members' stories of abuse and discussed the benefits some members derived from the judicious use of appropriately prescribed medications. The authors concluded: "It becomes clear that just as it is wrong to enable or support any alcoholic to become readdicted to any drug, it's equally wrong to deprive any alcoholic of medication which can alleviate or control other disabling physical and/or emotional problems" (Alcoholics Anonymous World Services, 1984, p. 300).

For patients who are concerned that they might not be accepted into AA because of their use of psychiatric medications, this AA literature can be helpful. The advisability of a patient enrolling in a 12-step program needs to be evaluated on an individual basis. A health care provider familiar with 12-step concepts can often facilitate patients' attempts to use these programs. The numerous advantages of self-help groups make them a

---

BOX 31.3

Topics for Education Groups for Patients with Dual Disorder

The effects of alcohol and drugs on the body
Alcohol, drugs, and medication—what can go wrong
- What is a healthy lifestyle?
- Triggers for relapse
- What is Alcoholics (or Narcotics) Anonymous?
- What is a sponsor in Alcoholics (or Narcotics) Anonymous?
- What is recovery from mental illness and substance abuse?
- What are tools of recovery?
- The disease of addiction
- The relapse cycle
- How to cope with feelings without using alcohol or other drugs
- Relapse prevention: what works?
- What are cognitive distortions?

- HIV prevention and education
- Leisure time management
- How to manage stress
- Relaxation training
- Assertiveness and recovery
- Common slogans to live by
- Pitfalls in treatment
- The process of recovery
- Creating a relapse prevention plan
- What are my goals? How does the use of alcohol and drugs affect them?
Coping with thoughts about alcohol and drugs
- Problem-solving basics
- Coping with anger
- Negative thinking and how to manage it
- Enhancing social support networks

potentially powerful support for continued recovery. Alternative mutual self-help programs similar to 12-step programs are available in some geographic areas. Rational Recovery and Secular Organization for Sobriety are groups that downplay the concept of powerlessness and the spiritual aspects associated with 12-step programs.

RELAPSE PREVENTION: CREATING A NEW LIFESTYLE

Relapse is the failure to maintain the behaviours needed to remain abstinent (Annis & Davis, 1995). One model of relapse prevention is based on the self-efficacy theory. It proposes that when a patient enters a situation in which the risk for resuming drinking or drug use is high, his or her expectations of the ability to cope with the situation without substances will predict his or her substance use (Annis & Davis, 1995). If a patient feels confident that he or she can cope with an emotionally charged situation, his or her likelihood of using substances in that situation is lower. See Box 31-4 for a list of common situations in which relapse often occurs.

Relapse prevention groups can be valuable sources of support for patients. These groups help patients to (1) analyze which situations are most likely to trigger relapses; (2) examine cognitive, emotional, and behavioural components of high-risk situations; and (3) develop cognitive, behavioural, and effective coping strategies and environmental supports. Role playing ways out of high-risk situations is a technique that these groups often use (Annis & Davis, 1995; Marlatt & Gordon, 1985). Homework assignments help patients create relapse prevention plans that address new coping strategies for these high-risk situations.

This model uses cognitive-behavioural techniques to help patients plan for stressors that can lead to relapse.

BOX 31.4

Categories of Relapse Episodes

I. Intrapersonal and environmental determinants
   A. Coping with negative emotional states
   B. Coping with negative physical and physiologic states
   C. Enhancement of positive emotional states
   D. Testing personal control
   E. Giving in to temptations or urges
II. Interpersonal determinants
   A. Coping with interpersonal conflict
   B. Coping with social pressure
   C. Enhancement of positive emotional states

From Marlatt, G. A., & Gordon, J. R. (1985). *Relapse prevention.* New York: Guilford Press. Used with permission.

The methods highlighted are practical, emphasize and strengthen patients' coping skills, and can be adapted to the needs of individual patients. Relapse prevention plans initiated in treatment are just pieces of paper if they are not implemented after discharge. The following section discusses elements in effective discharge planning for patients with dual disorders.

CONTINUUM OF CARE AND DISCHARGE PLANNING

Early intervention in crises is important for patients with dual disorders, but equally important is a focus beyond medication management and inpatient treatment episodes. Social interaction skills and coping skills learned in treatment need to be reinforced in community settings to create or enhance a stable living situation and possible vocational opportunities. Active planning and intervention are needed for housing and employment, or deterioration may occur, despite gains made during hospitalization.

Establishing a positive social network is a critical function of any program intended to treat dual disorders. Isolation and alienation from prior sources of support is a problem that most chronically mentally ill substance users share. Some patients relate poorly to their families, others are overly dependent on them, and others have difficulty establishing and maintaining social relationships. Some patients' only "families" are peers within the drug subculture who reinforce substance-abusing behaviour.

Opportunities to socialize, access to positive recreational activities, and a supportive peer group are stabilizing influences on patients who may otherwise drop out of treatment altogether. Part of a comprehensive relapse prevention plan is to establish or reinforce the patient's social support network so that he or she can obtain (1) opportunities for substance-free socializing, (2) crisis counselling to prevent readmission to a hospital, and (3) support for sobriety.

Supportive housing is also essential for patients with dual disorders. Supportive housing is especially crucial for patients who are being discharged from the hospital because the risk for relapse is greatest during the first few months after discharge. Halfway houses for substance users may de-emphasize medication compliance, and housing designed for the chronically mentally ill may not emphasize abstinence enough. Thus, an important part of the multidisciplinary team approach to discharge planning for patients with dual disorders is to help them find the best possible living situation.

Younger patients with severe mental illness may want and expect to find appropriate employment, but some of these patients may be unrealistic about potential professions. However, this desire can be a significant motivator and a useful tool in a treatment program. Referring patients to halfway houses or residential substance use treatment programs that stress vocational skill training can be beneficial. Use of community vocational rehabilitation services and of educational opportunities can be an important part of a discharge plan.

Case Management

Case managers are responsible for conducting outreach activities, linking patients with direct services, monitoring patients' progress through various milieus, educating patients about psychiatric and substance use disorders, reiterating treatment recommendations, and coordinating treatment planning across programs (Segal, 1988). Case managers can use four approaches for delivering services to patients with dual disorders (Segal, 1988):

- *Brokerage-generalist.* This short-term model seeks to identify the patient's needs and helps gain access to appropriate resources.

- *Assertive community treatment.* This model involves assertive advocacy, making contact with patients in their homes and natural settings, with the focus on practical problems of daily living.
- *Strength-based perspective.* This model emphasizes providing support for patients to assert direct control over their search for resources and to examine the patients' own strengths in acquiring these resources.
- *Clinical-rehabilitation.* In this model, the clinician provides counselling and is responsible for resource acquisition.

Table 31-4 lists how these models of case management address case management activities for the patient with dual disorders.

Family Support and Education

The families of patients with dual disorders need education and support. The focus of family support groups, such as those under the auspices of the National

---

Table 31.4	Models of Case Management for Patients With Dual Disorders			
Primary Case Management Activities	**Broker-Generalist**	**Strengths Perspective**	**Assertive Community Treatment**	**Clinical Rehabilitation**
Engages in outreach and case finding	No	Depends on agency mission and structure	Depends on agency mission and structure	Depends on agency mission and structure
Provides assessment and reassessment	Specific to immediate resource acquisition needs	Strengths based, applicable to any area of need	Broad-based comprehensive assessment	Broad-based, comprehensive assessment
Assists in goal planning	Brief, related to acquiring resources	Patient driven, teaches specific ways to set and achieve goals	Comprehensive and may include any area of patient's life	Comprehensive and may include any area of patient's life
Makes referrals to needed resources	Patient or case manager may make contact	Patient or case manager may make contact	As needed; resources may be integrated in services	Patient or case manager may make contact
Provides additional services such as therapy, skills teaching	Referral to others for these	Limited; teaches patient to identify strengths and about self-help groups	Provides many services in comprehensive package	Provides services consistent with model
Responds to crisis	Related to resource needs	Related to resource and mental health concerns: active in stabilization and referral	Assertive advocacy on several levels	Assertive advocacy on several levels
Provides direct services related to resource acquisition as part of case management (eg, drop-in centre; employment counselling)	Referral to resources that provide direct services	Provides services to prepare patient to gain own resources (eg, role playing, accompanying patient to services)	Provides many direct services as part of comprehensive package	Provides services as part of a rehabilitation services plan; skill teaching

Alliance for the Mentally Ill, has been both to educate and to help the family cope with a mentally ill relative. Al Anon and Nar Anon take a similar approach to providing peer support to families of substance users. These self-help groups aid family members in balancing confrontation of the problem, detachment from forcing a solution to it, and support of the treatment process.

Comprehensive Concurrent Treatment

Several traditional approaches are possible for treating dual disorders:
- Treat the mental illness first.
- Treat the substance use disorder first.
- Treat both conditions concurrently.

Recent literature suggests that a comprehensive concurrent approach is often beneficial once the presenting problem has been stabilized. Box 31-5 presents features of a dual disorder outpatient program.

Planning for Nursing Care

Numerous challenges face the nurse who provides care to patients with dual disorders. Comprehensive planning within a multidisciplinary team approach has been highly successful in the care of such patients. Community organizations can be valuable sources of support as well. (See Chapter 23 for available community resources.)

SUMMARY OF KEY POINTS

- The incidence of alcohol or drug abuse and one or more comorbid mental health disorders is very high.
- Dual disorders can consist of a primary mental illness and subsequent substance use, a primary substance use disorder and psychopathologic sequelae, dual primary diagnoses, or two disorders resulting from a common cause.
- In patients with dual disorders, relapse is common if both the substance use disorder and the mental health disorder are not addressed concurrently.
- Barriers to effective treatment of dual disorders include the nature of substance use, countertransference and the position of substance users in society, misunderstandings about and the stigmatization of mental illness, and underlying health issues.
- Assessment of dual disorders often depends on objective data obtained from interviews with family members, reviews of court records, laboratory test results, and physical examination findings.
- Alcohol and drug use can cause numerous mental health problems, including organic brain disorders, depression, hallucinations, agitation, confusion, and stupor. These substances interact with common prescription and over-the-counter drugs to cause adverse reactions.
- Alcohol and other drugs often exacerbate existing mental health disorders and can lead to noncompliance with prescribed medication regimens and other aspects of treatment.
- Elements of treatment for patients with dual disorders include possible hospitalization, crisis stabilization, engagement in long-term treatment, medication management, patient education, use of self-help groups, relapse prevention, continuation of care, case management, and family support.
- Relapse prevention is crucial in treating patients with dual disorders and entails analyzing high-risk situations for relapse; examining the cognitive, emotional, and behavioural components of high-risk situations; and using effective coping strategies and available environmental supports.

BOX 31.5

Features of a Dual Disorder Outpatient Program

Community meeting and goal setting: Patients set small, realistic goals for themselves for the day, which aids them in their ultimate goal of better living in recovery.
Anger management and social communication: Patients learn appropriate ways to express anger and how to socialize with others.
Group therapy: Patients discuss interpersonal issues, get feedback from their peers, and learn problem-solving skills.
Dual recovery anonymous meetings: Patient-run meeting (a modified Alcoholics Anonymous meeting) addresses the specific needs of the patient with dual disorders.
Leisure planning: Patients learn skills to enjoy leisure involving clean and sober fun.
Gardening, art therapy, music therapy, swimming: These methods provide alternatives to the use of alcohol and other drugs.
Health education: Patients learn about the effects of drugs and alcohol on the body and about other relevant medical topics.
Medication education: Patients learn about psychiatric medications, their uses, the side effects, and interactions with drugs or alcohol.
Relapse prevention planning: Patients talk about their last relapse; triggers, feelings, and stresses that contributed to the relapse; and the consequences and formulate relapse prevention plans.
Individual counselling: Patients receive individual counselling to develop goals and work on problem-solving techniques.
Psychiatric consultation: Patients are evaluated and followed up for medication and other psychiatric interventions.
Note: Patients are *not* discharged from the program if they are intoxicated. They are asked not to come to the program intoxicated but to return when they are sober to continue work on their recovery.

CRITICAL THINKING CHALLENGES

1 What criteria would you use to refer an intoxicated and depressed patient in a psychiatric emergency department to the following?
   a An alcohol detoxification centre
   b An inpatient psychiatric unit
   c An outpatient alcohol-treatment program
   d An outpatient community mental health clinic
2 How would you respond to a patient with dual disorders who states, "Once my medication is stable, I will be able to drink again."
3 In your opinion, what are the five most important concepts to cover in educating a patient with dual disorders?

WEB LINKS

www.camh.net This website of the Centre for Addiction and Mental Health, which is Canada's leading addiction and mental health teaching hospital, in Toronto, provides many links to education, research, treatment, policy, and so forth.

www.hc-sc.gc.ca The Health Canada site has links to best practices for concurrent mental health and substance abuse disorders. It also provides a National program directory listing programs that address concurrent mental health and substance abuse disorders.

www.ccsa.ca The website of the Canadian Centre on Substance Abuse includes information, policy material, and research on dual disorders.

www.corp.aadac.com The website of the Alberta Alcohol and Drug Abuse Commission provides basic information related to dual diagnosis.

www.heretohelp.bc.ca The website of the B.C. Partners for Mental Health and Addictions Information provides information, support, resources, and links related to dual diagnosis issues.

MOVIES

Poundmaker's Lodge: A Healing Place: 1987. *The National Film Board of Canada. Poundmaker's Lodge,* named after a 19th century Aboriginal leader, is a treatment centre in St. Albert, Alberta, where Aboriginal people troubled by addiction to drugs and alcohol can come together for mutual support, to partake of healing rituals like the sweat lodge, and to rediscover their traditions. The film places Aboriginal alcoholism and mental health issues in historical and sociocultural contexts. It shows the despair of a people dispossessed of land, culture, language, and dignity and their strength and courage in overcoming substance abuse.

VIEWING POINTS: In your opinion, what are some of the steps that nurses could take to help ensure that multicultural groups of all kinds receive more culturally appropriate treatment for difficulties with addictions and mental health issues?

Patrick's Story: 1999. *The National Film Board of Canada.* Patrick Bird was a 'casualty of colonialism,' having walked a dark boyhood journey of sexual abuse, neglect, foster homes, detention centres, loss, abandonment, drugs, alcohol, and self-mutilation. Through no fault of his own, Patrick was disconnected from his family, his childhood, and his Cree culture and left with few resources to cope with the pain and powerlessness. *Patrick's Story* explores what brought a young man to attempt suicide and what turned his life around.

VIEWING POINTS: In your opinion, how does this film highlight the relationship between substance abuse and mental health issues? What were your feelings as you watched this movie? In what ways does this movie offer a message of inspiration and hope?

REFERENCES

Alcoholics Anonymous World Services, Inc. (1984). *The A. A. member-medications and other drugs: A report from a group of physicians in A. A.* New York: Author.

American Psychiatric Association. (2000). *Diagnostic and statistical manual of mental disorders* (4th ed., Text revision). Washington, DC: Author.

Annis, H. M., & Davis, C. S. (1995). Relapse prevention. In R. K. Hester & W. R. Miller (Eds.), *Handbook of alcoholism treatment approaches* (2nd ed., pp. 170–181). Boston: Allyn & Bacon.

Ball, E. M., & McCann, R. A. (2001). Antisocial personality disorder. In J. L. Jacobson & A. M. Jacobson (Eds.), *Psychiatric secrets* (2nd ed.). Philadelphia: Hanley & Belfus.

B.C. Partners for Mental Health and Addictions Information. (2003). *Concurrenet disorders: Addictions and mental disorders.* Vancouver: Author.

Beauchamp, J. K., & Olson, K. R. (2000). Drug overdoses and dependence. In R. M. Wachter, L. Goldman, & H. Hollander (Eds.), *Hospital medicine.* Philadelphia: Lippincott Williams & Wilkins.

Beeder, A. B., & Millman, R. B. (1997). Treatment of patients with psychopathology and substance abuse. In J. H. Lowinson, P. Ruiz, R. B. Millman, & J. G. Langrod (Eds.), *Substance abuse: A comprehensive textbook* (3rd ed., pp. 675–690). Baltimore: Williams & Wilkins.

Bellack, A., & Gearon, J. (1998). Substance abuse treatment for people with schizophrenia. *Addictive Behaviors, 23*(6), 749–766.

Brehm, N. M., & Khantzian, E. J. (1997). A psychodynamic perspective. In J. H. Lowinson, P. Ruiz, R. B. Millman, & J. G. Langrod (Eds.), *Substance abuse: A comprehensive textbook* (3rd ed., pp. 106–117). Baltimore: Williams & Wilkins.

Canadian Mental Health Association, Ontario Division. (1997). *Concurrent disorders: Policy consultation document.* Toronto: Author.

Churchill, D. M. (2003). Toward an integrative approach to substance abuse: An inquiry into the recognition, diagnosis and treatment of substance abuse by social workers. *Dissertation Abstracts International, 63*(8-A), US: Univ Microfilms International.

Dackis, C., & Gold, M. S. (1997). Psychiatric hospitals for treatment of dual diagnosis. In J. H. Lowinson, P. Ruiz, R. B. Millman, & J. G. Langrod (Eds.), *Substance abuse: A comprehensive textbook* (3rd ed., pp. 467–485). Baltimore: Williams & Wilkins.

Drake, R. E. (2001). Implementing dual diagnosis services for clients with severe mental illness. *Psychiatric Services, 52*(4).

Evans, K., & Sullivan, J. (2001). *Dual diagnosis: Counselling the mentally ill substance abuser.* New York: Guilford Press.

Federal, Provincial and Territorial Advisory Committee on Population Health. (1999). *Statistical report on the health of Canadians.* Ottawa: Author.

Goldberg, J., Garno, J., Leon, A., et al. (1999). A history of substance abuse complicates remission from acute mania in bipolar disorder. *Journal of Clinical Psychiatry, 60*(11), 733–739.

Goodwin, D. W. (1997). Alcohol: Clinical aspects. In J. H. Lowinson, P. Ruiz, R. B. Millman, & J. G. Langrod (Eds.), *Substance abuse: A comprehensive textbook* (3rd ed., pp. 144–151). Baltimore: Williams & Wilkins.

Hwang, S. (2001). Mental illness and mentality among homeless people. *Acta Psychiatrica Scandinavicca, 103*(2), 81–82.

Hwang, S. (2002). Is homelessness hazardous to your health? Obstacles to the demonstration of a causal relationship. *Canadian Journal of Public Health, 93*(6), 407–410.

Joseph, H. (1997). Substance abuse and homelessness within the inner cities. In J. H. Lowinson, P. Ruiz, R. B. Millman, & J. G. Langrod (Eds.), *Substance abuse: A comprehensive textbook* (3rd ed., pp. 875–889). Baltimore: Williams & Wilkins.

Kertesz, S. G., Horton, N. J., Friedmena, P. D., & Samet, J. H. (2003). Slowing the revolving door: Stabilization programs reduce homeless persons' substance use after detoxification. *Journal of Substance Abuse Treatment, 24*(3).

Kushner, M. G., Sher, K. J., & Beitman, M. D. (1990). The relation between alcohol problems and the anxiety disorders. *American Journal of Psychiatry, 147*(6), 685–695.

Lehman, A. F., Myers, C. P., & Corty, E. (1989). Assessment and classification of patients with psychiatric and substance abuse syndromes. *Hospital and Community Psychiatry, 40*(10), 1019–1024.

Marlatt, G. A., & Gordon, J. R. (1985). *Relapse prevention.* New York: Guilford Press.

Marx, J. M., Hockberger, R., & Walls, R. (2002). *Rosen's emergency medicine: Concepts and clinical practice* (5th ed.; p. 1560). St. Louis: Mosby.

Messina, N., Wish, E., & Nemes, S. (1999). Therapeutic community treatment for substance abusers with antisocial personality disorder. *Journal of Substance Abuse Treatment, 17*(1–2), 121–128.

Miller, N. S. (1995). *Addiction psychiatry: Current diagnosis and treatment* (p. 112). New York: Wiley-Liss.

Miller, N. S. (1998). Management of withdrawal syndromes and relapse prevention in drug and alcohol dependence. *American Family Physician, 58*(1), 139–146.

Miller, W. R., & Kurtz, E. (1994). Models of alcoholism used in treatment: Contrasting AA and other perspectives with which it is confused. *Journal of Studies on Alcoholism, 55*(2), 159–166.

Olson, W. (2004). Delirium tremens. In F. Ferri (Ed.), *Ferri's clinical advisor, 2004: Instant diagnosis and treatment.* St. Louis: Mosby.

Petrakis, I., Gonzalez, G., Rosenheck, R., & Krystal, J. (2002). Comorbidity of alcoholism and psychiatric disorders: An overview. *Alcohol Research and Health, 26*(2), 81–89.

Portenoy, R. K., & Payne, R. (1997). Acute and chronic pain. In J. H. Lowinson, P. Ruiz, R. B. Millman, & J. G. Langrod (Eds.), *Substance abuse: A comprehensive textbook* (3rd ed., pp. 236–246). Baltimore: Williams & Wilkins.

Regier, D. A., Farmer, M. E., Rae, D. S., et al. (1990). Comorbidity of mental disorders with alcohol and other drug abuse: Results from the epidemiologic catchment area (ECA) study. *Journal of the American Medical Association, 264,* 2511–2518.

Ries, R. (1995). *Assessment and treatment of patients with coexisting mental illness and alcohol and other drug abuse* (pp. 29–89). Rockville, MD: U.S. Department of Health and Human Services.

Rosenthal, R. N., & Westreich, L. (1999). Treatment of persons with dual diagnosis of substance use disorders and other psychological problems. In *Addictions: A comprehensive guide* (pp. 439–476). New York: Oxford University Press.

Ross, H. E. (1995). DSM-III-R alcohol abuse and dependence and psychiatric comorbidity in Ontario: Results from the mental health supplement to the Ontario Health Survey. *Drug and Alcohol Dependence, 39*(2), 111–128.

Ross, H. E., Glaser, F. B., & Germanson, T. (1988). The prevalence of psychiatric disorders in patients with alcohol and other drug problems. *Archives of General Psychiatry, 45*(11), 1023–1031.

Royal Commission on Aboriginal Persons. (1996). *Report of the Roayl Commission on Aboriginal Persons.* Ottawa: Author.

Scott, J., Gilvarry, E., & Farrell, M. (1998). Managing anxiety and depression in alcohol and drug dependence. *Addictive Behaviors, 23*(6), 919–931.

Segal, B. (1988). Drugs and behavior. New York: Gardner Press.

Senate Committee on Social Affairs, Science and Technology. (2004). *Mental health, mental illness and addiction: Issues and options for Canada.* Ottawa: Author.

Shivani, R., Goldsmith, R., & Anthenelli, R. (2002). Alcoholism and psychiatric disorders: Diagnostic challenges. *Alcohol Research and Health, 26*(2), 90–98.

Sowers, W., & Golden, S. (1999). Psychotropic medication management in persons with co-occurring psychiatric and substance use disorders. *Journal of Psychoactive Drugs, 31*(1), 59–70.

Thomas, V., Melchert, T., & Banker, J. (1999). Substance dependence and personality disorders: Comorbidity and treatment outcome in an inpatient treatment population. *Journal of Studies of Alcohol, 60,* 271–277.

Wallen, M. C., & Weiner, H. D. (1989). Impediments to effective treatment of the dually diagnosed patient. *Journal of Psychoactive Drugs, 21*(2), 161–168.

Weiss, R. D., Marin, S. M., & Frances, R. J. (1992). The myth of the typical dual diagnosis patient. *Hospital and Community Psychiatry, 43*(2), 107–108.

Zweben, J. E. (1987). Can patients on medication be sent to 12-step programs? *Journal of Psychoactive Drugs, 19*(3), 299–300.

For challenges, please refer to the **CD-ROM** in this book.

32

Psychosocial Aspects of Medically Compromised Persons

Gail L. Konçable and Michel Tarko

LEARNING OBJECTIVES

After studying this chapter, you will be able to:

- Identify medically ill populations at risk for secondary mental illness.
- Analyze the effect on clients and their families of mental illness associated with the medical illness.
- Discuss comorbid psychosocial and biologic disorders seen in psychiatric settings and their treatments.
- Discuss neurobiologic and psychological disturbances associated with specific medical illnesses and the medications used to treat them.
- Develop a plan of care for clients who are experiencing mental illness associated with medical illness.
- Discuss biopsychosocial interventions that promote clients' mental health in physical illness.

KEY TERMS

allodynia ▪ comorbidity ▪ endorphins ▪ gate-control model ▪ HIV-1–sassociated cognitive-motor complex ▪ hyperalgia ▪ hyperesthesia ▪ hypothalamic-pituitary-adrenal (HPA) axis ▪ ischemic cascade ▪ kindling ▪ nociception ▪ neurotransmitters ▪ plasticity ▪ self-efficacy ▪ serotonin ▪ substance P

KEY CONCEPTS

Cognitive-behavioural model ▪ Neurochemical modulation

Psychiatric illness often accompanies medical illness and is a significant health care problem in the medically ill population. People who have chronic medical illnesses have a nearly 41% higher rate of psychiatric disorders than do people without chronic medical illness. In addition, the chronically medically ill have a 28% higher lifetime prevalence of psychiatric disorders than do people without psychiatric disorders. Studies spanning decades indicate that diabetes mellitus, cardiac disease, and associated metabolic disorders are more common among clients with psychiatric disorders than among the general population (Joffe, Brasche, & MacQueen, 2003). As many as 80% of chronically mentally ill clients have significant medical illness, which may or may not be related to psychopharmacologic therapy (Dixon, Postrado, Delahanty, Fischer, & Lehman, 1999; Goldsmith, 1999) Mood, anxiety, and substance use disorders are the most prevalent psychiatric conditions of clients with chronic or terminal illnesses, such as chronic pain, acquired immunodeficiency syndrome (AIDS), acute trauma, stroke, and cancer (Ford, Trestman, Steinberg, Tennen, & Allen, 2004). Because most medically ill people are elderly, biologic, psychological, and social changes may place them at greater risk for mental illness and increased potential mortality and morbidity.

Psychological Illness Related to Specific Physiologic Disorders

The biologic basis of mental disorders that are preceded by comorbid medical disorders is thought to be similar to the biologic basis of primary psychiatric disorders, in which neurochemical changes occur in the process of catecholamine metabolism (Arnsten, 1997). The neurochemicals (transmitters) that orchestrate thinking, learning, speaking, and motor responses also influence mood, perception, and emotional interpretation. Neurochemical modulation maintains a balance in the essential levels of these transmitters. When modulation is disrupted, either mechanically or chemically, biopsychosocial disorder occurs.

⬢ **KEY CONCEPT Neurochemical modulation** maintains a balance in the essential levels of the neurotransmitters that influence mood, perceptions, and emotional interpretation.

Unfortunately, mental illness is not commonly recognized or treated in general medical settings. Psychiatric symptoms may be masked by medical symptoms or misdiagnosed as somatoform disorders. The treatment regimen may contribute to psychosocial dysfunction because many medications prescribed for chronic illness alter affect (Goldsmith, 1999; Neese, 1991). Generally,

health care providers expect clients to exhibit depressed mood and anxiety as a normal response to illness. In fact, it is considered abnormal if a client does not grieve over the loss of health or does not express discouragement or anxiety about treatment and the possibility of death.

When psychosocial dysfunction remains unexamined and untreated, the course and outcome of associated medical illness may be affected. Mental illness may weaken the motivation for self-care, impair symptom reporting, and delay the search for treatment (Katon & Schulberg, 1992). These symptoms may precede or occur during acute hospitalization and continue after discharge and apparent physical recovery. As a result, hospitalization may be prolonged and recovery delayed, or impaired, at increased emotional and financial cost to the client and the family (Levenson, 1992). In severe cases, mood disorders associated with medical illness increase morbidity and mortality (Hill, Kelleher, & Shumaker, 1992; Paten, 1999; Polsky et al., 2005). Careful assessment to identify and evaluate symptoms of concomitant mental illness separately from those of medical illness is required, together with appropriate treatment, to achieve the client's best psychological and medical outcome.

Another aspect of psychiatric disorders and medical illness is the common comorbidity of physical disorders among people who require primary psychiatric care. Factors associated with increased hospital stays of psychiatric patients include physical disability and concomitant medical illness (Cohen & Cosimer, 1989; Collins, 1991). Mental health care professionals must carefully evaluate and monitor changes in coexisting medical conditions to prevent their exacerbation or serious complications that would necessitate acute medical treatment or prolonged hospital stay.

This chapter reviews issues related to mental illness in the medically ill population and common comorbid medical disorders in the psychiatric population. The psychosocial disturbances associated with chronic pain, human immunodeficiency virus (HIV), trauma, neurologic disorders, stroke, and chronic medical illnesses such as heart disease and cancer are presented. Suggestions for diagnostic appraisal and appropriate intervention are given. These medical conditions were chosen because they are responsible for most hospital admissions and frequently are associated with psychiatric comorbidity. Psychiatric mental health liaison clinicians are consulted to see patients with these conditions in all phases of their illness, from acute hospitalization and treatment to rehabilitation and return to the community.

Psychological Impact of Pain

Physiologic pain is a protective response to noxious stimuli that serves as a warning of injury. Clinical pain related to inflammation and pathologic processes is characterized by low-threshold sensitization. Despite major advances in treatments that lessen its force, pain remains one of the most powerful and complex human experiences. Assessing and treating pain are difficult because the pain response is subjective and a client's degree of pain cannot be observed directly. A client's complaints may be difficult to localize. Moreover, the person's discomfort may seem out of proportion to the observed conditions or influenced by disordered emotions, personality, or environmental conditioning. Severe or chronic pain may affect mentally healthy people in adverse ways. The prevalence and impact of pain have led to numerous approaches to therapy, including the use of antipsychotic drugs, antidepressants, antianxiety agents, and stimulants. Considerable evidence suggests that psychiatric medications and interventions can be effective in treating acute and chronic pain.

The gate-control model of pain response is based on physiologic evidence that pain perception (nociception) involves pathways in the dorsal horn of the spinal cord that relay noxious stimuli to the brain. In addition, certain other nerve fibers function as an antagonistic "gate" to augment or dampen the subjective experience of pain (Melzack, 1993; Robinson, 2003). The cognitive-biobehavioural model considers not only the client's emotive and cognitive perception of pain, but also the interaction of environmental influences, physical factors, and pain perceptions over time. From this perspective, clients' interpretation of pain, their coping resources, and their emotive psychological processes interact with the experience of pain and can influence the physiologic activities that characterize pain (Turk, 2004). Some pain theorists believe that the gate-control theory has been largely discredited (McCaffery & Pasero, 1999); others are working to refine the theory as more knowledge of pain becomes available.

> ◆ **KEY CONCEPT** The **cognitive-behavioural model** is the model of perception that includes emotion, cognition, environment, and physical and psychological factors.

BIOLOGIC BASIS OF THE PAIN RESPONSE

Pain is transmitted through specific neural pathways that carry information about touch and temperature (Fig. 32-1). Recent physiologic evidence obtained from magnetic resonance imaging and positron emission tomography has demonstrated that painful stimuli also cause significant activation in areas of the brain responsible for memory, emotion, and personality (Talbot et al., 1991) (Fig. 32-2). Pain receptors may be activated by mechanical, thermal, or chemical stimuli.

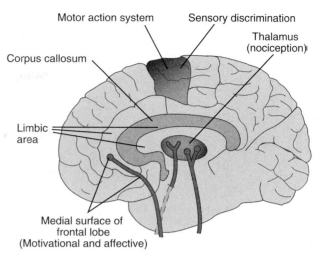

FIGURE 32.1 Pain stimuli activate regions of the brain that influence memory, emotion, and personality.

Neurotransmitters are chemicals circulating in the synaptic areas of neurons. They serve to initiate, block, or modulate nerve signal transmission and ultimately control neural function. Several neurotransmitters within primary pain pathways are involved in pain transmission (Box 32-1). When these neurochemicals are released, they initiate local inflammatory reactions and sensitize and stimulate central pain receptors. Substance P is the most common nociceptive transmitter that is released and transported along the central and peripheral pain synapses in the presence of noxious stimuli. Endorphins, neurotransmitters that have opiate-like behaviour, produce an inhibitory effect at opiate receptor sites and probably are responsible for pain tolerance. The release of endorphins is centrally mediated by serotonin (Zangen, Nakash, & Yadid, 1999). Serotonin, histamine, and bradykinin sensitize and stimulate the pain receptors to generate experienced pain. Direct demonstrations of changes in endorphin levels during pain and relief from pain are being reported (Ren, 1994; Sosnowski, 1994). The role of endorphins may go beyond pain modulation to include mood enhancement behaviour modification and influence the development of tolerance or dependence on narcotics.

Acute pain, one of the most common symptoms of clients in emergency and acute care settings, can result from a variety of physiologic abnormalities and trauma. It is characterized by sudden, severe onset and generally subsides as the injury heals. Postoperative incisional pain is an iatrogenic (physician-induced) tissue injury most often seen in medical settings. Careful assessment and treatment of pain in these settings have a great impact on healing and recovery.

Chronic pain, defined as pain on a daily basis or pain that is constant for more than 6 months (Atkinson & Slater, 1989), can be related to various pathologies and

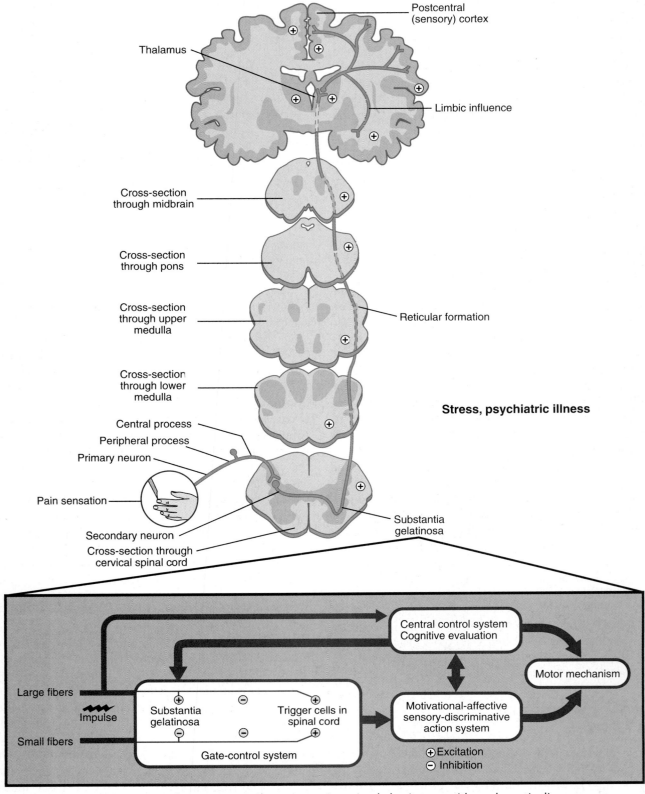

FIGURE 32.2   Ascending sensory pathways: anterior spinothalamic tract with a schematic diagram of the gate-control theory of pain mechanism.

BOX 32.1

Neurotransmitters Active in Pain Sensation and Induced Plasticity

C-Fiber Neuropeptides Released by Noxious Stimulation Peripherally
Substance P
Neurokinin A
Somatostatin
Calcitonin gene-related peptide (CGRP)
Galanin
Vasoactive intestinal polypeptide (VIP)
Cholecystokinin

Excitatory Amino Acids With Widespread Activity in the CNS (Thalamus and Somatosensory Cortices)
L-Glutamate
N-methyl-D-aspartate (NMDA)

Pain-Modulating Neurotransmitters
Endorphins
Enkephalin
Serotonin

Note: Many of these same neurotransmitters are released in large amounts during brain injury and contribute to neuronal cell death in a variety of neurologic and psychological disease processes.

---

takes the form of syndromes, such as headache, temporomandibular pain disorders, back pain, and arthritis. Clinical syndromes with chronic pain symptoms include neoplasia (cancer), thalamic stroke (central pain), neuropathies (diabetes), and reflex sympathetic dystrophy (Box 32-2). Nervous tissue injury leads to neuropathic pain that may be described as burning, aching, pricking, or lancinating. This central or neuropathic pain is the underlying mechanism for most chronic pain and leads to **hyperalgia** (increased sensation of pain), allodynia (lowered pain threshold), and **hyperesthesia** (increased nociceptor sensitivity). Permanent change in central pain interpretation frequently results in abnormal physiologic, biochemical, cellular, and molecular responses

BOX 32.2

Pain Syndromes Seen in the Primary Care Setting

Migraine headache: a cerebrovasomotor disorder in which a focal reduction of cerebral blood flow initiates an ischemic headache. May be preceded by a visual aura and followed by nausea, vomiting, and incapacitating head pain.

Low back pain: pain arising from the vertebral column or surrounding muscles, tendons, ligaments, or fascia. Causes range from simple muscle strain to arthritis, fracture, or nerve compression from a ruptured disk.

Chronic benign orofacial pain: temporomandibular joint pain.

Rheumatoid arthritis: more than 100 different types of joint disease produce inflammation of the joints. Associated with varying degrees of pain and stiffness and eventual loss of use of the affected joints.

Reflex sympathetic dystrophy: causalgia. A painful burning syndrome that occurs after peripheral nerve injury. Associated with hyperesthesia, vasomotor disturbances, and dystrophic changes due to sympathetic hyperactivity.

Cancer pain: pain from malignant tumors that is caused by local infiltration or metastatic spread involving specific organs, bones, or peripheral or cranial nerves, or the spinal cord. Pain therapy is aimed at providing sufficient relief to allow maximum possible daily functioning and a relatively pain-free death.

Neuropathic pain

Polyneuropathy: neuropathy involving multiple peripheral nerves

Diabetic neuropathy: neuropathy due to diabetes mellitus; marked by diminished sensation secondary to vascular changes

Inflammatory neuropathy: neuropathy related to the presence of chemical or microorganic pathogens

Traumatic neuropathy: neuropathy caused by avulsion or compression

Plexopathy: neuropathy involving a peripheral nerve plexus

Peripheral or central neuralgia: abrupt, intense, paroxysmal pain due to intrinsic nerve injury or extrinsic nerve compression

Herpetic neuralgia: pain associated with the dermatomal rash of acute herpes zoster

Radiculopathy: pain radiating along a peripheral nerve tract, such as sciatica

Vasoocclusive pain: thrombotic crisis of sickle cell anemia in joints and peripheral muscles that is caused by ischemia

Myofascial pain: pain in palpable bands (trigger points) of muscle. Associated with stiffness, limitation of motion, and weakness.

that misinterpret nonpainful sensations as painful (**plasticity**) (Melzack, Coderre, Katz, Vaccarino, 2000). This neural plasticity contributes to the development of errant firing and the pain syndromes of referred pain (pain felt in a part other than where it was produced) and phantom pain (pain that feels as though its source is a missing [amputated] limb).

PSYCHOLOGICAL ASPECTS OF THE PAIN RESPONSE

Pain is not only a sensation but also a perceptual phenomenon with an important affective component. When a client's pain persists for an extended period, a range of psychosocial influences, such as the client's mood, fears, expectancies, coping efforts, and financial and social resources, and the responses of significant others begin to influence the client's perception of the pain. Affective and anxiety disorders are prevalent among people with chronic pain. They may be a symptom of or a defense against psychological stress caused

by continuous nociceptive input (Koob, 1999). Biopsychosocial stimuli and responses may cause the client with chronic pain to become preoccupied with the pain and can contribute to depression. In addition, the presence of persistent noxious sensations contributes to neurochemical and neurohormonal imbalances that lead to depressed mood and anxiety. Whether the psychological pain is primary or secondary may be difficult to determine because the neurovegetative symptoms of depression may resemble the client's attempts to control the pain or the concomitant medical-physical conditions. Anorexia, sleep disturbance, and agitation or psychomotor retardation may be present. In addition, affective disturbances, such as sadness, loss of interest in life, feelings of worthlessness, self-reproach, excessive guilt, indecisiveness, and suicidal ideation, are all symptoms reported by clients with chronic pain (Turk, 2004). Substance use disorder may arise from the client's search for relief through overuse of drugs that lessen the pain sensation. A formal psychiatric assessment is essential when these symptoms exist.

ASSESSMENT OF THE CLIENT WITH CHRONIC PAIN

Appropriate diagnosis and treatment of pain as a primary presenting symptom must begin with a comprehensive history and physical examination. In talking with the nurse about the pain, a client will not only describe its characteristics, location, and severity but may also provide information about possible psychosocial and behavioural factors that are influencing the pain experience. No direct relationship may be evident between the severity or extent of detectable disease and the intensity of the client's pain. A number of assessment instruments have been developed to aid in evaluation, but a fundamental approach is necessary to determine the impact of pain on the client's life. All systems must be examined in the client to determine the degree to which biomedical, psychosocial, and behavioural factors interact to influence the nature, severity, and persistence of the client's pain and disability. Box 32-3 presents a pain assessment tool.

SENSORY AND PHARMACOLOGIC MODULATION OF PAIN

Chronic pain occurs with a wide variety of medical illnesses. Proper diagnosis of the underlying condition determines primary treatment, which could eliminate or significantly reduce the need for analgesic drugs. Unsuspected medical conditions, such as alcoholism, autoimmune disease, or cancer, must be considered if pain develops in the absence of a known cause. Caregivers must know the mechanisms of action of analgesic drugs to administer them safely and monitor their

---

IN A LIFE

Sue Rodriguez (1950–1994)
Amyotrophic Lateral Sclerosis (ALS)

Public Persona
After being diagnosed in 1991 with ALS (also known as Lou Gehrig's disease), Sue Rodriguez realized that she might want to end her life once she was severely incapacitated with the disease. She also recognized that, if this time came, she would be physically incapable of killing herself and would need assistance. Assisting a person to die is illegal, however, under Section 241(b) of the Canadian Criminal Code. Euthanasia (ie, deliberately ending the life of a suffering person) is also illegal. Sue Rodriguez challenged these laws all the way to the Supreme Court, but failed to change them. Ultimately, she defied the law in 1994 by deciding the time and the method of her death. She had an unnamed physician and a friend, Sven Robinson (who was a Member of Parliament at the time), by her side.

Personal Realities
One can only imagine how Sue Rodriguez struggled with the anguish of her terminal illness, the anxiety and despair of leaving behind a teenage son, and her desire to end her life with respect and dignity. The stress of going public with her beliefs and fighting for them was great, but she hoped that her actions would help others living with similar illnesses. She also wanted her son to respect the law and didn't want her last act on earth to be illegal. She asserted that if she could not obey the law in the end, at least she would know that she had done all that she could to change it . . . as would her son.

See http://archives.cbc.ca/IDD-1-69-1135/life_society/sue_rodriguez/.

BOX 32.3

Assessing Clients Who Report Pain

A. What is the extent of the client's disease or injury (physical impairment)?

B. What is the magnitude of the illness? That is, to what extent is the client suffering, disabled, and unable to enjoy usual activities?

C. Does the client's behaviour seem appropriate to the disease or injury, or is there any evidence of amplification of symptoms for any of a variety of psychological or social reasons or purposes?

D. How often and for how long does the client perform specific behaviours, such as reclining, sitting, standing, and walking?

E. How often does the client seek health care and take analgesic medication (frequency and quantity)?

The Multiaxial Assessment of Pain (MAP) (Rudy & Turk, 1991) includes evaluation of three axes: biomedical, psychosocial, and behavioural.

Pain Behaviour Checklist

Pain behaviours have been characterized as interpersonal communications of pain, distress, or suffering. Pain behaviour may be a more accurate indication of intensity and tolerance than verbal reports. Check the box of each behaviour you observe or infer from the client's comments.

☐ Facial grimacing, clenched teeth
☐ Holding or supporting of affected body area
☐ Questions such as, "Why did this happen to me?"
☐ Distorted gait, limping
☐ Frequent shifting of posture or position
☐ Requests to be excused from tasks or activities; avoidance of physical activity
☐ Taking of medication as often as possible
☐ Moving extremely slowly
☐ Sitting with rigid posture
☐ Moving in a guarded or protective fashion
☐ Moaning or sighing
☐ Using a cane, cervical collar, or other prosthetic device
☐ Requesting help in ambulation; frequent stopping while walking
☐ Lying down during the day
☐ Irritability

---

effects. Clients' responses to individual drugs vary, and many agents at different doses may be tried before pain relief is achieved. Table 32-1 presents treatment approaches to pain. The use of physical and psychological modulation techniques, as well as pharmacotherapy or physical therapy, is more successful than the latter therapies alone (Turk, 2004). Combination treatment often affects mood and anxiety levels as well. Clients educated to use cognitive strategies such as biofeedback, a positive emotional state, relaxation, physical therapy or exercise, meditation, guided imagery, suggestion, hypnosis, placebos, and positive self-talk are able to tolerate higher levels of pain than are clients without specific coping strategies (Turk & Feldman, 1992). Most of these techniques involve redirecting the client's attention away from the pain and helping the client learn strategies of self-efficacy (self-effectiveness). Some of the biopsychosocial outcomes that can be measured to determine effectiveness of prescribed therapies include improvements in biologic, psychological, and sociocultural variables (Fig. 32-3). The biologic basis for the effectiveness of these strategies may be their ability to increase brain endorphin production (Bandura, O'Leary, & Taylor, 1987).

Many barriers exist to effective pain management (Box 32-4). Reluctance on the part of health professionals and the client may contribute to persistent pain, which ultimately can adversely affect the client's quality of life. Clients with chronic pain experience not only decreased functional capability but also diminished strength and endurance, nausea, poor appetite, and poor, interrupted sleep. The psychological impact includes diminished leisure and enjoyment, anxiety and fear, depression, somatic preoccupation, and difficulty concentrating. Social impairment may exist in the form of diminished social and sexual relationships, altered appearance, and increased dependence on others. All these contribute to the suffering caused by the pain experience.

Maladaptive coping by clients with chronic pain leads them to fear pain and to acquire a negative attitude about pain and how it affects their lives. These negative views can adversely influence biopsychological and physiologic processes, thereby sustaining or even exacerbating the pain. Noncompliance by these clients with sequential prescription changes and combined treatments also can be problematic. Strategies to assess compliance are regular self-report, assessment of behavioural change, biochemical assay, clinical improvement, and outcome assessment. The nurse can enhance compliance by closely monitoring the therapeutic efficacy and untoward effects of the treatments being used, involving the client and family in treatment planning, educating the client and family about self-care, and instructing the client in noninvasive approaches to pain control.

Psychopathologic Complications of AIDS

The medical syndrome of AIDS is characterized by multiple opportunistic infections and is associated with malignancy. People with AIDS are often overwhelmed by devastating disorders that cause profound fatigue, insomnia, anorexia, emaciation, pain, and disfigurement. The psychological impact of AIDS is considerably worsened by

Table 32.1 Treatment Approaches to Pain

Principles of Pain Treatment	Second Step	Third Step	Fourth Step

▪ Establish the correct diagnosis.
▪ Recognize that pain reduction, rather than complete pain control, is a reasonable goal
▪ Control other symptoms besides pain. This includes treating the symptoms that were present before treatment (such as depression and anxiety) and the adverse effects associated with the pain therapy.
▪ Treat physical conditions that may initiate or exacerbate the pain.
 	
First Step
Analgesics for treatment of pain and:
Nonsteroidal antiinflammatory drugs (NSAIDs)
  Acetaminophen
  Acetylsalicylic acid
  Ibuprofen
Oral local anesthetics
  Flecainide
  Mexiletine
  Tocainide
Topical agents
  Capsaicin
  EMLA
  Lidocaine gel
Baclofen
Neuroleptics
  Pimozide
Corticosteroids
Calcitonin
Benzodiazepines
  Clonazepam
Drugs for sympathetically maintained pain
  Nifedipine
  Phenoxybenzamine
  Prazosin
  Propranolol
	Antidepressants, TENS, and psychosocial support, and/or:
	Tricyclic and tetracyclic antidepressants
	  Amitriptyline
	  Clomipramine
	  Desipramine
	  Doxepin
	  Imipramine
	  Maprotiline
	  Nortriptyline
	  Mirtazapine
	Selective and nonselective serotonin reuptake Inhibitors
	  Buproprione
	  Fluoxetine
	  Fluvoxamine
	  Nefazodone
	  Olanzopine
	  Paroxetine
	  Sertraline
	  Trazodone
	  Venlafaxine
	Anticonvulsants
	  Carbamazepine
	  Neurontin
	  Phenytoin
	Opioid analgesics
	  Codeine
	  Meperidine
	  Morphine
	Monoamine oxidase inhibitors
	  Isocarboxazid
	  Phenelzine sulfate
	  Tranylcypromine
	Herbal and alternative medicine
	  SamE
	  Ginseng
	  Swedish massage
	  Acupressure
	  Acupuncture
	  Zero balancing
	  Reflexology
	  Meditation
	  Prayer
	Note: Treat the adverse effects of all the agents used.
		Adrenergic agents, TENS, and psychosocial support, and/or:
		Clonidine
		Naloxone infusion, and/or:
		Other agents (mexiletine, diphenhydramine)
		Note: Add the third-step agents to partially helpful agents used in first step, or use alone and treat the adverse effects of all the agents used.
			Psychiatric intervention
			Psychotherapy with pain patients:
			
			Cognitive
			▪ Explain the nature of the pain sensation.
			▪ Describe realistic expectations about the degree and course of pain.
			▪ Describe realistic expectations of treatment and side effects.
			▪ Use the placebo effect by supporting the treatment efficacy.
			▪ Relieve anxiety.
			
			Behavioural
			▪ Make the initial doses large rather than small, to effect some relief.
			▪ Reassure that medication will be available, not contingent on proof of need.
			▪ Reinforce healthy behaviour/adaptation; do not reinforce obsession with pain.
			▪ Assure of regular evaluation not contingent on presence of pain.
			
			Ablative Procedure for Selected Patients
			
			Neuroblockade
			▪ Trigger point injection (TPI)
			▪ Epidural steroid injection (ESI)
			▪ Facet joint injection (FJI)
			▪ Nerve root blocks
			▪ Medical branch blocks
			▪ Peripheral nerve block
			▪ Sympathetic nerve block
			
			Spinal Cord Stimulation
			▪ Neurostimulator implants
			▪ TENS
			▪ Thalamic stimulation

TENS, transcutaneous electrical nerve stimulation
Note: If the client has failed to experience response to all standard pharmacologic treatments, psychiatric evaluation for underlying problems (such as severe depression and risk for suicide) should be emphasized.

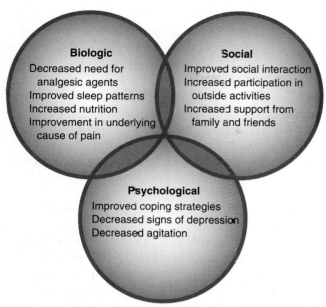

FIGURE 32.3 Biopsychosocial outcomes for patients with pain.

the social stigma associated with the infection and the special affinity of HIV for brain and central nervous system (CNS) tissue.

BIOLOGIC BASIS OF NEUROLOGIC MANIFESTATIONS OF HIV

In as many as 60% of those who have AIDS, neurologic complications occur that are directly attributable to infection of the brain. Important clinical manifestations

include impaired cognitive and motor function. This aspect of the syndrome is referred to as the **HIV-1–associated cognitive-motor complex**. Neuronal injury and frank nerve cell loss probably contribute to the neurologic deficits (Manji & Miller, 2004). Evidence suggests that the presence of HIV stimulates brain cells to release neurotoxins and excitatory amino acids in excess. The resultant neurochemical changes and disrupted cell membrane integrity cause cell death similar to that which occurs with other types of brain injury. These neurochemical changes and eventual catecholamine depletion contribute to the cognitive, motor, and psychiatric manifestations of HIV infection.

PSYCHOLOGICAL ASPECTS OF AIDS

The most common initial signs and symptoms of the AIDS dementia complex are changes in mentation and personality, followed by delirium, dementia, organic mood disorder, and organic delusional disorder. The onset of major depression and uncomplicated bereavement soon after diagnosis is common. Comorbid neurologic infections such as encephalitis and meningitis can predispose the client with AIDS to delirium. The clinical picture reflects the areas of the brain invaded by HIV; however, physiologic conditions such as addiction to alcohol or drugs, brain damage, chronic illness, hypoxia related to pneumonia, infections, space-occupying brain lesions, and systemic reactions to medications may contribute to the progression of mental changes. Loss of normal cortical function may lead to abnormal social behaviour, depression, psychosis, and anxiety. The psychological influences of stress and sleep and sensory deprivation can further contribute to the altered perception and mentation. Figure 32-4 shows the possible pathologic progression of HIV neuronal injury.

Psychiatric disorders contribute to the course of AIDS in several ways. Mood disorder may be reflected in the client who has an initial substance use disorder or an antisocial personality that predisposes him or her to a lifestyle that increases the client's risk for exposure to HIV. The neuropathology associated with the presence of HIV then contributes to the progression of the disease and deterioration. AIDS-associated psychopathology frequently is unrecognized, misdiagnosed, and incorrectly treated. Diagnosis can be difficult when risk factors are not known or when cognitive or psychiatric symptoms precede the onset of other manifestations of HIV infection. Early CNS involvement is detected through neuropsychological testing and magnetic resonance imaging. The degree of cognitive dysfunction may not be a valid indication of the degree of organic involvement. In addition, diagnostic findings on computed tomography scans, such as cerebral atrophy and prominent basal ganglia calcification, may not correlate with the severity of the client's dementia (Gabuzda & Hirsch, 1987).

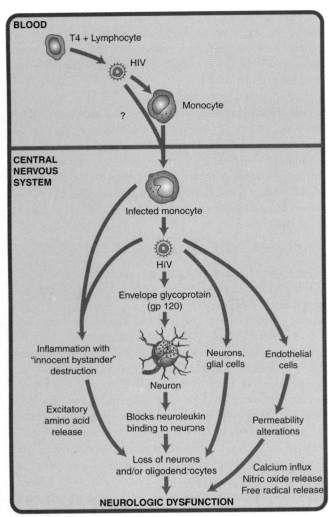

FIGURE 32.4 Possible pathologic progression of HIV neuronal injury.

ASSESSMENT OF THE CLIENT WITH AIDS

Early recognition of psychiatric disorders associated with AIDS is important to enhance our understanding of the behaviour of people with AIDS. Mental status changes and altered affect should be investigated through formal neurologic and psychological testing to determine the extent of impairment. Successful coping and cognitive adaptation are often further hindered by the presence of psychiatric disorders associated with HIV (Box 32-5). These mental illnesses include mood disorders, adjustment disorders, anxiety disorders, substance use disorders, and personality disorders. Organic mood disorder may be characterized by symptoms of a major depressive or manic episode. The depressed mood, feelings of guilt, anhedonia, and hopelessness can be accompanied by insomnia or hypersomnia, psychomotor retardation or agitation, and suicidal ideation. Low self-esteem, feelings of worthlessness and hopelessness, and impaired thinking or concentration are other likely findings. It is important to differentiate between major depression and complicated or uncomplicated grieving over the loss of health or of significant others to premature death because of HIV. When a client receives a diagnosis of AIDS, he or she may face social isolation, severe life-threatening complications, unfamiliar and perhaps ineffective treatments, and the prospect of premature death. As with any life crisis, the client and family members experience severe anxiety, fear, and depression. They may develop obsessive-compulsive rituals to allay anxiety related to the infection. In addition, these clients may experience panic disorders.

People who do not engage in high-risk behaviour and who are unlikely to have been exposed to HIV may nevertheless report physical and psychological manifestations associated with HIV. Anxiety about the disease can produce symptoms not unlike those of HIV infection. Phobias, delusions, and factitious (Munchausen syndrome) AIDS disorders have all been reported in uninfected people. In many cases, psychotherapy for the underlying psychological disorder is effective.

BIOPSYCHOSOCIAL TREATMENT INTERVENTIONS

Treatment of AIDS should attempt to maintain normal hydration, electrolyte balance, and nutrition, as well as a safe, comfortable environment. Antiviral agents, such as zidovudine, ribavirin, and phosphonoformate, cross the blood–brain barrier and achieve adequate anti-HIV concentrations in cerebrospinal fluid after systemic administration.

In addition, it is important to provide the client and the client's family, friends, and caregivers with emotional and educational support. Their sense of competence and control in relation to living with AIDS should be promoted (Littrell, 1996). Those close to the client may especially need psychotherapy if the patient is young. Treatment of psychiatric disorders should include the individual and family, as well as psychotropic medications, in a manner similar to the treatment of primary psychiatric disorders.

Early diagnosis and treatment are imperative to maximize the client's adherence to risk reduction regimens and to prevent the transmission of infection. Treatment plans can often be tailored to meet the needs of the client and family. The consultation-liaison psychiatric professional can recommend appropriate multidisciplinary interventions to meet the challenge of AIDS with compassion and dignity.

Psychological Illness Related to Trauma

Physiologic trauma activates the overall stress response of the autonomic nervous system (see Chapter 34). Massive catecholamine release causes certain cardiovascular,

BOX 32.5

Psychiatric Disorders Associated With HIV Infection

Organic Mental-Disorder

Dementia
  HIV dementia or AIDS–dementia complex
  Dementia associated with opportunistic infection
    Fungal
      Cryptococcoma
      Cryptococcal meningitis
      Candidal abscesses
    Protozoal
      Toxoplasmosis
    Bacterial
      Mycobacterium avium–intracellulare
    Viral
      Cytomegalovirus
      Herpesvirus
      Papovavirus progressive multifocal
        leukoencephalopathy
  Dementia associated with cancer
    Primary cerebral lymphoma
    Disseminated Kaposi's sarcoma

Delirium
Organic delusional disorder
Organic mood disorder
  Depression
  Mania
  Mixed
Affective disorders
  Major depression
  Dysthymic disorder
Adjustment disorders
  Adjustment disorder with depressed mood
  Adjustment disorder with anxious mood
Substance abuse disorder
Borderline personality disorder
Antisocial personality disorder
Bereavement
Anxiety disorders
  Obsessive-compulsive disorder
  Panic

---

muscular, gastrointestinal, and respiratory symptoms that release energy stores and support survival. Tissue destruction, musculoskeletal pain, physical disability, and body image changes all contribute to the physiologic and psychological stress response, which continues long after the injury is sustained. The overwhelming behavioural responses are hypervigilance, fear, and anxiety; psychological sequelae may include social isolation, agitation, personality disorders, posttraumatic stress disorder, and depression or, in extreme cases, dissociative identity disorders.

BIOLOGIC BASIS OF THE TRAUMA RESPONSE

The neurotransmitters responsible for behavioural responses to fear and anxiety are usually held in balance to maintain a level of arousal appropriate for environmental threat. Information from the sensory processing areas in the thalamus and cortex alerts the amygdala (the lateral and central nucleus). Events that are interpreted as threatening activate the hypothalamic-pituitary-adrenal (HPA) axis, initiating the stress response. Adrenal steroids are released and trigger the physiologic reactions just described. Complex neurochemical processes involving norepinephrine, γ-aminobutyric acid (GABA), and serotonin are overwhelmed by the catecholamine release. For example, norepinephrine receptors adjust to the increased level of hyperstimulation. Then, as the catecholamines are depleted, the norepinephrine receptors react to the relative catecholamine shortage. This response alters cognitive and affective function similar to the altered function that

occurs in anxiety disorders. Persistent, severe distress leads to a general dysregulation of the HPA axis and inappropriate and prolonged secretion of high levels of catecholamines. This chronic stress disorder has been linked to increased susceptibility to immunosuppressive medical illness, such as certain cancers, as well as to infection, myocardial disease, and neurologic degenerative disorders (Radley et al, 2004).

Adaptation to trauma is related to such factors as the severity of the trauma, the person's maturity and age when the trauma occurs, available social support, and the person's ability to mobilize coping strategies (Heim et al., 2000). During adaptation to prolonged stress, the patient's cognitive thought processes and coping behaviours cause dopamine to be released in the prefrontal cortex of the brain. These dopaminergic systems are presumed to play a major role in physiologic and emotional coping responses, storage of the trauma experience into memory, and possibly the development of posttraumatic stress disorder (McAllister et al., 2004). Serotonin is also thought to influence adaptation and mobilize coping strategies.

PSYCHOLOGICAL ASPECTS OF THE TRAUMA RESPONSE

Individual behaviour and perception are essential components of the stress reaction. Response to the challenge depends on prior experience, developmental history, and physical status. Individual differences in the extent of endocrine and autonomic activity also occur during stress. Psychological sequelae of sustained stress and trauma may be manifested as flashbacks, intrusive recurring thoughts, panic or anxiety attacks, paranoia, inappropriate startle reactions, nightmares, or the extreme of posttraumatic stress disorder. Catecholamine depletion and activation of the dopamine pathways may contribute to deterioration in social and intellectual functioning after severe physical or emotional trauma. The client may become so withdrawn and depressed that he or she stops participating in activities of daily living (ADLs). Toward the other extreme, the client may become agitated and combative, perceiving any treatment as a continued threat.

Extreme forms of maladaptation are manifested in kindling and dissociative identity disorder. Kindling is thought to be responsible for the spontaneous recurrence of depressive illness that is associated with loss and trauma at an early age. Permanent biochemical changes from the early trauma response precipitate the sudden onset of affective disorder in the absence of any present stressor (Nemeroff, 2004). Dissociation disorders are rare but take the form of somatization (physical symptoms), agnosia, multiple personalities, or amnestic fugue states in which the client escapes the stressor by subconscious loss of identity or adoption of a new identity. Although these disorders are not common, mood and anxiety disorders may occur after a trauma event. They are associated with slowed rehabilitation and deterioration in social functioning and ADLs after the trauma period has passed (Jorge, Robinson, Starkstien, & Arndt, 1994).

ASSESSMENT OF THE TRAUMATIZED CLIENT

Complete physical assessment after physical traumatic injury is imperative in life-threatening circumstances. Multiple trauma and head injury are the major causes of death and disability in young adults. Emergency care and intensive care providers are highly trained to recognize signs and symptoms of physiologic injury and to intervene to stabilize primary and secondary trauma in the general medical setting. Trauma scales and triage models have been developed to assist in immediate assessment and to measure neurologic and physical condition (Fig. 32-5) (Burkle, 1991). They have also been used to predict long-term outcome in clients for whom permanent cognitive and physical disability may limit recovery and challenge adaptive responses.

Psychological injury must be evaluated thoroughly through observation and interview to determine prevalent signs and symptoms of accompanying psychological disorders. This process includes evaluating the client's adjustment and coping skills, personal way of dealing with the trauma, social circumstances, and environmental and life stressors. Assessment must be ongoing to help the client deal with disfigurement, sudden disability, and changes in self-care. The evaluation should include assessment of the client's perception of experienced stress, feelings related to the stress, dominant mood, cognitive functioning, defense and coping mechanisms, and available support systems. In addition, assessment of the risk for self-inflicted injury or suicide is critical.

BIOPSYCHOSOCIAL TREATMENT INTERVENTIONS

Psychiatric clinicians provide an important aspect of emergency care. Interventions that establish trust, reduce anxiety, promote adaptive coping, and cultivate a sense of control help the client to begin recovery and maintain emotional health. Crisis intervention methods, stress management, cognitive behavioural therapies, psychotherapy, and psychotropic medications, alone or in combination, may be useful in achieving the best possible outcome.

When trauma causes the client's death, the family must be informed of the death and allowed to grieve, to prevent the development of a pathologic or prolonged grief response. Traumatic death is sudden and unexpected, and often the victim is young. Surviving family members usually have a severe emotional reaction to the death. Dysfunctional family dynamics may become evident during this period. The psychiatric liaison nurse can use family intervention strategies to enhance or improve relationships while the family's motivation to do all that is possible is high.

Psychological Illness Related to Central Nervous System Disorders

Neurologic impairment is most often related to brain cell (neuron) destruction. The primary causes of neuronal damage are traumatic injury, ischemia, infarction (cerebrovascular accident), abnormal neuron growth (brain tumor), and metabolic poisoning associated with systemic disease. Brain cell loss may also be the result of degenerative processes, such as those that occur in Alzheimer's or Parkinson's disease. Psychological illness often is a complication of organic neurologic disease and may be difficult to distinguish from the neuropathology itself. Therefore, appropriate intervention depends on skilled assessment to discriminate and detect mental status changes related to organic brain injury, as well as disorders of mood and thought.

BIOLOGIC BASIS OF NEUROLOGIC IMPAIRMENT

All mechanisms of brain cell injury destroy brain cells directly or initiate a cascade of cell breakdown from ischemia. This ischemic cascade begins with hypoxia

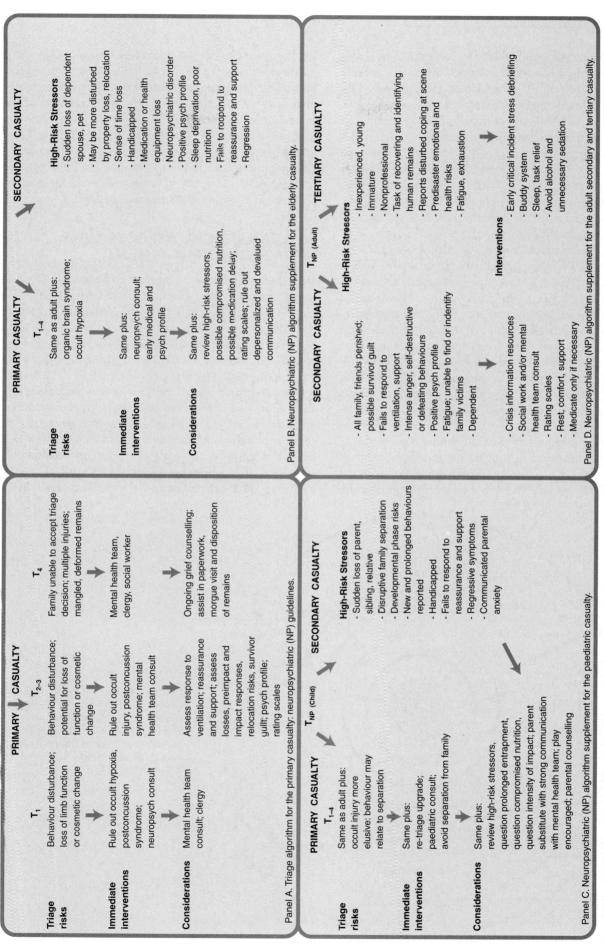

FIGURE 32.5   Triage algorithm for the primary casualty: neuropsychiatric guidelines. (Adapted from Burkle, F. M., Jr. [1991]. Triage of disaster-related neuropsychiatric casualties. *Psychiatric Aspects of Emergency Medicine*, 9[1], 87–104.)

and is followed by paralysis of the ion exchange across the cell membrane, edema, calcium influx, free-radical production, and lipid peroxidation (Fig. 32-6). The severity of brain injury is related to the degree and duration of ischemia. Complete ischemia results in brain infarction, commonly known as stroke. The resulting neurologic impairment is related to the size and location of the affected brain area (Fig. 32-7). More eloquent areas of the brain, such as the internal capsule, are extremely sensitive to ischemia. They are typically injured first and contribute to more generalized impairment, such as memory loss or altered judgment.

The primary psychological disorder experienced by people with brain injury is depression (Astrom, Adolfsson, & Asplund, 1993). Depressive symptoms related to organic brain injury are generated by altered biochemical neurotransmitter systems. Hyperactivity and dysregulation of the HPA axis probably contribute to the elevated cortisol and catecholamine levels after cerebral insult. In addition, changes in the metabolism of biogenic amines after brain cell death and ischemia may mediate both mood disturbances and cognitive dysfunction in clients who have had stroke (Luis, Vanderploeg, & Curtiss, 2003).

In cognitive brain function, dopamine is essential for normal neurotransmission of motor messages, motivation, and level of anxiety and mood; epinephrine establishes learning and memory; and serotonin regulates the level of alertness, the categorization of information, and the perception of well-being. These neurotransmitter pathways are temporarily interrupted or permanently disrupted during the acute injury. Secondary injury caused by swelling and compression may further compromise neurons in surrounding areas, causing marginal neurotransmitter function. In addition, circulating catecholamines can lead to oversecretion of dopamine or serotonin, which disrupts the necessary balance in production and uptake of the transmitters.

PSYCHOLOGICAL ASPECTS OF NEUROLOGIC IMPAIRMENT

Depressive disorder is a common complication of brain injury, particularly ischemic stroke. About 20% of clients with acute stroke have the symptom cluster of the (*Diagnostic and Statistical Manual of Mental Disorders*, 4th edition, text revision *DSM-IV-TR*; American Psychiatric Association, 2000) criteria for major depression (see Chapter 19). Other symptoms, such as sleep disturbances, cognitive dysfunction, poor concentration, difficulty making decisions, somatic discomfort, poor appetite, social withdrawal, and fatigue or agitation, often accompany the mood disturbance. The high-risk period extends for 2 years after the stroke, and left untreated, the depression generally lasts for at least 6 months (Verdelko, Henon, Lebert, Pasquiere, Leys,

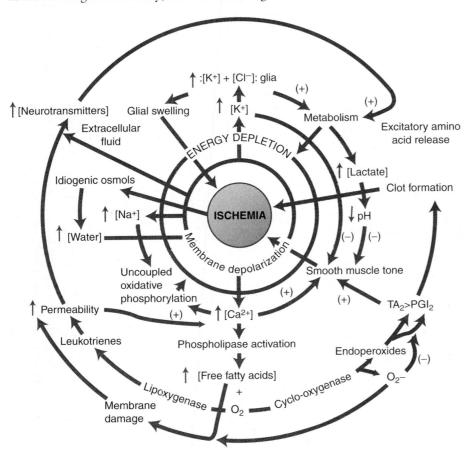

FIGURE 32.6 Ischemic cascade causes secondary brain injury and altered neurotransmitter function. (Based on Raichle, M.E. [1983]. The pathophysiology of brain ischemia. *Annals of Neurology, 13*[1], 2–10.)

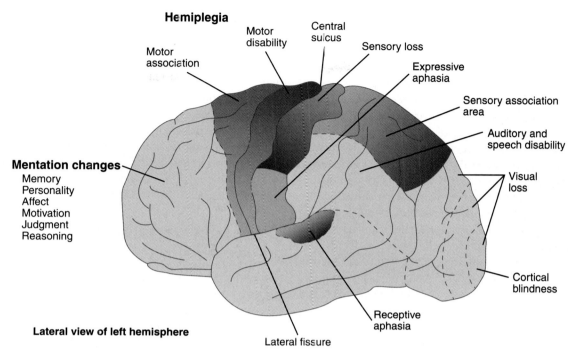

FIGURE 32.7   Functional cerebral anatomy and stroke.

2004). Table 32-2 compares *DSM-IV-TR* diagnostic criteria for depression and cerebrovascular accident–related emotional sequelae.

Minor and moderate depression may go unrecognized and undiagnosed when clients who have had a stroke describe somatic symptoms and demonstrate lack of motivation in ADLs. Depression is more likely to develop in such clients if they have altered speech or aphasia, severe hemiparesis, or both. However, clients who have had a stroke experience depression more frequently than do other disabled and chronically ill clients, although the level of functional disability is the

Table 32.2	Comparison of *DSM-IV-TR* Diagnostic Criteria for Depression and Stroke-Related Affective Sequelae		
Major Depression	**Dysthymia***	**Stroke Residual Sequelae**	**Other Symptoms Associated With Depression**
Depressed mood	Depressed mood	Depressed mood	Decreased sexual desire or
Anhedonia	Appetite change	Anhedonia	sexual functioning
Weight change	Sleep disturbance	Weight loss	Loss of insight
Low energy or fatigue	Low energy or fatigue	Low energy or fatigue	Autonomic symptoms (eg,
Motor disturbance	Low self-esteem	Paralysis or paresis	sweating, tachycardia)
Sleep disturbance	Decreased concentration	Sleep disturbance	Somatic anxiety symptoms
Feelings of worthlessness or guilt	Hopelessness	Feelings of guilt	Psychic anxiety symptoms
Decreased concentration		Decreased concentration	Somatic preoccupation
Thoughts of death or suicide		No psychotic symptoms	(hypochondriasis)
No independent psychosis		Diminished self-care	Pain, especially chronic pain
Some psychotic symptoms		Pain, usually chronic	Diminished self-care
		Social withdrawal	Social incapacitation
		Isolation	
		Hopelessness	
		Somatic preoccupation	

*Cameron, O. G. (1990), Guidelines for diagnosis and treatment of depression in patients with medical illness, *Journal of Clinical Psychiatry, 51*, 7(Suppl.), 49–54.

same (Verdelko et al., 2004). This phenomenon is thought to possibly be related to the combination of permanent disability and altered neurotransmitter systems that persist after cerebral infarction.

Although the mechanism of neuronal injury is one of degeneration in Parkinson's disease and other neuromuscular diseases, the neurochemical changes in the brain are similar with respect to the loss of dopamine secretion and receptor sites in the internal capsule motor pathways. About 40% of clients with Parkinson's disease experience depression (Rojo, et al., 2003). Although major depression may occur, most have less severe forms that contribute to impairment in daily functioning possibly as much as does the underlying disease. Depression is the main factor negatively affecting quality of life and a source of distress for the client and the family and caregivers. There is evidence suggesting that altered serotonergic function may be responsible, at least in part, for the depressive symptoms in Parkinson's disease and that altered noradrenergic function may underlie some of the associated anxiety symptoms. Clinical trials have demonstrated the selective serotonin reuptake inhibitors and combined selective serotonin and norepinephrine reuptake inhibitors are more effective than traditional tricyclic antidepressants in reducing or relieving depression and anxiety in clients with neurologic disease (Mayeux, Stern, Cote, & Williams, 1984; Murai et al., 2001; Schiffer et al., 1996). In addition, the serotonergic system is disrupted as the neuronal synapses are destroyed or injured. This generalized loss of dopaminergic activity and decreasing functional ability also probably contribute to depressed mood in clients who have had a stroke.

Mental illness related to organic brain injury is consistently dependent on the degree of functional impairment, particularly loss of the ability to communicate and administer self-care. Depressed mood may become evident in the acute recovery phase or during rehabilitation. Depression often negatively affects survival and recovery. It impedes progress throughout the rehabilitation process and ultimately prevents an optimal outcome. Early evaluation assists in the detection of mental illness after brain injury.

ASSESSMENT OF THE CLIENT WITH NEUROLOGIC PROBLEMS

A thorough neurologic examination is important in determining the location and degree of disability but even more critical in establishing the locus of retained function. Many scales exist that accurately assess neurologic function and that are easy to administer and generally accepted as reliable tools to detect the degree and limitations of disability. Cognition and mentation can be more discretely measured by the Folstein Mini-Mental State examination (Folstein, Folstein, & McHugh, 1975), and functionability for self-care can be

measured using the Barthel Index (Mahoney & Barthel, 1965). The evaluation of mood using the Centre for Epidemiological Studies Depression Scale (CES-D) or the Beck Depression Inventory (Beck et al., 1961) provides important information for designing intervention strategies for the at-risk client who has had a stroke. Findings of depressive symptoms indicate the need for a more definitive neuropsychological referral. The dexamethasone suppression test (DST) has also been used to diagnose clinical depression. However, it is not completely reliable, and frequent false-positive test results limit its clinical utility (Carroll et al., 1981).

BIOPSYCHOSOCIAL TREATMENT INTERVENTIONS

Isolation, lack of companionship, bereavement, and poverty are associated with depressive symptoms in the general population and compound the relative risk of depression developing after brain damage. In addition, a personal or family history of major depression increases the risk for depressed mood. Prevention strategies should be used as early as possible for clients known to have these risks. These strategies include the assessment and provision of social support resources while the client is hospitalized and as an important component of discharge planning to rehabilitation services; the prescription of therapies to enhance competence in the performance of ADLs, with a focus on the use of retained function, rather than on adaptation to disabilities only; formal psychosocial testing and psychopharmacologic treatment when appropriate (Palomaki et al., 1999; Robinson et al., 2000); and the education of the client and family to increase their awareness of signs and symptoms of depressed mood so that they will know when to seek medical attention and treatment to avert major depression, if possible. In addition, the presence of depressed mood and other symptoms of the depressive cluster indicate the need for cognitive, behavioural, biologic, and social interventions to support appropriate psychopharmacologic treatment.

Psychological Illness Related to Acute and Chronic Medical Illness

Systemic medical illness is associated with a higher prevalence of concurrent psychiatric disorders. Disorders such as cancer, heart disease, endocrine abnormalities, and organ failure are often associated with more functional disability than most chronic medical illnesses and may be the basis of medically unexplained somatic symptoms. Among the psychiatric disorders, substance use disorder, anxiety, and depressive disorder occur most frequently in clients with chronic medical illnesses.

Table 32.3	Prevalence of Psychiatric Disorders in Medically Ill Compared With People Who Are Not Medically Ill		
Prevalence of Psychiatric Disorders*		**Medically Ill (%)**	**Not Medically Ill (%)**
Six-month prevalence		24.7	17.5
Substance abuse		8.5	
Anxiety		11.9	
Affective disorder		9.4	
Lifetime prevalence		42.4	33.0
Substance use		26.2	
Anxiety		18.2	
Phobias		12.1	
Panic disorder		1.5	
Obsessive-compulsive disorder		2.4	
Affective disorder		12.9	

*Prevalence rates are sex- and age-adjusted.
Adapted from National Institute of Mental Health Epidemiologic Catchment Area Program, Burkle, F. M., Jr. (1991), Triage of disaster-related neuropsychiatric casualties *Psychiatric Aspects of Emergency Medicine*, 9(1), 87–104.

Within the anxiety disorders, phobias are most common, with panic disorder and obsessive-compulsive disorder less common (Hoster, Conway, & Mevkongas, 2003). Table 32-3 compares the prevalence rates of depressive and anxiety disorders in people who are medically ill with the rates in people who are not.

BIOLOGIC ASPECTS OF MENTAL ILLNESS RELATED TO MEDICAL DISEASE

The nervous, endocrine, and immune systems and their components are designed to communicate and interact through biochemical means. The cerebral cortex and limbic system initiate neuroendocrine HPA axis activity by thought processes in response to environmental stimuli. Various hormonal messengers travel between the hypothalamic, pituitary, and adrenal systems to initiate secondary peripheral responses. The immune system responds to signals from the HPA axis and returns messages as well. Its protective activities rely on neurochemicals to initiate the infection defense and stress response. At all levels, the circulating hormone levels serve as feedback messengers to inhibit HPA activity after sufficient response has occurred.

Dysregulation of the hypothalamic, pituitary, and adrenal systems at all levels leads to malfunction of the other systems. Abnormal nervous system firing in the hippocampus alerts the adrenal and immune systems unnecessarily, and vice versa. The principal neurochemical messengers in this regulation are thought to be nor-epinephrine, endorphins, cortisol, and dopamine. This trio of systems detects metabolic and cellular disease processes that eventually cause signs and symptoms of medical diseases, and body resources are activated to stop these pathologic processes. Psychiatric conditions occur during the course of these medical illnesses and in some instances may contribute to the genesis of the physiologic disease.

A psychiatric disorder may be the first manifestation of a primary disease, such as depressive syndrome in Huntington's chorea, multiple sclerosis, Parkinson's disease, HIV, Cushing's disease, and systemic lupus erythematosus. Depressive symptoms are an intrinsic part of the primary pathophysiology of endocrine disorders, metabolic disturbances, malignancies, viral infections, inflammatory disorders, and cardiopulmonary conditions. Tables 32-4 and 32-5 list medical conditions associated with anxiety disorders and depression, respectively.

Endocrine system pathologic processes involve abnormal HPA axis function, which affects neurotransmitter balance (Stratakis & Chrousos, 1995). Depression and anxiety are often present in patients with hyperthyroidism and hypothyroidism, Cushing's disease (hyperadrenalism), and Addison's disease (hypoadrenalism).

Malignancies have also been associated with anxiety and depression. Depressive syndromes have been associated with cancer, and biologic relationships between the two disorders may exist such that the onset of depression may herald undetected carcinoma. Diagnoses range from major depression to adjustment disorder with depressed mood.

Systemic infections and generalized inflammatory disorders such as rheumatoid arthritis that acutely and chronically stress the immune system or that may be the result of immune dysfunction are associated with psychological disorders. In addition, renal, pancreatic, and hepatic transplant recipients, who are artificially immunosuppressed because of treatment with prophylactic anti-infectious agents, experience primary neuropsychiatric symptoms related to metabolic imbalances and neuropsychiatric side effects from treatment.

Table 32.4	**Medical Conditions Associated With Anxiety Disorders**	
Psychiatric Disorder	**Medical Illness**	**Incidence (%)**
Panic disorder	Parkinson's disease	20
	Primary biliary cirrhosis	10
	Chronic obstructive pulmonary diseases	24
	Cardiomyopathy	83
	Post–myocardial infarction	16
	Chronic pain	16
	Focal seizures	*
Social phobia	Parkinson's disease	17
Obsessive-compulsive disorder	Sydenham's chorea	13
Phobia	Multiple sclerosis	*
Generalized anxiety	Primary biliary cirrhosis	10
	Graves' disease	62

*Incidence not significant but reportable.

Cardiac disease deserves special attention because it has been associated with precipitated depressive syndromes and anxiety disorders. The fact that more than 70% of clients who have an acute myocardial infarction (MI) remain depressed for as long as 1 year after the event indicates that the mental illness may not be simply an adjustment disorder. Gender differences in risk for anxiety and depression after MI have been found. In a 5-year prospective study, women had increased risk for both anxiety and depression in the first 2 years after MI, whereas men had increased risk for depression that began 2 years after MI (Bjerkeset, Nordahl, Mykletun, Holmen, & Dahl, 2005). The incidence of depression is also high in cardiac transplant recipients (54%) but is much lower in clients who undergo cardiac bypass surgery (6% to 15%). In a study by Hill and coworkers (1992), 75% of cardiac clients who received therapy for their depression experienced response to treatment.

In addition to the disease process contributing to psychological complications, the drugs used to treat chronic disease may induce mental illness. Psychotropic and nonpsychotropic medications can be potent generators of depression and anxiety (Table 32-6). The indications and pharmacologic activity of these medications often have biopsychosocial implications. In addition, medically ill elderly clients are particularly susceptible to medication effects at lower doses. Depressive and anxiety-related symptoms may in fact have an additive effect on client function, well-being, and recovery when combined with medical illness. When a drug is suspected of causing mental changes, the recommended course of action is to withdraw the drug and find an effective alternative. When an alternative is not available, the dosage should be decreased to an effective level at which symptoms resolve.

PSYCHOLOGICAL ASPECTS OF MEDICAL ILLNESS

In all cases of medical illness, it is natural for clients to respond to the loss of health with hopelessness, particularly when the illness is demoralizing, life threatening, and without a clear prognosis. People who are chronically ill are distressed by loss of function and limitations on their daily activities. They are often forced to comply with treatments that add discomfort but no apparent benefit. Medical clients commonly experience weight loss, insomnia, and motor retardation, but perhaps not to the degree of "conspicuous" psychiatric illness. In addition, chronic life stress and mental illness may have set in motion a series of biologic processes ultimately resulting in the medical disorder, which may be further exacerbated by the stress of hospital admittance. A vicious cycle of medical and mental disorders may arise.

Mental illness in medically ill people is potentially lethal because normal affects and cognitive functioning may be essential to recovery and compliance with the medical treatment plan. In addition, the use of excessive analgesics and reluctance to perform self-care and rehabilitative activities hinder recovery and expose the person to other potential complications. The detection and diagnosis of any secondary mental illnesses in clients with medical illnesses is critical. The physiologic and pharmacologic factors that contribute to the mental illness must be explored and ruled out before effective intervention can begin.

ASSESSMENT OF THE CLIENT WITH MEDICAL ILLNESS

Unfortunately, it may be very difficult for the clinician, evaluating a medically ill client in whom psychiatric symptoms develop, to ascertain whether these symptoms

Table 32.5	Medical Illnesses Associated With Symptoms of Depression
Endocrinopathies	Hypothyroidism and hyperthyroidism
	Hypoparathyroidism and hyperparathyroidism
	Cushing's syndrome (steroid excess)
	Adrenal insufficiency (Addison's disease)
	Hyperaldosteronism
Malignancies	Abdominal carcinomas, especially pancreatic
	Brain tumors (temporal lobe)
	Breast cancer
	Gastrointestinal cancer
	Lung cancer
	Prostate cancer
	Metastases
Neurologic disorders	Ischemic stroke
	Subarachnoid hemorrhage
	Parkinson's disease
	Normal-pressure hydrocephalus
	Multiple sclerosis
	Closed head injury
	Epilepsy
Metabolic imbalance	Serum sodium and potassium reductions
	Vitamin B_{12}, niacin, vitamin C deficiencies; iron deficiency (anemias)
	Metal intoxication (thallium and mercury)
	Uremia
Viral/bacterial infection	Infectious hepatitis
	Encephalitis
	Tuberculosis
	AIDS
Hormonal imbalance	Premenstrual, premenopausal, postpartum periods
Cardiopulmonary	Acute myocardial infarction
	Post–cardiac arrest
	Post–coronary artery bypass graft
	Post–heart transplantation
	Cardiomyopathy
Inflammatory disorders	Rheumatoid arthritis

Table 32.6	Medications Associated With Mental Illness in Medically Ill Patients
Analgesics and nonsteroidal antiinflammatory drugs (NSAIDs)	Ibuprofen
	Indomethacin
	Opiates
	Pentazocine
	Phenacetin
	Phenylbutazone
Antihypertensives	Clonidine
	Hydralazine
	Methyldopa
	Propranolol
	Reserpine
Antimicrobials	Ampicillin (gram-negative agents)
	Clotrimazole
	Cycloserine
	Griseofulvin
	Metronidazole
	Nitrofurantoin
	Streptomycin
	Sulfamethoxazole (sulfonamides)
Neurologic agents	l-Dopa
	Levodopa
Antiparkinsonian drugs	Amantadine
Anticonvulsants	Carbamazepine
	Phenytoin
Antispasmodics	Baclofen
	Bromocriptine
Cardiac drugs	Digitalis
	Guanethidine
	Lidocaine
	Oxprenolol
	Procainamide
Psychotropic drugs	Benzodiazepines
Stimulants/sedatives	Amphetamines
	Barbiturates
	Chloral hydrate
	Chlorazepate
	Diethylpropion
	Ethanol
	Fenfluramine
	Haloperidol
Steroids and hormones	Adrenocorticotropic hormone
	Corticosteroids
	Estrogen
	Oral contraceptives
	Prednisone
	Progesterone
	Triamcinolone
Antineoplastic drugs	Bleomycin
	C-Asparaginase
	Trimethoprim
	Vincristine
Other miscellaneous drugs	Anticholinesterases
	Cimetidine
	Diuretics
	Metoclopramide

are the result of direct psychobiologic changes brought about by the illness (Box 32-6). People at obvious risk have a family history or personal history of mental illness or were experiencing psychological problems before symptoms of the medical illness were present. The main problem for the clinician is to determine which signs and symptoms are part of the medical illness and its treatment and which signify the presence of a psychological disorder. A complete health assessment and physical examination, including a psychological examination and a cognitive-affective assessment, will help determine the priority and severity of symptoms and interventions. In

BOX 32.6

Research for Best Practice

Describing the Experience of Having Congestive Heart Failure

THE QUESTION: The researchers believe that the incidence and prevalence of congestive heart failure (CHF) are increasing among Canadians. Few studies, however, delineate the experience of clients with CHF, and there are inconsistent findings regarding whether gender differences influence quality of life, treatment approaches, and survival. In this study, it was asked: What is the experience of people living with CHF?

METHODS: The authors used a case study approach with six women and men, ranging in age from 37 to 82, who were clients at an Ontario CHF clinic. Semistructured interviews along with quality-of-life measures, medical history data, medical management, and New York Heart Association scores, were used to achieve an in-depth description of participants' experiences with CHF. Cross-case analyses were used to reveal themes and determine hypotheses.

FINDINGS: Thirteen themes were found: burden to others, frustration, loss, acceptance, hope for the future, fatigue, maintenance of independence, fear, physical symptoms, confusion due to lack of knowledge, isolation, depression, and shock and disbelief. The majority of these themes are psychosocial in nature. Constello and Boblin generated three hypotheses from their thematic analysis: (1) the psychosocial impact of CHF overrides the physical impact; (2) sex differences exist, with men more likely to experience social isolation and loss than women, and women more likely to report fear; and (3) the experience of CHF is influenced by age, with physical experiences and depression reported more with younger age groups. Future research into these hypotheses is recommended.

IMPLICATIONS FOR NURSING: Six interventions based on client needs identified in the study are suggested by the researchers. The interventions include: client education, encouragement of self-care, telephone/electronic support, exercise and cardiac rehabilitation, group support that includes families, and pharmacologic management.

From Constello, J., & Boblin, S. (2004). What is the experience of men and women with congestive heart failure? *Canadian Journal of Cardiovascular Nursing, 14*(3), 9–20.

some instances, the primary diagnosis may be depression, although the symptoms may be similar to those of medical illness in the absence of diagnostic findings. Factors to be considered in diagnosing mental illness in medical clients are outlined in Box 32-7.

Several important cognitive-affective symptoms best differentiate the effects of depression from those of medical illness. These include feelings of failure, low self-esteem, guilt feelings, loss of interest in people, feelings of being punished, suicidal ideation, dissatisfaction, difficulty with decisions, and crying (Neese, 1991). The severity of the vegetative symptoms generally increases with the severity of the depressive disorder, as well as the severity of the medical illness. Decreased appetite, sleep disturbances, and loss of energy are not considered indicators of depression in the medically ill client because these symptoms are common in medical illness as well. The Beck Depression Inventory and the CES-D are easy to administer and may indicate the need for a psychiatric referral.

CLINICAL FEATURES OF SPECIAL SIGNIFICANCE

Two problems of special significance, psychosis and suicidal thoughts, are related in that clients with delusions or hallucinations tend to be at greater risk for suicide attempts or more likely to resist treatment (eg, to refuse to eat or take medication) for their medical condition. It is important to distinguish between a mentally competent client's right to refuse life-saving medical treatment

and a depressed client's desire to die. A clinical evaluation of the effect of depression on the client's capacity to make competent decisions is imperative. If optimal medical and psychiatric treatments have been provided and the client has been found competent enough to make decisions about further medical care, it may be appropriate to honor the client's desire to die.

Clients with chronic medical illness and clients with primary mental illness may pose similar problems in psychiatric hospitals when their medical condition fails. The use of advance directives helps in addressing these problems.

BOX 32.7

Factors to Consider in Diagnosing Depression in Medical Clients

- One of more specific medical illnesses
- Defining criteria for one of the depressive syndromes
- Family psychiatric history
- Past psychiatric history of the client
- Client's response to treatment, if any, for any prior depressive episode
- Sex of the client
- Client's age at onset of depression
- Depression that preceded the medical illness
- Psychosocial precipitants before onset of depression
- Duration of depressive illness
- Biologic markers of depression
- Relative frequence in the population of diagnoses under consideration
- Diagnosis by commission, not omission

BIOPSYCHOSOCIAL TREATMENT INTERVENTIONS

It is essential to provide optimal treatment of clients' medical illnesses without neglecting their mental distress. Most reports suggest that clinicians should be more aggressive in the pharmacologic treatment of mental illness in the medically ill. The basic rules for medicating clients include using the minimum dose initially, advancing the dose slowly, and performing frequent blood level monitoring. The doses required to achieve therapeutic blood levels may be lower or even half the usual therapeutic dose and take longer to titrate. It is important to understand the pharmacokinetics (absorption, distribution, metabolism, and elimination) of the treatment of choice, to prevent further systemic effects. Selective serotonin reuptake inhibitors (SSRIs) and selective serotonin and norepinephrine reuptake inhibitors (SNRIs) are used equally as the treatment for depression in the medically ill client population. Because the side effects of psychopharmacologic agents can be especially troublesome in medically ill people, treatment must be changed or stopped if drug or illness interactions occur, or if treatment of the mental illness appears to be unsuccessful. SSRIs are increasingly popular in treating medically ill clients because their side-effect profile is more tolerable within a wider therapeutic range. Most clients experience response to antidepressant therapy with a decrease in the severity of their vegetative symptoms in 4 to 8 days.

Both supportive individual psychotherapy and family therapy are helpful. Assisting the client and family in understanding the nature and relationship of the medical and psychiatric diagnoses may strengthen the support system, alter the perception of caregiver burden, and identify appropriate coping strategies. Mutually agreed-upon goals and therapy actively involve the client in progress toward recovery. At some point, the clinician may need to help the client identify psychodynamic conflicts and maladaptive coping strategies that may be contributing to his or her distress. Cognitive intervention should address those areas of the client's life that can be controlled, despite major lifestyle changes, to reinforce a feeling of competence. It also is important to convey the fact that although medical and mental illness are difficult to prevent, they are often treatable.

Intervening in Mental and Medical Illness

The relationship between stress and illness is becoming more apparent as studies increasingly disclose the effects of stress on the body. Chronic illness is viewed as a stressor and is associated with increased psychological distress, and interventions can minimize that distress. Nurses are committed to preventing illness and promoting healthy living. Thus, it is essential that they be aware of the physiologic and psychological impact of chronic stress, understand the coping process, and know appropriate alternative strategies for coping with illness. In addition, nurses can evaluate the effectiveness of strategies being used and revise care plans to improve outcomes for the client.

Clients with primary mental illness in need of medical care are at particular risk when somatic complaints are viewed as part of the primary process. Undiagnosed pathophysiologic processes may become advanced while being attributed to somatization. A thorough medical history and physical examination are standard practice for clients in all settings.

Ideally, a multidisciplinary team of care providers that includes a psychiatric liaison nurse should work together to deliver optimum treatment of complex medical and mental illness. All clients with chronic medical illnesses are at risk for psychological distress and should be approached with this understanding. Clinicians should include a general cognitive-affective status evaluation in their assessment of all medically ill clients and make appropriate psychiatric liaison consultation to offset the negative impact of mental illness on recovery.

A psychosocial review of systems is useful in admission assessment to detect psychosocial stress or risk. This review provides the minimum information needed for each client—neglect of even one area could compromise client care. Information on substance use, stressful life events, expectations, fears, meanings, social support, sexual concerns, work, finances, education, psychiatric history, mood, cognition, culture, and functional status is obtained from the review. This information is useful in determining relevant nursing diagnoses and developing the plan of care.

Stress management training, systematic relaxation, supportive education, and stress monitoring should be built into the plan of care, regardless of the medical diagnosis. Assessment of anxiety and depression are ongoing, and crisis intervention with psychotherapy may be necessary to reduce the severity of mental distress. Physiologic stress factors, such as increased heart rate, blood pressure, and respiration, and signs of restlessness and sadness can be measured to determine the effectiveness of the intervention. Secondary mental illness can be approached using the same strategies that are effective for primary mental dysfunction. Interventions overlap across criteria, and all interventions provide some element of supportive therapy or social support.

Mental health can and should be monitored in clients who have physical illnesses. Certain kinds of pathologic processes place clients at greater risk for mental illness. These processes can be identified and interventions prescribed to prevent psychiatric disorders from developing or to minimize their severity. Cognitive and behavioural strategies have a place in the treatment regimen and offer the practitioner an opportunity to expand the boundaries of traditional client-oriented practice in effective ways.

Alternatives to traditional medical intervention are increasingly employed as adjunct therapy in clients with pain related to cancer, neuropathy, or degenerative disorders. Natural and herbal therapies, therapeutic massage, zero balancing, thought-field therapy, imaging, prayer, and meditation have all been found to be useful in easing the mental and physical discomfort of the client with medical illness. In addition, these therapies are more satisfying to clients who otherwise must receive toxic medication as part of their conventional medical treatment (see Table 32-1).

SUMMARY OF KEY POINTS

◘ Psychiatric disorders are more common in people with systemic or chronic medical illnesses than in other people. Comorbid depression is common in certain medical diseases, such as endocrine and metabolic disturbances, viral infections, inflammatory disorders, and cardiopulmonary diseases. Specific anxiety disorders are associated with other medical conditions, such as Parkinson's disease, focal seizures, primary binary cirrhosis, and chronic pain.

◘ Psychiatric illness that accompanies medical illness is seldom recognized and treated. Psychiatric symptoms may precede the onset of disease symptoms, and it may be difficult to distinguish between the symptoms of the two conditions.

◘ The biologic basis of mental illness associated with medical illness (eg, catecholamine depletion, disorders in metabolism or production of neurotransmitters) is similar to that of primary psychiatric illness, and biopsychosocial treatment strategies are effective.

◘ Mental illness in medically ill people is potentially lethal because normal affective-cognitive function may be critical to recovery and compliance with the medical treatment plan. Therefore, it is imperative that mental health is included in the standard health assessment of all medically ill people and that appropriate referrals be made.

CRITICAL THINKING CHALLENGES

1 You are caring for a client who has had a stroke and who refuses breakfast and a morning bath. Applying what you know about the neurologic damage caused by stroke and the frequency of depression in such clients, develop a care plan addressing the client's biopsychosocial needs.

2 As you care for a client with AIDS, you notice that his partner is pacing and hyperventilating. Using your knowledge of relationships, systems, and the interconnectedness of physical and psychological illness, how would you approach him?

3 Discuss the pain syndromes you may see in the primary care setting.

4 A client is being seen for chronic pain. Discuss how you would go about assessing barriers to pain management with this client.

5 You are a psychiatric–mental health liaison nurse and have been asked to prepare a program for the medical-surgical nursing staff on psychiatric aspects of medical illnesses. What topics would you include, and what would be your rationale for including each?

MOVIES

Philadelphia: 1993. This is the story of Andy Beckett, played by Tom Hanks. Beckett is an exceptionally gifted and successful Philadelphia lawyer who is gay. Beckett did not declare his sexual orientation to the law firm that aggressively recruited and employed him. When he becomes HIV positive and develops AIDS, he is fired by the firm, allegedly for incompetence. Beckett sues them for wrongful dismissal.

VIEWING POINTS: As you observe the film, consider the dynamics of his trials and tribulations as a gay man living with AIDS in a heterosexist corporate world. Take note of prejudice and discrimination, but also of tolerance, understanding, and compassion. The movie was criticized for providing its main character with a much more understanding family than is typically the case for peoples with AIDS. What do you think about this? The movie *Philadelphia* may be seen as a modern-day David and Goliath story. Do you think it is essentially a story of hope?

The Barbarian Invasions (Restricted, In French with English subtitles): 2003. This movie, a sequel to *The Decline of the American Empire*, deals with a universal topic: mortality from cancer. The ethos of impending death hovers across the entire film, yet it is neither a grim nor a depressing experience. The Director, Denis Arcand, has infused a great deal of wit throughout the film, and it meshes well with the anticipated pathos.

VIEWING POINTS: As one watches the film, one could easily make the argument that *The Barbarian Invasions* is as much about life (love, despair, humor) as it is about death. Does thinking about death help us live in a better way?

REFERENCES

American Psychiatric Association. (2000). *Diagnostic and statistical manual of mental disorders* (4th ed., Text revision). Washington, DC: Author.

Arnsten, A. F. (1997). Catecholamine regulation of the pre-frontal cortex. *Journal of Psychopharmacology, 11,* 151–162.

Astrom, M., Adolfsson, R., & Asplund, K. (1993). Major depression in stroke patients: A 3-year longitudinal study. *Stroke, 24,* 976–982.

Atkinson, J. H. Jr., & Slater, M. A. (1989). Psychiatric medications and pain management in emergency medicine. *Topics in Emergency Medicine, 11*(3), 1–110.

Bandura, A., O'Leary, A., & Taylor, C. B. (1987). Perceived self-efficacy and pain control-opioid and nonopioid mechanisms. *Journal of Personality and Social Psychology, 53,* 563–571.

Beck, A. T., Ward, C. H., Mendelson, M., et al. (1961). An inventory for measuring depression. *Archives of General Psychiatry, 4,* 561–571.

Bjerkeset, O., Nordahl, H., Mykletun, A., Holmen, J., & Dahl, A. (2005). Anxiety and depression following myocardial infarction: Gender differences in a 5-year prospective study. *Journal of Psychosomatic Research, 58,* 153–161.

Burkle, F. M. Jr. (1991). Triage of disaster-related neuropsychiatric casualties. *Psychiatric Aspects of Emergency Medicine, 9*(1), 87–104.

Cameron, O. G. (1990). Guidelines for diagnosis and treatment of depression in patients with medical illness. *Journal of Clinical Psychiatry, 51*(7 Suppl.), 49–54.

Carroll, B. J., Feinberg, M., Greden, J. F., et al. (1981). A specific laboratory test for the diagnosis of melancholia: Standardization, validation and clinical utility. *Archives of Clinical Psychiatry, 38,* 15–22.

Cassem, E. H. (1990). Depression and anxiety secondary to medical illness. *Psychiatric Clinics of North America, 13*(4), 597–612.

Cohen, C., & Cosimer, G. (1989). Factors associated with increased hospital stay by elderly psychiatric patients. *Hospital and Community Psychiatry, 40*(7), 741–743.

Collins, J. G. (1991). Acute pain management. *International Anesthesiology Clinics, 29*(1), 23–36.

Constello, J., & Boblin, S. (2004). What is the experience of men and women with congestive heart failure? *Canadian Journal of Cardiovascular Nursing, 14*(3), 9–20.

Dixon, L., Postrado, L., Delahanty, J., Fischer, P. J., & Lehman, A. (1999). The association of medical comorbidity in schizophrenia with poor physical and mental health. *Journal of Nervous and Mental Disease, 187*(8), 496–502.

Folstein, M. F., Folstein, S. E., & McHugh, P. R. (1975). Mini-Mental state: A practical method for grading the cognitive state of patients for the clinician. *Journal of Psychiatric Research, 12,* 189–198.

Ford, J. D., Trestman R. L., Steinberg, K., Tennen, E., & Allen, S. (2004). Prospective association of anxiety, depressive, and addictive disorders with high utilization of primary, specialty and emergency medical care. *Social Science & Medicine, 58*(11), 2145–2148.

Gabuzda, D. H., & Hirsch, M. S. (1987). Neurologic manifestations of infection with human immunodeficiency virus: Clinical features and pathogenesis. *Annals of Internal Medicine, 107,* 383–391.

Gold, P. W., Licinio, J., Wong, M. L., & Chrousos, G. P. (1995). Corticotropin releasing hormone in the pathophysiology of melancholic and atypical depression and in the mechanism of action of antidepressant drugs. *Annals of the New York Academy of Sciences, 771,* 716–729.

Goldsmith, R. J. (1999). Overview of psychiatric comorbidity: Practical and theoretical considerations. *Psychiatric Clinics of North America, 22*(2), 331–349.

Heim, C., Newport, D. J., Heit, S., et al. (2000). Pituitary-adrenal and autonomic responses to stress in women after sexual and physical injury in childhood. *Journal of the American Medical Association, 5,* 592–597.

Hill, D. R., Kelleher, K., & Shumaker, S. A. (1992). Psychosocial interventions in adult patients with coronary heart disease and cancer: A literature review. *General Hospital Psychiatry, 14*(6 Suppl.), 28S–42S.

Hosier, M. C., Conway, K. P., Meukangas, K. R. (2003). Associations between anxiety disorders and physical illness. *European Archives of Psychiatry and Clinical Neuroscience, 253*(6), 313–320.

Joffe, R. T., Brasche, J. S., MacQueen, G. M. (2003). Psychiatric aspects of endocrine disorders in women. *Psychiatric Clinics of North America 261*(3), 683–691.

Jorge, R. E., Robinson, R. G., Starkstien, S. E., & Arndt, S. V. (1994). Influence of major depression on 1-year outcome in patients with traumatic brain injury. *Journal of Neurosurgery, 81,* 726–733.

Kandel, E. R., & Schwartz, J. H. (1987). *Principles of neural science* (2nd ed.). New York: Elsevier.

Katon, W., & Schulberg, H. (1992). Epidemiology of depression in primary care. *General Hospital Psychiatry, 14,* 237–247.

Katz, N. (1994). Role of invasive procedures in chronic pain management. *Seminars in Neurology, 14*(3), 225–237.

Koob, G. F. (1999). Corticotrophin-releasing factor, norepinephrine and stress. *Biological Psychiatry, 46,* 1167–1180.

Levenson, J. L. (1992). Psychosocial interventions in chronic medical illness: An overview of outcome research. *General Hospital Psychiatry, 14*(6 Suppl.), 43S–49S.

Littrell, J. (1996). How psychological states affect the immune system: Implications for interventions in the context of HIV. *Health & Social Work, 21*(4), 287–296.

Luis, C. A., Vanderploeg, R. D., & Curtiss, G. (2003). Predictors of postconcussion symptom complex in community dwelling male veterans. *Journal of the International Neuropsychological Society, 9*(7), 1001–1015.

Mahoney, F. T., & Barthel, D. W. (1965). Functional evaluation: Barthel index. *Maryland Medical Journal, 14,* 61–65.

Manji, H., & Miller, R. (2004). The neurology of HIV infection. *Journal of Neurology Neurosurgery and Psychiatry, 75*(Suppl), 29–38.

McAllister, J. W., Flashman, L. A., Sparling, M. B., & Saykin, A. J. (2004). Working memory deficits after traumatic brain injury: catecholeminergic mechanisms and prospects for treatment. *Brain Injury, 18*(4), 331–350.

McCaffery, M., & Pasero, C. (1999). *Pain clinical manual* (2nd ed.). St. Louis: Mosby.

Melzack, R. (1993). Pain: Past, present and future. *Canadian Journal of Experimental Psychology, 47*(4), 615–629.

Melzack, R., Coderre, T. J., Katz, J., Vaccarino, A. L. (2001). Central neuroplasticity and pathological pain. Annals of New York Academy of Science, *933,* 157–174.

Murai, T., Muller, U., Werheid, K., et al. (2001). In vivo evidence for differential association of striatal dopamine and midbrain serotonin systems with neuropsychiatric symptoms in Parkinson's disease. *Journal of Clinical Neuroscience, 13,* 222–228.

Neese, J. B. (1991). Depression in the general hospital. *Nursing Clinics of North America, 26*(3), 613–622.

Nemeroff, C. B. (2004). Neurobiological consequences of childhood trauma. *Journal of Clinical Psychiatry, 65*(Suppl 1) 18–28.

Palomaki, H., Kaste, M., Berg, A., Lonnqvist, R., Lonnqvist, J., Lehtihalmes, M., & Hares, J. (1999). Prevention of poststroke depression: 1 Year randomised placebo controlled double blind trial of mianserin with 6 month follow up after therapy. *Journal of Neurology, Neurosurgery and Psychiatry, 66,* 490–494.

Paten, S. B. (1999). Long-term medical conditions and major depression in the Canadian population. *Canadian Journal of Psychiatry, 44*(2), 151–157.

Polsky, D., Doshi, J. A., Marcus, S., Oslin, D., Rothbard, A., Thomas, N., & Thompson, C. L. (2005). Long-term risk for depressive symptoms after a medical diagnosis. *Archives of Internal Medicine, 165*(11), 1260–1266.

Radley, J. J., Sisti, H. M., Has, J., Rocker, A. B., McCall, T., Hef, P. R., McEwen, B. S., & Morrison, J. H. (2004). Chronic behaviour stress induces apical dendritic reorganization in pyramidal neurons of the medial prefrontal cortex. *Neuroscience, 125*(1), 1–6.

Raichle, M. E. (1983). The pathophysiology of brain ischemia. *Annals of Neurology, 13*(1), 2–10.

Ren, K. (1994). Wind-up and the NMDA receptor: From animal studies to human pain. *Pain, 59,* 157–158.

Robinson, R. G. (2003). Poststroke depression: Prevalence, diagnosis, treatment, and disease progression. *Biological Psychiatry, 54*(3), 376–387.

Robinson, R, Schultz, S., Castillo, C., et al. (2000). Nortriptyline versus fluoxetine in the treatment of depression and in short-term recovery after stroke: A placebo controlled, double-blind study. *American Journal of Psychiatry, 157,* 351–359.

Rojo, A., Aguilar, M., Garolera, M. T., Cubo, E., Navas, I., Quintano, S. (2003). Depression in Parkinson's disease: Clinical correlates and outcomes. *Parkinsonism Related Disorders, 10*(1) 23–28.

Rudy, T. E., & Turk, D. C. (1991). Psychological aspects of pain. *International Anesthesiology Clinics, 29*(1), 9–21.

Sosnowski, M. (1994). Pathophysiology of acute pain. *Pain Digest, 4,* 100–105.

Stoudemire, A., Moran, M. G., & Fogel, B. S. (1990). Psychotropic drug use in the medically ill: Part 1. *Psychosomatics, 31*(4), 377–391.

Stoudemire, A., Moran, M. G., & Fogel, B. S. (1991). Psychotropic drug use in the medically ill: Part 2. *Psychosomatics, 32*(1), 34–46.

Stratakis, C. Chrousos, G. (1995). Neuro-endocrinology and pathophysiology of the stress system. *Annals of New York Academy of Science, 771,* 1-18.

Talbot, J. D., Marrett, S., Evans, A. C., et al. (1991). Multiple representations of pain in human cerebral cortex. *Science, 251*(3), 1355–1358.

Turk, D. C. (2004). Understanding pain sufferers: The role of cognitive successes. *Spine Journal 4*(1), 1–7.

Turk, D. C., & Feldman, C. S. (1992). Facilitating the use of noninvasive pain management strategies with the terminally ill. *Hospice Journal, 8*(1–12), 193–214.

Verdelko, A., Henon, H., Lebert, F., Pasquiere, F., & Leys, D. (2004). Depressive symptoms after stroke and relationship with dementia: A three year follow-up study. *Neurology, 62*(6), 905–911.

Zangen, A., Nakash, R., Yadid, G. (1999). Serotonin-mediated increases in the extracellular levels of beta-endorphins in the arcuate nucleus and nucleus accumbens: A microdialysis study. *Journal of Neurochemistry, 73*(6), 2569–2574.

For challenges, please refer to the **CD-ROM** in this book.

Forensic Psychiatric and Mental Health Nursing

Cindy Peternelj-Taylor

LEARNING OBJECTIVES

After studying this chapter, you will be able to:

- Describe the complexity of mental health challenges experienced by the forensic population.
- Examine issues that are critical to the development of therapeutic relationships with forensic clients.
- Consider the challenges and opportunities that exist for nursing given the diversity of settings in which forensic nurses practice.
- Analyze issues inherent in professional role development for nurses practicing with forensic clients.
- Evaluate the societal norms that affect contemporary care and treatment of forensic clients.
- Discuss strategies for ongoing education, research, and practice development in forensic nursing.

KEY TERMS

dynamic security ▪ forensic nursing ▪ static security ▪ compassionate release ▪ boundary violations

▶ KEY CONCEPTS

custody and caring ▪ othering ▪ manipulation ▪ vulnerable

Forensic nurses practice at the shifting interface of the criminal justice system and the health care system, and their ability to provide competent and ethical care is often compromised by social and political animosity regarding crime, criminality, and mental disorder. Regrettably, for a variety of reasons and life circumstances, a large number of vulnerable and at-risk individuals find themselves seeking health care under the auspices of the criminal justice system. It is no wonder that forensic nurses have been described as pioneers, exploring new horizons for nursing (Holmes, 2005).

As members of an emergent specialty of nursing, forensic nurses are responsible for providing care and treatment to forensic clients in a variety of secure institutional facilities, including jails, prisons, correctional facilities, young offender institutions, forensic psychiatric hospitals, and forensic psychiatric units within general hospitals. They are also involved in community-based court diversion schemes and community treatment orders, and they assist forensic clients with reintegration into the community. This chapter, therefore, focusses on nursing care of individuals who have violated the law in some way: those remanded in custody while awaiting trial (charged but not yet sentenced), those who have been remanded in custody for a psychiatric evaluation, those who are found unfit to stand trial or not criminally responsible on account of a mental disorder, and those who have been charged, remanded in custody, and sentenced by the courts. A variety of terms are used to refer to this evolving specialty area of practice, including forensic psychiatric nursing, community forensic mental health nursing, and correctional or prison nursing. For simplicity, *forensic nursing* is used throughout this chapter and refers to nurses who integrate psychiatric and mental health nursing "philosophy and practice within a sociocultural context that includes the criminal justice system to provide comprehensive care to clients, families, and communities" (Peternelj-Taylor & Hufft, 2006, p. 379).

CRIMINALIZATION OF THE MENTALLY ILL

Throughout Canada, jails, prisons, and young offender institutions, by default, have become repositories for individuals with mental illness. In the past decade alone, the number of individuals with significant mental health needs within the federal correctional system in Canada has more than doubled, with treatment often nonexistent, or unsatisfactory when compared with the community standard (Office of the Correctional Investigator [OCI], 2005). This trend is also noted in the United States, where correctional institutions are commonly referred to as "primary mental health facilities" (Human Rights Watch, 2003) or the "new psychiatric hospitals" (Aufderheide & Brown, 2005). The criminal-

ization of the mentally ill has frequently been attributed to the deinstitutionalization movement that occurred in the 1960s and the 1970s, and continues today (Peternelj-Taylor & Johnson, 1995; Sealy & Whitehead, 2004; Statistics Canada, 2003). Unfortunately, the ongoing failure of provincial and federal governments to provide sufficient mental health funding to fully realize the goals of deinstitutionalization (eg, independent living within the community) has resulted in a fragmented mental health system. Individuals who experience chronic mental illness are often well known by the police, the courts, jails, and correctional facilities. Critics conclude that for many individuals caught up in this web, their only crime is that they are "guilty of mental illness" (Kanapaux, 2004).

THE PARADOX OF CUSTODY AND CARING

Forensic settings are controversial. They arouse strong convictions from various sectors who debate their proper place in society. Nursing practice within this domain is particularly complex because it brings together the "coupling of two contradictory socio-professional mandates: to punish and to provide care" (Holmes, 2005, p. 3). This paradox is disconcerting because a clear distinction between these two mandates is not always easily demarcated. Forensic settings provide society with two fundamental services: social necessities and social goods. Social necessities are considered essential to a community's existence; conversely, social goods are perceived as kindnesses, and although not necessarily essential, they are of benefit to the community nonetheless. Forensic settings meet their social necessity mandate through social control of those in their care. The protection of the community at large is perceived as a direct consequence of the processes of confinement and control. Forensic settings also provide social goods in the form of health care to those who are confined. In essence, forensic nurses are charged with the predicament of providing social good (eg, health care) within institutions dedicated to the provision of social necessities (eg, confinement) (Osborne, 1995; Peternelj-Taylor & Johnson, 1995; Peternelj-Taylor, 2004).

> **KEY CONCEPT** Nurses in forensic settings must meet the competing demands of **custody** (confinement and security) **and caring** (nursing care).

This coexistence of social control and nursing care creates a paradox for nurses (Holmes, 2005), one that is laden with clinical issues and moral dilemmas not commonly encountered in more traditional health care settings. This paradox requires special attention and discernment because it permeates every aspect of forensic nursing. It is likely the single factor that differentiates

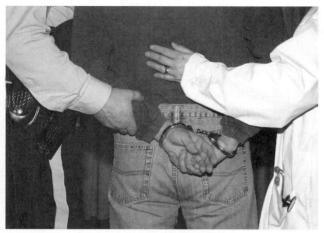

FIGURE 33.1 **Custody and caring.** (Courtesy of the Division of Media and Technology, University of Saskatchewan.)

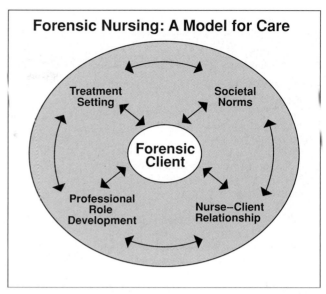

FIGURE 33.2 **Forensic nursing: a model for care.** (From Peternelj-Taylor, C. (2004). *NURS 486—Forensic Nursing in Secure Environments.* College of Nursing, University of Saskatchewan.)

forensic nursing from mental health nursing in a more general sense (Peternelj-Taylor, 2000). It is within this paradox, where the competing demands for custody and caring are embraced, that the moral climate of forensic institutions is shaped (Austin, 2001) (Fig. 33-1).

FORENSIC NURSING: A MODEL FOR CARE

Nurses working with forensic clients will find a familiar psychiatric and mental health nursing role, one that is "like 'stepping through the looking glass'—everything is the same, yet different" (Smith, 2005, p. 54). To illustrate the uniqueness of forensic nursing, a model of care is presented. It highlights the contextual and clinical practice issues affecting the articulation of a professional nursing role with forensic clients, regardless of setting. The five components of this model are the forensic client, nurse–client relationship, professional role development, treatment setting, and societal norms. Although each component of the model is discussed separately, in reality the components are dynamic and interactive in nature. Peternelj-Taylor and Hufft (2006) conclude that health care goals must be consistent with the reality of the client's life circumstances, as well as the realities and the limitations of the setting in which nursing practice takes place. It may well be that not all forensic nurses will engage fully with each component of the model of care presented. However, the model as presented herein reflects the nature and scope of forensic nursing in Canada (Fig. 33-2).

Characteristics of the Forensic Client

As a group, forensic clients present with a multitude of long-neglected physical and mental health care challenges, often complicated by significant substance abuse problems. The health and psychosocial issues that they experience are often complex and multifaceted, contributing to the challenges encountered in their attempts to engage in treatment and reintegration. Frequently their lives have been marked by illiteracy, poverty, and homelessness. Cultural minorities, in particular, are overrepresented in correctional institutions (Anno, Graham, Lawrence, & Shansky, 2004; Canadian Public Health Association [CPHA], 2004). Morbidity and mortality data suggest that those who are incarcerated experience higher rates of disease and disability when compared with nonincarcerated populations, which highlights the need for nursing leadership in primary, secondary, and tertiary levels of intervention (Box 33-1). As individuals, forensic clients often experience discrimination, stigmatization, and marginalization; they often lack supportive relationships commonly associated with emotional and mental well-being. And, they are totally dependent on the system (whether it is the correctional system or the health care system) to meet their health care needs. Given the magnitude of these commingling issues, many forensic clients are at risk for dual, multiple, and overlapping sources of vulnerability. Yet, referring to those who have committed crimes against society, as "vulnerable" seems somewhat contrary to conventional wisdom (Peternelj-Taylor, 2005a).

Vulnerability and Vulnerable Populations

Broadly defined, vulnerability refers to a multifaceted concept that represents the commingling of resources, risk factors, and health status among a particular

BOX 33.1

Health Status of Federally Incarcerated Individuals in Comparison to the General Canadian Population

Characteristics of Incarcerated Individuals

SOCIOECONOMIC MEASURES
- Twice as likely not to have finished high school
- Nine times as likely to have been unemployed

HEALTH BEHAVIOURS
- More than twice as likely to smoke
- Thirty times more likely to inject drugs
- Two to 10 times more likely to have an alcohol or substance abuse disorder

CHRONIC CONDITIONS
- 40% more likely to be treated for diabetes if male and three times likely if female
- 68% more likely to be treated for cardiovascular conditions if male and more than two times more likely if female
- 43% more likely to be treated for asthma if male and almost three times more likely if female
- 50% more likely to need the use of mechanical aids

INFECTIOUS DISEASES
- More than twice as likely to have been infected with hepatitis B virus
- More than 20 times more likely to have been infected with hepatitis C virus
- More than 10 times more likely to have been infected with human immunodeficiency virus
- Much more likely to be infected with tuberculosis

MENTAL HEALTH DISORDERS
- More than twice as likely to have had a mental disorder
- Three times more likely to have schizophrenia in males and 20 times more likely in females
- Four times more likely to have a mood disorder

MORTALITY
- At a 45% increased risk for death
- Eight times more likely to die of homicide
- Almost four times more likely to die of suicide

From Canadian Public Health Association. (2004). *A Health Care Needs Assessment of Federal Inmates*, 95(suppl.1), S49. Copyright 2004 by the Canadian Public Health Association. Reprinted with permission.

population or aggregate of people, which places them at risk for altered health status (de Chesnay, 2005; Flaskerud & Winslow, 1998). de Chesnay (2005) looks at this concept in two ways:

- Individual focus (vulnerability)—which is concerned with such notions as "susceptibility" or "at risk for health problems"
- Aggregate view (vulnerable populations)—which is applied to those at risk for physical, psychological, or social health challenges, and also includes vulnerability by virtue of one's status or group membership.

KEY CONCEPT Persons or populations are considered **vulnerable** when attributes, factors, or assigned status places them at greater risk for injury or poor health when compared with others.

Even though nurses have historically "ministered" to vulnerable populations (Drake, 1998), nursing has failed to acknowledge forensic clients (particularly those who are incarcerated) as a vulnerable population (Flaskerud et al., 2002; Moynihan, 2006). Clearly, forensic clients represent a significant portion of society's at-risk population. As such, understanding the concepts of vulnerability and vulnerable populations is essential to contemporary forensic nursing practice.

Clients Experiencing Mental Illness

There is great variation in the nature and severity of mental illnesses experienced by individuals who come into conflict with the law. In 1992, the Corrections and Conditional Release Act (Bill C-30) was proclaimed. This ended the Lieutenant Governor's Warrant System, whereby clients who were found "not guilty by reason of insanity" were held at the pleasure of the Lieutenant Governor for an unspecified period of time. It created review boards that are mandated to oversee the care and disposition of persons found unfit to stand trial or not criminally responsible on account of mental disorder (Statistics Canada, 2003). Under current Canadian law, an individual who comes into conflict with the law and is mentally ill can be found as follows:

- Unfit to stand trial (UST), when it is recognized that the accused is not fully capable of instructing legal counsel, or not capable of understanding the nature and the consequences of a trial (can later be found "fit" and tried in court and convicted, or deemed not criminally responsible on account of mental disorder)
- Not criminally responsible on account of mental disorder (NCRMD), based on the accused person's mental state at the time the offence was committed. Although it is not a finding of guilt, the court may give the following dispositions: detention in hospital, conditional discharge, or an absolute discharge. Individuals detained in hospital are not required to submit to treatment; the disposition is meant to detain the person and make care available. If treatment is required, owing to the individual's deteriorating mental status, treatment is then provided as per provincial or territorial mental health policies.

- In some jurisdictions, community treatment orders (CTOs) and Court Diversion are options that may be exercised to treatment programs through community or provincial mechanisms, instead of going to trial (Statistics Canada, 2003).

In all cases, the mentally disordered offender challenges the collective wisdom of both the health care system and the criminal justice system, creating a "crossover" of sorts, particularly when the individual has been found responsible for his or her crimes despite the mental illness. The incarceration experience represents a significant stressful life event, even for those who do not have a mental disorder; separation from family and friends, limitations on privacy, overcrowding, and fear of assault severely affect the individual's quality of life. For those with mental illness, prisons are dangerous places; they are often victimized by other offenders, they are at greater risk for attempting suicide (including self-harming); and they are confined to segregation for their own protection. Unfortunately, such experiences can completely overwhelm the resources of individuals with mental illness. When compared with the individuals in the community, offenders experience greater rates of schizophrenia, depression, bipolar disorder, anxiety disorders, and substance abuse disorders (Appelbaum, Hickey, & Packer, 2001; CPHA, 2004; Phillips & Caplan, 2003).

The most recent report from the OCI (2005) recommended a major overhaul to existing mental health services provided by federal corrections. Specific recommendations included (1) comprehensive clinical intake assessment; (2) improvement to the existing treatment centres; (3) intermediate mental health units within existing penitentiaries to provide ongoing assessment and treatment; and (4) community mental health services to support offenders on conditional release. Investing in assessment, treatment, and community supervision will contribute to the mental well-being of the individual clients and enhance public safety by maximizing safe reintegration into the community (OCI, 2005).

Special Populations in the Forensic Setting

Although it could be argued that all forensic clients have special needs requiring the attention of special services and interventions by forensic nurses, groups more likely to require unique approaches include women, older adults, young offenders, cultural minorities, and families.

Female Forensic Clients

The past decade has seen a marked increase in the number of women confined to forensic settings; and even though women represent a small percentage of the overall forensic population, they currently account for its largest growth in Canada and other Western nations (CPHA, 2004; Harrison & Beck, 2005). In general, women most likely to find themselves within forensic settings are women who have grown up in poor communities, have limited education and job skills, and are the primary caregivers for dependent children. For many women, the fear of losing custody of their children is ever present (Blanchard, 2004; Harner, 2004; Maeve, 2003). Female forensic clients are frequently victims as well as perpetrators of crime, having experienced physical, emotional, and sexual abuse, as children and as adults, at the hands of fathers, husbands, boyfriends, acquaintances, and strangers (Green et al., 2005; Maeve, 2003; Peternelj-Taylor, 2005d). Aboriginal women are overrepresented within correctional systems, and their adaptation is complicated by forced separation from family and community, creating significant barriers to timely reintegration into their home communities (OCI, 2005).

Common health concerns of incarcerated women include significant substance abuse problems; higher rates of blood-borne infections such as HIV, AIDS, hepatitis B and C viruses; significant mental health concerns including anxiety related disorders (eg, post-traumatic stress disorder), concerns related to personality disorders (eg, poor interpersonal functioning and self-injurious behaviours), and serious mental illness (including depression and schizophrenia); pregnancy and gynaecologic problems; obesity; and chronic disorders such as diabetes, hypertension, epilepsy, and respiratory diseases (CPHA, 2004; Green et al., 2005; Maeve, 2003; Peternelj-Taylor, 2005d; Roth & Pressé, 2003).

Elderly Forensic Clients

For an increasing number of older Canadians, growing old in prison or in a forensic psychiatric facility is a harsh reality. Elderly forensic clients are considered those aged 50 years and older; the transformation to "elderly" is thought to be accelerated by 10 to 12 years within this group of clients (Anno et al., 2004; Gallagher, 2001).

Depending on the nature of imprisonment or hospitalization, the individual may experience stressors related to general survival (particularly those who are incarcerated), coping with financial pressures, and withdrawal from drugs or alcohol, as well as the cumulative impact of high-risk behaviours, negative lifestyle practices, and inadequate health care, coupled with psychosocial issues related to confinement and isolation (Anno et al., 2004; Beckett, Peternelj-Taylor, & Johnson, 2003). Elderly forensic clients experience both physical and mental health care needs that set them apart from their younger counterparts, as well as those typical age-related problems experienced by their nonincarcerated peers. Common physical concerns evident in this population include cardiovascular disease, pulmonary disorders, diabetes, arthritis, cancer, and Alzheimer's disease and other dementias. Common mental health needs include stress, social isolation, depression, and suicide (CPHA, 2004; Correctional Services of Canada [CSC], 2005; Gal, 2002; Beckett et al., 2003).

The health care needs of older forensic clients clearly challenge traditional correctional resources and budgets, and questions related to the ability of correctional facilities to adequately care for older offenders are real (Beckett et al., 2003; Gallagher, 2001). For increasing numbers of elderly and infirm forensic clients, the fear of dying while confined is a terse reality. Although compassionate release to community-based long-term care facilities, known as *parole by exception* in Canada, is allowed under the Corrections and Conditional Release Act, ongoing fears about community safety, bed shortages in long-term care facilities, and the stigma surrounding the circumstances of the forensic client's hospitalization or incarceration are considered on an individual basis. This option, however, is available to only a very few long-term and infirm forensic clients, and palliative care within forensic settings is a poignant reality (Beckett et al., 2003; Fowler-Kerry, 2003; Duggleby, 2005).

Young Offenders

Young people who come into conflict with the law are a vastly underserved population with greater than average health care needs, and because of this, they are particularly vulnerable to adverse outcomes. Frequently, their behavioural problems associated with their criminal charges mask their overall health care needs and thwart treatment efforts. It is not uncommon for youth who find themselves in custody to experience symptoms consistent with schizophrenia, anxiety disorders, behaviour disorders, and substance abuse disorders, although they may not have a formal diagnosis as such. Additionally, youth frequently demonstrate health patterns related to their family environments, as family commonly struggle with mental and physical health problems and substance abuse issues, and present with criminal histories and records (Shelton, 2000, 2001, 2004; Shelton & Pearson, 2005).

Canada holds the dubious honour of incarcerating more youth per capita than any other country in the Western world, including the United States (Department of Justice, 2006). Aboriginal youth in particular are overrepresented among youth in custody at every stage of the Canadian criminal justice system. Latimer and Foss (2004) report that Aboriginal youth are almost eight times more likely to be in custody than their non-Aboriginal counterparts. Using a 1-day snapshot approach to data collection, the incarceration rate for Aboriginal youth during the data collection period was 64.5 per 10,000 population, whereas the incarceration rate for non-Aboriginal youth was 8.2 per 10,000.

These figures are particularly alarming when one considers that Aboriginal youth represent about 5% of the Canadian population.

The mental health care concerns reported by Latimer and Foss (2004) are equally alarming and include high rates of fetal alcohol spectrum disorder, significant substance use issues, suicidal ideation, self-harm, and histories of attempted suicide and high rates of physical, sexual, and emotional abuse contributing to a large portion of the youth being involved with a child protection agency at the time of their admission.

Tragically, most forensic nurses will come into contact with youth through the criminal justice system because very few hospitals are set up to deal with the complexity of needs experienced by the young offenders. However, confinement in and of itself will not facilitate improvement in the mental health of this vulnerable group (Shelton, 2001), and intersectoral approaches, which bring together justice, law, social services, education, and health care, are necessary to address the complexity of issues facing the young offender.

Culturally Diverse Clients

The ethnic diversity of Canada as a whole is reflected in the demographic profile of Canadian forensic facilities. However, as might be predicted, clients representing ethnic and racial minorities are disproportionately represented. Although Aboriginal offenders make up only 2% of Canada's adult population, they represent about 17% of the federal incarcerated population (CPHA, 2004; CSC, 2005). Comparable rates of hospitalization in forensic settings operated by the health care system are unavailable.

Overrepresentation of Aboriginal people within the criminal justice system is attributed to a number of complex factors related to effects of rapid culture change, cultural oppression, and marginalization (Kirmayer, Brass, & Tait, 2000), resulting in high rates of poverty, substance abuse, and victimization within families and communities of origin (CSC, 2005; Latimer & Foss, 2004). There has been a growing awareness among the health care and criminal justice systems of the need to provide culturally sensitive and appropriate programming. In the past, programs were developed on the assumption of sameness; this approach not only negated the forensic client's ethnic identity and culture of origin, but also created barriers in the formation of therapeutic relationships and treatment programs, which ultimately interfered with successful community rehabilitation (Amellal, 2005; Hufft & Kite, 2003).

Families

In recent years, the needs of family members, the "forgotten clients" (Goldkuhle, 1999), have necessitated expanded roles for forensic nurses and community-based partnerships. Family members, children, and friends are a hidden forensic population; they are not accounted for and are rarely discussed by policy makers or health service providers. Frudenberg (2001) concludes that incarceration has unintended consequences on families: higher rates of female-headed households, family disruption, family break-up, forced kinship care, and foster care. Additionally, family members have often experienced various types of violence (eg, child abuse, domestic violence, elder abuse); children in paricular are more likely to experience physical, emotional, and cognitive problems and engage in self-destructive patterns that increase their likelihood of spending time within the forensic system (ie, prisons) when compared with children of nonincarcerated parents (Goldkuhle, 1999; Frudenberg, 2001).

Kent-Wilkinson (1999) advocates the use of a forensic family genogram, when working with forensic clients. A genogram is both an assessment and an intervention tool, one that can assist nurses in identifying individual and family patterns (e.g., mental health history, criminal behaviour, substance abuse) and contribute to more comprehensive assessments, interventions, and appropriate community referrals for family members. Collaborating with family members is critical to the safe reintegration of the forensic client into the community and is a role that is increasingly being embraced by forensic nurses, particularly those affiliated with community-based mental health programs. Many factors affect the forensic client's readjustment to the community, including family dynamics, stress, and the family's degree of involvement. It is not uncommon for families to experience guilt and remorse regarding the forensic client's criminal acts (Encinares & Lorbergs, 2001). In some cases, the behaviours of family members can sabotage treatment and reintegration plans, and nursing staff are often the brunt of sarcasm and hostility (Encinares & Golea, 2005).

Nurse–Client Relationship

Nursing by its very nature is relational; it is through the nurse–client relationship that nurses gain a deeper understanding and appreciation of the human condition. In fact, the ability to establish and maintain a therapeutic relationship with a forensic client is among the most important competencies required by forensic nurses (Peternelj-Taylor, 2002, 2004). In the forensic milieu, the emphasis of the therapeutic relationship as a primary intervention strategy is dependent on how the nurse's role is defined and on the context of the setting in which nursing practice takes place. For example, for forensic nurses practicing in an inpatient forensic psychiatric unit, working at a sex offender treatment program, or counselling HIV positive clients in a prison setting, the therapeutic relationship is fundamental to

the identification and resolution of problems. In other areas of forensic nursing practice, for example, in an ambulatory care clinic in a correctional facility, the therapeutic relationship may be more in the background (Registered Nurses Association of Ontario, 2002). Regardless of the setting or the nature of the relationship, it cannot be assumed that a therapeutic relationship will be present, simply by virtue of one's nursing role (Peternelj-Taylor, 2004; Schafer & Peternelj-Taylor, 2003).

Engagement in a therapeutic relationship can be especially difficult for nurses when the client is accused (or convicted) of committing a morally reprehensible act. Clearly, some forensic clients possess characteristics that could easily evoke negative responses from their caregivers. They engage in threatening behaviours, they break rules and test boundaries, and they are unappreciative of nurses' efforts in providing health care (Austin, 2001; Maeve & Vaughn, 2001; Schafer, 2002). Nurses, as members of society, are not immune to attitudes, beliefs, and stereotypes, and these may negatively colour their perceptions, their therapeutic response, and their professional roles with forensic clients. The belief that every client has the potential to change and the right to treatment is one not shared by all forensic nurses (Peternelj-Taylor & Johnson, 1995; Rose, 2005). Martin (2001) warns that nurses "need to be cautious that their approach to patients does not reinforce the stigma and discrimination of the wider community" (p. 29).

To be successful, forensic nurses need to honestly and candidly explore their own preconceived ideas, attitudes, beliefs, and stereotypes regarding the forensic client. All too often, nurses can get caught up in the sensationalism that surrounds a particular forensic client (often fuelled by media hype), or the setting in which practice takes place, and ultimately they can lose sight of the person in need of care. Furthermore, it is not uncommon for nurses who are employed in forensic settings to experience additional stressors unique to their work, which ultimately affect their ability to establish and maintain therapeutic relationships with the clients in their care. Some examples are issues related to personal safety (ie, threat of violence by forensic clients), ethical dilemmas, understaffing, secondary trauma and related post-traumatic stress disorder, and competing and conflicting expectations held between health care and correctional authorities (Appelbaum et al., 2001; Holmes, 2005; Peternelj-Taylor, 2004).

Common Relationship Issues Experienced by Forensic Nurses

Although barriers to therapeutic relationships can be found in all areas of nursing, it is the "special circumstance" (Austin, 2001) of forensic settings, where the moral climate is shaped by the divergent and competing demands for custody and caring, that contributes to forensic settings being described as "hotbeds" for potential problems. This is in part due to the complexity of health care needs experienced by forensic clients, the seductive pull of helping and the intensity of relationships that can develop, the professional isolation experienced by forensic nurses, and the cultural and philosophical differences that exist between forensic clients, forensic nurses, and other members of the treatment team (Hufft & Kite, 2003; Peternelj-Taylor, 2002, 2005a; Schafer & Peternelj-Taylor, 2003).

Othering

It is within these habitats of special circumstance that nurses meet forensic clients, and how the client is perceived is often illustrated by how nurses "language" their care. For example, are the clients seen as inmates? As cons? As psychopaths? As murders? As psychos? As borderlines? Such labels not only evoke stereotypical images but also, more importantly, cast the individual into the role of the "other" (Peternelj-Taylor, 2004, 2005b). This negative form of engagement, known as *exclusionary othering*, can affect all aspects of nursing care and promote underinvolvement in a client's care. *Inclusionary othering*, on the other hand, is promoted as a way of learning about the other, as an individual, and not simply a crime or a label. One way of coming to know the forensic client is through role taking and trying to understand the world from the client's perspective. Although this may be a tall order when working with forensic clients, nurses can learn about othering by

gaining an appreciation for what it means to be othered (Canales, 2000).

> **KEY CONCEPT Othering** is about the way one perceives and engages with another person. It can be exclusionary and negative (ie, the other is different from and thus "less than" me) or inclusionary and tolerant or accepting (ie, the other is different from me, so I need to learn about his or her world view).

Boundary Violations

The complexities and uncertainties surrounding boundaries and boundary violations in practice can be difficult for forensic nurses to manage, leading to ongoing confusion in practice. The inability to differentiate the professional relationship from a social relationship by attempting to have one's personal needs met through the nurse–client relationship is consistently discussed as a precursor to boundary violations in the nursing literature (Pilette, Berck, & Achber, 1995; Peternelj-Taylor & Yonge, 2003) (see Chapter 8). In forensic settings, nurses are often painted as "victims of circumstances" when boundaries are transgressed with a forensic client. However, it is important to remember that, from an ethical perspective, the nurse is the one responsible for managing boundaries within the nurse–client relationship, not the client. Mixed messages regarding treatment boundaries can be especially disconcerting for forensic clients, who frequently have problems with boundaries in general (Box 33-2).

BOX 33.2 RESEARCH FOR BEST PRACTICE

Therapeutic Relationships and Boundary Maintenance: Forensic Clients' Perspective

Schafer, P., & Peternelj-Taylor, C. (2003). Therapeutic relationships and boundary maintenance: The perspective of forensic patients enrolled in a treatment program for violent offenders. *Issues in Mental Health Nursing, 24,* 605–625.

THE PURPOSE: The focus of this qualitative study was the exploration of therapeutic relationships and boundary maintenance from the perspective of forensic clients enrolled in a treatment program for violent offenders.

METHODS: A naturalistic inquiry was conducted with 12 male participants (aged 22–42 years), who were each interviewed three times. The semistructured interviews were audiotaped and transcribed verbatim. Eight participants were interviewed a fourth time as a way of soliciting their feedback regarding the analysis of the data. Constant comparative method of data analysis was used.

FINDINGS: Analysis of the data revealed a core process, the development of therapeutic relationships, indicating that the development of relationships was a complex process. Five interrelated themes emerged from the interview data: (1) adjusting to the house (captured the client's transition to the treatment environment); (2) knowing the fundamental structures of the house (represented the participants perceptions of influential contextual factors); (3) evaluating the primary therapist as a guide (illustrates the complex processes that the partic-

ipants engaged in, in order to judge whether the nurses were "for them, or against them"); (4) experiences that promote or hinder the relationship; and finally (5) ways of being with the primary therapist (illustrated four different types of relationships that developed).

IMPLICATIONS FOR NURSING: This research indicates that understanding gender relationships, power, patterns of interacting, and self-awareness is critical to the formation of therapeutic relationships and maintenance of boundaries. Because clinical competence can only be achieved within the context of the relationship, clinical supervision in forensic nursing that emphasizes professional development is recommended. Likewise, forensic nurses need to develop the required resources to conceptualize clients' behaviours as clinical challenges, and to use this knowledge to promote the therapeutic interests of the clients. Finally, the custodial roles that nurses engage in can hinder the development of therapeutic relationships (in some cases), and as such, should be examined within the context of the treatment environment.

Manipulation

The potential for manipulation is a very real factor in secure environments, one that requires thoughtful consideration by nurses in the provision of nursing care. In some cases, individuals in forensic settings will attempt to manipulate health care services for some secondary gain (eg, medication, escape from the prison environment, social diversion) and issues pertaining to safety cannot be ignored (Peternelj-Taylor, 2004). As Austin (2001) notes, "cautioning, scepticism, and the questioning of patients' motives and actions, are part of the daily experience of forensic nurses" (Austin, 2001, p. 13).

> **KEY CONCEPT Manipulation** is a concern in secure environments because it can involve the use of deceit to reach a goal that could not be pursued openly (eg, escape).

However, when a forensic client is labelled a manipulator, nurses and others will generally respond more punitively and fail to engage the client in a therapeutic dialogue surrounding the meaning of his or her behaviours; as such, the opportunity for mutual problem solving, around the manipulative behaviours, is lost to the relationship (Peternelj-Taylor, 2004; Schafer, 2002). In short, forensic nurses need to be astutely aware that there exists the potential for manipulation in all interactions with forensic clients, and they need to find the right balance between assuming the worst and knowing that it can always happen (Smith, 2005).

Professional Role Development

Historically, role development for forensic nurses has been difficult, owing to the myth that nurses who work with forensic clients are "second class nurses" unable to secure employment elsewhere (Peternelj-Taylor & Johnson, 1995; Pullan & Lorbergs, 2001). Given the breadth and scope of forensic nursing as illustrated within this chapter, it should be evident that forensic nurses are highly skilled and knowledgeable professionals, committed to the health and well-being of the clients in their charge, as well as the community at large.

Professional Nursing Identity

One of the greatest challenges that nurses experience when working in forensic environments is to remain true to their professional nursing roles and avoid been seduced or co-opted into assuming custodial roles, where expectations and responsibilities are more clearly defined (Holmes & Federman, 2003, 2006; Maeve, 2003; Peternelj-Taylor & Johnson, 1995; Smith, 2005). In forensic settings operated by the criminal justice system, forensic nurses must have a strong nursing identity, in order to maintain their professional authority and responsibility, without succumbing to the temptation to align themselves with correctional staff. However,

forensic nurses who work within the health care system should also heed this lesson, for they too can assume a more custodial stance, especially when they believe that community treatment orders or dispositions in hospital are lenient forms of punishment. So, even when the care of forensic clients is the responsibility of the health care system, incongruent attitudes among health care staff *may* prevail (Rose, 2005). Lawson (2005) states that when we "set ourselves up as judge and jury" (p. 149) we minimize our ability to be therapeutic.

Professional Development for Forensic Nurses

In 1981, Petryshen published a classic paper entitled "Nursing the Mentally Disordered Offender." Since then, forensic nursing in Canada has undergone significant transformations in education, research, and practice developments related to the provision of nursing care to forensic clients.

Education

Forensic nursing content is slowly finding its way into undergraduate and graduate nursing curricula across the country, primarily through existing courses in psychiatric mental health or community health nursing. Kent-Wilkinson (2006) concludes that successful programs have often been pioneered by forensic nurse experts, based on their clinical and teaching experiences. Furthermore, technologic advances in nursing education have contributed to the growth of this specialty as a result of opportunities inherent through online learning. Smith (2005) also supports the need for continuing professional development for nurses who practice in forensic settings, as a way of reinforcing the therapeutic identity of nurses, and thereby assisting them with nursing policy development.

Research

Canadian nurses have been writing about forensic nursing issues for many years, yet the literature remains largely theoretical and anecdotal, and forensic nursing research in Canada remains largely underdeveloped at this time. Embracing a research agenda with forensic clients will guide nursing practice in this highly specialized area, provide new insights into primary, secondary and tertiary health care (including reintegration into the community), and contribute to nursing science through the advancement of nursing knowledge regarding vulnerable populations in general. The pursuit of an active research agenda is fundamental to keeping forensic nursing as a specialty alive and well (Peternelj-Taylor, 2000, 2005a).

Practice Developments

To date, standards for forensic nursing at the provincial or national level are nonexistent. A fledgling group, the

BOX 33.3

Tips for Security Awareness in Forensic Settings

- When working in institutional settings, never bring anything in or take anything out for a client, regardless of how insignificant the request may seem.
- Always let coworkers know your whereabouts at all times; interview clients in designated interview rooms, or in places visible to other staff members. When working in the community, always leave your itinerary, the anticipated length of your visits, and how you can be reached.
- Observe policies and procedures related to security awareness specific to the forensic setting in which you are working. Ask questions in order to understand the rationale behind the policies.

- Do not share personal information about yourself, or other staff, with clients.
- Clients will sometimes engage in sexually inappropriate banter or gestures. Report this immediately, no matter how embarrassed you may be.
- Be aware of the location of staff in relation to clients. Use a buddy system (eg, another staff member) when uncomfortable approaching a client, especially when entering the client's living space.
- In all cases, open communication is critical to safe and competent nursing practice. Report all suspicious behaviour as soon as possible.

Forensic Nurses' Society (see Web Links), is aiming to become an emerging interest group with the Canadian Nurses Association and to affiliate with the International Association of Forensic Nurses. The proposed mandate of the Society is twofold: to provide a network for forensic nurses and a forum to discuss evidence-based practice within the subspecialty areas identified by the International Association of Forensic Nurses. Becoming a special interest group of the Canadian Nurses Association would formally recognize forensic nursing as a specialty; however, certification as a designated specialty remains uncertain (see Chapter 6).

Treatment Setting

Unlike more traditional practice settings, the interpersonal climate, organizational culture, and social context of forensic settings result in forensic environments being identified among the most severe and extreme environments known to society. Power, control, and implicit authority are manifested in the physical and interpersonal environments of both correctional systems and health care systems and can be incompatible with the achievement of treatment goals (Austin, 2001; Holmes, 2005; Phillips & Caplan, 2003)

Security Awareness

When working with forensic clients, issues surrounding safety and security are considered critical competencies, and nurses often struggle to find the right balance between their caring and custodial roles. The therapeutic treatment needs of their clients must always be considered within the context of maintaining security. Forensic settings (apart from community-based programs) are typically highly controlled environments, with the whereabouts of clients constantly monitored through a variety of institutional routines, mechanisms, rules, and regulations (Austin, 2001; Drake, 1998; Peternelj-Taylor & Johnson, 1995). Surveillance of staff

and clients is deemed critical to the safe operation of all forensic facilities. Because of this, however, nursing staff often experience additional stressors because they too are subject to the judgment of others: those who watch over, are watched over in turn (Holmes, 2005). For example, in correctional environments, health care is not generally viewed as a priority, and nursing interventions are often poorly understood and viewed with suspicion (Smith, 2005).

Forensic nurses quickly become aware of two forms of security awareness: static security and dynamic security. Static security awareness includes such things as the structural or environmental artefacts common to secure environments, for example, the use of two-way radios, personal protection alarms, video monitoring, electronic door locks, internal barriers, and perimeter fences or walls. Dynamic security awareness, on the other hand, is concerned with institutional policies, staffing patterns, methods of operation, and relational security. Finding the right balance between the security needs of the forensic setting (and the community at large) and the client's treatment needs is a balancing act at best. Practical points for competent and safe practice are found in Box 33-3.

In forensic settings operated under the jurisdiction of the health care system (eg, forensic psychiatric hospitals and forensic psychiatric units), forensic nurses assume broader roles in the maintenance of security. This can be particularly disconcerting because they may be expected to handcuff clients before a court visit, or search them for contraband before and after personal visits (or absences from the unit), while at the same time engage them in a therapeutic nurse–client relationship. This overt attention to custodial roles can jeopardize the fragility of the developing therapeutic relationship, and systems often need to be in place that see nurses from other units, or those not responsible for direct nursing care, to assist with these necessary custodial measures (Woods, 2004).

Risk Assessment and Management
Forensic nurses practicing in forensic settings work with clients with a proven capacity for violence. In

recent years, risk assessment and management have become increasingly important competencies required of forensic nurses. Risk assessment is critical because it guides intervention and treatment. Simply stated, the greater the assessed risk, the higher levels of intervention and supervision that are required; conversely, the lower the assessed risk, the lower levels of intervention and supervision that are required, regardless of whether the forensic client is seeking treatment within a secure environment, or as a community treatment program (Woods, 2004). Although a detailed discussion of risk assessment and management is beyond the scope of this chapter, it is mentioned here because increasingly forensic nurses, with additional training and experience, are using actuarial (or statistical) and clinical risk assessment tools to formulate treatment plans that increasingly include risk management (Encinares & Golea, 2005; Encinares & Lorbergs, 2001; Encinares, McMaster, & McNamee, 2005).

SOCIETAL NORMS

Humane care is defined by society and subject to changing convictions regarding the worthiness of the forensic client. The very existence and continual expansion of correctional facilities is a striking example of society's failure to address complex health and social issues.

In a recent advocacy campaign, the Canadian Association of Elizabeth Fry Societies declared "Women don't belong in cages: Prisons are the real crime." However, society continues to operate under the misguided belief that imprisonment will not only deter others from committing crimes but also contribute further to community safety. Prime Minister Harper's administration is proposing to "get tough on crime." Unfortunately, this mandate is not about investing in people, nor is it about investing in primary crime prevention strategies. Instead, it is a reinvestment into prisons—society's *answer* to poverty, homelessness, and mental illness. An investment that minimizes the impact of interpersonal violence and illicit drug–related activities on individuals and communities, and ignores the lack of health care services available to vulnerable and marginalized groups. It fails to look at alternative measures for dealing with crime (Peternelj-Taylor, 2005d).

To understand the comprehensive needs of individuals whose lives have become enmeshed within the criminal justice system requires an understanding of the failings of multiple systems designed to keep individuals, families, and communities healthy and safe. Maeve (2003) concludes, "nursing is uniquely positioned to intervene with the socially significant health issues associated with crime, incarceration, and release" (p. 39). In doing so, they must be politically astute in their attempts to affect social change, particularly in light of public animosity regarding individuals who come into conflict

with the law. Most of all, it requires an enduring conviction that caring for forensic clients, as vulnerable members of society, is the appropriate and decent thing to do.

SUMMARY OF KEY POINTS

- The provision of nursing care to individuals who have transgressed the law is a challenging and rewarding psychiatric and mental health nursing experience, one that balances the conflicting convictions of custody and caring.
- Components of care in forensic nursing include the forensic client, nurse–client relationship, professional role development, treatment setting, and societal norms.
- The ability to engage the forensic client in a therapeutic relationship is critical to competent forensic nursing care. Relationship issues experienced by forensic nurses include othering, boundary violations, and manipulation.
- Forensic nurses are uniquely situated to provide nursing care to forensic clients in a variety of community and institution-based treatment settings.
- Intersectoral approaches, which bring together justice, law, social services, education, and health care, are deemed necessary to address the multitude of issues facing forensic clients, their families, and their communities.

CRITICAL THINKING CHALLENGES

1 In recent years, correctional facilities have experienced great challenges in caring for elderly and infirm forensic clients, and on occasion, clients are transferred to community-based long-term care facilities for compassionate reasons. What challenges might accompany the implementation of such a policy?

2 Canada has the dubious honour of incarcerating more youth than any other Western country. What are the implications of this phenomenon for forensic nurses?

3 The ability to engage the forensic client in a therapeutic relationship is a critical competency for forensic nurses. How might nurses overcome their negative reactions to a client who has committed a heinous crime?

4 The nursing profession as a whole has become more attune to the importance of boundaries in the therapeutic relationship. How would you approach a colleague who you suspected was struggling to maintain professional boundaries with a forensic client?

5 Working with forensic populations often brings nurses face to face with many complex health and social issues previously not considered. Given the

fact that each and every forensic nurse is a member of many communities, how might a forensic nurse effect change at the community level?

WEB LINKS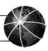

www.ccsd.ca Children and Youth: Crime Prevention Through Social Development, hosted by the Canadian Council on Social Development, explains the theory and practice of crime prevention through social development; highlights current projects in this field, and provides opportunities for people accessing the site to get involved.

www.csc-scc.gc.ca The Correctional Service of Canada (CSC) contributes to the protection of society by actively encouraging and assisting offenders to become law-abiding citizens, while exercising reasonable, safe, secure, and humane control. CSC's website is an excellent resource for current information about corrections in Canada, including policy, legislation, research, and various publications, including *Forum on Corrections Research*.

www.elizabethfry.ca The Canadian Association of Elizabeth Fry Societies (CAEFS) is an association made up of 25 self-governing, community-based Elizabeth Fry Societies from across Canada that work with and for women and girls in the justice system, particularly those who are, or may be, criminalized.

www.forensicnurse.ca The Forensic Nurses' Society is evolving with the intention of becoming an emerging special interest group with the Canadian Nurses Association, and to affiliate with the International Association of Forensic Nurses. The society hopes to provide a network for forensic nurses in Canada and represent the diverse areas of forensic nursing.

www.iafn.org The International Association of Forensic Nurses (IAFN), founded in 1992, brought together a diverse group of nurses whose practice interfaced in someway with the law. In 1995, forensic nursing was officially recognized as a specialty area by the American Nurses Association (ANA) and, in 1997, the IAFN and the ANA published the *Scope and Standards of Forensic Nursing*. In 2005, the IAFN launched the *Journal of Forensic Nursing*, a peer-reviewed publication dedicated to advancing the science of forensic nursing.

www.johnhoward.ca The John Howard Society of Canada is an organization of provincial and territorial Societies composed of, and governed by, people whose goal is to understand and respond to problems of crime and the criminal justice system. Their motto "Effective, just and humane responses to the causes and consequences of crime" is actualized through the organizations' many roles, including advocacy, research, and community education.

www.justice.gc.ca The Department of Justice, Canada, provides a very informative and interactive quiz entitled *Myths and Realities about Youth Justice*. From here, students can also access additional resources regarding the Youth Criminal Justice Act, policies and procedures around diversion, sentencing and reintegration, and current research related to youth and the criminal justice system in Canada.

www.prisonersofage.com Prisoners of Age is a project that features photographs and interviews with elderly inmates and correctional personnel, conducted in Canadian and American prisons since 1996. The poignant photos and interviews provide a glimpse into the lives of aging prisoners, their crimes, and the many challenges they experience.

www.sfu.ca The Centre for Restorative Justice at Simon Fraser University provides a wealth of information (including examples) applicable to forensic nursing and an excellent introduction to this approach to justice, including the values and principles that underpin it.

MOVIES

Dead Man Walking: 1995. This acclaimed film features the relationship between a death-row inmate, Matthew Poncelet (Sean Penn), and a local nun, Sister Helen Prejean (Susan Sarandon), whom he consults with for spiritual guidance in the days before his execution. The viewer experiences Prejean's personal distress as she attempts to reconcile her anti–death penalty views with the truth of Poncelet's brutal crimes and the pain of the victims' families and communities.

VIEWING POINTS: Although capital punishment was abolished in Canada in 1976, the film illustrates the conflicting convictions and dilemmas that nurses often experience when working with clients who have committed reprehensible crimes.

Gothika: 2003. This supernatural thriller features Dr. Miranda Grey (Halle Berry), a respected criminal psychologist, who finds herself a patient on the psychiatric unit of the penitentiary where she practices. Accused of killing her husband, her claims of innocence and loss of memory are seen by her former coworkers as a descent into madness. Although a tagline, "You can't trust someone who thinks you're crazy," held promise for revealing aspects of therapeutic relationships in prison, portrayals of clients and setting are very stereotypical. The movie will no doubt contribute to the public's impression that individuals who are mentally ill are violent.

VIEWING POINTS: How do the nurses and other health care professionals interact with Dr. Grey and the other clients? What static and dynamic security measures are illustrated within the forensic psychiatric unit at Woodward Penitentiary for Women?

The Shawshank Redemption: 1994. This is a thought-provoking movie about prison life in the 1940s. The lead character, Andy Dufresne (Tim Robbins), is wrongfully convicted of killing his wife and her lover and is sentenced to two consecutive life terms. Although the harsh realities of prison culture, including the abuse of power, are brutally portrayed in this film, *The Shawshank Redemption* is really about the human spirit, friendship, and the redeeming nature of hope, as illustrated in the movie's tagline, "Fear can hold you prisoner. Hope can set you free."

VIEWING POINTS: Observe how the concept of institutionalization is illustrated within the movie. How might a forensic nurse use "hope" as an intervention strategy within his or her practice?

REFERENCES

Amellal, D. (2005, Oct.). A diversified correctional approach. *Let's Talk, 30*(2). Retrieved February 20, 2006 from http://www.csc-scc.gc.ca/text/pblct/letstalk/2005/30-2/5_e.shtml.

Appelbaum, K. L., Hickey, J. M., & Packer, I. (2001). The role of correctional officers in multidisciplinary mental health care in prisons. *Psychiatric Services, 52*(10), 1343–1347.

Anno, B. J., Graham, C., Lawrence, J. E., & Shansky, R. (2004). *Correctional health care: Addressing the needs of elderly, chronically ill, and terminally ill inmates* (Accession No. 018735). Washington, DC: National Institute of Corrections.

Aufderheide, D. H., & Brown, P. H. (2005, Feb.). Crisis in corrections: The mentally ill in America's prisons. *Corrections Today,* 30–33.

Austin, W. (2001). Relational ethics in forensic psychiatric settings. *Journal of Psychosocial Nursing and Mental Health Services, 39*(9), 12–17.

Beckett, J., Peternelj-Taylor, C., & Johnson, R. (2003). Growing old in the correctional system. *Journal of Psychosocial Nursing and Mental Health Services, 41*(9), 12–18.

Blanchard, B. (2004). Incarcerated mothers and their children: A complex issue. *Forum on Correctional Research, 16*(1), 45–46.

Canadian Public Health Association. (2004). *A Health Care Needs Assessment of Federal Inmates, 95*(Suppl. 1), S1–S63.

Canales, M. K. (2000). Othering: Toward an understanding of difference. *Advances in Nursing Science, 22*(4), 16–31.

Correctional Services of Canada. (2005, Feb.). *Issues and challenges facing CSC.* Retrieved April 12, 2005, from http://www.csc-scc.gc.ca/text/pblct/guideorateur/6_e.shtml.

de Chesnay, M. (2005). *Caring for the vulnerable: Perspectives in nursing theory, practice and research.* Boston: Jones & Bartlett.

Department of Justice. (2006). *The youth criminal justice act: Summary and background.* Retrieved February 20, 2006, from http://www.justice.gc.ca/en/ps/yj/ycja/explan.html.

Drake, V. K. (1998). Process, perils, and pitfalls of research in prison. *Issues in Mental Health Nursing, 19*, 41–52.

Duggleby, W. (2005). Fostering hope in incarcerated older adults. *Journal of Psychosocial Nursing and Mental Health Services, 43*(9), 15–20.

Encinares, M., & Golea, G. (2005). Client centered-care for individuals with dual diagnoses in the justice system. *Journal of Psychosocial Nursing and Mental Health Services, 43*(9), 29–36.

Encinares, M., & Lorbergs, K. (2001). Framing nursing practice within a forensic outpatient service. *Journal of Psychosocial Nursing and Mental Health Services, 2001, 39*(9), 35–41.

Encinares, M., McMaster, J. J., & McNamee, J. (2005). Risk assessment of forensic patients: Nurses' role. *Journal of Psychosocial Nursing and Mental Health Services, 43*(3), 30–36.

Fowler-Kerry, S. (2003). Palliative care within secure forensic environments. *Journal of Psychiatric and Mental Health Nursing, 10*, 367–369.

Flaskerud, J. H., & Winslow, B. J. (1998). Conceptualizing vulnerable populations health-related research. *Nursing Research, 47*(2), 69–78.

Flaskerud, J. H., Lesser, J., Dixon, E., Anderson, N., Conde, F., Kim, S et al. (2002). Health disparities among vulnerable populations: Evolution of knowledge over five decades in *Nursing Research* publications. *Nursing Research, 51*(2), 74–85.

Frudenberg, N. (2001). Jails, prisons, and the health of urban populations: A review of the impact of the correctional system on community health. *Journal of Urban Health: Bulletin of the New York Academy of Medicine, 78*(2), 214–235.

Gal, M. (2002). The physical and mental health needs of older offenders. *Forum on Corrections Research, 14*(2), 15–19.

Gallagher, E. M. (2001). Elders in prison: Health and well-being of older inmates. *International Journal of Law and Psychiatry, 24*, 325–333.

Goldkuhle, U. (1999). Professional education for correctional nurses: A community-based partnership model. *Journal of Psychosocial Nursing and Mental Health Services, 37*(9), 38–44.

Green, B. L., Miranda, J., Daroowalla, A., & Siddique, J. (2005). Trauma exposure, mental health functioning, and program needs of women in jail. *Crime & Delinquency, 51*, 133–151.

Harner, H. M. (2004). Relationships between incarcerated women: Moving beyond stereotypes. *Journal of Psychosocial Nursing, 42*(1), 38–46.

Harrison, P. M., & Beck, A. J. (2005, April). Prison and jail inmates at midyear 2004 (Report NCJ 208801). *Bureau of Justice Statistics Bulletin,* 1–14. Retrieved May 1, 2005, from http://www.ojp.gov/bjs/pub/pdf/pjim04.pdf/.

Holmes, D. (2005). Governing the captives: Forensic psychiatric nursing in corrections. *Perspectives in Psychiatric Care, 41*(1), 3–13.

Holmes, D., & Federman, C. (2003). Constructing monsters: Correctional discourse and nursing practice. *International Journal of Psychiatric Nursing, 8*(1), 942–962.

Holmes, D., & Federman, C. (2006). Organizations as evil structures. In T. Mason (Ed.), *Forensic psychiatry: Influences of evil* (pp. 15–30). Totowa, NJ: Humana Press.

Hufft, A., & Kite, M. M. (2003). Vulnerable and cultural perspectives for nursing care in correctional systems. *Journal of Multicultural Nursing & Health, 9*(1), 18–26.

Human Rights Watch. (2003). *Ill equipped: U.S. prisons and offenders with mental illness.* New York, NY: Author. Retrieved March 14, 2004, from http://www.hrw.org/reports/2003/usa1003.

Kanapaux, W. (2004). Guilty of mental illness. *Psychiatric Times, XXI* (1). Retrieved October 17, 2005, from http://www.psychiatric-times.com/p040101a.html.

Kent-Wilkinson, A. (1999). Forensic family genogram: An assessment and intervention tool. *Journal of Psychosocial Nursing and Mental Health Services, 37*(9), 52–56.

Kent-Wilkinson, A. (2006). Forensic nursing education: Developments, theoretical conceptualizations, and practical applications for curriculum. In R. M. Hammer, B. Moynihan, & E. M. Pagliaro (Eds.), *Forensic nursing: A handbook for practice* (pp. 781–820). Sudbury, MA: Jones & Bartlett.

Kirmayer, L. J., Brass, G. M., & Tait, C. L. (2000). The mental health of Aboriginal peoples: Transformations of identity and community. *Canadian Journal of Psychiatry, 45*(7), 607–616.

Latimer, J., & Foss, L. C. (2004, Feb.). *A One-Day Snapshot of Aboriginal Youth in Custody Across Canada: Phase II*, Department of Justice Canada. Retrieved February 18, 2006, from http://www.justice.gc.ca/en/ps/rs/rep/2004/snap2/index.html.

Lawson, L. (2005). Furthering the search for truth and justice. *Journal of Forensic Nursing, 1*(4), 149–150.

Maeve, K. M. (2003). Nursing care partnerships with women leaving jail: Effects on health and crime. *Journal of Psychosocial Nursing and Mental Health Services, 41*(9), 30–40.

Maeve, K. M., & Vaughn, M. S. (2001). Nursing with prisoners: The practice of caring, forensic nursing or penal harm nursing? *Advances in Nursing Science, 24*(2), 47–64.

Martin, T. (2001). Something special: Forensic psychiatric nursing. *Journal of Psychiatric and Mental Health Nursing, 8*, 25–32.

Moynihan, B. (2006). Vulnerable populations. In R. M. Hammer, B. Moynihan, & E. M. Pagliaro (Eds.), *Forensic nursing: A handbook for practice* (pp. 217–231). Sudbury, MA: Jones & Bartlett.

Office of the Correctional Investigator. (2005). *Annual report of the Correctional Investigator 2004–2005.* Retrieved December 15, 2005, from http://www.oci-bec.gc.ca/reports/AR200405_download_e.asp.

Osborne, O. (1995). Public sector psychosocial nursing. *Journal of Psychosocial Nursing and Mental Health Services, 33*(8), 4–6.

Peternelj-Taylor, C. (2000). The role of the forensic nurse in Canada: An evolving specialty. In D. Robinson & A. Kettles (Eds.), *Forensic nursing and multidisciplinary care of the mentally disordered offender* (pp. 192–212). London: Jessica Kingsley Publishers.

Peternelj-Taylor, C. (2002). Professional boundaries: A matter of therapeutic integrity. *Journal of Psychosocial Nursing and Mental Health Services, 40*(4), 22–29.

Peternelj-Taylor, C. (2003). Incarceration of vulnerable populations. (2003). *Journal of Psychosocial Nursing and Mental Health Services, 41*(9), 4–5.

Peternelj-Taylor, C., & Yonge, O. (2003). Exploring boundaries in the nurse-client relationship: Professional roles and responsibilities. *Perspectives in Psychiatric Care, 39*(2), 55–66.

Peternelj-Taylor, C. (2004). An exploration of othering in forensic psychiatric and correctional nursing. *Canadian Journal of Nursing Research, 36*(4), 130–146.

Peternelj-Taylor, C. (2005a). Conceptualizing nursing research with offenders: Another look at vulnerability. *International Journal of Law and Psychiatry, 28*, 348–359.

Peternelj-Taylor, C. (2005b). Engaging the "other." *Journal of Forensic Nursing, 1*(4), 179, 191.

Peternelj-Taylor, C. (2005c). Mental health promotion in forensic and correctional environments. *Journal of Psychosocial Nursing and Mental Health Services, 43*(9), 8–9.

Peternelj-Taylor, C. (2005d). "Ordinary" women, extraordinary life circumstances. *Journal of Forensic Nursing, 1*(2), 84–85.

Peternelj-Taylor, C. A., & Hufft, A. G. (2006). Forensic nursing. In W. K. Mohr (Ed.), *Psychiatric-mental health nursing* (6th ed., pp. 377–393). Philadelphia: Lippincott Williams & Wilkins.

Peternelj-Taylor, C. & Johnson, R. (1995). Serving time: Psychiatric mental health nursing in corrections. *Journal of Psychosocial Nursing and Mental Health Services, 33*(8), 12–19.

Petryshen, P. (1981). Nursing the mentally disordered offender. *Canadian Nurse, 77*(6), 26–28.

Phillips, R. T. M., & Caplan, C. (2003). Administrative and staffing problems for psychiatric services in correctional and forensic settings. In R. Rosner (Ed.), *Principles and practice of forensic psychiatry* (2nd ed., pp. 505–512). New York: Chapman & Hall.

Pilette, P. C., Berck, C. B., & Achber, L. C. (1995). Therapeutic management of helping boundaries. *Journal of Psychosocial Nursing and Mental Health Services, 33*(1), 40–47.

Pullan, S. E., & Lorbergs, K. A. (2001). Recruitment and retention: A successful model in forensic psychiatric nursing. *Journal of Psychosocial Nursing and Mental Health Services, 39*(9), 18–25.

Registered Nurses Association of Ontario. (2002). *Establishing therapeutic relationships.* Toronto: Author. Retrieved October 12, 2004, from http://www.rnao.org/bestpractices/completed_guidelines/BPG_Guide_C2_TR.asp.

Rose, D. (2005). Respect for patient autonomy. *Journal of Forensic Nursing, 1*(1), 23–27.

Roth, B., & Pressé, L. (2003). Nursing interventions for parasuicidal behaviors in female offenders. *Journal of Psychosocial Nursing and Mental Health Services, 41*(9), 20–29.

Schafer, P. E. (2002). Nursing interventions and future directions with patients who constantly *break rules and test boundaries.* In A. M. Kettles, P. Woods & M. Collins (Eds.), *Therapeutic interventions for forensic mental health nurses* (pp. 56–71). London: Jessica Kingsley Publishers.

Schafer, P. E., & Peternelj-Taylor, C. (2003). Therapeutic relationships and boundary maintenance: The perspective of forensic patients enrolled in a treatment program for violent offenders. *Issues in Mental Health Nursing, 24*, 605–625.

Sealy, P., & Whitehead, P. C. (2004). Forty years of deinstitutionalization of psychiatric services in Canada: An empirical assessment. *Canadian Journal of Psychiatry, 49*(4), 249–257.

Shelton, D. (2000). Health status of young offenders and their families. *Journal of Nursing Scholarship, 32*(2), 173–178.

Shelton, D. (2001). Emotional disorders in young offenders. *Journal of Nursing Scholarship, 33*(3), 259–263.

Shelton, D. (2004). Experiences of detained young offenders in need of mental health care. *Journal of Nursing Scholarship, 36*(2), 129–133.

Shelton, D., & Pearson, G. (2005). ADHD in juvenile offenders: Treatment issues nurses need to know. *Journal of Psychosocial Nursing and Mental Health Services, 43*(9), 38–46.

Smith, S. (2005, Feb.). Stepping through the looking glass: Professional autonomy in correctional nursing. *Corrections Today,* 54–56, 70.

Statistics Canada. (2003). *Special study on mentally disordered accused and the criminal justice system.* Canadian Centre for Justice Studies (no. 85-559-XIE). Ottawa: Ministry of Industry. Retrieved December 1, 2005, from http://www.statcan.ca/english/freepub/85-559-XIE/85-559-XIE2002001.pdf.

Woods, P. (2004). The person who uses forensic mental health services. In I. Norman & I. Ryrie (Eds.), *The art and science of mental health nursing: A textbook of principles and practice* (pp. 594–623). Maidenhead, UK: Open University Press.

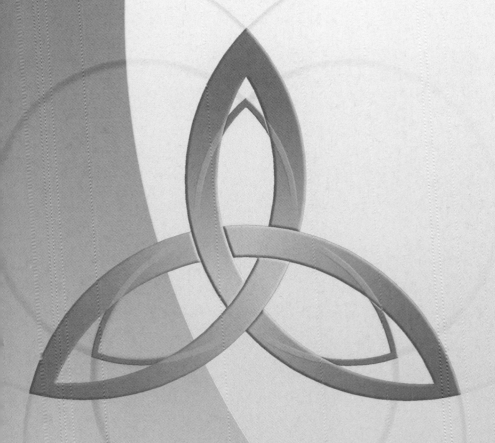

VIII

Care Challenges in Psychiatric and Mental Health Nursing

Stress, Crisis, and Disaster Management

Gerri Lasiuk, Lorraine D. Williams,
and Mary Ann Boyd

LEARNING OBJECTIVES

After studying this chapter, you will be able to:

- Discuss the conceptualization of stress as a response, as a stimulus, and as a transaction.
- Use the stress, coping, and adaptation model presented in this chapter to assess individuals' stress and coping abilities.
- Differentiate problem-focussed and emotion-focussed coping.
- Discuss the relationship between stress and adaptation.
- Define stress, crisis, and disaster; compare and contrast each of these to a psychiatric emergency.

KEY TERMS

- allostasis ▪ allostatic load ▪ bereavement ▪ cognitive appraisal ▪ constraints ▪ demands ▪ dissupport ▪ emotion-focussed coping ▪ emotions ▪ grief ▪ homeostasis ▪ mourning ▪ problem-focussed coping ▪ reappraisal ▪ social functioning ▪ social network ▪ social support ▪ stressor ▪ stress-diathesis model

KEY CONCEPTS

- adaptation ▪ coping ▪ crisis ▪ disaster ▪ person–environment relationship ▪ stress

Although *stress* has been the focus of considerable scientific, clinical, and general interest over the past century, most of us would be hard pressed to explain what it is. As Hans Selye phrased it, "stress, like relativity, is a scientific concept which has suffered the mixed blessing of being too well known, and too little understood" (1980, p. 127). This chapter explores the concepts of stress, crisis, and disaster and describes how nurses can use the nursing process to identify and address needs of persons experiencing these events.

STRESS

Conceptualizations of Stress

The word *stress* has its roots in the Latin word *strictus*, meaning tight or narrow, and the Middle English word *stresse*, which refers to hardship or distress (Harper, 2001). Although this latter definition carries forward into our current everyday language, in research and clinical realms, the word stress has specific meanings. In the literature, stress is conceptualized as (1) a response, (2) a stimulus, and (3) a transaction (Semmer, McGrath, & Beehr, 2005). These different ways of thinking about stress reflect our evolving understanding of this complex phenomenon.

Stress as a Response

Walter Cannon and Hans Selye, two pioneers in the study of stress, both conceptualized stress as a response to changing environmental conditions. Cannon, a noted Harvard physiologist, is considered by many to be the father of modern stress research. In his book *The Wisdom of the Body* (1939), he coined the term **homeostasis** to describe the body's ability to maintain a stable internal environment despite changing environmental conditions. His thesis was that environmental changes are perceived as threats to personal integrity or safety and signal a compensatory response mediated by the sympathetic branch of the autonomic nervous system (ANS). He also believed that strong emotions like fear and anger are fundamental to the stress response and that they have evolved because of their high survival value. "Fear" he wrote, "has become associated with the instinct to run, to escape; and anger or aggressive feeling, with the instinct to attack" (p. 227). This notion, later dubbed the *fight or flight* response, remains a key concept in any discussion of stress.

Working at McGill University in Montreal, Hans Selye (1956, 1974) developed his general adaptation syndrome (GAS). Selye differentiated *stress* (a nonspecific response of the body to any demand placed on it) from *stressors* (events that initiate the response) and argued that stressors can be physical (eg, infection, intense heat or cold, surgery, debilitating illnesses), psychological (eg, psychological trauma, interpersonal

problems), or social (eg, lack of social support). They can also be short-term (acute) or long-term (chronic). According to Selye, the perception of a stressor triggers an automatic, total-body response. The first stage of this response is the *alarm reaction*, during which virtually all body systems (eg, sense organs, brain, heart and blood vessels, lungs, digestive system, immune system) respond into a coordinated effort to deal with the stressor. If these efforts are successful, the body returns to its normal state. If, on the other hand, the stressor continues for hours or days, the organism moves into the *stage of resistance*, and efforts to adapt to the stressor continue. In circumstances in which the stressor is ongoing or extreme, the body moves into the *stage of exhaustion*. In this final stage, the individual's resources deplete, and exhaustion and death ensue. Selye hypothesized that many diseases, including hypertension, peptic ulcer, and autoimmune illnesses, are caused by prolonged adaptive reactions in which corticosteroids play a pathogenic role.

Although there is no doubt that Selye made significant contributions to our understanding of the human stress experience, new research refutes the idea of a nonspecific response to diverse environmental stimuli. Those who challenge Selye's theory point out that many neuroendocrine responses are not general at all, but very specific. They further argue that all stressors do not necessarily produce the same response in every individual; what is a stressor for one person may not be a stressor for another (Lazarus & Folkman, 1984). The conceptualization of stress solely as a response is also criticized for its circular reasoning (ie, an event is stressful because it elicits a stress response).

Stress as a Stimulus

Those who conceptualize stress as a stimulus (eg, Dohrenwend & Dohrenwend, 1974; Holmes & Rahe, 1967) view it as an event that elicits a stress response (however that is defined). In this approach to understanding stress, researchers looked for associations between significant life events (eg, marriage, divorce, relocation, death) and stress. One of the most widely used tools in this type of research is the Recent Life Changes Questionnaire (RLCQ; Holmes & Rahe, 1967), which appears in Table 34-1. A major problem with conceptualizing stress in this manner is that it can only be identified in retrospect, that is, only after a response occurs. Other criticisms include the failure of its proponents to discriminate between the effects of positive and negative events and to address the effects of chronic or recurrent events (see Jones & Kinman, 2001, for a full discussion).

The mid-1970s to the early 1990s was a critical period in stress research. During this time, a debate raged in the literature between two camps of stress researchers. One camp favoured the view that critical life events (ie, the presence of an objective event) mediate the experience of

Table 34.1   Recent Life Changes Questionnaire

Social Area	Life Changes	LCU Values*
Family	Death of spouse	105
	Marital separation	65
	Death of close family member	65
	Divorce	62
	Pregnancy	60
	Change in health of family member	52
	Marriage	50
	Gain of new family member	50
	Marital reconciliation	42
	Spouse begins or stops work	37
	Son or daughter leaving home	29
	In-law trouble	29
	Change in number of family get-togethers	26
Personal	Jail term	56
	Sex difficulties	49
	Death of a close friend	46
	Personal injury or illness	42
	Change in living conditions	39
	Outstanding personal achievement	33
	Change in residence	33
	Minor violations of the law	32
	Begin or end school	32
	Change in sleeping habits	31
	Revision of personal habits	31
	Change in eating habits	29
	Change in church activities	29
	Vacation	29
	Change in school	28
	Change in recreation	28
	Christmas	26
Work	Fired at work	64
	Retirement from work	49
	Trouble with boss	39
	Business readjustment	38
	Change to different line of work	38
	Change in work responsibilities	33
	Change in work hours or conditions	30
Financial	Foreclosure of mortgage or loan	57
	Change in financial state	43
	Mortgage (home, car, etc)	39
	Mortgage or loan less than $10,000 (stereo, etc)	26

Directions: Sum the LCUs for your life change events during the past 12 months.
  250 and 400 LCUs per year: Minor life crisis
  Over to LCUs per year: Major life crisis
*LCU, Life change unit. The number of LCUs reflects the average degree or intensity of the life change.
(From Rahe, R. H. [2000]. Recent Life Changes Questionnaire [RLCQ] [1997]. Holmes, T. H. In American Psychiatric Association. Task Force for the Handbook of Psychiatric Measures. *Handbook of psychiatric measures.* Washington, DC: American Psychiatric Association, pp. 235–237)

stress. Supporters of this view "urged researchers to measure pure events, uncontaminated by perceptions, appraisals, or reactions" (Dohrenwend & Shrout, 1985, p. 782). On the other side of the argument, Richard Lazarus and his colleagues (Lazarus, DeLongis, Folkman, & Gruen, 1985) maintained that it is the appraisal of an event (ie, the subjective evaluation of an event or situation) that is critical to the stress experience. Although the debate centred on measurement and other methodologic problems, Lazarus (1999) contends that

the real issue was the fundamental nature of stress and the person–environment relationship. In the end, the latter group prevailed, and the view of stress as a transaction has became the dominant explanatory model.

Stress as a Transaction

In their seminal work, *Appraisal and Coping,* Lazarus and Folkman (1984) conceptualize stress as a transaction or relationship between the person and the environment that is appraised by the person as taxing or exceeding their resources and threatening well-being. The central premise here is that **stress** is "neither an environmental stimulus, a characteristic of the person, nor a response, but a relationship between demands and the power to deal with them without unreasonable or destructive costs" (Coyne & Holroyd, 1982, p. 108).

> **⬢ KEY CONCEPT** Stress is the relationship between the person and the environment that is appraised as exceeding the person's resources and endangering his or her well-being.

This view of stress is consistent with the notion of **allostasis**. The word allostasis, which literally means *maintaining stability through change*, was coined by Sterling and Eyer (1988) to describe how the cardiovascular system adjusts to resting and active states of the body. Allostasis is a useful concept for understanding the relationship of the body's normal rhythms to changing environmental conditions. For example, the hypothalamus regulates the sleep and wakefulness and the production of adrenocortical hormones in response to the light–dark cycle. Alterations in the light–dark cycle related to air travel result in dysregulation of adrenocortical hormone and contribute to disruption of sleep, activity, appetite, and cognitive function. Another example is the perception of immediate danger, which triggers the release of both adrenalin and adrenocortical hormones necessary to mount a defencive response (ie, fight or flight). The perception of an experience as stressful triggers physiologic and behavioural responses that lead to allostasis and adaptation. Over time, allostatic load accumulates, and chronic overexposure to neural, endocrine, and immune stress mediators can have adverse effects on various organ systems, resulting in disease.

The term **allostatic load** (McEwen, 1998) refers to the cumulative negative effects on the body of continually having to adapt to changing environmental conditions and psychosocial challenges. It is mediated both by the efficiency of the body's response and the number of stressors an individual experiences. Allostatic load is more than "chronic stress"; it involves genetics and early development, as well as learned behaviours reflecting lifestyle choices of diet, exercise, smoking, and alcohol consumption. Allostatic load is the sum total of "wear and tear" on the body that accumulates as the result of maintaining normal body rhythms in the face of changing environmental conditions, managing the normal challenges of daily life, and maintaining the adverse physiologic consequences of harmful lifestyle choices (eg, fat-rich diet, excessive alcohol, or smoking).

Person–Environment Relationship

The **person–environment relationship** is defined here as the dynamic interaction between a person and his or her environment. It assumes that an individual brings to every event or situation a set of values and beliefs that he or she develops over a lifetime under the influence of genetic, personal, social, and environmental factors. These contribute to one's worldview, which shapes the meaning and significance of a particular situation. What is important to one individual may not be for another; as an example, one may value a college education, whereas another may value living with neighbours in a small, isolated community.

Values and Commitment

When an individual values a particular outcome, he or she will be more committed to activities that foster that outcome. Commitment to a particular goal is an important factor in the stress response, as the following example illustrates. Students who earn As generally experience more exam stress than do students who earn Bs and Cs. Before they write an exam, "A students" often express the fear that they will fail and are devastated when they earn Bs or Cs. Although it seems paradoxical that students who consistently earn higher grades are more stressed than those who perform less well, the test-taking situation is actually more threatening to the better students because they place a higher value on academic achievement than do the other students.

Personality and Behaviour Patterns

As well as values, beliefs, and goals, individuals have characteristic patterns of response to similar situations. These attitudes and behaviours develop over time and become almost reflexive. For example, the timid preschool-aged child who refuses to attend nursery school often fears going to kindergarten and may later have difficulty leaving home for college.

In the mid-1970s, cardiologists Meyer Friedman and Ray Rosenman observed an association between what they called *type A* personality characteristics and the development of cardiovascular disease (Friedman & Rosenman, 1974). The type A personality is typically competitive, aggressive, ambitious, and impatient. Alert, tense, and restless, these individuals think, speak, and act quickly. They also tend to be aggressive, hostile, and have a sense of time urgency that keeps them in a chronic state of physiologic arousal. These individuals have a high need to control events around them and are frustrated when they are unsuccessful in doing so. In contrast, individuals with *type B* personality characteristics are more relaxed, easy-going, and content. They take minor irritations in their stride and approach challenges as problems to be solved. Individuals who exhibit type B characteristics move through life at a comfortable pace and have realistic expectations of what they can achieve in a given period.

Although early research seemed to support a link between type A personality characteristics and atherosclerosis leading to coronary heart disease (CHD), later research did not bear this out. There were failures to replicate earlier findings and even negative results. For example, Dimsdale (1988) reported lower post–myocardial infarction mortality rate among individuals with type A characteristics than those with type B characteristics. Logan Wright's (1988) research later identified five factors that contribute to CHD: inherited risk; risks associated with lifestyle choices (eg, smoking, overeating); anger directed inward; anger directed outward (ie, time urgency and chronic autonomic arousal), and classic type A characteristics. The current consensus seems to be that although the type A trait cluster has some heuristic value, chronic negative emotions are probably the most significant predictors of CHD.

Other research examining the relationship of personality and stress focusses on *hardiness*, a cluster of personality traits that buffer or moderate the effects of stress (Kobasa, 1979). In her study of a large group of individuals undergoing the same stressful event, Kobasa identified three factors that separated those who became ill from those who did not. These factors are control, commitment, and expectancy of change. Individuals who have some sense of being able to control events in their life, who are committed to something (eg, values, their goals, other people), and who view change as a part of life are less likely to become ill than individuals who do not demonstrate these things. It should be noted here that Kobasa's notion of control as conferring protection against stress relates closely to Julian Rotter's (1966) concept of internal locus of control. Rotter, a social learning theorist, proposed that there are two dimensions of locus of control—internal and external. Individuals within an internal locus of control believe that they can influence the outcome of events in the world. They accept that they are responsible for their behaviour, appraise situations rationally, and choose a course of action that will have favourable consequences. In contrast, individuals who have an external locus of control believe that their fate is under the control of some external agent (eg, fate, luck, authority figures). The latter tend to be passive and do not see themselves as having the agency to affect desired outcomes. Not surprisingly, individuals with an internal locus of control perceive stressful events differently than those who have an external locus of control. These individuals perceive situations less catastrophically and assess their coping resources as being more effective. As we shall see later, a person's appraisal of a situation and of his or her coping abilities directly influences the experience of stress.

Interaction With Environment

The external environment is everything outside of the person, including physical surroundings and social interactions. Crowding, temperature, and noise are all aspects of the physical environment, as is exposure to hazardous material in the soil, air, and water (Matthies, Höger, & Guski, 2000). Social aspects of the environment include living arrangements and interpersonal relationships.

Social Networks. People live within a **social network** consisting of relationships among a defined set of people with whom they have regular face-to-face contact (Clegg, 2001). An individual develops and maintains their social identity and acquires emotional support, material aid, services, information, and new social contacts through their relationships with others (Majer, Jason, Ferrarie, Venable, & Olson, 2002). One's social network can increase resources, enhance the ability to cope with change, and influence the course of illness (Jones & Johnston, 2000).

Contacts within a social network are categorized into three levels:

1. *Level I*—6 to 12 people with whom the person has intimate contact (eg, one's closest family and friends)
2. *Level II*—30 to 40 people whom the person sees regularly (eg, more distant family and friends, neighbours, and coworkers)
3. *Level III*—the several hundred people with whom an individual has direct contact, but incidental contact in the course of their day-to-day life (eg, acquaintances, the grocer, mail carrier)

The various levels of an individual's social network may intersect each other; for example, a close friend or sister may also be a close confidant and a workout buddy. The larger the network is, the more support that is available to the person. An ideal network is dense and interconnected so that individuals within the network are also in contact with one another. Dense networks are better able to respond in times of stress and crisis and to provide emotional support to a person in distress.

Intensity and reciprocity are two concepts important to understanding social networks. *Intensity* is the degree or closeness of a relationship. Some relationships are naturally more intense than others are, and ideally, an individual's social network reflects a balance between intense and less intense relationships. Intense relationships can restrict a person's opportunity to interact with other network members, but without at least a few intense relationships, a person lacks intimacy. *Reciprocity* is the extent to which there is balanced give and take in a relationship. Network members provide and receive support, aid, services, and information from each other; sometimes members are on the giving side; at other times, they receive. Reciprocity represents a necessary equilibrium between the two states.

Social Support. One of the important functions of the social network is to provide **social support**, the positive and harmonious interpersonal interactions that occur in social relationships. It is important to keep in mind that

Table 34.2	Examples of Functions of Social Support
Function	**Example**
Emotional support	Attachment, reassurance, being able to rely on and confide in a person
Tangible support	Direct aid such as loans or gifts, services such as taking care of someone who is ill, doing a job or chore
Informational support	Providing information or advice, and giving feedback about how a person is doing

From Schaefer, C., Coyne, J., & Lazarus, R. (1982). The health-related functions of social support. *Journal of Behavioral Medicine, 44,* 381–406.

social support is a dynamic process that occurs within the structure of a social network. Social support serves three functions:

1. Emotional support, which fosters an individual's sense of being loved and cared for
2. Tangible support, which translates into additional resources
3. Informational support, which helps a person view situations in a new light (Table 34-2)

There is a growing body of empirical evidence demonstrating that social support enhances health and reduces mortality. It also helps people make needed behaviour changes. Through social support, individuals feel helped, valued, and in personal control, which in turn reduces physiologic arousal and strengthens the immune system. Directly and indirectly, social support buffers stressful life events in two ways: (1) during stressful events, network members collect and analyze information, offer guidance, and help the person under stress interpret the world; and (2) by treating the person under stress as a unique, special human being, members of the social network provide comfort and a sanctuary or place of refuge (Roberts, 2000).

Individuals who are relatively healthy are more likely to have stronger support systems and are able to respond effectively to negative life events than are those who are ill. As well, some life events, such as marriage, divorce, and bereavement, actually change the level of social support by adding to or subtracting from a person's social network. For example, when a person loses a spouse who was also their main source of support, the stress is greater because their loss is compounded. Social support then, is a dynamic process that is in constant flux and varies with life events and health status (Yeager & Roberts, 2003). Not all interpersonal interactions within a network are supportive; an individual can have a large, complex social network but little social support.

The concept of **dissupport** derives from the observation that some relationships can be harmful, stressful, and even damaging to an individual's self-esteem. Social dissupport is the opposite of social support, and refers to relationships that hinder growth, are emotionally destructive, and deplete resources. Even more complex are those relationships that are both supportive and dissupportive, such as those that provide tangible support (eg, money) but that are emotionally destructive at the same time. The following behaviours are examples of social dissupport (adapted from Malone, 1988):

- Verbal, physical, or emotional abuse
- Discounting an individual, his or her opinions, behaviours, or values
- Discouraging an individual from openly expressing his or her feelings
- Withholding advice or blocking a person's access to useful information
- Consuming an individual's material resources

Demands and Constraints. Within the social network are external and internal demands and personal and environmental constraints. The physical environment imposes external demands, such as crowding, crime, noise, and pollution, whereas the social environment imposes others, such as behavioural and role expectations. Internal **demands** include physical and psychological needs and wants. **Constraints**, on the other hand, are limitations that are both personal and environmental. Personal constraints include internalized cultural values and beliefs that dictate actions or feelings and psychological deficits that are products of the person's unique development. Environmental constraints are finite resources, such as money and time, that are available to people.

Demands and constraints are unique to the individual and contribute to the experience of stress (Lazarus, 2001). They also interact with one another; for example, work demands, such as shift work, may interact with physical demands, such as a need for sleep, which in turn exacerbates stress. Caregivers are particularly burdened by excessive demands and constraints because the ill person's needs take priority over their own. Without additional resources, the caregiver is prone to chronic stress and even burnout.

Sociocultural Factors. Cultural expectations and role strain serve as demands, constraints, or both in the experience of stress. Stress may result when a person violates cultural group values to meet role expectations—for example, the woman who stays in an abusive relationship to avoid the stress associated with violating the cultural norm of lifelong marriage, no matter what the circumstances. The shame and guilt associated with norm violation and the anticipated isolation from being ostracized can seem worse than the physical and psychological pain of the abusive situation.

The social, psychological, and financial benefits associated with employment are highly valued by many cultures. In all cultures, work is assigned significance beyond economic compensation. It is often the central focus of adulthood, and for many, it contributes to personal identity, financial resources, and social status. As well, it structures and regulates time, provides opportunity for interacting with others, and may be a source of personal satisfaction. Even though work is demanding, unemployment can actually be more stressful because of the associated isolation and loss of social status and income.

Gender expectations can be a source of demands and constraints for women, who perform multiple roles. In most cultures, women who work outside the home remain primarily responsible for child care and household maintenance. Some are adept at separating these roles and compartmentalizing problems at work from those at home. When there is a healthy balance between work and home, women experience a low level of psychological stress. However, when the balance is disturbed, daily stressors contribute to health problems (Stuart & Garrison, 2002).

Appraisal

Appraisal involves judging the quality or value of something. Lazarus (2001) uses the term **cognitive appraisal** to describe the process of examining the demands and constraints of a situation or event in relation to one's personal resources. According to Lazarus, cognitive appraisal has two levels: primary and secondary. During **primary appraisal,** the person determines whether an event or situation has relevance for them. In essence, they consider what they have at stake in a particular situation, which directly influences the quality and intensity of their emotional response. In **secondary appraisal,** the individual asks, "What are my options for dealing with this situation?" Within this frame, stress is the perception of threat or harm (primary appraisal) for which an individual has no effective response (secondary appraisal). It is influenced, not by a single stressor, but by a person–environment relationship that is appraised by the individual as both meaningful and threatening to life, integrity, or well-being. The person's commitment to a particular outcome affects their stress response in that the more committed they are to a goal, the greater their vulnerability to stress.

Stress Responses

The perception of a threat triggers an automatic, total-body response. Structures in the brain receive and integrate simultaneous inputs from a number of sources and coordinate a series of physiologic and behavioural responses that enhance an individual's chances of survival.

CRNE Note

Because stress and coping contribute significantly to health-illness, they are relevant to all individuals, not just those diagnosed with mental illnesses. Nursing assessment should focus on the client's appraisal of the stressful event. Understanding a person's beliefs, values, commitment, and typical response patterns will help the nurse identify and support effective coping skills.

Physiologic Responses

The physiologic response to stress initiates in the central nervous system (CNS) but quickly involves all body systems, as Table 34-3 illustrates. CNS structures important to the stress response are the hypothalamus, the anterior and posterior pituitary glands, the brain stem, and the spinal cord (Kindlen, 2003). The hypothalamus is responsible for maintaining the body's internal environment and for mounting a response in the face of a threat. It orchestrates these functions through dense neural connections with the posterior pituitary gland, brain stem, and spinal cord and through its endocrine links with the anterior pituitary gland. The hypothalamus responds to the perception of danger by activating the sympathetic branch of the ANS, which mediates vigilance, arousal, activation, and mobilization (Sapolsky, 2004, p. 22; Fig. 34-1). It also secretes corticotropin-releasing hormone (CRH) to signal the anterior pituitary gland to release adrenocorticotropic hormone (ACTH), which stimulates the adrenal medulla to secrete catecholamines. Also through CRH, the hypothalamus excites firing of the locus coeruleus (LC) in the brain stem to increase norepinephrine in the CNS. The hypothalamus also synthesizes arginine vasopressin or antidiuretic hormone (AVP/ADH), which is released by the posterior pituitary gland; AVP/ADH acts to increase blood pressure by causing vasoconstriction and water retention.

The activities of the hypothalamic–pituitary–adrenocortical (HPA) axis and the sympathic-adrenal medullary system operate within different time periods to provide the body with a wide range of defencive responses. Because the neural response of the ANS is instantaneous, it is the body's first line of defence against stressors. The release of AVP/ADH and catecholamines is slightly slower and augments ANS effects. In the short term, these responses mobilize energy reserves (mainly in the form of glucose) and prepare the body to deal with the stressor by running away or fighting it off. If the stressor is prolonged, the body must make longer-term metabolic adjustments that ensure a sufficient supply of energy. Through the release of growth hormone–releasing hormone (GH-RH) and CRH, the hypothalamus stimulates the release of growth hormone (GH) and ACTH from the anterior

Table 34.3	Effects of Sympathetic Nervous System Arousal		
Organ	**Effect of Sympathetic Stimulation**	**Organ**	**Effect of Sympathetic Stimulation**
Eye		Kidney	Decreased output and renin secretion
Pupil	Dilated		
Ciliary muscle	Slight relaxation (far vision)	Bladder	
Glands	Vasoconstriction and slight secretion	Detrusor	Relaxed (slight)
Nasal		Trigone	Contracted
Lacrimal		Penis	Ejaculation
Parotid		Systemic arterioles	
Submandibular		Abdominal viscera	Constricted
Gastric		Muscle	Constricted (adrenergic α)
Pancreatic			Dilated (adrenergic β_2)
Sweat glands	Copious sweating		Dilated (cholinergic)
Apocrine glands	Thick, odoriferous secretions	Skin	Constricted
Heart		Blood	
Muscle	Increased rate	Coagulation	Increased
	Increased force of contraction	Glucose	Increased
		Lipids	Increased
Coronaries	Dilated (β_2); constricted (α)	Basal metabolism	Increased up to 100%
Lungs		Adrenal medullary secretion	Increased
Bronchi	Dilated	Mental activity	Increased
Blood vessels	Mildly constricted	Piloerector muscles	Contracted
Gut			Increased glycogenolysis
Lumen	Decreased peristalsis and tone	Skeletal muscle	Increased strength
Sphincter	Increased tone (most times)	Fat cells	Lipolysis
Liver	Glucose released		
Gallbladder and bile ducts	Relaxed		

From Guyton, A. C., & Hall, J. E. (2000). *Textbook of medical physiology* (10th ed.) (p. 775). Philadelphia: WB Saunders.

pituitary and the secretion of glucocorticoids (eg, cortisol) from the adrenal cortex. Cortisol is essential to the body's sustained stress response because it mobilizes lipid stores and skeletal protein for energy, which allows the conservation of glucose energy for neural tissue. It also acts on the liver to elevate and stabilize blood glucose levels through gluconeogenesis and lipolysis. As well as having these metabolic effects, cortisol is an anti-inflammatory. By reducing the dilation and permeability of blood vessels that is part of the inflammatory response, cortisol aids in the maintenance of blood pressure and minimizes fluid loss to the tissue. At the same time, chronically elevated cortisol prolongs healing and leaves the body vulnerable to infection.

Emotional Responses

The association between emotion and cognition is a controversial topic. One group of researchers and clinicians take the position that emotions are primary and influence the form and content of cognition. Others believe that cognition is primary and gives rise to emotion. Consistent with his transactional conceptualization of stress, Lazarus (1991) takes a more integrative approach. He contends that cognition and emotion are essentially simultaneous and interdependent, linked in an ongoing flow of negotiation related to environmental stimuli. This leads him and his colleagues to define **emotion** as "complex, organized psychophysiological reactions consisting of cognitive appraisals, action impulses, and patterned somatic reactions" (cited in Folkman & Lazarus, 1991, p. 209). Table 34-4 outlines what Lazarus (1999) calls the stages of emotion.

Cognitive appraisal is fundamental to the experience of emotion because it colours the meaning of a situation or event. Based on their research, Lazarus and his colleagues suggest that there are core relational themes associated with each emotion. See Table 34-5 for a summary of this work. Anxiety, for example, is typically associated with uncertainty or a nonspecific threat, whereas happiness reflects an appraisal of the person–environment condition that is beneficial. Patterned somatic reactions are the individual's own unique experience of the physiologic changes associated with an emotion. For one person, a rush of energy is the salient feature of anger, whereas for another person, it is trembling and a feeling of weakness. These physical reactions motivate or inhibit action impulses. For example, the person who feels energized may attack an aggressor, whereas the person who experiences trembling and weakness is likely to withdraw.

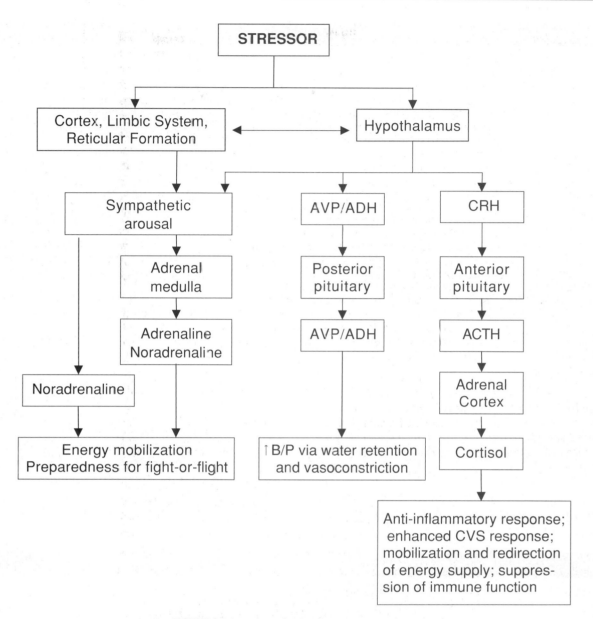

FIGURE 34.1   Physiologic responses to stress.

Coping

According to Lazarus (1998), the following three principles are vital to an understanding of coping: (1) it continually changes over the course of an encounter; (2) it must be assessed independently of its outcomes; and (3) it consists of what an individual thinks and does in response to the perceived demands of a situation. With those principles in mind, Lazarus defines **coping** as "constantly changing cognitive and behavioural efforts to manage specific external and/or internal demands that are appraised as taxing or exceeding the resources of the person" (p. 201). The individual's efforts to cope reflect his or her continuous appraisals and reappraisals of the person–environment relationship in light of changing conditions and the effects of their coping efforts. The individual who appraises his or her coping responses as effective is likely to feel competent and to repeat those same coping responses in the future. Conversely, if the individual appraises his or her coping efforts as ineffective, the individual will probably feel helpless and overwhelmed. Positive coping leads to adaptation, characterized by well-being, and maximum social functioning. The inability to cope leads to maladaptation and illness, a diminished self-concept, and deterioration in social functioning. These ideas are captured in the stress, coping, and adaptation model presented in Figure 34-2.

Table 34.4	Stages of Emotion	
Stages	**Definition**	**Example**
Anticipation	A change in the person–environment relationship, warning of an upcoming harm or benefit. Expectations are created about the outcome that can exacerbate the emotion. Positive expectations increase the likelihood of disappointment; negative expectations can make a negative outcome seem positive.	A person anticipates a promotion because of the boss's increased attention. Instead, the person is reprimanded for unsatisfactory work. He is extremely disappointed. *Or* a person buys a lottery ticket and does not expect to win. When the person does not win, she shrugs and says that buying the ticket was fun.
Provocation	Any occurrence in the environment or within a person that is judged as having changed the person–environment relationship in the direction of harm or benefit.	An unexpected relative arrives at an inopportune time.
Unfolding	Flow of emotion within an encounter. It usually involves an interaction with another, who in turn is provoked and reacts emotionally.	A jealous husband accuses his wife of infidelity. She in turn becomes angry at her husband.
Outcome	An emotional state that reflects an appraisal of what has happened as it relates to a person's well-being.	A wife is very sad after a violent argument with her husband.

Adapted from Lazarus, R. S. (1999). *Stress and emotion: A new synthesis.* New York: Springer.

KEY CONCEPT Coping is an individual's constantly changing cognitive and behavioural efforts to manage specific external or internal demands that are appraised as taxing or exceeding the individual's resources.

There are two types of coping: problem focussed, which actually changes some element of the person–environment relationship; and emotion focussed, which changes the meaning of the situation. In **problem-focussed coping**, the person responds to a stressor by eliminating or altering the event or situation that is causing it (eg, the student who reduces their exam anxiety by studying). In **emotion-focussed coping**, the individual reduces stress by diverting his or her attention away from the situation or by changing the meaning the individual

Table 34.5	Core Relational Themes for Each Emotion
Emotion	**Relational Meaning**
Anger	A demeaning offense against me and mine
Anxiety	Facing an uncertain, existential threat
Fright	Facing an immediate, concrete, and overwhelming physical danger
Guilt	Having transgressed a moral imperative
Shame	Having failed to live up to an ego ideal
Sadness	Having experienced an irrevocable loss
Envy	Wanting what someone else has
Jealousy	Resenting a third party for the loss of or a threat to another's affection
Disgust	Taking in or being too close to an indigestible object or idea (metaphorically speaking)
Happiness	Making reasonable progress toward the realization of a goal
Pride	Enhancement of one's ego-identity by taking credit for a valued object or achievement, either our own or that of someone or a group with whom we identify
Relief	A distressing goal-incongruent condition that has changed for the better or gone away
Hope	Fearing the worst but yearning for better
Love	Desiring or participating in affection, usually but not necessarily reciprocated
Compassion	Being moved by another's suffering and wanting to help

Adapted from Lazarus, R. S. (1999). *Stress and emotion: A new synthesis.* New York: Springer.

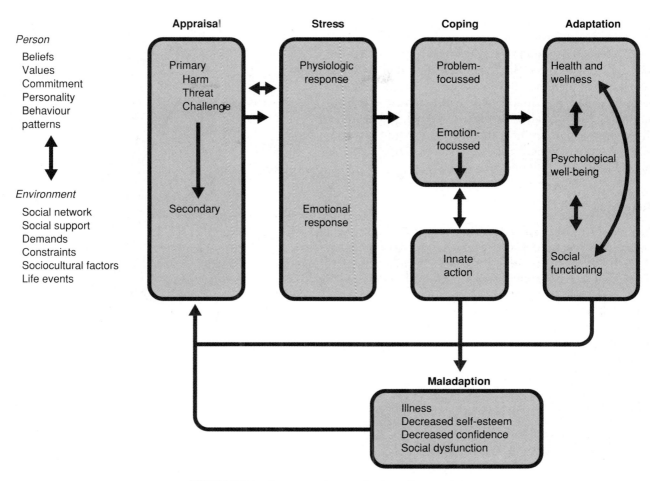

Person

Beliefs
Values
Commitment
Personality
Behaviour
patterns

Environment

Social network
Social support
Demands
Constraints
Sociocultural factors
Life events

Appraisal

Primary
Harm
Threat
Challenge

Secondary

Stress

Physiologic
response

Emotional
response

Coping

Problem-
focussed

Emotion-
focussed

Innate
action

Adaptation

Health and
wellness

Psychological
well-being

Social
functioning

Maladaption

Illness
Decreased self-esteem
Decreased confidence
Social dysfunction

FIGURE 34.2   Stress, coping, and adaptation model.

assigns to it. Table 34-6 contrasts problem-focussed and emotion-focussed coping.

Coping involves the continuous re-evaluation or reappraisal of the changing person–environment relationship. **Reappraisal** incorporates feedback about the effects of coping and allows for continual adjustment to new information. In this way, the stress response becomes part of the dynamic relationship between the person and the environment. No single coping strategy is effective in all situations. Throughout our lives, we develop a repertoire

Table 34.6	**Ways of Coping: Problem-Focussed Versus Emotion-Focussed**
Problem-Focussed Coping	**Emotion-Focussed Coping**
When noise from the television interrupts a student's studying and causes the student to be stressed, the student turns off the television and eliminates the noise.	A husband is adamantly opposed to visiting his wife's relatives because they keep dogs in their house. Even though the dogs are well cared for, their presence in the relative's home violates his need for an orderly, clean house and causes the husband sufficient stress that he copes by refusing to visit. This becomes a source of marital conflict. One holiday, the husband is given a puppy and immediately becomes attached to the dog, who soon becomes a valued family member. The husband then begins to view his wife's relatives differently and willingly visits their house more often.
An abused spouse is finally able to leave her husband because she realizes that the abuse will not stop, even though he promises never to hit her again.	A mother is afraid that her teenaged daughter has been in an accident because she did not come home after a party. Then the woman remembers that she gave her daughter permission to stay at a friend's house. She immediately feels better.

of coping strategies and learn which ones are most effective in different situations. These strategies become deeply ingrained into patterned responses. Ideally, individuals are realistic in their appraisal of the demands of them, are flexible in their use of coping resources, and remain open to learning new coping strategies. Poor reality testing, impaired judgment, inflexibility, and an unwillingness to acquire new resources can render individuals vulnerable to stress-related problems and illness.

Adaptation

Adaptation reflects an individual's capacity to survive and flourish in a constantly changing environment (Lazarus, 1999). Adaptation (or lack of it) affects three important areas: health, psychological well-being, and social functioning. A period of stress may compromise any or all of these areas. If a person copes successfully with stress, he or she returns to a previous level of adaptation. Successful coping results in an improvement in health, well-being, and social functioning. Unfortunately, at times, maladaptation occurs.

> **KEY CONCEPT Adaptation** is the individual's capacity to survive and flourish in a constantly changing environment; it affects three important areas: health, psychological well-being, and social functioning.

Adaptation, health, well-being, and social functioning are so closely interdependent that it is impossible to separate them. For instance, psychiatric symptoms can cause problems in work performance and in turn contribute to a negative self-concept. Although each area will be discussed separately, as Figure 34-3 demonstrates, alterations in one area affect all other areas.

Health and Illness

For more than 50 years, we have had empirical evidence of a link between stress and illness. Animal experiments in the 1950s and 1960s demonstrated that a number of stressors (eg, isolation, crowding, exposure to a predator, and electrical shock) increased morbidity and mortality from tumours and infections (Saddock & Saddock, 2003). In human research, acute academic exam stress has been linked to a reduction in natural killer cells and increased activation of latent viruses (Glaser, Rice, Sherridan, & Fertel, 1987). More recent studies demonstrate a correlation between exam stress and an increase in cytokines—proteins (produced by lymphocytes and other cells) that promote or inhibit an immune response (Lui, Coe, Swenson, Kelly, Kita, & Busse, 2002). As well, Segerstrom and Miller's (2003) meta-analysis of 30 years of research on the effects of chronic stress associated with caring for a relative with

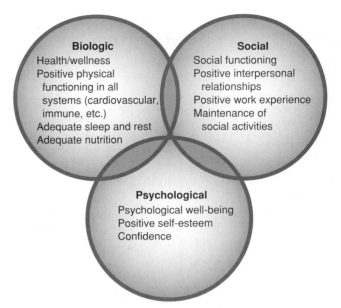

FIGURE 34.3 Biopsychosocial adaptation.

dementia found a reduction in most measures of immune function.

The **stress-diathesis model** provides a widely accepted explanation about the relationship between stress and mental health-illness (Stanley & Burrows, 2005). The model proposes that pre-existing genetic, biologic, and psychological vulnerabilities interact with negative or stressful life events to cause illness. Furthermore, the model predicts an inverse relationship between vulnerability and stress such that the more vulnerable the individual, the smaller the stressor required to cause illness. Several lines of research conclude that the tendency to "nervousness, emotionality, 'neuroticism,' negative affect, anxiety, and being 'high strung' runs in families and has a high genetic component, with 50% of these characteristics arising from genetic or biologic vulnerability" (Stanley & Burrows, 2005, p. 90). In a large community-based study, Kendler, Neale, Kessler, Heath, & Eaves (1992) found that generalised anxiety disorder and depression share a common genetic predisposition and that episodes of illness are related to environmental stressors.

Ineffective coping has other negative implications for health. For instance, if emotion-focussed coping is used when a problem-focussed approach is appropriate, stress is not relieved. In addition, if a coping strategy violates gender, ethnic, or cultural norms, stress is often exaggerated. Some coping strategies actually increase the risk for mortality and morbidity, such as the excessive use of alcohol, drugs, tobacco, or overeating. Although these strategies may provide some short-term stress relief, they often cause long-term secondary stress. The corollary is that healthy coping strategies such as exercising, adequate sleep, leisure activities, and good nutrition reduce stress reduction and promote health and well-being.

Psychological Well-Being

A person's feelings about the resolution of a stressful encounter depend on whether he or she views the outcome as satisfactory. Appraising a situation as challenging, rather than harmful or threatening, is more likely to result in increased self-confidence and a sense of well-being. An encounter that a person accurately appraises as harmful or threatening is more likely to have a positive outcome if the person views it as manageable.

Outcome satisfaction for one person does not necessarily represent outcome satisfaction for another. For instance, suppose that two students receive the same passing score on an examination. One may feel a sense of relief, but the other may feel anxious or disappointed because they appraise the score as too low. An individual's emotional response to an outcome reflects the meaning they assign to it. Those who consistently have positive outcomes from stressful experiences are more likely to have positive self-esteem and self-confidence. Unsatisfactory outcomes, on the other hand, are associated with negative mood states, such as depression, anger, guilt leading to decreased self-esteem, and feelings of helplessness.

Social Functioning

Social functioning, the performance of daily activities within the context of interpersonal relationships and roles, can be seriously impaired during stressful episodes. For instance, the stress of a divorce may interfere with work performance. If coping leads to a positive outcome, then social functioning returns to normal or improves. Social functioning will continue to be impaired if the person views the outcome as unsuccessful and experiences negative emotions.

Health Effects of Extreme Stress

Although historical and literary references to the lasting effects of extreme stress (eg, natural disasters, combat, and physical/sexual assault) date back to the 3rd century BC (Birmes, Hatton, Brunet, & Schmitt, 2003), post-traumatic stress disorder (PTSD) did not appear in the *Diagnostic and Statistical Manual of Mental Disorders (DSM)* until 1980 (APA, 1980). The importance of officially sanctioning the health effects of extreme stress cannot be overstated. First, the diagnostic label put a name to the effects of horrific life events and created a conceptual framework for the systematic study of the trauma associated with extreme stress. Second, it stipulated that an external stressor (rather than a weakness in the individual) initiates the development of the disor-

der. Third, identifying the potentially serious and long-lasting responses to extreme stress validated and legitimized the experiences of affected individuals. Finally and perhaps most importantly, the construct of PTSD endorsed the view that individuals exist within a unique environmental context and that through continuous and reciprocal interaction, the individual and the environment influence and are influenced by each other (van der Kolk & McFarlane, 1996). The significance of this stance is that it encourages health care providers to approach the person-in-context holistically and to view *psychiatric disorders* as embodied human experiences. The diagnostic criteria for PTSD have undergone several revisions since they were first published 26 years ago; the most current version appears in the *DSM-IV-TR* (APA, 2000; see Appendix A).

Individuals typically respond to extreme stress with intense fear, helplessness, or horror (APA, 2000), which alters their sense of self, their basic trust in other people, and their belief in the world as a safe, predictable place. As discussed earlier in this chapter, the perception of a threat triggers the ANS to mount a defensive response. Instantaneously, hormones and neurotransmitters course through the body in a coordinated effort to deal with the stressor. When the danger subsides, the body returns to its normal state. Under conditions of extreme stress or when the threat is prolonged (eg, being held captive, ongoing domestic violence, and repeated childhood physical and sexual abuse) the stress response systems do not return to normal levels. As Judith Herman (1992, p. 34) explains,

> [when] neither resistance not escape is possible, the human system of self-defense becomes overwhelmed and disorganized. Each component of the ordinary response to danger, having lost its utility, tends to persist in an altered and exaggerated state long after the danger is over.

The cumulative effects of stress-responsive hormones and neuromodulators can leave survivors of extreme stress permanently changed.

Clinicians and researchers group these changes into three clusters of signs and symptoms, labelled *hyperarousal, intrusion,* and *constriction. Hyperarousal* keeps survivors in a heightened state of physiologic arousal. Ever vigilant and living at the edge of terror, they are irritable, startle easily, and sleep poorly. *Intrusion* is the imprinting of the extremely stressful event on the mind and body. We see this in media images of September 11—frozen faces, staring in wide-eyed disbelief. Extremely stressful events are set into memory differently than are ordinary experiences. "Traumatic memories lack verbal narrative and context; rather, they are encoded in the form of vivid sensation and images" (Herman, 1992, p. 38), which may later reoccur as *flashbacks* (during waking states) and as traumatic nightmares (during sleep). Flashbacks are triggered by reminders of the traumatic event. These reminders may be sights, sounds, odours, tastes, or physical sensations that transport the survivor back into the stressful event. A flashback is not an ordinary memory, it is a vivid reliving of the trauma that floods the survivor with the full emotional force of the original event. *Constriction* is the numbing that is required for surrender. Unable to fight off or escape the threat, survivors dissociate from the event so that they can endure it. Constriction alters perception, sensation, and time sense. In a dissociated state, individuals report feeling detached from their bodies or viewing the event dispassionately, as though it was happening in a movie.

Several lines of research support the claim that survivors of extreme stress have poorer physical and mental health and a lower health-related quality of life (Schnurr & Green, 2004). For example, the National Comorbidity Study (Kessler, Sonnega, Bromet, Hughes, & Nelson, 1995), the largest American study of psychiatric comorbidity to date, reports that 79% of women and 88% of men diagnosed with PTSD also meet diagnostic criteria for at least one other psychiatric disorder. The disorders most prevalent among men with lifetime PTSD are alcohol abuse/dependence (51.9%), major depressive episode (47.9%), conduct disorder (43.3%), and drug abuse/dependence (34.5%). The most common disorders among women diagnosed with PTSD are major depressive episode (48.5%), simple phobia (29.0%), social phobia (28.4%), and alcohol abuse/dependence (27.9%). Among Vietnam veterans diagnosed with PTSD, generalized anxiety disorder, alcohol abuse, and major depression are the most common co-occurring psychiatric problems (Kulka et al., 1990). Researchers have also found a direct relationship between the number of childhood adversities and the presence of adult diseases, including ischemic heart disease, cancer, chronic lung disease, skeletal fractures, and liver disease (Felitti et al., 1998). Because survivors of extreme stress often attempt to cope with or avoid their distress through drug and alcohol use, self-mutilation, suicide, and disordered eating, they are often seen in psychiatric–mental health treatment settings (Springs & Freidrich, 1992).

This wide range of physical, psychological, emotional, and spiritual effects of extreme stress led Herman (1992) to challenge the sufficiency of the PTSD diagnostic construct, to capture the full range of human response to trauma. Based on her extensive clinical work with Holocaust survivors and survivors of sexual assault, she argues that as the nature, severity, and duration of extremely stressful events vary, so do individual responses. Herman believes that it is more accurate to conceptualize the human response to extreme stress as a continuum. This continuum, illustrated by Figure 34-4, is anchored at one end by an acute stress reaction that resolves on its own without treatment, and on the other by what Herman calls "complex posttraumatic stress disorder," with "classic or simple" PTSD residing somewhere between the

Acute Stress Disorder	Simple PTSD	Complicated PTSD (DESNOS)

FIGURE 34.4 The spectrum of human responses to extreme stress (adapted from Herman, 1992).

two. Herman's conceptualization of complex PTSD is captured in the criteria for Disorders of Extreme Stress Not Otherwise Specified (DESNOS; APA, 2000).

These diagnostic distinctions are especially important in clinical settings because they orient health practitioners to the fact that they encounter survivors of extreme stress everyday in their practice. Survivors are individuals—patients, clients, health care consumers—of every age, who seek health services in every area of specialty. In some instances, health care professionals will know that the individual before them is a survivor, but in most brief encounters, they will not. Given the intimacy and (often) invasiveness of procedures and treatments, it should not be a surprise that for many survivors, health-serving environments are very frightening places. What are simple and routine encounters for health professionals can be very distressing for survivors because much about health-serving environments is reminiscent of the original trauma, including a sense of powerlessness, lack of control, invasion of personal boundaries, exposure, vulnerability, and pain. A simple touch, even when it is gentle, can trigger a flashback.

Although most health professionals will not develop the specialized knowledge and skills needed to work intensively with trauma survivors through their healing, it is important for all practitioners to know about the long-term health effects of extreme stress. A group of Canadian researchers (Schachter, Stalker, & Teram, 2001) recently conducted a multidisciplinary, multisite research project exploring ways that health professionals can work sensitively with adult survivors of childhood sexual abuse (CSA). The results of that work are published in a handbook titled *Handbook on Sensitive Practice for Health Professionals: Lessons From Women Survivors of Sexual Abuse* (available online at http://www.phac-aspc.gc.ca). The *Handbook* is written for practitioners and students of all health disciplines, who have no special training in psychotherapy and who have limited experience working with survivors of CSA. It offers principles and guidelines for providing sensitive care to survivors of all types of trauma.

Nursing Care of Individuals Affected by Stress

Assessment of Individuals Affected by Stress

Nursing assessment of individuals experiencing stress attends to biologic, psychological, emotional, and

IN A LIFE

Maria Campbell (1940)

Maria Campbell, the eldest daughter of seven children, was born in Park Valley, Saskatchewan, to parents of Scottish, Indian, and French descent. She is best known for her autobiography, *Halfbreed*, which recounts the first 33 years of her life. The book tells of how Maria lost her mother when she was only 12 years old, leaving her to care for her younger siblings. In an effort to keep her family together, young Maria married an abusive white man who reported her to child welfare authorities, and her siblings were placed in foster homes. Devastated, Maria moved to Vancouver, where her husband deserted her, and she turned to a life of drugs and prostitution. Alone and desperate, she attempted suicide twice and was hospitalized for psychiatric care. It is in the hospital that Maria joined Alcoholics Anonymous and began a journey of healing.

In the book, Maria Campbell not only tells her own story, but she speaks of the discrimination and racism that affect all Métis people. In the book's introduction, she says, "I write this for all of you, to tell you what it is like to be a halfbreed woman in this country. I want to tell you about the joys and sorrows, the oppressing poverty, the frustrations and the dreams." (1973, p. 8). Although Campbell's story is one of stress and crises, it is also a story of courage and resilience. She is no longer a scared, little girl but a strong, independent woman full of hope for herself and her people.

Today Campbell continues to write, teaches at the University of Saskatchewan, and is a political activist for Métis rights. She is the recipient of many writing awards and has Honorary Doctorate degrees from the University of Regina and York University.

Campbell, M. (1973). *Halfbreed*. Halifax, NS, Canada: Goodread Biographies.

---

environmental (physical and social), as well as coping, resources. In particular, the nurse should explore recent changes (positive or negative) in the individual's life (eg, trauma, loss, developmental milestones).

If an individual's signs and symptoms meet the diagnostic criteria for an Axis I or II disorder (APA, 2000), the stress response is conceptualized as being part of the disorder. However, if an individual is experiencing significant emotional or behavioural symptoms in response to an identifiable stressful situation and the diagnostic criteria do not account for the response, a diagnosis of adjustment disorder (APA, 2000) may be appropriate (see Table 34-7). This residual category describes responses to a stressful situation that do not meet criteria for an Axis I disorder. There are six subtypes: with depressed mood, with anxiety, with anxiety and depressed mood, with disturbance of conduct, with mixed disturbance of emotions and conduct, and unspecified. The diagnosis of adjustment disorder specifies that the onset of the emotional or behavioural disturbances must begin within 3 months of the stressful situation and cannot last for more than 6 months after the stressor abates.

The overall goals of care for those individuals actively experiencing a stress response are to eliminate or moderate the stressor (if possible), to reduce untoward effects of the stress response, and to facilitate the maintenance or development of positive coping skills. The goals of care for individuals who are at high risk for stress (eg, are experiencing significant life changes, have pre-existing vulnerabilities, or have limited coping mechanisms) are to recognize the potential for stress and to strengthen or develop positive coping skills.

Table 34.7 Key Diagnostic Characteristics of Adjustment Disorder

Diagnostic Criteria	Target Symptoms and Associated Findings
• Emotional or behavioural symptoms in response to an identifiable stressor occurring within 3 months of the onset of the stressors.	• Subjective distress or impairment in functioning
• Clinically significant symptoms or behaviours (1) are characterized by distress that is in excess of what would be expected from exposure to the stressor, or (2) cause a significant impairment in social or occupational (academic) functioning.	• Decreased performance at work or school
• Stress-related disturbance does not meet the criteria for another specific Axis I disorder and is not merely an exacerbation of a pre-existing Axis I or Axis II disorder.	• Temporary changes in relationships
• Symptoms do not represent bereavement.	
• Symptoms do not persist for more than 6 months after the stressor has terminated.	• Decreased compliance with recommended medical regimen

Acute: disturbance lasts more than 6 months
Chronic: disturbance lasts for 6 months or longer

309.0	With depressed mood
309.24	With anxiety
309.28	With mixed anxiety and depressed mood
309.3	With disturbance of conduct
309.4	With mixed disturbance of emotions and conduct
309.9	Unspecified

Biologic Assessment

Biologic data are essential for analyzing an individual's physical responses to stress, coping efforts, and adaptation. This information comes from the health history, physical examination, and diagnostic testing (as indicated; see Chapter 10). Nurses should pay particular attention to:

- Signs and symptoms of sympathetic arousal (Table 34-8)
- Alterations in vegetative functions (eg, appetite and eating patterns, sleep, energy level, sexual activity)
- Chronic illness or conditions with a strong stress component (eg, hypertension, migraine, chronic pain syndromes, irritable bowel syndrome)
- Evidence of immune system suppression (eg, frequent infections)

Table 34.8   Physiologic Stress-Related Symptoms

System	Symptom
Cardiovascular	Headache
	Chest pain
	Increased pulse
	Palpitations
	Fainting (blackouts, spells)
	Increased blood pressure
Respiratory	Shortness of breath
	Smoking history
	Increased rate and depth of breathing
	Chest discomfort (pain, tightness, ache)
Gastrointestinal	Nausea
	Vomiting
	Abdominal pain (cramps, stomach ache)
	Change in appetite
	Change in stool
	Obesity/frequent weight changes
Musculoskeletal	Pain
	Weakness
	Fatigue
Genitourinary	Menstrual changes
	Urinary discomforts (pain, burning, urgency, hesitancy)
	Sexual difficulty (pain, impotence, altered libido, anorgasmia)
Dermatologic	Itching
	Rash
	"Sweats"
	Eczema

Adapted from Carpenito-Moyet, L. (2004). *Nursing diagnosis: Application to clinical practice* (10th ed.). Philadelphia: Lippincott Williams & Wilkins.

- Physical appearance (eg, deficits in grooming and hygiene; nonverbal indications of muscle tension, anxiety, or depression)
- Alterations in activity and exercise patterns

As well, the biologic assessment of stress and coping considers the use of pharmacologic agents, including prescribed and nonprescribed medications, over-the-counter and herbal preparations, alcohol, tobacco, and illicit drugs. Many individuals begin or increase the frequency of using these agents as a way of coping with stress. In turn, over-reliance on relaxants or mood-altering substances can become a secondary stressor and contribute to maladaptation. Understanding patterns of use (eg, frequency, dose, circumstances, and effects) is important to assessing their role in stress management. The more important the substances are to a person's handling of stress, the greater the potential for abuse and addiction. Box 34-1 lists some potential nursing diagnoses within the North American Nursing Diagnosis Association (NANDA, 2005) taxonomy for individuals experiencing or at risk for stress response.

Interventions for the Biologic Domain

Individuals experiencing or at risk for untoward stress responses may benefit from a number of biologic interventions.

BOX 34.1

Potential Nursing Diagnoses in the Biologic Domain

Within the North American Nursing Diagnosis Association taxonomy, the following are some potential nursing diagnoses for individuals experiencing or at risk for stress response:

- Anxiety
- Body image, Disturbed
- Comfort, Impaired
- Constipation
- Diarrhea
- Energy field, Disturbed
- Fatigue
- Fear
- Fluid volume, Deficit/Risk for deficient
- Health maintenance, Ineffective
- Infection, Risk for
- Sleep pattern, Disrupted
- Therapeutic regime management, Ineffective
- Knowledge, Deficit
- Noncompliance
- Nutrition, More/less than body requirements
- Pain, Acute/Chronic
- Post-trauma syndrome
- Self-care deficit, Hygiene/Feeding
- Sexual dysfunction

(From North American Nursing Diagnosis Association [NANDA]. [2005]. *NANDA nursing diagnoses: Definitions and classification, 2005–2006.* Philadelphia: Author.)

- The importance of (re-)establishing regular routines for activities of daily living (eg, eating, sleeping, self-care, and leisure time) cannot be overstated. As well as ensuring adequate nutrition, sleep and rest, and hygiene, a routine may help to structure an individual's time and give them a sense of personal control or mastery.
- Exercise can reduce the emotional and behavioural responses to stress. In addition to the physical benefits of exercise, regular exercise can provide structure to a person's life, enhance self-confidence, and increase feelings of well-being. Under stress, many individuals are not receptive to the idea of exercise, particularly if it has not been a part of their life. Exploration of their usual activity patterns, as well as knowledge and beliefs about the value of exercise, will help to identify where the nurse may intervene.
- Activities such as yoga, mediation, deep breathing, and progressive muscle relaxation can help individuals mediate some the physical stress response, improve sleep, and reduce pain. As well, nurses should consider referring clients for hypnosis or biofeedback when indicated.
- Health teaching in such areas as nutrition, sleep hygiene, and medication management may also be part of nursing interventions in this domain.

Psychological Domain

Psychological Assessment

Information about the psychological and emotional dimensions of stress will be forthcoming throughout the assessment process. In particular, the nurse should do the following:

- Observe for behavioural and affective indicators of stress response (eg, energy level and general presentation; appearance, grooming, and hygiene; psychomotor agitation and retardation; facial expression; speech characteristics).
- Explore reports of recent changes in mood or current emotional distress (eg, anxiety, fear, irritability, anger, tension, pressure, depression).
- Note alterations or impairment in mental status (eg, suicidal ideation; self-deprecatory thoughts; impulsivity; ruminations; impaired concentration, problem-solving, or memory).
- Explore the individual's appraisal of significant life events (eg, losses, physical or sexual abuse or assault, motor vehicle crashes, natural disasters, combat experience), the effect of those experiences, and the individual's commitment to particular outcomes. A tool like the RLCQ (Holmes & Rahe, 1967; refer to Table 34-1) can be helpful.
- Ask about alterations in day-to-day function or inability to fulfill responsibilities (eg, family, work, school).
- Explore the individual's current resources and effectiveness of usual coping strategies (see Table 34-9).

Box 34-2 lists potential nursing diagnoses in the psychological domain.

Interventions for the Psychological Domain

The Nursing Interventions Classification (NIC; McCloskey & Bulechek, 2000) provides interventions in the behavioural domain that support psychological functioning and facilitate lifestyle changes. The NIC includes six classes of useful nursing interventions: behaviour therapy, cognitive therapy, communication enhancement, coping assistance, patient education, and psychological comfort promotion. The interventions are listed in Table 34-10.

BOX 34.2

Potential Nursing Diagnoses in the Psychological Domain

The nurse should consider the following as potential nursing diagnoses in the psychological domain:
- Adjustment, Impaired
- Anxiety
- Body image, DisturbedConflict, Decisional
- Confusion, Acute/Chronic
- Coping, Ineffective/Defencive
- Denial, Ineffective
- Development, Risk for delayed
- Diversional activity, Deficit
- Environmental interpretation, Impaired
- Failure to thrive
- Growth and development, Delayed
- Hopelessness
- Identity, Disturbed

- Knowledge, Deficit
- Memory, Impaired
- Post-trauma syndrome
- Powerlessness
- Relocation syndrome
- Role performance, Ineffective
- Self-esteem, Chronic low/Situational low
- Self-mutilation
- Sensory perception, Disturbed
- Sexual dysfunction
- Spiritual distress
- Suicide, Risk for
- Thought process, disturbed
- Violence, Self/Other directed

(From North American Nursing Diagnosis Association [NANDA]. [2005]. *NANDA nursing diagnoses: Definitions and classification, 2005-2006.* Philadelphia: Author.)

Table 34.9   Problem-Focussed and Emotion-Focussed Behaviours

Behaviour	Focussed Type	Definition	Effective	Ineffective
Goal setting	Problem focussed	The conscious process of setting time limitations on behaviour	When goals are attainable and manageable; eg, making an appointment with boss to discuss pay raise	When the appraisal of the situation is missed or inaccurately evaluated
Information seeking	Problem focussed	Process of learning about all aspects of a problem that provides perspective and reinforces self-control	When situations are complex and additional information is needed; eg, attending a parent effectiveness class because of being unsure about discipline techniques	When the needed information is already obtained and the activity delays action
Mastery	Problem focussed	Learning of new procedures or skills that facilitate self-esteem, reinforce self-control	When there are new procedures to learn; eg, self-care activities, insulin injection, catheter care	When the situation does not require learning new procedures, or they have nothing to do with the stressful situation
Help seeking	Problem focussed	Reaching out to others for support; sharing feelings provides an emotional release, reassurance, and comfort	When similar problems are shared by others; eg, in Alcoholics Anonymous, weight-loss programs, psychosocial programs	When using help seeking to avoid action in the current situation
Minimization	Emotion focussed	The seriousness of the problem is minimized	Useful way of providing needed time for appraisal; eg, a person is told that her child is in an automobile accident and forces herself to think the accident is minor until additional information is received	When the appraisal of the situation is missed or inaccurately evaluated
Projection, displacement, and suppression of anger	Emotion focussed	When anger is attributed to or expressed toward a less-threatening person or thing	When threat is reduced, the individual can deal with the situation; eg, the boss reprimands a worker for submitting a report late—the worker in turn hits his fist on the copying machine as he walks by	When reality is distorted and relationships disturbed, which further compound the problem; suppression of anger may result in stress-related physical symptoms
Anticipatory preparation	Emotion focussed	Mental rehearsal of possible consequences of behaviour or outcomes of stressful situations	Provides the opportunity to develop perspective as well as to prepare for the worst; eg, when waiting for exam results, the patient develops a plan of action if the results are negative	When anticipation creates unmanageable stress as in anticipatory mourning
Attribution	Emotion focussed	Finding personal meaning in the problem situation, which may be through religious faith or individual belief	May offer consolation; eg, fate, the will of the divine; luck	When all sense of self-responsibility is lost

Adapted from Carpenito-Moyet, L. (2004). *Nursing diagnosis: Application to clinical practice* (10th ed.). Philadelphia: Lippincott Williams & Wilkins.

Table 34.10   Interventions for Stress Reduction and Coping Enhancement

Behaviour Therapy*	Cognitive Therapy	Communication Enhancement	Coping Assistance Interventions	Patient Education	Psychological Comfort Promotion
Reinforce or promote desirable behaviours or alter undesirable behaviours	Reinforce or promote desirable cognitive functioning or alter undesirable functioning	Facilitate effective verbal and nonverbal interactions	Help build on existing strengths, foster adaptation to change, achieve a higher level of function	Facilitate new learning	Promote comfort using psychological techniques

Generalist Interventions

Behaviour Therapy*	Cognitive Therapy	Communication Enhancement	Coping Assistance Interventions	Patient Education	Psychological Comfort Promotion
Assertiveness training	Anger management	Active listening skills	Anticipatory guidance	Learning facilitation	Anxiety reduction
Behaviour management	Bibliotherapy	Communication enhancement	Body image enhancement	Learning readiness enhancement	Calming technique
Behaviour modification	Reality orientation	Socialization enhancement	Counselling	Parent education	Distraction
Limit setting			Grief work facilitation	Teaching: disease process	Simple guided imagery
Patient contracting			Decision-making support	Teaching: group individual	Simple relaxation therapy
Self-modification assistance			Care of the dying	Teaching: activity exercise, diet, medication, procedure/ treatment, psychomotor skills, safe sex	
Self-responsibility assistance			Emotional support		
Smoking cessation assistance			Hope instillation		
Substance use prevention			Humour		
Activity therapy			Role enhancement		
			Recreation therapy		
			Self-awareness enhancement		
			Self-esteem enhancement		
			Spiritual support		
			Support system enhancement		
			Values clarifications		

Specialist (Advanced Practice) Interventions†

Behaviour Therapy*	Cognitive Therapy	Communication Enhancement	Coping Assistance Interventions	Patient Education	Psychological Comfort Promotion
Psychotherapy	Psychotherapy	Psychotherapy	Psychotherapy, individual and group	Same as generalist	Psychopharmacologic agents prescribed
Consultation	Consultation	Consultation	Consultation		Autogenic training
Animal-assisted therapy	Cognitive restructuring	Complex relationship building	Genetic counselling		Biofeedback
Substance use treatment	Cognitive stimulation	Music therapy	Grief therapy		Hypnosis
Art therapy	Memory training	Art therapy	Guilt work		Meditation
	Reminiscence therapy	Play therapy	Sexual counselling		
		Animal-assisted therapy	Touch therapy		

*Behavioural interventions: care that supports psychological functioning and facilitates lifestyle changes.
†Specialist interventions require additional training. Specialist interventions are in addition to those at the generalist level.
McCloskey, J., & Bulechek, G. (2000). *Nursing interventions classification (NIC)* (3rd ed.). St. Louis: Mosby–Year Book.

Social Domain

Social Assessment

Information from a social assessment is invaluable to understanding an individual's coping resources. The ability to make healthy lifestyle changes is strongly influenced by one's social support system. Even the expression of stress is related to social factors, particularly ethnic and cultural expectations and values.

Social assessment also includes identification of the person's social network. The nurse should elicit the following information:

- Size and extent of the network, both relatives and nonrelatives, and the length and quality of the relationships
- Functions the network serves (eg, intimacy, social integration, nurturance, reassurance of worth, guidance and advice, access to new contacts)
- Degree of reciprocity between the individual and others in the network (ie, Who provides support to the client? Who does the client support?)
- Degree of interconnectedness among network members

The Malone Social Network Inventory (MSNI) (Malone, 1988, p. 20), shown in Table 34-11, is a guide for exploring an individual's social relationships using an open-ended interview. The MSNI elicits the following information:

- Who is in the network
- The nature relationship (eg, spouse, child, minister)
- A brief description of what each relationship provides

- The degree of helpfulness
- The expected degree of helpfulness

The client ranks each relationship on a 5-point Likert-type scale (1 is low and 5 is high) as to its degree of helpfulness. Next, the client identifies how helpful he or she would like each relationship to be. The gap between how helpful a relationship is and how helpful the client would like it to be yields what Malone calls a *dissonance score*—the higher the score, the higher the dissonance. The relationships with the high dissonance scores may become the focus of therapeutic intervention.

Box 34-3 lists potential nursing diagnoses within the social domain.

Interventions for the Social Domain

Individuals who are coping with stressful situations often benefit from interventions that facilitate social functioning and promote the health and welfare of social network members. The NIC (McCloskey & Bulechek, 2000) includes the following generalist interventions in family care: caregiver support, family integrity promotion, family involvement, family mobilization, family process maintenance, family support, respite care, and home maintenance assistance. Parenting education can also be useful to effective family functioning. The nurse should also consider referring the client to family therapy when that is indicated.

Evaluation and Treatment Outcomes

The treatment goals established in the plan of care guide evaluation. The goals of individual care relate to

Table 34.11	Malone Social Network Inventory				
Initials	Relationship	What Relationship Provides	Current	Helpfulness Rating 1 (lowest)–5 (highest)	Desired

From Malone, J. (1988). The social support social dissupport continuum. *Journal of Psychosocial Nursing and Mental Health Services, 26*(12), 18–22.

Potential Diagnoses in the Social Domain

Potential nursing diagnoses within the social domain include:

- Anxiety, Death
- Attachment, Impaired, or Risk for impaired
- Caregiver role strain
- Communication, Impaired
- Conflict
- Coping, Ineffective
- Family processes: alcoholism, Dysfunctional
- Grieving
- Loneliness
- Parenting, Impaired
- Role performance, Ineffective
- Sexual dysfunction
- Social interaction, Impaired
- Sorrow, Chronic
- Sexuality patterns, Ineffective
- Violence, Other directed

(From North American Nursing Diagnosis Association [NANDA]. [2005]. *NANDA nursing diagnoses: Definitions and classification, 2005–2006.* Philadelphia: Author.)

improved health, well-being, and social function. Depending on the level of intervention, there may also be goals for the family and other members of the client's social network. Family outcomes may relate to improved communication or social support (eg, reduced caregiver stress). Social network outcomes focus on strengthening the social network and improving its function.

CRISIS

Our current understanding of the biopsychosocial implications of crisis has its roots in Eric Lindemann's (1944) study of bereavement among friends and relatives of the Coconut Grove nightclub fire in Boston in 1942. Four hundred and thirty-nine individuals died in that fire, which at the time, was the worst single building fire in U.S. history. In the course of his research, Lindemann learned that family and friends of those who died experienced somatic symptoms, feelings or anger and guilt, and preoccupation with the deceased. From this work, he developed a model that describes grief as progressing through three stages: shock and disbelief; acute mourning; and resolution. Lindemann concluded that grief is both a natural response to loss and necessary to survivors' mental health. He later extended his ideas about crisis to more common, yet significant, life events (eg, the birth of a child, marriage, death). He hypothesized that the changes associated with these events cause emotional strain and require individuals to adapt to a new reality. These adaptive efforts either lead to mastery (psychological growth) or impaired functioning. Lindemann was convinced that by helping individuals through

the bereavement process, mental health professionals could prevent later psychological and emotional problems. This thinking reflected two important trends that were germinating in psychiatry around the globe: the recognition of the potential for and the value of early intervention to prevent emotional and psychological problems and the movement from hospital-based to community-based psychiatric treatment.

Although Lindemann did much of the foundational work in the area of crisis, Gerald Caplan is widely acknowledged as the master architect of crisis intervention. A psychiatrist and close colleague of Lindemann's, Caplan (1961) equated mental health with a strong, mature ego, which he defined as: (1) the capacity to withstand stress and maintain equilibrium; (2) accurate perception of reality; and (3) a balanced repertoire of coping strategies based on sound reality testing. Under the aegis of the Harvard School of Public Health, Caplan established the Harvard Family Guidance Center—an interdisciplinary crisis research and consultation project that studied the impact of four stressors: premature birth, birth of children with congenital abnormalities, birth of twins, and tuberculosis. Caplan is believed to be the first to apply the term *crisis* in psychiatry; to relate the concept of homeostasis to crisis intervention; and to describe the stages of a crisis.

Caplan defined **crisis** as occurring "when a person faces an obstacle to important life goals that is, for a time, insurmountable through the utilization of customary methods of problem solving" (1961, p. 18). More specifically, a crisis is a response in which psychological equilibrium is disrupted; usual coping methods are ineffective in restoring that equilibrium; and, there is evidence of functional impairment (Caplan 1961; Flannery & Everly, 2000). This disequilibrium causes a rise in inner tension and anxiety that, if it continues, engenders emotional upset and an inability to function (Caplan, 1961). Figure 34-5 summarizes the phases of crisis response.

Although crises force individuals into uncharted territory, Caplan (1961) recognized that most individuals achieve resolution without professional help within 4 to 6 weeks. He viewed this time as a period of transition in which the individual, family, or group is more vulnerable to harm and at the same time, more open to outside intervention. This prompted him to advocate for community-based crisis services aimed at identifying maladaptive responses and intervening early to assist those involved to transform problems into opportunities for personal growth and new learning.

> **KEY CONCEPT** A **crisis** response occurs when an individual encounters an obstacle or problem, important to their life goals that cannot be solved by customary problem-solving methods. It is acute, time-limited, and may be developmental, situational, or interpersonal in nature.

A problem arises that contributes to increase in anxiety levels. The anxiety stimulates the implementation of usual problem-solving techniques of the person.

↓

The usual problem-solving techniques are ineffective. Anxiety levels continue to rise. Trial-and-error attempts are made to restore balance.

↓

The trial-and-error attempts fail. The anxiety escalates to severe or panic levels. The person adopts automatic relief behaviours.

↓

When these measures do not reduce anxiety, anxiety can overwhelm the person and lead to serious personality disorganization, which signals the person is in crisis

FIGURE 34.5 Phases of Crisis Response.

Types of Crises

Situational Crisis

A situational crisis is any event that overwhelms an individual's coping resources and upsets their equilibrium. The precipitating event may be positive or negative, physiological, psychological, or social in nature. Examples of situational crises include illness, the death of a loved one, separation or divorce, job loss, school problems, physical or sexual assault, or an unplanned pregnancy. Situational crises also result from less common occurrences such as accidents, natural or human-caused disasters, and acts of terrorism. Box 34-4 discusses the death of a loved one, a situational crisis that all of us will encounter in our lifetime.

Developmental Crisis

Theorists, such as Erik Erikson, propose that human development proceeds sequentially through a series of stages, each with a new set of social roles, and responsibilities. Stage theorists hold that demands from the social environment exert pressure on an individual to move on to the next developmental stage and that a failure to meet these new expectations precipitates a developmental crisis. Successful resolution of this crisis is necessary for movement into the next stage. Developmental crises are an expected part of maturation and are a time during which individuals acquire new skills and resources.

The concept of developmental crisis assumes that psychosocial development progresses in an orderly, easily identifiable process. Other developmental theories, for example those proposed by Miller (1994) and Gilligan (1994), refute the notion that human development advances in stages (see Chapter 7). That being said, the concept of developmental crisis is useful for describing unfavourable person–environment relationships that relate to maturational events, such as leaving home for the first time, completing school, or the birth of one's first child.

Crisis or Not? The Effects of Balancing Factors

Donna Aguilera (1998) contends that whether or not a stressful event evolves into a crisis depends on three interdependent *balancing factors*—perception of the event, available situational supports, and coping mechanisms. As Figure 34-6 illustrates, the timely and successful resolution of a crisis is more likely if an individual has a realistic view of the situation; has adequate supports available; and has effective coping mechanisms.

Nursing Care of Individuals Experiencing Crisis

Crisis Intervention

Crisis intervention is the provision of emergency psychological care to victims to assist them to return to an adaptive level of functioning and to prevent or moderate the potentially negative effects of psychological trauma (Everly & Mitchell, 1999). Although there are several models of crisis intervention, virtually all of them incorporate the follow principles (Flannery & Flannery, 2000):

1. **Early intervention**. By their nature, crises are acute and distressing events that overwhelm an individual's coping resources. Inability to resolve a crisis in a timely manner renders those affected at risk for long-term health problems. Crisis intervention services are typically community based and operate 24 hours per day. Crisis teams provide

BOX 34.4

Death of a Loved One: A Crisis Event

One of the most common crisis-provoking events is the loss of a loved one through death. Although death is a certainty for all of us, Western culture "denies and defies death. Death is often seen as a defeat, a failure, and an outcome to be avoided at all costs. As a result, the bereaved often feel profoundly isolated" (Roberts & Berry, 2002, p. 53).

Definition of Terms

Bereavement is typically understood to be the objective event or occurrence of having suffered a loss (Rando, 1993).

Grief is the subjective experience (eg, thoughts, feelings, behaviours, and body sensations) that accompanies the perception of a loss (Rando, 1993). Table 34-11 identifies some of the common physical, behavioural, emotional, and social responses to grief.

Mourning is the external manifestations of grief, which are highly influenced by gender, ethnicity, culture, religion, and the cause of death (Wolfelt, 1999).

Tasks of Mourning

Worden (2003) describes the four tasks of mourning, which are necessary to the process of adapting to loss and re-establishing equilibrium. Unlike other theorists who conceptualize mourning in terms of *stages* or *phases*, which connote linearity, Worden emphasizes the issues that bereaved individuals must face and successfully negotiate as they come to terms with their new reality:

1. *Accepting the reality of the loss.* The first task of grieving is to accept the reality and full consequence of the loss. A part of this is recognizing the permanence of death and that life as it was is over forever.
2. *Working through the pain of grief.* It is important for the bereaved individual to experience and acknowledge the pain of grief. Denial or suppression of this pain prolongs grieving.
3. *Adapting to an environment in which the deceased is absent.* This adaptation requires the bereaved individual to adjust to a new reality, which involves developing a new self-identity (ie, as a widow or single person) and taking on of new social roles and responsibilities.
4. *Developing a new relationship with the deceased and re-engaging with life.* In coming to terms with the loss, the bereaved individual does not forget the deceased, but rather establishes a new relationship with the deceased. This involves healing the wound of the severed attachment so that new ones can be formed. Resolution of grief is manifest by the gradual return of feelings of well-being and the ability to continue with life. The bereaved person does not deny his or her former life or forget the loved one, but finds a way to weave memories of the past into their current reality.

It is important to keep in mind that although the experience of loss is universal, individual responses vary widely, and there is no one clearly defined course or process of bereavement or grieving. Grief is influenced by age, development, gender, history of loss and/or trauma, history of depression, the nature and quality of the relationship with the deceased, and type of loss (eg, anticipated, violent, traumatic). Recent research underscores that the experience and expressions of grief are influenced by such factors as familial relationships and expectations, social and cultural factors, and religion (Center for the Advancement of Health, 2003).

Complicated Grief

Complicated grief is also termed abnormal, pathologic, chronic, or exaggerated grief. It refers to grief that does not seem to be advancing the bereaved individual toward acceptance and reorganization. Grief is complicated when an individual does not accomplish one or more of the tasks of mourning. Examples of this include denying the reality of one's loss; prolonged and intense emotions that do not seem to lessen over time; the apparent absence of mourning; and the inability to reinvest in life.

Role of Health Care Teams in Supporting Grief

As members of the health care team, nurses participate in supporting bereaved individuals through the process of grieving. The goals of this care are to assist bereaved individuals with the tasks of mourning and to prevent complicated grief. Activities may include sitting in silence with the bereaved, active listening, assistance with practical needs, and referral for ongoing support.

---

telephone triage and counselling, but may also travel to the scene of the crisis, where they work closely with other emergency service personnel (eg, police, ambulance, fire fighters, hospital emergency departments).

2. **Stabilization.** An immediate goal of all crisis intervention efforts is to prevent the situation from worsening. Stabilization involves mobilizing resources and support networks with the aim of minimizing harm and quickly restoring some semblance of order and routine.

3. **Facilitate understanding.** An important part of crisis intervention is helping individuals to develop an accurate understanding of the situation and its potential consequences. This usually involves listening to individuals' accounts of their experience and assisting them to identify and articulate their feelings about what is happening. Facilitating a clear understanding of a situation helps individuals to develop a realistic appraisal of the demands on them and aids the integration of the crisis into their cognitive schema.

4. **Focus on problem solving.** A primary task of crisis intervention is the identification and prioritization of immediate problems. Once achieved, interventions focus on assisting those involved to find short-term solutions.

5. **Encourage self-reliance.** Encouraging and supporting individuals to participate in identifying and solving problems facilitates their return to independent function and the development of a sense of mastery.

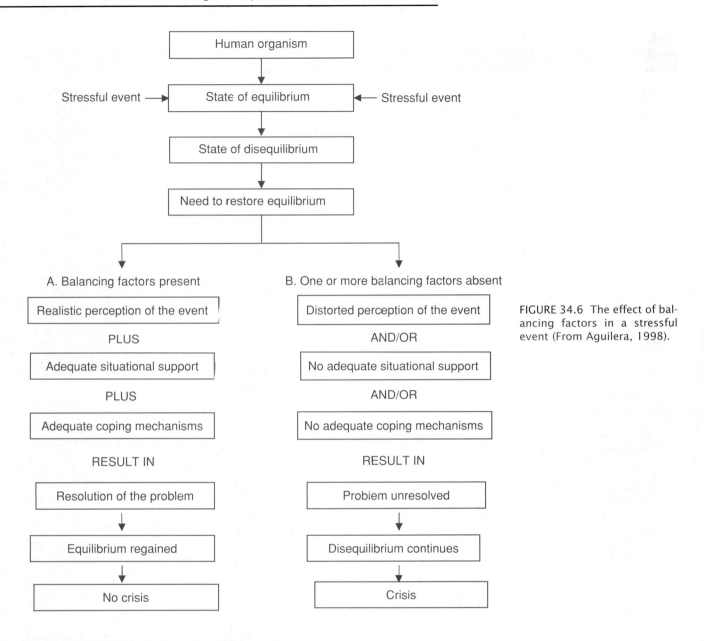

FIGURE 34.6 The effect of balancing factors in a stressful event (From Aguilera, 1998).

CRNE Note

The goals of crisis intervention are to assist individuals to return to an adaptive level of functioning and to prevent or moderate the potentially negative effects of extreme stress. Principles of crisis intervention include early intervention, stabilization, facilitating understanding, a focus on problem solving, and encouragement of self-reliance.

The case study in Box 34-5 uses Robert's Seven Stage Crisis Intervention Model (Fig. 34-7) (Roberts, 1991) to illustrate the application of these principles to a clinical situation.

Telephone Help Lines. Most health authorities have telephone help lines operated by governmental and nongovernmental organizations. These lines, typically staffed by mental health professionals or trained volunteers, offer support for problems such as child abuse, suicide, and farm stress. These lines permit immediate access to a spectrum of support and intervention services for individuals who are experiencing a crisis or need help to manage life-stressors.

Short-Stay Hospitalization and Community-Based Emergency Housing. Some health authorities designate a few beds on their psychiatric units for short-stay, crisis stabilization. Individuals are admitted to these beds for a brief period of inpatient care (typically 72 hours) when they have no supports in the community, need to have their medications assessed or stabilized, or require some other health service. As well, communities often have community-based, emergency housing. For example, some communities have shelters

BOX 34.5

Case Study Demonstrating Robert's Seven-Stage Crisis Intervention Model

The mobile mental health crisis unit in a large Canadian city receives a call from Theresa, the maternal aunt of 19-year-old Billy, an Aboriginal male whose 12-year-old brother died 4 months ago from sniffing gasoline. On hearing of his brother's death, Billy quit college and went on a 5-day drinking binge. At the time of the call, he was lying on his bed in the dark. Theresa tells the crisis nurse that Billy has been eating very little for the past several weeks and has been sleeping 12 to 14 hours per day. He rarely leaves his room and speaks only when addressed directly. What little conversation he does offer is preoccupied with his brother and their parents who died in a car crash a number of years earlier. Theresa has tried everything she can think of to convince Billy to get help; she is worried about leaving him alone for fear he will harm himself.

Stage 1: Conduct Crisis and Biopsychosocial Assessment (including lethality assessment). Joanne, the crisis intervention nurse, performs a focussed assessment and, using direct questions, ascertains important details about the situation (eg, caller name, address, and telephone number; the nature of the emergency; the presence/potential for injury or loss of life; availability of weapons or other potentially dangerous items). Within 2 or 3 minutes, she determines that Billy has experienced major losses (one of them very recently), that his behaviour is suggestive of acute mourning and/or depression; that he is at high risk for self-harm; and that his aunt, who is his primary social support, has exhausted her resources for dealing with the situation. The nurse tells Theresa that she and a colleague are on their way to talk with Billy and that they will be bringing police assistance. The nurse decides to involve the police for two reasons. The first is that by their nature, crises are unpredictable situations and have some potential for violence. A police presence sometimes deters aggressive acting out; if it does not, it ensures that there are trained personnel to effectively contain it. The second reason is that the police have authority, under provincial mental health legislation, to transport individuals for psychiatric assessment, even against their will. In order to do this, they must have evidence that the individual is in imminent danger to himself or herself or someone else.

Stage 2: Establish Rapport and a Working Therapeutic Relationship. Joanne establishes rapport with Theresa on the telephone by listening carefully to her, validating her concerns, and offering concrete and specific assistance. When the nurse and other members of the crisis team arrive at the home, Joanne stays with Theresa, while her colleague Don begins talking with Billy through his locked bedroom door. Don uses his well-developed interpersonal skills (see Chapter 8) to make a connection with the young man and to convince him to come out of his room and talk face to face. That will require high-level interpersonal skills (see Chapter 8). When it becomes apparent that Billy is not a danger to himself or others, the police leave.

Stage 3: Identify Dimensions of Presenting Problem. Fortunately, when the crisis team speaks with Billy, they learn that he has not done anything to harm himself. He is experiencing a great deal of emotional pain for which he has few words, has lost his sense of meaning in life, and has only a vague plan of shooting himself. He does not have immediate access to a firearm. In his conversation with Don, Billy acknowledges that the loss of his parents was devastating, but it was his brother's death that caused his "world to crash apart."

Stage 4: Explore Feelings and Emotions. Don encourages Billy to talk about his experience and offers him words for the things he is feeling. Eventually, Billy agrees to include his aunt and Joanne in the conversation.

Stage 5: Generate and Explore Alternatives. Billy, Theresa, Don, and Joanne sit around the kitchen table with cups of tea discussing the supports available to the family.

Stage 6: Develop a Plan. Theresa states that praying to the Creator everyday and speaking to a local elder help her to get through many difficult times. Billy says that he will pray with her every day, signs a written safety contract, and agrees to see an intake worker at the mental health centre for an assessment tomorrow. The safety contract specifies a number of things that Billy will do if he begins to feel overwhelmed again, including, praying, talking to Theresa, and calling the crisis line.

Stage 7: Follow-up Plan. Joanne calls Theresa the next afternoon and learns that she and Billy had spent the evening talking and praying together. He had eaten breakfast and showered this morning before attending his appointment at the mental health centre. The intake worker referred Billy to a men's grief support group and was going to speak with the student counselling service at his college to arrange one-to-one counselling.

for children and youth who cannot remain at home, shelters for victims of domestic violence, and short- and long-term accommodations for individuals with serious and persistent mental illness. These settings provide users with food, a place to stay, emotional support, and referrals to other community services.

DISASTER: NATURAL AND HUMAN CAUSED

Natural (eg, hurricanes, tsunamis, and earthquakes) and human-caused disasters (eg, transportation disas-

ters, chemical or nuclear waste spills, and acts of terrorism) can strike with little warning. Often, it is the unpredictability of such events that causes fear, confusion, and a sense of helplessness that can have lasting effects on the health and well-being of those involved. Those exposed to disasters experience multiple stressors, including threats to personal safety and integrity; loss of property; exposure to suffering and death; economic devastation; lawlessness; and social disorganization. By definition, disasters overwhelm institutions, health care, and social services and require from months to years for both individuals and communities

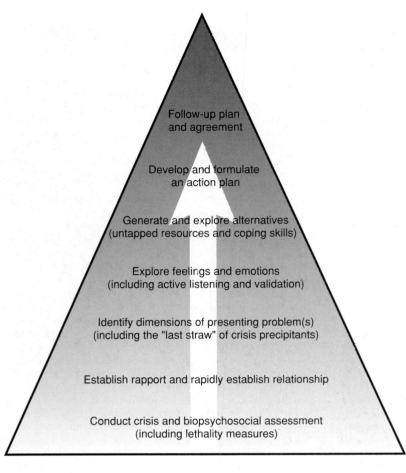

FIGURE 34.7 Robert's Seven-Stage Crisis Intervention Model (1991).

to recover (Fullerton, Ursano, Norwood, & Holloway, 2003).

> ⬟ **KEY CONCEPT Disaster** is a sudden, overwhelming, and catastrophic event that causes widespread damage, social disorganization, mass casualties, and human suffering.

Characteristics of Disasters

Disasters are not alike, each is defined by a constellation of characteristics that has implications for surviving individuals and communities. These include natural versus human causation; proximity and degree of personal impact; magnitude and scope; visible end or "low point"; and probability of recurrence (DeWolfe, 2000). Individually and collectively, these characteristics affect the nature, intensity, and duration of the stress associated with a disaster.

Natural Versus Human Causation

The research is not clear as to whether natural or human-caused disasters have a greater impact on the psychological well-being of those affected. What seems to be the case is that there are cognitive, emotional, psychological, and social reactions unique to each (Weisaeth, 1994). In disasters with a human element (eg, suicide bombings and other acts of terrorism, chemical or nuclear spills, or transportation disasters), survivors struggle to come to terms with the deliberate intent to harm and human error. The belief that an event was both senseless and preventable; a sense of betrayal by another human being; and an identifiable agent who is the target of anger and blame can complicate and prolong survivors' recovery period. In Canada, we have seen an example of this delayed healing in the events following the bombing of Air India Flight 182, which occurred on June 23, 1985 over the Atlantic Ocean south of Ireland. All 329 passengers and crew died, including 82 children. The explosion, caused by a bomb planted in checked baggage, was the single largest terrorist attack before those of September 11, 2001 and the largest mass murder in Canadian history. The Canadian government's trial of those accused of the bombing ended in March 2005, with the acquittal of Ripudaman Singh Malik and Ajaib Singh Bagri. The trial lasted almost two decades and cost nearly $130 million. The only person convicted of any involvement in the bombing was Inderjit Singh Reyat, who pled guilty in 2003 to building the explosive device used on Flight 182; he was sentenced to 10 years in jail. Many of the surviving families say publicly that they are still searching for answers and a sense that justice has been done.

In the case of natural disasters, the cause is seen as being without evil intent and beyond human control. Some survivors find it easier to accept that the destruction and loss of life as a random occurrence or an *act of God*. In all disasters, no matter what the cause, individuals' belief in the world as a safe and predictable is irrevocably changed. A central part of the recovery process involves reconstructing a sense of self and a set of beliefs about how the world operates within this new reality.

Degree of Personal Impact

Research evidence consistently demonstrates that the greater the exposure individuals have to a disaster and its effects, the greater the postdisaster response (Solomon & Green, 1992). Injury and death of loved ones, the loss of one's home and belongings, and widespread destruction of one's community all affect an individual's postdisaster response. The complex interaction of grief and trauma exacerbate the effects of each and can prolong recovery (Kohn & Levav, 1990). Individuals directly exposed to the devastation associated with disaster tend to experience more anxiety, depression, sadness, posttrauma symptoms, somatic symptoms, and, in some studies, substance abuse.

Magnitude and Scope of the Disaster

As with degree of personal impact, there is *a dose–response relationship* between the magnitude of devastation and psychological impact. When a disaster destroys an entire community, all semblance of normalcy disappears, and survivors' lives are turned upside down. Not surprisingly, there are higher levels of anxiety, depression, PTSD, somatic symptoms, and generalized distress associated with widespread community destruction (Solomon & Green, 1992). When at least some elements of community life remain intact (eg, schools, churches, or businesses), they serve as a foundation for the recovery process. Social networks establish or re-establish more readily when gathering places remain standing and institutional structures are functional.

Compare, for example, the effects of hurricane Katrina with the ice storm that affected parts of Ontario, Quebec, and New Brunswick in January 1998. Katrina, a category 4 hurricane, made landfall along the Central Gulf Coast near New Orleans, Louisiana on August 29, 2005. Its storm surge soon breached the levee system that protected New Orleans from Lake Pontchartrain, and areas of the city were subsequently flooded. More than 1,100 hundred individuals died in Katrina's wake; whole communities were razed, and thousands of individuals were displaced. Although the Canadian ice storm caused massive power outages lasting for several weeks in some areas, the infrastructure remained intact.

Visible End or "Low Point"

When disasters have a clearly identifiable ending, it signals to survivors that the threat has passed and that the situation has reached its low point. A clear end point enables the community to begin tallying its losses and marks the beginning of the recovery process. When the end point of a disaster is ambiguous (eg, as it was with hurricane Katrina or with the 2005 Canadian National train derailment near Squamish, British Columbia that spilled toxic sodium hydroxide into the Cheakamus River), it may take weeks or months before survivors feel that the disaster is over. In disasters involving chemical or nuclear contamination, the impact period is even more uncertain and protracted because visible evidence of damage (eg, birth defect, increased rates of cancer and other diseases, and implications for the natural environment) may not be apparent for decades (Green & Solomon, 1995). This prolonged impact period with no clear end impedes survivors' recovery.

Probability of Recurrence

When the disaster has a seasonal pattern (eg, forest fires, floods, hurricanes, or tornadoes) survivors may worry that they will be hit again before the season ends. During the *off season*, communities rebuild, vegetation grows back, and visual reminders of the disaster gradually recede, all of which facilitate recovery. When the probability of a recurrence is perceived as high (eg, following earthquakes and floods), recovery can be slowed. For example, aftershocks following an earthquake and media coverage of the increased risk for flooding due to high water tables or overwhelmed sewage systems can keep affected individuals anxious and preoccupied. As well, delays in disaster relief payments or insurance settlements can frustrate survivors and hinder rebuilding.

Individual Survivor Characteristics

Although disasters indiscriminately affect everyone and everything in their path, the experience will be slightly different for every individual. The meaning assigned to the disaster, personality characteristics, worldview, social supports, and spiritual beliefs all affect individuals' appraisals of the situation, their coping abilities, and their recovery. Previous trauma and losses can either enhance coping or compromise it. Well-developed personal coping resources, an intact and dense social network, and timely and adequate disaster relief all greatly assist recovery. In contrast, pre-existing health problems, concurrent stressors, and weak social support all increase vulnerability to the negative effects of disaster (van der Kolk & McFarlane, 1996).

Once again, research findings are inconsistent with regard to who fares worse during a disaster. There is some evidence that individuals in the 40- to 60-year-old range (the so-called *sandwich generation*) may be at higher risk for stress-related illness because of the competing demands of parenting, employment, and caring for aging parents (Green & Solomon, 1995). Although those individuals who are not in long-term relationships may be more vulnerable to some aspects of stress, marital conflict often escalates following a disaster. On the other hand, as the research described in Box 34-6 demonstrates, a distressing event can motivate positive life changes.

Phases of Disaster

Although the experience of disaster is unique to each individual and community, there are some identifiable phases, influenced by interacting elements of the person–environment relationship (DeWolfe, 2000). Disasters may or may not include all of the following.

Warning or Threat Phase

Disasters vary with respect to the amount of warning that communities have before they occur. For instance, earthquakes usually strike without warning, whereas floods and hurricanes may have hours to days of warning. The lack of warning before an impending disaster is associated with greater feelings of vulnerability and lack of control, which may exacerbate subsequent psychological trauma. As well, individuals may feel guilt or blame themselves if they do not respond adequately to warnings and suffer losses as a result.

Impact Phase

Depending on the nature of the disaster, the impact phase can be short or protracted. As well, the greater the magnitude of personal loss associated with the disaster, the greater the psychosocial effects. Typically, individuals are initially immobilized by shock and confusion and cannot fully comprehend what is happening to their world around them. This quickly abates as they turn their attention to the immediate survival needs of themselves and their loved ones.

Rescue or Heroic Phase

During the first minutes and hours of a disaster, the preservation of life and property is paramount. For some individuals, the epinephrine-driven autonomic arousal enables heroic rescue efforts, and altruism is evident among survivors and emergency personnel alike. There are two potentially negative aspects associated with this phase of disaster. The first is that although activity levels may be high, actual productivity is often low. Second, stress impairs cognitive function and the ability to appraise risk, which can result in injury and death.

Remedy or Honeymoon Phase

In the days and weeks following a disaster, government and volunteer assistance may be readily available. The relief of having survived and the camaraderie of sharing a life-threatening experience can draw individuals and communities closer together. When this happens, survivors experience a short-lived sense of optimism that life will soon return to normal.

Inventory Phase

As time passes and the reality of the situation settles in, individuals begin to realize the full impact of their losses and the limits of disaster assistance. At the same time,

---

BOX 34. 6

Research For Best Practice

Positive Responses to Traumatic Events

Davis, C. G., & MacDonald, S. L. Threat appraisals, distress and the development of positive life changes after September 11th in a Canadian sample. *Cognitive Behaviour Therapy, 33*(2), 63–78

THE QUESTION: Does the magnitude of perceived threat and the intensity of resultant emotional distress predict positive life changes?

METHODS: Adults in Ottawa, Ontario were surveyed to determine whether the magnitude of perceived personal threat in response to the terrorist attacks of September 11, 2001 correlated with the intensity of their emotional distress and whether stronger first-day emotional reactions would predict positive life changes.

FINDINGS: Although the participants in this study were not directly harmed by the attacks of September 11th, participants appraised the events as personally threatening and reported feeling significantly distressed. This study found that the higher the appraisal of personal threat and the more distress an individual reported immediately after the attacks, the more likely the individual was to report having made positive life changes (eg, closer to family, refocussed priorities) several weeks later. Initial distress and greater perceived threat also correlated positively with whether people provided help after the disaster. Follow-up data 11 months later revealed significant stability of these positive life changes.

IMPLICATION FOR NURSING: Although stress, crises, and disaster affect all of us, human beings have an innate capacity to rebound and recover from traumatic events. Many trauma experts (eg, Staab, Foa, and Friedman) agree that for most of us, adversity fosters resilience, not psychopathology. Research on individuals with positive responses after a traumatic event indicates that their preferred coping mechanisms are to (1) focus on brief time intervals (eg, think only about the next step); (2) maintain a view of oneself as competent and a view of others as willing and able to provide support; and (3) focus on the current implications of the trauma and to avoid regretting past decisions and actions.

most individuals are suffering the effects of lack of sleep compounded by the enormous demands of moment-by-moment survival. The unrealistic optimism of the honeymoon phase fades into discouragement and fatigue.

Disillusionment Phase

When the immediate danger passes and disaster relief agencies and volunteers begin to leave, survivors may feel abandoned and angry. If parts of a community are not affected by the disaster, they quickly return to *business as usual*, which further discourages and alienates survivors. As well, resentments flare up if survivors believe that they have not received the same amount of assistance or compensation as others. Issues like this foster divisiveness, jealousy, and hostility in communities and undermine community cohesion and support. As disaster survivors begin to accept the loss of life as it was, stressors accumulate in the forms of family conflict, financial hardship, bureaucratic red tape, rebuilding and relocation, and a lack of recreation or leisure time. As the wear and tear take its toll, stress-related health problems emerge.

Reconstruction and Recovery Phase

The postdisaster reconstruction and recovery phase goes on for years. Eventually survivors realize that they are primarily responsible to solve the problems associated with rebuilding their homes, their businesses, and their lives. New buildings and roads serve as permanent reminders of loss. At the point that individuals can begin to see meaning, personal growth, and opportunity in relation to their disaster experience, they are well on the road to recovery.

Individuals and communities recover from disaster at different rates depending on the nature of the disaster and the degree of exposure. This process is never linear or sequential because of the many interacting variables involved. In Canada, all levels of government participate in preparing for and responding to disasters. Health-serving agencies work closely with municipal governments to develop, update, and practice disaster response plans. Because of the vital role that nurses play in health care delivery, nurses make important contributions in every aspect of disaster relief, both here at home and abroad.

CRNE Note

Disasters are defined by a number of interacting factors, including natural versus human causation; proximity and degree of personal impact; magnitude and scope; visible end or low point; and probability of recurrence. Individually and collectively, these factors influence the nature, intensity, and duration of the stress associated with a disaster.

SUMMARY OF KEY POINTS

- Stress occurs when a person–environment relationship is appraised as being unfavourable. Stress responses are simultaneously emotional and physiologic, leading to an innate tendency to act.
- Many personal factors, such as personality patterns, beliefs, values, and commitment to an outcome, interact with environmental demands and constraints that produce a person–environment relationship.
- Within the social network, social support can help a person cope with stress.
- Effective coping can be either problem focussed or emotion focussed. The outcome of successful coping is enhanced health, psychological well-being, and social functioning.
- A crisis is a severely stressful situation that causes exaggerated stress responses. The nursing process is similar for the person experiencing a stress response, except that increased attention is paid to safety issues.
- Disaster is a sudden, overwhelming catastrophic event that causes great damage, destruction, mass casualties, and human suffering that require assistance from all available resources.

CRITICAL THINKING CHALLENGES

1 Compare and contrast Selye's stress response to Lazarus's model of stress, coping, and adaptation.
2 Explain why one individual may experience the stress of losing a job differently from another.
3 Briefly explain the physiologic stress response.
4 A woman at the local shelter announced to her peers that she was returning to her husband because she could see that it was partly her fault that he beat her. Is this an example of problem-focussed or emotion-focussed coping? Justify your answer.
5 After the death of his mother, a 24-year-old single man with schizophrenia moves into an apartment. He continues to take his medication but feels sad about his mother's death. He is not adjusting well to living alone and tells his nurse that he no longer wants to go to work. In tears, he admits that he is lonely and can no longer manage the day-to-day demands of his apartment. The nurse generates the following nursing diagnosis: Ineffective Coping related to inadequate support system. Develop a plan of care for this young man.
6 Define *stress*, *crisis*, and *disaster*. Compare and contrast each of these to a psychiatric emergency.
7 Identify Worden's (1991) tasks of mourning and discuss the nurse's role in relation to them.
8 You are a nurse working with a mobile, mental health crisis team. An elderly woman calls to say that she has just been robbed at knifepoint on her way home from shopping. How would you proceed with assessing this patient?

WEB LINKS

www.tc.unl.edu This site offers a review of the principles of stress management.

www.stress-management-isma.org The International Stress Management Association seeks to advance the education of professionals and students and to facilitate methodically sound research in several professional interdisciplinary stress management fields.

www.isma.org.uk This is the United Kingdom home page of the International Stress Management Association (ISMA). ISMA is a leading professional body for stress management. Its website has articles from its journal.

www.icn.ch This website includes the International Council of Nurses position statement on Nurses and Disaster Preparedness.

www.pep.bc.ca This website contains a 26-step *to-do list* for emergency preparedness published by the government of British Columbia.

http://www.yorku.ca This website contains a report, *Ethics and SARS: Learning Lessons from the Toronto Experience*, by a working group of the University of Toronto Joint Centre for Bioethics and discusses ethical concerns that nurses face during crisis and disaster situation, including the duty to care.

MOVIES

Schindler's List: 1993. The film presents the true story of Oskar Schindler, a member of the Nazi party, womanizer, and war profiteer, who saved the lives of more than 1,000 Jews during the Holocaust. The movie shows how during long periods of political turmoil and terror, life can become somewhat normalized. Yet, fear underlies people's daily lives. Crises erupt at different times during the very long period of chronic stress.

VIEWING POINTS: Differentiate the periods of chronic stress from crisis in this film. Observe the reactions of different characters under stress. Is the behaviour different from what you would expect? Observe your own feelings throughout the movie. Did you experience stress?

Outbreak: 1995. In this film, Col. Sam Daniels, an infectious disease specialist, is called to Zaire to study the outbreak of a deadly illness. He finds a virus that spreads so quickly it could wipe out an entire nation in just a few weeks.

VIEWING POINTS: Although this movie is a work of fiction, its message takes on new meaning in the current era of SARS, Ebola virus, and avian influenza A (H5N1). During disasters, decision makers need to balance individual freedoms against the common good. Identify some of the ethical issues related to quarantine. What do nurses and other health professionals need to consider as they balance their own personal safety against the duty to treat the sick?

Paradise Road: 1997. Based on a true story, this movie chronicles the experiences of a group of women from different countries and social levels in a Japanese concentration camp. Adrienne Pargiter, a graduate of the Royal Academy of Music, organizes a vocal band in spite of their captors' resistance.

VIEWING POINTS: Resilience refers to human capacity to adapt and even thrive in the face of adversity and trauma. What factors contributed to the women's resilience in this film? At what points in the story did the different women transcend from victim to survivor?

REFERENCES

Aguilera, D. C. (1998). *Crisis intervention: Theory and methodology*, St. Louis: Mosby.

American Psychiatric Association. (1980). *Diagnostic and statistical manual of mental disorders* (3rd ed.). Washington, DC: Author.

American Psychiatric Association (APA). (2000). *Diagnostic and statistical manual of mental disorders* (4th ed., Text revision). Washington, DC: Author.

Birmes, P., Hatton, L., Brunet, A., & Schmitt, L. (2003). Early historical literature for post-traumatic symptomatology. *Stress and Health, 19*, 17–26.

Cannon, W. B. (1939). *The wisdom of the body.* New York: WW Norton.

Caplan, G. (1961). *An approach to community mental health.* New York: Grune & Stratton.

Carpenito-Moyet, L. (2004). *Nursing diagnosis: Application to clinical practice* (10th ed.). Philadelphia: Lippincott Williams & Wilkins.

Center for the Advancement of Health. (2003). *Report on bereavement and grief research.* Retrieved December 7, 2005, from http://www.cfah.org/pdfs/griefreport.pdf.

Clegg, A. (2001). Occupational stress in nursing: A review of the literature. *Journal of Nursing Management, 9*(2),101–106.

Coyne, J. C., & Holroyd, K. (1982). Stress, coping and illness: A transactional perspective. In T. Milton, C. Green, & R. Meagher, *Handbook of clinical health psychology* (pp. 103–127). New York: Plenum Press.

Davis, C. G., & Macdonald, S. L. (2004). Threat appraisals, distress and the development of positive life changes after September 11th in a Canadian sample. *Cognitive Behaviour Therapy, 33*(2), 68–78.

DeWolfe, D. J. (2000). *Training manual for mental health and human service workers in major disasters* (2nd ed.). Rockville, MD: Substance Abuse and Mental Health Services Administration (DHHS/PHS).

Dimsdale, J. E. (1988). A perspective on Type A behavior and coronary disease. *New England Journal of Medicine, 318*(2), 110–112.

Dohrenwend, B. S., & Dohrenwend, B. P. (1974). *Stressful life events: Their nature and their effects.* New York: Wiley & Sons.

Dohrenwend, B. P., & Shrout, P. E. (1985). "Hassles" in the conceptualization and measurement of stress variables. *American Psychologist, 40*(7), 780–785.

Everly, G. S., & Mitchell, J. T. (1999). *Critical incident stress management: A new era and standard of care in crisis intervention* (2nd ed.). Ellicott City, MD: Chevron.

Felitti, V. J., Anda, R. F., Nordenberg, D., Williamson, D. F., Spitz, A. M., et al. (1998). Relationship of childhood abuse and household dysfunction to many of the leading causes of death in adults: The

Adverse Childhood Experiences (ACE) Study. *American Journal of Preventive Medicine, 14*(4), 245–258.

Flannery, R, B., & Everly, G. S. (2000). Crisis intervention: A review. *International Journal of Emergency Mental Health, 2*(2), 119–25.

Folkman, S., & Lazarus, R. S. (1991). The concept of coping. In A. Monatand & R. S. Lazarus (Eds.), *Stress and coping: An anthology* (3rd ed.) (pp. 209–227). New York: Columbia University Press.

Friedman, M., & Rosenman, R. (1974). *Type A and your heart.* New York: Knopf.

Fullerton, C. S., Ursano, R. J., Norwood, A. E., & Holloway, H. H. (2003). Trauma, terrorism, and disaster. In R. J. Ursano, C. S. Fullerton, & A. E. Norwood (Eds.), *Terrorism and disaster* (pp. 1–20). Cambridge, MA: Cambridge University Press.

Gilligan, C. (1994). Joining the resistance, psychology, politics, girls and women. In M. Berger (Ed.), *Women beyond Freud: New concept of feminine psychology* (pp. 99–145). New York: Brunner Mozel.

Glaser, R., Rice, J., Sherridan, J., & Fertel, R. (1987). Stress-related immune suppression: Health implications. *Brain, Behavior and Immunity, 1*(1), 7–20.

Green, B. L., & Solomon, S. D. (1995). The mental health impact of natural and technological disasters. In J. R. Freedy, & S. E. Hobfoll (Eds.), *Traumatic stress: From theory to practice.* New York: Plenum Press.

Guyton, A. C., & Hall, J. E. (2000). *Textbook of medical physiology* (10th ed.). Philadelphia: WB Saunders.

Hall, M. J., Norwood, A. E., Ursano, R. J., & Fullerton, C. S. (2003). The psychological impacts of bioterrorism. *Biosecurity & Bioterrorism, 1*(2), 139–144.

Harper, D. (2001). *Online etymology dictionary.* Retrieved June 30, 2005, from http://www.etymonline.com.

Herman, J. (1992). *Trauma and recovery.* New York: Basic Books.

Holmes, T., & Rahe, R. (1967). The Social Readjustment Patient Scale. *Journal of Psychosomatic Research, 11*(2), 213–218.

Hoven, C. W., Duarte, C. S., Mandell, D. J. (2003). Children's mental health after diagnostics: The impact of the World Trade Center attack. *Current Psychiatry Reports, 5*(2) 101–107.

Jones, F., & Kinman, G. (2001). Approaches to studying stress. In F. Jones & J. Bright (Eds.), *Stress, myth, theory and research* (pp. 17–45). Harlow, UK: Prentice-Hall.

Jones, M. C., & Johnston, D. W. (2000). Reducing distress in first level and student nurses: A review of the applied stress management literature. *Journal of Advanced Nursing, 32*(1), 66–74.

Kendler, K. S., Neale, M. C., Kessler, R. C., Heath, A. C., & Eaves, L. G. (1992). Major depression and generalized anxiety disorder. Same genes, (partly) different environments. *Archives of General Psychiatry, 49*(9), 716–722.

Kessler, R. C., Sonnega, A., Bromet, E., Hughes, M., & Nelson, C. B. (1995). Posttraumatic stress disorder in the National Comorbidity Survey. *Archives of General Psychiatry, 52*(12), 1048–1060.

Kindlen, S. (2003). Injury and illness. In S. Kindlen (Ed.), *Physiology for health care and nursing* (2nd ed.). Edinburgh, UK: Churchill Livingstone.

Kinzbrunner, B. M., Weinreb, N, J., & Policzer, J. S. (2002). *End of life care.* New York: McGraw-Hill.

Kobasa, S. C. (1979). Stressful life events, personality and health: An inquiry into hardiness. *Journal of Personality and Social Psychology, 37*(1), 1–11.

Kohn, R., & Levav, I. (1990). Bereavement in disaster: An overview of the research. *International Journal of Mental Health, 19*(2), 61–76.

Kulka, R. A., Schlenger, W. E., Fairbank, J. A., Hough, R. L., Jordan, B. K., Marmar, C. R., & Weiss, D. S. (1990). *Trauma and the Vietnam War generation: Report of findings from the National Vietnam Veterans Readjustment Study.* New York: Brunner/Mazel.

Lazarus, R. (1991). *Emotion and adaptation.* New York: Oxford University Press.

Lazarus, R. S. (1998). *The life and work of an eminent psychologist: An autobiography of Richard S. Lazarus.* New York: Springer.

Lazarus, R. S. (1999). *Stress and emotion: A new synthesis.* New York: Springer.

Lazarus, R. S. (2001). Relational meaning and discrete emotions. In K. R. Scherer, A. Schorr, & T. Johnstone (Eds.), *Appraisal processes in emotion: Theory, methods, research* (pp. 37–67). New York: Oxford University Press.

Lazarus, R. S., DeLongis, A., Folkman, S., & Gruen, R. (1985). Stress and adaptation outcomes: The problem of confounded measures. *American Psychologist, 40*(7), 770–779.

Lazarus, R., & Folkman, S. (1984). *Stress, appraisal and coping.* New York: Springer.

Lindemann, E. (1944). Symptomatology and management of acute grief. *American Journal of Psychiatry, 151*(6 Suppl), 155–160.

Lindemann, E. (1956). The meaning of crisis in individual and family. *Teachers College Record, 57,* 310.

Lui, L. Y., Coe, C. L., Swenson, C.A., Kelly, E. A., Kita, H., & Busse, W. W. (2002). School examinations enhance airway inflammation to antigen challenge. *American Journal of Critical Care Medicine, 165*(8), 1062–1067.

McEwen, B. S. (1998). Protective and damaging effects of stress mediators. *New England Journal of Medicine, 338*(3), 171–179.

Majer, J. M., Jason, L. A., Ferrarie, J. R., Venable, L. B., & Olson, B. D. (2002). Social support and self-efficacy for abstinence: Is peer identification an issue? *Journal of Substance Abuse Treatment, 23*(3), 209–215.

Malone, J. (1988). The social support and dissupport continuum. *Journal of Psychosocial Nursing and Mental Health Services, 26*(12), 18–22.

Matthies, E., Höger, R., & Guski, R. (2000). Living on polluted soil: Determinants of stress symptoms. *Environment and Behavior, 32*(2), 270–286.

McCloskey, J., & Bulechek, G. (2000). *Nursing interventions classification* (NIC) (3rd ed.). St. Louis: Mosby–Year Book.

Miller, J. (1994). Women's psychological development connections, disconnections, and violations. In M. Berger (Ed.), *Women beyond Freud: New concept of feminine psychology* (pp. 79–97). New York: Brunner Mozel.

Miller, R. A., & Rahe, R. H. (1997). Life changes scaling for the 1990s. *Journal of Psychosomatic Research 43*(3), 279–292.

North American Nursing Diagnosis Association (NANDA). (2005). *NANDA nursing diagnoses: Definitions and classification, 2005–2006.* Philadelphia: Author.

Rando, T. (1993). *Treatment of complicated mourning.* Champaign, IL: Research Press.

Roberts, A. R. (1991). Conceptualizing crisis theory and the crisis model. In A. R. Roberts (Ed.), *Contemporary perspectives on crisis intervention and prevention* (pp. 3–17). Englewood Cliffs, NJ: Prentice-Hall.

Roberts, A. R. (2000). *Crisis intervention handbook: Assessment, treatment, and research* (2nd ed.). New York: Oxford University Press.

Roberts, K. F., & Berry, P. H. (2002). Grief and bereavements. In K. K. Kuebler, P. H. Berry, & D. E. Heidrich (Eds.), *End of life care: Clinical practice guidelines,* (pp. 53–63). Philadelphia: WB Saunders.

Rotter, J. B. (1966). Generalized expectancies for internal versus external control reinforcement. *Psychological Monographs, 80* (whole no. 609).

Saddock, B. J., & Saddock, V. A. (2003). *Kaplan & Saddock's synopsis of psychiatry* (9th ed.). Philadelphia: Lippincott Williams, & Wilkins.

Sapolsky, R. M. (2004). *Why zebras don't get ulcers* (3rd ed.). New York: Henry Holt.

Schachter CL, Stalker CA, & Teram E. (2001). *Handbook on sensitive practice for health professionals: Lessons from women survivors of sexual abuse.* Ottawa: Family Violence Prevention Unit, Health Canada. Available at: http://www.phac-aspc.gc.ca.

Schaefer, C., Coyne, J., & Lazarus, R. (1982). The health-related functions of social support. *Journal of Behavioral Medicine, 4*(4), 381–406.

Schnurr, P. P., & Green, B. L. (Eds.). (2004). Trauma and health: Physical health consequences of exposure to extreme stress. Washington, DC: American Psychological Association.

Segerstrom, S. C., & Miller, G. E. (2003). Psychological stress and the immune system in humans: A meta-analytic view of 30 years of inquiry. *Psychological Bulletin 130*(4), 601–630.

Selye, H. (1956). *The stress of life*. New York: McGraw-Hill.

Selye, H. (1974). *Stress without distress*. Philadelphia: JB Lippincott.

Selye, H. (1980). The stress concept today. In I. L. Kutash, L. B. Schlesinger, et al. (Eds.), *Handbook on stress and anxiety* (pp. 127–143). San Francisco: Jossey-Bass.

Semmer, N. K., McGrath, J. E., & Beehr, T. A. (2005). Conceptual issues in research on stress and health. In C. L. Cooper (Ed.), *Handbook of stress medicine and health* (2nd ed.) (pp. 1–43). Boca Raton, FL: CRC Press.

Solomon, S. D., & Green, B. L. (1992). Mental health effects of natural and human-made disasters. *PTSD Research Quarterly, 3*(1), 1–8.

Springs, F. E., & Friedrich, W. N. (1992). Health risk behaviors and medical sequelae of childhood sexual abuse. *Mayo Clinic Proceedings, 67*(6), 527–532.

Stanley, R. O., & Burrows, G. D. (2005). The role of stress in mental illness: The practice. In C. L. Cooper (Ed.), *Handbook of stress medicine and health* (2nd ed.) (pp. 87–100). Boca Raton, FL: CRC Press.

Sterling, P., & Eyer, J. (1988). Allostasis: A new paradigm to explain arousal pathology. In S. Fisher & J. Reason (Eds.), *Handbook of life stress, cognition and health* (pp. 629–649). New York: John Wiley & Sons.

Stuart, T. D., & Garrison, M. E. (2002). The influence of daily hassles and role balance on health status: A study of mothers of grade school children. *Women's Health, 36*(3), 1–11.

van der Kolk, B. A., & McFarlane, A. (1996). The black hole of trauma. In B. A. van der Kolk, A. McFarlane, & L. Weisaeth (Eds.), *Traumatic stress: The effects of overwhelming experience on mind, body, and society* (pp. 3–23). New York: Guilford Press.

Weisaeth, L. (1994). Psychological and psychiatric aspects of technological disasters. In R. J. Ursano, B. G. McCaughey, & C. S. Fullerton (Eds.) *Individual and community responses to trauma and disaster: The structure of human chaos*. New York: Cambridge University Press.

Wolfelt, A. D. (1999). Dispelling 5 common myths about grief. Retrieved August 10, 2005, from http://www.womensweb.ca/mental/suicide/myths2.php.

Worden, J. W. (2003). *Grief counseling and grief therapy: A handbook for the mental health practitioner* (electronic edition). New York: Brunner-Routledge.

Worden, J. W. (1991). Grief counselling and grief therapy (2nd ed). New York: Springer.

Wright, L. (1988). The Type A behavior pattern and coronary artery disease. *American Psychologist, 43*(1), 2–14.

Yeager, K. R. & Roberts, A. R. (2003). Differentiating among stress, acute stress disorder, crisis episodes, trauma, and PTSD: Paradigm and treatment goals. *Brief Treatment and Crisis Intervention, 3*(1), 145–167.

For challenges, please refer to the **CD-ROM** in this book.

Management of Aggression and Violence

Sandy Harper-Jaques and Marlene Reimer

LEARNING OBJECTIVES

After studying this chapter, you will be able to:

- Explore feelings about the experience and expression of anger.
- Discuss the biopsychosocial factors that influence the expression of aggressive and violent behaviour.
- Discuss biopsychosocial theories used to explain anger, aggression, and violence.
- Identify behaviour or actions that escalate and de-escalate violent behaviour.
- Recognize the risk for "nurse abuse" (attacks on nurses).
- Generate options for responding to the expression of anger and violent behaviour in clinical nursing practice.
- Apply the nursing process to the management of anger, aggression, and violence in clients.

KEY TERMS

catharsis • emotional circuit • restraint • seclusion • violence

KEY CONCEPTS

aggression • anger • assertiveness

Definitions of anger, aggression, and violence vary and are influenced by experience, beliefs, culture, and gender. Individuals and groups develop their own views of acceptable and unacceptable words and actions. Theoretic distinctions can be made among anger, aggression, and violence, but clinically, their expression may be blurred. Each phenomenon may occur alone or in combination with one or both of the others.

Most societies develop norms for acceptable and unacceptable behaviour; some groups at some point in time have accepted all forms of aggression and violence. Today, images and stories about aggressive and violent acts throughout the world are rampant. Like other places, health care settings are not immune to expressions of anger, aggression, and violence.

In any setting, aggression and violence are a reflection of the values of the individual, family, community, and society. Many people tend to minimize the frequency and severity of aggressive and violent acts; for example, couples who interact violently downplay the severity and effects of the episodes (Belknap, 2003). The expression of anger, aggression, and violence by clients and, sometimes, their families is a tremendous challenge for nurses. This chapter discusses prominent theories about the nature of these phenomena and offers varying, sometimes controversial, models, theories, and evidence, with each discussion attempting to explain the phenomena of anger, aggression, and violence. Clinicians can use each particular model as a basis for assessment, nursing diagnosis, planning, intervention, and evaluation. The chapter also explores how the nurse can apply the nursing process in managing angry, aggressive, or violent clients and in preventing or de-escalating situations that may lead to aggression or violence.

Anger

Anger is "a strong, uncomfortable emotional response to a provocation that is unwanted and incongruent with one's values, beliefs or rights" (Thomas, 1998). Anger is usually described as a temporary state of emotional arousal, in contrast to hostility, which is associated with a more enduring negative attitude (Thomas, 2001) (see Chapter 36). Although anger is portrayed as a bad emotion that always leads to aggression, this is often not the case. Thomas (2001) asserts that the expression of anger may prevent aggression and help to resolve a situation.

Language pertaining to anger is imprecise and confusing. The word *anger* is used to describe a wide range of feelings, from annoyance at having to wait at a red light when in a hurry to a severe emotional reaction to the news that a family member has been physically assaulted. Some of the words used interchangeably with anger include annoyance, frustration, temper, resentment, hostility, hatred, and rage. In addition, the word *angry* is used to describe both a transient emotional state and a personality trait (Thomas, 1993). This imprecision is related to varying beliefs and theories, including the following (Gerloff, 1997; Shannon, 2000):

- Anger is a fixed quantity that is either dammed up or floods the system.
- Anger and aggression are linked. Anger is the feeling, and aggression is the behaviour; both result from an innate instinct.
- Anger is the instinctive response to a threat or to the inability to meet goals or desires.
- If outward expression of anger is blocked, then it turns inward and develops into depression.
- Anger arises out of feelings of hurt or anxiety.

Box 35-1 invites the reader to explore variations in responses to anger through the use of an experiential exercise.

> **KEY CONCEPT Anger** is an affective state experienced as the motivation to act in ways that warn, intimidate, or attack those who are perceived as challenging or threatening. It occurs when there is a threat, delay, thwarting of a goal, or conflict between goals.

EXPERIENCE OF ANGER

Anger offers a signal to those experiencing it that something is wrong in themselves, others, or their relationships with others (Lerner, 2001). Thomas (2001) suggests that the experience of anger can serve as a warning that demands are greater than available resources. If one accepts that human beings are rational and capable of appraising situations, the subjective component of the experience of anger becomes an important area for study. With the exception of anger that arises from specific neurologic damage or biochemical imbalances, angry episodes can be viewed as

---

BOX 35.1

Self-Awareness Exercise: Personal Experience of Anger

People's reactions differ when they experience anger. Some people report a sense of power, control, and calmness different from their usual experience; others report feeling shaky, tearful, and on the verge of collapse. Still others describe physical sensations of nausea and dizziness.

Think about the last time that you felt angry. List the body sensations and other emotions that you experienced. Now ask a friend, colleague, or family member to do the same. Compare lists. What are the similarities and differences between you? How will awareness of these differences help you in your clinical practice?

Table 35.1	Styles of Anger Expression	
Style	**Characteristic**	**Gender Socialization**
Anger suppression	Emphasizing the need to keep angry feelings to oneself	In North America, girls are discouraged from expressing anger.
Anger expression	Expressing anger in an attacking or blaming way	In North America, boys are encouraged to express their anger, to not "lie down" or "give in" to others.
Anger discussion	Discussing the anger with a friend or family member Approaching a person with whom one is angry and discussing the concern directly	Popular and professional literature offers techniques in assertive expression.

social events (Thomas, 1998). The meaning of angry episodes develops from the beliefs held about anger and the interpretation given to the episode (Shannon, 2000). According to Ellis (1977), people choose to experience anger, basing this choice on the related thinking processes. Following Ellis's model, the thinking process would be as follows:

- I wanted something.
- I didn't get what I wanted, and I feel frustrated.
- It's awful not to get what I want.
- Others should not frustrate me.
- Others are bad for frustrating me.
- Bad people should be punished.

The experience of anger is a normal human emotion; it is the inappropriate expression of anger that may be threatening to the self or others.

EXPRESSION OF ANGER

Difficulties in expressing anger have often been associated with psychiatric health problems. Anger turned inward has been implicated as a contributor to mood disorders, especially depression (Koh, Kim, & Park, 2002). Several medical disorders have also been positively correlated with the suppression of anger, including essential hypertension, migraine headaches, psoriasis, rheumatoid arthritis, and Raynaud's disease.

Behavioural expressions of anger vary. In the 19th century, anger was viewed as sinful, dangerous, and destructive—an emotion to be contained, controlled, and denied. This negatively viewed emotion was to be dominated and conquered, and the ideal family life was free of anger. Husbands and wives were discouraged from expressing anger toward each other; parenting manuals promoted the suppression of anger in children (Thomas, 1993). This view contributed to the development of a powerful taboo against feeling and expressing anger. People who have accepted this persistent taboo may have difficulty even knowing when they are angry (Shannon, 2000).

During the early 20th century, Freud and Lorenz advocated the use of **catharsis**, the release of ideas through talking and expressing appropriate emotion, in the expression of anger. However, catharsis has been shown empirically to promote, not reduce, anger (Thomas, 1998).

In recent years, interest has arisen in developing communication techniques that promote the expression of anger in nondestructive ways (Gerloff, 1997; Shannon, 2000). These varying beliefs have added to the confusion about anger. Differences in expectations about how men and women should express anger also contribute to the confusion. Table 35-1 gives examples of different styles of anger expression.

Varying beliefs about appropriate ways to express anger become apparent when a client and a nurse enter into a therapeutic relationship. Genetic predisposition, emotional development during infancy and childhood, and family environment influence the variations in expression for both the nurse and the client (Thomas, 2001). Previous experiences in expressing anger and reactions from others will also be influential.

Aggression and Violence

In this chapter, aggression is defined as "verbal statements against someone that are intended to intimidate or threaten the recipient." **Violence** is defined as "a physical act of force intended to cause harm to a person or an object and to convey the message that the perpetrator's point of view is correct and not the victim's" (Harper-Jaques & Reimer, 1992, p. 312). Aggression and violent behaviour reflect a continuum from suspicious behaviour to extreme actions that threaten the safety of others or result in injury or death (see Table 35-2 for examples).

> **KEY CONCEPT Aggression** is verbal statements that are intended to threaten.

Aggression does not occur in a vacuum. Both the client and the context must be considered. Therefore, a multidimensional framework (Fig 35-1) is essential for understanding and responding to these behaviours (Morrison & Carney Love, 2003).

Table 35.2	Examples of Behaviours on the Continuum of Aggression and Violence	
Term	**Description**	**Clinical Example**
Suspicious behaviour	Hypervigilance to external cues Attends more to cues that fit with current thinking patterns	A female client with a long history of delusional disorder (including the belief that her family wants to "lock her away") questions the motives of a community mental health nurse when she asks the client about her medication regimen. The client misperceives the nurse's inquiry as evidence of a conspiracy against her.
Verbal hostility	Verbal comments that are sarcastic, coercive, or blaming and often expressed with the intent to hurt others May be used as a means of getting attention or inviting others to take action	When administration of PRN medication is delayed, a client's mother comes to the nursing station and starts to yell. She states that the nurses don't care, are lazy, and should work harder. She also demands that someone give her daughter the analgesic. (Family members have been reported to use demanding behaviours to have needs met.)
Physical violence	Act of striking out, throwing an object, pushing, etc., that appears to be intended to cause harm to a person or object	A young man attending a mental health clinic has missed his appointment with the psychiatrist. When he finds out he cannot be scheduled to see her for another week, he yells at the receptionist, bangs his fist on the desk, and then picks up a chair and throws it at her.

Models of Anger, Aggression, and Violence

This section discusses some of the main theoretical explanations for anger, aggression, and violence. A single model or theory cannot fully explain anger, aggression, and violence; instead, the nurse must choose the most useful models for explaining a particular client's experience and for planning interventions.

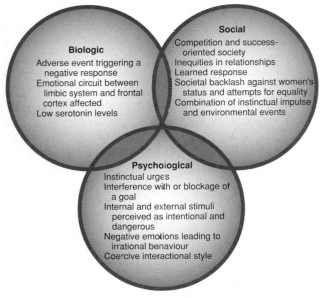

FIGURE 35.1 Biopsychosocial etiologies for clients with aggression.

BIOLOGIC THEORIES

From a biologic viewpoint, a tendency to have more frequent angry episodes may partially originate from developmental deficits, anoxia, malnutrition, toxins, tumours, or neurodegenerative diseases or trauma affecting the brain. Clients with a history of damage to the cerebral cortex are more likely to exhibit increased impulsivity, decreased inhibition, and decreased judgment than are those who have not experienced such damage. The interaction of neurocognitive impairment and social history of abuse or family violence increases the risk for violent behaviour (Scarpa & Raine, 1997). The odds of violent behaviour also increase when separate risk factors, such as schizophrenia, substance abuse, and not taking prescribed medications, coexist in the same person (Citrome & Volavka, 1999). Before reading additional research evidence, try the anger exercise in Box 35-2. What does daily experience suggest about biologically based aspects of the experience and expression of anger?

Cognitive Neuroassociation Model

The cognitive neuroassociation model is one explanation for the interplay of biologic and other internal influences (Berkowitz, 1989; Miller, Pedersen, Earleywine, & Pollock, 2003). Initially, an adverse event (such as pain from tripping over a skateboard) triggers a primitive negative response. Peripheral receptors communicate this response to the spinal cord through the spinothalamic tract to the hypothalamus. The hypothalamus, which synthesizes input from throughout the nervous system, is part of the limbic system. The limbic system mediates primitive emotion and basic drives to produce behaviours for survival, such as the fight-or-flight response (Harper-Jaques & Reimer, 1992).

At first, cognitive appraisal is not involved in these rudimentary feelings of fear or anger, other than identifying the stimulus as aversive; however, higher-order cognitive processing quickly begins to take over. The brain associates the current experience of physiologic sensations with memories, ideas, and previously experienced expressive-motor reactions. It then interprets and differentiates the experience. Depending on prior experience and associations, the response may be intensified or suppressed. It is this latter part of the process that is most amenable to modification through psychotherapy.

CRNE Note

In caring for a potentially aggressive client, the nurse should recognize that biochemical imbalance contributes to the person's inability to control aggression.

Neurostructural Model and the Emotional Circuit

The brain structures most frequently associated with aggressive behaviour are the limbic system and the cerebral cortex, particularly the frontal and temporal lobes. Harper-Jaques and Reimer (1992) propose the phrase **emotional circuit** to describe the interrelationship between the emotional processes of the limbic system and the neurocognitive processes of the frontal

lobe and other parts of the cortex. They hypothesize that the functioning of this system determines the meaning a person gives to a particular situation. Thus, meaning is influenced by physiologic capability to perceive incoming messages, prioritize among competing stimuli, and interpret these messages in relation to stored ideas, beliefs, and memories.

Neurochemical Model and Low Serotonin Syndrome

In recent decades, knowledge has exploded about the complex role of neurotransmitters in human behaviour. Serotonin is a major neurotransmitter involved in mood, sleep, and appetite. Low serotonin levels are associated not only with depression, but also with irritability, increased pain sensitivity, impulsiveness, aggression, vulnerabilty to alcoholism, and obsessive-complusive behaviour (Heinz, Mann, Weinberger, & Goldman, 2001).

Serotonin is sensitive to fluctuations in dietary intake of its precursor, tryptophan, which is found in high-carbohydrate foods. Once it crosses the blood–brain barrier, tryptophan is synthesized into serotonin within the 5-hydroxytryptophan (5-HTP) neurons by interaction with the enzyme tryptophan hydroxylase. Normally, the amount of tryptophan available in the plasma is below saturation (ie, below the amount that could be used if available). Tryptophan intake and the availability of binding sites on the plasma proteins affect synthesis of serotonin. Thus, assessing overall dietary intake is relevant, particularly of good tryptophan sources, such as wheat, flour, corn, milk, and eggs. Preliminary research evidence suggests that tryptophan depletion may increase anger levels in individuals already prone to aggressive behaviour (Schmeck et al., 2002).

People with a history of aggressive behaviour have been found to have a lower-than-average level of serotonin. Studies of humans with known aggressive tendencies, such as violent offenders, have repeatedly shown lower-than-average concentrations of 5-hydroxyindoleacetic acid (5-HIAA), the major metabolite for serotonin (Soloff, Lynch, & Moss, 2000) and prefrontal cortex dysfunction (Best, Williams, & Coccaro, 2002). Similarly, the plasma concentration of tryptophan is lower in people with alcoholism who have a history of aggressive behaviour than in people with alcoholism and no such history. Criminals whose acts of violence were committed impulsively have lower levels of 5-HIAA than do criminals whose acts of violence were premeditated. Implusivity and difficulty controlling anger are characteristic of borderline personality disorder, another condition associated with lower than normal serotonin levels (Paris, 2005). Hyperarousal, such as may occur through being constantly vigilant against possible attack (eg, in guerrilla warfare), also may contribute to aggressive behaviour.

This evidence for a biologic component to aggressive behaviour does not mean that only biologic means of treatment can be effective. Feedback between human behaviour and biochemistry is continuous; verbal suggestions and even early life stressors can affect biochemistry, just as biochemistry affects behaviour (Heinz et al., 2001; Pardo, Pardo, & Raichle, 1993). Environmental and learned behaviours influence the type and degree of aggression expressed, even by those for whom there is a biologic component (Soloff et al., 2000).

PSYCHOLOGICAL THEORIES

Several psychological explanations exist for aggressive and violent behaviours. This section discusses psychoanalytic, behavioural, and cognitive theories.

Psychoanalytic Theories

Psychoanalytic theorists view emotions as instinctual urges. They view suppression of these urges as unhealthy and as possible contributors to the development of psychosomatic or psychological disorders (Thomas, 1998). Freud struggled to understand the nature and expression of human aggressive behaviour. In his early works, he linked aggression with libidinal factors; however, this association did not explain destructive actions during wars and armed conflict. In his later writings, Freud identified aggression as a separate instinct, like the sexual instinct. He viewed aggression as an innate human quality that could be expressed when a person was provoked or abused. In doing so, he challenged the commonly held belief that human beings are essentially good.

Freud explained aggressive or violent behaviour as a combination of instinctual impulses and events in the environment that stimulated release of the instinctual urge. Freud's view fostered the use of catharsis. Therapeutic approaches, such as primal scream and nursing interventions that direct the client to "let it out" by pounding a pillow find their origins in this theory (Tavris, 1989; Thomas, 1990). However, recent studies have not shown catharsis to be helpful in reducing anger. Venting can also have negative consequences when the action taken is hurtful to or blaming of others or damages property.

Erich Fromm (1900–1980), an American psychoanalyst best known for his application of psychoanalytic theory to social and cultural problems, believed that animals and humans share a form of aggression he called *benign*. This genetically programmed response was designed as a defense to protect oneself against a threat. The distinction between humans and animals was that human beings could reason. This capability provided them with options that are not available to animals. Thus, unlike animals, human beings are capable of behaving aggressively for reasons other than self-preservation. Fromm (1973) defined aggression in humans as any behaviour that causes or intends to cause damage to another person, animal, or object. Humans may foresee both real and perceived threats. Perceived threats that are based on distorted perceptions may lead to aggressive and violent behaviours; for example, the cognitive and information-processing deficits of clients with psychosis or schizophrenia (see Chapter 17) are frequently implicated in episodes of aggression and violence.

Behavioural Theories

The goal of behaviourists is to predict and control behaviour. Introspection has no role in these theories. One behavioural theory, drive theory, suggests that violent behaviour originates externally. A person experiences anger and acts violently in response to interference with or blocking of a goal. Laboratory experiments and the reality of everyday experience have proved the limitations of this theory (Thomas, 1990). Not all situations in which one's goal is blocked lead to anger or violence.

Another behavioural theory is social learning theory. In his research, Bandura (1973) drew attention to the role of learning and rewards in the expression of anger and violence. He studied interactions between mothers and children. The children learned that anger and aggressive behaviour helped them get what they wanted from their mothers. Children's observation of aggressive behaviour between family members and in their communities fosters a context for learning aggressive behaviour. It may also lead to an assumption that aggressive behaviour is appropriate. According to this view, people learn to be aggressive by participating in an aggressive environment.

Cognitive Theories

Cognitive theorists are interested in how people transform internal and external stimuli into useful information. They emphasize understanding how a person takes new information and fits it into an already developed schema. Beck (1976) proposed that cognitive schema such as judgments, self-esteem, and expectations influence angry responses. In a situation perceived as intentional, dangerous, and unprovoked, the recipient's reaction will be intensified. The person's reaction will be further intensified if he or she views the offender as undesirable. In psychological disorders, cognitive processing may be compromised (Rubinsztein, Sahakian, & Dolan, 2002; Sergi & Green, 2003).

Rational-emotive theory, one type of cognitive theory, considers cognition, affect, and behaviour to be interrelated psychological processes (Ellis, 1977). This theory regards anger as an inappropriate negative emotion because it stems from irrational beliefs. Change is directed at altering irrational beliefs by identifying and working to change them and their associated psychological processes.

SOCIOCULTURAL THEORIES

Western society is characterized by a competitive, success-oriented ideology that values the individual and individual accomplishments over collaboration and a sense of community. Self-esteem, particularly for men, may be based on social and economic status and influence over others and the environment (Thomas, 2003).

The pursuit of status produces inequities in relationships, whereby one person is superior and the other is subordinate. A hazard inherent in the pursuit of status is the view that a person is entitled to have influence and control, and that the "entitled person" has the right to use whatever means necessary to obtain status (Jenkins, 1990). These means may include force or disregarding the rights and needs of others. The entitled person may also begin to consider other people responsible for his or her thoughts, feelings, or actions.

Violence against women is one example of the way in which men have used a belief in entitlement to justify such actions as threatening, hurting, or murdering women. In 2001 the United Nations (UN) Commission on Human Rights issued a resolution on the elimination of violence against women. This resolution implores governments of countries who are members of the UN to develop policies and provide funding for violence prevention and treatment programs. This resolution has provided governments with a rationale to challenge men's position of entitlement. The challenge has evolved from an examination of the status quo and a call for society to view women as equal partners with men. Women now have greater access to education, increased economic independence, and opportunities to control the frequency and number of pregnancies. These changes have led some to suggest that the continuing prevalence of violence toward women (Tajaden & Thoennes, 2000) is a backlash against their increased efforts toward achieving equality.

INTERACTIONAL THEORY

Morrison (1998) challenges research and theories suggesting that aggression and violence are biologically or psychologically based. She asserts that these views lead to excusing the person's behaviour. She proposes that violence among people in psychiatric settings is the same as violence in other settings. Therefore, the client's behaviour should be considered a social problem and responded to on that basis. This challenge is grounded in several studies that examined the interactional style of the aggressive and violent individual. People with interactional styles that were argumentative or coercive were more likely to engage in aggressive or violent interchanges. Such people are often described as having a "chip on their shoulders." Morrison clearly states her view that the antecedent variables (ie, history of violence, psychiatric diagnosis, length of hospitalization) and the mediating variable of interactional style are the primary reasons for the behaviour.

NURSING MANAGEMENT: HUMAN RESPONSE TO ANGER AND AGGRESSION

Aggression and violence often arise from one party's belief that his or her view of a situation is the only correct one. The first party considers other views wrong and in need of changing. A second party's refusal to give in to the view of the first may lead to violence (Capra, 2002). Box 35-3 illustrates such a scenario in the clinical setting.

Clients may use aggression and violence as ways to get what they want. They may resort to violence to force change or to regain or maintain control. Rewards from violence include attention from nursing staff and status and prestige among the client group (Harris & Morrison, 1995). For example, the client who behaves violently is observed more frequently and has more opportunities to discuss concerns with nurses.

Nurses bring their own perceptions and reactions to clinical settings. They respond to the behaviours of the clients and families for whom they care. Clients and

---

BOX 35.3

Clinical Vignette: Paul's Anger

Paul, a new client on the unit, appears to be experiencing auditory hallucinations. The nurse approaches Paul, careful not to invade his personal space, and begins to walk with him. In an attempt to assess his current mental status, the nurse points out that he seems restless and asks if the voices have returned. Paul responds, "They are telling me this place isn't safe. The angel in the corner is signalling to me. She wants me to leave!" Paul starts to walk toward the door. In an attempt to offer an alternative point of view and orient him to the present, the nurse understands that what the client is seeing and hearing are hallucinations. The nurse attempts to increase Paul's feeling of safety by identifying his perceptions as hallucinations and reassuring him of his safety. "No I won't stay and you can't make me." Paul pushes the nurse aside and runs to the door.

What Do You Think?

If you were the nurse in this situation, what would be your next response? How would you acknowledge Paul's concerns and encourage him to stay?

families, in turn, react to nurses (Leahey & Harper-Jaques, 1996). Nurses' beliefs about themselves as individuals and professionals will influence their responses to aggressive behaviours. For example, the nurse who considers any expression of anger or aggression inappropriate will approach an agitated client in a manner different from that used by the nurse who considers agitated behaviour to be meaningful.

The nurse's ability to maintain personal control is challenged when faced with angry, provoking clients. Some clients who are experiencing emotional problems have an uncanny ability to verbally target a nurse's vulnerable characteristics. It is a usual response to become defensive when one feels vulnerable. However, when nurses lose control of their own responses, the potential for punitive interventions or the use of threats or sarcasm is greater. Duxbury (2002) asked clients about their views on inpatient aggression and violence. Clients (N = 80) reported staff factors that they believed contributed to aggression and violence: namely, staff being too controlling and ineffective communication among staff.

Contrary to popular belief, most clients who have mental health problems do not behave aggressively or violently. Nurses in all areas of clinical practice need to understand angry emotions, know how to prevent aggression and violence, and respond assertively. To better prepare themselves to respond to different types of behaviour, many nurses take assertiveness training courses and workshops. Many nursing schools also teach assertiveness. Nurses should understand the phenomena of anger, aggression, and violence as meaningful behaviours that warrant attention, rather than as disruptive behaviours to control.

> ⬟ **KEY CONCEPT Assertiveness** is a set of behaviours and a communication style that is open, honest, direct, and confident. Assertiveness enables the expression of emotions, including anger, in a manner that assumes responsibility. It allows placement of boundaries and prevents acceptance of inappropriate aggression from others.

To develop a means of predicting aggressive and violent behaviours, some researchers have examined demographics, client characteristics, and unit climate. Others have attempted to determine the relationship between medical diagnosis and violence. A third area of inquiry has been the role of the client's history in predicting violence.

Several research reports suggest that particular characteristics are predictive of violent behaviours. Low self-esteem that may be further eroded during hospitalization or treatment may influence a client to use force to meet his or her needs or to experience some sense of empowerment. Many people who have chronic mental health problems "fight" the experience and refuse to accept medical treatment. When admitted to the hospital, they may experience turmoil from both the illness and the anger at the additional loss of control that hospitalization mandates.

Impaired communication, disorientation, and depression have been found to be consistently associated with aggressive behaviour among nursing home residents with dementia (Talerico, Evans, & Strumpf, 2002). Specific diagnoses have not been identified as predictive of violence, although some reports suggest that clients who have reduced impulse control (ie, diagnoses such as schizophrenia, bipolar disorder, organic brain syndrome, brain injury, or attention deficit hyperactivity disorder) are at increased risk for violent episodes (Tasman, 1997).

Predictors of Violence

When assessing a client, his or her history is probably the most important predictor of potential for violence. Important markers include previous episodes of rage and violent behaviour, escalating irritability, intruding angry thoughts, and fear of losing control. Brain injury, substance use or abuse, and temporal lobe epilepsy have also been discussed as possible predictors of violence (Harper-Jaques & Reimer, 1992; Mesulam, 2000). Whether a relationship exists between temporal lobe epilepsy and aggressive behaviour remains a matter of controversy (Citrome & Volavka, 1999). Aggressive behaviour that occurs in the interictal period (ie, between seizures) may also be related to the intense frustration that people who have epilepsy often experience and could lead to violent behaviour. Certain antiepileptic drugs, particularly barbiturates, may contribute to irritability and aggressive behaviour. However, mood-stabilizing medications such as carbamazepine (Tegretol) and divalproex sodium (Depakote) have reduced aggressive behaviour. The nurse should include any history of seizures, current medications, and compliance with pharmacotherapy in client assessments. Some physiologic and behavioural cues to anger are listed in Table 35-3.

An additional assessment option was investigated by Swett and Mills (1997). Shortly after client admission, nurses used the Nurses' Observational Scale for Inpatient Evaluation (NOSIE) to rate clients. The authors report that a high score on the irritability factor of the NOSIE may be useful to clinicians in predicting which clients may be assaultive.

Analysis and Outcome Identification

The nurse analyzes all assessment data across the biologic, psychological, and social domains to understand the dangers that the client's behaviour poses for self or

Table 35.3 Physiologic and Behavioural Cues to Anger	
Internal Signs	**External Signs**
▪ Increased pulse, respirations, and blood pressure ▪ Chills and shudders ▪ Prickly sensations ▪ Numbness ▪ Choking sensations ▪ Nausea ▪ Vertigo	▪ Increased muscle tone ▪ Changes in body posture; clenched fists; set jaw ▪ Changes to the eyes: eyebrows lower and draw together, eyelids tense, eyes assume a "hard" appearance ▪ Lips pressed together to form a thin line, or in a square shape ▪ Flushing or pallor ▪ Goose bumps ▪ Twitching ▪ Sweating

others. The most common nursing diagnoses for clients experiencing intense anger and aggression are Risk for Self-Directed Violence and Risk for Other-Directed Violence (North American Nursing Diagnosis Association [NANDA], 2005). Outcomes focus on aggression control.

Planning and Implementing Interventions

This section emphasizes the development of a partnership between the nurse and client, who work together to find solutions to prevent the recurrence of explosive episodes and to de-escalate volatile situations. However, sometimes the client's condition (eg, advanced dementia) or the situation will prevent the development of a partnership. In such instances, the nurse must take charge. The nurse who intervenes from within the context of the therapeutic relationship must be cognizant of the fit of a particular intervention. The nurse's action is based on his or her response to the client. The client's affective, behavioural, and cognitive response to the intervention provides information about its effects and guides the nurse's next response (Wright & Leahey, 2005) (Fig. 35-2). The following assumptions are important to consider in planning interventions with this client population (Harper-Jaques & Masters, 1994):

- The nurse and client collaborate to find solutions and alternatives to aggressive and violent outbursts.
- Anger is a normal emotion. All people have the right to express their anger. All people have a responsibility to express their anger in a way that does not, emotionally or physically, threaten or harm others.
- In most instances, the person who behaves aggressively or violently can assume responsibility for the behaviour.
- The nurse views the client from the perspective of acknowledging that the client has solved problems before and is only temporarily in need of help.
- The nurse understands that norms for behaviour are created within the context of a particular envi-

ronment and are influenced by the client's history and culture.

Nurses who work collaboratively with potentially violent clients must also keep in mind that they can take certain actions to minimize personal risk:

- Using nonthreatening body language
- Respecting the client's personal space and boundaries
- Positioning themselves so that they have immediate access to the door of the room in case they need to leave the room
- Choosing to leave the door open to an office while talking to a client
- Knowing where colleagues are and making sure those colleagues know where they are
- Removing or not wearing clothing or accessories that could be used to harm them, such as scarves, necklaces, or dangling earrings

When a violent outburst appears imminent or occurs, immediate intervention is required and should be

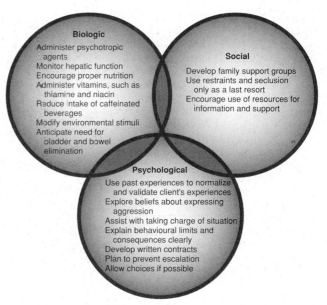

FIGURE 35.2 Biopsychosocial interventions for clients with aggression.

directed by a designated leader (Box 35-4). Preassigning a crisis intervention leader at the change of shift or during a staff meeting can reduce confusion and time-consuming delays during a crisis. The crisis leader assumes responsibility for requesting additional staff, assigning staff duties, and designing and directing interventions (Brasic & Fogelman, 1999; Carpenito-Moyet, 2001).

The nurse who works with potentially aggressive clients does so with respect and concern. The goal is to work with clients to find solutions. The nurse approaches these clients calmly, being mindful to use nonthreatening body language and to avoid violation of boundaries. In dealing with aggression, as in other aspects of nursing practice, the nurse will find that at times the best intervention is silence. It is easy to equate intervention with activity, the sense that "I must do something." But quiet calmness on the nurse's part may be enough to help a client regain control of his or her behaviour and perspective on the situation.

Trying to clarify what has upset the client is important. The nurse can use therapeutic communication techniques to prevent a crisis or defuse a critical situation (see Box 35-5). During daily interactions with clients, nurses intervene in many creative and useful ways. The intervention alone does not serve as the solution; it is the process or art of offering the intervention within the context of the nurse–client relationship that is successful. These interventions will not be successful with all clients all the time. However, it is not the nurse's or client's fault when an intervention is ineffective. The intervention simply did not fit the situation at that particular time.

Biologic Domain

Biologic Assessment

The nurse may encounter clients whose aggressive tendencies have been exacerbated by a biochemical imbalance. However, nurses must recognize that biologic alterations are neither necessary nor sufficient to account for most aggressive behaviours. In taking the client's history, the nurse listens for evidence of industrial exposure to toxic chemicals, missed doses of medications, alcohol intoxication, and withdrawal, or premenstrual dysphoric disorder. Similarly, a history of even minor structural changes resulting in trauma, hemorrhage, or tumour may contribute to lowering a client's anger threshold, and thus requires investigation.

Aggressive episodes that are mainly biologic in origin share certain characteristics (Corrigan, Yudofsky, & Silver, 1993):

- The client has a history or evidence of central nervous system (CNS) lesion or dysfunction.
- Onset of the episode is sudden and relatively unprovoked.
- The outburst is less controlled than those associated with external influences.
- The episode has a clear beginning and ending.
- The client expresses remorse after the episode.

Sensory Impairment. Sensory impairment and difficulties in communicating have been reported as one precipitant of agitation in older adults (Allen, 1999). The most common impairments are hearing loss and reduced visual acuity. A common component of nursing assessment documents is visual and hearing impairments. If a client cannot provide information about his or her hearing and vision, the nurse should ask a family member or friend. If there are impairments, the nurse should ensure that hearing aids are working for clients who use them and assess clients for access to glasses or contact lenses.

Interventions for the Biologic Domain

Administering and Monitoring Medications. Several classes of drugs are used in the management of aggressive behaviour. Important points for the nurse to consider in making decisions about client and family teaching, medication administration, and consultation with physicians and pharmacists are as follows:

- Evidence supports the use of *atypical antipsychotics*, such as clozapine (Clozaril), risperidone (Risperdal), and olanzapine (Zyprexa), in reducing agitation (Chakos & Lieberman, 2001). As with other psychotropic medications, the action of the atypical antipsychotics is not fully understood. It is thought that they block dopamine and serotonin receptors. Extrapyramidal side effects are few, which makes these drugs easier to tolerate than the typical antipsychotics (see the drug profile on risperidone [Risperdal] in Chapter 16 for more information).
- *Selective serotonin reuptake inhibitors* (SSRIs) (eg, fluoxetine [Prozac], paroxetine [Paxil]) are increasingly being used for their antiaggressive effects, as

well as for their antidepressant effects. Their effects on aggressive behaviour usually occur before their effects on depression.

- *β-adrenergic receptor blockers*, such as propranolol (Inderal), may be used for their effect in decreasing the peripheral manifestations of rage that are associated with excitement of the sympathetic nervous system (Silver et al., 2000).
- *Lithium carbonate* has been effective in treating aggressive behaviour associated with brain injury (Burke, Loeber, & Birmaker, 2002).
- *Divalproex sodium* and *carbamazepine* have been shown to reduce aggressive behaviour.
- Psychotropic drugs often interact with antiepileptic and antispasmodic agents, altering pharmacokinetics. For example, chlorpromazine may increase the risk for seizures in clients taking antiepileptic drugs (Fahs, Potiron, Senon, & Perivier, 1999).
- The liver metabolizes most psychotropic drugs (except lithium). The nurse should be alert to possible hepatic dysfunction in clients with a history of alcohol or drug abuse.

Managing Nutrition. Clients with long-standing poor dietary habits (eg, indigent clients, clients with alcoholism) often have deficiencies of thiamine, niacin, and folic acid (Young, 2002). Prolonged use of alcohol can block as much as 70% of thiamine uptake. Increased irritability, disorientation, and paranoia may result. Encouraging clients to eat more whole grains, nuts, fruits, vegetables, organ meats, and milk, instead of "junk" foods, is important. The nurse may need to help clients with obtaining the resources needed to buy and prepare healthier food choices.

Caffeine is a potent stimulant (Lorist & Tops, 2003). Some inpatient psychiatric units have reduced clients' accessibility to coffee and other caffeinated beverages as a means of trying to reduce aggressive behaviour. Results have been mixed.

Psychological Domain

Psychological Assessment

The nurse interested in working with clients to prevent and manage aggressive and violent behaviours should observe them for disturbances in thought processing. Clients may have disordered thoughts for various reasons, including associated psychiatric diagnoses. Some common diagnostic categories that the nurse needs to look for in the client's history are major depressive episode, bipolar disorder, delusional disorders, posttraumatic stress disorder, schizophrenia, and depersonalization. The nurse should also look for a current or past history of substance abuse because clients who abuse drugs, alcohol, or solvents may also exhibit disordered thought processing. Intoxication can trigger erratic thought processes and unpredicted violence. Some form of thought disorder may remain after a person is detoxified, becoming a permanent feature of the person's way of processing ideas. In addition, the nurse must look for acute and chronic medical conditions, such as brain tumour, encephalitis, electrolyte imbalance, and hepatic failure, which may also alter thought-processing (Citrome & Volavka, 1999). The thought processes of greatest interest to the nurse in assessing a client's potential for aggression and violence are perception and delusion.

Perception. Perception is awareness of events and sensations and the ability to make distinctions between them. Clients with disordered perceptions may misinterpret objects or events. Such misperception is called an *illusion*. For example, a client may assume that a person walking toward him or her is going to strike out and thus take action to defend against this illusionary foe. The nurse can explore a client's perception by asking such questions as, "I noticed you were looking very cautious as I approached you. I wonder what you are thinking?"

Delusions. Clients may maintain false or unreasonable beliefs, known as delusions, despite attempts to dissuade them from their point of view. The nurse may not notice any abnormalities in the client's behaviour or appearance until the client begins to discuss delusional ideas. Discussion of the delusions may precipitate aggressive or violent behaviour. To explore these false beliefs, the nurse could, with the client's consent, ask questions respectfully. The nurse should match the pacing of such questions to the client's responses. Attempts to dissuade the client from his or her beliefs are usually ineffective.

Interventions for the Psychological Domain

Psychological interventions help clients gain control over their expression of anger and aggressive behaviour. In some instances, these interventions eliminate the need for chemical (medications) or mechanical restraints. De-escalating potential aggression is always preferable to challenging or provoking a client. Anger control assistance, as set forth by the *Nursing Interventions Classification* (NIC) (McCloskey & Bulechek, 2000), is useful and can prevent deterioration of a client's control of behaviour (Box 35-6). For example, nurses at a psychiatric centre in New York state (Visalli, McNasser, Johnstone, & Lazzaro, 1997) developed an anger management assessment tool and a handout for use by

---

BOX 35.6

Therapeutic Dialogue: The Potentially Aggressive Client

Paul is a 23-year-old client in the high observation area of an inpatient unit. He is pacing back and forth. He is pounding one fist into his other hand. In the past 24 hours, Paul has been more cooperative and less agitated. The behaviour the nurse observes now is more like the behaviour that Paul displayed 2 days ago. Yesterday the psychiatrist told Paul that he would be granted more freedom in the unit if his behaviour improved. The psychiatrist has just seen Paul and refused to change the restrictions on Paul's activities.

Ineffective Approach

Nurse: Paul, I can understand this is frustrating for you.
Paul: How can you understand? Have you ever been held like a prisoner?
Nurse: I do understand Paul. Now you must calm down or more privileges will be removed.
Paul: [voice gets louder] But I was told that calm behaviour would mean more privileges. Now you are telling me calm behaviour only gets me what I have got! Can't you talk to the doctor for me?
Nurse: No, Paul I can't talk to the doctor. [Paul appears more frustrated and agitated as the conversation continues.]

Effective Approach

Nurse: Paul, you look upset (observation). What happened in your conversation with the psychiatrist? (seeking information)

Paul: Yesterday he said calmer behaviour would mean more freedom in the unit. I have tried to be calmer and not to swear. You said you noticed the difference. But today he says "no" to more freedom.
Nurse: Some people might feel cheated if this happened to them. (Validation). Is that how you feel?
Paul: Yeah, I feel real cheated. Nothing I do makes a difference. That's the way it is here and that's the way it is when I am out of the hospital.
Nurse: Sounds like experiences like this leave you feeling pretty powerless. (Validation).
Paul: I don't have any power, anywhere. Sometimes when I have no power I get mean. At least then people pay attention to me.
Nurse: In this situation with your doctor, what would help you feel that you had some power? (Inviting client partnership).
Paul: Well if he would listen to me; if he would read my chart.
Nurse: I am a bit confused by the psychiatrist's decision. I won't make promises that your privileges will change but would it be okay with you if I talk with him?
Paul: That would make me feel like someone is on my side.

Critical Thinking Challenge

- In the first scenario, how did the nurse escalate the situation?
- Compare the first scenario with the second. How are they different?

clients. In a 1-year follow-up study, they reported a reduction in the use of seclusion and restraint and an increase in the successful use of alternative interventions to respond to aggression.

Affective Interventions. Affective interventions are designed to reduce or increase intense emotions that may hinder the client from finding alternatives to the use of aggression or violence (Wright & Leahey, 2005). They include validating, listening to the client's illness experience, and exploring beliefs.

VALIDATING. Clients who experience intense anger and rage can feel isolated. The nurse can reduce the clients feelings of isolation by acknowledging these intense feelings. By drawing on past experience with other client's, the nurse can also reassure the client that others have felt the same way.

LISTENING TO THE CLIENT'S ILLNESS EXPERIENCE. Often, clients and their family members are invited to provide details about past medical treatments, medications, hospitalizations, and therapies. What is overlooked is the experience of the health problem or the experience of interactions with professionals. Inviting clients and families to talk about their previous experience with the health care system may highlight both their concerns and resources. See Box 35-7 for an example of how a nurse uses this intervention to improve a client's care.

EXPLORING BELIEFS. Exploring the client's beliefs about the expression of angry feelings can be useful. Discussion of beliefs that prevent the client from seeking alternate ways of handling distressing emotions and situations may help him or her to take charge of the situation.

Cognitive Interventions. Cognitive interventions are usually those that provide new ideas, opinions, information, or education about a particular problem. The nurse offers a cognitive intervention with the goal of inviting the client to consider other possibilities (Wright & Leahey, 2005). Examples include giving commendations, offering information, providing education, and using thought stopping and contracting.

CRNE Note

The best time to teach the client techniques for managing anger and aggression is when the client is not experiencing the provoking event. Cognitive therapy approaches are useful and can be prioritized according to responses.

GIVING COMMENDATIONS. Often, in clinical settings, the focus becomes "problem saturated" (White, 1988/89) and what the client does well is overlooked. A commendation focuses on the client's behaviour pattern over time and highlights his or her strengths and resources (Limacher & Wright, 2003). For example,

---

BOX 35.7

Clinical Vignette: Mary's Rage

Mary, a 22-year-old single woman, was a regular client at the crisis centre. During previous visits, she came alone or with her mother and demanded immediate attention. This time she comes with her mother. The receptionist groans and rolls her eyes as she describes this family to the new intake nurse. "They are obnoxious. It is best to handle them fast and get them out of here!"

Before the interview, the nurse reviews Mary's extensive file. She notes that on many occasions Mary was aggressive and violent while in the centre. The mother has complained to the local health authority about the centre on at least two occasions.

During the interview, the nurse asks mother and daughter the following questions:
- What was the most useful thing that has happened during previous contacts at the centre?
- What was the least useful thing about previous contacts at the centre?

The family looks surprised to be asked these questions. They state that previous visits were useful only in providing them with written proof that Mary could not work. That information required by the social service agency ensured continuation of Mary's disability checks. Furthermore, Mary and her mother state that they often left the centre feeling that the nurses were not interested in their concerns and believed that if Mary tried harder, her hallucinations would decrease. They add that they often waited 1 to 2 hours to be seen, whereas other clients were seen more quickly. Mary admits that she sometimes made a lot of noise in the waiting room to be seen sooner.

The nurse then asks, "What would need to happen during your visit today to make you feel that coming here was worthwhile?" The mother expresses interest in receiving information about hallucinations and how she could help Mary when she experiences them. Mary says she wants to know how to handle angry feelings.

---

ple, commending a client's decision to request medication or to remove herself from an overstimulating environment highlights the woman's ability to assume responsibility for thoughts and feelings that have previously invited aggressive behaviour.

OFFERING INFORMATION. Nurses can offer information or arrange opportunities for clients to receive information from other professionals. Clients may sometimes become agitated and threaten to harm the nurse because they do not know what is expected of them or they do not remember why they need to be in treatment. The nurse can tell them about unit expectations or the reasons for hospitalization. The nurse can also determine the client's information needs by asking questions. One option in providing information, education, and support is to develop a family support group, which can provide a forum for responding to general concerns and questions at the same time.

In the mental health setting, the nurse must make behavioural limits and consequences clear. When possible, the nurse should match consequences to the client's interests and desires. For example, Jane was slamming doors and banging down dishes in the kitchen of the group home. The nurse approached her to discuss other means of expressing her anger. During the conversation, the nurse reminded Jane that further agitated behaviour would mean that Jane would not participate in a shopping trip planned that day. The trip was important to Jane, so she chose to discuss her concern with the nurse.

PROVIDING EDUCATION. Nurses can offer education to clients and families about various topics. Greater understanding about mental health problems and altered mental status may help to prevent aggression by clarifying misunderstandings. Nurses can also teach clients and families about anger management. Two examples of teaching programs on anger management are provided by Thomas (2001) and Frey and Weller (2000).

THOUGHT STOPPING. In thought stopping, the nurse asks the client to identify thoughts that heighten feelings of anger and invites the client to "turn the thoughts off" by focussing on other thoughts or activities (Burns, 1999). Ideas of other activities include talking to someone, reading, baking, or thinking about a future event.

CONTRACTING. A contract is a written document that the nurse and client develop. The document clearly states acceptable and unacceptable behaviours, consequences and rewards, and the role of both the client and nurse in preventing and managing aggressive behaviour (Morrison, 1998).

Behavioural Interventions.

Behavioural interventions are designed to assist the client to behave differently (Wright & Leahey, 2005). Examples of such interventions include assigning behavioural tasks, using bibliotherapy, interrupting patterns, and providing choices.

ASSIGNING BEHAVIOURAL TASKS. Sometimes, the nurse may assign a behavioural task as a way to help the client maintain or regain control over aggressive behaviours. Behavioural tasks might include writing down a list of grievances that the client will discuss with the nurse or observing how other people take charge of anger and aggression. For example, the nurse may ask the client to observe clients or staff on the unit, people at a shopping mall, or particular movies or television shows to evaluate how other people in real or fictitious situations handle anger.

USING BIBLIOTHERAPY. In bibliotherapy, the nurse may ask the client to read a particular pamphlet or article on anger management. The nurse and client then discuss what the client read to decide which, if any, of the ideas the client can use when angry.

INTERRUPTING PATTERNS. Although clients are not usually aware of it, escalation of feelings, thoughts, and behaviour from calmness to violence usually follows a particular pattern. Disruption of the pattern can some-

times be a useful means for preventing escalation and can help the client regain composure. Nurses can suggest several strategies to interrupt patterns:

- Counting to 10
- Removing oneself from interactions or stimuli that may contribute to increased distress
- Doing something different (eg, reading, exercising, watching television)

PROVIDING CHOICES. When possible, the nurse should provide the client with choices, particularly clients who have little control over their situation because of their condition. For example, the client who is experiencing a manic episode and is confined to her room may have few options in her daily schedule. However, she may be allowed to make choices about food, personal hygiene, and which pajamas to wear.

Social Domain

Social Assessment

The nurse should evaluate factors related to the social domain that may be contributing to aggression or violence in a client. For example, are conditions in the client's home, family, or community leading to aggression or violent episodes? Are financial or legal troubles placing stress on the client that places him or her at risk?

Interventions for the Social Domain

Reducing Stimulation. Theorists have hypothesized that people differ as to the level of stimulation that they need or prefer (Kolanowski et al., 1994). Normally, people adjust their environments accordingly: Some people like their music loud, whereas others want it soft; some people seek out the thrill of high-risk sports, whereas others prefer to be spectators. Within the context of a brain disorder or an unusually restrictive environment, such adjustments may not be within the client's control. The client with a brain injury, progressive dementia, or distorted vision may be experiencing intense and highly confusing stimulation, even though the environment, from the nurse or family's perspective, seems calm and orderly.

For people whose perceptions or thoughts are disordered from brain damage, degeneration, or other thought-processing difficulties, modification of the environment may be one of the main interventions. Likewise, introducing more structure into a chaotic environment can help decrease the risk for aggressive behaviour (Citrome & Volavka, 1999). The nurse can make stimuli meaningful or can simplify and interpret the environment in many practical ways, such as by identifying people or equipment that may be unfamiliar, providing cues as to what is expected (eg, posting signs with directions, putting toothbrush and toothpaste by the sink), and removing or silencing unnecessary stimuli (eg, turning off paging systems). A good place to start is with the NIC environmental management interventions (Box 35-8).

Considering the environment from the client's viewpoint is essential. For instance, if the surroundings are unfamiliar, the client will need to process more information. Lack of a recognizable pattern or structure further taxes the client's capacity to encode information. Appropriate interventions include clarifying the meaning and purpose of people and objects in the environment, enhancing the client's sense of control and the predictability of the environment, and reducing other stimuli as much as possible (Stolley, Gerdner, & Buckwalter, 1999).

BOX 35.8

Environmental Management: Violence Prevention

Definition: Monitoring and manipulating the physical environment to decrease the potential of violent behaviour directed toward self, others, or environment

Activities

- Remove potential weapons (eg, sharps, ropelike objects) from the environment.
- Search environment routinely to maintain it as hazard free.
- Search client and belongings for weapons or potential weapons during inpatient admission procedures as appropriate.
- Monitor the safety of items that visitors bring to the environment.
- Instruct visitors and other caregivers about relevant client safety issues.
- Limit client use of potential weapons (eg, sharps, ropelike objects).
- Monitor client during use of potential weapons (eg, razors).
- Place client with potential for self-harm with a roommate to decrease isolation and opportunity to act on self-harm thoughts, as appropriate.
- Assign single room to client with potential for violence toward others.
- Place client in a bedroom located near a nursing station.
- Limit access to windows, unless locked and shatterproof, as appropriate.
- Lock utility and storage rooms.
- Provide paper dishes and plastic utensils at meals.
- Place client in the least restrictive environment that still allows for the necessary level of observation.
- Provide ongoing surveillance of all client access areas to maintain client safety and therapeutically intervene, as needed.
- Remove other individuals from the vicinity of a violent or potentially violent client.
- Maintain a designated safe area (eg, seclusion room) for client to be placed when violent.
- Provide plastic, rather than metal, clothes hangers, as appropriate.

Adapted from McCloskey, J., & Bulechek, G. (2000). *Nursing interventions classification (NIC)* (3rd ed.). St. Louis: Mosby.

Anticipating Needs. The nurse can anticipate many needs of clients. In assuming responsibility for clients with cognitive impairment, the nurse needs to know when the client last voided and the pattern of bowel movements. Regular toileting routines are not just interventions to prevent incontinence. Similarly, the anticipation of basic needs such as thirst and hunger is important, especially when working with adults or children who cannot readily express their needs. Other discomforts can arise from such conditions as ingrown toenails and adverse medication reactions.

The urge to void can be a powerful stimulus to agitated behaviour. It is not uncommon in a neurologic observation unit to see a young man with a recent head injury become violent just before spontaneously voiding. From a biologic perspective, such a client is probably normally sensitive or even hypersensitive to a full bladder. He probably also has sufficient cognitive function to recognize his need to void. Even some level of social inhibition may be operational in that he recognizes that voiding while lying on his back in bed, with strangers around, is inappropriate. But if he cannot speak or ask for help, he may become increasingly panic stricken. Thrashing around in bed, unable to communicate his need, he may strike out at staff.

The following scenario is the true account of how one graduate student dealt with another common situation. A 75-year-old woman was pacing around the nursing station of a psychogeriatric unit in a nursing home, crying for her mother. Various people spoke kindly to her, trying to explain that her mother was not there. Donna, a graduate student, was studying the wandering behaviours of clients with Alzheimer's disease on the unit. Hypothesizing that there is purpose behind these actions, she walked alongside the woman. After talking a bit with her about the client's mother, Donna asked the client what she would like to do if her mother were there. Gradually the client confided that she needed her mother to help her find the bathroom. Donna then offered to help the woman, walking her to the bathroom. After voiding copiously, the client seemed greatly relieved and settled down.

Using Seclusion and Restraint. Seclusion and restraint are controversial interventions to be used judiciously and only when other interventions have failed to control the client's behaviour. The availability of effective psychotropic medications since the 1950s has reduced the need for these interventions of last resort. Reasons usually cited for using them are to protect the client from injury to self or others, to help the client reestablish behavioural control, and to minimize disruption of unit treatment regimens. The controversy over these interventions and their potential to be applied punitively heightens the need for clear institutional standards for their use. The development and use of clear practice standards can reduce the likelihood that these interventions will be misused (AARN statement, 2003). Lewis (2002) challenges the use of restraint as a primary intervention in forensic settings. Lewis presents nontouch interventions as an alternative to restraint. In contrast, Hibbs (2000) proposes the use of cognitive interventions with clients while they are restrained. These interventions are designed to challenge thought patterns that contribute to aggressive behaviours.

Evaluation is also important in tracking the use of seclusion and restraint. An interdisciplinary approach is reported by Hancock and colleagues (2001) and Morrison and colleagues (2000). Through a process of joint planning and implementation with health professionals from several disciplines, use of restraint was reduced by 83%.

INTERACTIONAL PROCESSES

When the nurse develops a collaborative relationship with the client, he or she can assist the client to not exhibit aggressive behaviour. Johnson, Martin, Guha, and Montgomery (1997) explored the experience of thought-disordered individuals before an aggressive incident. Three themes emerged from interviews with 12 clients who had a diagnosis of a thought disorder and a history of aggressive incidents:

- The strong influence of the external environment
- The use of aggressive behaviours to feel empowered briefly in a situation
- The occurrence of aggressive incidents, despite knowledge of strategies to control anger

The skills the nurse uses in interactions with the client may invite escalation or de-escalation of a tense situation (Morrison, 1998). When the nurse uses communication skills to draw out the client's experience, together the nurse and client coevolve an alternative view of the problem. Some nursing writers (Leahey & Harper-Jaques, 1996; Vosburgh & Simpson, 1993; Wright & Leahey, 2005) have highlighted the importance of attending to notions of reciprocity and circularity when providing nursing care. For example, the nurse explores the meaning of the expression of aggressive behaviours with the client and the client's beliefs about the ability to control aggressive impulses. Or the nurse and client could discuss the effects of the nurse's behaviours on the client and the effects of the client's behaviours on the nurse. Such an approach facilitates the development of an accepting and equal nurse–client relationship. The client is a partner invited to assume responsibility for inappropriate actions. This approach is in contrast to a hierarchical nurse–client relationship that emphasizes the nurse's role in controlling the client's behaviours and defining changes the client must make. In a collaborative approach, the nurse values the client's experience and acknowledges his or her strengths. The nurse asks the client to use those strengths to either maintain or resume control of behaviour.

In Western cultures, events are typically thought of in a linear fashion (Wright & Leahey, 2005). The nurse who uses a linear causality frame of reference to think about client aggression and violence will view the problem as follows:

PACING → leads to → THREATENING
BEHAVIOURS
(Event A)   (Event B)

From this linear perspective, the nurse labels the client as the problem, and other factors assume secondary importance. The nurse might decide, first, to gain control over the client's behaviour. The nurse may base this decision on his or her affective response and previous experience (ie, that threatening behaviours frighten other clients and disrupt the unit routine). The nurse's response to a client's behaviour could be to ask the client to stop yelling, to inform the client that the behaviour is inappropriate, or to suggest the use of medication if the client does not calm down. When one thinks based on linear causality, he or she assumes that event A (pacing) causes event B (threatening behaviour).

When one thinks using circular causality, he or she attempts to understand the link between behaviours and to determine how the threatening behaviour will influence a continuation or cessation of pacing. The nurse who engages in circular thinking will also know that his or her responses to the client will influence the situation. The nurse's responses will be in the domains of cognition (ideas, concepts, and beliefs), affect (emotional state), and behaviour (Tomm, 1980). The nurse will be aware of the reciprocal influences of the nurse's and client's behaviours (Wright & Leahey, 2005). In viewing the situation from a circular perspective, the nurse is interested in understanding how people are involved, rather than in discovering who is to blame. This perspective does not ignore individual responsibility for aggressive or violent actions, and it does not blame the victim. It does invite the nurse to consider the multiple influences on the expression of aggressive and violent behaviour (Robinson, Wright, & Watson, 1994).

RESPONDING TO ASSAULT

In recent years, compelling scientific evidence that violence portrayed in the media is harmful to children has fostered debate about violence and its effects. As a result, television networks have taken both voluntary and legislated actions to limit violent programming during hours when children are generally watching programs. However, these gains in limiting access to violence have been countered by the growing availability of violent video games and websites.

Given today's societal context, it is not surprising that aggression and violence directed toward nurses is often ignored. Aggression and violence by clients can threaten the safety of nurses, other clients, other health care professionals, family members, and visitors. Nurses are the targets of client violence more often than any other health care professional (DelBel, 2003). Family members may also direct aggression and violence toward nurses, especially when they disagree with staff about the client's treatment plan or have been kept waiting for long periods (Duncan, Estabrookes, & Reimer, 2000).

In health care settings, nurses assume an active role in preventing and managing aggressive and violent behaviours. Involuntary (as opposed to voluntary) admission to a psychiatric facility or altered mental status in any setting may constrain the development of a trusting relationship between nurse and client. Nurses are more likely than physicians to be involved with clients who are aggressive or potentially violent because of the amount of time they are in close contact with clients. Nurses also have a major role in setting limits and defining boundaries.

Concern and investigation of assaults on nurses has been growing. In a survey of all registered nurses working in acute care institutions in one Canadian province, 17% reported one or more incidents of physical assault (defined as being spit on, bitten, hit, or pushed) in the last five shifts worked (Duncan et al., 2000). Assaults may occur in situations in which the client perceives the nurse's actions as restricting, controlling, or aggressive (eg, the use of physical restraints) (Morrison, 1998).

The reported rates of assaults on nurses vary greatly. The reported incidence is higher in long-term care, general hospitals, and psychiatric facilities, but nurses who work in ambulatory care settings or community clinics are not immune to assault (Gerberich et al., 2005). Variations in statistics result from differences in definitions of violence, reporting practices, and data collection and analysis, as well as underreporting.

Assaults on nurses by clients can have immediate and long-term consequences. Reported assaults range from verbal threats and minor altercations to severe injuries, rape, and murder. Any assault can produce severe consequences for the victim. Nonphysical violence toward nurses by clients or others can have long-lasting effects, such as post-traumatic stress disorder (Gerberich et al., 2005).

Lanza's research (1992) indicates that nurses experience a wide range of responses (Table 35-4) similar to those of victims of any other type of trauma. However, because of their role as caregivers, nurses may suppress the normal range of feelings after an assault, believing that it is wrong to experience strong feelings of anger and fear in this situation. This belief may relate to the conflict nurses experience in having to care for clients who have hurt them.

Steps can be taken at a clinical and management level to reduce the risk for assaults on nurses by clients. Clinically, nurses must be provided with training programs in the prevention and management of aggressive behaviour. These programs, like courses on cardiopulmonary resuscitation (CPR), impart both knowledge and skills. Like CPR training, the courses need to be made available to nurses regularly so that they have opportunities to reinforce and update what they have learned. Nurses who have participated in preventive training programs as students or as professionals are less likely to be involved in situations with aggressive or violent clients. Those with no training are at greater risk (Brasic & Fogelman, 1999). Less experienced staff with poor communication skills are at higher risk for assault (Wright, Dixon, & Tompkins, 2003).

Table 35.4	Nurses' Responses to Assault	
Response Type	**Personal**	**Professional**
Affective	• Irritability • Depression • Anger • Anxiety • Apathy	• Erosion of feelings of competence, leading to increased anxiety and fear • Feelings of guilt or self-blame • Fear of potentially violent clients
Cognitive	• Suppressed or intrusive thoughts of assault	• Reduced confidence in judgment • Consideration of job change
Behavioural	• Social withdrawal	• Possible hesitation in responding to other violent situations • Possible over-controlling • Possible hesitation to report future assaults • Possible withdrawal from colleagues • Questioning of capabilities by coworkers
Physiologic	• Disturbed sleep • Headaches • Stomach aches • Tension	• Increased absenteeism from somatic complaints

EVALUATION AND TREATMENT OUTCOMES

Treatment outcomes can be considered at both individual and aggregate levels. The desired outcome at the individual level is for the client to regain or maintain control over aggressive or potentially aggressive thoughts, feelings, and actions. *Aggression control* is the term used in the *Nursing Outcomes Classification* (*NOC*) (Moorhead, Johnson, & Maas, 2003). The nurse may observe that the client shows decreased psychomotor activity (eg, less pacing), has a more relaxed posture, speaks more directly about feelings of anger and personal needs, requires less sedating medication, shows increased tolerance for frustration and the ability to consider alternatives, and makes effective use of other coping strategies. Evidence of a reduction in risk factors may include decreased noise and confusion in the immediate environment, calmness on the part of nursing staff and others, and a climate of clear expectations and mutual acceptance and respect. In units, day hospitals, or group home settings, indicators of positive treatment outcomes might be a reduction in the number and severity of assaults on staff and other clients, fewer incident reports, and increased staff competency in de-escalating potentially violent situations.

CONTINUUM OF CARE

Anger and aggression occur in all settings. During periods of extreme aggression, in which people are a danger to themselves or others because of a mental disorder, they are admitted to an acute psychiatric unit. Removing individuals from their environment and hospitalizing them in a locked psychiatric unit provides enough safety that the aggressive behaviour dissipates. Because uncontrolled anger and aggression interfere with their ability to function, people who have problems in these areas require referral to appropriate resources before these destructive behaviours erupt.

Additional understanding of the phenomena of anger, aggression, and violence as they occur in the clinical setting is needed. Research studies that have illuminated this problem from a nursing perspective need to be continued and expanded. Specific areas of study need to examine the links among biology, neurology, and psychology. In addition, further explorations of the reciprocal influence of client interactional style and treatment setting culture will assist in the development and management of humane treatment settings. Finally, and perhaps most importantly, nurses must research the effectiveness of particular nursing interventions (see Box 35-9).

BOX 35.9   RESEARCH FOR BEST PRACTICE

How Nurses Experience Clients' Aggression

Duxbury, J. (1999). An exploratory account of registered nurses' experiences of client aggression in both mental health and general nursing settings. *Journal of Psychiatric and Mental Health Nursing, 6*(2), 107–114.

THE QUESTION: Is the way nurses choose to intervene in preventing or managing aggressive behaviours shaped by dominant theoretical models of aggression? For example, in the biomedical model, treatment focuses on containing aggression through a reactive approach.

METHODS: A qualitative study was undertaken to examine registered nurses' experiences of violent incidents with clients in mental health settings and general nursing environments. Data were collected from 34 mental health nurses from acute inpatient settings and 32 nurses from acute medical-surgical units using the critical incident technique (CIT). Each participant received a blank sheet of paper with the question, "In your own words, please describe one or more incident(s) which has involved a client being violent." Content analysis was performed on this qualitative data to identify themes and explore differences between the two settings.

FINDINGS: The most common types of aggressive behaviours were verbal and physical. Most nurses attributed aggressive behaviour to internal factors, with noticeable emphasis on controlling interventions. Nurses identified environmental and interactional factors much less frequently, suggesting that the biomedical model predominated. Experiences of the two groups of nurses were similar, but their patterns of response differed somewhat. Mental health nurses were more likely to manage the situation themselves, whereas general nurses were more likely to seek outside assistance (eg, medical staff, mental health teams, police). These findings should not be generalized to other environments, but they provide some insight into the experiences and behaviours of nurses in acute care settings. Unfortunately, in this study, the full set of questions needed for CIT was not used, so it is not known what was significant about these incidents from the nurses' point of view. The author also acknowledges that the wording of the one question may have influenced the lack of emphasis on prevention and de-escalation in the responses.

IMPLICATIONS FOR NURSING: Research findings such as these can remind nurses that how they think they practice may not actually be how they practice and that theoretical models may influence their actions. These nurses recognized the importance of internal factors in contributing to aggressive behaviour; however, they revealed less attention to environmental considerations. Of most significance was the lack of emphasis on interactional factors. Nurses must recognize that their behaviour greatly affects how clients feel and behave. This research study is suitable for conceptual utilization, that is, expanding ways of thinking about nursing practice.

SUMMARY OF KEY POINTS

◉ Biopsychosocial theories used to explain anger, aggression, and violence include the following types:

—Neurobiologic, including the cognitive neuroassociation model, neurostructural model (the emotional circuit), and neurochemical model (low serotonin syndrome)

—Psychological, including psychoanalytic theories, behavioural theories (eg, drive theory, social learning theory) and cognitive theories (eg, rational-emotive theory)

—Sociocultural theories

—Interactional theory

◉ Biologic factors to assess in clients who display aggressive and violent behaviours include exposure to toxic chemicals, use of medications, substance abuse, premenstrual dysphoric disorder, trauma, hemorrhage, and tumour.

◉ Biologic intervention choices include administering medications and managing nutrition.

◉ Psychological factors to assess in clients who display aggressive and violent behaviours include thought processing (eg, perception, delusion) and sensory impairment.

◉ Psychological intervention choices can be affective (eg, validating, listening, exploring beliefs), cognitive (eg, giving commendations, offering information, providing education, using thought stopping or contracting), or behavioural (eg, assigning tasks, using bibliotherapy, interrupting patterns, providing choices).

◉ Social intervention choices include reducing stimulation, anticipating needs, and using seclusion or restraints.

◉ Client aggression and violence are serious concerns for nurses in all areas of clinical practice. Training in and policies and procedures for the prevention and management of aggressive episodes should be available in all work settings.

CRITICAL THINKING CHALLENGES

1 Mary Jane, a 24-year-old single woman, has just been admitted to an inpatient psychiatry unit. She was transferred to the unit from the emergency room, where she was treated for a drug overdose. She is sullen when she is introduced to her roommate and refuses to answer the questions the nurse has that are part of the admission procedure. The nurse tells Mary Jane that he will come back later to see how she is. A few minutes later, Mary Jane approaches the nursing station and asks in a demanding tone to talk with someone and complains that she has been completely ignored since she came into the unit. What frameworks can the nurse use to understand Mary Jane's behaviour? At this point in time, what data does he have to develop a plan of care? What interventions might the nurse choose to use to help Mary Jane behave in a manner that is consistent with the norms of this inpatient unit?

2 Discuss the influence of gender and cultural norms on the expression of anger. When a nurse is caring for a client from a culture that the nurse is not familiar with, what could the nurse ask to ensure that her/his expectations of the client's behaviour are consistent with the gender and cultural norms of the client?

3 Under what circumstances should people who are aggressive or violent be held accountable for their behaviour? Are there any exceptions?

4 When a nurse minimizes verbally abusive behaviour by a client, family member, or health care colleague, what implicit message does she or he send?

5 In what way does our understanding of sociocultural theories influence the relationships that we, as nurses, develop with clients and families? Does this understanding also influence the relationships between nurses and other health care professionals?

6 Paul is sitting quietly reading a newspaper. Jane sits down next to him and starts talking to him about the weather. Paul responds by pushing Jane off the couch. How do you understand Paul's behaviour? Could Paul's action have been prevented?

WEB LINKS

www.canadian-health-network.ca   The Canadian Health Network provides *useful web-based information on many health-related topics. This website offers information on violence and its impact on health.*

www.cna-nurses.ca   The Canadian Nurses Association Position Statement on Violence *discusses the important role nurses play in dealing with and eliminating violence.*

www.phac-aspc.gc.ca/ncfc-cnif/family_violence.html   The website of the National Clearing House on Family Violence [NCFV] *offers information about family violence and links to literature for use in learning more about violence and offering resources to clients.*

www.who.int/mediacentre/events/violence_health   *The World Health Organization World Report on Violence and Health describes the magnitude and impact of violence throughout the world. A broad spectrum of violence is examined, with a separate chapter of the report devoted to each of the following seven topics: child abuse, youth violence, violence by intimate partners, sexual violence, elder abuse, suicide, and collective violence. There are also country and regional data available.*

MOVIES

Caddyshack: 1980. Bill Murray plays a groundskeeper at a posh golf club. His determination and anger toward some gophers lead to interesting outcomes!

VIEWING POINTS: How does the groundskeeper's thinking about the gophers change during the movie? How does his thinking influence his behaviour? How does his thinking influence his ability to examine the consequences of his behaviour?

The Insider: 1999. Russell Crowe plays a tobacco industry insider with scientific evidence that cigarettes are made to increase their addictive qualities. Al Pacino plays a news program producer who tries to get the story. Throughout the movie, many attempts are made to suppress the story.

VIEWING POINT: What is the goal of the people who use aggression and violence in this film?

Girl Interrupted: 2000. This movie tells the story of a young woman who is committed to a mental hospital after a suicide attempt.

VIEWING POINTS: In what way do the behaviours of the staff encourage aggression and violence? How do nurses intervene to help the clients regain or maintain control of aggressive behaviours.

REFERENCES

Allen, L. A. (1999). Treating agitation without drugs. *American Journal of Nursing, 99*(4), 36–42.

Bandura, A. (1973). *Aggression: A social learning analysis.* New York: Prentice-Hall.

Beck, A. T. (1976). *Cognitive therapy and emotional disorders.* New York: International Universities Press.

Belknap, R. A. (2003). Understanding abuse and violence against women: A two-day immersion course. *Nurse Educator, 28*(4), 170–174.

Berkowitz, L. (1989). Frustration-aggression hypothesis: Examination and reformulation. *Psychological Bulletin, 106*(1), 59–73.

Best, M., Williams, J. M., & Coccaro, E. F. (2002). Evidence for a dysfunctional prefrontal circuit in clients with an impulsive aggressive disorder. *Proceedings of the National Academy of Sciences, 99*(12), 8448–8453.

Brasic, J. R., & Fogelman, D. (1999). Clinician safety. *Psychiatric Clinics of North America, 22*(4), 923–940.

Burke, J. D., Loeber, R., & Birmaher, B. (2002). Oppositional defiant disorder and conduct disorder: A review of the past 10 years, Part II. *Journal of American Academy of Adolescent Psychiatry, 41*(11), 1275–1293.

Burns, D. (1980). *Feeling good: The new mood therapy.* New York: Avon Books.

Capra, F. (2002). *The hidden connections: Integrating the biological, cognitive and social dimensions of life into a science of sustainability.* New York: Doubleday.

Carpenito-Moyet, L. J. (2004). *Nursing diagnosis: Application to practice* (10th ed.). Philadelphia: Lippincott Williams & Wilkins.

Carpenito-Moyet (2003). *Position statement on the use of restraints in client care settings.* Edmonton, Alberta: Alberta Association of Registered Nurses.

Carpenito-Moyet (2002). *Guidelines for Code White Response: A component of prevention & management of aggressive behaviour in health care.* Occupational Health & Safety Agency for Health Care in British Columbia (BC), Workmen's Compensation of BC, Health Association in BC.

Chakos, M., & Lieberman, J. A. (2001). Effects of clozapine, olanzapine, risperidone, and haloperidol on hostility among clients with schizophrenia. *Psychiatric Services, 52*(11), 1510–1514.

Citrome, L., & Volavka, J. (1999). Violent clients in the emergency setting. *Psychiatric Clinics of North America, 22*(4), 789–801.

Corrigan, P. W., Yudofsky, S. C., & Silver, J. M. (1993). Pharmacological and behavioral treatment for aggressive psychiatric inpatients. *Hospital and Community Psychiatry, 44*(3), 125–133.

DelBel, J. C. (2003). Escalating workplace aggression. *Nursing Management, 34*(9), 30–34.

Duncan, S., Estabrookes, C. A., & Reimer, M. A. (2000). Violence against nurses. *Alberta RN, 56*(2), 13–14.

Duxbury, J. (1999). An exploratory account of registered nurses' experiences of client aggression in both mental health and general nursing settings. *Journal of Psychiatric and Mental Health Nursing, 6*(2), 107–114.

Duxbury, J. (2002). An evaluation of staff and client views of and strategies employed to manage inpatient aggression and violence on one mental health unit: A pluralistic design. *Journal of Psychiatric & Mental Health Nursing, 9*(3), 325–327.

Ellis, A. (1977). *Anger: How to live with and without it.* Secaucus, NJ: Citadel Press.

Fahs, H., Potiron, G., Senon, J. L., & Perivier, E. (1999). Anticonvulsants in agitation and behavior disorders in demented subjects. *Encephale, 25*(2), 169–174.

Frey, R. E. C., & Weller, J. (2000). Rehab rounds: Behavioral management of aggression through teaching interpersonal skills. *Psychiatric Services, 51*, 607–609.

Fromm, E. (1973). *The anatomy of human destructiveness.* New York: Holt, Rinehart and Winston.

Gerberich, S. G., Church, T. R., McGovern, P. M., Hansen, H. E., Nachreiner, N. M., Geisser, M. S., Ryan, A. D., Mongin, S. J., & Watt, G. D. (2004). An epidemiological study of the magnitude and consequences of work related violence: The Minnesota nurses' study. *Occupational Environmental Medicine, 61*, 495–503.

Gerloff, L. (1997). Anger management. *Arkansas Nursing News, 14*(1), 5–7.

Hancock, C. K., Buster, P. A., Oliver, M. S., Fox, S. W., Morrison, E., & Burger, S. L. (2001). Restraint reduction in acute care: An interdisciplinary approach. *Journal of Nursing Administration, 31*(2), 74–77.

Harper-Jaques, S., & Masters, A. (1994). Powerful words: The use of letters with sexual abuse survivors. *Journal of Psychosocial Nursing and Mental Health Services, 32*(8), 11–16.

Harper-Jaques, S., & Reimer, M. (1992). Aggressive behavior and the brain: A different perspective for the mental health nurse. *Archives of Psychiatric Nursing, 6*(5), 312–320.

Harris, D., & Morrison, E. F. (1995). Managing violence without coercion. *Archives of Psychiatric Nursing, 9*(4), 203–210.

Heinz, A., Mann, K., Weinberger, D. R., Goldman, D. (2001). Serotonergic dysfunction, negative mood states, and response to alcohol. *Alcoholism: Clinical and Experimental Research, 25*(4), 487–495.

Hibbs, A. (2000). Cognitive therapy: A complementary strategy for expressed anger during the restraint of an aggressive individual. *British Journal of Forensic Practice, 2*(2), 19–29.

Jenkins, A. (1990). *Invitations to responsibility.* Adelaide, NSW, Australia: Dulwich Centre Publications.

Johnson, B., Martin, M. L., Guha, M., & Montgomery, P. (1997). The experience of thought disordered individuals preceding an aggressive incident. *Journal of Psychiatric and Mental Health Nursing, 4*, 213–220.

Koh, K. B., Kim, C. H. & Park, J. K. (2002). Predominance of anger in depressive disorders compared with anxiety disorders and somatoform disorders. *Journal of Clinical Psychiatry, 63*(6), 486–492.

Kolanowski, A., Hurwitz, S., Taylor, L. A., et al. (1994). Contextual factors associated with disturbing behavior of institutionalized elders. *Nursing Research, 43*(2), 73–79.

Lanza, M. L. (1992). Nurses as client assault victims: An update, synthesis, and recommendations. *Archives of Psychiatric Nursing, 6*(3), 163–171.

Leahey, M., & Harper-Jaques, S. (1996). Family–nurse relationship: Core assumptions and clinical implications. *Journal of Family Nursing, 2*(2), 133–151.

Lerner, H. (2001). *The dance of anger: A woman's guide to changing the patterns of intimate relationships.* New York: Harper & Row.

Lewis, D. M. (2002). Responding to a violent incident: Physical restraint or anger management as therapeutic interventions. *Journal of Psychiatry and Mental Health Nursing, 9*(1), 57–63.

Limacher, L. H., & Wright, L. M. (2003). Commendations: Listening to the silent side of a family intervention. *Journal of Family Nursing, 9*(2), 130–150.

Lorist, M. M., & Tops, M. (2003). Caffeine, fatigue, and cognition. *Brain and Cognition, 53*(1), 82–94.

McCloskey, J., & Bulechek, G. (2000). *Nursing interventions classification (NIC)* (3rd ed.). St. Louis: Mosby.

McElheran, N., & Harper-Jaques, S. (1994). Commendations: A resource intervention for clinical practice. *Clinical Nurse Specialist, 8*(1), 7–10.

Mesulam, M. (2000). *Principles of behavioral and cognitive neurology* (2nd ed.). Oxford: Oxford University Press.

Miller, N., Pedersen, W. C., Earleywine, M., & Pollock, V. E. (2003). Artificial theoretical model of triggered displaced aggression. *Personality Social Psychology Review, 7*(1), 57–97.

Moorhead, S., Johnson, M., & Maas, M. (2003). *Nursing outcomes classification* (3rd ed.). Philadelphia: Elsevier.

Morrison, E. F. (1998). The culture of caregiving and aggression in psychiatric settings. *Archives of Psychiatric Nursing, 12*(1), 21–31.

Morrison, E. F., & Carney Love, C. (2003). An evaluation of four programs for the management of aggression in psychiatric settings. *Archives of Psychiatric Nursing, 17*(4), 146–155.

Morrison, E. F., Fox, S., Burger, S., Goodloe, L., Blosser, J., & Gitter, K. (2000). A nurse led, unit based program to reduce restraint use in acute care. *Journal of Nursing Care Quality, 14*(3), 72–80.

North American Nursing Diagnosis Association (NANDA). (2005). *Nursing diagnoses: Definitions and classification 2005–2006.* Philadelphia: Author.

Pardo, J. V., Pardo, P. J., & Raichle, M. E. (1993). Neural correlates of self-induced dysphoria. *American Journal of Psychiatry, 150*(5), 713–719.

Paris, J. (2005). Borderline personality disorder. *Canadian Medical Association Journal, 172*(12), 1579–1583.

Robinson, C., Wright, L., & Watson, W. (1994). A non-traditional approach to family violence. *Archives of Psychiatric Nursing, 8*(1), 30–37.

Rubinsztein, E. R., Sahakian, B. J., & Dolan, R. J. (2002). The neural basis of mood congruent processing biases in depression. *Archives of General Psychiatry, 59*(7), 597–604.

Scarpa, A., & Raine, A. (1997). Psychophysiology of anger and violent behavior. *Psychiatric Clinics of North America, 20*(2), 375–394.

Schmeck, K., Sadigorsky, S., Englert, E., Demisch, L., Dierks, T., Barta, S., & Poustka, F. (2002). Mood changes following acute tryptophan depletion in healthy adults. *Psychopathology, 35*(4), 234–240.

Sergi, M. J., & Green, M. F. (2003). Social perception and early visual processing in schizophrenia. *Schizophrenia Research, 59*(2–3), 233–241.

Shannon, J. W. (2000). *Understanding and managing anger: Diagnosis, treatment and prevention.* Presentation by Mind Matters Seminar, April 2000, Calgary, Alberta, Canada.

Silver, J. M., Yudofsky, S. C., Slater, J. A., Gold, R. K., Stryer, B. L., Williams, D. T., Wolland, H., & Endicott, J. (2000). Propranolol treatment of chronically hospitalized aggressive clients. *Journal of Neuropsychiatry & Clinical Neuroscience, 12*(3), 413.

Soloff, P. H., Lynch, K. G., & Moss, H. B. (2000). Serotonin, impulsivity, and alcohol use disorders in the older adolescent: A psychobiological study. *Alcoholism: Clinical and Experimental Research, 24*(11), 1609–1619.

Stolley, J. M., Gerdner, L. A., & Buckwalter, K. C. (1999). Dementia management. In G. M. Bulechek & J. C. McCloskey (Eds.), *Nursing interventions: Effective nursing treatments* (3rd ed., pp. 533–548). Philadelphia: WB Saunders.

Swett, C., & Mills, T. (1997). Use of NOSIE to predict assaults among acute psychiatric clients. Nurses' Observation Scale for Inpatient Evaluation. *Psychiatric Services, 48*(9), 1177–1180.

Tajaden, P., & Thoennes, N. (2000). *Findings from national violence against women survey.* Washington, DC: U.S. Department of Justice.

Talerico, K. A., Evans, L. K., & Strumpf, N. E. (2002). Mental health correlates of aggression in nursing home residents with dementia. *Gerontologist, 42*(2), 169–177.

Tasman, A. (1997). *Psychiatry.* Philadelphia: WB Saunders.

Tavris, C. (1989). *Anger: The misunderstood emotion.* New York: Simon & Schuster.

Thomas, S. P. (1990). Theoretical and empirical perspectives on anger. *Issues in Mental Health Nursing, 11*, 203–216.

Thomas, S. P. (1993). *Women and anger.* New York: Springer.

Thomas, S. P. (1998). Assessing and intervening with anger disorders. *Nursing Clinics of North America, 33*(1), 121–133.

Thomas, S. P. (2001). Teaching healthy anger management. *Perspectives in Psychiatric Care, 37*(2), 41–48.

Thomas, S. (2003). Men's anger: A phenomenological exploration of its meaning in a middle class sample of American men. *Psychology of Men & Masculinity, 4*(2), 163–175.

Tomm, K. (1980). Towards a cybernetic systems approach to family therapy at the University of Calgary. In D. Freeman (Ed.), *Diagnosis and assessment in family therapy* (pp. 101–122). London: Aspen.

United Nations High Commission on Human Rights. (2001). Human rights resolution 2001.49. *Elimination of violence against women.* Available at http://www.unhchr.ch.

Visalli, H., McNasser, G., Johnstone, L., & Lazzaro, C. A. (1997). Reducing high-risk interventions for managing aggression in psychiatric settings. *Journal of Nursing Care Quality, 11*(3), 54–61.

Vosburgh, D., & Simpson, P. (1993). Linking family theory and practice: A family nursing program. *Image—The Journal of Nursing Scholarship, 25*(3), 231–235.

White, M. (1988/89, Summer). The externalizing of the problem and the re-authoring of lives and relationships. *Dulwich Centre Newsletter,* 3–21.

Wright, L. M., & Leahey, M. (2005). *Nurses and families: A guide to family assessment and intervention* (3rd ed.). Philadelphia: FA Davis.

Wright, N. M. J., Dixon, A. J., & Tompkins, C. N. E. (2003). Managing violence in primary care: An evidence-based approach. *British Journal of General Practice, 53*, 557–562.

Young, S. N. (2002). Clinical nutrition. 3. The fuzzy boundary between nutrition and psychopharmacology. *Canadian Medical Association Journal, 166*(2), 205–209.

For challenges, please refer to the **CD-ROM** in this book.

36

Caring for Abused Persons

Mary R. Boyd and Elizabeth A. McCay

LEARNING OBJECTIVES

After studying this chapter, you will be able to:

- Describe biopsychosocial theories of abuse.
- Discuss theories explaining why some persons become abusive and why some persons remain in violent relationships.
- Describe biopsychosocial consequences of abuse.
- Describe the diagnostic criteria for posttraumatic stress disorder (PTSD).
- Discuss the three major symptom categories found in PTSD and their associated etiologic factors.
- Describe the diagnostic criteria for dissociative identity disorder (DID).
- Integrate biopsychosocial theories into the analysis of human responses to abuse and its survival.
- Formulate nursing care plans for survivors of abuse.

KEY TERMS

acute stress disorder (ASD) ▪ alexithymia ▪ behavioural sensitization ▪ complex post-traumatic stress disorder (PTSD) ▪ cycle of violence ▪ dissociation ▪ dissociative identity disorder (DID) ▪ emotional abuse ▪ extinction ▪ factitious disorder by proxy (Munchausen syndrome by proxy) ▪ fear conditioning ▪ intergenerational transmission ▪ neglect ▪ physical abuse ▪ posttraumatic stress disorder (PTSD) ▪ sexual abuse ▪ traumatic bonding

⬟ KEY CONCEPTS

empowerment ▪ self-esteem

Violence demonstrated in the abuse of women, men, children, and elders is a national health problem that causes significant impairment in survivors. Abuse of any type permanently changes the survivor's construction of reality and the meaning of his or her life. It wounds deeply, endangering core beliefs about self, others, and the world. It usually destroys the survivor's self-esteem.

Nurses encounter survivors of abuse in all health care settings. For this reason, they must be knowledgeable about abuse. They must understand its indicators, causes, assessment techniques, and effective nursing interventions. Unfortunately, few nurses ask about abuse because doing so is uncomfortable (Gallop et al., 1998; McCay et al., 1997). It requires nurses to acknowledge evil in human nature and their own vulnerability to that evil. Protection and recovery from abuse require survivors to remember and discuss terrible events. However, secrecy and silence protect perpetrators and seriously endanger survivors. Nurses communicate a powerfully disturbing message with their silence: that the most traumatic event of a patient's life is too upsetting for others to hear. If nurses do not allow and encourage survivors to tell their stories, the abuse experiences will continue to haunt patients as symptoms of mental disorders.

This chapter focuses on the nursing process with women, men, children, and elders who are survivors of abuse. It provides basic nursing information needed to address the multiple, complex problems of these patients.

> ◆ **KEY CONCEPT** **Self-esteem** is how one feels about oneself. Its components are self-acceptance, self-worth, self-love, and self-nurturing.

TYPES OF ABUSE

Most abuse that women, men, children, and elderly people experience is intimate violence; that is, the perpetrator is a loved and trusted partner or family member. As a result, the world and home are no longer safe, people seem dangerous, and life may become a tortured existence of warding off ever-present threats. Empowerment is a foreign concept to those who are being abused.

> ◆ **KEY CONCEPT** **Empowerment** is promotion of the continued growth and development of strength, power, and personal excellence.

Woman Abuse

Woman abuse, domestic violence, spouse abuse, partner abuse, wife abuse, and battered wives are all terms used interchangeably to denote violence directed toward women. However, some of these terms do not specifically refer to the abuse of a woman by an intimate partner. For example, the term *domestic violence* may be used in cases in which one person directs abuse against an entire family. The terms *spouse abuse* and *partner abuse* could indicate that the couple in whom abuse occurs, either heterosexual or homosexual, lives together but is unmarried. However, these terms also imply that women abuse their male partners at the same frequency and with similar consequences as men direct violence against women (Ryan & King, 1998), which is simply not true. In most cases (90% to 95%), victims of battering are women, and the perpetrators are men (Swann, 2001). According to a recent Statistics Canada Report, the violence experienced by women that was inflicted by their spouse or common-law partner was more severe and more frequent than the violence experienced by men in similar circumstances (Canadian Centre for Justice Statistics, 2005). When women use force against their male partners, they often do so in self-defence, and the injuries they receive are more severe than those they inflict (Swann, 2001). For these reasons, *woman abuse* has been chosen as the most appropriate term to use in this chapter in designating violence, including rape, directed toward a woman by an intimate partner.

Woman abuse is a significant health problem that crosses all ethnic, racial, and socioeconomic lines. Estimates of the annual prevalence of woman abuse range from 2 million to approximately 4 million cases (Brady & Dansky, 2002). Specific rates of victimization were assessed in the 2004 General Social Survey (GSS) on Victimization of 25,000 women and men. Survey results indicated that 7% of women and 6% of men reported being the victim of violence in the relationship with their intimate partner (Canadian Centre for Justice Statistics, 2005). Specifically, it is estimated that 653,000 women and 546,000 men were victims of intimate partner violence at the time of the 2004 GSS survey (Canadian Centre for Justice Statistics, 2005). It is possible that these figures may be low because underreporting contributes to conservative estimates. Many women are afraid or reluctant to identify their abusers. In some cases, they fear retaliation against themselves or their children. In other cases, they continue to hold strong feelings for their partners, despite the abuse.

It is important to recognize that women of all ages and sociocultural backgrounds may have experienced abuse. Regardless, certain factors have been found to be associated with increased risk for violence in women. Women who are at higher risk of abuse are younger (18 to 24 years of age), elderly (65 years of age or older), or pregnant and have a history of childhood victimization or of witnessing maternal abuse (Statistics Canada, 1993; as cited in Health Canada, 2002b). Women living with disabilities may also be at higher risk for abuse than nondisabled women because these women frequently depend on others to assist with a wide range of activities, which increases vulnerability (Health Canada, 2002b).

Evidence suggests that single, divorced, and separated women may actually be at greater risk for abuse than are married women (Fishwick, Campbell, & Taylor, 2004). Moreover, this group is at particularly high risk for severe violence. Danger assessments show that abusive ex-partners often exhibit obsessive threatening behaviour after their relationships end and pose significant dangers to women. Forty-three percent of women seen in emergency departments (EDs) attributed their abuse to a past partner. These findings emphasize that ending a relationship often does not end violence (Fishwick et al., 2004). This information is important for health care providers, who frequently pressure women to end abusive relationships.

Rates of woman abuse vary among women of different racial backgrounds. Research supports that Aboriginal women are at high risk for violence in their intimate relationships. The GSS data indicate that 24% of Aboriginal women had experienced intimate partner violence within the 5-year period before the 2004 survey (Canadian Centre for Justice Statistics, 2005). Even higher rates of woman abuse have been reported for Aboriginal women by other studies. For example, a study in Ontario documents that 8 of 10 Aboriginal women experienced violence at the hands of their intimate partner (Health Canada, 1996, as cited in Health Canada, 2002b). Specifically, 87% reported physical abuse, and 55% reported sexual abuse. Further, physical abuse of women in Northern Aboriginal communities is thought to be pervasive, with estimates ranging from 75% to 90% (Health Canada, 1996, as cited in Health Canada, 2002b).

The perpetuation of violence begins early in dating relationships. The prevalence of dating violence is unknown because, as with other forms of violence, it usually takes place in private and is not reported. A few studies provide some data on the extent of the problem. One study found that of 1,870 cases of domestic assaults, 51.5% were classified as boyfriend or girlfriend violence. About 20% to 50% of men and women in dating relationships have admitted physically abusing a dating partner. These figures do not include date rape. One study found that behaviours that would qualify as date rape or sexual assault occurred at a rate of 15.4%, or 38 per 1,000 women (Barnett, Miller-Perrin, & Perrin, 1997). More recent sources suggest that prevalence of dating violence ranges from 9% to 46% of adolescent females and males involved as victims or perpetrators (King & Ryan, 2004). Some studies report that dating violence is mutual and reciprocal. One study conducted in an ethnically and economically diverse urban community found that dating violence affected 45.5% of participating girls and boys (Watson, Cascardi, Avery-Leaf, & O'Leary, 2001). A qualitative study of 40

adolescent girls aged 15 and 16 years provides some insight into these high rates of dating violence (Banister, Jakubec, & Stein, 2003). The study findings highlight the tremendous power imbalance that exists in dating relationships for adolescent girls, which frequently results in a tolerance of violence simply to maintain the relationship (Banister, Jakubec, & Stein, 2003). A longitudinal study of dating violence in adolescent boys residing in Montreal (LaVoie et al., 2002) illustrates the importance of familial factors for adolescent boys in dating violence. Specifically, harsh parenting and antisocial behaviour were found to be predictive of dating violence in 717 boys aged 16 to 17 years living in a less affluent area of Montreal (LaVoie et al., 2002).

To understand woman abuse, one must understand the dynamics of violent intimate relationships. Woman abuse is not just physical or sexual abuse. Rather, it is a chronic syndrome characterized by emotional abuse, degradation, restrictions on freedom, destruction of property, threatened or actual child abuse, threats against one's family, stalking, and isolation from family and friends. Violence of this nature has at its core a pattern of coercive control and domination over all aspects of a woman's life (Flitcraft, 1995, 1997). Threats of violence against the woman and her loved ones are among the tactics that the batterer uses to enforce the woman's submission and secrecy (King & Ryan, 2004). Many battered women report that physical violence is much less damaging than the accompanying emotional abuse. Relentless emotional and psychological violence destroys and isolates women (Boyd & Mackey, 2000a). The varieties of abuse used to exert power and control over women are represented in Figure 36-1. It has been observed that women in abusive relationships frequently feel that they have no personal control, whereas men frequently feel in control of the situation (Maes, Delmeire, Mylle, & Altamura, 2001; as cited in Carter-Snell & Hegadoren, 2003).

Battering

Battering is the single greatest cause of serious injury to women. Estimates of injury related to battering seen in EDs range from 14% to 50% (Campbell, Torres, McKenna, Sheridan, & Landenburger, 2004). In a cross-sectional survey of 3,287 Canadian women living in shelters, 73% had gone to the shelter as a consequence of abuse (Statistics Canada, 2003a). GSS data indicate that women are three times more likely to be physically injured than men in the context of intimate partner violence (Health Canada, 2002b). Woman abuse contributes to a high rate of completed and attempted suicides in women; 81% of women reporting suicide attempts have experienced abuse by an intimate partner (Thompson et al., 1999). Moreover, many women who experience abuse experience post-traumatic stress

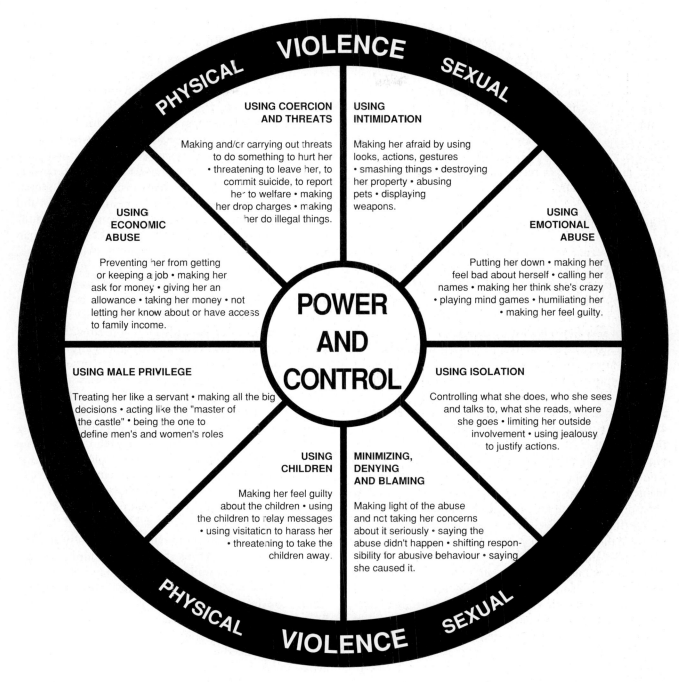

FIGURE 36.1 Power and control wheel. (Courtesy of Domestic Abuse Intervention Project, 202 East Superior Street, Duluth, MN.)

disorder (PTSD) (Norris, Foster, & Weisshaar, 2002). In a study of 65 women receiving treatment from three Canadian urban mental health centres, women reporting early-onset sexual abuse were more likely to meet criteria for complex PTSD than women reporting late-onset PTSD (McLean & Gallop, 2003). In addition, individuals with PTSD are 15 times more likely to attempt suicide than are individuals in the general population (Thompson et al., 1999).

In some instances, battered women may even be killed by their abusers (Health Canada, 2002b), especially when they take deliberate action to leave an abusive relationship. In 1996, 75% of 1,800 homicides perpetrated by intimate partners had female victims (Sisley et al., 1999). Indeed, the realistic fear of being killed is one factor that keeps many women from leaving abusive partners, even after years of severe abuse.

Battering also poses a significant danger to unborn children. Estimates of the prevalence of battering during pregnancy vary from 4% (Sisley et al., 1999) to as high as 22% (Parker, Bullock, Bohn, & Curry, 2004). Differences in prevalence rates may be attributed to differences in definitions of abuse used by study authors. According to a Statistics Canada survey, 21% of women who were battered by a former or existing partner were pregnant (Statistics Canada, 1993, as cited in Health Canada, 2002b). Abuse during pregnancy is a significant risk factor for several foetal and maternal complications, including low birth weight, low maternal weight gain, infections, and anaemia. Moreover, abuse of women often results in their use of alcohol and other drugs, which, in turn, may harm unborn children (Parker et al., 2004).

Rape and Sexual Assault

Rape and sexual assault are common in Canada, with 24,049 sexual assaults being reported in 2000 and women constituting the majority (86%) of sexual assault victims (Statistics Canada, 2001). Younger women are at increased risk for sexual assault: in 2000, 54% of female victims of sexual assault were younger than 18 years of age. In a study of sexual assault among undergraduate women attending Canadian Universities, 28% of women reported that they had been sexually victimized in a dating relationship (DeKeseredy & Schwartz, 1998). Sexual assault includes any form of nonconsenting sexual activity, ranging from fondling to penetration. Most sexual assaults are underreported for the same reason that domestic violence is underreported—women are embarrassed and ashamed and fear being blamed for the assault. These reactions to sexual assault persist, even though rape is a felony (Abbey et al., 2003).

Rapists can be classified into three categories: the power rapist, the anger rapist, and the sadistic rapist (Petter & Whitehill, 1998). Power rapists account for 55% of sexual assaults. They often attack people their own age and use intimidation and minimal physical force to control their victims. Their assaults are generally premeditated. Anger rapists account for 40% of sexual assaults. These rapists tend to target either very young or elderly victims. They may use extreme force and restraint that results in physical injury to the victim. Sadistic rapists account for 5% of sexual assaults; however, they are the most dangerous. Their crimes are premeditated, and they often torture and kill their victims. Sadistic rapists derive erotic gratification from their victims' suffering (Petter & Whitehill, 1998).

Coerced Sex and Increased Risk for Human Immunodeficiency Virus

Woman abuse is also a risk factor for human immunodeficiency virus (HIV) infection among women. Among women who test positive for HIV, the lifetime prevalence of adult coerced sexual activity perpetrated by a male partner has been estimated to be 74% or higher (Morrill, Kasten, Urato, & Larson, 2001). In an earlier study of women in treatment for alcohol and other drug use and at high risk for HIV infection, 42% reported that their sexual partner physically abused them, 45% reported that sexual partners threatened them with violence, and 21% reported that they had sex because they were afraid they would be hurt if they refused (Brown, Recupero, & Stout, 1995).

An abusive partner may increase risk for HIV infection in several ways. Women who have abusive partners may not be able to avoid sexual contact. Fear of a partner's violent behaviour may prevent women from insisting on use of condoms. A woman's insistence on condom use can imply that either partner is being unfaithful and can result in abuse. Victimized women are also four times more likely to have sex with a risky partner than are women who have not been abused (Morrill et al., 2001).

The rate of HIV infection appears to be rapidly increasing in Aboriginal women living in northern Alberta (Mill, 1997). A qualitative study of eight Aboriginal women infected with HIV indicates that these women endured abusive familial relationships that lead to the adoption of high-risk life on the street, which frequently included prostitution, intravenous drug use, and revictimization, increasing the risk for HIV infection (Mill, 1997). Similar findings are reported by McKeown and colleagues (2004) in a sample of 18 First Nations women, further supporting the relationship between childhood abuse and the risk for HIV infection in this population.

Stalking

Stalking is a crime of intimidation. Stalkers intimidate and terrorize their victims through threatening behaviour, which includes waiting, watching, and calling, that causes fear or substantial emotional distress (Canadian Centre for Justice Statistics, 2005). In the 2004 General Social Survey of 25,0000 women and men, 11% of women and 7% of men aged 15 and older reported that they were stalked to the extent that the experience evoked fear for themselves or someone else close to them (Canadian Centre for Justice Statistics, 2005). As with other abuse, most knew the stalker, whereas one fourth were stalked by strangers (Canadian Centre for Justice Statistics, 2005). Women were more likely than men to be harassed by an ex-spouse, ex-boyfriend, or ex-partner. Individuals who were stalked by an intimate ex-partner were stalked for longer periods of time. For example, those who were stalked by an ex-spouse were pursued for well over 1 year, and women were stalked by an ex-spouse two times more often than men (Canadian Centre for Justice Statistics, 2005).

In Canada, stalking, or in legal terms criminal harassment, is against the law (Canadian Centre for Justice Statistics, 2005). It is notable that in 2001, charges were laid for 57% of reported stalking incidents involving women, whereas charges were laid for only 39% of stalking incidents involving men (Statistics Canada, 2003a). The Department of Justice, Canada is involved in an ongoing process of review to strengthen the laws pertaining to violence and sexual assault, including criminal harassment (Department of Justice, Canada, 2005).

Abuse of Men

Although sexual assault and violence have typically focussed on women, the literature is now indicating that the rate of violence and sexual assault is now higher in men than traditionally believed (Stermac, Del Bove, & Addison, 2004). As noted earlier, the GSS data indicated that 6% of men are victims of intimate partner violence (IPV), only 1% less than the rate of IPV reported for women (Department of Justice, Canada, 2005). The consequences of violence and sexual assault can also be devastating for men. For example, more than half of a sample of male rape victims referred to a forensic setting met criteria for PTSD, and many male victims reported profound emotional distress and sexual dysfunction (Huckle, 1995). A recent study examined 141 cases from a sexual assault database located in a large urban Ontario city (Stermac, Del Bove, & Addison). The data suggest that male victims of sexual assault are more likely to be young, street-involved, with increased vulnerability such as either a cognitive or physical disability (Stermac, Del Bove, & Addison, 2004). The authors suggest that future research is needed to understand better this previously unrecognized vulnerable group.

Child Abuse

Child abuse can take several forms, and the definition of each type varies by state. All forms of child abuse rob children of rights they should have. Those rights include the rights to be and behave like a child; to be safe and protected from harm; and to be fed, clothed, and nurtured so that the child can grow, develop, and fulfill his or her unique potential.

The prevalence of child abuse is unknown. The Canadian Incidence Study of Reported Child Abuse and Neglect (CIS) of 7,000 child welfare investigations over a 3- month period in 1998 estimated that there were 135,573 child maltreatment investigations in 1998. Child welfare workers confirmed abuse in 45% of the reported cases of maltreatment (Trocme & Wolfe, 2001, as cited in Department of Justice Canada, 2003). Of course, this figure does not include cases that were unreported. Of the total number of reported child abuse cases, estimates are that 43% represent neglect, 31% physical abuse, and 10% sexual abuse (Trocme & Wolfe, 2001, as cited in Department of Justice Canada). Emotional maltreatment was the primary reason for the investigation in 19% of cases, and emotional maltreatment was confirmed in

54% of those reported. Police statistics also provide valuable information about the prevalence of violence against children and youth. Specifically, the Incident-based Uniform Crime Reporting Survey (UCR2) documents the number of physical and sexual assaults reported to the police in a designated period of time. In 2003, data from 122 police units compiled in the UCR2 indicated that 25% of reported physical and sexual assaults pertained to children and youth younger than 18 years of age, who compose 21% of Canada's population (Canadian Centre for Justice Statistics, 2005).

It is also extremely important to acknowledge the child abuse that occurred in the residential schools for Aboriginal children within the last century (Law Commission of Canada, 2000). The Law Commission of Canada noted that Aboriginal children were the only children who were designated to live in an institution, away for family and community, because of their race. Frequently these children were prohibited from speaking their mother tongue and were deliberately deprived of all connection with their culture and identity, placing this group of children at high risk for abuse (Law Commission of Canada, 2000). The report acknowledges the profound level of harm to the children, families, and communities that occurred as a result of these children being displaced and mistreated.

Child Neglect

Child neglect is the most common form of child abuse reported (Gary, Campbell, & Humphreys, 2004; Gary & Humphreys, 2004) and frequently is chronic (Department of Justice, Canada, 2003). There are several types of **neglect**, such as failure to protect a child, physical neglect, and medical neglect. Failure to protect a child includes failure to prevent various kinds of accidental injury, such as ingestion of poison, electric shocks, falls, and burns (Barnett et al., 1997). Physical neglect includes failure to provide food, clothing, shelter, or cleanliness (Department of Justice, Canada, 2003). Indicators of physical neglect include diaper dermatitis, lice, scabies, dirty appearance, clothes inappropriate for the weather, and unclean and unsafe living environment. Medical neglect includes failure to provide for the child's medical needs, including failure to seek appropriate care or to comply with prescribed treatments (Wallace, 1999).

Physical Abuse

Physical abuse may include severe spanking, hitting, biting, burning, kicking, shoving, choking, or any other type of physical action directed toward the child that results in nonaccidental injury (Department of Justice, Canada, 2003). Injuries to children caused by physical abuse range from mild to severe and life-threatening.

Types of injuries include skin and soft tissue injuries; internal injuries; dislocations and fractures; tooth loss; burns; abrasions or bruises made by fists or belts; hair loss from pulling the hair; wounds from guns, knives, razors, or other sharp objects; retinal haemorrhage; and conjunctival haemorrhage (Gary et al., 2004; Gary & Humphreys, 2004; Wallace, 1999). Often, clothing hides these injuries, and practitioners must look for other signs of abuse, such as fear, aggressive or withdrawn behaviour, poor social relations, learning problems, delinquent behaviour, and wearing clothing that is meant to cover injuries but is inappropriate for the weather. In addition, when treating a child with such injuries, professionals should suspect abuse when explanations are implausible and inconsistent with injuries, involved parties give different versions of the incident, or treatment seeking is delayed (Wallace, 1999).

Sexual Abuse

Behaviours that constitute child **sexual abuse** range from mild, covert behaviours to overt sexual acts. Examples of sexual abuse include exhibitionism, voyeurism, touching the child's sexual organs, and oral, anal, and vaginal sex (Department of Justice, Canada, 2003; Gary et al., 2004; Gary & Humphreys, 2004; Urbancic, 2004; Wallace, 1999). Childhood sexual exploitation is also included with the discussion of childhood sexual abuse, specifically, using children for the purpose of pornography or prostitution. (Department of Justice, Canada, 2003). There are three categories of sexual abuse: incest, sexual abuse perpetrated by a nonfamily member, and pedophilia. Incest is defined in the Criminal Code of Canada (1985) in this way: Everyone commits incest who, "Knowing that another person by blood relationship is his or her parent, child, brother, sister, grand parent or grand child, as the case may be, has sexual intercourse with that person" (5.155). This definition limits illegal sexual activity to sexual intercourse; it does not include fondling, oral sex, and masturbation. These acts, when committed against children, are covered under other laws not restricted to blood relatives. Pedophilia describes those who have a sexual fixation on young children that usually translates into sexual acts with the victims. The following conditions qualify as pedophilia:

- For at least 6 months, the person has recurrent intense sexual urges and sexually arousing fantasies involving sexual activity with a prepubescent child.
- The person has acted on or is extremely distressed by these urges.
- The person is at least 16 years old and at least 5 years older than the child (Wallace, 1999).

Research shows that about 8% to 10% of child sexual abuse offenders are strangers; 47% are family members; 40% are acquaintances. The high-risk years for child sexual abuse are ages 4 to 9 years (Wallace, 1999).

Several factors may mediate the effects of child sexual abuse. In general, younger children with a history of emotional difficulties may be more traumatized than will be older and more stable children. Repeated abuse for long periods with more violence and bodily penetration results in greater traumatization. Sexual abuse by someone that the child knows and trusts causes more severe trauma. The child abused by a family member experiences a devastating breach of trust, loss of a safe home, and threats to fundamental survival requirements (Boyd & Mackey, 2000a). Finally, negative reactions by significant others, health care professionals, or others may exacerbate the effects of trauma (Wallace, 1999).

Emotional Abuse

Emotional abuse includes acts or omissions that psychologically damage the child (Gary et al., 2004). The emotionally abused child does not have visible injuries to alert others. Nevertheless, emotional abuse severely affects a child's self-esteem and often leaves permanent emotional scars. Survivors of abuse frequently report that emotional abuse is worse than physical abuse (Wallace, 1999).

There are several types of emotional abuse. *Rejecting* involves refusing to acknowledge the child's worth and the legitimacy of his or her needs. The child receives the message that he or she is no good and is unwanted. *Isolating* involves cutting the child off from normal social experiences, preventing the child from forming friendships, and hindering the development of social skills. *Terrorizing* involves creating a climate of fear and making the child believe that the world is a capricious and hostile place. *Ignoring* means being psychologically unavailable to the child and, therefore, starving him or her emotionally. Normal self-development depends on emotional connection to others. *Corrupting* involves mis-socializing the child to engage in destructive and antisocial behaviours and reinforcing deviance. This type of abuse makes the child unfit for normal social experience and sets him or her up for additional rejection (Barnett et al., 1997; Wallace, 1999).

Factitious Disorder by Proxy: Munchausen Syndrome by Proxy

Factitious disorder by proxy is another form of child abuse (see Chapter 21). This disorder includes "the intentional production or feigning of physical or psychological signs or symptoms in another person who is under the individual's care for the purpose of indirectly assuming the sick role" (American Psychiatric Association [APA], 2000, p. 781). The signs of this disorder include repeated hospitalizations and medical evaluations of the child without definitive diagnosis; symptoms or medical signs that are inappropriate or inconsistent;

symptoms that disappear when the child is away from the parent; a parent who encourages medical tests for the child; parental uneasiness as the child recovers; and a parent who is less concerned with the child's health than with spending time with caregivers (Bartsch, Risse, Schutz, Weigand, & Weiler, 2003). One source estimates that approximately 10% of children who are victims of factitious disorder by proxy will die at the hands of their parents (Wallace, 1999).

Secondary Abuse: Children of Battered Women

Children of battered women are often overlooked as abuse victims unless they demonstrate evidence of physical or sexual abuse themselves (Rhea, Chafey, Dohner, & Terragno, 1996). However, these children often show signs of PTSD (Berman, Hardesty, & Humphreys, 2004; Campbell & Lewandowski, 1997). Children may witness their mother being choked, threatened with a weapon, or threatened with death (Berman et al., 2004; Boyd & Mackey, 2000a; Campbell & Lewandowski, 1997). These children fear for both their own and their mother's safety (Boyd & Mackey, 2000a). The 2004 GSS data indicate that children witnessed spousal violence in 33% of cases (Canadian Centre for Justice Statistics, 2005). Research has substantiated the traumatic long-term effects of witnessing violence. For example, children who have witnessed violence in the home were more likely to demonstrate increased levels of depression, emotional problems, and delinquency (Fitzgerald, 2004, as cited in Canadian Centre for Justice Statistics, 2005). In addition, children who grow up in violent families experience living with secrecy, relocations as the mother leaves home to seek safety, economic hardship, maternal depression that may reduce her ability to nurture, and frightening interactions with the police and court systems (Berman et al., 2004; Boyd & Mackey, 2000a; Campbell & Lewandowski, 1997). Moreover, many children who witness violence begin to accept it as a normal part of relationships and a way to deal with problems (Sisley et al., 1999). A National Longitudinal Survey of Children and Youth in 1994 to 1995 found that children who witnessed violence in the home were more likely to be physically aggressive 2 to 4 years later (Statistics Canada, 2003b).

Elder Abuse

Elder abuse is increasingly recognized as a serious problem in Canada and other countries. As the population continues to age, it is likely that the problem will worsen. As with other types of abuse, the prevalence of elder abuse is unknown. The 1999 GSS data provide evidence that approximately 7% of the sample of 4,000 adults aged 65 years and older had experienced either emotional or financial abuse inflicted by an adult child, spouse, or caregiver within 5 years of the survey, whereas only 1% of the older adults surveyed reported physical or sexual abuse (Department of Justice, Canada, 2005), and 2% reported more than two types of abuse. In contrast, the 2000 UCR2 data from 122 police units across Canada indicated that the most common crime committed by family members against older people was common assault. The three frequent types of violent crimes were documented by family members against the elderly: common assault (54%), verbal threats (21%), and assault with a weapon resulting in bodily harm (13%) (Department of Justice, Canada, 2005). Estimated rates of neglect are not available in Canada, whereas in the United States the estimated prevalence rate of neglect is the most frequent type of abuse at 58.5%, with estimated rates of physical abuse (15.7%), financial or material mistreatment (12.3%), emotional abuse (7.3%), and sexual abuse (0.04%) reported at considerably lower rates (Comijs et al., 1998; Wallace, 1999). The nature of neglect and of physical, sexual, and emotional abuse is similar to that described for women and children. Financial or material mistreatment may include improper or illegal acts to obtain and use an elderly person's resources for personal benefit (Wallace, 1999).

Risk factors for elder abuse include older age, impairment in activities of daily living (ADLs), cognitive disability or other mental illness, dependency on the caregiver, isolation, stressful events, and a history of intergenerational conflict between the elder and the caregiver (Sengstock, Ulrich, & Barrett, 2004).

THEORIES OF ABUSE

Many theories have attempted to explain violence between intimate partners and in the family. The theories reviewed here have been categorized as biologic, psychological, and social. In all likelihood, family violence is truly a biopsychosocial phenomenon that no one of these theories can fully explain (Fig. 36-2). A separate section presents additional theories that are more specific to the phenomenon of woman abuse.

Biologic Theories

Neurologic Problems

Aggressive behaviour may be associated with several neurologic conditions, including traumatic brain injury, seizure disorder, and dementia (see Chapter 35). Neurodevelopmental factors and traumatic brain injury can produce seizure disorders, attentional dysfunction, or focal neurobehavioural syndromes, all of which are associated with aggressive behaviour. The most common association between seizures and aggressive behaviour

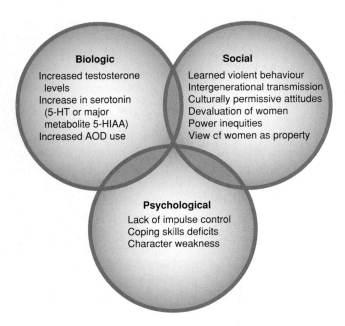

Biologic
Increased testosterone levels
Increase in serotonin (5-HT or major metabolite 5-HIAA)
Increased AOD use

Social
Learned violent behaviour
Intergenerational transmission
Culturally permissive attitudes
Devaluation of women
Power inequities
View of women as property

Psychological
Lack of impulse control
Coping skills deficits
Character weakness

FIGURE 36.2   Biopsychosocial etiologies for violent behaviour.

occurs during the postictal period (the period immediately after the seizure), during which the individual may be confused and react aggressively.

Damage to the orbitofrontal cortex often causes impulsive, labile, irritable, and socially inappropriate behaviour. Individuals with such damage often respond aggressively to trivial stimuli. In addition, damage to the neocortex, limbic system, and hypothalamus may result in aggressive behaviour. These systems have hierarchic control over one another. Damage to higher centres may disinhibit aggression from lower centres. Aggressive behaviour also may be related to disruptions in neurotransmitter systems. Disruption in serotonin, dopamine, and gamma-aminobutyric acid (GABA) systems has been linked with several psychiatric disorders, including depression, schizophrenia, impulsive behaviour, suicide, and aggression (Rosenbaum, Geffner, & Benjamin, 1997).

Links With Substance Abuse

The use of alcohol and other drugs (AOD) is commonly associated with violent incidents. Alcohol has been found to be present in approximately one half to two thirds of sexual assaults (Ulman, 2003). Although AOD use alone is rarely sufficient to account for violence, the Ontario Mental Health Supplement indicated that parental substance use is significantly associated with an increased risk for childhood physical and sexual abuse (Walsh, MacMillan, & Jamieson, 2003). Other factors, such as low family income, stress, and abuse in the family of origin, are often more important (Collins & Messerschmidt, 1993; Wallace, 1999). The relationship

of AOD to violence may result from three factors: (1) AOD-induced cognitive impairment, (2) the user's expectations that AOD increases the tendency toward aggression, and (3) socioculturally grounded beliefs that people are unaccountable for their behaviour while intoxicated (Abbey et al., 2003).

Studies have demonstrated that drinking alcohol may change perceptions about accountability for behaviour (Abbey et al., 2003). The belief that intoxicated behaviour will be judged less harshly may encourage and provide an excuse for those who abuse substances to engage in normally unacceptable behaviour. Research shows that people attempt to justify their criminal behaviour by blaming alcohol after the fact (Abbey et al., 2003). However, the rules about AOD and accountability appear to be applied differently to men and women. One early study that examined the effects of intoxication on attributions of blame in a rape incident found that both men and women judged the rapist as less responsible if intoxicated, whereas they held the victim more responsible if intoxicated (Richardson & Campbell, 1982). On the other hand, a more recent study has indicated that in cases of sexual assault, the consumption of alcohol or drugs is seven times more likely to lead to arrest (Scott & Beaman, 2004).

Psychosocial Theories

Psychopathology Theory

Psychopathology theory seeks to understand violence by examining characteristics of individual men and women (Wallace, 1999). Theorists from this perspective focus on personality traits, internal defence systems, and mental disorders. An outdated theory that was particularly damaging labelled women masochistic, paranoid, or depressed (Bograd, 1999). One underlying assumption of this labelling was that some women enjoy abuse and deliberately provoke attacks because they need to suffer.

Research on batterers has shown that there is not a common profile or a typical batterer. Studies have found evidence of personality disorders, including antisocial, borderline, narcissistic, and dependent. A Canadian study of 997 men who were recruited from outpatient forensic settings and the community indicated that abusive or severely abusive men were more likely to have antisocial personality disorders, demonstrate impulsive behaviour, and have dysfunctional attitudes regarding spousal abuse compared with nonabusive men (Hanson, Cadsky, Harris, & Lalonde, 1997). Abusive men were also more likely to have a history of violence during childhood.

Although research has not consistently found one common mental disorder or set of characteristics in violent individuals, a recently identified typology of men who batter shows promise (Emery & Laumann-Billings, 1998). Type I batterers are violent in many situations, have many victims, and display antisocial characteristics. Type II batterers abuse only their family, commit less severe violence, are generally less aggressive, and demonstrate remorse. These men tend to be dependent, jealous, and unlikely to have personality or other disorders. Type III batterers display dysphoric-borderline or schizoid characteristics, such as emotional volatility, depression, feelings of inadequacy, and social isolation (Emery & Laumann-Billings, 1998). Type III batterers also tend to be violent only within their families.

Social Learning Theory

Violent families create an atmosphere of tension, fear, intimidation, and tremendous confusion about intimate relationships (Boyd & Mackey, 2000a). Children in violent homes often learn violent behaviour as an approved and legitimate way to solve problems, especially within intimate relationships. Social learning theory posits that men who witness violence in their homes often perpetuate violent behaviour in their families as adults (Dewey, 2004; Emery & Laumann-Billings, 1998; Wallace, 1999). Moreover, women who grow up in violent homes learn to accept violence and expect it in their own adult relationships (Boyd & Mackey, 2000a). These concepts are often referred to as the **intergenerational transmission** of violence. Consistent with the theory of intergenerational transmission of violence, research findings from a telephone survey of 1,249 adults living in the city of Vancouver provide evidence that all forms of violence occurring in families of origin are predictive of relationship violence (Kwong, Bartholomew, Henderson & Trinke, 2003).

Findings of extreme violence in the parental homes of battered individuals and individuals who grew up witnessing violence are common and support the intergenerational transmission of violence theory (Dewey, 2004). However, not all those who batter or are abused come from violent homes. Estimates are that approximately 40% of those who experienced abuse or witnessed abuse in childhood will consequently abuse their wives or children (Dutton, 1998).

Social Theories

Covering the many sociologic theories of violence is beyond the scope of this chapter. Sociologic theories posit that abuse occurs because of cultural norms that permit and even glamorize violent behaviour (Dewey, 2004). From a societal perspective, the acceptance of violence as normal appears widespread among young people. In one study, as many as 70% of a group of female college students listed at least one form of

violence as acceptable in dating relationships. Even more disturbing is that 80% of these women mentioned situations in which physical force between partners was tolerable. Slapping was cited most often (49%), whereas punching was seen as acceptable by 21% of these women (Girshick, 1993). In addition, as many as 34% of women marry someone who abused them in a dating relationship (Barnett et al., 1997). In keeping with these findings, a qualitative study by Canadian researchers revealed that young adolescent girls (ages 15 and 16 years) were so eager to have a male dating partner that they were willing to tolerate physical violence and verbal abuse, just to "keep the guy" (Banister, Jakubec, & Stein, 2003).

Family violence is also related to qualities of the community in which the family is embedded. Poverty, absence of family services, social isolation, lack of cohesion in the community, and stress contribute to family violence (Dewey, 2004). The relationship of poverty, social isolation, and child abuse has been well established (Emery & Laumann-Billings, 1998; Health Canada, 1998). Economic disadvantage creates tremendous stress for families, increasing the risk for child abuse and maltreatment. It should be kept in mind that economically impoverished families may seek social services more frequently, and as such, the reporting of abuse may be increased in these families (Health Canada, 1998). However, not all poor families abuse their children. One difference between poor families who do and do not abuse their children lies in the degree of social cohesion and mutual caring found in their communities (Emery & Laumann-Billings, 1998). Neighbourhoods with high levels of child abuse frequently have severe social disorganization and lack of community identity. In addition, they have higher rates of juvenile delinquency, drug trafficking, and violent crime (Emery & Laumann-Billings, 1998).

One of the most accepted theories of elder abuse is the family stress theory. The theory hypothesizes that providing care for an elder induces stress within the family. Family stress includes economic hardship, loss of sleep, and intrusions into family activities and routines. Moreover, caring for a dependent elder takes an enormous physical toll on the caregiver. If there is no relief, the caregiver may become overwhelmed, lose control, and abuse the elder (Sengstock et al., 2004; Wallace, 1999). With the aging of the Canadian population, the demands on family members to provide care are rising, as are the associated stress of caregiving and the increased risk for elder abuse (Canadian Centre for Justice Statistics, 2005). Other characteristics of caregivers that may predispose them to abuse elderly parents include alcohol or drug abuse, dementia, restricted outside activities, unrealistic expectations, and a blaming, hypercritical personality.

Theoretic Dynamics Specific to Woman Abuse

Feminist Theories

Feminist theory focuses on issues of gender, inequality, power and privilege, patriarchy, and the subordination of women as explanations for woman abuse (Landenburger, Campbell, & Rodriguez, 2004). According to the feminist perspective, woman abuse results from a patriarchal society that perpetuates attitudes that support violence against women (Lloyd & Emery, 2000; Wallace, 1999). Three major characteristics of such a patriarchal society are the devaluation of women, power inequities, and the view of women as property (Barnett et al., 1997; Wallace, 1999).

Feminists charge that patriarchal society is the product of a predominately white, male-dominated majority that believes that women are inherently inferior to men. Such societies value women primarily for their reproductive capacity and potential to please men (Sampselle et al., 1992; Wallace, 1999).

Feminists also point to a power inequity in society as a contributing factor to woman abuse. Women have made many advances in recent years; however, men continue to control most institutions (Lloyd & Emery, 2000). Women continue to earn less than men for paid work and are less likely to advance to positions of authority and power (Nolen-Hoeksema, 2002; Sampselle et al., 1992). Moreover, marriage often victimizes women in ways other than through violence. Although men now contribute to household work, most women who hold jobs outside the home continue to perform most household and child care tasks (Lloyd & Emery, 2000). This power inequity is reflected in higher depression rates among married women than among married men (Nolen-Hoeksema, 2002). In cases of divorce, most women become single parents with a standard of living significantly lower than that of their former spouse (Wallace, 1999). The study findings from a feminist grounded theory study of 40 single mothers who recently left abusive partners in Ontario and New Brunswick reveals that the majority of participants continued to experience ongoing harassment, even though these single mothers had left their abusive partners (Ford-Gilboe, Wuest, & Merritt-Gray, 2005). The central challenges faced by these women included decreased resources, persistent persecution, and ongoing chronic health problems that were, in fact, a consequence of leaving the abusive relationship (Ford-Gilboe, Wuest & Merritt-Gray, 2005).

Until the early 1900s, women legally were the property of men in the United States (Sampselle et al., 1992). Ownership of women continues in many parts of the world and continues to influence attitudes toward women. The entertainment and advertising industries perpetuate the image of women as property by depicting them as objects and often portraying the dismembering of women's bodies (Kilbourne, 1987, 1999). The focus on women's body parts in advertising dehumanizes women, and that dehumanization is often the first step in making women acceptable targets of violence. For example, a 3-month study of newspaper coverage of disabled men and women in Canada and Israel indicated that women received less media coverage then men, yet the media coverage of women demonstrated a higher level of victimization and violence, overall (Gold & Auslander, 1999). Moreover, the explicit portrayal in the media of women in various states of undress and in seductive postures suggests that they are vulnerable and openly welcome sexual advances. Frequently, the message is, "Buy the product and get the woman" (Kilbourne, 1987).

Theory of Borderline Personality Organization and Violence

Dr. Donald Dutton is an international expert in the field of domestic violence, who has advocated extensively for more comprehensive interventions to respond to domestic violence. He is currently on faculty at the University of British Columbia. His 1998 book, *The Abusive Personality*, is a seminal work that addresses the relationship of borderline personality organization (BPO) to the type of batterer who is chronically and intermittently abusive but abusive only within his family (see Chapter 24). Dutton's work combines aspects from social learning theory, reinforcement principles from learning theory, and evidence that early trauma can alter personality through changes that occur biologically or through learning. He bases his theory on his own research and that of others, such as Bandura (social learning theory) (1977) and van der Kolk (traumatic stress and its consequences) (1996).

Dutton (1998) describes three characteristics or cycles of BPO that shift with time and seem to coincide with the cycle of violence first proposed by Walker in 1979 and described later in this chapter. These characteristics can apply to men or women with BPO; however, because this discussion focuses on men's aggression toward their female partners, it addresses the individual with BPO as male. Phase I of the male borderline personality, or "cyclic personality," consists of an internal buildup of tensions, in which the man feels depressed and irritable but does not know how to verbalize his inner dysphoria. In fact, he may not even be able to recognize or label the painful feelings, a condition called **alexithymia** (Dutton, 1998). The inability to recognize or express painful feelings and ask for what he needs traps the man in a downward spiral of bad feelings, compounded by an inability to maintain his own self-integrity. He is dependent on his partner for his sense of self. Therefore, the loss of the partner carries the risk that he will lose himself. According to Dutton, the reason that men with BPO become so abusive in their intimate relationships, but not in other relationships, is linked to their extreme dependency on their partners for sense of self and their inability to tolerate aloneness. This type of dependency is often called a "masked or hostile dependency." To maintain this relationship, the man with BPO must control his partner; therefore, his controlling behaviour masks his dependency. The man with BPO expects his partner to do the impossible. When she fails, he erupts in extreme anger because his sense of self is threatened. He converts dysphoria into abuse through (1) the belief that the partner should be able to soothe the bad feelings and (2) conversion of feelings of terror into rage. His use of projection, a defence mechanism, leads him to believe that it is her fault. The explosive combination of ego needs, an inability to communicate them, chronic irritability, jealousy, and projective blaming combine to ensure a violent relationship (Dutton, 1998).

As this phase continues, the man with BPO becomes verbally abusive, and the partner withdraws. The man wants closeness, not withdrawal, but he does not have the skills to ask for it. In addition to increasing anger, the man with BPO becomes increasingly demanding. At this stage, the dichotomous thinking or splitting characteristic of BPO is evident, and the man sees the partner as "all bad"—unfaithful, unloving, and malevolent. The unexpressed rage builds until the man with BPO erupts with violence. The violence drives the partner further away, increasing the man's feelings of abandonment. As a result, the abusive man promises anything to get the partner back. (This phase coincides with Walker's contrition phase in the cycle of violence.) The opposite side of splitting is now in evidence, as the man describes his partner as "all good"—"a madonna" (Dutton, 1998, p. 96). This example of splitting is sometimes referred to as "madonna/whore."

It is hypothesized that the abuser's BPO results from early physical abuse. Researchers suggest that early physical abuse causes long-term problems in modulating emotion and aggression and may lead to chronic anger (Dutton, 1998). The difficulty in modulating emotion often manifests first in affective numbing and constriction or in alexithymia. Hyperarousal follows emotional numbing, a process that culminates in violence (Dutton, 1998). These symptoms are manifestations of PTSD, described later in this chapter. Abusive men also score higher than do control subjects on other measures of trauma, such as depression, anxiety, sleep disturbances, and dissociation (Dutton, 1998). However, the form that the violence takes appears to be learned. That is, boys tend to identify with the aggressor and act out, whereas girls often identify with the victim and turn to self-destructive acts, such as substance abuse and self-mutilation (Dutton, 1998).

One other aspect of this cycle appears to ensure its continuation—that of positive reinforcement. The type of violence perpetrated by men with BPO has been labelled "deindividuated violence"; that is, the violence is responsive only to internal cues from the perpetrator and unresponsive to cues from the victim (Dutton, 1998). The violence feeds on itself because it is rewarding; it reduces the perpetrator's aversive arousal and tension. As a result, batterers often continue the assault until they are exhausted. Expressing rage through violent acts is the only way they know to reduce their tension or aversive arousal, and it becomes addictive (Dutton, 1998).

The cycle described by Dutton helps explain the descriptions of violent men provided by more than 200 women with whom he has worked. The following are examples of their descriptions of violent partners: "He's like Jekyll and Hyde" "He's completely different sometimes," and "His friends never see the other side of him; they think he's just a nice guy, just one of the boys" (Dutton, 1998, p. 53).

Theories of Why Women Stay in Violent Relationships

A more appropriate question than "Why do women stay in violent relationships?" is "How does she ever manage to leave given all the strikes against her?" (Anderson & Saunders, 2003). There are many reasons women stay in violent relationships. One of the strongest reasons is economic (Wallace, 1999). Despite years of progress, women still earn less than men for equal work. Many women lack the education or skills that would allow them to earn an adequate living outside the home. For these women, leaving their abusive partners means that they and their children would be homeless and without any source of support for even basic necessities. Furthermore, many shelters for battered women have long waiting lists and provide only temporary housing.

The socialization of women to assume major responsibility for marriages and child rearing is often another barrier to leaving abusive relationships. Society teaches women that their proper place is at home and their primary responsibility is caring for their husbands and children (Chodorow, 1974; Gilligan, 1982; Wallace, 1999). Many women believe that making their marriage a success is their responsibility. Therefore, when they are abused, they assume that it is their fault and that their duty is to remain and try harder for their children's sakes (Boyd & Mackey, 2000a; Lloyd & Emery, 2000). Moreover, many women who were abused in childhood or witnessed abuse of their mothers think that abuse is part of a normal relationship (Boyd & Mackey, 2000a).

Women also face political and legal obstacles in leaving abusive partners. Although the legal response to wife battering is improving, police response remains inadequate in many areas of the United States (Boyd & Mackey, 2000a). If a man is arrested for assault and no action is taken to prevent future violence, he may be released shortly and retaliate against his partner. Fear for their lives and the lives of their children and other relatives often keep women from attempting to leave abusive relationships (Anderson & Saunders, 2003; Boyd & Mackey, 2000a).

Even more difficult to understand is why some women stay in violent dating relationships. About 30% to 50% of dating couples continue their relationships despite violence (Barnett et al., 1997). One factor is that dating violence often does not occur until the relationship has been sustained for a long time. By then, many women feel that they have invested too much in the relationship to end it. Research has shown that the length of the relationship and the commitment level are positively correlated with physical and sexual abuse. Similarly, an analysis of the Canadian National Survey on woman abuse in universities and colleges demonstrates that deference (degree of conformity to social norms) and availability (time spent in the relationship) are important concepts that predict woman abuse in dating relationships (Alvi & Selbee, 1997).

Survivors may go though a process consisting of several phases in leaving an abusive relationship (Anderson & Saunders, 2003). Women may leave and return several times as they are learning new coping skills. The phases may involve cognitive and emotional "leaving" before actually leaving the relationship. The phases may include (1) enduring and managing the violence while disconnecting from self and others; (2) acknowledging the abuse, reframing it, and counteracting it;

and (3) disengaging and focussing on her own needs (Anderson & Saunders, 2003). The phase immediately following separation from an abusive partner is extremely important as the woman attempts to establish a new life. Based on the findings from a qualitative study of 15 women residing in eastern Canada, a four-stage process of "reclaiming the self" emerged as the main psychological process central to leaving an abusive partner (Wuest & Merritt-Gray, 2001), which is consistent with the stages described by Anderson and Saunders (2003) (Box 36-1).

Cycle of Violence

Many cases of woman abuse reflect a recognized cycle of violence (Wallace, 1999). The cycle consists of three recurring phases that often increase in frequency and severity (Walker, 1979). The cycle is fully described in Figure 36-3.

Traumatic Bonding

The formation of strong emotional bonds under conditions of intermittent maltreatment has been reported in several studies with human and animal subjects. For example, people taken hostage may show positive regard for their captors. Abused children often show strong attachment to their abusing parents. Cult members show strong loyalty to malevolent cult leaders (Dutton, 1995). Therefore, the relationship between battered women and their partners may be just one example of traumatic bonding—the development of strong emotional ties between two people, one of whom intermittently abuses the other. Traumatic bonding suggests that a power imbalance and intermittent abuse help to form extremely strong emotional attachments.

BOX 36.1 RESEARCH FOR BEST PRACTICE

Regenerating the Family

THE QUESTION: What is known about how families engage in health promotion in everyday life after leaving an abusive partner?

METHODS: The researchers used a grounded theory approach to develop a substantive theory of family health promotion in the context of intimate partner violence. Forty mothers and 11 children from New Brunswick and Ontario were interviewed twice to gain an understanding of health promotion strategies used by mother-headed families after leaving an abusive male partner. Audiotaped interviews were transcribed verbatim, and the data were analyzed using the constant comparative method.

FINDINGS: The process of regenerating family emerged as a health promotion strategy that involved acquiring an understanding of the abusive past; building a comfortable family environment characterized by trust and

security rather than oppression and fear; and developing new respectful and caring ways of relating to each other. Attempts to re-establish a healthy family climate frequently occur in the context of dealing with ongoing harassment and intrusion from the abusive male partner.

IMPLICATIONS FOR NURSING: The findings of this study may be used to direct the clinical practice of nurses because they offer support to families in the aftermath of leaving an abusive partner. Nurses may better appreciate the importance of helping families to limit the intrusion following separation from the abusive partner, as well as to actively support families' efforts to develop comfortable nonthreatening environments. The researchers suggest that children may need specific help with understanding their private versus public stories.

Wuest, J., Merritt-Gray, M., & Ford-Gilbee, M. (2004). Regenerating family: Strengthening the emotional health of mothers and children in the context of intimate partner violence. *Advances in Nursing Science, 27*(4), 257–74.

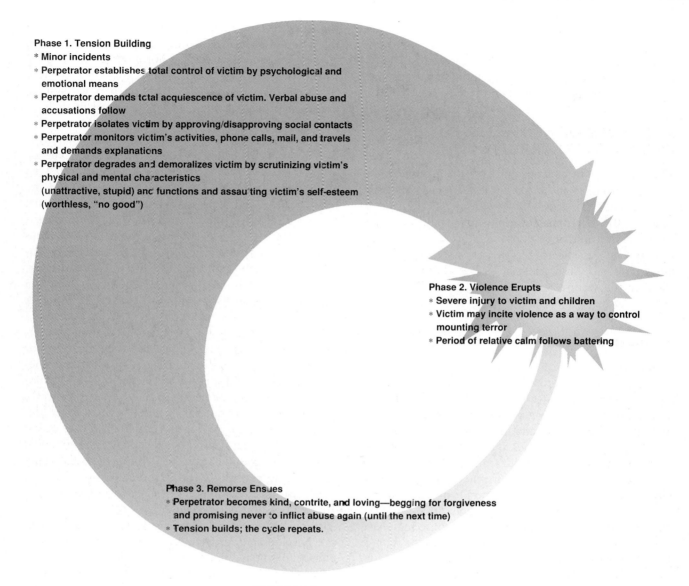

Phase 1. Tension Building
* Minor incidents
* Perpetrator establishes total control of victim by psychological and emotional means
* Perpetrator demands total acquiescence of victim. Verbal abuse and accusations follow
* Perpetrator isolates victim by approving/disapproving social contacts
* Perpetrator monitors victim's activities, phone calls, mail, and travels and demands explanations
* Perpetrator degrades and demoralizes victim by scrutinizing victim's physical and mental characteristics (unattractive, stupid) and functions and assaulting victim's self-esteem (worthless, "no good")

Phase 2. Violence Erupts
* Severe injury to victim and children
* Victim may incite violence as a way to control mounting terror
* Period of relative calm follows battering

Phase 3. Remorse Ensues
* Perpetrator becomes kind, contrite, and loving—begging for forgiveness and promising never to inflict abuse again (until the next time)
* Tension builds; the cycle repeats.

FIGURE 36.3   The cycle of violence.

Traumatic bonding theory (Dutton & Painter, 1993) explains why the cycle of violence is so powerful in entrapping a woman in a violent relationship. Researchers from British Columbia generated hypotheses based on Dutton's theory of traumatic bonding and attachment theory to assess the relevance of attachment theory to 63 women who had recently left abusive relationships (Henderson, Bartholomew, & Dutton, 1997). As predicted, women who demonstrated attachment patterns consistent with a negative view of the self composed the majority of the sample (88%).

The woman in a power imbalance perceives herself to be in a powerless position in relation to her partner, whom she perceives as extremely powerful. As the power imbalance intensifies, she feels increasingly worthless, less capable of fending for herself, and therefore, more in need of her partner. This cycle of dependency and lowered self-esteem is continually repeated,

eventually creating a strong affective bond to the partner (Dutton, 1995).

Intermittent reinforcement or punishment is one of the strongest learning paradigms in behavioural theory, especially in maintaining a particular behaviour (Dutton, 1995). An example that is often used to illustrate this concept is the gambler who persistently puts coins in a slot machine. Despite substantial losses, the gambler persists because the next time just might be the big payoff. Therefore, the gambler is not rewarded every time, but intermittently. To apply this to battered women, women may stay because this time the man may actually mean what he says and stop the abuse. After all, he has been kind and loving intermittently.

Research suggests that traumatic bonding is especially important when a woman attempts to leave her abusive partner (Dutton, 1995). When a woman leaves an abusive relationship, especially after a battering incident, she is emotionally drained and vulnerable. As time passes, her fear of her abuser diminishes, and needs supplied by the partner become evident. At this time, she is particularly susceptible to the abuser's attempts to persuade her to return to the relationship (Dutton & Painter, 1993)

SURVIVORS OF ABUSE: HUMAN RESPONSES TO TRAUMA

The experience of violence and abuse is overwhelming for most survivors and often has devastating long-term consequences (Wilson, 2001; Wilson, Friedman, & Lindy, 2001). Victimization does not produce a single uniform syndrome or response. Research on the effects of victimization reflects considerable consistency in the biopsychosocial responses to overwhelming trauma, whether the victim is a child, adult, or elder (Hendricks-Matthews, 1993).

Biologic Responses

Victims of violence experience mild to severe physical consequences. Mild injuries may include bruises and abrasions of the head, neck, face, trunk, and extremities. Severe injuries include multiple traumas, major fractures, major lacerations, and internal injuries, including chest and abdominal injuries and subdural haematomas (Campbell et al., 2004; Health Canada, 2002b). Loss of vision and hearing can result from blows to the head. Physical or sexual violence may result in head injuries that can produce changes in cognition, affect, motivation, and behaviour. Victims of sexual abuse may have vaginal and perineal trauma that is sufficient to require surgical repair (Barnett et al., 1997; Health Canada, 2002b). Anorectal injuries may also be present, including disruption of anal sphincters, retained foreign bodies, and mucosal lacerations. The following section covers the most common responses to violence and abuse:

- Depression (the dysregulated stress response theory of depression)
- Acute stress disorder (ASD)
- Post-traumatic stress disorder (PTSD)
- Dissociative identity disorder (DID)

Depression

Depression, one of the most common responses to abuse, is a biologically based disorder that can result from the effects of chronic stress on neurotransmitter and neuroendocrine systems. The body's response to stress is a complex, integrated system of reactions, encompassing body and mind. Threat or stress engages the stress system, which consists of the hypothalamic–ituitary–adrenal (HPA) axis and the sympathetic nervous system (Thase, Jindal, & Howland, 2002; Wong & Yehuda, 2002). Engagement of the HPA axis is associated with the release of corticotropin-releasing hormone (CRH) from the pituitary gland. CRH stimulates the pituitary gland to secrete adrenocorticotropic hormone (corticotropin), which stimulates the adrenal cortex to secrete cortisol. Stress also engages the sympathetic nervous system, causing the locus ceruleus and the adrenal medulla to release norepinephrine.

The CRH and locus ceruleus and norepinephrine systems participate in a mutually reinforcing feedback loop (Thase et al., 2002; Wong & Yehuda, 2002). That is, increases in CRH stimulate increased firing of the locus ceruleus and increased release of norepinephrine. Similarly, stressors that activate norepinephrine neurons increase CRH concentrations in the locus ceruleus (Charney et al., 1993). These systems prepare the threatened person to respond to danger by enhancing the person's arousal, attention, perception, energy, and emotion and by suppressing the immune response (Wong & Yehuda, 2002).

The stress response is meant to be of limited duration (Thase et al., 2002). However, when resistance or escape is impossible, the human stress system becomes overwhelmed and disorganized (Herman, 1997). Exposure to severe stressors early in life has been shown to compromise the regulation of HPA activity for a lifetime (Carter-Snell & Hegadoren, 2003; Thase et al., 2002). Accordingly, Carter-Snell and Hegadoren (2003) theorize that the increased occurrence of sexual abuse in girls may contribute to the increased prevalence of stress disorders reported in women. Most types of abuse are extreme forms of chronic stress. A protracted or dysregulated stress response has been associated with the development of major depression, especially the melancholic type (Chrousos & Gold, 1992; Henry, 1992). Melancholic features include dysphoric hyperarousal that is reflected in agitation, early morning awakening, anorexia, anxiety, excessive guilt, and hypervigilance (APA, 2000). Survivors of abuse report many of these symptoms.

Acute Stress Disorder and Post-traumatic Stress Disorder

The experience of trauma exerts tremendous physical and psychological stress on survivors. The cluster of signs and symptoms that frequently occur after major trauma is now labelled **acute stress disorder** (ASD) and **post-traumatic stress disorder** (PTSD). Originally, the diagnosis of PTSD was given only to men who demonstrated symptoms after combat experiences. In such cases, PTSD has been given several names, including *shell shock* after World War I, *traumatic neurosis* after World War II, and PTSD after the Vietnam War (Kaplan & Sadock, 1998). Lasiuk and Hegadoren (2006) in their historical overview of the PTSD concept describe the often misunderstood link between the condition "hysteria" described in early 19th century Europe, war trauma, and PTSD. Subsequent research has demonstrated that symptoms of ASD and PTSD occur not only after war but also after many types of severe trauma, including physical abuse, sexual abuse, and rape.

ASD is a new disorder in the updated *Diagnostic and Statistical Manual of Mental Disorders*, 4th edition, text revision (*DSM-IV-TR*) (APA, 2000). It is diagnosed when a barrage of stress-related symptoms occurs within 1 month of a traumatic event and persists for at least 2 days, causing significant distress. If symptoms persist beyond 1 month, the diagnosis changes to PTSD. Research has indicated that symptoms of ASD predict the development of PTSD (Raphael & Matthew, 2002). The diagnostic criteria for ASD are similar to those for PTSD.

Because ASD is a new diagnostic category in *DSM-IV-TR*, its prevalence is unknown. Community-based studies show a lifetime prevalence for PTSD of 1% to 14% (APA, 2000). Researchers studying at-risk people, including survivors of abuse, have found prevalence rates ranging from 3% to 64% (APA, 2000; Epstein, Saunders, Kilpatrick, & Resnick, 1998). A comprehensive review of research on the epidemiology of PTSD suggests several gender differences (Norris et al., 2002). Men are more exposed to traumatic events than are women. However, women are about twice as likely as men to experience PTSD, and the median time from onset to remission for women is 4 years, compared with 1 year for men (Lasiuk & Hegadoren, in press). Several factors may contribute to these differences. One factor is that men and women experience different types of traumatic events. More men report exposure to events such as fire or disaster, life-threatening accidents, physical assault, combat, being threatened with a weapon, and being held captive. More women report child abuse, sexual molestation, and sexual assault. Sexual violence is associated with a high risk for the development of PTSD. Another factor is differing reactions to traumatic events. To meet criteria for a diagnosis of PTSD, the traumatized individual must experience terror, horror, or helplessness in response to the trauma (Criterion A2 in *DSM-IV-TR*) (APA, 2000, p. 467). More women than men meet this criterion, suggesting that women may be more distressed than men by traumatic events. However, neither types of events nor perceptions of threat fully account for the difference in prevalence rates of PTSD in men and women (Norris et al., 2002).

Other factors that may contribute to higher prevalence of PTSD in women include higher rates of anxiety and depressive disorders and traumatic events before the age of 15 years (Breslau et al., 1997; Carter-Snell & Hegadoren, 2003; Orsillo, Raja, & Hammond, 2002). In one study of childhood exposure to trauma, a greater percentage of women (27%) than men (8%) reported rape, assault, or ongoing physical or sexual abuse. More men (28%) than women (11%) with childhood trauma reported serious accidents or injury. Exposure to accidents or injury in childhood did not lead to PTSD in respondents of either gender; whereas, rape and abuse resulted in a high rate of early PTSD in women (63%), but no cases in men (Breslau et al., 1997).

PTSD may develop any time after the trauma. The delay may be as short as 1 week or as long as 30 years (Kaplan & Sadock, 1998). Symptoms may fluctuate in intensity with time and usually are worse during periods of stress. Some 30% of patients with PTSD recover completely, 40% continue to have mild symptoms, 20% continue to have moderate symptoms, and 10% remain unchanged or become worse (Kaplan & Sadock, 1998).

Young children and elderly people have special difficulty with traumatic events. Young children may not have developed adequate coping mechanisms to deal with severe stressors, and older people are likely to have rigid coping mechanisms, making successful coping with the trauma more difficult (Kaplan & Sadock, 1998).

Women with PTSD frequently have comorbid anxiety, depressive disorders, or both, and the association among childhood abuse, PTSD, and substance abuse is also becoming well established (Boyd, 2000, 2003; Boyd & Mackey, 2000b; Brady & Dansky, 2002; Stewart, Ouimette, & Brown, 2002). The neurobiology of ASD and PTSD involves the stress response previously described. In addition, stress is manifested in three broad symptom categories associated with ASD and PTSD: hyperarousal, intrusion, and avoidance and numbing (APA, 2000; Rothschild, 1998).

Hyperarousal

After a traumatic experience, the stress system seems to go on permanent alert, as if the danger might return at any time (Rasmusson & Friedman, 2002; Wong & Yehuda, 2002). In this state of physiologic hyperarousal, the traumatized person is hypervigilant for signs of danger, startles easily, reacts irritably to small annoyances, and sleeps poorly. These symptoms are characteristic of increased noradrenergic function (O'Donnell, Hegadoren, & Coupland, 2004), particularly in the locus ceruleus and limbic system (hypothalamus, hippocampus, and amygdala), and of increased dopamine activity, particularly in the prefrontal cortical dopamine system (Rasmusson & Friedman; Wong & Yehuda). Dopamine hyperactivity is associated with the hypervigilance seen in PTSD. Many people with PTSD do not return to their normal baseline level of alertness. Instead, they seem to have a new baseline of elevated arousal, as if their "thermostat" had been reset (Bremner, Southwick, & Charney, 1999).

Behavioural sensitization may be one mechanism underlying the hyperarousal seen in PTSD. This phenomenon, sometimes referred to as *kindling*, occurs after exposure to severe, uncontrollable stressors. The sensitized person reacts with a magnified stress response to later, milder stressors (Bremner, Southwick, et al., 1999; Charney et al., 1993; Krystal et al., 1989). Research shows that a single or repeated exposure to a severe stressor potentiates the capacity of a subsequent stressor to increase synaptic levels of norepinephrine and dopamine in the forebrain (Charney et al., 1993). This finding would account for the fact that some survivors with PTSD experience intense fear, anxiety, and panic in response to minor stimuli. One example of behavioural sensitization is that PTSD after combat exposure is more likely to develop in veterans who are survivors of childhood abuse than in those who have not experienced prior trauma (Southwick, Bremner, Krystal, & Charney, 1994).

The state of hyperarousal causes other problems for survivors. The loss of neuromodulation leads to loss of affect regulation, so that the survivor is irritable and overreacts to others (van der Kolk & Fisler, 1993). This type of behaviour may cause others to avoid the survivor. The continual arousal may desensitize the survivor to real threat and decrease the probability that she will respond to perceived danger (Messman-Moore & Long, 2003). This development may cause the person to miss clues of danger and place himself or herself in situations that can lead to revictimization.

Intrusion

Long after abuse has stopped, survivors relive it as though it were continually recurring. Flashbacks and nightmares, which the survivor experiences with terrifying immediacy, are vivid and often include fragments of traumatic events exactly as they happened (Bremner, Southwick, et al., 1999). Moreover, a wide variety of stimuli that may have been associated with the trauma can elicit flashbacks and dreams. Consequently, survivors avoid such stimuli (Bremner, Southwick, et al., 1999).

Three related but somewhat different explanations may account for the vivid, disturbing flashbacks and dreams that individuals with PTSD have: disturbances of memory, classic conditioning (fear conditioning), and extinction.

Memory function is altered in PTSD. Memory deficits include short-term memory and potentiation of recall of traumatic experiences and dissociative flashbacks. Human beings are bombarded constantly by sensory stimuli yet attend to and remember only a fraction of it (Bremner, Southwick, et al., 1999; Southwick et al., 1994). People seem to remember best those events that have emotional effects and occur when they are alert, aroused, and responsive to their internal and external environment. Because noradrenergic activity is elevated in individuals with PTSD when exposed to emotional and traumatic stimuli, memory encoding may be improved, leading to intrusive thoughts and memories (O'Donnell, Hegadoren & Coupland, 2004).

During stress, there is a massive release of neurotransmitters, particularly norepinephrine, epinephrine, and opioid peptides. This flood of "stress hormones" may lead to structural changes in the brain that potentiate long-term memory. In most situations, this type of memory has survival value: remembering events that occur during danger may protect oneself during similar future situations. However, in PTSD, the memories occur when the individual is not in danger. Research supporting this hypothesis demonstrated that if norepinephrine is administered to animals immediately after training, long-term memory is enhanced. Epinephrine and endogenous opioids may influence memory consolidation (transforming short-term memory to long-term memory) by affecting norepinephrine (Bremner, Southwick, et al., 1999; Southwick et al., 1994).

The hippocampus and amygdala are involved in memory consolidation. The hippocampus is involved in object memory and placement of memory traces in space and time (Bremner, Southwick, et al., 1999; Cohen, Perel, DeBellis, Friedman, & Putnam, 2002). High levels of stress have been shown to damage the hippocampus and decrease its volume, producing memory deficits such as amnesia and deficits in autobiographical memory (memory of one's life story) (Bremner, Southwick, et al., 1999). The amygdala integrates sensory information for storage in and retrieval from memory. The amygdala also attaches emotional significance to sensory information and transmits this information to all the other systems involved in the stress response. Over-reactivity of the amygdala might explain the recurrent and intrusive traumatic memories and the excessive fear associated with traumatic reminders characteristic of PTSD (Cohen et al., 2002). Moreover, electrical stimulation of the amygdala and hippocampal area has been associated with dream-like and memory-like hallucinations that are similar to flashbacks reported by patients with PTSD (Bremner, Narayan, et al., 1999).

Classic conditioning, or **fear conditioning**, occurs when a neutral stimulus (the conditioned stimulus [CS]) is paired with an aversive unconditioned stimulus (US) that elicits an unconditioned fear response (UR). After repeated pairing, the CS alone will elicit the fear response, which is now the conditioned response (CR). For example, certain sights, sounds, or smells that occurred in close proximity to the traumatic event may elicit a fear response in the future. The result of this process is that an individual becomes fearful and anxious in response to a wide variety of stimuli (Bremner, Southwick, et al., 1999; Southwick et al., 1994); therefore, a wide variety of stimuli can elicit symptoms of PTSD.

The amygdala and hippocampus also appear to be important players in fear conditioning (Bremner, Southwick, et al., 1999; O'Donnell, Hegadoren & Coupland,

2004; Southwick et al., 1994). Other important brain sites include the thalamus, locus ceruleus, and sensory cortex. Interaction between the cortex and the amygdala may be necessary for specific stimuli to elicit traumatic memories (Bremner, Southwick, et al.; Charney et al., 1993).

Several neurochemical systems are involved in regulating fear conditioning, including norepinephrine, dopamine (DA), opiate, and corticotropin-releasing systems. In addition, N-methyl-D-aspartate (NMDA), one of the major excitatory neurotransmitters in the brain, appears necessary for this type of learning to occur. NMDA antagonists applied to the amygdala prevent the development of fear-conditioned responses (Bremner, Southwick, et al., 1999; Charney et al., 1993).

Extinction is the loss of a learned conditioned emotional response after repeated presentations of the conditioned fear stimulus without a contiguous traumatic event. In other words, the individual no longer responds with fear to the conditioned response. For example, many children are afraid of the dark; however, after many uneventful nights, children gradually lose their fear. Failure of the neuronal mechanisms involved in extinction also may explain the continued ability of conditioned stimuli to elicit traumatic memories and flashbacks in PTSD (Bremner, Southwick, et al., 1999; Charney et al., 1993). Recent research on brain dysfunction associated with PTSD resulting from childhood abuse of women has shown that damage to the medial prefrontal cortex interferes with extinguishing fear responses. In addition, individuals with damage to the medial prefrontal cortex show emotional dysfunction and an inability to relate in social situations that require correct interpretation of the emotional expressions of others. These findings suggest that dysfunction of this area of the brain may play a role in pathologic emotions that follow exposure to extreme stressors, such as childhood sexual abuse (Bremner, Narayan, et al., 1999).

Avoidance and Numbing (Dissociative Symptoms)

Survivors try to avoid people or situations that might provoke memories of the trauma. This restriction in their activities may interfere with normal functioning. Survivors also report anhedonia (loss of ability to sense pleasure) and may report that they feel as if parts of themselves have died. These disturbing symptoms may lead them to engage in acts of self-mutilation to feel alive or ultimately to suicide (van der Kolk & Fisler, 1993).

A person who is completely powerless may go into a state of surrender. In that state, the person escapes the situation by altering his or her state of consciousness, that is, by dissociating (Herman, 1997). **Dissociation** is defined as a disruption in the normally occurring linkages between subjective awareness, feelings, thoughts, behaviour, and memories (APA, 2000; Briere & Elliott, 1994).

Dissociation is a complex psychophysiologic process that produces alterations in sense of self, accessibility of memory and knowledge, and integration of behaviour (Putnam, 1994; Rothschild, 1998). In simpler words, a person who dissociates is making himself or herself "disappear." That is, the person has the feeling of leaving their body and observing what happens to them from a distance. During trauma, dissociation enables a person to observe the event while experiencing no pain, or only limited pain, and to protect themselves from awareness of the full impact of the traumatic event (van der Kolk, 1996). A study of Montreal school-aged girls indicates that sexual abuse was associated with eight times the level of dissociation and four times the level of PTSD in the girls who had been sexually abused compared with matched controls without sexual abuse (Collin-Vezina & Herbert, 2005). Examples of dissociation include (1) derealization and depersonalization (the experience of self or the environment as strange or unreal); (2) periods of disengagement from the immediate environment during stress, such as "spacing out"; (3) alterations in bodily perceptions; (4) emotional numbing; (5) out-of-body experiences; and (6) amnesia for abuse-related memories (Briere & Elliott, 1994; Rothschild, 1998). Fear activates the endogenous opioid system, producing stress-induced analgesia (SIA) (Bremner, Southwick, et al., 1999; van der Kolk, 1996). SIA may be associated with avoidance and numbing. The purpose of SIA is to protect against pain in dangerous situations so that the individual (animal or human) can defend itself (fight) or escape the situation (flight). In severely stressed animals, opiate withdrawal symptoms can be produced by removing the stressor or by injecting naloxone, an opiate antagonist. In people with PTSD, SIA can become conditioned to stimuli resembling the original trauma. Research with humans showed that as long as 20 years after the original trauma, people with PTSD developed SIA equivalent to 8 mg of morphine in response to such stimuli. Excessive opioid and norepinephrine secretion can interfere with memory. Freezing or numbing responses may prevent animals from remembering situations of overwhelming stress. Trauma-related dissociative reactions after prolonged exposure to severe, uncontrollable stress may be analogous to this effect in animals (van der Kolk, 1996).

Dissociative Identity Disorder

Dissociation exists on a continuum, with most people experiencing short, situation-specific episodes, such as daydreaming (Putnam, 1994). Among survivors of abuse, dissociative symptoms may be part of the symptom picture of ASD and PTSD, or they may be the

Table 36.1	Key Diagnostic Characteristics for Dissociative Identity Disorder	

Diagnostic Criteria	Target Symptoms and Associated Findings
• Presence of two or more distinct personality states or identities • At least two identities or personality states recurrently take control of the person's behaviour • Inability to recall important information that is too extensive to be explained by ordinary forgetfulness • Not due to direct physiologic effects of substances or general medical condition • In children, symptoms not attributable to imaginary playmates or other fantasy play	• Post-traumatic symptoms (nightmares, flashbacks, startle responses) • Post-traumatic stress disorder • Self mutilation • Suicidal behaviour • Aggressive behaviour • Repetitive relationships characterized by physical and sexual abuse ***Associated Physical Examination Findings*** • Scars from self-inflicted injuries or physical abuse • Migraine and other types of headaches, irritable bowel syndrome and asthma ***Associated Laboratory Findings*** • Physiologic functioning may vary across personality states • High scores on measures of hypnotizability and dissociative capacity

predominant symptom (Lasiuk & Hegadoren, in press). In such cases, the disorder is **dissociative identity disorder** (DID) (formerly multiple personality disorder) (Rothschild, 1998). The hallmarks of DID are two or more distinct identities with unique personality characteristics and an inability to recall important information about self or events that is too extensive to be explained by ordinary forgetfulness (APA, 2000). Other memory disturbances linked with dissociation include intermittent and disruptive intrusions of traumatic memories into awareness and difficulties in determining whether a given memory reflects an actual event or information acquired through another source (Putnam, 1994). The diagnostic criteria for DID are found in Table 36-1.

Two other dimensions of dissociation that are associated with DID include passive influence experiences and hallucinatory experiences. A passive influence experience is a situation in which a person feels as if he or she were controlled by a force from within. These experiences may include a sense that one is being made to do something against one's will that may be distasteful or harmful to self and others (Putnam, 1994).

Many survivors of abuse report dissociative perceptual disturbances, such as visual hallucinations, extrasensory perceptions, and peculiar time distortions (Anderson, Yasenik, & Ross, 1993; Hendricks-Matthews, 1993). The hallucinatory experiences in dissociative disorders are distinct in several ways from those that occur in psychotic disorders. They are often experienced as internalized, rather than externalized, voices and may be associated with specific experiences or people. The affected person hears the voices distinctly; the voices often have particular attributes such as gender, age, and affect. The voices may be supportive and comforting or berating (Putnam, 1994). Hallucinatory experiences may also involve the appearance of "shadowy figures" ghosts or spirits, or rapidly moving objects. The person is generally aware that the voices or images are not real (Putnam, 1994).

The overall prevalence of DID is unknown. Estimates are that 1% of the American population may be affected and as many as 5% to 20% of people in psychiatric hospitals (National Women's Health Information Center [NWHIC], 2003). The cause of DID is unknown. However, the patient history invariably involves a traumatic event in childhood. Four types of causative factors have been identified: a traumatic event, a psychological or genetic vulnerability to develop the disorder, formative environmental factors, and the absence of external support (Kaplan & Sadock, 1998). Examples of psychological vulnerability include being suggestible or easily hypnotized. Formative environmental events may include a lack of role models who demonstrate healthy problem solving or practices to relieve anxiety or stress. Many who experience DID lack supportive others, such as parents, siblings, other relatives, and supportive people outside the family (e.g., teachers) (Kaplan & Sadock, 1998).

Complex Trauma

In her book *Trauma and Recovery*, Judith Herman proposed a new diagnosis: "complex post-traumatic stress disorder" (1997, p. 119). Her proposal was based on experience that none of the diagnostic categories in the APA's *Diagnostic and Statistical Manual* (3rd ed., rev., APA, 1987) were appropriate for survivors of extreme, prolonged trauma, especially interpersonal trauma (i.e., severe, prolonged child abuse), including the diagnosis of PTSD. She noted that survivors of prolonged, repeated trauma experience characteristic personality changes, including problems of relatedness, identity, and vulnerability to repeated harm, inflicted by others or self. Complex PTSD was considered for inclusion in the fourth edition of the *DSM* as "disorders of extreme stress not otherwise specified (DESNOS)" (van der Kolk, 1996, p. 203). DESNOS was eventually incorporated into the *DSM-IV-TR* under the "Associated Features and Disorders" section. The symptoms include impaired affect modulation (difficulty modulating anger or sexual behaviours; self-destructive and suicidal behaviour); impulsive/risk-taking behaviour; alterations in attention and consciousness (amnesia, dissociation); somatization; chronic characterologic changes, including alterations in relations with others (inability to trust or maintain relationships, tendency to be revictimized or to victimize others); and alterations in systems of meaning (despair, hopelessness, loss of previously sustaining beliefs) (APA, 2000; van der Kolk, 1996).

These symptoms are similar to those of borderline personality disorder (BPD). Many people with BPD were severely abused in childhood. Splitting self and others into *all-good* or *all-bad* may result from a developmental arrest: a fragmentation of self, based on modes of organizing experience that were common in earlier developmental stages. Self-mutilation, often labelled as masochism or manipulative behaviour, may be a way of regulating psychological and biologic equilibrium when ordinary means of self-regulation have been disturbed by trauma. Psychotic episodes in patients with BPD are similar to flashbacks, intrusive recollections of traumatic memories that were stored on a somatosensory level (van der Kolk, 1996). Research findings demonstrate that the diagnoses of both BPD and complex PTSD were significantly higher in a group of women with early-onset sexual abuse compared with late-onset sexual abuse, suggesting that women with a history of childhood sexual abuse might be better understood within the rubric of complex PTSD (McLean & Gallop, 2003).

Substance Abuse and Dependence

Childhood abuse, PTSD, and substance abuse are known to be associated. Investigators have reported that as many as 84% of female inpatient substance abusers had a history of sexual or physical assault (Brady & Dansky, 2002; Stewart et al., 2002). High rates of abuse have also been found in samples of outpatient, rural women (Boyd, 2000, 2003). The Vancouver Injection Drug User Study of sexual violence among intravenous drug users indicates that 68% of women and 19% of men had a lifetime history of sexual violence (Braitstein et al., 2003).

Survivors who experience PTSD, depression, and other forms of dysphoric hyperarousal or emotional distress often abuse substances, including alcohol and other sedative drugs that lessen stress and reduce hyperarousal and distress by inhibiting noradrenergic activity (Brady & Dansky, 2002; Stewart et al., 2002). Sexually abused adolescents and adults may use alcohol and other drugs as alternatives to psychological dissociation (Roesler & Dafler, 1993). Increasing numbers of women reportedly abuse cocaine to wipe out dysphoric feelings caused by abuse. These women report that the intense high of cocaine totally obliterates painful feelings, if only for a short time (Boyd, 2000). Substance abuse in a person with PTSD is particularly problematic. The comorbidity worsens the symptoms and courses of both disorders, increases suicidality, and makes treatment more difficult (Boyd, 2000; Hana & Grant, 1997).

Psychological Responses

Low Self-Esteem

The consequences of abuse are devastating, and the term "low self-esteem" seems inadequate. Women who are abused as children often experience "alienation from self and others" (Boyd & Mackey, 2000a). Alienation from self includes painful feelings that go to the "core of a woman being"—experiencing self as fundamentally flawed and having no purpose in life. Alienation from others, especially significant others, is associated with painful feelings of loneliness, depression, anger, shame, and guilt and with feeling hurt, unloved, and unwanted (Boyd & Mackey, 2000a). Women who experience alienation from self and others often turn to substance abuse to cope with their intense pain (Boyd & Mackey, 2000b).

Low self-esteem or alienation may be attributable to the direct effects of physical or sexual abuse or to the accompanying psychological abuse. One technique that perpetrators use to control and disempower women is to erode their sense of self-worth with a constant barrage of criticism. Perpetrators frequently tell women that they are stupid, ugly, inadequate wives and mothers, inadequate sexually, and incompetent. Other contributing factors include a sense of being different from other people, the need to maintain secrecy, lack of trust, and self-blame (Boyd & Mackey, 2000a).

Low self-esteem may be one factor contributing to a battered woman's reluctance to disclose her abuse. Because of low self-esteem, battered women, even many who are successful outside the home, underestimate their ability to do anything about the abuse (Boyd & Mackey, 2000a). As such, it is not surprising that "reclaiming the self" was identified as the main psychological process central to leaving an abusive partner in a qualitative study of women who had recently left abusive male partners (Wuest & Merritt-Gray, 2001).

Guilt and Shame

A history of abuse is often associated with excessive guilt and shame. These feelings stem from survivors' mistaken beliefs that they are somehow to blame for their abuse

(Boyd & Mackey, 2000a; Campbell et al., 2004; Long & Smyth, 1998). Feelings of humiliation and shame may prevent women from seeking medical care and reporting abuse to authorities. The experience of being battered is so degrading and humiliating that women are often afraid to disclose it. Many women fear that they will not be taken seriously or will be blamed for inciting the abuse or for staying with their abusers (Boyd & Mackey, 2000a; Campbell et al., 2004; Long & Smyth, 1998). In keeping with this observation, research findings indicate that resilient women with a history of childhood sexual abuse and no history of substance abuse felt less blame and stigma associated with being sexually abused compared with women with a history of childhood sexual abuse who were currently receiving treatment for substance abuse (Dufour & Nadeau, 2001).

Anger

Chronic irritability, unexpected or uncontrollable feelings of anger, and difficulties with the expression of anger are frequent experiences for survivors of abuse (Campbell et al., 2004). They may express anger toward the perpetrator, fate, those who have been spared suffering, or someone whom the victim believes could have prevented the abuse (Barnett et al., 1997).

Feelings of anger may signal that a person is an incest survivor. However, some incest survivors have difficulty expressing anger and mask it with compliance and perfectionism (Campbell et al., 2004; Hendricks-Matthews, 1993).

Social and Interpersonal Responses

Problems With Intimacy

The abused child experiences intrusion, abandonment, devaluation, or pain in the relationship with the abuser, instead of the closeness and nurturing that are normal for intimate relationships, such as those between parent and child (Briere & Elliott, 1994; Long & Smyth, 1998; Urbancic, 2004). As a result, many survivors have difficulty trusting and forming intimate relationships.

Sexual problems are common among survivors of abuse. Among the most common and chronic problems are fear of intimate sexual relationships, feelings of repulsion toward sex, lack of enjoyment of sex, dysfunctions of desire and arousal, and failure to achieve orgasm. Some survivors engage in compulsive promiscuity and prostitution, reflecting their internalization of the message that the only thing that they are good for is sex (Hendricks-Matthews, 1993; Long & Smyth, 1998; Urbancic, 2004).

Revictimization

Many women who have been sexually abused as children are revictimized on multiple occasions later in life.

Among women with a history of sexual assault, rates of revictimization range from 15% to 79% (Arata, 2002; Breitenbecher, 2001; Messman-Moore & Long, 2003). A community-based Toronto study of sexual violence surveyed 420 women and found that 26.4% had an experience of sexual assault in childhood and adulthood (Randall & Haskell, 1995). Numerous factors have been related to revictimization, including PTSD symptoms, dissociation, alexithymia, use of alcohol and other drugs, boundary issues, and sexual behaviour (Breitenbecher, 2001; Messman-Moore & Long). Proneness to revictimization may result from a general vulnerability in dangerous situations that may be associated with dissociation. Dissociation makes women unaware of their environment and also may make them look confused or distracted. Thus, women in a dissociative state may be easy targets (Cloitre, Scarvalone, & Difede, 1997; Messman-Moore & Long, 2003).

Alexithymia may also add to a woman's risk for revictimization. Difficulty in labelling and communicating feelings may make it difficult for a woman to set limits on sexual advances. Moreover, these women may not be able to read accurately the emotional cues of others, which diminishes their ability to respond effectively in interpersonally dangerous situations (Cloitre et al., 1997).

Women with abuse histories frequently have difficulty with boundaries. During childhood abuse, they experienced boundary violations as normal and connected with their expectations of intimate relationships. Confusion over boundaries may result in confusion about appropriate behaviour in adult intimate relationships (Cloitre et al., 1997; Messman-Moore & Long, 2003).

The sexual behaviour pattern of survivors may place them at risk for revictimization. One effect of sexual victimization is that the child's sexuality is shaped by "traumatic sexualization." Traumatic sexualization occurs when a child is rewarded for sexual behaviour with affection, attention, privileges, and gifts. As a result, the child may learn that her self-worth is tied to her sexuality, and she may use sexual behaviour to manipulate others (Breitenbecher, 2001; Messman-Moore & Long, 2003).

Nursing and the Human Response to Disorder

Nurses encounter survivors of abuse in many health care settings. The percentage of ED visits that are attributed to domestic violence ranges from 4% to 18% (Campbell et al., 2004); however, reports have been as high as 80% (McGrath et al., 1997). A critical ethnographic study of 30 nurses working in the ED departments of two urban hospitals in Canada provides direction for the care of abused women in the ED (Varcoe, 2001). Specifically, issues that obscure the needs of abused women, such as the perceived need to focus on rapid processing of patients and stereotypical judgments, were identified (Varcoe, 2001). Approximately 50% of female patients admitted to psychiatric facilities are victims of either child or adult abuse (Seeman, 2002). Other settings in which the nurse encounters battered women include primary care settings, obstetric-gynecology settings, paediatric units, well-child clinics, geriatric units, and nursing homes.

The paediatric ED provides a unique opportunity to identify and respond to child survivors, as well as battered mothers (Campbell et al., 2004). As many as 59% of mothers of child abuse victims are battered women, and child abuse occurs disproportionately in homes with woman abuse (Wright, Wright, & Isaac, 1997). Identifying battered mothers may be the most important means of identifying child abuse. Conversely, when a nurse suspects child abuse, he or she cannot ignore the possibility that the mother is also a victim. Identifying children who are traumatized by witnessing the battering of their mothers also is essential. However, despite the opportunity the paediatric ED affords, disturbingly few battered women are identified there. Health care providers in paediatric EDs have reported several obstacles to identification, including lack of training, time constraints, powerlessness, lack of comfort, lack of control over the victim's circumstances, and fear of offending the patient (Wright et al., 1997). Another important setting for effective identification of battered women is in the postpartum setting. Researchers implemented a domestic violence assessment in two hospitals in the city of Vancouver and found that the screening rate for domestic violence increased from 42% to 60% for a period of 18 months (Janssen, Holt, & Sugg, 2002).

Nurses may encounter elder abuse in virtually any setting. Examples include EDs, medical-surgical units, psychiatric units, and homes during home care visits. In addition, nurses may encounter elder abuse in nursing homes. Events such as unnecessary chemical (medications) or physical restraints used to control an elder's behaviour may be abusive and should be investigated.

Although some aspects of care are specific to adult, child, or elderly survivors of abuse, many elements are common in the nursing care of all survivors, regardless of age or setting. The goals of all nursing interventions in cases of abuse are to stop the violence and ensure the survivor's safety. Victimization removes all power and control from a woman, child, or elder. Therefore, as appropriate for age and ability, all nursing interventions should empower survivors to act on their own behalf and must be done in a collaborative partnership. To that end, nurses must be willing to offer support and information and not impose their own values on survivors by encouraging them to leave abusive relationships. Strong psychological and economic bonds tie many women to their perpetrators. Moreover, adult survivors who are capable of making decisions are the

experts on their situations. They are the best judges of when leaving the relationship is appropriate (Canadian Nurses Association, 1992; Walker, 1994).

However, removing children and elders from their families or caregivers often is necessary to ensure immediate safety. If the home of an abused or neglected child or elder cannot be made safe, the nurse must support other professionals involved in placing the child or elder in a foster or nursing home (Gary & Humphreys, 2004; Sengstock et al., 2004). However, intervening in cases of elder abuse is not a clear-cut issue. Nurses must allow elders whose decision making is not impaired (*competence* is a legal term) an appropriate degree of autonomy in deciding how to manage the problem, even if they choose to remain in the abusive situation (Allan, 1998). Forcing an elder to do something against his or her wishes is itself a form of victimization.

Intervention strategies for elders depend on whether the elder accepts or refuses assistance and whether he or she can make decisions. If the elder refuses treatment, the nurse must remain nonjudgmental and provide information about available services and emergency numbers. The Canadian approach to adult protection legislation, concerned with preventing abuse and neglect, has been guided by reforms in adult guardianship and substitute decision making. There are three adult protection models now in existence across Canada. Please see Gordon's (2001) article for a comprehensive review of adult protection legislation in Canada.

Biologic Domain

Biologic Assessment. Research indicates that health care providers often fail to respond therapeutically to survivors of abuse. In many instances, they neglect to identify abuse as the cause of traumatic injuries or mental health problems (Blakely & Ribeiro, 1997; Campbell et al., 2004; Henderson, 2001). Even more damaging, many health care professionals treat abuse survivors derogatorily, blaming them for the abuse or for staying in abusive situations. Unfortunately, nursing staff may revictimize survivors with BPD. Often these women have been severely traumatized, and their behaviour is difficult and disruptive. In some cases, caregivers react negatively, labelling this behaviour attention seeking and manipulative. When nurses react to the patient in a negative, punitive manner, they retraumatize these women (Gallop, McCay, Guha, & Khan, 1999). It is not uncommon to see this behaviour punished by staff avoidance, time in seclusion rooms, and overmedication. BPD symptoms should be interpreted as ineffective coping strategies, developed in response to severe trauma, rather than as deliberate attempts to manipulate staff (Hattendorf & Tollerud, 1997).

To improve providers' responses, the Canadian Nurses Association (CNA) recommends that students

Sheldon Kennedy (1970–)
Professional Hockey Player

Public Personna
Canadian-born Sheldon Kennedy played professional hockey in the National Hockey League (NHL). He was an outstanding and talented hockey player who began training in the Canadian Hockey League (CHL) at a young age. As a junior-level hockey player in Winnipeg, he was coached by Graham James, one of the most nationally famous and highly respected coaches.

Personal Realities
In 1996, Kennedy came forward with sexual abuse allegations against his former CHL coach, Graham James. Kennedy said the assaults took place between the ages of 14 and 19 and occurred on a weekly basis. On September 3, 1996, Kennedy reported the sexual abuse by James to the Calgary city police. In January 1997, Graham James was sentenced to 3½ years in prison for the sexual abuse. Kennedy then went public with his story, including the revelation of the many times he contemplated suicide. Shortly afterward, the NHL sponsored Kennedy to enrol in a substance abuse program for his drinking and drug problems.

Kennedy's courage has brought hope to many. He has created the Sheldon Kennedy Foundation that helps increase awareness of sexual abuse, raises money through events such as a cross-country skate, and contributes to programs such as the Anaphe Ranch in British Columbia, a healing place for Canadian children who have been abused. In honour of his efforts, the government of Saskatchewan declared August 21, 1998 Sheldon Kennedy Day.

From information gathered at http://www.silent-edge.org/, http://www.gov.sk.ca/, and http://www.snn-rdr.ca/.

acquire the necessary knowledge and skill acquisition to prevent violence, as well as to detect and intervene with individuals who are survivors of abuse and violence (Health Canada, 2002a). The CNA (1992) states that nurses can play a significant role in addressing family violence because nurses are frequently the first professionals to interact with individuals affected by family violence. Nurses should assess everyone for violence—both women and men, no matter what age or presenting problem. An awareness of violence and a high index of suspicion are the most important elements in assessing the problem (Campbell et al., 2004). If suspected abuse is never assessed, it will never be uncovered.

Establishing a trusting nurse–patient relationship is one of the most important steps in assessing any type of abuse. Survivors are unlikely to disclose sensitive information unless they perceive the nurse to be trustworthy and nonjudgmental. Important considerations in establishing open communication are ensuring confidentiality and providing a quiet, private place in which to conduct assessment. The law mandates that nurses report child abuse to the authorities, and nurses must make that responsibility clear before beginning the assessment. Child abuse is usually reported to the children aid society.

LETHALITY ASSESSMENT FIRST. The most important assessment and the one to be done first is a lethality assessment (CNA, 1992; Walker, 1994). The nurse must ascertain whether the survivor is in danger for his or her life, either from homicide or suicide and, if children are in the home, whether they are in danger (Campbell et al., 2004). The nurse should take immediate steps to ensure the survivor's safety. In the case of suspected child abuse assessed in a health care agency, an interdisciplinary team consisting of physicians, psychologists, nurses, and social workers usually makes this decision. In other settings, the nurse may be the person to make that decision. Nurses do not have to obtain proof of abuse, only a reasonable suspicion. The Danger Assessment Screen developed by Jacquelyn Campbell and colleagues is a useful tool for assessing the risk that either the adult survivor or perpetrator will commit homicide (Box 36-2).

Most survivors do not report abuse to health care workers without being asked specifically about it. Only 13% of women seen in the ED after a battering incident either told or were asked by staff about abuse (Sisley et al., 1999). A survey of the ED in 230 Canadian hospitals indicated that the implementation of domestic violence policies may be as low as 10% or 20% (Hotch, Grunfeld, Mackay, & Ritch, 1996). Survivors may be reluctant to report abuse because of shame and fear of retaliation, especially if the victim depends on the abuser as caregiver. In addition, children may be afraid that they will not be believed. Asking specific abuse screening questions has been shown to increase the detection of abuse substantially (from 3% to 15%) (Sisley et al., 1999). For that reason, nurses must develop a repertoire of age-appropriate, culturally sensitive abuse-related questions.

Appropriate questions to ask in assessing abuse in women are found in the Abuse Assessment Screen in Box 36-3. Other questions that might be useful in eliciting disclosure are: "When there are fights at home, have you ever been hurt or afraid?" "It looks like someone has hurt you. Tell me about it." "Some women have described problems like yours and have told me that their partner has hurt them. Is that happening to you?" (Campbell et al., 2004; CNA, 2002). When survivors are disclosing abuse, they need privacy and time to tell their story. They need to know that the nurse is listening, believes them, and is concerned for their safety and well being (Long & Smyth, 1998).

Most survivors are not offended when health care workers ask about abuse directly, as long as they conduct the interview nonjudgmentally. Survivors may perceive failure to ask about abuse as evidence of lack of concern, adding to feelings of entrapment and helplessness.

BOX 36.2

Danger Assessment

Several risk factors have been associated with homicides (murders) of both batterers and battered women in research that has been conducted after the killings have taken place. We cannot predict what will happen in your case, but we would like you to be aware of the danger of homicide in situations of severe battering and to see how many of the risk factors apply to your situation. (The "he" in the questions refers to your husband, partner, ex-husband, ex-partner, or whoever is currently physically hurting you.)

1. Has the physical violence increased in frequency during the past year?
2. Has the physical violence increased in severity during the past year, or has a weapon or threat with weapon been used?
3. Does he ever try to choke you?
4. Is there a gun in the house?
5. Has he ever forced you into sex when you did not wish to do so?
6. Does he use drugs? By drugs, I mean "uppers" or amphetamines, speed, angel dust, cocaine, "crack," street drugs, heroin, or mixtures.
7. Does he threaten to kill you, or do you believe he is capable of killing you?
8. Is he drunk every day or almost every day? (In terms of quantity of alcohol.)
9. Does he control most or all of your daily activities? For instance, does he tell you whom you can be friends with, how much money you can take with you shopping, or when you can take the car? (If he tries, but you do not let him, check here___.)
10. Has he ever beaten you while you were pregnant? (If never pregnant by him, check here___.)
11. Is he violently and constantly jealous of you? (For instance, does he say, "If I can't have you, no one can.")
12. Have you ever threatened or tried to commit suicide?
13. Has he ever threatened or tried to commit suicide?
14. Is he violent toward the children?
15. Is he violent outside the home?

TOTAL YES ANSWERS:___.

THANK YOU. PLEASE TALK TO YOUR NURSE, ADVOCATE, OR COUNSELLOR ABOUT WHAT THE DANGER ASSESSMENT MEANS IN TERMS OF YOUR SITUATION.

Adapted from Campbell, J., & Humphreys, J. (Eds.) (1993). *Nursing care of survivors of family violence* (p. 259). St. Louis: Mosby.

The high prevalence of abuse and the reluctance of survivors to volunteer information about it mandate routine screening of every patient for abuse by explicit questioning. Perhaps even more important, the nurse must complete such screening in privacy, away from the woman's partner, the child's parents or legal guardians, or the elderly person's relative or companion (Campbell et al., 2004; Sisley et al., 1999). If a partner, parent, other relative, or companion accompanies the patient to the health care facility, protocols should be in place to separate the patient from these individuals until assessment is completed. One approach is to ask the other person to wait in the reception area, explaining that assessments are always done in private.

After assessment is completed in a health care agency, the nurse should offer the adult survivor use of the telephone. The agency appointment may be the only time that the survivor can make calls in private to family, who might offer support, or to the police, lawyers, or shelters. Scheduling future appointments may provide the survivor with a legitimate reason to leave the perpetrator temporarily and continue to explore her options.

HISTORY AND PHYSICAL EXAMINATION. All survivors who report or for whom the nurse suspects abuse should receive a complete history and physical examination. Throughout, the nurse must remain nonjudgmental and communicate openly and honestly (CNA, 1992; Campbell et al., 2004; Long & Smyth, 1998). A Canadian grounded theory study of woman survivors of child sexual abuse indicates that feeling safe with a health care provider who is sensitive and willing to listen can facilitate disclosure (Schachter, Radomsky, Stalker, & Teram, 2004). It is not the nurse's responsibility to judge any situation, whether that is a woman's

BOX 36.3

Abuse Assessment Screen

1. Have you ever been emotionally or physically abused by your partner or someone important to you?
   YES ___
   NO ___
2. Within the past year, have you been hit, slapped, kicked or otherwise physically hurt by someone?
   YES ___
   NO ___
   If YES, by whom: _____
   Number of times: ___
   Mark the area of injury on body map.
3. Within the past year, has anyone forced you to have sexual activities?
   If YES, who: _____
   Number of times: ___
4. Are you afraid of your partner or anyone you listed above?
   YES ___
   NO ___

decision to remain in an abusive relationship, the abusive actions of children's parents, or abuse perpetrated by caregivers of the elderly. Therefore, nurses must continually monitor their own feelings toward the abuser and survivor, especially in cases of child abuse. Working with child survivors often causes distress and feelings of anger and inadequacy. Seeking supervision may prevent negative feelings from influencing the nurse–patient relationship in a nontherapeutic manner and perhaps retraumatizing the survivor (Long & Smyth, 1998).

The history should include past and present medical history, ADLs, and social and financial support. The nurse should obtain a detailed history of how injuries occurred. As with any history, the nurse begins with the complaint that brought the patient to the health care agency. The nurse assesses whether explanation for the injuries or symptoms is plausible, given their nature. Discrepancies between the history and physical examination findings may suggest abuse or neglect. The nurse moves from safe to more sensitive topics, such as the nature of the injuries. Walker (1994) suggests using what she calls the "four-incident technique" to elicit a complete abuse history. The nurse asks the survivor to describe four battering incidents: the first incident that she remembers, the most recent incident, the worst incident, and a typical incident. This series of questions is designed to elicit a complete picture of the cycle of violence and its progression. If the child is too young or an elder is too impaired to give a history, the nurse should interview one or both parents of the child or the caregiver of the elder. If the survivor is a child or dependent elder who cannot describe what happened or make decisions about personal safety and care, the health care team may take steps to place the survivor in protective custody and defer additional assessment to the appropriate agency. The physical examination should include a neurologic examination, radiographs to identify any old or new fractures, and examination for sexual abuse. Nurses assessing the elderly need to be familiar with normal aging and signs and symptoms of common illnesses in the elderly to distinguish those conditions from abuse (Allan, 1998). Similarly, nurses need to know healthy child development to detect deviations that abuse or neglect may cause. For children, assessing developmental milestones, school history, and relationships with siblings and friends is important (Walker, 1994). Any discrepancies between history and physical examination and implausible explanations for injuries and other symptoms should alert the nurse to the possibility of abuse. Box 36-4 lists indicators of actual or potential abuse that need to be thoroughly assessed for all survivors.

The nurse should thoroughly document all findings. Injuries should be photographed if possible, but this can be done only with written permission from an adult survivor or one of the child's parents. If the survivor will not permit photographing, the nurse should document the injuries on a body map. Survivors may need assurance that their medical records will not be released to anyone without written permission and that documentation of injuries will be important if legal action is taken. If the survivor does not admit abuse, the nurse cannot note abuse in the record. However, the nurse can document that the description of injuries is inconsistent with the injury pattern.

Biologic indicators, such as elevated pulse and blood pressure, sleep and appetite disturbances, exaggerated startle responses, flashbacks, and nightmares, may suggest PTSD or depression. Signs and symptoms of dissociation include memory difficulties, a feeling of unreality about oneself or events, a feeling that a familiar place is strange and unfamiliar, auditory or visual hallucinations, and evidence of having done things without remembering them (Carlson & Putnam, 1993). If any of these signs or symptoms is present, the survivor requires a thorough diagnostic workup for PTSD and DID.

CRNE Note

In accordance with the Canadian Standards of Psychiatric and Mental Health Nursing, people in abusive relationships have a right to self-determination. Care involves offering choice and respecting individual preference.

The nurse should assess every adult or adolescent who discloses victimization for substance abuse. The Michigan Alcoholism Screening Test (MAST) (Selzer, 1971) and the Drug Abuse Screening Test (DAST) (Skinner, 1982) are two screening instruments for use in any health assessment. An adolescent version of the MAST is available. If the results of these tests or the answers to any alcohol-related or drug-related questions are positive, the nurse should evaluate the survivor further for an alcohol or drug disorder.

Nursing Diagnoses for Biologic Domain
Selected nursing diagnoses focussing on the human responses that nurses manage in the biologic domain may include Post-Trauma Syndrome, Delayed Growth and Development, Impaired Memory, and Rape-Trauma Syndrome.

Interventions for Biologic Domain
Restoring health is a primary concern for survivors of abuse. When injuries are severe and surgery is required, the survivor may require hospital admittance.

TREATING PHYSICAL SYMPTOMS. Treatment of trauma symptoms may include cleaning and dressing burns or other wounds and assisting with casting of broken bones

BOX 36.4

History and Physical Findings Suggestive of Abuse

Presenting Problem
- Vague information about cause of problem
- Delay between occurrence of injury and seeking of treatment
- Inappropriate reactions of significant other or family
- Denial or minimizing of seriousness of injury
- Discrepancy between history and physical examination findings

Family History
- Past family violence
- Physical punishment of children
- Children who are fearful of parent(s)
- Father and/or mother who demands unquestioning obedience
- Alcohol or drug abuse
- Violence outside the home
- Unemployment or underemployment
- Financial difficulties or poverty
- Use of elder's finances for other family members
- Finances rigidly controlled by one member

Health and Psychiatric History
- Fractures at various stages of healing
- Spontaneous abortions
- Injuries during pregnancy
- Multiple visits to the emergency department
- Elimination disturbances (eg, constipation, diarrhoea)
- Multiple somatic complaints
- Eating disorders
- Substance abuse
- Depression
- Post-traumatic stress disorder
- Self-mutilation
- Suicide attempts
- Feelings of helplessness or hopelessness
- Low self-esteem
- Chronic fatigue
- Apathy
- Sleep disturbances (eg, hypersomnia, hyposomnia)
- Psychiatric hospitalizations

Personal and Social History
- Feelings of powerlessness
- Feelings of being trapped
- Lack of trust
- Traditional values about home, partner, and children's behaviour
- Major decisions in family controlled by one person
- Few social supports (isolated from family, friends)
- Little activity outside the home
- Unwanted or unplanned pregnancy
- Dependency on caregivers
- Extreme jealousy by partner
- Difficulties at school or work
- Short attention span
- Running away
- Promiscuity
- Child who has knowledge of sexual matters beyond that appropriate for age
- Sexualized play with self, peers, dolls, toys
- Masturbation
- Excessive fears and clinging in children

Neurologic System
- Difficulty with speech or swallowing
- Hyperactive reflexes
- Developmental delays
- Areas of numbness
- Tremors

Mental Status
- Anxiety, fear
- Depression
- Suicidal ideation
- Difficulty concentrating
- Memory loss
- Verbal aggression
- Themes of violence in artwork and school work

Distorted Body Image
- History of chronic physical or psychological disability
- Inability to perform activities of daily living
- Delayed language development

Physical Examination Findings

General Appearance
- Fearful, anxious, hyperactive, hypoactive
- Watching partner, parent, or caregiver for approval of answers to questions
- Poor grooming or inappropriate dress
- Malnourishment
- Signs of stress or fatigue
- Flinching when approached or touched
- Inappropriate or anxious nonverbal behaviour
- Wearing clothing inappropriate to the season or occasion to cover body parts

Vital Statistics
- Elevated pulse or blood pressure
- Other signs of autonomic arousal (exaggerated startle response, excessive sweating)
- Underweight or overweight

Skin
- Bruises, welts, edema, or scars
- Burns (cigarette, immersion, friction from ropes, pattern like electric iron or stove)
- Subdural haematoma
- Missing hair
- Poor skin integrity: dehydration, decubitus ulcers, untreated wounds, urine burns or excoriation

Eyes
- Orbital swelling
- Conjunctival haemorrhage
- Retinal haemorrhage
- Black eyes
- No glasses to accommodate poor eyesight

Ears
- Hearing loss
- No prosthetic device to accommodate poor hearing

Mouth
- Bruising
- Lacerations
- Missing or broken teeth
- Untreated dental problems

(continued)

BOX 36.4   (Continued)

History and Physical Findings Suggestive of Abuse

Abdomen
- Abdominal injuries during pregnancy
- Intra-abdominal injuries

Genitourinary System or Rectum
- Bruising, lacerations, bleeding, edema, tenderness
- Untreated infections

Musculoskeletal System
- Fractures or old fractures in various stages of healing
- Dislocations
- Limited range of motion in extremities
- Contractures

Medications
- Medications not indicated by physical condition
- Overdose of drugs or medications (prescribed or over the counter)
- Medications not taken as prescribed

Communication Patterns/Relations
- Verbal hostility, arguments
- Negative nonverbal communication, lack of visible affection
- One person answers questions and looks to other person for approval
- Extreme dependency of family members

(see Box 36-5 for more information). Malnourished and dehydrated children and elders may require nursing interventions such as intravenous therapy or nutritional supplements that alleviate the alteration in nutrition and fluid and electrolyte balance.

CRNE Note

It is essential to assess the risk for danger to people who are experiencing abusive relationships. Remember that their basic needs must be met (safety, housing, food, child care) before their psychological traumas can be addressed.

PROMOTING HEALTHY DAILY ACTIVITY. Teaching sleep hygiene and promoting exercise, leisure time, and nutrition will help battered survivors regain a healthy physical state and learn self-care. Taking care of oneself may be difficult, yet important, for survivors who have spent years trying to separate themselves from their bodies (dissociate) to survive years of abuse (Walker, 1994). A history of IPV threatens the physical and mental health of women and children in many ways (Ford-Gilbo, Wuest, & Merritt-Gray, 2005). Techniques such as going to bed and arising at consistent times, avoiding naps and caffeine, and scheduling periods for relaxation just before retiring may be useful in promoting sleep. Aerobic exercise is a useful technique for relieving anxiety and depression and promoting sleep.

BOX 36.5

Special Concerns for Victims of Sexual Assault

Assessment Focus

The history and physical examination of the survivor of sexual assault differ significantly from other assessment routines because the evidence obtained may be used in prosecuting the perpetrator (Sheridan, 2004). Therefore, the purpose is twofold:
- To assess the patient for injuries
- To collect evidence for forensic evaluation and proceedings.

Usually, someone with special training, such as a nurse practitioner who has taken special courses, examines a rape or sexual assault victim. Generalist nurses may be involved in treating the injuries that result from the assault, including genital trauma, such as vaginal and anal lacerations, and extragenital trauma, such as injury to the mouth, throat, wrists, arms, breasts, and thighs (Sheridan, 2004).

Key Interventions

Nursing intervention to prevent short- or long-term psychopathology after sexual assault is crucial. Psychological trauma following rape and sexual assault includes immediate anxiety and distress and the development of PTSD,

depression, panic, and substance abuse (Resnick et al., 1999).

Key interventions include:
- Early treatment because initial levels of distress are strongly related to later levels of PTSD, panic, and anxiety (Resnick et al., 1999).
- Supportive, caring, and nonjudgmental nursing interventions during the forensic rape examination are also crucial. This examination often increases survivors' immediate distress because they must recount the assault in detail and submit to an invasive pelvic or anal examination.
- Anxiety-reducing education, counselling, and emotional support, particularly in regard to unwanted pregnancies and sexually transmitted diseases, including HIV. All survivors should be tested for these possibilities. Treatment may include terminating a pregnancy; administering medications to treat gonorrhoea, chlamydia, trichomoniasis, and syphilis; and administering medications that may decrease the likelihood of contracting HIV infection.
- Interventions that are helpful for survivors of domestic violence; these also apply to survivors of sexual assault.

ADMINISTERING AND MONITORING MEDICATIONS. Survivors with a comorbid mood or anxiety disorder including PTSD may require pharmacologic interventions. Although only nurses with advanced preparation and prescriptive authority may prescribe medications, all nurses must be familiar with medications used to treat mood and anxiety disorders and the side effects of these drugs. Medications may be contraindicated for young and elderly survivors.

The autonomic nervous system is involved in many of the symptoms of depression and PTSD. Therefore, the use of agents that decrease its activity, such as the benzodiazepines, beta-blockers, and antidepressants, can help treat these symptoms (Friedman, 2001; Sutherland & Davidson, 1999). Tricyclics and other antidepressants are effective in treating depression and some symptoms of PTSD, such as nightmares, sleep disorders, and startle reactions. They are less effective in treating other PTSD symptoms, such as numbing (Friedman, 2001; Sutherland & Davidson, 1999). The benzodiazepines are useful in treating anxiety and sleep disturbances in PTSD, but because they can cause dependence, they are contraindicated in women who also have a substance abuse disorder.

Approved for treating PTSD, the selective serotonin reuptake inhibitor (SSRI) sertraline (Zoloft) has improved PTSD symptoms in women but not in men (Henney, 2000) (see Chapters 19 and 20 for information on monitoring medications and their side effects).

MANAGING CARE OF PATIENTS WITH COMORBID SUBSTANCE ABUSE. Survivors who have a comorbid substance abuse disorder need referral to a treatment center for alcohol and drug disorders. The treatment center should have programs that address the special needs of survivors. Alcohol-dependent and drug-dependent survivors frequently stop treatment and return to alcohol and drug abuse if their abuse-related problems are not addressed appropriately (Boyd, 2000; Ouimette, Moos, & Brown, 2003). As might be expected, research findings suggest that attitudes, such as self-blame and stigmatization, seem to be important variables related to substance abuse for women with a history of childhood sexual abuse (Dufour & Nadeau, 2001).

Survivors, especially those with substance abuse problems, are at high risk for HIV infection and AIDS. If women do not know their HIV status, they should be encouraged to get tested. Those with positive test results should receive counselling and begin taking appropriate medication. Those without HIV need to be taught about the high-risk behaviours for HIV infection and how to protect themselves from contracting HIV infection.

Psychological Domain

Psychological Assessment

A mental status evaluation should be part of every health assessment. Symptoms such as anhedonia, difficulties concentrating, feelings of worthlessness or guilt, and thoughts of death or suicide suggest depression or PTSD. A thorough assessment of suicidal intent is crucial.

Nursing Diagnoses for Psychological Domain

Selected nursing diagnoses focussing on the human responses that nurses manage in the psychological domain may include Ineffective Coping, Hopelessness, Chronic Low Self-Esteem, Anxiety, Risk for Self-Directed Violence, and Risk for Other-Directed Violence.

Interventions for Psychological Domain

ASSISTING WITH PSYCHOTHERAPY FOR COUNSELLING. Psychotherapy may include individual, group, family, or marital therapy. Only psychiatric nurse specialists at the master's or doctoral levels who have had training in these therapeutic methods may conduct psychotherapy. In addition, the nurse therapist should have training in conducting therapy specifically with survivors of abuse. That training should include care of PTSD, DID, depression, and substance abuse. The goal of therapy is to integrate the patient's traumatic memories with the remainder of the patient's personal history and identity, manage painful affect, and restructure the meaning of the traumatic experiences (Wilson, 2001). The ultimate goal is for the survivor to integrate the trauma in memory as a past event that no longer has the power to terrorize.

Family or marital therapy may be unwise unless the perpetrator of abuse has obtained therapy for himself or herself and demonstrated change. Otherwise, survivors are placed in a very difficult situation. If they disclose abuse in family or marital therapy, perpetrators may retaliate with violence, but if they do not disclose the abuse, the crucial issue will not be addressed (Landenburger et al., 2004).

Several issues must be addressed for all survivors in psychotherapy or counselling (Campbell et al., 2004). All nurses can implement these interventions, using skills appropriate to their educational level and training. Nurses must address the guilt, shame, and stigmatization that survivors experience. They can approach these issues in several ways. Assisting survivors to verbalize their experience in an accepting, nonjudgmental atmosphere is a first step. Nurses must challenge directly attributions of self-blame for the abuse and feelings of being dirty and different. Helping survivors to identify their strengths and validating thoughts and feelings may help to increase self-esteem. An anonymous case report by a nursing student describes the importance of therapy for nurses who have a history of childhood sexual abuse in promoting their own healing journey and ultimately their capacity to help others (Anonymous, 1998).

WORKING WITH CHILDREN. Children may need to learn a "violence vocabulary" that allows them to talk about their abuse and assign responsibility for abusive behaviour. Children also need to learn that violence is not okay, and it is not their fault (Berman et al., 2004). Allowing children to discuss their abuse in the safety of a supportive, caring relationship may alleviate anxiety and fear (Berman et al., 2004).

Re-enacting the abuse through play is another technique that may be helpful in assisting children to express and work through their anxiety and fear. Play therapy uses dolls, human or animal figures, or puppets to work through anxiety or fears (Hill, 2003). Other techniques used with children to reduce fear include reading stories about recovery from abusive experiences (literal or metaphoric), using art or music to express feelings, and psychodrama. In addition, teaching strategies to manage fear and anxiety, such as relaxation techniques, coping skills, and imagery, may give the child an added sense of mastering his or her fear (Barnett et al., 1997). In a comprehensive review of child maltreatment literature, MacMillian (2000) indicates that research supports the use of abuse-specific cognitive-behaviour therapy as a treatment to improve outcome for school-aged children.

MANAGING ANGER. Anger and rage are part of the healing process for survivors (Walker, 1994). Expression of intense anger is uncomfortable for many nurses. However, they should expect anger expression and develop comfortable ways to respond. Moreover, an important nursing intervention is teaching and modelling anger expression appropriately. Inappropriate expressions of anger might drive supportive people away. Anger management techniques include appropriately recognizing and labelling anger and expressing it assertively, rather than aggressively or passive-aggressively. Assertive ways of expressing anger include owning the feeling by using "I feel" statements and avoiding blaming others. Teaching anger management and conflict resolution may be especially important for children who have seen nothing but violence to resolve problems (Lowenthal, 2001).

TEACHING SKILLS AND CLARIFYING IDENTITY. Other nursing interventions include teaching self-protection skills, healthy relationship skills, and healthy sexuality. Again, this teaching may be especially important for children who have no role models for healthy relationships. Children also need to know what constitutes controlling and abusive behaviour and how to get help for abuse.

Children who have been sexually abused may become confused about their sexuality. They may regard sex as dirty and as something that can be used against other people. Discussions about healthy sexuality and feelings about sex may help these children regain a healthy perspective on sex-related matters (Peled, Jaffe, & Edleson, 1995).

Group therapy with survivors offers a powerful method to counter self-denigrating beliefs and to confront issues of secrecy and stigmatization (Urbancic, 2004). Moreover, one of the therapeutic factors in group therapy—universality, or the discovery that others have had similar experiences—may be a tremendous relief, especially to child survivors.

PROVIDING EDUCATION. Education is a key nursing intervention for survivors. As appropriate to age or condition, survivors must understand the cycle of violence and the danger of homicide that increases as violence escalates or the survivor attempts to leave the relationship. Survivors also need information about resources, such as shelters for battered women, legal services, government benefits, and support networks (CNA, 1992; Walker, 1994). Before giving the survivor any written material, the nurse must discuss the possibility that if the perpetrator were to find the information in the survivor's possession, he or she might use it as an excuse for battering.

Survivors also need education appropriate for age and cognitive ability about the symptoms of anxiety, depression, dissociation, and PTSD. They must understand that these symptoms are common in anyone who has sustained significant stressors and are not signs of being "crazy" or weak. If survivors require medication for these symptoms, they must know how to monitor symptoms so that the effectiveness of pharmacologic management can be determined (Box 36-6).

One of the most important teaching goals is to help survivors develop a safety plan (CNA, 1992; Walker, 1994). The first step in developing such a plan is helping the survivor recognize the signs of danger. Changes in tone of voice, drinking and drug use, and increased criticism may indicate that the perpetrator is losing control. Detecting early warning signs helps survivors to escape before battering begins (Campbell et al., 2004; Urbancic, 2004; Walker, 1994).

BOX 36.6

Psychoeducation Checklist: Abuse

When caring for the patient who has been abused, be sure to address the following topics in the teaching plan:
☐ Cycle of violence
☐ Access to shelters
☐ Legal services
☐ Government benefits
☐ Support network
☐ Symptoms of anxiety, dissociation, and post-traumatic stress disorder
☐ Safety or escape plan
☐ Relaxation
☐ Adequate nutrition and exercise
☐ Sleep hygiene
☐ HIV testing/counselling

The next step is to devise an escape route (CNA, 1992; Walker, 1994). This involves mapping the house and identifying where the battering usually occurs and what exits are available. The survivor needs to have a bag packed and hidden, but readily accessible, that has what is needed to get away. Important things to pack are clothes, a set of car and house keys, bank account numbers, birth certificate, insurance policies and numbers, marriage license, valuable jewellery, important telephone numbers, and money (CNA, 1992; Walker, 1994). The survivor must carefully hide the bag so that the perpetrator cannot find it and use it as an excuse for assault. If children are involved, the adult survivor should make arrangements to get them out safely. That might include arranging a signal to indicate when it is safe for them to leave the house and to meet at a prearranged place (Walker, 1994). A safety plan for a child or dependent elder might include safe places to hide and important telephone numbers, including 911 and those of the police and fire departments and other family members and friends.

FINDING STRENGTH AND HOPE. Providing hope and a sense of control is important for survivors of trauma (Campbell et al., 2004). Nurses can help survivors find hope and view themselves as survivors by assisting them to identify specific strengths and aspects of their lives that are under their control. This type of intervention may empower women to find options to remaining in an abusive relationship. The research by Ford-Gilboe, Wuest, and Merritt-Gray (2005) indicates that women were able to promote the health of their families after leaving an abusive partner, offering hope and a means of understanding for nurses working with women who are struggling to find the strength to choose health.

USING BEHAVIOURAL INTERVENTIONS. Treatment for depression, anxiety, and PTSD symptoms can be divided into two categories: exposure therapy and anxiety management training (Rothbaum & Foa, 1996). Only professionals trained in exposure therapy techniques can use them; however, nurses need to be familiar with this approach. The goal of exposure therapy, which includes flooding and systematic desensitization, is to promote the processing of the traumatic memory by exposing the survivor to the traumatic event through memories or some cue that reactivates trauma memories. Through repeated exposure, the event loses its ability to cause intense anxiety (Coffey, Dansky, & Brady, 2003).

COPING WITH ANXIETY. Anxiety management is a crucial intervention for all survivors. There is a high comorbidity among trauma, PTSD, and anxiety disorders (Orsillo et al., 2002). During treatment, survivors will experience situations and memories that provoke intense anxiety and must know how to soothe themselves when they experience painful feelings. Moreover, most survivors struggle with control issues, especially involving their bodies. Anxiety management skills offer one way to maintain some control over their bodies (Lundberg-Love, 1997).

Anxiety management training may include progressive relaxation, deep breathing, imagery techniques, and cognitive restructuring. Progressive relaxation entails systematically tensing and then relaxing the major muscle groups. Visualization consists of imagining a scene that is especially relaxing (eg, spending a day at the beach), while practicing relaxation and deep breathing. Any interventions that reduce dysphoric symptoms can help survivors feel more in control of their situation.

Anxiety disorders, including PTSD and depression, are associated with cognitive distortions that cognitive therapy techniques can challenge (Zust, 2000). Self-defeating thoughts in anxiety disorders involve perceptions of threat and danger, and those in depression involve negative self-perceptions (Blackburn & Davidson, 1990). Nurses can teach survivors how to identify and challenge these self-defeating thought patterns. Cognitive therapy techniques may be especially useful in helping survivors to stop blaming themselves for their abuse.

Nurses must become accustomed to measuring gains in small steps when working with survivors. Making any changes in significant relationships has serious consequences and can be done only when the adult survivor is ready. Carter-Snell & Hegadoren (2003) point out that women are frequently the primary caregiver and as such may have limited resources to devout to therapy. Therefore, the context of each individual woman's life needs to be kept in mind. It is easy for nurses to become angry or discouraged, and they must be careful not to communicate these feelings to survivors (Campbell et al., 2004; Urbancic, 2004). Discussing such feelings with other staff provides a way of dealing with them appropriately. In such discussions with supervisors or other staff, the nurse must protect the patient's confidentiality by discussing feelings around issues, not particular patients. The nurse should frame the discussion in such a way that individual patients cannot be identified.

Social Domain

Social Assessment

An evaluation of social networks and daily activities may provide additional clues of psychological abuse and controlling behaviour (Gary & Humphreys, 2004; Wallace, 1999). When a nurse assesses social isolation, evaluating the reasons behind it is crucial. Many perpetrators isolate their family from all social contacts, including other relatives. Some survivors isolate themselves because they are ashamed of the abuse or fear nonsupportive responses. An evaluation of social support is important for other reasons. Having supportive family or friends is crucial in short-term planning for developing a safety plan and is also important to long-term recovery. A survivor cannot leave an abusive situation if she has nowhere to go. Supportive family and friends may be willing to provide shelter and safety.

Nurses can assess restrictions on freedom that may suggest abuse and control by asking such questions as: "Are you free to go where you want?"; "Is staying home your choice?" and "Is there anything that you would like to do that you cannot?"

The degree of dependency on the relationship is another important variable to assess. Women who have young children and are economically dependent on the perpetrator may feel that they cannot leave the abusive relationship. Those who are emotionally dependent on the perpetrator may experience an intense grief reaction that further complicates their leaving (Campbell et al., 2004; Wallace, 1999). Elders and children are often dependent on the abuser and cannot leave the abusive situation without alternatives.

Nursing Diagnoses for Social Domain

Selected nursing diagnoses focussing on the human responses that nurses manage in the social domain may include Hopelessness, Powerlessness, and Ineffective Role Performance.

Interventions for Social Domain

WORKING WITH ABUSIVE FAMILIES. Family interventions in cases of child abuse focus on behavioural approaches to improve parenting skills (Gary & Humphreys, 2004). A behavioural approach has multiple components. *Child management skills* help parents manage maladaptive behaviours and reward appropriate behaviours. *Parenting skills* teach parents how to be more effective and nurturing with their children. *Leisure skills* training is important to reduce stress in the household and promote healthy family time. *Household organization* training is another way to reduce stress by teaching effective ways to manage the multiple tasks that families have to perform. Such tasks include meal planning, cooking, shopping, keeping physician's appointments, and planning family activities (Gary & Humphreys, 2004).

Anger control and stress management skills are important parts of behavioural programs for families. Anger control programs teach parents to identify events that increase anger and stress and to replace anger-producing thoughts with more appropriate ones. Parents learn self-control skills to reduce the expression of uncontrolled anger. Stress-reduction techniques include relaxation techniques and methods for coping with stressful interactions with their children (Lowenthal, 2001). These skills may be especially important in families in which elder abuse is occurring. Both caregivers and abused elders may need to learn assertive ways to express their anger and healthy ways to manage their stress. Helping caregivers find ways to get some relief

from their caregiving burdens may be crucial in reducing abuse that comes from exhaustion in trying to manage multiple roles. Examples might be to identify agencies that offer respite care or agencies that offer day care for elders and support groups in which caregivers can share experiences and gain support from others dealing with similar issues.

WORKING IN THE COMMUNITY. Nurses may be involved in interventions to reduce violence at the community level. Many abusive parents and battered women are socially isolated. Assistance in developing support networks may help reduce stress and, therefore, reduce abuse. Community contacts vary for each survivor but might include crisis hot lines, support groups, and education classes (Gary & Humphreys, 2004).

Community health nurses may play a vital role in the detection, treatment, and referral of child sexual abuse (Blakeley & Ribeiro, 1997). Specifically, nurses may make home visits to abusive parents. Home visits provide support to families and provide them with knowledge about child development and management (Barnett et al., 1997). Abuse of any kind is a volatile situation, and nurses may place themselves or the survivor in danger if they make home visits. Nurses should carefully assess this possibility before proceeding. If necessary, the nurse and adult survivor may need to arrange a safe place to meet.

Evaluation and Treatment Outcomes

Evaluation and outcome criteria depend on the setting for interventions. For instance, if the nurse encounters a survivor in the ED, successful outcomes might be that injuries are appropriately managed and the patient's immediate safety is ensured. For long-term care, outcome criteria and evaluation might center on ending abusive relationships. Examples of other outcome criteria that would indicate successful nursing intervention are recognizing that one is not to blame for the violence, demonstrating knowledge of strengths and coping skills, and re-establishing social networks.

Evaluation of nursing care for abused children depends on attaining goals mutually set with the parents. An end to all violence is the optimal outcome criterion; however, attainment of smaller goals indicates progress toward that end. Outcomes such as increased problem-solving and communication skills within the family, increased self-esteem in both children and parents, and increased use of nonphysical forms of discipline may all indicate progress toward the total elimination of child abuse.

Follow-up efforts are important in evaluating the outcomes of elder abuse. The optimal outcome is to end all abuse and keep the elderly person in his or her own living environment, if appropriate. Although the abuse may have been resolved temporarily, it may flare up again. Ongoing support for the caregiver and assistance with caregiving tasks may be necessary if the elder is to remain at home. Nursing home or assisted living may be the most desirable option if the burden is too great for the family and the likelihood of ongoing abuse or neglect is high.

Another important outcome of nursing intervention with survivors is appropriate treatment of any disorder resulting from abuse (eg, ASD, PTSD and other anxiety disorders, DID, major depression, substance abuse). Follow-up nursing assessments should monitor symptom reduction or exacerbation, adherence to any medication regimen, and side effects of medication. The ultimate outcome is to end violence and enable the survivor to return to a more productive, safe, and nurturing life without being continually haunted by memories of the abuse.

Treatment for the Batterer

Participants in programs that treat batterers are usually there because the court has mandated the treatment. Programs are often outpatient groups that meet weekly for an extended period of time, often 36 to 48 weeks. Some advocate longer programs, believing that chronic offenders require 1 to 5 years of treatment to change abusive behaviour.

Groups often use cognitive-behavioural techniques or a psychoeducational, skill-building approach (Healey, Smith, & O'Sullivan, 1998). This approach offers the batterer tools that help him see that his violent acts are not uncontrollable outbursts but rather foreseeable behaviour patterns that he can learn to interrupt. Cognitive-behavioural interventions target three elements: (1) what the batterer thinks about just before a battering incident; (2) the batterer's physical and emotional response to these thoughts; and (3) what the batterer does that progresses to violence (yelling, throwing things). The group teaches members to recognize and interrupt negative feelings about their partners and to reduce physiologic arousal through relaxation techniques.

Psychoeducational topics are often similar to those covered by the Duluth Curriculum, which is a model program. Topics may include nonviolence; nonthreatening behaviour; respect; support and trust; honesty and accountability; sexual respect; and partnership, negotiation, and fairness. Other programs also offer more in-depth counselling, arguing that psychoeducational approaches do not address the true problem (Healey et al., 1998). If the problem were simply a deficit in skills, the batterer would be dysfunctional in work or relationships outside the family. Batterers need resocialization that convinces them that they do not have the right to abuse their partners. Other programs add a moral aspect by taking a value-laden approach against violence and confronting the batterer's behaviour as unacceptable and illegal.

Accountability for violent acts is an important early goal in treating batterers (Healey et al., 1998). Most batterers deny responsibility for their actions and refuse to look at battering as a choice. Therefore, it is important that batterers become accountable for their actions. Interventions aim at getting the batterer to acknowledge his violence across the full range of abusive acts that he has committed, for example, verbal abuse, intimidation, controlling behaviour, and sexual abuse. Batterers may use several tactics to avoid accountability, and all must be addressed. Those tactics include denying the abuse ever happened ("I never touched her"); minimizing the abuse by downplaying the violent acts or underestimating its effects ("It was just a slap" or "she bruises easily"); and blaming the abuse on the victim ("she pushed me too far"), alcohol or other drugs ("I was high"), or other life circumstances ("I had too many pressures at work").

A recent qualitative study conducted in Nova Scotia of six group facilitators engaged in providing programs to men who batter revealed the many complexities of providing effective treatment for these men (Augusta-Scott & Dankwort, 2002). Discussions with the group facilitators suggested that a form of narrative therapy, in which the men were invited to discover what would be personally meaningful about engaging in treatment, might be a necessary prerequisite to effective treatment (Augusta-Scott & Dankwort, 2002).

Because batterers typically minimize or deny their violent behaviour, it is often necessary to interview the survivor to gain a complete picture of the batterer's behaviour. A trained victim advocate usually contacts partners. There are other reasons for contacting partners. This may be the first contact the partner has had with professionals, and she may benefit by telling her story. Many partners do not know that services are available to them, and this is an opportunity to tell her what is available. In addition, advocates often explain the batterer program and emphasize that it takes a long time and requires the batterer to take responsibility for his violent behaviour. Partners need to hear that many batterers are not willing to change their behaviour. Another important point that partners need to know and discuss with professionals is that batterers often use entry into treatment as a justification for pressuring partners to remain in the relationship, but that this behaviour is a good indicator that abuse will continue.

There are four points in treating batterers when it is essential to contact the partner for safety reasons: (1) when the batterer begins attending the program; (2) if and when he is terminated from treatment for noncompliance; (3) when he has completed treatment; and (4) if he is an imminent threat to the partner's safety (Healey et al., 1998).

Batterer intervention must be culturally competent (Healey et al., 1998). Many factors can affect violence against women, including socioeconomic status, racial or ethnic identity, country of origin, and sexual orientation, and those differences must be addressed. Another factor that must be addressed is alcohol and other drug use. Intervention programs may require batterers to undergo substance abuse treatment concurrently, and batterers are required to remain sober and submit to random drug testing.

Treatment programs alone are not sufficient to stop many batterers (Healey et al., 1998). To be effective, programs must operate within a comprehensive intervention effort that includes criminal justice support. The criminal justice response includes arrest, incarceration, adjudication, and probation supervision that includes issuing a warrant if the batterer does not attend the batterer program or supervision. The combination of criminal justice response and batterer treatment may convey a more powerful message to the batterer about the seriousness of his actions than a batterer program alone. Unfortunately, many offenders never show up for batterer intervention, and arrests for violation of probation may be rare because of overload and staffing shortages. Inaction by the criminal justice system is serious; it sends the message that there is little concern for violence against women and that batterers can get away with it. Several approaches to batterer intervention are controversial (Healey et al., 1998).

Anger management attributes battering to out-of-control anger and teaches anger management techniques. There are several arguments against this approach. It does not address the real issue—batterers' desire to control their partners. Batterers are able to control their behaviour in other difficult situations but choose anger and intimidation to control their partners. Anger management may merely teach batterers nonviolent methods to exert control. Couples counselling may endanger the survivor. Women will not be free to disclose, and any disclosures may give the batterer reason to retaliate. Self-help groups modelled on Alcoholics Anonymous are inappropriate for initial intervention for several reasons. Without trained facilitators who will confront denial and excuses, batterers may never accept accountability for their violence. On the other hand, an untrained facilitator may use an excessively confrontational approach that is abusive and models antagonistic behaviour.

How effective is batterer treatment? Results from an extended follow-up of court-ordered batterer intervention programs show that many men continue to be assaultive during or on completion of treatment. Based on partners' reports, 32% had reassaulted their partners by 15 months after treatment; 38% had done so by 30 months, and 42% had done so at 48 months. Twenty-five percent of the men repeatedly reassaulted their partners through 48 months of follow-up. However, the results did show that reassaults de-escalated somewhat with time (Gondolf, 2001).

SUMMARY OF KEY POINTS

- The abuse of women, men, children, and elders is a national health problem that requires awareness and sensitivity from nurses.
- The abuse of women may be physical, emotional and psychological, or social.
- Child abuse may be neglectful, physical, sexual, or emotional. Other forms of child abuse include Munchausen syndrome by proxy and witnessing abuse of their mothers or significant caregivers.
- The abuse of Aboriginal children in residential schools was particularly harmful because these children were segregated from their families and communities, frequently for years at a time.
- Elder abuse may be physical, emotional, neglectful, or financial.
- Among the many theories that have been proposed to explain abuse are psychopathology, social learning, sociologic, feminist, neurobiologic, borderline personality disorder, and substance abuse.
- A well-documented cycle of violence consists of three phases of increasing frequency and severity.
- Child abuse leaves many scars that can lead to such problems in adulthood as depression, anxiety, self-destructive behaviour, poor self-esteem, and lack of trust.
- Responses to abuse include depression, acute stress disorder (ASD), post-traumatic stress disorder (PTSD), and dissociative identity disorder (DID).
- Nurses need to be familiar with signs and symptoms of abuse and to be vigilant when assessing patients.
- Nurses can help victims of abuse to view themselves as survivors.

CRITICAL THINKING CHALLENGES

1 Abuse is a pervasive problem, and anyone can be a victim (women, men, children, elders, gays, lesbians). Why do so few nursing units and nurses make it routine to ask questions about abuse?
2 Abuse is not just a "women's issue." The prevalence of abuse might decrease if men make it a "men's issue" as well. What is preventing this from happening?
3 What are your thoughts and feelings about women who are victims of abuse in which both partners (victim and perpetrator) abuse alcohol and other drugs?
4 What are your thoughts and feelings about women who will not leave an abusive relationship?

5 What are some reasons that women remain in abusive relationships?

6 Why do some women become involved in more than one abusive relationship?

7 How do you handle your feelings toward abusive parents or relatives who abuse elders?

8 What are the issues in mandatory reporting of violence toward women, particularly violence that occurs in the home?

WEB LINKS

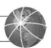

www.phac-aspc.gc.ca The National Clearinghouse on Family Violence (NCFV) is Canada's national resource center for information about family violence. The NCFV collects, develops, and disseminates resources on prevention, protection, and treatment. By increasing awareness, the NCFV encourages Canadian communities to become involved in reducing the occurrence of family violence. Their website includes provincial, national, local, and international links.

www.chp-pcs.gc.ca The website of the Canada Health Portal, a public health agency of Canada, provides a listing of services and programs to meet the needs of older adult victims of violence in Canada. Two hundred and eighty programs and services are listed by province, from the east to the west coast.

www.canada.justice.gc.ca The website of the Department of Justice, Canada provides a comprehensive overview of violence in Canada, including Family Violence, Spousal Abuse, Child Abuse, Abuse of Older Adults, and Dating Violence. The site includes Canadian statistics, relevant literature, and policy and legal implications, as well as links to additional sites.

MOVIES

Marion Bridge: 2002. Winner of the 2002 best Canadian film at the Toronto International Film Festival, *Marion Bridge* is the story of Agnes' return home to the Maritimes to help care for her dying mother. The audience shares the tension as family secrets emerge and Agnes and her two sisters, Theresa and Louise, struggle with their past and present.

VIEWING POINTS: What are the ways that the members of this family have used to cope with the abuse in their lives? What does their story reveal about both positive and negative ways of coping? Do you think that ideal images of love, such as the one Agnes treasured in the song, "Marion Bridge," are helpful or harmful?

Loyalties: 1987. In this critically acclaimed movie set in Alberta, the friendship between an English physician's wife and her children's Aboriginal "nanny" sets the scene for a conflict of loyalties. This story captures well the shame, hope and fear of a family living with a dark secret.

VIEWING POINTS: Consider the alternative ways in which the situation of these two families could have evolved differently. What factors influence the outcome of such a situation?

Once Were Warriors: 1994. A mother of five re-evaluates her 18-year marriage to her alcoholic, hot-tempered husband when his barroom violence tragically encroaches into their home life. Produced and filmed in New Zealand, this film also presents how urbanization has undermined the culture and strength of the indigenous Maori people.

VIEWING POINTS: What evidence can you find in this film that may reflect intergenerational transmission of violence? In what ways do you think that culture can influence attitudes toward abuse (both positive and negative)? What are positive and negative cultural influences in this film?

REFERENCES

Abbey, A., Zawacki, T., Buck, P., Clinton, A., & McAuslan, P. (2003). Sexual assault and alcohol consumption. What do we know about their relationship and what types of research are needed? *Aggression & Violent Behaviour, 277,* 1–33.

Allan, M. A. (1998). Elder abuse: A challenge for home care nurses. *Home Health Care Nurse, 16*(2), 103–110.

Alvi, S., & Selbee, K. (1997). Dating status variations and woman abuse: A test of the dependence, availability and deterrence (DAD) model. *Violence Against Women, 3(6),* 610–628.

American Psychiatric Association (APA). (1987). *Diagnostic and statistical manual of mental disorders* (3rd ed., revised.). Washington, DC: Author.

American Psychiatric Association (APA). (2000). *Diagnostic and statistical manual of mental disorders* (4th ed., Text revision). Washington, DC: Author.

Anderson, D. K., & Saunders, D. G. (2003). Leaving an abusive partner: An empirical review of predictors, the process of leaving, and psychological well-being. *Trauma, Violence, & Abuse, 4*(2), 163–191.

Anderson, G., Yasenik, L., & Ross, C. A. (1993). Dissociative experiences and disorders among women who identify themselves as sexual abuse survivors. *Child Abuse and Neglect, 17*(5), 677–686.

Anonymous. (1998). Battling back from childhood sexual abuse and surviving the journey. *Journal of Psychosocial Nursing & Mental Health Services, 36*(12), 13–17.

Arata, C. M. (2002). Child sexual abuse and sexual revictimization. *Clinical Psychological: Science and Practice, 9,* 135–164.

Augusta-Scott, T., & Dankwort, J. (2002). Partner abuse groups interventions;—Lessons from educational & narrative therapy approaches. *Journal of Interpersonal Violence, 17*(7), 783–805.

Bandura, A. (1977). *Social Learning Theory.* New York: General Learning Press.

Banister, E. M., Jakubec, S. L., & Stein, J. A. (2003). "Like what am I supposed to do?" Adolescent girls' health concerns in their dating relationships. *Canadian Journal of Nursing Research, 35*(2), 16–33.

Barnett, O. W., Miller-Perrin, C. L., & Perrin, R. D. (1997). *Family violence across the lifespan: An introduction.* Thousand Oaks, CA: Sage.

Bartsch, C., Risse, M., Schutz, H., Weigand, N., & Weiler, G. (2003). Munchausen syndrome by proxy (MSBP): An extreme form of child abuse with a special forensic challenge. *Forensic Science International, 137*(2–3), 147–151.

Berman, H., Hardesty, J., & Humphreys, J. C. (2004). Children of abused women. In J. C. Campbell & J. C. Humphreys (Eds.), *Family violence and nursing practice* (pp. 160–185). Philadelphia: Lippincott Williams & Wilkins.

Blackburn, I., & Davidson, K. (1990). *Cognitive therapy for depression and anxiety.* Boston: Blackwell Scientific Publications.

Blakeley, J., & Ribeiro, V. (1997). Community health and pediatric nurses' knowledge, attitudes, and behaviors regarding child sexual abuse. *Public Health Nursing, 14*(6), 339–345.

Bograd, M. (1999). Strengthening domestic violence theories: Intersections of race, class, sexual orientation, and gender. *Journal of Marital and Family Therapy, 25*(3), 275–289.

Boyd, M. R. (2000). Predicting substance abuse and comorbidity in rural women. *Archives of Psychiatric Nursing, 14*(2), 64–72.

Boyd, M. R. (2003). Vulnerability to alcohol and other drug disorders in rural women. *Archives of Psychiatric Nursing, 17*(1), 33–41.

Boyd, M. R., & Mackey, M. (2000a). Alienation from self and others: The psychosocial problem of rural alcoholic women. *Archives of Psychiatric Nursing, 14*(3), 134–141.

Boyd, M. R., & Mackey, M. (2000b). Running away to nowhere: Rural women's experience of becoming alcohol dependent. *Archives of Psychiatric Nursing, 14*(3), 142–149.

Brady, K. T., & Dansky, B. S. (2002). Effects of victimization and posttraumatic stress disorder on substance use disorders in women. In F. L. Hall, T. S. Williams, J. A. Panetta, & J. M. Herrera (Eds,), *Psychiatric illnesses in women* (pp. 449–466). Washington, DC: American Psychiatric Publishing.

Braitstein, P., Li, K., Tyndall, M., Spittal, P., O'Shaughnessy, M., Schilder, A., Johnston, C., Hogg, R., & Schechter, M. (2000). Sexual violence among a cohort of injection drug users. *Social Science & Medicine, 24*(6), 781–797.

Breitenbecher, K. H. (2001). Sexual victimization among women: A review of the literature focusing on empirical investigations. *Aggression and Violent Behavior, 6*, 415–432.

Bremner, J. D., Narayan, M., Staib, L. H., Southwick, S. M., McGlashan, T., & Charney, D. S. (1999). Neural correlates of memories of childhood sexual abuse in women with and without posttraumatic stress disorder. *American Journal of Psychiatry, 156*, 1787–1795.

Bremner, J. D., Southwick, S. M., & Charney, D. S. (1999). The neurobiology of posttraumatic stress disorder: An integration of animal and human research. In P. A. Saigh & J. D. Bremner (Eds.), *Posttraumatic stress disorder: A comprehensive text.* Boston: Allyn and Bacon.

Breslau, N., Davis, G. C., Andreski, P., et al. (1997). Sex differences in posttraumatic stress disorder. *Archives of General Psychiatry, 54*(11), 1044–1048.

Briere, J. N., & Elliott, D. M. (1994). Immediate and long-term impacts of child sexual abuse. *The Future of Children, 4*(2), 54–69.

Brown, P. J., Recupero, P. R., & Stout, R. (1995). PTSD substance abuse comorbidity and treatment utilization. *Addictive Behaviors, 20*, 251–254.

Campbell, J. C., & Humphreys, J. (Eds.). (1993). *Nursing care of survivors of family violence.* St. Louis: Mosby.

Campbell, J. C., & Lewandowski, L. A. (1997). Mental and physical effects of intimate partner violence on women and children. *Psychiatric Clinics of North America, 20*(2), 353–354.

Campbell, J. C., McKenna, L. S., Torres, S., et al. (1993). Nursing care of abused women. In J. C. Campbell & J. C. Humphreys (Eds.), *Nursing care of survivors of family violence* (pp. 248–289). St. Louis: Mosby.

Campbell, J. C., Torres, S., McKenna, L. S., Sheridan, D. J., & Landenburger, K. (2004). Nursing care of survivors of intimate partner violence. In J. C. Campbell & J. C. Humphreys (Eds.), *Family violence and nursing practice* (pp. 307–360). Philadelphia: Lippincott Williams & Wilkins.

Canadian Centre for Justice Statistics. (2005). *Family violence in Canada: A statistical profile 2005.* Ottawa: Statistics Canada.

Canadian Nurses Association. (1992). *Family violence clinical guidelines for nurses.* Ottawa: National Clearing House on Family Violence.

Carlson, E. B., & Putnam, F. W. (1993). An update on the Dissociative Experiences Scale. *Dissociation, 6*(1), 16–27.

Carter-Snell C., & Hegadoren K. (2003). Stress disorders and gender: Implications for theory and research. *Canadian Journal of Nursing Research, 35*(2), 34–55.

Charney, D. S., Deutch, A. Y., Krystal, J. H., et al. (1993). Psychobiologic mechanisms of posttraumatic stress disorder. *Archives of General Psychiatry, 50*(4), 294–305.

Chodorow, N. (1974). Family structure and feminine personality. In M. R. Rosaldo & L. Lamphere (Eds.), *Woman, culture, and society* (pp. 43–66). Stanford: Stanford University Press.

Chrousos, G. P., & Gold, P. W. (1992). The concepts of stress and stress system disorders. *Journal of the American Medical Association, 267*(9), 1244–1252.

Cloitre, M., Scarvalone, P., & Difede, J. (1997). Posttraumatic stress disorder, self- and interpersonal dysfunction among sexually retraumatized women. *Journal of Traumatic Stress, 10*(3), 437–452.

Coffey, S. F., Dansky, B. S., & Brady, K. T. (2003). Exposure-based, trauma-focused therapy for comorbid posttraumatic stress disorder-substance use disorder. In P. Ouimette & P. J. Brown (Eds.), *Trauma and substance abuse: Causes, consequences, and treatment of comorbid disorders* (pp. 127–146). Washington, DC: American Psychiatric Association.

Cohen, J. A., Perel, J. M., DeBellis, M. D., Friedman, M. J., & Putnam, F. W. (2002). Treating traumatized children: Clinical implications of the psychobiology of posttraumatic stress disorder. *Trauma, Violence, & Abuse, 3*(2), 91–108.

Collin-Vezina, D., & Hebert, M. (2005). Comparing dissociation and PTSD in sexually abused school-aged girls. *Journal of Nervous & Mental Disease, 193*(1), 47–52.

Collins, J. J., & Messerschmidt, P. M. (1993). Epidemiology of alcohol-related violence. *Alcohol Health and Research World, 17*(2), 93–100.

Comijs, H. C., Pot, A. M., Smit, J. H., et al. (1998). Elder abuse in the community: Prevalence and consequences. *Journal of the American Geriatric Society, 46*(7), 885–888.

Criminal Code of Canada, r.s.c. (1985). c–C-46, s/55.

DeKeseredy, W. S,. & Schwartz, M. D. (1998). Woman abuse on campus: Results from the Canadian National Survey. London: Thousand Oaks Sage Publications.

Department of Justice, Canada. (2003). *Child Abuse: A fact sheet from the Department of Justice.* Ottawa: Department of Justice, Canada.

Department of Justice, Canada. (2005). *Abuse of older adults: A fact sheet from the Department of Justice.* Ottawa: Department of Justice, Canada.

Dewey, J. (2004). Theories of aggression and family violence. In J. C. Campbell & J. C. Humphreys (Eds.), *Family violence and nursing practice* (pp. 3–28). Philadelphia: Lippincott Williams & Wilkins.

Dufour, M. H., & Nadeau, L. (2001). Sexual abuse: A comparison between resilient victims and drug-addicted victims. *Violence and Victim, 16*(6), 655–672.

Dutton, D. G. (1995). *The domestic assault of women.* Vancouver: UBC Press.

Dutton, D. G. (1998). *The abusive personality.* New York: Guilford.

Dutton, D. G., & Painter, S. (1993). Emotional attachments in abusive relationships: A test of traumatic bonding theory. *Violence and Victims, 8*(2), 105–120.

Emery, R. E., & Laumann-Billings, L. (1998). An overview of the nature, causes, and consequences of abusive family relationships: Toward differentiating maltreatment and violence. *American Psychologist, 53*(2), 121–135.

Epstein, J. N., Saunders, B. E., Kilpatrick, D. G., & Resnick, H. S. (1998). PTSD as a mediator between childhood rape and alcohol use in adult women. *Child Abuse & Neglect, 22*(3), 223–234.

Fishwick, N. J., Campbell, J. C., & Taylor, J. Y. (2004). Theories of intimate partner violence. In J. C. Campbell & J. C. Humphreys

(Eds.), *Family violence and nursing practice* (pp. 29–57). Philadelphia: Lippincott Williams & Wilkins.

Flitcraft, A. (1997). Learning from the paradoxes of domestic violence. *Journal of the American Medical Association, 277*(17), 1400–1401.

Flitcraft, A. H. (1995). Clinical violence intervention: Lessons from battered women. *Journal of Health Care for the Poor and Underserved, 6*(2), 187–197.

Ford-Gilboe, M., Wuest, J., & Merritt-Gray, M. (2005). Strengthening the capacity to limit intrusion: Theorizing family health promotion in the aftermath of women abuse. *Qualitative Health Research, 15*(4), 477–501.

Friedman, M. J. (2001). Allostatic versus empirical perspective in pharmacotherapy for PTSD. In J. P. Wilson, M. J. Friedman, & J Lindy (Eds.), *Treating psychological trauma and PTSD* (pp. 94–124). New York: Guilford.

Gallop, R., McCay, E., Austin, W., Bayer, M. & Peternelji-Taylor, C. (1998). Working with psychiatric clients who have been sexually abused. *Journal of the American Psychiatric Nursing Association, 4*, 9–17.

Gallop, R., McCay, E., Guha, M., & Khan. P. (1999). The experience of hospitalization and restraint of women who have a history of childhood sexual abuse. *Health Care Women International, 20*(4), 401–416.

Gary, F. A., Campbell, D. W., & Humphreys, J. (2004). Theories of child abuse. In J. C. Campbell & J. C. Humphreys (Eds.), *Family violence and nursing practice* (pp. 58–73). Philadelphia: Lippincott Williams & Wilkins.

Gary, F. A., & Humphreys, J. C. (2004). Nursing care of abused children. In J. C. Campbell & J. C. Humphreys (Eds.), *Family violence and nursing practice* (pp. 252–287). Philadelphia: Lippincott Williams & Wilkins.

Gilligan, C. (1982). In a different voice: Psychological theory and women's development. Cambridge, MA: Harvard University Press.

Girshick, L. B. (1993). *Teen dating violence. Violence update.* Thousand Oaks, CA: Sage.

Gold, N., & Auslander, G. (1999). Gender issues in newspaper coverage of people with disabilities: A Canada-Israel comparison. *Women and Health, 29*(4), 75–96.

Gondolf, E. W. (2001). *An extended follow-up of batterers and their partners.* Atlanta: Centers for Disease Control and Prevention. Available at http://www.iup.edu.

Gordon, R. M. (2001). Adult protection legislation in Canada: Models, issues, and problems. *International Journal of Law and Psychiatry. 24*(2–3), 117–134.

Guille, L. (2004). Men who batter and their children: An integrated review. *Aggression and Violent Behaviour, 9*(2) 129–163.

Hana, E. Z., & Grant, B. F. (1997). Gender differences in *DSM-IV* alcohol use disorders and major depression as distributed in the general population: Clinical implications. *Comprehensive Psychiatry, 38*(4), 202–212.

Hanson, R. K., Cadsky, O., Harris A., & Lalonde, C. (1997). Correlates of battering among 997 men: Family history, adjustment and attitudinal differences. *Violence and Victims, 12*(3), 191–208.

Hattendorf, J., & Tollerud, T. R. (1997). Domestic violence: Counseling strategies that minimize the impact of secondary victimization. *Perspectives in Psychiatric Care, 33*(1), 14–23.

Healey, K., Smith, C., & O'Sullivan, C. (1998). *Batterer intervention: Program approaches and criminal justice strategies.* Washington, DC: U.S. Department of Justice, National Institute of Justice. Available at http://www.ojp.usdoj.gov.

Health Canada. (1998). *The consequences of child maltreatment: A reference guide for health practitioners.* Ottawa: Family Violence Prevention Unit, Health Canada.

Health Canada. (2002a). *Nursing education and violence prevention, detection and intervention.* Ottawa: National Clearing House on Family Violence.

Health Canada. (2002b). *Woman abuse: Information from the National Clearing House on family violence.* Ottawa: Health Canada.

Henderson, A. (2001). Factors influencing nurses' responses to abused women: What they say they do and why they say they do it. *Journal of Interpersonal Violence, 16(12)*, 1284–1306.

Henderson, A. J. Z., Bartholomew, K., & Dutton, D. G. (1997). He loves me; he loves me not: Attachment and separation resolution of abused women. *Journal of Family Violence, 12*(2), 169–191.

Hendricks-Matthews, M. K. (1993). Survivors of abuse: Health care issues. *Primary Care, 20*(2), 391–406.

Henney, J. E. (2000). Sertraline approved for posttraumatic stress disorder. *Journal of the American Medical Association, 283*(5), 596.

Henry, J. P. (1992). Biological basis of the stress response. *Integrative Physiological and Behavioral Science, 1*, 66–83.

Herman, J. (1997). *Trauma and recovery: The aftermath of violence-from domestic abuse to political terror.* New York: Basic Books.

Hill, A. (2003). Issues facing brothers of sexually abused children: Implication for professional practice. *Child & Family Social Work, 8*(4), 281–291.

Hotch, D., Grunfeld, A., Mackay, K., & Ritch, L. (1996). Policy and procedures for domestic violence patients in Canadian emergency departments: A national survey. *Journal of Emergency Nursing, 22*(4), 278–282.

Huckle, P. L. (1995). Male rape victims referred to a forensic psychiatric service. *Medicine Science & Law, 35*(3), 187–192.

Janssen, P. A., Holt, V. L., & Sugg, N. K. (2002). Introducing domestic violence assessment in a postpartum clinical setting. *Maternal Child Health Journal, 6*(3), 195–203.

Kaplan, H. I., & Sadock, B. J. (1998). *Kaplan and Sadock's synopsis of psychiatry.* New York: Williams & Wilkins.

Kilbourne, J. (1987). *Still killing us softly.* Cambridge, MA: Cambridge Documentary Films.

Kilbourne, J. (1999). *Can't buy my love: How advertising changes the way we think and feel.* New York: Simon & Schuster.

King, M. C., & Ryan, J. M. (2004). Nursing care and adolescent dating violence. In J. C. Campbell & J. C. Humphreys (Eds.), *Family violence and nursing practice* (pp. 288–306). Philadelphia: Lippincott Williams & Wilkins.

Krystal, J. H., Kosten, T. R., Southwick, S., et al. (1989). Neurobiological aspects of PTSD: Review of clinical and preclinical studies. *Behavior Therapy, 20*, 177–198.

Kwong, M. J., Bartholomew, K., Henderson, A. J. Z., & Trinke, S. J. (2003). The intergenerational transmission of relationship violence. *Journal of Family Psychology, 17*(3), 288–301.

Landenburger, K., Campbell, D. W., & Rodriguez, R. (2004). Nursing care of families using violence. In J. C. Campbell & J. C. Humphreys (Eds.), *Family violence and nursing practice* (pp. 220–251). Philadelphia: Lippincott Williams & Wilkins.

Lasiuk, G., & Hegadoren, K. (2006). Posttraumatic stress disorder. Part 1: Historical development of the concept. *Perspectives in Psychiatric Care, 42*(1), 13–20.

Lasiuk, G., & Hegadoren, K. (in press). Posttraumatic stress disorder. Part 2: Development of the construct within the North American Psychiatric Taxonomy. *Perspectives in Psychiatric Care.*

LaVoie, F., Herbert, M., Tremblay, R., Vitaro, F., Vezina, L., & McDuff, P. (2002). History of family dysfunction and perpetuation of dating violence by adolescent boys: A Longitudinal study. *Journal of Adolescent Health, 30*, 375–383.

Law Commission of Canada. (2000). *Restoring dignity: Responding to child abuse in Canadian institutions.* Ottawa: Minister of Public Works and Government Services.

Lloyd, S. A., & Emery, B. C. (2000). The context and dynamics of intimate aggression against women. *Journal of Social and Personal Relationships, 17*(4–5), 503–521.

Long, A., & Smyth, A. (1998). The role of mental health nursing in the prevention of child sexual abuse and the therapeutic care of survivors. *Journal of Psychiatric and Mental Health Nursing, 5*, 129–136.

Lowenthal, B. (2001). Teaching resilience to maltreated children. *Reclaiming Children and Youth, 3*, 169–173.

Lundberg-Love, P. K. (1997). Current treatment strategies of adult incest survivors and their partners. In R. Geffner, S. B. Sorenson, & P. K. Lundberg-Love (Eds.), *Violence and sexual abuse at home: Current issues in spousal battering and child maltreatment* (pp. 293–311). New York: Haworth Maltreatment & Trauma Press.

MacMillan, H. L. (2000). Child maltreatment: What we know in the year 2000. *Canadian Journal of Psychiatry, 45*(8), 702–709.

McCay, E., Gallop, R., Austin, W., Bayer, M., & Peternelji-Taylor, C. (1997). Validation of the sexual abuse comfort scale. *Journal of Psychiatric and Mental Health Nursing, 4*, 361–367.

McGrath, M. E., Bettacchi, A., Duffy, S. J., et al. (1997). Violence against women: Provider barriers to intervention in emergency departments. *Academy Emergency Medicine, 4*, 297–300.

McLean, L. M., & Gallop R. (2003). Implications of childhood sexual abuse for adult borderline personality disorder and complex posttraumatic stress disorder. *American Journal of Psychiatry, 160*(2), 369–371.

McKeown, I., Reid, S., & Orr, P. (2004). Experiences of sexual violence and relocation in the lives of HIV infected Canadian women. *International Journal of Circumpolar Health, 63*(Suppl 2), 399–404.

Messman-Moore, T. L., & Long, P. J. (2003). The role of childhood sexual abuse sequelae in the sexual revictimization of women: An empirical review and theoretical reformulation. *Clinical Psychology Review, 23*, 237–571.

Mill, J. E. (1997). HIV risk behaviors become survival techniques for aboriginal women. *Western Journal of Nursing Research, 19*(4), 466–489.

Morrill, A. C., Kasten, L., Urato, M., & Larson, M. J. (2001). Abuse, addiction, and depression as pathways to sexual risk in women and men with a history of substance abuse. *Journal of Substance Abuse, 13*, 169–184.

National Women's Health Information Center. (2003). Women with disabilities: Dissociative disorders. Available at http://www.4woman.gov.

Nolen-Hoeksema, S. (2002). Gender differences in depression. In I. H. Gotlib & C. L. Hammen (Eds.), *Handbook of depression* (pp. 492–509). New York: Guilford.

Norris, F. H., Foster, J. D., & Weisshaar, D. L. (2002). The epidemiology of sex differences in PTSD across developmental, social, and research contexts. In R. Kimmerling, P. Ouimette, & J. Wolfe (Eds.), *Gender and PTSD* (pp. 3–42). New York: Guilford.

O'Donnell, T., Hegadoren, K., & Coupland, N. (2004). Noradrenergic mechanisms in the pathophysiology of post-traumatic stress disorder. *Neuropsychobiology, 50*(4), 273–283.

Orsillo, S. M., Raja, S., & Hammond, C. (2002). Gender issues in PTSD with comorbid mental health disorders. In R. Kimerling, P. Ouimette, & J. Wolfe (Eds.), *Gender and PTSD* (pp. 207–231). New York: Guilford.

Ouimette, P., Moos, R. H., & Brown, P. J. (2003). Substance use disorder—posttraumatic stress disorder comorbidity: A survey of treatments and proposed practice guidelines. In P. Ouimette & P. J. Brown (Eds.), *Trauma and substance abuse: Causes, consequences, and treatment of comorbid disorders* (pp. 91–110). Washington, DC: American Psychiatric Association.

Parker, B., Bullock, L., Bohn, D., & Curry, M. A. (2004). In J. C. Campbell & J. C. Humphreys (Eds.), *Family violence and nursing practice* (pp. 77–96). Philadelphia: Lippincott Williams & Wilkins.

Peled, E., Jaffe, P. G., & Edleson, J. L. (1995). *Ending the cycle of violence*. Thousand Oaks, CA: Sage.

Petter, L. M., & Whitehill, D. L. (1998). Management of female sexual assault. *American Family Physician, 58*(4), 920–926.

Putnam, F. W. (1994). Dissociative disorders in children and adolescents. In S. J. Lynn & J. W. Rhue (Eds.), *Dissociation: Clinical and theoretical perspectives* (pp. 175–189). New York: Guilford.

Raphael, B., & Matthew, M. (2002). Acute posttraumatic interventions. In F. Lewis-Hall, T. S. Williams, J. A. Panetta, & J. M. Herrera (Eds.), *Psychiatric illnesses in women* (pp. 139–158). Washington, DC: American Psychiatric Press.

Randall, M., & Haskell, L. (1995). Sexual violence in women's lives. Findings from the Women's Safety Project, a community-based survey. *Violence Against Women,1*(1), 6–31.

Rasmusson, A. M., & Friedman, M. J. (2002). Gender issues in the neurobiology of PTSD. In R. Kimerling, P. Ouimette, & J. Wolfe (Eds.), *Gender and PTSD* (pp. 43–75). New York: Guilford.

Resnick, H., Acierno, R., Holmes, M., Kilpatrick, D. G., & Jager, N. (1999). Prevention of post-rape psychopathology: Preliminary findings of a controlled acute rate treatment study. *Journal of Anxiety Disorders, 13*(4), 359–370.

Rhea, M. H., Chafey, K. H., Dohner, V. A., & Terragno, R. (1996). The silent victims of domestic violence—Who will speak? *Journal of Child and Adolescent Psychiatric Nursing, 9*(3), 7–15.

Richardson, D., & Campbell, J. L. (1982). Alcohol and rape: The effect of alcohol on attributions of blame for rape. *Personality and Social Psychology Bulletin, 8*(3), 468–476.

Roesler, T. A., & Dafler, C. A. (1993). Chemical dissociation in adults sexually victimized as children: Alcohol and drug use in adult survivors. *Journal of Substance Abuse Treatment, 10*, 537–543.

Rosenbaum, A., Geffner, R., & Benjamin, S. (1977). A biopsychosocial model for understanding relationship aggression. In R. Geffner, S. B. Sorenson, & R. K. Lundburg-Love (Eds.), *Violence and sexual abuse at home* (pp. 57–80). New York: Haworth Maltreatment & Trauma Press.

Rothbaum, B. O., & Foa, E. B. (1996). Cognitive-behavioral therapy for posttraumatic stress disorder. In B. A. van der Kolk, A. C. McFarlane, & L. Weisaeth (Eds.), *Traumatic stress: The effects of overwhelming experience on mind, body, and society* (pp. 491–509). New York: Guilford.

Rothschild, B. (1998). Post-traumatic stress disorder: Identification and diagnosis. *Swiss Journal of Social Work*. Available at http://www.healing-arts.org.

Ryan, J., & King, M. C. (1998). Scanning for violence: Educational strategies for helping abused women. *AWHONN Lifelines, 2*(3), 36–41.

Sampselle, C. M., Bernhard, L., Kerr, R. B., et al. (1992). Violence against women: The scope and significance of the problem. In C. M. Sampselle (Ed.), *Violence against women: Nursing research, education, and practice issues* (pp. 3–16). New York: Hemisphere.

Schachter, C. L., Radomsky, N. A., Stalker, C. A., Teram, E. (2004). Women survivors of child sexual abuse. How can health professionals promote healing? *Canadian Family Physician, 50*, 405–412.

Scott, H. S., & Beaman, R. (2004). Demographic and situational factors affecting injury, resistance, completion, and charges brought in sexual assault cases: What is best for arrest? *Violence & Victims, 19*(4), 479–494.

Seeman, M. V. (2002). Single-sex psychiatric services to protect women. *Medscape General Medicine, 4*(3) [formerly published in Medscape *Women's Health eJournal* 7(4), 2002]. Available at http://www.medscape.com.

Selzer, M. L. (1971). The Michigan Alcoholism Screening Test: The quest for a new diagnostic instrument. *American Journal of Psychiatry, 127*, 89–94.

Sengstock, M. C., Ulrich, Y. C., & Barrett, S. A. (2004). Abuse and neglect of the elderly. In J. C. Campbell & J. C. Humphreys (Eds.), *Family violence and nursing practice* (pp. 97–149). Philadelphia: Lippincott Williams & Wilkins.

Sheridan, D. (2004). Legal and forensic nursing responses to family violence. In J. C. Campbell & J. C. Humphreys (Eds.), *Family violence and nursing practice* (pp. 386–406). Philadelphia: Lippincott Williams & Wilkins.

Sisley, A., Jacobs, L. M., Poole, G., et al. (1999). Violence in America: A public health crisis-domestic violence. *Journal of Trauma, Injury, and Critical Care, 46*(6), 1105–1112.

Skinner, H. A. (1982). The Drug Abuse Screening Test. *Addictive Behavior, 7*, 363–371.

Southwick, S. M., Bremner, D., Krystal, J. H., & Charney, D. S. (1994). Psychobiologic research in post-traumatic stress disorder. *Psychiatric Clinics of North America, 17*(2), 251–264.

Statistics Canada (2001). *Canadian Crime Statistics 2000.* Ottawa: Canadian Centre for Justice Statistics, Statistics Canada.

Statistics Canada (2003a). *Family violence in Canada: A statistical profile.* Ottawa: Federal Family Violence Initiative, Statistics Canada.

Statistics Canada. (2003b). *The Daily. Witnessing violence: Aggression & anxiety in young children.* Ottawa: Health Reports, Statistics Canada.

Stermac, L., Del Bove, G., & Addison, M. (2004). Stranger and acquaintance sexual assault of adult males. *Journal of Interpersonal Violence, 19*(8), 901–915.

Stewart, S. H., Ouimette, P., & Brown, P. J. (2002). Gender and the comorbidity of PTSD with substance use disorders. In R. Kimerling, P. Ouimette, & J. Wolfe (Eds.), *Gender and PTSD* (pp. 232–270). New York: Guilford.

Sutherland, S. M., & Davidson, J. T. (1999). Pharmacological treatment of posttraumatic stress disorder. In P. A. Saigh & J. D. Bremner (Eds.), *Posttraumatic stress disorder: A comprehensive text* (pp. 327–353). Boston: Allyn & Bacon.

Swann, S. C. (2001). Women's use of violence in intimate relationships: Myths and facts. Paper presented at the Effects of Domestic Violence in Children: A Fathers Role Conference, Southern Connecticut State University, New Haven, Connecticut.

Thase, M. E., Jindal, R., & Howland, R. H. (2002). Biological aspects of depression. In I. H. Gotlib & C. L. Hammen (Eds.), *Handbook of depression* (pp. 192–218). New York: Guilford.

Thompson, M. P., Kaslow, N. J., Kingree, J. B., et al. (1999). Partner abuse and posttraumatic stress disorder as risk factors for suicide attempts in a sample of low-income, inner-city women. *Journal of Traumatic Stress, 12*(1), 59–71.

Ulman, S. E. (2003). A critical review of field studies on the link of alcohol and adult sexual assault in women. *Aggression and Violent Behavior, 8,* 471–486.

United States Department of Justice. (2002). Strengthening antistalking statutes. Available at http://www.ojp.usdoj.gov.

Urbancic, J. C. (2004). Sexual abuse in families. In J. C. Campbell & J. C. Humphreys (Eds.), *Family violence and nursing practice* (pp. 186–219). Philadelphia: Lippincott Williams & Wilkins.

Van der Kolk, B. A. (1996). The complexity of adaptation to trauma self-regulation, stimulus discrimination, and characterological development. In B. A. van der Kolk, A. C. McFarlane, & L. Weisaeth (Eds.), *Traumatic stress: The effects of overwhelming experience on mind, body, and society.* New York: Guilford.

Van der Kolk, B. A., & Fisler, R. E. (1993). The biologic basis of post-traumatic stress. *Primary Care, 20*(2), 417–432.

Van der Kolk, B. A., McFarlane, A. C., & Weisaeth, L. (Eds.). (1996). *Traumatic stress: The effects of overwhelming experience on mind, body, and society.* New York: Guilford.

Varcoe, C. (2001). Abuse obscured: An ethnographic account of emergency nursing in relation to violence against women. *Canadian Journal of Nursing Research, 32*(4), 95–115.

Walker, L. (1979). *The battered woman.* New York: Harper & Row.

Walker, L. (1994). The abused women: A survivor therapy approach [Film]. Available from Newbridge Communications, Inc., 333 East Street, New York, NY 10016.

Wallace, H. (1999). *Family violence: Legal, medical, and social perspectives* (2nd ed.). Boston: Allyn & Bacon.

Walsh, C., MacMillan, H. L., & Jamieson, E. (2003). The relationship between parental substance abuse and child maltreatment: findings from the Ontario Health Supplement. *Child Abuse & Neglect, 27*(12), 1409–1425.

Watson, J. M., Cascardi, M., Avery-Leaf, S., & O'Leary, K. D. (2001). High school students' responses to dating aggression. *Violence and Victims, 16,* 339–348.

Wilson, J. P. (2001). An overview of clinical considerations and principles in the treatment of PTSD. In J. P. Wilson, M. J. Friedman, & J. Lindy (Eds.), *Treating psychological trauma and PTSD* (pp. 59–93). New York: Guilford.

Wilson, J. P., Friedman, M. J., & Lindy, J. D. (2001). A holistic, organismic approach to healing trauma and PTSD. In J. P. Wilson, M. J. Friedman, & J. Lindy (Eds.), *Treating psychological trauma and PTSD* (pp. 28–56). New York: Guilford.

Wong, C. M., & Yehuda, R. (2002). Sex differences in posttraumatic stress disorder. In F. Lewis-Hall, T. S. Williams, J. A. Panetta, & J. M. Herrera (Eds.), *Psychiatric illnesses in women* (pp. 57–96). Washington, DC: American Psychiatric Press.

Wright, R. J., Wright, R. O., & Isaac, N. E. (1997). Response to battered mothers in the pediatric emergency department: A call for an interdisciplinary approach to family violence. *Pediatrics, 99*(2), 186–192.

Wuest, J., & Merritt-Gray, M. (2001). While leaving abusive male partners, women engaged in a 4 stage process of reclaiming self. *Canadian Journal of Nursing Research, 32,* 79–94.

Wuest, J., Merritt-Gray, M., & Ford-Gilboe, M. (2004). Regenerating family: Strengthening the emotional health of mothers and children in the context of intimate partner violence. *Advances in Nursing Science, 27*(4), 257–274.

Zust, B. L. (2000). Effect of cognitive therapy on depression in rural battered women. *Archives of Psychiatric Nursing, 14*(2), 51–63.

For challenges, please refer to the **CD-ROM** in this book.

Self Harm and Suicidal Behaviour: Children, Adolescents, and Adults

B. Lee Murray and Emily J. Hauenstein

LEARNING OBJECTIVES

After studying this chapter, you will be able to:

- Define suicide, suicidal ideation, self-harm, parasuicide, and suicidal behaviour.
- Describe population groups that have high rates of suicide.
- Discuss the rights of patients and other legal issues in the care of suicidal patients.
- Determine factors that affect the nurse's responsibility in assessment and intervention with suicidal individuals, including adolescents.
- List screening measures for depression, suicide intent, and psychiatric diagnostic measures.
- Discuss the process of a comprehensive suicide risk assessment.
- Describe factors that increase the risk for suicide completion.
- Describe the no self-harm contract (contracting for safety).
- Describe the nurse's responsibilities in promoting short- and long-term recovery in suicidal adult inpatients.
- Discuss the patient's and nurse's responsibilities in discharging the patient to the community.

KEY TERMS

self-harm behaviour • suicidal behaviour • beneficence • confidentiality • informed consent • involuntary hospitalization • least restrictive environment • no self-harm contract • parasuicide • suicide • suicide contagion • suicidal ideation • voluntary hospitalization • assessment of risk • compassion fatigue

⬟ KEY CONCEPTS

hopelessness • powerlessness • helplessness

The definition of **suicide** is simple: the voluntary and intentional act of killing oneself. The complexities associated with suicide, however, are grounded in an individual's perceptions and experiences of life, specifically those relating to sexuality, mental illness, family factors, age, and gender. Two dimensions of suicide, which need to be considered, are completed suicide and attempt of suicide. An **attempt of suicide** can be characterized as living through an experience of suicide despite having expected or intended to die. Though the individual may receive support, help, and hospitalization and be grateful for such services, the intent to end life was present. Conversely, a **completed suicide** is the engagement of suicidal behaviour where death has occurred. Acts of suicide, despite the actual outcome, are defined as **suicidal behaviour**. Likewise, thought of suicide is known as **suicide ideation**. **Parasuicide** is self-injurious behaviour, or self-harm, which may mimic suicidal behaviour but the primary motivating force of action is not to kill oneself (Kreitman, 1970; Zor et al., 2005). Death may occur, however, as a result of parasuicidal actions (Welch, 2001; Zor et al., 2005). Of importance here is to understand that parasuicide is *not* suicide (Kreitman, 1979), where the will is to kill oneself intentionally. Our understanding of parasuicide is incomplete, and its prevalence is believed to be grossly underestimated because most studies report only hospital contacts (Meehan, Lamb, Saltzman & O'Carroll, 1992). As well, research studies on suicide and parasuicide have not clearly defined these phenomena (Guo, Scott, & Bowker, 2003), and parasuicide may not be distinguished from attempted suicide.

Self-harm exists in the suicide and parasuicide paradigms. **Self-harm** is characterized as any behaviour or act that causes harm to the body. The nature of the self-harm itself is dependent on the intent of the individual.

Many lives are deeply affected by suicide and the struggle with what to do when a patient, colleague, friend, or loved one is suicidal. Self-harm and suicidal behaviours are very challenging for nurses and other health care professionals to address. It is important to try to understand the meaning of the self-harm and suicidal behaviours, particularly because such behaviours can be understood as a means of communicating to others one's despair.

Suicide, like mental illness, is stigmatized in contemporary society. The stigma against suicide has deep roots in some religions, such as Christianity, in our collective thinking, and until a few decades ago, it was considered a crime in Western nations. Such stigma can prevent people from voicing their suicidal thoughts or asking for help: they are afraid they will be seen as weak, "mad," or coming from bad families (Tadros & Jolley, 2001). When a suicidal act fails, the visibility of medical intervention can trigger stigmatization by others (Joachim & Acorn, 2000).

Stigma may be also experienced by the survivors of someone who completed suicide if blame for the loss is affixed to them; such stigma can significantly complicate their bereavement (Cvinar, 2005). Reports and portrayals of suicide in the media may further contribute to stigmatization (Coverdale, Naim, & Claasen, 2002).

Suicide remains a significant public health problem in Canada, despite efforts at both policy and clinical levels (eg, to identify risk and protective factors and appropriate interventions). Suicide prevention is difficult because suicide is "the outcome of complex interactions among neurobiological, genetic, psychobiological, social, cultural, and environmental risk and protective factors" (Guo, Scott & Bowker, 2003, p. 2), and our knowledge about it remains limited (Tondo & Baldessarini, 2001). Parasuicide further complicates understanding the prevalence of suicide. It also places significant demands on the health care system (Stewart, Manion, Davidson, & Cloutier, 2001).

Nurses are in a unique position to contribute to preventative efforts. With knowledge of early risk assessment and interventions, understood within the context of a person's family, social world, and broader community, as well as knowledge of how to engage with and respond to the actively suicidal person, nurses can make a difference. They can prevent escalation or chronicity of the behaviour (Murray, 2003). Nurses can do much to demystify suicide and destigmatize those at risk through individual and public education. The content of this chapter provides the information needed to understand suicidal and parasuicidal behaviours, as well as the tools to respond appropriately to them.

EPIDEMIOLOGY OF SUICIDAL BEHAVIOUR

Suicide occurs in all age groups, social classes, and cultures. The World Health Organization (WHO) (2002) reports that 815,000 people killed themselves in 2000. This suggests that one death by suicide occurs every 40 seconds. As attempted suicides are estimated to occur 10 to 20 times more often than completed suicides, there is worldwide about one attempt every 3 seconds. In Canada, suicide is the fifth leading cause of death. It is the leading cause of death for men aged 25 to 29 years and 40 to 49 years, for women aged 30 to 34 years, and the second leading cause of death for those aged 10 to 24 years. Canada's suicide rate, compared worldwide, is in the mid to high range (WHO, 2002): 11.9 deaths per 100,0000 deaths (in 2001) (Statistics Canada, 2004). Prevalence rates may be still underestimated: suicide can be disguised as a motor vehicle collision or homicide, especially in young people (Kohlmeier, McMahan, & DiMaio, 2001; Ohberg & Lonnqvist, 1998). The most common method used for completed suicide is

BOX 37.1

Risk and Protective Factors for Suicide

Risk Factors

Demographic or social factors
- Being an older adult
- Being male
- Poverty
- Being Aboriginal
- Being single (widow > divorced > separated > single)
- Social isolation, including new or worsening estrangement, and rural location
- Economic or occupational stress, loss, or humiliation
- New incarceration
- History of gambling
- Easy access to firearms

Clinical factors
- Past and current major psychiatric illness (especially depression)
- Personality disorder (borderline, narcissistic, antisocial)
- Impulsive or violent traits by history
- Current medical illness
- Family history of suicide
- Previous suicide attempts or other self-injurious or impulsive acts
- Current anger, agitation, or constricted preoccupation
- Current abuse of alcohol or drugs
- Easy access to lethal toxins (including prescribed medication)
- Formulated plan, preparations for death or suicide note
- Low ambivalence about dying vs. living

Factors specific to youth
- All of the above
- Lack of family support
- History of abuse
- School problems
- Social ostracism, humiliation
- Conduct disorder
- Struggle with sexual orientation
- Recent marriage, unwanted pregnancy

Precipitants
- Recent stressors (especially losses of emotional, social, physical, or financial security)

Protective Factors

- Intact social supports
- Active religious affiliation or faith (may also be a risk factor if shame/guilt about behaviour is involved)
- Marriage and presence of dependent children
- Ongoing supportive relationship with a caregiver
- Absence of depression or substance abuse
- Access to medical and mental health resources
- Impulse control
- Proven problem-solving and coping skills

Presence of risk and protective factors should be noted in the patient's chart as part of the risk assessment

Adapted from http://www.medceu.com/course-no-test.cfm?CID=308.

---

suffocation (39%), followed by poisoning (26%) and firearms (22%) (Mishara, 2003).

Suicide is more common among groups with specific risk factors and has been associated with loss, unemployment, transience, recent life events (eg, divorce, moving, problems with children), interpersonal distress, and earlier attempts (Appleby, Cooper, Amos, & Faragher, 1999). Research indicates that, universally, suicide is strongly associated with depression (O'Connell, Chin, Cunningham, & Lawlor, 2004). The best predictor for suicide is a previous attempt (Nemeroff, Compton, & Berger, 2001), whereas a significant protective factor is being married with dependent children (Tondo & Baldessarini, 2001). See Box 37.1 for a list of risk and protective factors.

KEY CONCEPT Hopelessness is a perception of having no hope that one's life situation or circumstance will change or improve. It is characterized by feelings of inadequacy and an inability to act on one's own behalf.

Helplessness is the perception of having limited ability or ambition to change one's current life situation. It is characterized by a sense of being unable to help oneself and a sense that there is a lack of support or protection.

Powerlessness is the perception of having no power or control over one's life circumstance; feeling that the world will never be fair; feeling helpless and totally ineffectual; or feeling one lacks legal or other authority.

Age

Prepubertal Children

Suicide is rare among children who are younger than 10 years. There were no reports of self-harm resulting in completed suicide in children this age in 2002 and only two completed suicides from 1993 to 1997 (Statistics Canada, 2002). However, suicides by children this age may be significantly underestimated. Mishara (1999) reported that medical examiners are reluctant to categorize self-inflicted death as suicide because of the belief that children do not fully understand the ramifications of their self-harm behaviour. Mishara, however, found that by grade 3, children have a comprehensive understanding of suicide, and younger children understand what it means to kill themselves.

Preadolescents and Adolescents

More teenagers die from suicide than from cancer, heart disease, birth defects, stroke, pneumonia, influenza, and chronic lung disease combined. In 2002, 35 Canadian children aged 10 to 14 years (10.5% of all deaths within this age group) died due to intentional self-harm (Statistics Canada, 2005). The Public Health Agency of Canada (2000) reported suicide to be the second leading cause of death for youth aged 15 to 24 years (585 deaths), that is, 24% of all deaths in this age group. In 2002, 215 youth aged 15 to 19 years and 277 aged 20 to 24 years died as a result of self-harm (Statistics Canada, 2005). Preadolescent and adolescent males are nearly twice as likely to complete suicide than their female counterparts.

Although the number of completed suicides may seem disturbingly high, the rate of attempted suicide is equally alarming. Langlois and Morrison (2002) reported that in 1999, 40.8, 152.2, and 117.9 per 100,000 Canadian youth aged 10 to 14, 15 to 19, and 20 to 29 years, respectively, attempted suicide.

Adults

Worldwide trends indicate that suicide increases with age. Rates among those aged 60 years and older are about three times higher than for people aged 15 to 29 years (Statistics Canada, 2005). By age 55 to 64 years, suicide is the eighth leading cause of death (Public Health Agency of Canada, 2002). Although suicide is the second leading cause of death for individuals 25 to 34 years old (21.8% of deaths) (Statistics Canada, 2002), it is the fourth leading cause for those aged 35 to 54 (8.5% of deaths). As age increases, suicide rates as a cause of death within the age group declines, indicative of an increase in pathologic deaths occurring from cancers, heart attacks, and so on.

Many young adults who complete suicide have a psychiatric diagnosis (Kishi, Robinson, Kosier, 2001; Brieger, Ehrt, Bloeink, & Marneros, 2002). Other factors linked to suicide include childhood physical and sexual abuse and other psychosocial issues (Appleby, Cooper, Amos, & Faragher, 1999; Foster, Gillespie, McClelland, & Patterson, 1999; Gunnell, et al., 1999). Recent data show high suicide risk in young widowed men (Luoma & Pearson, 2002).

Older Adults

Although other causes of death are more prominent, suicide risk is high among the older adults (O'Connell, Chin, Cunningham, & Lawlor, 2004). Unfortunately, suicidal older adults have received far less attention in the scientific literature than their younger counterparts (Conwell & Duberstien, 2001). Nationally, the ratio of suicide attempts to completions in older adults is 4:1. Older adults generally have a stronger intent to die, plan their suicide more carefully, and are more likely to use lethal means of killing themselves than are younger people (Conwell & Duberstein, 2001). The often frail health of older adults may contribute to the rate of completed suicides, and because many older adults live alone, the chance of a suicide being thwarted is often less than among younger people.

Although Canadian older adults have a higher rate of completing suicide, they have the lowest rate of suicide other than children aged 5 to 14 years (WHO, 2002). Of all suicides in Canada in 2001, 11.8% were by people older than 65 years of age. Suicide is less stigmatized for this age group and may be viewed as more acceptable.

For older adults, suicide is associated with less education, widowhood, previous attempts, depressive disorder, social isolation, financial difficulties, and substance abuse (Conwell & Duberstein, 2001; Conwell et al., 2002; Kishi et al., 2001). Specifically, elderly widowed men have the highest risk for suicide (Tondo & Baldessarini, 2001). As in other age groups, major depressive disorder (MDD) is a significant factor in suicide. In 2001, Conwell and Duberstein reported that 71% to 95% of elderly people who completed suicide had a major psychiatric disorder at the time of death. However, comorbid physical illnesses often make recognition of MDD difficult.

> ◆ **KEY CONCEPT Lethality** refers to the probability that a person will complete suicide. Lethality is determined by the seriousness of the person's intent and the likelihood that the planned method will result in death. High lethality includes firearms, hanging, carbon monoxide poisoning, drowning, suffocation, or jumping from a great height.
>
> **Risk/rescue ratio** refers to the lethality of means and the likelihood of rescue. Suicidal risk carries with it a progression of seriousness from suicidal ideation to completed suicide. Risk is lowest when intent is weak and the method used has low lethality. The likelihood of rescue is dependent on communication of intent and lower lethality of means.

Gender

Worldwide, males complete suicide at a rate three times that of females, although women are four times more likely to attempt suicide than men (Health Canada, 2003). The reasons for the differences are not entirely understood. One hypothesis contends that completion rates differ because men are more likely to use highly lethal methods such as firearms (Tondo & Baldessarini, 2001). In a study of marital status and suicide risk among men and women, O'Connor & Noel (1997) found that single men are more likely to attempt suicide than their married counterparts; conversely, married women are suicidal more frequently than single women. Similarly, Quan, Arboleda-Fisrez, Fick, Stuart, & Love (2002) report that widowers had a five times higher risk for suicide than did married males, whereas the rates for suicide among married and widowed women remained similar. In an epidemiologic study of relationships and suicides, Eng, Rimm, Fitzmaurice, and Kawachi (2002) found that unmarried, unsociable men between 42 and 77 years with minimal social networks and no close relatives were at significantly greater risk for suicide.

Psychiatric disorders and unemployment are precipitating factors for risk for suicide in both men and women; however, they affect each gender differently. MDD is often comorbid with substance abuse in men, and as many as 33% of patients with alcoholism commit suicide (Angst, Angst, & Stassen, 1999; Berglund & Ojehagen, 1998). Aggression, hopelessness, emotion-focussed coping, and having little purpose in life have been associated with suicidal behaviour in men (Edwards & Holden, 2001; Prigerson & Slimack, 1999), as has social isolation (Alexander, 2001) and less participation in religious activities (Nisbet, Duberstein, Conwell, & Seidlitz, 2000). Economic deprivation and unemployment are more likely to precipitate suicide in men, but not necessarily in women (Hawton, Harriss, Hodder, Simkin, & Gunnell, 2001; Kposowa, 2001). Conversely, women who complete suicide often have several comorbid psychiatric disorders (Hall, Platt, & Hall, 1999). Women who have MDD and comorbid schizophrenia or anxiety and those with bipolar disorder are at high risk for suicide (Rihmer & Pestality, 1999; Saarinen, Lehtonen, & Lonnqvist, 1999). Current or previous exposure to violence, sexual assault, or both also increases women's risk for suicide (Koplin & Agathen, 2002; Nelson et al., 2002), and having a small child reduces it (Qin, Agerbo, Westergård-Nielson, Eriksson, & Mortenson, 2000). Although unemployment has long been associated with suicide in men, recent research has shown that for the long-term, unemployed women also are at serious risk for suicide: unemployed women had a suicide rate three times that of employed women in a follow-up study of 9 years (Kposowa, 2001).

Aboriginal Peoples

"I am here today because my ancestors, starving as they often were, fought to survive. Why did the old people strive to live . . . and the young people now want to die?" (NANYouth, 2004)

Before Aboriginal people first made contact with Europeans, suicide was rare (White & Jodoin, 2003). Since that time, Aboriginal rates of suicide have steadily increased, especially in the past few decades. As of 1999, suicide and self-harm were the leading cause of death of First Nations people up to the age of 44 years (Health Canada, First Nations Inuit Health Branch, 2003). Today the rate of suicide among Aboriginal people is three times that of the national rate (Royal Commission on Aboriginal Peoples, 1995) and is the single greatest cause of injury death in this population (White & Jodoin, 2003). More than 60% of Aboriginal people, as compared with 40% of nonnative people, are intoxicated at the time of suicide (NANYouth, 2004).

It is important to note that there is a chance that Aboriginal suicide rates are underreported. White and Jodoin (2003) postulate two reasons why the rates may be misrepresentative. First, data collected by Statistics Canada pertain only to status Aboriginals living in the 10 provinces and in the 3 territories. Therefore, nonstatus First Nations, Métis, and Inuit people living elsewhere in

---

IN A LIFE

The Mushuau Innu of Davis Inlet

In 1993, the world was stunned to see a video of six children sniffing gas and screaming that they wanted to die. Combined with the report from the previous year of a house fire that killed six children while their parents were drinking, long-needed attention was finally drawn to Davis Inlet and the plight of the Mushuau Innu who lived there.

Approximately 680 Mushuau Innu lived in Davis Inlet and now live in Natuashish, Labrador. Fifty percent of the population is younger than 16 years of age. The community has one of the highest suicide rates in the world: 178 per 100,000, and is also plagued with severe poverty, high infant mortality rates, alcohol and solvent abuse, violence, and parental neglect (Samson, 2003). The community is keenly aware of these problems and for the past 30 years has been working with other Innu communities, health care professionals, the Government of Canada, and the Government of Labrador and Newfoundland to address them.

Although in 2001, the Innu and federal and provincial governments jointly developed the Labrador Innu Comprehensive Healing Strategy, overall progress is slow. The long-term goals remain to address all aspects of Mushuau Innu life, including education, governance, health, and spirituality.

For further information about the Mushuau Innu, see http://www. ainc-inac.gc.ca/irp/

Canada are excluded in the national suicide data. Second, the rate of accidental deaths among Aboriginal people is four to five times higher than in the general population, and a percentage of these deaths may be from suicide (White & Jodoin, 2003). The Royal Commission on Aboriginal People (1995) speculates that up to 25% of the deaths reported as accidents are actually undisclosed suicides. Suicide attempts, as well as thoughts of suicide, need to be considered when addressing the issues affecting suicide and Aboriginal peoples.

Suicide is the leading cause of death among Aboriginal youth, with rates of 10, 100, and 145 per 100,000 for youth aged 10 to 14, 15 to 19, and 20 to 24 years, respectively (Kirmayer et al., 1993, Suicide Education and Information Centre [SEIC]). Of all age groups, Aboriginal youth aged 15 to 29 years are at the highest risk for completing suicide. Although aboriginal youth living in cities have the same rates of suicide as their non-native peers, Aboriginal youth living on reserves are six times more likely to complete suicide than their non-native peers (NANYouth, 2004). Although the rate of suicide is higher for Aboriginal people as compared with other Canadians, not every Aboriginal community in Canada experiences such high rates of suicide (White & Jodoin, 2003). Marked differences can be noted between provinces, regions, and even between communities in the same geographic region (SEIC, September 2003).

In studying suicide among British Columbia's Aboriginal communities, Chandler and Lalonde (1998) discovered that some communities have suicide rates 800 times the national average, and in other communities, suicide was virtually unknown. They also identified six protective factors that may explain the differences in suicidal rates between communities (see Box 37-2). According to a Health Canada report (2003), community wellness strategies may have the best chance of making a difference in suicidal rates between Aboriginal communities. Guidelines were suggested in developing such a strategy (see Box 37-3).

BOX 37.2

Community Protective Factors Against Risk for Suicide

Cultural continuity is identified in terms of six protective factors that may explain the differences in suicidal rates between Aboriginal communities. Those factors listed in terms of importance are:
- Self-government
- Land claims
- Education services
- Police and fire services
- Health services
- Cultural Facilities

(From Chandler, M. J., & Lalonde, C. [1998]. Cultural continuity as a hedge against suicide in Canada's First Nations. *Transcultural Psychiatry, 35*[2], 191–219.)

BOX 37.3

Aboriginal Community Wellness Strategies

- Locally initiated, owned, and accountable programs
- Suicide prevention should be the responsibility of the entire community.
- Focus on behavioural patterns of children and young people is crucial and requires the involvement of family and community.
- Suicide prevention must be addressed from a biologic, psychological, sociocultural, and spiritual perspective.
- Long-term crisis and intervention programs must be developed.
- Suicide intervention strategies must be evaluated as needed.

(From Health Canada, First Nations and Inuit Health Branch. [2003]. *A statistical profile on the health of First Nations in Canada.* Ottawa: Government of Canada.)

Sexual Orientation

In recent years, sexual orientation as a risk factor for suicide has been highly debated. Russell and Joyner (2001) point to the common belief that dealing with the stigma of homosexuality may lead gay, lesbian, bisexual, and transgendered (GLBT) people to depression or even suicide. During adolescence, when the major focus of a youth's life is on peers and sexuality, a GLBT youth's search for self-identity may heighten depression and suicidal behaviour (Rotheram-Borus & Fernandez, 1995). "Coming out" is a risk factor because of negative reactions of others, particularly peers and family. Acknowledging one's sexual orientation at an early age or never disclosing one's sexual orientation can put GLBT youth at a higher risk of suicide (Remafedi, Farrow, & Deisher, 1991). Someone who comes out at an early age is at an increased risk for harassment and assaults, whereas someone who does not feel safe enough to disclose his or her sexual orientation may feel extremely isolated (Morrison & L'Heureux, 2001). In both cases, there can be feelings of helplessness, hopelessness, powerlessness, and isolation, which increase the risk for depression and suicide (Beck, Steer, Kovacs, & Garrison, 1985). GLBT youth are also at a higher risk for suicide if they self- present with high levels of gender nonconformity (Remafedi, Farrow, & Deisher, 1991), report high levels of inner conflict regarding their sexual orientation (Savin-Williams, 1990), or report sexual abuse (Gibson, 1994). It is important to note that the risk factors associated with being GLBT are in addition to those common to all ages and sexual orientations.

Regional Variations

Eastern and central regions of the Far North have some of the highest mortality rates from suicide in Canada (Statistics Canada, 2003a). Québec had the highest regional rate of suicide in Canada at 132.5 per 100,000, with the rate being 18.5 in the Yukon, 20.8 in the Northwest Territories, and 80.2 in Nunavut. Nunavik and the northern regions of Canada, ranging from British Columbia to Labrador, have suicide rates higher than the national average of 11.3 (Statistics Canada, 2003a). These higher suicide rates are due to a combination of factors. The population of the north of Canada is predominantly Aboriginal; most people live in rural or semirural environments where hunting (and ready access to firearms) is common; and social isolation can occur due to low population per square mile.

Suicide rates vary by province: Alberta, 14.1; British Columbia, 9.4; Manitoba, 11.4; New Brunswick, 13.2; Newfoundland/Labrador, 6.7; Nova Scotia, 9.0; Ontario, 7.7; Prince Edward Island, 10.0; Québec, 16.5; and Saskatchewan, 11.3 (Statistics Canada, 2003b). Within each province, rates of suicide are not consistent because urban centres tend to have lower suicide rates than the national average, for example, Toronto (7.6), Winnipeg (10.5), and Vancouver (10.9). As with the north, various demographic, social, cultural, and geographic factors affect rates of suicide.

Guns and Suicide

Almost 80% of all firearm deaths are suicides, and firearms are used in nearly 20% of all suicide fatalities (Canada Safety Council, 2004). Recent legislation by the Canadian government requiring the registration of all firearms is an attempt to decrease deaths (homicide and suicide) related to firearms. Research supports this legislation; a Québec study run by Le Centre de Prevention du Suicide (Simon, 1996) concluded that there is no evidence that if a firearm is not readily available, another method will be used. The Canadian Safety Council reported that, although accessibility of firearms is usually associated with rural areas (ie, hunting), urban areas show the highest rates of completed suicides by firearms.

Suicidal Ideation and Self-Harm

Rather than being seen as an overt expression of a desire to die, the majority of suicidal acts are seen as "cries for help" or attempts to postpone dealing with an unbearable situation (Health Canada, 1994). Understanding the motivation for such acts is important because 30% to 60% of suicides have been preceded by an attempt and 10% to 14% of those who attempt suicide eventually kill themselves (Tondo & Baldessarini, 2001). As well, long-term follow-up studies of people with parasuicidal behaviour found that 10% to 13% ultimately take their lives (Sakinofsky, Roberts, Brown, Cummings, & James, 1990).

Previous self-harm behaviour, then, is among the best predictors of future suicide attempts and completions. In addition, MDD, physical, cognitive, psychological, and social risk factors contribute to suicidal ideation. Physical factors include medical illness and alcohol and drug use (Grant & Hasin, 1999; Hendin, 1999; Kishi et al., 2001; Vilhjalmsson, Kristjansdottir, & Sveinbjarnardottir, 1998). Cognitive risk factors include problem-solving deficits and hopelessness (D'Zurilla, Chang, Nottingham, & Faccini, 1998). Psychological risk factors include internal distress and low self-esteem (Holden, Kerr, Mendonca, & Velamoor, 1998). Social risk factors include financial hardship, legal stress, family difficulties, and poor social support (Vilhjalmsson et al., 1998). Childhood trauma (including physical and sexual abuse) has been linked to both parasuicide and suicidal ideation in adulthood (Molnar, Berkman, & Buka, 2001).

Suicidal ideation and self-harm are more common among adolescents than other age groups. Contributing factors of such behaviour in adolescents include family discord, neglect, physical abuse, adolescent unemployment, residential transience, chronic behaviour problems, and recent interpersonal stress (Appleby, Cooper et al., 1999; Grilo et al., 1999; Gunnell et al., 1999). Substance abuse increases the likelihood that suicidal ideation will result in parasuicide (Gould et al., 1998).

Self-harm behaviour in adolescents is often a way to communicate needs or wants, and often, the need is for attention or care (Murray, 2003). As such, self-harm is an unacceptable means to acceptable ends and may communicate that the adolescent believes something is wrong, life is tough, and things are becoming unbearable. Parasuicide behaviour (such as cutting or self-mutilation) may also relieve or release certain emotions and feelings and may produce a tangible, physical pain substituting unfamiliar, unbearable psychological suffering (Harris, 2000; Levenkron, 1998; Machoian, 2001). In addition, such behaviours may be related to punishment of self or others (Rew, Thomas, Horner, Resnick, & Beuhring, 2001; Walsh & Rosen, 1988). Self-punishment is often identified with self-loathing, anger, guilt, and shame (Murray, 2003).

Behaviour escalates if the purpose of the self-harm is not achieved (Machoian, 2001). Therefore, feeling unheard or misunderstood often results in the escalation of self-harm behaviour. Furthermore, escalation occurs when self-harm behaviour is not understood in the context of why it is happening and when the purpose of the behaviour is not explored (Murray, 2003). Even if the purpose of self-harm behaviour is recognized, ignoring or minimizing the behaviour may escalate its intensity and frequency with increased attempts to get the message across (Murray, 2003).

ETIOLOGY OF SUICIDAL BEHAVIOUR

Suicidal behaviour occurs in the context of an individual's physiologic, psychological, and social situation and is usually

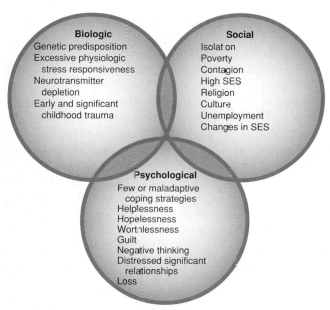

FIGURE 37-1   Biopsychosocial etiologies of suicide.

triggered by stressors that are unmanageable and exceed typical coping efforts. Vulnerabilities are enhanced by engagement in risky behaviours, often used in an effort to cope with stress. Risky behaviours related to suicide include fast, dangerous driving, tempting death, promiscuity, use of alcohol or drugs, and purchase of a handgun. Appropriate interventions guided by a comprehensive assessment of risk at this point can reduce the likelihood of suicidal behaviour. A comprehensive assessment identifies the physical, psychological, and social factors that contribute to feelings of self-harm (Fig. 37-1). These include changes in central nervous system (CNS) neurotransmitters, engaging in negative thinking and risky behaviours, and deterioration of social relationships. The convergence of physiologic, psychological, and social factors can be directly linked to suicidal behaviour.

Biologic Theories

Most will agree that suicide, like many other aspects of humanness, does not solely lie within a single sphere of the biopsychosocial model. However, in order to facilitate learning, suicide will be discussed in relation to each of these spheres.

Biologic theories of suicide attempt to enlighten the phenomenon of suicide by recognizing and interpreting physiologic, neurophysiologic, and hormonal changes. Psychopathologic changes are evident in most suicidal people. MDD, sometimes comorbid with other psychiatric illnesses, is prevalent. Moreover, because suicide rates tend to be higher in families in which suicide has occurred, genetic and familial factors will be explored in this section. Finally, a biologic explanation of increased suicide risk among those who experienced childhood sexual abuse is considered.

MDD tends to develop when a person who is vulnerable to it (because of genetic or other factors) is subjected to repeated or sustained stress. Stress responsiveness in these people ultimately changes neurotransmitter and hormonal functioning to affect a depressed state (Hauenstein, 1996). Those who complete suicide have extremely low levels of the neurotransmitter serotonin, 5-hydroxytryptamine (5-HT) (Mann, Oquendo, Underwood, & Arango, 1999) or lower levels of the neurotransmitter dopamine (Pitchot et al., 2001).

Considerable evidence exists showing a familial trend in suicide (McGuffin, Marusic, & Farmer, 2001; Qin, Agerbo, & Mortenson, 2003). First-degree relatives of individuals who have completed suicide have a two to eight times higher risk for suicide than do individuals in the general population (McGuffin et al., 2001). Suicide of a first-degree relative is highly predictive of a medically serious suicide attempt in another first-degree relative (Modai et al., 1999). This risk is slightly heightened in females (Qin et al., 2003). The children of depressed mothers with a history of suicide attempts have higher rates of suicidal behaviour (Klimes-Dougan et al., 1999; Pfeffer, Normandin, & Kakuma, 1998). The genetic link to suicide is evident in studies of twins. Qin and colleagues (2003) showed that suicidal behaviour in one monozygotic twin increased the risk 11-fold for suicidal behaviour in the co-twin. Another study showed that a serious attempt by one twin increased the risk in a dizygotic co-twin more than twofold and in a monozygotic co-twin almost fourfold (Statham et al., 1998). In this study, genetic factors alone accounted for about half the increased risk for suicidal behaviour. Among adolescent female twins, genetic factors played a part in 35% of suicide attempts (Glowinski et al., 2001). Adoption studies have shown that among adults who experience mood disorders and were adopted as children, the suicide rate among the biologic relatives of the adoptees is much higher than the rate among the adoptive relatives. Genetic abnormalities in the serotonergic neurotransmitter system may be responsible for the heightened familial risk for suicide (Mann, Brent, & Arango, 2001). Collectively, these studies demonstrate that the biologic risk for suicide appears independent of environmental factors.

Child abuse has been described as a specific vulnerability for psychopathology and suicide (MacMillan et al., 2001). Enhanced vulnerability to MDD and suicide associated with child abuse are attributable to changes in the hypothalamic–pituitary–adrenal axis caused by intractable stress and altered serotonin and dopamine metabolism (Skodol, Siever, & Livesley, 2002). Evidence from twin studies suggests that the link between childhood sexual abuse and biologic alterations contributing to psychopathology may be independent of other environmental influences. Several studies show that adult psychopathology is greater in abused twins when compared with nonabused co-twins (Bulik, Prescott, & Kendler, 2001; Kendler et al., 2000; Nelson et al., 2002). Additional specific features of the abuse, including severity, contributed to worse outcomes in the abused twins.

Psychological Theories

Coming to understand suicide as it is related to the human psyche is important. MDD, generalized anxiety, personality disorders, and other psychiatric illnesses occur frequently in the suicidal person. For instance, major affective illnesses or mood disorders (major depressive and bipolar manic-depressive disorders) are associated with about half of all suicides (Tondo & Baldessarini, 2001). Alcohol and substance use disorders are found in approximately 25% of suicides and the lifetime risk for suicide associated with substance abusers is similar to that associated with diagnosis of depression (Roy, 1989; Clark et al., 1998). Anxiety disorders, even after controlling for comorbid depression and substance abuse, account for 15% to 20% of suicides, whereas psychotic disorders such as schizophrenia account for a further 10% to 15% of suicides (Roy, 1989). Furthermore, the risk for suicide is increased by a factor of six in personality disorders like borderline and antisocial personality (Foster, Gillespie, McClland, & Patterson, 1999). Those with multiple comorbid problems such as affective or psychotic disorders combined with drug or alcohol abuse are at the highest risk for suicide (Angst et al., 1999; Appleby et al., 1999; Baldessarini et al., 1999; Guze & Robins, 1970; Roy, 1989).

Psychodynamic theories designate conflicts, losses, and changes in relationships as contributors to suicidal risk and view suicide as a depressive or psychotic act, sometimes associated with fantasies of escape, reward, reunion, and resurrection (Hendin, 1991). Suicide can be conceptualized psychologically as an excessive reaction arising from intense preoccupation with humiliation and disappointment (Leenaars, 1998). It can be driven by intolerable aloneness and isolation (Adler & Buie, 1996), punitive and aggressive impulses of revenge, spite or self-sacrifice, wishes to kill and be killed, or yearning for release into a better experience through death (Tondo and Baldessarini, 2001). Cognitive approaches also attribute suicide to learned helplessness and hopelessness as an automatic and pervasive pathologic scheme for organizing and interpreting experience (Beck, Kovacs, & Weissman, 1979; Rosenberg, 1993). The widely used cognitive theory of depression espoused by Aaron Beck and his associates (Beck, Rush, Shaw, & Emery, 1979) accounts for how negative thoughts occur, how they tend to be repetitive and intrusive,

and how they can lead to suicidal behaviour (see Chapter 14).

People who engage in suicidal behaviour often have difficult relationships with the people in their lives (Jamison, 1999). Attachment theory explains social isolation and disrupted interpersonal relationships as being a part of the spectrum of suicide (Lopez & Brennan, 2000). In this theory, adult behaviour is shaped by early interactions with the primary caregiver during infancy. Disturbed attachment results in the inability to form meaningful relationships or in constant concern about the viability of a lasting relationship. Suicide is, then, the result of conflicted or distant adult relationships and the social isolation that arises (Eng et al., 2002).

Social Theories

Social factors are particularly important to the etiology of suicide. As humans we are inherently a part of the social fabric in which we exist. To be alive is to be in the world. Suicide, then, is the desire to estrange oneself from the world. Some suicidal people describe a desire to "feel nothing for a while," a temporary respite from life and the world. This section will review Emile Durkheim's theory of suicide and then focus on key social factors that contribute to suicide.

Studying the social factors that contribute to rates of suicide, Emile Durkheim, at the end the 19th century, developed a theoretical framework outlining the social causes of suicide. Durkheim classified suicide under four headings: egoistic suicide, altruistic suicide, anomic suicide, and fatalistic suicide. These classifications of suicide are based on the degree of imbalance between social integration and moral regulation (Kendall, Lothian-Murray, & Linden, 2004).

The degree of social integration, Durkheim believed, is a variable affecting rates of suicide. *Egoistic suicide* occurs among individuals who are not significantly bound to society. Some believe that the social isolation of single people is causally related to their higher rates of suicide when compared with their married counterparts. Conversely, *altruistic suicide* occurs when individuals become overly connected to society, for example, a patriotic soldier who kills himself or herself after a defeated battle because he or she is shamed.

Durkheim also acknowledges that extreme cases of social stability and social consensus contribute to rises in suicide rates. A society lacking a sense of purpose, social regulation, or community values experiences *anomic suicide*. This type of suicide occurs during times of financial depression. Contrastingly, in areas of overregulation and oppression, *fatalistic suicides* occur. Although Durkheim discussed little about fatalistic suicide, many use the suicide of slaves as an exemplar.

Contemporary sociologic investigations seek social structure models of influence on suicide. A theory explicated by Cohen, Mason, and Bedimo (2003) contends that socioeconomic status is a driving factor in what happens to an individual, affecting the physical and social structures available to him or her. For example, poverty represented by substandard housing affects other important neighbourhood social structures, such as schools, voluntary organizations, and jobs. People who may wish to teach in these schools, help out, or conduct business in the neighbourhood are deterred by the neighbourhood deterioration. Poverty also reduces exposure to opportunities for individual advancement. Poverty affects health outcomes directly, because of environmental hazards, or indirectly, through inadequate access to health care.

Substantial data exist to support this model of suicide. Cohen and colleagues (2003) found that the percentage of boarded-up buildings in a neighbourhood was positively associated with suicide. Socioeconomic deprivation and unemployment were found to be associated with suicide in several studies (Cubbin, LeClere, & Smith, 2000; Goodman, 1999; Hawton et al., 2001; Kposowa, 2001; Steenland, Halperin, Hu, & Walker, 2003). Unemployment may also pose an indirect risk for suicide through family tension arising from loss of income and a normal social role. This loss may then lead to indignity, isolation, hopelessness, alcohol abuse, and violence (Platt, 1993).

Tondo and Baldessarini (2001) agree that rates of suicide are significantly higher at the poorer end of the socioeconomic continuum. However, they note increases in suicide among the extremely wealthy. Although this may appear paradoxical, wealth brings with it a distinct set of worries and concerns. Importantly, suicide is at its greatest rates when a substantial change in social status occurs.

Suicide and Religion

Rates of suicide vary considerably among religions and between regions with a predominant religion, despite most religions' opposition to suicide. Neeleman (1998) suggests that those who have higher rates of participation in religious practices may have lower risk for suicide.

Suicide Contagion

A social phenomenon seen among adolescents is suicide contagion. Several studies have shown that when one teenager takes his or her life, several more may follow (Gould & Kramer, 2001; Poijula, Wahlberg, & Dyregrov, 2001). Poijula and colleagues (2001) found an increase in suicides in three secondary schools in the year after a suicide occurred. However, rates did not increase in schools that used crisis intervention at the time of the suicide.

Suicide by imitation seems to be influenced, in part, by its portrayal through mass media (Goldney, 1989; Phillips & Carstensin, 1986; Schmidtke & Hafner, 1988). However, mass media's influence can be minimized by avoiding sensationalized reports of suicide that supply details as to the methods used (Jobes, Berman, O'Carroll, Eastgard, & Knickmeyer, 1996). Key factors in imitative behaviour are identification with a victim by age, sex, and location, although other influences, such as economic status, attitudes toward suicide, and problem-solving strategies, affect imitative behaviour (Berman, 1988).

Social circumstances also affect parasuicidal behaviour. Research indicates that changes in the life circumstances of people with parasuicidal behaviour can reduce the risk for suicide. Sakinofsky, Roberts, Brown, Cummings, and James (1990) studied 228 parasuicidal people for 1 year to determine whether resolution of their problems reduced further suicidal behaviour. Three months after their attempts, those who had overcome their difficulties were significantly less depressed and hostile and felt less isolated than they initially reported. Their self-esteem had risen; they did not feel as powerless as before, and they experienced significant improvements in marital and family relationships. Those who had not resolved their issues continued to fare poorly in all respects.

EFFECTS OF SUICIDE

Effect on Survivors

Worldwide, about 1 million people die from suicide each year (WHO, 2004). Each suicide has an impact on an average of six or seven survivors, so that 6 million people lose someone close to them as a result of suicide each year (Tondo & Baldessarini, 2001). Suicide has devastating effects on everyone it touches, especially family and close friends. Undue and prolonged suffering can be caused by the sudden shock, the unanswered questions of "why," and potentially the discovery of the body (Knieper, 1999). Suicide bereavement is different than that experienced by families whose loved one's death is not self-inflicted. The grieving over the way the death occurred, the social processes affecting the survivors, and the effect of the suicide on the family converge to establish a grieving process that is unique (Jordan, 2001).

Often family survivors of suicide reported more stigmatization, shame, and rejection than did matched families whose family member died in other ways. They also reported that police, medical examiners, and the media exacerbated their grief by their insensitivity. For this reason, it is important for nurses to listen and be present, patient, compassionate, and understanding with survivors of suicide. Simplistic explanations and clichés should be avoided. Survivors of suicide need help in following their own search for understanding of what has happened. In the end, their personal search for meaning regarding the death is important. Their coping abilities will mediate their grief responses. It is an ongoing task, but recovery from a loved one's suicide is made easier by good coping skills and social support that help one deal with the psychological trauma (Mitchell, Gale, Garand, & Wesner, 2003; Reed, 1998).

Economic Effects

Suicide affects society by consuming both human lives and economic resources (Clayton & Barceló, 2000). Estimating the cost of suicide is difficult. In Canada, the average cost of hospitalization for suicide and attempted suicide was $5,500 per admission, ranging from $3,000 to $31,000 (HereToHelp, 2003). In 1997, suicide and attempted suicide cost the Canadian health care system $100 million (HereToHelp, 2003). In New Brunswick in 1996, for the 94 reported suicide deaths, the direct costs were $535,158, including health care services, autopsies, and funerals. The indirect cost per suicide death due to lost productivity had a value of $79,353,354, a mean cost of $849,877 (Clayton & Barceló, 2000).

LEGAL CONSIDERATIONS IN CARING FOR SUICIDAL PEOPLE

In Canada, evolving social and religious attitudes have been reflected in the decriminalization of attempted suicide. In 1972, attempted suicide was removed from the provisions of the criminal code. Counselling or assisting suicide, however, remains a criminal act (Section 241, Criminal Code of Canada).

Canadians have legal rights that health care providers must consider during suicide prevention and treatment. Providers cannot deprive patients of their right to self-determination unless no other course is available to ensure a patient's safety. They must preserve rights to privacy and anonymity unless they cannot protect a patient without disclosing his or her suicidal intent to others. Patients have the right of beneficence, which is the right to be free from harm. Physically restraining or hospitalizing a patient against his or her will has the potential for both physical and emotional harm and should be used only under the threat of imminent suicide or psychosis. Nurses must understand patients' legal rights and be able to explain them clearly. This means that nurses need to be familiar with their provincial mental health legislation (see Chapter 3).

Confidentiality

Disclosing information without the patient's permission violates his or her rights to privacy and anonymity and may damage the therapeutic relationship. Patients lose trust when the nurse shares their suicidal intent with others unless the nurse has specifically explained the limits of confidentiality. When informing the patient of existing limits of confidentiality, the nurse must be very clear and specific. The CNA clearly articulates the concept of confidentiality as safeguarding information acquired within a professional relationship, except when doing so would cause significant harm (CNA, 2002).

The CNA code of ethics is consistent with provincial legislation. Namely, the patient has a right to confidentiality unless he or she is at risk for harming self or others or discloses sexual abuse of minors. In those situations, the nurse can enlist the help of others (eg, outside of the health care team) to protect the patient's or others' safety.

Protecting the patient's right to confidentiality is a special concern when a minor child has suicidal intent. As with adult patients, the nurse is required to describe the right to confidentiality and its limits. The nurse must always consider informing parents or legal guardians of a child who has suicidal intent. The parents of a minor child retain the privilege to determine the right care for their child, and they need sufficient information to make good decisions. Before beginning any suicide risk assessment, nurses must let a child know that disclosure of self-harm may be shared with parents. Honesty about what the nurse can and cannot keep confidential ultimately increases a child's trust and often results in a more therapeutic relationship.

Informed Consent

Obtaining fully **informed consent** from the patient protects his or her right to self-determination. However, nurses must inform suicidal patients about limits to their self-determination and make efforts to obtain their cooperation. From the time that the nurse encounters a suicidal patient until a suitable placement is made, the nurse must share with the patient his or her right to be placed in the **least restrictive environment** that will ensure safety. The least restrictive environment is the setting that puts the fewest constraints on the patient's rights while still ensuring the patient's safety. By informing patients about their choices, the nurse gains the patient's trust and decreases the likelihood that involuntary hospitalization will be necessary.

The ethical requirement of **beneficence**, doing no harm, is critical when restraining patients against their will. Caring for patients who are suicidal and determined to get away is difficult without touching and actively restraining them. Still, nurses must do their best to disclose to patients the specifics of planned treatments, including restraints, and attempt to obtain their consent to proceed. Respect for the patient needs to be maintained throughout the process. (For further discussion of these issues, see Chapter 5).

Documentation

The nurse must thoroughly document encounters with suicidal patients. This action is for the patient's ongoing treatment and the nurse's protection. The nursing notes must reflect that the nurse took every reasonable action to provide for the patient's safety. If a no self-harm contract has been instituted, the record must contain specific aspects of the contract.

Involuntary Admission and the Provincial Health Acts

When a patient will not or cannot (because of noncompetent status) agree to enter the hospital voluntarily, **involuntary hospitalization** may be initiated. Considerable controversy surrounds the notion of involuntary hospitalization and treatment. See Chapter 3 for discussion of provincial legislation that empowers physicians and peace officers to detain, without consent, a person whom they consider to be of danger to themselves or others (Health Canada, 1994). Changing social attitudes toward human rights, together with the influence of the 1982 Canadian Charter of Rights and Freedoms, has led to more stringent criteria for involuntary committal. For example, Ontario's Mental Health Act requires that a physician assess the situation and state, in writing, that because of a mental disorder, the individual is at risk for serious bodily harm to self or other unless admitted (Health Canada, 1994). Legislative changes in many provinces have reinforced the individual's right to refuse admission and treatment except in narrowly defined circumstances.

Special considerations for the hospitalization of children and adolescents are given in Box 37-4. Health care practitioners must make every effort to obtain the patient's permission to enter the hospital voluntarily, for both legal and therapeutic reasons. Legally, **voluntary hospitalization** protects the rights of patients, permitting them some freedom in negotiating discharge from the hospital. Therapeutically, voluntary admission reinforces patients' control of the situation as partners in their own care and preserves dignity.

NURSING ASSESSMENT AND INTERVENTIONS

Suicidal behaviours are seriously underreported and often not recognized by health care professionals. Estimates are that approximately 40% of people who complete suicide have visited a health care provider within 1 to 6 months of a suicide attempt (Foster et al., 1999; Link et al., 1999). Nurses can play important roles in

---

BOX 37.4

Child and Adolescent Hospitalization

Hospitalizing a child or adolescent is different from hospitalizing an adult. The decision to admit a child to the hospital rests with the parents and the mental health professional. The requirements for the least restrictive environment still pertain to children and adolescents, but minors do not have the same civil rights as do adults. Moreover, making decisions about the safety of children and adolescents is frequently difficult. Their competence to enter into contracts is often questionable, and their ability to manage their own behaviour is hard to assess. For these reasons, many mental health professionals err on the side of hospitalization for young people with active suicidal ideation.

Hospitalization of suicidal children tends to be prolonged because many have underlying psychosocial issues. Childhood suicidal behaviour may occur in the context of extreme family discord, and children in these dysfunctional families may be the victims of abuse or neglect (Grilo et al., 1999; Lipschitz et al., 1999; Renaud et al., 1999). Nursing care is directed toward connecting with the child/adolescent and family in order to complete a comprehensive assessment of risk and family function. Interventions are then based on the results of the assessment and identifying what needs to change in the child/adolescent's life situation.

---

suicide prevention because they practice in diverse health care settings and thus work with many different kinds of patients. Acutely suicidal behaviour is a true psychiatric emergency. Nurses must act immediately and vigorously to prevent the patient's death.

Biopsychosocial Domain

Nursing interventions based on a comprehensive assessment of risk provide a holistic approach to nursing care of the suicidal patient. The process of risk assessment will be discussed, followed by a discussion of nursing interventions in relation to the biologic, psychological, and social aspects of the suicidal person.

Comprehensive Assessment of Risk

Comprehensive assessment provides a clear picture of self-harm behaviour and guides possible interventions (see Box 37-5 for questions to guide a comprehensive assessment of risk). A model developed by Murray integrates a number of theories to establish a comprehensive assessment of risk. The model emphasizes an approach that views patients in context of their family, their social world, and the broader community (Murray & Wright, in press). It encourages engagement and the development of a connectedness with the client and his or her family, using the language of a Brief Solutions and Family Therapy approach (Berg, 1994; Corcoran, 1998; DeShazer, 1988; Eggert & Thompson, 2002; Minuchin & Fishman, 1981; O'Hanlon & Werner-Davis, 1989),

BOX 37.5

Questions to Guide a Comprehensive Assessment of Risk

The most successful approach is to ask open-ended questions and explore further with curious questions.

Stressors

What is troubling you most at the moment?
   Explore with curious questions in terms of all areas of the patient's life.
   Explore each area, asking the patient to tell you more.
The idea is to get a clear picture of the patient's life situation and presenting stressors as the patient perceives them.

Symptoms

Can you tell me about your sleep patterns?
   Explore using curious questions:
      Are you having difficulty sleeping?
      Do you want to stay in bed and sleep through the day?
Can you tell me about your eating habits?
   Explore using curious questions:
      Have you lost your appetite?
      Do you eat in an attempt to cope with difficulties?
What do you do for enjoyment?
   Explore with curious questions:
      Do you find you no longer enjoy activities you thought were enjoyable?
      How often do you use drugs or alcohol to cope?

Prior Behaviour

Have you ever thought of harming yourself?
   Explore with curious questions:
      Can you tell me about that? (time, place, situation, feelings, meaning)
   What was the self-harm about?
   What happened?
   What did you expect to happen?
   What did you want to happen?

Current Plan

Do you currently have a plan to harm yourself?
   Explore with curious questions:
      What would you do?
      Do you have access to the pills? (other methods)
      Have you picked a specific day or time?

Resources and Support

Do you have someone you recognize as supportive?
   Explore with curious questions:
      Who can you talk to about your concerns?
      Who can you confide in?
      Offer suggestions of a number of people the patient may not have thought of (eg, parent's friend, colleague, clergy, coach, etc.).

emphasizing the power and resiliency of families as key components for change and resolution. An intergenerational perspective and use of the genogram (deGraaf, 1998; McGoldrick, 1992) are also an integral part of the approach. This perspective recognizes family patterns over time and traces the history of abuse, alcoholism, trauma, and loss (Gould & Kramer, 2001; Maine, Shute, & Martin, 2001). Recognition of developmental factors that contribute to individual and family struggles and of family interactional patterns and boundaries also assists in providing a broad and complete assessment (see Chapter 16 for information on family assessment).

Applied Suicide Intervention Skills Training (ASIST)/ Living Works Inc. (Ramsey, Tanny, Taierney, & Lang, 1994) provides the framework for risk assessment, emphasizing assessment of stressors, symptoms, prior suicidal behaviour, current plan, and resources and support. An overall Rogerian approach (Rogers, 1980) guides the interactions with the patient and their family with a nonblaming, nonjudgmental, and unconditional positive regard to understand and process what the suicidal ideation or behaviour is really about. Integration of the model also assists in understanding the onset, purpose, maintenance, and escalation of the suicidal behaviour and assesses specific risk factors related to the self-harm behaviour.

A comprehensive assessment of stressors is vital to guide appropriate interventions. Assessment includes collection of adequate data to provide a clear picture of the patient's life and relevant stressors. As much as possible, the patient's perspective of their stressors and their life situations should be explored. This includes a good understanding of their family, peers, and social relationships as well as workplace issues. Past loss issues need to be explored with the patient to identify any possible precipitating factors related to change or loss. It is also important to discuss issues of abuse and to be aware that these issues must be approached with the appropriate degree of sensitivity.

Symptoms may be explored in context of a depression assessment, keeping in mind the broad spectrum of depressive symptoms (see Chapter 19 for assessment of depression). Such symptoms include isolating or withdrawing from friends and family, sleep and eating disturbances, and not enjoying or participating in activities that were enjoyed in the past. Engaging in risky behaviour such as rebellion, noncompliance, or drugs or alcohol use are commonly associated with suicide (Ramsey et al., 1994).

The nurse or another experienced professional should assess the patient for other psychiatric disorders, especially those most commonly associated with suicidal behaviour (eg, MDD, panic disorder, severe anxiety disorder, schizophrenia, substance abuse, borderline personality disorder, and antisocial personality disorder) (Brieger et al., 2002; Catallozzi, Pletcher, & Schwarz, 2001; Preuss et al., 2002; Prigerson & Slimack, 1999;

Radomsky, Haas, Mann, & Sweeney, 1999). Severity of MDD is associated with a greater likelihood of suicide completion (Alexopoulos et al., 1999; Grant & Hasin, 1999). For adolescents, a key question is whether any family member has attempted or completed suicide (Cerel, Fristad, Weller, & Weller, 1999; Klimes-Dougan et al., 1999; McKeown et al., 1998). Alcoholism is another prominent factor in suicide. Patients with alcoholism account for 25% of completed suicides (Berglund & Ojehagen, 1998).

In 1997, Beck revised the Scale for Suicide Ideation (Beck, Brown, & Steer, 1998; Beck, Kovacs, & Weissman, 1979) to include only eight items, and renamed it the Suicide Intent Scale. This scale is short and useful in determining whether a patient has a strong intent to die. However, even with low levels of intent, a completed suicide may occur.

CRNE Note

A comprehensive suicide assessment is always considered a priority. Taking the time to engage and connect with the patient before the assessment is crucial (Murray, 2003). It is important for nurses to integrate an assessment process that delineates stressors, symptoms, prior suicidal behaviour, current plan, and available identified resources and support (Ramsey et al., 1994).

Assessing Self-Harm

Assessing the context of each act of prior self-harm behaviour begins to paint a picture of motivation behind the behaviour. Exploration of prior behaviour also gives a message of interest and concern on the part of the health professional. A nonblaming, nonjudgmental approach allows further exploration and understanding of the patient's situation as the patient begins to trust the therapeutic relationship.

Assessment also includes exploration of self-harm behaviour that has been observed by the patient. Self-harm behaviour can be imitative, especially if it is interpreted as a way of coping with frustration and anger or a way of punishing self or others (Rew et al., 2001). Depending on the reaction of others, people may misunderstand self-harm behaviour as an acceptable way to cope with a difficult or intolerable life. Others' reaction of self-harm behaviour needs to be explored, whether or not the response was the expected or desired one. Understanding this can be the first step in helping the patient meet needs and wants in more healthy ways.

Having a Current Plan

Suicide requires intent, a plan, knowledge of how to carry out the act, and few obstacles to completing it.

Patients who complete suicide have developed a workable method of killing themselves. They are less likely to have young children or other immediate responsibilities and may not be concerned with religious prohibitions concerning the act. The relationship between the availability of a method of suicide and suicide completion is strong (Cantor & Baume, 1998). It is important for the nurse to ask whether the patient has a current plan for suicide. Further exploration of the plan gives the nurse a more accurate assessment of risks and guides appropriate interventions.

In contrast to those who carefully prepare to take their own lives are those who decide impulsively to end their lives. The latter are usually adolescents, people who abuse alcohol or drugs, or people with personality disorders. Patients with psychoses may respond impulsively to "voices" that direct them to kill themselves. Patients with psychoses are at considerable risk because of their inability to separate psychotic thinking from reality.

Resources and Support

Lack of resources and support may put patients at the greatest risk for self-harm behaviour. Suicidal people often feel socially isolated and struggle to identify and accept support from people in their immediate environment; therefore, it is important to explore supportive people in the patient's life. Interest in the patient's life and attention received during a thorough assessment are therapeutic and can also provide connectedness and engagement with the patient and family. This connectedness provides the therapeutic environment necessary to engage the patient and family in meaningful change (Jobes, 2000). See Box 37-6, Research for Best Practice.

Nursing Diagnoses and Outcome Identification

Several nursing diagnoses may be useful when dealing with a suicidal patient, including Risk for Suicide, Interrupted Family Processes, Ineffective Health Maintenance, Risk for Self-Directed Violence, Impaired Social Interaction, Ineffective Coping, Chronic Low Self-Esteem, Disturbed Sleep Pattern, Social Isolation, and Spiritual Distress.

Planning and Implementing Nursing Interventions

Thorough assessment becomes part of the intervention process. The health professional's genuine interest, concern, and exploration begin to establish a needed trusting relationship. Using this approach, health care professionals help patients identify what and who needs

BOX 37.6

RESEARCH FOR BEST PRACTICE

THE QUESTION: What is experience of suicide assessment and intervention for an adolescent when it is conducted by a clinical nurse specialist (CNS) using a described risk assessment model?

METHODS: Adolescent participants were interviewed using a phenomenologic approach to explore their lived experience of suicide risk assessment and intervention.

FINDINGS: The major themes that emerged from the data were change, hope, and connection. Participants described the initial assessment interview as *helpful, beneficial, reducing their anxiety,* and giving them a sense of *getting things under control.* They described a **change** in their thinking, other intrapersonal changes, and a change in interpersonal relationships over time as a result of the assessment. They spoke of their **hope** that things could or would change and how they shifted from a sense of giving up hope to hopefulness. They also spoke of recognizing their ability to deal with problems and issues, and of the importance of not feeling alone. The participants spoke of feeling **connected** to the CNS and of feeling that someone cared.

IMPLICATIONS FOR NURSING: Nurses' use of an assessment model that focuses on understanding the suicidal person's world and the meaning of his or her behaviour was experienced as helpful by adolescents. The first step in establishing a meaningful relationship with the adolescent is connecting with them and engaging them in the relationship. This requires genuine interest on the part of the nurse and an ability to set aside one's own values and beliefs while allowing adolescents to tell their story from their point of view. Active listening, and open-ended questioning is necessary for a meaningful exchange of ideas and solutions. The challenging behaviour of adolescents needs to be viewed in context of their family, social and school environment, and broader community. A focus on the adolescent's strengths and resources often promotes a shift toward cooperation and away from problematic, inappropriate, self-harm behaviours. The nurse's expectation and confidence in the adolescent's ability to act appropriately promotes responsible participation, self-direction, and self-control.

Murray, B. L., & Wright, K. (in press). Integration of a Suicide Risk Assessment and Intervention Approach: The perspective of youth. *Journal of Psychiatric and Mental Health Nursing,*

to change in their environment. This approach uncovers concrete areas of improvement or change. This empowerment addresses their feelings of hopelessness, helplessness, and powerlessness.

Understanding the purpose and meaning of the self-harm behaviour guides the intervention strategies. It also gives the patient and their family a sense of hope that things can change, that someone understands their situation and is willing to assist them in making changes. If behaviour is understood as a means of communication, then interventions need not only change behaviours, but also the "cry for help" that underpins the acts. Therefore, ignoring self-harm behaviour is not helpful, although family members may not know what to do and may hope it will go away (Hall, Oliver, & Murphy, 2001). This response may actually escalate the behaviour. Punishment and overreaction are also not helpful.

If some or many of the risk factors for suicide (see Box 37-1) are present in a member of a high-risk group, the nurse must determine what is necessary to ensure the patient's ongoing safety, which is the nurse's first priority. Until the nurse has identified a patient's safety needs and implemented a plan to ensure the patient's safety, the nurse must not leave the acutely suicidal person alone for any reason, not even briefly.

A nurse should not try to treat a potentially suicidal patient without help or consultation. Even the most experienced mental health professional may lose a patient in treatment because of suicide. The reader is referred to http://www.suicideinfo.ca/csp/assets/help-card.pdf for a short checklist of things to do when a patient is suicidal.

No Self-Harm (Contracting for Safety)

The nurse should consider a no self-harm contract only after a thorough assessment of the patient (Simon, 1999). The nurse must consider several factors in making a no self-harm contract with a patient. The patient must be competent to enter into such a contract; patients under the influence of drugs or alcohol or experiencing psychoses are not competent to make no self-harm contracts. Patients who have made previous suicide attempts or who are extremely isolated are not good candidates for no self-harm contracts. Legal and professional scholars disagree on the ability of children and adolescents to make decisions of this gravity on their own behalf. Involving parents in the decision about the appropriate mode of environment for their suicidal child is important. Advantages and disadvantages of no self-harm contracts and several examples of contracts can be found in a review by Range and colleagues (2002).

Inpatient Care and Acute Treatment

Suicidal patients were once hospitalized for extended periods to ensure that the suicidal crisis had passed and to provide sufficient time to establish a solid base of treatment for the underlying psychiatric disorder. This is no longer the case. Hospitals are overly restrictive environments that may inhibit the patient's development of the self-reliance needed to return to the community.

Objectives of hospitalization are to maintain the patient's safety, reduce or eliminate the suicidal crisis, decrease the level of suicidal ideation, initiate treatment for the underlying disorder, evaluate for substance abuse, and reduce the patient's level of social isolation.

If the nurse and another professional determine that the patient is acutely suicidal and at considerable risk for completing suicide, he or she must decide whether to hospitalize the patient for the patient's safety. Safety in such cases is commonly determined by whether a patient may be a threat to self or others. Provincial law requires the patient to be hospitalized only when he or she cannot make reasoned decisions to ensure his or her safety. The law also requires that the restriction of the patient occurs only when it provides a therapeutic effect. In considering hospitalization of a patient, the nurse must consider how hospitalization will be useful in ensuring safety and relieving the patient's suicidal crisis.

Interventions for the Biologic Domain

Ensuring Safety

During the early part of the hospitalization, the most important way to reduce stress is to help the patient feel more secure and hopeful. Nurses can do so by ensuring the patient's safety with as little intrusion as possible on the person's exercise of free will. Achieving this goal can be difficult. The major deterrent to patients' completing suicide in psychiatric hospitals is their engagement in a therapeutic relationship and regular observation by nurses. Each hospital has its own specific protocol for maintaining patients' safety. In addition to nursing standards of care, hospital staffing and other policies that affect the degree to which a suicidal patient can be restrained may influence the procedures mandated for caring for patients.

Maintaining a safe environment includes observing the patient regularly for suicidal behaviour, removing dangerous objects, and providing counselling opportunities for the patient. Part of ensuring patient safety is helping patients to re-establish personal control by including them in decisions about their care and restricting their behaviour only as necessary. Ongoing and effective communication with the patient is key to allowing patients to disclose and discuss their life situation and the resulting emotions and behaviour. Patients often feel shaky in the first hours of psychiatric hospitalization, and it is comforting to know that a caring person is nearby. Observational periods can be used to help the patient express a broad range of feelings and strengthen their belief in their own abilities to keep themselves safe. The nurse can help the patient who is not skilled in self-expression or self-management skills to describe feelings more effectively and cite ways of managing safety needs. Then, at the next observation time, the nurse may have the opportunity to reinforce the patient's own safety behaviour. Thus, the observation period can be transformed from something negative ("The patient can't be trusted," "I am out of control") to something positive ("The patient is becoming safer," "Maybe I can keep myself safe after all") (Cardell & Pitula, 1999). As the patient becomes more confident in understanding and controlling self-harm behaviour, the frequency of observation periods can be reduced.

Seclusion and restraint are two modalities sometimes used in the inpatient settings to maintain patient safety. However, these restrictive interventions are extremely stressful for patients and may interfere with their recovery. Moreover, seclusion and restraint often are used to compensate for inadequate staffing numbers. Unduly restraining patients to prevent their suicide interferes with the development of trusting relationships between patients and health care providers. The stress associated with restraints contributes to the biochemical disarray of their underlying psychiatric disorders. Restraints prevent patients from managing their own dysphoric and anxiety symptoms and reinforce their sense of hopelessness and helplessness. Restraints also enhance patients' fears that they are "crazy" and incapable of controlling their impulses. These methods reinforce a patient's perception of being out of control and lessen his or her ability to form a partnership with mental health providers.

Assisting With Somatic Therapies

Suicidal patients who are seriously depressed will likely receive somatic therapies, and patients' response to them must be monitored. The major somatic therapies used in the treatment of suicidal behaviour are antidepressant medications and electroconvulsive therapy (ECT). ECT may be useful for selected inpatients with intractable suicidal ideation and severe depression. ECT often eliminates suicidal behaviour in people who do not experience response to medication, or who do not tolerate antidepressant medications, such as elderly people and those with comorbid medical disorders. Although the decision to use ECT must be made carefully, ECT can be a life-saving procedure for the acutely suicidal patient. Nurses need be able to support patients in accepting and understanding this treatment (see Chapter 13).

The objective of medication for suicidal behaviour is to raise serotonin rapidly to a level that reduces suicide risk (Nemeroff et al., 2001). To that end, third-generation and newer antidepressant medications should be used for those who are in imminent danger of harming themselves. These include fluoxetine (Prozac), sertraline (Zoloft), paroxetine (Serzone), bupropion (Wellbutrin), venlafaxine (Effexor), and citalopram (Celexa). These drugs generally are nontoxic and cause few side effects, especially after being taken for 1 to 2 weeks. They often are faster acting than the older drugs, but their onset of action varies. Especially useful are fluoxetine and paroxetine, which may be taken once a day. Sertraline also can be taken once a day, but achieving the proper dose can sometimes be difficult. Patients who take an overdose of these medications have much better outcomes than those who abuse first- and second-generation antidepressants.

The first- and second-generation antidepressants, including tricyclics and monoamine oxidase inhibitors, are equally effective for severe depression (Sutherland, Sutherland, & Hoehns, 2003). However, for those with suicidal behaviour, they may not be the best choice because these are highly toxic medications that people with suicidal intent can use to kill themselves. Resuscitation of a patient who has taken large amounts of one of these medications can be difficult because they are cardiotoxic. Medical sequelae may be long term if the patient is saved. Also, the side effects of these early antidepressants may result in the patient stopping the use of prescribed medication while still having suicidal thoughts. The need for laboratory assessment for therapeutic drug levels is another disadvantage of these drugs. Blood monitoring requires the patient's cooperation when his or her motivation may be at its lowest.

Assisting With Treatment for Substance Use

Suicidal behaviour is often associated with substance use disorders, especially among men. When substance use is an issue for the suicidal patient, the use must be addressed or inpatient treatment of suicidal behaviour is only palliative, and the danger of the patient repeating a suicidal attempt is high. For men, substance use disorder may be the primary psychiatric disorder, with depression a side effect of it. For women, depression commonly is the primary psychiatric disorder, and substance use disorders result from attempts to medicate the underlying depressive condition. The nurse should help the patient understand the role that alcohol and drugs play in his or her suicidal behaviour. Treatment for substance use disorders should be part of the treatment plan, as appropriate, including referral to specific inpatient or community-based programs.

Interventions for the Psychological Domain

It is important for nurses to use the hospitalization period to find out what may have precipitated or contributed to the suicidal crisis. Often, the precipitating factors and how the patient's coping process began to break down become evident. After identifying extreme stressors experienced by the patient, the nurse and patient can help determine ways for the patient to avoid those stressors in the future or, if they cannot be avoided, to manage them more effectively.

During hospitalization, the nurse should evaluate the patient's ways of thinking about problems and generating solutions. Some patients, by virtue of their depressive illness or social learning, have an unusually negative view of life. They often think such thoughts as, "I am no good," "Everything I do is useless," "I have no future," or "Nobody has ever liked me, and nobody ever will." Often patients are unable to recognize the connection between their stressors and their suicidal behaviour. Many patients have had very difficult and abusive experiences in their lives, and their ability to cope is threatened. It is important for the nurse to help the patient identify what needs to change in his or her life and how that change can come about most effectively. The prevention of further suicidal behaviour is dependent on the patient's belief that he or she can make changes with the necessary support and resources and that there is hope for the future (see Box 37-7 for examples of effective and ineffective dialogue with a patient).

Interventions for the Social Domain

Improving Communication

Some suicidal patients can identify family and friends who are willing to help, but in many cases, patients are concerned about burdening these people or do not feel comfortable sharing their concerns with others. Helping the suicidal patient express these concerns and arrive at ways of reducing them is important. In other cases, because of trauma and abuse, the patient may have difficulty identifying anyone in his or her life as supportive. These patients are usually at a high risk for suicide because of their perception of aloneness and lack of connection with any significant other. The nurse needs to assist the patient in identifying people in the patient's life that may be supportive and also by making appropriate referrals to professionals with expertise in the area. Within the confines of therapeutic boundaries, the nurse can also be one of the supportive people in the patient's life if the nurse is successful in establishing a professional relationship with the patient.

Networking and Discharge Planning

A final concern may be the patient's embarrassment about the hospitalization and his or her emotional state. Through education, the nurse can do much to destigmatize the situation for both the patient and significant others. Before discharge, it is ideal for the patient to be able to name people who can act as a support. When supportive people are present, with the patient's permission, the nurse can work with them to begin to develop a network for the patient to rely on to remain safe. It is important for the patient and supportive family and friends to have a plan to contact another person, either a confidante or a mental health care provider, when they have questions or distressing thoughts or feel unable to manage or control suicide thoughts and behaviours.

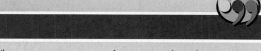

BOX 37.7

Therapeutic Dialogue: Suicide

When Caroline sought medical care for a cold from her nurse practitioner, the nurse observed more than a cough and runny nose. Caroline appeared downcast and unusually sad. As the nurse and patient talked, the subject of family life came up, whereupon Caroline began to cry softly. As words tumbled out, she said that she had been unhappy at home for a long time. When she was very young, she recalled being happy, but things changed when her brother was born, 4 years after her. Her father began to abuse her sexually, starting when Caroline was 5 years old and continuing until he moved out of the house when she was 12 years old. Caroline suspects her mother knew of the abuse, although she did nothing about it.

Two years ago, Caroline's father completed suicide. Caroline feels relieved about his death but frustrated that she never got a chance to tell him how angry she was with him. Caroline's relationship with her mother has not improved. Caroline says that her mother favours her brother and is always telling her she won't amount to anything. Caroline begins to cry harder.

Ineffective Approach

Nurse: Clearly, many things are troubling you. Don't you think that things seem worse now because you have a cold?
Caroline: Well, that could be. What are you going to do to make me feel better?
Nurse: Give you some medicine to help you sleep and clear your nose. I think you should see a psychiatrist, too.
Caroline: I don't need a psychiatrist. I came here for my cold.
Nurse: I know you did, but you seem to be depressed.
Caroline: What are you, some kind of social worker? I am just tired.
Nurse: I am a nurse, and you seem down to me. Are you thinking about suicide?
Caroline: I don't think you know what you're talking about. I want to go now. Could you give me my medicine?

Effective Approach

Nonjudgmental, curious questions; painting a picture helps you and the patient.
Nurse: It seems as though many things have been piling up on you. Does it seem that way to you, too?
Caroline: It sure does. I've just been trying to get through one day at a time, but now with this cold and no sleep, I feel like I can't go on.

Nurse: When you say you can't go on, what do you mean by that?
Caroline: Lately, I have been thinking about running away to some place where I can't be found and maybe starting over. But then I think, where would I go? Where would I stay? Who would take care of me?
Nurse: When you think that your plan for escape won't work, what happens?
Caroline: (Starting to cry again.) Then I think that maybe it would be better if I just did what my father did. I really don't think anyone would miss me.
Nurse: So you think you might take your life, like your Dad did?
Caroline: Yeah, and what really scares me is lately I have been thinking about that a lot. I keep saying to myself, "You're just tired," but I am so exhausted now that I can't chase the thoughts away.
Nurse: So, do you think about suicide every day?
Caroline: It seems like I never stop thinking about it.
Nurse: Is there anything you can do to make the thoughts go away?
Caroline: Nothing. (Silence.)
Nurse: What would you do?
Caroline: I think I would get as many pills as I could find, drink a lot of alcohol, and maybe smoke some pot and just go to sleep.
Nurse: Do you have enough pills at home to kill yourself?
Caroline (wan smile): I was hoping that the sleeping medicine you would give me might do the job.
Nurse: It sounds like you need some help getting through this time in your life. Would you like some?
Caroline: I honestly don't know—I just want to sleep for a long time.

Critical Thinking Challenge

- In the first interaction, the nurse made two key blunders. What were they? What effect did they have on the patient? How did they interfere with the patient's care?
- What did Caroline do that might have contributed to the nurse's behaviours in the first interaction?
- In the second interaction, the nurse did several things that ensured reporting of Caroline's suicidal ideation. What were they? What differences in attitude might differentiate the nurse in the first interaction from the nurse in the second?

Educating the Patient and Family

The objectives of patient and family education are to increase the patient's understanding of the origins of his or her suicidal behaviour; establish effective treatment for depression; provide for ongoing and seamless outpatient treatment; devise a plan for managing future suicidal ideation; identify supportive others in the community; establish a plan to make contact with these people and community resources; and continue with drug and alcohol treatment. These objectives are demanding for both nurse and patient during brief hospitalization.

In addition to trying to reduce the stigma that the patient and family may associate with suicide, the nurse

must educate them about depression, suicidal behaviour, and treatments. When possible, the nurse should schedule educational sessions to include significant others, so that they will better understand the patient's illness and also learn what is necessary in providing outpatient care.

Evaluation and Treatment Outcomes

The most desirable treatment outcome is the patient's return to the community. Because most hospitalizations for suicidal behaviour are brief, discharge planning must begin immediately after the patient is admitted.

The nurse needs to explain to the patient that hospitalization is likely to be short term, and immediately begin to form a partnership with the patient and family to ensure a smooth transition to the community. *Partnering* means empowering the patient to engage in self-care as soon as possible by helping to provide the tools he or she needs to manage

Identifying Continuing Sources of Social Support

Appropriate referrals to professionals in the community and available resources and support are important. The community nurse or therapist requires adequate information to continue with effective interventions after discharge. In addition, engaging family and friends in the patient's ongoing care and finding sources of help in the community, such as church groups, clubhouses, drop-in centres, or other social groups, is a necessary task. A patient's inability to name any significant others or social groups often means a poor outpatient course.

Establishing an Outpatient Care Plan

At the time of discharge, the patient is still considered very ill. Most suicides occur during the first week after discharge, and many happen within the first 24 hours (Appleby, Shaw, et al., 1999). Before the patient's release, a specific, concrete plan for outpatient care must be in place. The care plan includes scheduling an appointment for outpatient care, providing for continuing medication until the first outpatient treatment visit, ensuring postrelease contact between the patient and significant others, providing for access to emergency psychiatric care, and arranging the patient's environment so that it provides both structure and safety.

At discharge, the patient should have enough medication on hand to last until the first community nurse visit. At that time, the community nurse can assess the patient's level of stability and determine whether a full prescription can be given safely to the patient. At that visit, the patient and community nurse can establish a plan of care that specifies the intensity of outpatient care. Very unstable patients may need two to three outpatient visits per week in the early days after hospitalization to maintain their safety in the community.

The patient and significant others must have a plan for the patient's ongoing supervision. This plan must be established in such a way that the patient does not feel undermined in his or her ability to manage self-care but is reassured that help will be available when needed. The family members or friends involved must feel that they are resources for the patient but not responsible for the patient's life or death. In the end, it is the patient, not supporters, who must bear responsibility for his or her safety. The patient who feels connected to but not dependent on significant others will be most likely to maintain safety in the community.

The patient's outpatient environment should be made as safe as possible before discharge. The nurse must share the care plan with family members so that they can remove any objects in the patient's environment that could be of assistance in completing suicide. The nurse must explain this measure to the patient to reinforce his or her sense of self-control. It is important to be reasonable in deciding what to remove from the environment. Patients who are truly determined to kill themselves after discharge may ultimately complete suicide.

Finally, there should be some continuity between inpatient and outpatient care. The nurse must tell the patient specifically how to obtain emergency psychiatric care. He or she should place written instructions near the patient's telephone. It is helpful for the community nurse, in addition to visits, to call periodically during the few first weeks after discharge to determine whether the patient is improving. This contact will help the patient to feel valued and connected to others. Lack of continuity is thought to contribute to significant suicide mortality after hospital discharge (Hulten & Wasserman, 1998).

Short-Term Outcomes

Short-term outcomes for the suicidal patient include maintaining the patient's safety, averting suicide, and mobilizing the patient's resources. Whether the patient is hospitalized or cared for in the community, his or her emotional distress must be reduced. This often is accomplished in an environment that restricts suicidal behaviour and provides sustained emotional support. The treatment during the suicidal crisis should also set the stage for meeting long-term objectives.

Long-Term Outcomes

Long-term outcomes must focus on maintaining the patient in psychiatric treatment, enabling the patient and family to identify and manage suicidal crises effectively, and widening the patient's support network.

Avoiding Compassion Fatigue

There is a cost to caring. It can be difficult to listen and engage deeply with clients' stories of fear, pain, and suffering. Professional work centred on relief of emotional suffering involves empathy as a key tool. Over time, being empathetic can become exhausting, even when the caregiver is diligently maintaining self-care skills. Secondary traumatization and burnout, the two components of compassion fatigue, affect most caregivers at some point during their professional career, leaving them challenged to reach out for help (Figley, 1995).

Compassion fatigue is a very real concern and one that may result in diminished capacity to function at work, at home, and within personal relationships. Its symptoms can parallel client symptoms of post-traumatic stress disorder (see Chapter 36). These symptoms include intrusive thoughts or images of patients' situations or trauma, difficulty separating work from personal life, lower frustration tolerance, hypervigilance, decreased feelings of confidence, diminished sense of purpose or enjoyment of career, and sleep disturbances or nightmares. The nurse may begin to avoid the stress through absenteeism. These symptoms signal that a nurse's mental health is at risk. Caring for suicidal patients who are close to one's own age or having a history of being abused or neglected in childhood enhances the risks. The suicidal behaviour of a patient with whom the nurse can particularly identify can be especially upsetting.

To care successfully for suicidal patients or others prone to crises, the nurse must engage in an active program of self-care, beginning with proper rest, exercise, and nutrition, that facilitates managing stress physiologically. Self-monitoring of symptoms is the next step. Like their patients, nurses need to develop cognitive coping skills and engage in stress reduction exercises. Debriefing (ie, sharing experiences and feelings concerning caring for a suicidal patient with other care team members) can help alleviate symptoms of stress. Some health regions in Canada have organized Critical Incident Stress Management (CISM) teams to provide Critical Incident Stress Debriefing (CISD) education regarding compassion fatigue, as well as in-services regarding self-care and stress management strategies for their health professionals.

SUMMARY OF KEY POINTS

- Suicidal behaviour is a means of communication that something is wrong in one's life, that life is difficult or intolerable.
- Suicide is a common and major public health problem that accompanies 15% of all cases of major depression.
- Suicide completion is more common in Caucasian men, especially elderly men.
- Rising rates of adolescent suicide correspond with the increasing availability of firearms and alcohol.
- More than half of all suicides are completed on the first attempt.
- Parasuicide is more common among women than men.
- Men have a higher rate of completed suicide because of the use of more lethal means (guns, hanging).
- People who attempt suicide most commonly do not seek medical or psychiatric assistance.
- People who engage in parasuicide are likely to do so repeatedly.
- Suicidal behaviour may be associated with genetic and biologic origins.
- People who threaten suicide have rights that must be preserved.
- The no self-harm contract (ie, contracting for safety) is one means of increasing the suicidal patient's safety in the community.
- When a patient must be hospitalized, voluntary hospitalization is the method of choice.
- The major objectives of brief hospital care are to maintain the patient's safety, re-establish the patient's biologic equilibrium, strengthen the patient's cognitive coping skills, and develop an outpatient support system.
- The nurse who cares for suicidal patients is vulnerable to compassion fatigue and must take steps to maintain personal mental health.

CRITICAL THINKING CHALLENGES

1 A religious woman who lives with her three children, husband, and mother in rural Québec comes to her primary care provider. She is tearful and very depressed. What factors should be investigated to determine her risk for suicide and need for hospitalization?

2 You are the primary health care nurse on a First Nations reservation. You want to implement a youth suicide prevention program. Discuss how you would proceed and some potential problems you might face.

3 Analyse lyrics of popular music that have a message about suicide and consider their possible effects on listeners. For instance, REM's *Everybody Hurts (Automatic for the People)* and David Bowie's *Rock and Roll Suicide*.

WEB LINKS

www.siec.ca The Canadian-based Suicide Information and Education Centre provides a link to the Suicide Prevention Training Program. The goal of this program is to provide skills training to increase caregiver competence. This site provides a library and resource centre with information on suicide and suicidal behaviour.

www.save.org Suicide Awareness\Voice of Education (SA\VE). This site provides information about suicide and access to texts and books. It also provides information on what to do in the event a loved one is suicidal.

www.daretolive.com The Dare to Live: Teen Suicide Prevention page is designed for teenagers. It provides information about suicide that is written for and directed to helping teens who are considering suicide.

www.suicideprevention.ca The Canadian Association for Suicide Prevention (CASP) website provides resources and information on mental heath and suicide prevention in both French and English.

www.suicideinfo.ca The Suicide Information and Education Collection is a special library and resources centre providing information on suicide and suicidal behaviour.

www.nimh.nih.gov The U.S. National Institute of Mental Health website provides statistical facts about suicide, recent reports on mental health and suicide, current research on suicide, and a bibliography.

www.goodcharlotterocks.com This is a Good Charlotte website that confronts the issue of suicide with a music video.

M O V I E S

Dead Poets Society: 1989. At the beginning of the first class, the replacement English teacher, Mr. Keating (played by Robin Williams), has one of the boys read the introduction to the poetry textbook, which describes how to place the quality of a poem on a scale, and give it a number, a process that was popular in literary circles at the time. Keating, much to the astonishment (and delight) of the students, has them physically remove the introduction. The rest of the movie is a process of awakening, in which the boys (and the audience) discover that authority can and must always act as a guide, but the only place where one can find out one's true identity is within oneself. This free thinking brings trouble for one of the boys, Neil, who decides to pursue acting, rather than medicine, the career his father chose for him. Neil eventually kills himself in his father's office when his father moves him from Welton to a military school. As a consequence of Neil's suicide, John Keating becomes the scapegoat of the schools's headmaster, Mr. Nolan, and has to leave Welton Academy. His students, however, find a way to show him that his messages about life have been understood.

VIEWING POINTS: How do life pressures and societal attitudes toward the successful life contribute to suicide? What are the particular pressures within your own school or local society?

Night Mother: 1986. Sissy Spacek stars as Jessie Cates, who has decided to end her desperately unhappy life by shooting herself with her father's gun. While putting her house in order, she tries to explain her decision to her mother Thelma, played by Anne Bancroft. Thelma tries to talk Jessie out of suicide.

VIEWING POINTS: What factors have contributed to Jessie's decision to end her life? What approach would you have taken to help Jessie?

Permanent Record: 1988. When David Sinclair, a popular and talented high school student, commits suicide, it leaves everyone, especially his best friend and bandmate, Chris, with a lot of questions. Chris takes over many of David's responsibilities, from the school production of "HMS Pinafore" to caring for his family, and soon finds himself under the same pressures.

VIEWING POINTS: Identify the factors that contributed to David's suicide and the impact of suicide on family and friends.

REFERENCES

Adler, G., & Buie, D. H., Jr. (1996). Aloneness and borderline psychopathology: Possible relevance of child development issues. In J. T. Maltsberger & M. J. Goldblatt (Eds.), *Essential papers on suicide* (pp. 356–378). New York: New York University Press.

Ahrens, B., Linden, M., Zaske, H., Berzewski, H. (2000). Suicidal behaviour: Symptom or disorder? *Comprehensive Psychiatry, 41*(2 Suppl 1), 116–121.

Alexopoulos, G. S., Bruce, M. L., Hull, J., Sireej, J. A., & Kakumo, T. (1999). Clinical determinant of suicidal ideation and behaviour in geriatric depression. *Archives of General Psychiatry, 56*(11) 1048–1053.

Angst, J., Angst, F., & Stassen, H. S. (1999). Suicide risk in patients with major depressive disorder. *Journal of Clinical Psychiatry, 60* (Suppl 2), 57–62.

Appleby, L., Cooper, J., Amos, T., & Faragher, B. (1999). Psychological autopsy study of suicides by people aged under 35. *British Journal of Psychiatry, 175*, 168–174.

Appleby, L., Shaw, J., Amos, T., et al. (1999). Suicide within 12 months of contact with mental health services: National clinical survey. *British Medical Journal, 318*(7193), 1235–1239.

Assembly of First Nations (2002). *Top misconceptions about Aboriginal peoples.* Retrieved August 9, 2005 from http://www.afn.ca.

Baldessarini, R. J., Tondo, L., & Hennen, J. (1999). Effects of lithium treatment and its discontinuation on suicidal behaviour in bipolar manic-depressive disorders. *Journal of Clinical Psychiatry 60* (suppl 2), 77–84.

Beck, A. T., Kovacs, M., & Weissman, A. (1979). Assessment of suicidal intention: The scale for suicidal ideation. *Journal of Consulting and Clinical Psychology, 47*(2), 343–352.

Beck, A. T., Rush, A. J., Shaw, B. F., & Emery, G. (1979). *Cognitive therapy in depression.* New York: Guilford Press.

Beck, A. T., Steer, R. A., Kovacs, M. & Garrison, B. (1985). Hopelessness and eventual suicide: A 10 year prospective study of patients hospitalized with suicide ideation. *American Journal of Psychology, 142*, 559–563.

Beck, A. T., Ward, C. H., Mendelson, M., et al. (1961). An inventory for measuring depression. *Archives of General Psychiatry, 4*, 561–571.

Berg, I. K. (1994). *Family-based services: A solution-focused approach.* New York: W. W. Norton.

Berglund, M., & Ojehagen, A. (1998). The influence of alcohol drinking and alcohol use disorders on psychiatric disorders and suicidal behaviour. *Alcoholism: Clinical & Experimental Research, 22*(Suppl 7), 3335–3455.

Berman, A. L. (1988). Fictional depiction of suicide in television films and imitation effects. *American Journal of Psychiatry, 145*, 982–986.

Brieger, P., Ehrt, U., Bloeink, R., & Marneros, A. (2002). Consequences of comorbid personality disorders in major depression. *Journal of Nervous and Mental Disease, 190*(5), 304–309.

Bulik, C. M., Prescott, C. A., & Kendler, K. S. (2001). Features of childhood sexual abuse & the development of psychiatric and substance use disorders. *British Journal of Psychiatry, 179,* 444–449.

Canadian Nurses Association (2002). *Code of Ethics for Registered Nurses.* Ottawa: Author.

Canada Safety Council. (2004). *Canada's silent tragedy.* Retrieved August 18, 2005, from http://www.safety-council.org/info/community/suicide.html.

Cantor, C. H., & Baume, P. J. (1998). Access to methods of suicide: What impact? *Australian & New Zealand Journal of Psychiatry, 32*(1), 8–14.

Cardell, R., & Pitula, C. R. (1999). Suicidal inpatients' perceptions of therapeutic and non-therapeutic aspects of constant observation. *Psychiatric Services, 50*(8), 1066–1070.

Catallozzi, M., Pletcher, J. R., & Schwarz, D. F. (2001). Prevention of suicide in adolescents. *Current Opinion in Pediatrics, 13,* 417–422.

Cerel, J., Fristad, M. A., Weller, E. B., & Weller, R. A. (1999). Suicide-bereaved children and adolescents: A controlled longitudinal examination. *Journal of the American Academy of Child and Adolescent Psychiatry, 38*(6), 672–679.

Chandler, M. J., & Lalonde, C. (1998). Cultural continuity as a hedge against suicide in Canada's First Nations. *Transcultural Psychiatry, 35*(2), 191–219.

Clark, D. C., & Goebel-Fabbri, A. E. (1998). Lifetime risk of suicide in major affective disorders. In D. Jacobs (Ed.), *Harvard Medical School guide to assessment and intervention in suicide* (pp. 270–286). San Francisco: Jossey-Bass.

Clayton, D., & Barceló, A. (2000). The cost of suicide mortality in New Brunswick, 1996.

Cohen, D. A., Mason, K., Bedimo, A., Sckibner, R., Basolo, V., Farley, T. A. (2003). Neighborhood physical conditions and health. *American Journal of Public Health, 93*(3), 467–471.

Conwell, Y., & Henderson, R. E. (1996). Neuropsychiatry of suicide. In B. S. Fogel, R. B. Schiffer, & S. M. Rao (Eds.), *Neuropsychiatry.* Baltimore: Williams & Wilkins.

Conwell, Y., & Duberstein, P. R. (2001). Suicide in elders. *Annals of the New York Academy of Sciences, 932,* 132–150.

Conwell, Y., Duberstein, P. R. & Caine, E. D. (2002). Risk factors for suicide in later life. *Biological Psychiatry, 52,* 193–204.

Corcoran, J. (1998). Solution-focused practice with middle and high school at-risk youths. *Social Work in Education. 20*(4), 232–242.

Coverdale, J., Naim, R., Claasen, D. (2002). Depictions of mental illness in printmedia: A prospective national sample. *The Australian and New Zealand Journal of Psychiatry 36*(5), 697–700.

Cubbin, C., LeClere, F. B., Smith, G. S. (2000). Socioeconomic status and injury mortality: Individual & neighbourhood determinants. *Journal of Epidemiology & Community Health, 54*(7), 517–524.

Cvinar, J. (2005). Do suicide survivors suffer social stigma? A review of the literature. *Perspective in Psychiatric Care, 41*(1) 14–21.

D'Zurilla, T. J., Chang, E. C., Nottingham, E. J., & Faccini, L. (1998). Social problem-solving deficits and hopelessness, depression, and suicidal risk in college students and psychiatric inpatients. *Journal of Clinical Psychology, 54*(8), 1091–1107.

deGraaf, T. K. (1998). A family therapeutic approach to transgenerational traumatization. *Family Processes, 37,* 233–242.

DeShazer, S. (1988). *Clues: Investigating solutions in brief therapy.* New York: W. W. Norton.

Edwards, M. J., & Holden, R. R. (2001). Coping, meaning in life, and suicidal manifestations: Examining gender differences. *Journal of Clinical Psychology, 57,* 1517–1534.

Eggert, L. L., & Thompson, E. A. (2002). Preliminary effects of brief school-based prevention approaches for reducing youth suicide: Risk behaviours, depression and drug involvement. *Journal of Child and Adolescent Psychiatric Nursing, 15*(2), 48–64.

Erg, P. M., Rimm, E. B., Fitzmaurice, G., & Kawachi, I. (2002). Social ties and change in social ties in relation to subsequent total and cause-specific mortality and coronary heart disease incidence in men. *American Journal of Epidemiology, 155*(8), 700–709.

Ennis, J., Barnes, R. A., Kennedy, S., & Trachtenberg, D. (1989). Depression in self-harm patients. *British Journal of Psychiatry, 154,* 41–47.

Ferreira de Castro, E., Cunha, M. A., Pimenta, F., & Costa, I. (1998). Parasuicide and mental disorders. *Acta Psychiatrica Scandinavica, 97*(1), 25–31.

Figley, C. (1995). *Compassion Fatigue.* New York: Brunnwe/Mazel.

Foster, T., Gillespie, K., McClelland, R., & Patterson, C. (1999). Risk factors for suicide independent of *DSM-III-R* Axis I disorder: Case-control psychological autopsy study in Northern Ireland. *British Journal of Psychiatry, 175,* 175–179.

Gaudet, M. (1994). *Overview of mental health legislation in Canada.* Ottawa: Mental Health Division, Health Canada.

Gibson, P. (1994). Gay male and lesbian youth suicide. In M. Feinleif, (Ed.), *Report of the Secretary's Task Force on Youth Suicide* (pp. 131–142). Washington DC: Department of Health and Human Services.

Glowinski, A. L., Bucholz, K. K., Nelson, E. C., et al. (2001). Suicide attempts in an adolescent female twin sample. *Journal of the American Academy of Child and Adolescent Psychiatry, 40*(11), 1300–1307.

Goldney, R. D. (1989). Suicide: Role of the media. *Australian and New Zealand Journal of Psychiatry, 23,* 30–34.

Goodman, E. (1999). The role of socioeconomic status gradients in explaining differences in U.S. adolescents' health. *American Journal of Public Health, 89,* 1522–1528.

Gould, M. S., & Kramer, R. A. (2001). Youth suicide prevention. *Suicide and Life-Threatening Behaviour, 31,* 6–31.

Gould, M. S., King, R., Greenwald, S., et al. (1998). Psychopathology associated with suicide and attempts among children and adolescents. *Journal of the American Academy of Child & Adolescent Psychiatry, 37*(9), 915–923.

Government of Canada, (1985). *Criminal Code of Canada.* Ottawa: Author.

Grant, B. F., & Hasin, D. S. (1999). Suicidal ideation among the United States drinking population: Results from the National Longitudinal Alcohol Epidemiologic Survey. *Journal of Studies on Alcohol, 60*(3), 422–429.

Gunnell, D., Lopatatzidis, A., Dorling, D., et al. (1999). Suicide and unemployment in young people: Analysis of trends in England and Wales, 1921–1995. *British Journal of Psychiatry, 175,* 263–270.

Guo, B., Scott, A., & Bowker, S. (2003). *Suicide prevention strategies: Evidence from systematic reviews. HTA 28.* Edmonton: Alberta Heritage Foundation for Medical Research.

Guze, S. B. & Robins, E. (1970). Suicide and primary affective disorders. *British Journal of Psychiatry, 117,* 437–438.

Hall, S., Oliver, C., & Murphy, G. (2001). Early development of self-injurious behaviour: An empirical study. *American Journal on Mental Retardation, 106,* 395–400.

Hall, R. C., Platt, D. E., & Hall, R. C. (1999). Suicide risk assessment: A review of risk factors for suicide in 100 patients who have made severe suicide attempts: Evaluation of suicide risk in a time of managed care. *Psychosomatics, 40*(1), 18–27.

Harris, J. (2000). Self-harm: Cutting the bad out of me. *Qualitative Health Research, 10,* 164–173.

Hauenstein, E. (1996). A nursing practice paradigm for depressed rural women: Theoretical basis. *Archives of Psychiatric Nursing,* X(5), 283–292.

Hawton, K., Harriss, L., Hodder, K., Simkin, S., Gunnell, D. (2001). The influence of the economic and social environment on deliberate self-harm & suicide: An ecological & person-based study. *Psychological medicine, 31*(5), 827–836.

Health Canada. (2003). *Acting on what we know: Preventing youth suicide in First Nations.* Retrieved August, 18, 2005 from, http://www.hc-sc.gc.ca/fnih-spni/pubs/suicide/prev_youth-jeunes/index_e.

Health Canada (1994). *Suicide in Canada: Update of the Report of the Task Force on Suicide in Canada.* Ottawa: Government of Canada.

Health Canada, First Nations and Inuit Health Branch. (2003). *A statistical profile on the health of First Nations in Canada.* Ottawa: Government of Canada.

Hendin, H. (1991). Psychodynamics of suicide, with particular reference to the young. *American Journal of Psychiatry, 148,* 1150–1158.

Hendin, H. (1999). Suicide, assisted suicide, and medical illness. *Journal of Clinical Psychiatry, 60*(Suppl 2), 46–50.

HereToHelp. (2003). *Economic costs of mental disorders and addicts.* B.C. Partners for Mental Health and Addictions Information. Retrieved August 10, 2005, from http://www.Heretohelp.bc.ca/publications/factsheets/economiccosts.shtml.

Holden, R. R., Kerr, P. S., Mendonca, J. D., & Velamoor, V. R. (1998). Are some motives more linked to suicide proneness than others? *Journal of Clinical Psychology, 54*(5), 569–576.

Hulten, A., & Wasserman, D. (1998). Lack of continuity—a problem in the care of young suicides. *Acta Psychiatrica Scandinavica, 97*(5), 326–333.

Jamison, K. R. (1999). *Night falls fast: Understanding suicide.* New York: Knopf.

Joachim, G., & Acorn, S. (2000). Stigma of visible and invisible chronic conditions. *Journal of Advanced Nursing, 32*(1), 243–248.

Jobes, D. A., Berman, A. L., O'Carroll, P. W., Eastgard, S., & Knickmeyer S. (1996). The Kurt Cobain suicide crisis: Perspectives from research, public health, and the news media. *Suicide and Life-Threatening Behaviour, 26,* 260–271.

Jobes, D. (2000). Collaborating to prevent suicide: A clinical research perspective. *Suicide and Life-Threatening Behaviour, 30,* 164–173.

Jordan, J. R. (2001). Is suicide bereavement different? A reassessment of the literature. *Suicide and Life-Threatening Behaviour, 31*(1), 91–102.

Kendall, D., Lothian-Murray, J., & Linden, R. (2004). *Sociology: In our time* (3rd ed.). Scarborough, ON: Thompson Canada Inc.

Kendler, K. S., Bulik, C. M., Silberg, J., Hettema, J. M., myers, J., Prescott, C. A. (2000). Childhood sexual abuse & adult psychiatric & substance use disorders in women: An epidemiological & cotwin control analysis. *Archives of General Psychiatry, 57*(10), 953–959.

Kirmayer, L. J., Gill, K., Fletcher, C., Ternar, Y., Boothroyd, L., Quesney C., Smith A., Ferrara, N., & Hayton, B. (1993). Emerging trends in research on mental health among Canadian Aboriginal peoples. Retrieved from the McGill University website, http:// upload.mcgill.ca.

Kishi, Y., Robinson, R. B., & Kosier, J. (2001). Suicidal ideation among patients during the rehabilitation period after life threatening physical illness. *Journal of Nervous and Mental Disease, 189*(9), 623–628.

Klimes-Dougan, B., Free, K., Rounsaville, D., et al. (1999). Suicidal ideation and attempts: A longitudinal investigation of children of depressed and well mothers. *Journal of the American Academy of Child & Adolescent Psychiatry, 38*(6), 651–659.

Knieper, A. J. (1999). The suicide survivor's grief and recovery. *Suicide and Life-Threatening Behaviour, 29*(4), 353–364.

Kohlmeier, R. E., McMahan, C. A., & DiMaio, V. J. M. (2001). Suicide by firearms: A fifteen year experience. *American Journal of Forensic Medicine and Pathology, 22*(4), 337–340.

Koplin, B., & Agathen, J. (2002). Suicidality in children and adolescents: A review: *Current Opinion in Pediatrics, 14,* 713–717.

Kposowa, A. J. (2001). Unemployment & suicide: A cohort analysis of social factors predicting suicide in the U.S. National longitudinal mortality study. *Psychological Medicine, 31*(1), 127–38.

Kral, M. (2003). Unikkaartuit: Meanings of wellbeing, sadness, suicide, and change into Inuit communities. Final report to the national health research and development programs. Ottawa: National Research Council of Canada.

Kreitman, N. S. (1970). *Parasuicide.* New York: John Wiley and Sons.

Kreitman, N. S. (1969). Parasuicide. *British Journal of Psychiatry, 115,* 1227–1228.

Langlois, S., & Morrison, P. (2002). Suicide deaths and suicide attempts. *Health Reports, 13*(2), 9–22.

Leenaars, A. A. (1998). *Suicide notes: Predictive clues and patterns.* New York: Human Sciences Press.

Levenkron, S. (1998). *Cutting: Understanding and overcoming self-mutilation.* London: W. W. Norton.

Link, B. G., Phelan, J. C., Bresnahan, M., Stueve, A., & Pescosolido, B. (1999). Public conceptions of mental illness: Labels, causes, dangerousness, and social distance. *American Journal of Public Health, 89*(9), 1328–1333.

Lopez, F. G., & Brennan, K. A. (2000). Dynamic processes underlying adult attachment organization: Toward an attachment theoretical perspective on the health and effective self. *Journal of Counseling Psychology, 47*(3), 283–300.

Luoma, J., & Pearson, J. L. (2002). Suicide and marital status in the United States, 1991–1996: Is widowhood a risk factor? *American Journal of Public Health, 92*(9), 1518–1522.

Machoian, L. (2001). Cutting voices: Self-injury in three adolescent girls. *Journal of Psychosocial Nursing and Mental Health Services, 39,* (11), 22–29.

MacMillian, H. L., Fleming, J. E., Streiner, D. L., et al. (2001). Childhood abuse and lifetime psychopathology in a community sample. *American Journal of Psychiatry, 158*(11), 1878–1883.

Maine, S., Shute, R. & Martin, G. (2001). Educating parents about youth suicide: Knowledge, response to suicidal statements, attitudes, and intention to help. *Suicide and Life-Threatening Behaviour, 31*(3), 320–332.

Mann, J. J., Brent, D. A., & Arango, V. (2001). The neurobiology and genetics of suicide and attempted suicide: A focus on the serotonergic system. *Neuropsychopharmacology, 24*(5), 467–477.

Mann, J. J., Oquendo, M., Underwood, M. D., & Arango, V. (1999). The neurobiology of suicide risk: A review for the clinician. *Journal of Clinical Psychiatry, 60*(Suppl 2), 7–11.

McGoldrick, M. (1992). The legacy of loss. In F. Walsh & M. McGoldrick (Eds.), *Living beyond loss: Death in the family* (pp. 104–129). New York: Norton.

McGuffin, P., Marusic, A., & Farmer, A. (2001). What can psychiatric genetics offer suicidology. *Journal of Crisis Intervention and Suicide, 22*(2), 62–65.

McKeown, R. E., Garrison, C. Z., Cuffe, S. P., et al. (1998). Incidence and predictors of suicidal behaviours in a longitudinal sample of young adolescents. *Journal of the American Academy of Child & Adolescent Psychiatry, 37*(6), 612–619.

Meehan, P. J., Lamb, J. A., Saltzman, L. E., & O'Carroll, P. (1992). Attempted suicide among young adults: Progress toward a meaningful estimate of prevalence. *American Journal of Psychiatry, 149*(1), 41–44.

Minino, A. M., Arias, E., Kochanek, K. D., Murphy, S. L., & Smith, B. L. (2002). Deaths: Final data for 2000. *National Vital Statistics Reports, 50,* 1–120.

Minuchin, S., & Fishman, C. (1981). *Family therapy techniques.* Cambridge, MA: Harvard University Press.

Mishara, B. L. (1999). Conceptions of death and suicide in children ages 6–12 and their implications for suicide prevention. *Suicide and Life-Threatening Behaviour, 29,* 105–119.

Mitchell, A. M., Gale, D. D., Garand, L., & Wesner, S. (2003). The use of narrative data to inform the psychotherapeutic process with suicide survivors. *Issues in Mental Health Nursing, 24,* 91–106.

Modai, I., Valevski, A., Solomish, A., Kurs, R., Hines, I. L., Ritsner, M., Mendel, S., (1999). Neural network detection of files of suicidal patients and suicidal profiles. *Medical Informatics & the Internet in Medicine, 24*(4), 249–56.

Molnar, B., Berkman, L. F., & Buka, S. L. (2001) Psychopathology, childhood sexual abuse and other childhood adversities: Relative links to subsequent suicidal behaviour in the U.S. *Psychological Medicine, 31*(6), 965–977.

Morrison, L. L., & L'Heureux, J. (2001). Suicide and gay/lesbian/bisexual youth: Implications for clinicians. *Journal of Adolescence 24*, 39–49.

Murray, B. L., & Wright, K. (2006). Integration of a suicide risk assessment and intervention approach: The perspective of youth. *Journal of Psychiatric Mental Health Nursing, 13*(2), 157–164.

Murray, B. L., (2003) Self-harm among adolescents with developmental disabilities: What are they trying to tell us? *Journal of Psychosocial Nursing, 41*(11), 37–45.

NANYouth. (2004). Aboriginal suicide statistics. Retrieved August 10, 2005, from the Nishnawbe Aski Nation website, http://www.nandecade.ca/article/71.asp.

Neeleman, J. (1998). Regional suicide rates in The Netherlands: Does religion still play a role? *International Journal of Epidemiology, 27*, 466–472.

Nelson, E. C., Heath, A C., Madden, P. A. F., et al. (2002). Association between self-reported childhood sexual abuse and adverse psychosocial outcomes: Results from a twin study. *Archives of General Psychiatry, 59*, 139–145.

Nemeroff, C. B., Compton, M. T., & Berger, J. (2001). The depressed suicidal patient: Assessment and treatment. *Annals of American Academy of Sciences, 932*, 1–23.

Nisbet, P. A., Duberstein, P. R., Conwell, Y., & Seidlitz, L. (2000). The effect of participation in religious activities on suicide versus natural death in adults 50 and older. *The Journal of Nervous and Mental Disease, 188*(8), 543–546.

O'Connell, H., Chin, A., Cunningham, C., & Lawlor, B. A. (2004). Recent developments: Suicide in older people. *British Medical Journal, 329*, 895–899.

OConnor, R. C., & Noel, P. S. (1997). Suicide and gender. *Mortality, 2*(3), 239–254.

O'Hanlon, W. H., & Werner-Davis, M. (1989). *In search of solutions: A new direction in psychotherapy* New York: W. W. Norton.

Ohberg, A., & Lonnqvist, J. (1998). Suicides hidden among undetermined deaths. *Acta Psychiatrica Scandinavica, 98*(3), 214–218.

Pfeffer, C. R., Normandin, L., & Kakuma, T. (1998). Suicidal children grow up: Relations between family psychopathology & adolescents' lifetime suicidal behaviour. *Journal of Nervous Mental Disease, 186*, 269–275.

Phillips, D. P., & Carstensen, L. L. (1986). Clustering of teenage suicides after television news stories. *New England Journal of Medicine, 315*, 685–689.

Pitchot, W., Hansenne, M., Moreno, A., et al. (2001). Reduced dopamine function in depressed patients is related to suicidal behaviour but not its lethality. *Psychoneuroendocrinology, 26*, 689–696.

Platt, S. (1993). The social transmission of parasuicide: Is there a modeling effect? *Crisis, 14*, 23–31.

Poijula, S., Walberg, K. E., Dyregrov, A. (2001). Adolescent suicide and suicide contagion in three secondary schools. *International Journal of Emergency Mental Health, 3*(3), 163–168.

Preuss, U. W., Schuckit, M. A., Smith, T. L., et al. (2002). Comparison of 3190 alcohol-dependent individuals with and without suicide attempts. *Alcoholism: Clinical and Experimental Research, 26*(4), 471–477.

Prigerson, H. G., & Slimack, M. J. (1999). Gender differences in clinical correlates of suicidality among young adults. *Journal of Nervous and Mental Disease, 187*(1), 23–31.

Public Health Agency of Canada. (2000). *Leading causes of death and hospitalization in Canada.* Retrieved August 15, 2005 from the PHAC website, http://www.phac-aspc.gc.ca/publicat/lcd-pcd97/ index.html.

Qin, P., Agergbo, E., & Mortensen, P. B. (2003). Suicide risk in relationship to socioeconomic, demographic, psychiatric, and familial factors: A national register-based study of all suicides in Denmark, 1981–1997. *American Journal of Psychiatry, 160*(4), 765–772.

Qin, P., Agerbo, E., Westergard-Nielson, N., Erikson, T., & Mortenson, P. B. (2000). Gender differences in risk factors for suicide in Denmark. *British Journal of Psychiatry, 177*, 546–550.

Quan, H., Arboleda-Flórez, J., Frick, G. H., Stuart, H. L., Love, E. J. (2002). Association between physical illness and suicide among the elderly. *Social Psychiatry & Psychiatric Epidemiology, 37*, 190–197.

Radloff, L. (1977). The CES-D Scale: A self-report depression scale for research in the general population. *Applied Psychological Measurement, 1*, 385–401.

Radomsky, E. D., Haas, G. L., Mann, J. J., & Sweeney, J. A. (1999). Suicidal behaviour in patients with schizophrenia and other psychotic disorders. *American Journal Psychiatry, 156*(10), 1590–1595.

Ramsey, R. F., Tanny, B. L., Taierney, R. J., & Lang, W. A. (1994). *Suicide intervention handbook.* Calgary, Canada: Living Works Education Inc.

Range, L. M., Campbell, C., Kovac, S. H., et al. (2002). No-suicide contracts: An overview and recommendations. *Death Studies, 26*, 51–74.

Remafedi, G., Farrow, J., Deisher, R. (1991) Risk factors for attempted suicide in gay and bisexual youth. *Pediatrics, 87*, 869–875.

Rew, L., Thomas, N., Horner, S., Resnick, M., & Beuhring, T. (2001). Correlates of recent suicide attempts in a tri-ethnic group of adolescents. *Journal of Nursing Scholarship, 4*, 361–367.

Rihmer, Z., & Pestality, P. (1999). Bipolar II disorder and suicidal behavior. *Psychiatric Clinics of North America, 22*(3), 667–673.

Rogers, C. (1980). *A way of being.* Boston: Houghton Mifflin.

Rosenberg, N. K. (1993). Psychotherapy of the suicidal patient. *Acta Psychiatrica Scandinavica, 371*, 54–56.

Rotheram-Borus, M. J., & Fernandez, M. I. (1995). Sexual orientation and developmental challenges experienced by gay and lesbian youths. *Suicide and Life-Threatening Behaviour, 23*(Suppl), 26–34.

Roy, A. (1989). Suicide. In H. I. Kaplan & B. J. Sadock (Eds.), *Comprehensive textbook of psychiatry* (pp. 1414–1427). Baltimore: Williams & Wilkins.

Royal Commission on Aboriginal Peoples. (1995). *Choosing life: Special report on suicide among Aboriginal people.* Ottawa: Communication Group.

Russel, S. T., & Joyner, K. (2001). Adolescent sexual orientation and suicide risk: Evidence from a nation study. *American Journal of Public Health, 91*(8), 1276–1281.

Saarinen, P. I., Lehtonen, J., & Lonnqvist, J. (1999). Suicide risk in schizophrenia: An analysis of 17 consecutive suicides. *Schizophrenia Bulletin, 25*(3), 533–542.

Safety Canada. (2004). Canada's silent tragedy. Retrieved from the Canadian Safety Council website, http://www.safety-council.org.

Sakinofsky, I., Roberts, R. S., Brown, Y., Cummings, C., & James, P. (1990). Problem resolution and repetition of parasuicide: A prospective study. *British Journal of Psychiatry, 156*, 395–399.

Samson, C. (2003). Sexual abuse and assimilation: Oblates, teachers and the Innu of Labrador. *Sexualities, 6*(1), 46–53.

Savin-Williams, R. (1990). *Gay and lesbian youth: Expressions of identity.* New York: Hemisphere.

Schmidtke, A., & Hafner, H. (1988). The Werther effect after television films: New evidence for an old hypothesis. *Psychological Medicine, 18*, 665–676.

Simon, R. (1996). Suicide and firearms: Restricting access in Canada. Presented to the American Association of Suicidology, April.

Simon, R. I. (1999). The suicide prevention contract: Clinical, legal and risk management issues. *Journal of the American Academy of Psychiatry & the Law, 27*(3), 445–450.

Skodol, A. E., Siever, L. J., & Livesley, W. J. (2002). The borderline diagnosis. II. Biology, genetics, and clinical course. *Biological Psychiatry, 51*, 951–963.

Statham, D. J., Heath, A. C., Madden, P. A., et al. (1998). Suicidal behaviour: An epidemiological and genetic study. *Psychological Medicine, 28*(4), 839–855.

Statistics Canada. (1994). *Death statistics in Canada: Causes of death 1992.* Retrieved August 7, 2005 from the Statistics Canada website, http://www.acbr.com/fas/causdeat.htm.

Statistics Canada. (2001, June). Depression. In *Health indicators*. Retrieved August, 7, 2005 from the Statistics Canada website, http://www.statcan.ca/english/freepub/82-221-XIE/01103/high/depres.htm.

Statistics Canada. (2002). *Causes of death*. Retrieved August 10, 2005 from the Statistics Canada website, http://www.statcan.ca/english/freepub/84-208-XIE/2002/tables.htm.

Statistics Canada. (2003a). Depression. In *Health indicators: Highlights*. Retrieved August, 7, 2005 from the Statistics Canada website, http://www.statcan.ca/english/freepub/82-221-XIE/01103/high/region/hdepres.htm.

Statistics Canada. (2003b). Suicide by province. In *Health indicators*. Retrieved from the Statistics Canada website, http://www.statcan.ca/english/freepub/82-221-XIE/2005001/tables/html/14193_01.htm.

Statistics Canada. (2004). The people: Major causes of death. In *Canada e-book*. Retrieved from the Statistics Canada website, http://www.statcan.ca.

Statistics Canada. (2005). Chapter XX: External causes of morbidity and mortality (V01-Y89), by age group and sex. Retrieved August 10, 2005, from the Statistics Canada website, http://www.statcan.ca/english/freepub/84-208-XIE/2002/tables/table20.htm.

Steenland, K., Halperin, W., Hu, S., & Walker, J. T. (2003). Deaths due to injuries among employed adults: The effects of socioeconomic class. *Epidemiology, 14*(1), 74–79.

Stewart, S. E., Manion, I. G., Davidson, S., & Cloutier, P. (2001). Suicidal children and adolescents with first emergency room presentations: Predictors of six-month outcome. *Journal of the American Academy of Child and Adolescent Psychiatry, 40*(5), 580–587.

Suicide Information and Education centre. (2003). *Suicide among Canada's Aboriginal peoples*. Retrieved August, 10, 2005 from the Centre for Suicide Prevention website, http://www.suicideinfo.ca.

Sutherland, J. E., Sutherland, S. J., & Hoehns, J. D. (2003). Achieving the best outcome in treatment of depression. *Journal of Family Practice, 53*(3), 118–126.

Tadros, G., & Jolley, D. (2001). The stigma of suicide [correspondence]. *British Journal of Psychiatry, 179*(2), 178.

Tondo, L., & Baldessarini, R. J. (2001). *Suicide: Historical, descriptive, and epidemiological considerations*. Retrieved August 02, 2005 from Medscape website, http://www.medscape.com/viewprogram/352_pnt.

Tondo, L. (2000). *Prima del tempo. Capire e Prevenire il suicidio*. Rome: Carocci.

Vilhjalmsson, R., Kristjansdottir, G., & Sveinbjarnardottir, E. (1998). Factors associated with suicide ideation in adults. *Social Psychiatry and Psychiatric Epidemiology, 33*(3), 97–103.

Walsh, B. W., & Rosen, P. M. (1988). *Self-mutilation: Theory research and treatment*. New York: Guilford Press.

Welch, S., S. (2001). A review of the literature on the epidemiology of parasuicide in the general population. *Psychiatric Services, 52*(3), 368–375.

White, J., & Jodoin, N. (2003). *Aboriginal youth: A manual of promising suicide prevention strategies*. Retrieved August 12, 2005 from, http://www.suicideinfo.ca/csp/go.aspx?tabid=144.

World Health Organization. (2002). *Self-directed violence*. Retrieved August 10, 2005 from the World Health Organization website, http://www.who.int/violence_injury_prevention/violence/world_report/factsheets/en/selfdirectedviolfacts.pdf.

Zimmerman, S. L. (2002). States' spending for public welfare and their suicide rates, 1960 to 1995. What is the problem? *Journal of Nervous and Mental Disease, 190*(6), 349–360.

Zor, F., Mustafa, D., Mehmet, B., Semih, D., Duman, H., & Sengezer, M. (2005). Psychological evaluation of self-inflicted burn patients: Suicide or parasuicide? *Burns, 31*, 178–181.

Zung, W. W. K. (1965). A self-rating depression scale. *Archives of General Psychiatry, 12*, 63–70.

For challenges, please refer to the **CD-ROM** in this book.

DSM-IV-TR Classification: Axes I and II Categories and Codes

DISORDERS USUALLY FIRST DIAGNOSED IN INFANCY, CHILDHOOD, OR ADOLESCENCE

Mental Retardation

Note: These are coded on Axis II.

- 317   Mild Mental Retardation
- 318.0   Moderate Mental Retardation
- 318.1   Severe Mental Retardation
- 318.2   Profound Mental Retardation
- 319   Mental Retardation, Severity Unspecified

Learning Disorders

- 315.00   Reading Disorders
- 315.1   Mathematics Disorders
- 315.2   Disorder of Written Expression
- 315.9   Learning Disorder NOS

Motor Skills Disorder

- 315.4   Developmental Coordination Disorder

Communication Disorders

- 315.31   Expressive Language Disorder
- 315.31   Mixed Receptive-Expressive Language Disorder

- 315.39   Phonological Disorder
- 307.0   Stuttering
- 307.9   Communication Disorder NOS

Pervasive Developmental Disorders

- 299.00   Autistic Disorder
- 299.80   Rett's Disorder
- 299.10   Childhood Disintegrative Disorder
- 299.80   Asperger's Disorder
- 299.80   Pervasive Developmental Disorder NOS

Attention-Deficit and Disruptive Behavior Disorders

- 314.xx   Attention-Deficit/Hyperactivity Disorder
  - .01   Combined Type
  - .00   Predominantly Inattentive Type
  - .01   Predominantly Hyperactive-Impulsive Type
- 314.9   Attention-Deficit/Hyperactivity Disorder NOS
- 312.8   Conduct Disorder
  - *Specify type:* Childhood-Onset/ Adolescent-Onset
- 313.81   Oppositional Defiant Disorder
- 312.9   Disruptive Behavior Disorder NOS

Feeding and Eating Disorders of Infancy or Early Childhood

- 307.52   Pica
- 307.53   Rumination Disorder
- 307.59   Feeding Disorder of Infancy or Early Childhood

Tic Disorders

- 307.23   Tourette's Disorder
- 307.22   Chronic Motor or Vocal Tic Disorder

NOS = not otherwise specified.

An x appearing in a diagnostic code indicates that a specific code number is required.

An ellipsis (. . .) is used in the names of certain disorders to indicate that the name of a specific mental disorder or general medical condition should be inserted when recording the name (eg, 293 Delirium Due to Hypothyroidism).

*Indicate the General Medical Condition.

**Refer to Substance-Related Disorders for substance-specific codes.

***Indicate the Axis I or Axis II Disorder.

American Psychiatric Association. (2000). *Diagnostic and statistical manual of mental disorders.* (4th ed., Text revision). Washington, DC: Author.

307.21   Transient Tic Disorder
         Specify if: Single Episode/Recurrent
307.20   Tic Disorder NOS

Elimination Disorders

—.-   Encopresis
787.6   With Constipation and Overflow Incontinence
307.7   Without Constipation and Overflow Incontinence
307.6   Enuresis (Not Due to a General Medical Condition)
         Specify type: Nocturnal Only/Diurnal Only/Nocturnal and Diurnal

Other Disorders of Infancy, Childhood, or Adolescence

309.21   Separation and Anxiety Disorder
         Specify if: Early Onset
313.23   Selective Mutism
313.89   Reactive Attachment Disorder of Infancy or Early Childhood
         Specify type: Inhibited/Disinhibited
307.3   Stereotypic Movement Disorder
         Specify if: With Self-Injurious Behavior
313.9   Disorder of Infancy, Childhood, or Adolescence NOS

DELIRIUM, DEMENTIA, AND AMNESTIC AND OTHER COGNITIVE DISORDERS

Delirium

293.0   Delirium Due to. . .*
—.-   Substance Intoxication Delirium**
—.-   Substance Withdrawal Delirium**
—.-   Delirium Due to Multiple Etiologies (code each of the specific etiologies)
780.09   Delirium NOS

Dementia

294.xx   Dementia of the Alzheimer's Type, With Early Onset
  .10   Without Behavioral Disturbance
  .11   With Behavioral Disturbance
294.xx   Dementia of the Alzheimer's Type, With Late Onset
  .10   Without Behavioral Disturbance
  .11   With Behavioral Disturbance
294.xx   Vascular Dementia
  .40   Uncomplicated
  .41   With Delirium
  .42   With Delusions
  .43   With Depressed Mood
         Specify if: With Behavioral Disturbance
294.1x   Dementia Due to HIV Disease
294.1x   Dementia Due to Head Head Trauma
294.1x   Dementia Due to Parkinson's Disease

294.1x   Dementia Due to Huntington's Disease
294.10   Dementia Due to Pick's Disease
290.10   Dementia Due to Creutzfeldt-Jakob Disease
294.1   Dementia Due to . . . [Indicate the General Medical Condition not listed above]
—.-   Substance-Induced Persisting Dementia**
—.-   Dementia Due to Multiple Etiologies (code each of the specific etiologies)
294.8   Dementia NOS

Amnestic Disorders

294.0   Amnestic Disorder Due to . . .*
         Specify if: Transient/Chronic
—.-   Substance-Induced Persisting Amnestic Disorder**
294.8   Amnestic Disorder NOS

Other Cognitive Disorders

294.9   Cognitive Disorder NOS

MENTAL DISORDERS DUE TO A GENERAL MEDICAL CONDITION NOT ELSEWHERE CLASSIFIED

293.89   Catatonic Disorder Due to . . .*
310.0   Personality Change Due to . . .*
         Specify type: Labile/Disinhibited/Aggressive/Apathetic/Paranoid/Other/Combined/Unspecified
293.9   Mental Disorder NOS Due to . . .*

SUBSTANCE-RELATED DISORDERS

The following specifiers may be applied to Substance Dependence:

With Physiological Dependence/Without Physiological Dependence
Early Full Remission/Early Partial Remission
Sustained Full Remission/Sustained Partial Remission
On Agonist Therapy/In a Controlled Environment

The following specifiers apply to Substance-Induced Disorders as noted:

With Onset During Intoxication/^{W} With Onset During Withdrawal

Alcohol-Related Disorders

Alcohol Use Disorders

303.90   Alcohol Dependence
305.00   Alcohol Abuse

Alcohol-Induced Disorders

303.00   Alcohol Intoxications
291.8   Alcohol Withdrawal
         Specify if: With Perceptual Disturbances

291.0   Alcohol Intoxication Delirium
291.0   Alcohol Withdrawal Delirium
291.2   Alcohol-Induced Persisting Dementia
291.1   Alcohol-Induced Persisting Amnestic Disorder
291.x   Alcohol-Induced Psychotic Disorder
  .5   With Delusions[I,W]
  .3   With Hallucinations[I,W]
291.8   Alcohol-Induced Mood Disorder[I,W]
291.8   Alcohol-Induced Anxiety Disorder[I,W]
291.8   Alcohol-Induced Sexual Dysfunction[I]
291.   Alcohol-Induced Sleep Disorder[I,W]
291.9   Alcohol-Related Disorder NOS

Amphetamine (or Amphetamine-Like)-Related Disorders

Amphetamine Use Disorders

304.40   Amphetamine Dependence*
305.70   Amphetamine Abuse

Amphetamine-Induced Disorders

292.89   Amphetamine Intoxication
              Specify if: With Perceptual Disturbances
292.0   Amphetamine Withdrawal
292.81   Amphetamine Intoxication Delirium
292.xx   Amphetamine-Induced Psychotic Disorder
  .11   With Delusions[I]
  .12   With Hallucinations[I]
292.84   Amphetamine-Induced Mood Disorder[I,W]
292.89   Amphetamine-Induced Anxiety Disorder[I]
292.89   Amphetamine-Induced Sexual Dysfunction[I]
292.89   Amphetamine-Induced Sleep Disorder[I,W]
292.9   Amphetamine-Related Disorder NOS

Caffeine-Related Disorders

Caffeine-Induced Disorders

305.90   Caffeine Intoxication
292.89   Caffeine-Induced Anxiety Disorder[I]
292.89   Caffeine-Induced Sleep Disorder[I]
292.9   Caffeine-Related Disorder NOS

Cannabis-Related Disorders

Cannabis Use Disorders

304.30   Cannabis Dependence*
305.20   Cannabis Abuse

Cannabis-Induced Disorders

292.89   Cannabis Intoxication
              Specify if: With Perceptual Disturbances
292.81   Cannabis Intoxication Delirium
292.xx   Cannabis-Induced Psychotic Disorder
  .11   With Delusions[I]
  .12   With Hallucinations[I]
292.89   Cannabis-Induced Anxiety Disorder
292.9   Cannabis-Related Disorder NOS

Cocaine-Related Disorders

Cocaine Use Disorders

304.20   Cocaine Dependence*
305.60   Cocaine Abuse

Cocaine-Induced Disorders

292.89   Cocaine Intoxication
              Specify if: With Perceptual Disturbances
292.0   Cocaine Withdrawal
292.81   Cocaine Intoxication Delirium
292.xx   Cocaine-Induced Psychotic Disorder
  .11   With Delusions[I]
  .12   With Hallucinationsi
292.84   Cocaine-Induced Mood Disorder[I,W]
292.89   Cocaine-Induced Anxiety Disorder[I,W]
292.89   Cocaine-Induced Sexual Dysfunction[I]
292.89   Cocaine-Induced Sleep Disorder[I,W]
292.9   Cocaine-Related Disorder NOS

Hallucinogen-Related Disorders

Hallucinogen-Use Disorders

304.50   Hallucinogen Dependence*
305.30   Hallucinogen Abuse

Hallucinogen-Induced Disorders

292.89   Hallucinogen Intoxication
292.89   Hallucinogen Persisting Perception Disorder
              (Flashbacks)
292.81   Hallucinogen Intoxication Delirium
292.xx   Hallucinogen-Induced Psychotic Disorder
  .11   With Delusionsi
  .12   With Hallucinationsi
292.84   Hallucinogen-Induced Mood Disorder[I]
292.89   Hallucinogen-Induced Anxiety Disorder[I]
292.9   Hallucinogen-Related Disorder NOS

Inhalant-Related Disorders

Inhalant Use Disorders

304.60   Inhalant Dependence*
305.90   Inhalant Abuse

Inhalant-Induced Disorders

292.89   Inhalant Intoxication
292.81   Inhalant Intoxication Delirium
292.82   Inhalant-Induced Persisting Dementia
292.xx   Inhalant-Induced Psychotic Disorder
  .11   With Delusions[I]
  .12   With Hallucinations*

292.84   Inhalant-Induced Mood Disorder[I]
292.89   Inhalant-Induced Anxiety Disorder[I]
292.9   Inhalant-Related Disorder NOS

Nicotine-Related Disorders

Nicotine Use Disorder

305.10 Nicotine Dependence*

Nicotine-Induced Disorder

292.0   Nicotine Withdrawal
292.9   Nicotine-Related Disorder NOS

Opioid-Related Disorders

Opioid Use Disorders

304.00   Opioid Dependence*
305.50   Opioid Abuse

Opioid-Induced Disorders

292.89   Opioid Intoxication
         Specify if: With Perceptual Disturbances
292.0   Opioid Withdrawal
292.81   Opioid Intoxication Delirium
292.xx   Opioid-Induced Psychotic Disorders
  .11   With Delusions[I]
  .12   With Hallucinations[I]
292.84   Opioid-Induced Mood Disorder[I]
292.89   Opioid-Induced Sexual Dysfunction[I]
292.89   Opioid-Induced Sleep Disorder[I,W]
292.9   Opioid-Related Disorder NOS

Phencyclidine (or Phencyclidine-Like)-Related Disorders

Phencyclidine Use Disorders

304.90   Phencyclidine Dependence*
305.90   Phencyclidine Abuse

Phencyclidine-Induced Disorders

292.89   Phencyclidine Intoxication
         Specify if: With Perceptual Disturbances
292.81   Phencyclidine Intoxication Delirium
292.xx   Phencyclidine-Induced Psychotic Disorders
  .11   With Delusions[I]
  .12   With Hallucinations[I]
292.84   Phencyclidine-Induced Mood Disorder[I]
292.89   Phencyclidine-Induced Anxiety Disorder[I]
292.9   Phencyclidine-Related Disorder NOS

Sedative-Hypnotic- or Anxiolytic-Related Disorders

Sedative-Hypnotic- or Anxiolytic Use Disorders

304.10   Sedative, Hypnotic, or Anxiolytic Dependence*
305.40   Sedative, Hypnotic, or Anxiolytic Abuse

Sedative, Hypnotic, or Anxiolytic-Induced Disorders

292.89   Sedative, Hypnotic, or Anxiolytic Intoxication
292.0   Sedative, Hypnotic, or Anxiolytic Withdrawal
         Specify if: With Perceptual Disturbances
292.81   Sedative, Hypnotic, or Anxiolytic Intoxication Delirium
292.81   Sedative, Hypnotic, or Anxiolytic Withdrawal Delirium
292.82   Sedative-, Hypnotic-, or Anxiolytic-Induced Persisting Delirium
292.83   Sedative-, Hypnotic-, or Anxiolytic-Induced Persisting Amnestic disorder
292.xx   Sedative-, Hypnotic-, or Anxiolytic-Induced Psychotic Disorder
  .11   With Delusions[I,W]
  .12   With Hallucinations[I,W]
292.84   Sedative-, Hypnotic-, or Anxiolytic-Induced Mood Disorder[I,W]
292.89   Sedative-, Hypnotic-, or Anxiolytic-Induced Anxiety Disorder[W]
292.89   Sedative-, Hypnotic-, or Anxiolytic-Induced Sexual Dysfunction[I]
292.89   Sedative-, Hypnotic-, or Anxiolytic-Induced Sleep Disorder[I,W]
292.9   Sedative-, Hypnotic-, or Anxiolytic-Induced Disorder NOS

Polysubstance-Related Disorder

304.80   Polysubstance Dependence*

Other (or Unknown) Substance-Related Disorders

Other (or Unknown) Substance Use Disorders

304.90   Other (or Unknown) Substance Dependence*
305.90   Other (or Unknown) Substance Abuse

Other (or Unknown) Substance-Induced Disorders

292.89   Other (or Unknown) Substance Intoxication
         Specify if: With Perceptual Disturbances
292.0   Other (or Unknown) Substance Withdrawal
         Specify if: With Perceptual Disturbances

292.81 Other (or Unknown) Substance-Induced Delirium
292.82 Other (or Unknown) Substance-Induced Persisting Dementia
292.83 Other (or Unknown) Substance-Induced Persisting Amnestic Disorder
292.xx Other (or Unknown) Substance-Induced Psychotic Disorder
   .11 With Delusions[I,W]
   .12 With Hallucinations[I,W]
292.84 Other (or Unknown) Substance-Induced Mood Disorder[I,W]
292.89 Other (or Unknown) Substance-Induced Anxiety Disorder[I,W]
292.89 Other (or Unknown) Substance-Induced Sexual Dysfunction[I]
292.89 Other (or Unknown) Substance-Induced Sleep Disorder[I,W]
292.9   Other (or Unknown) Substance-Induced Disorder NOS

SCHIZOPHRENIA AND OTHER PSYCHOTIC DISORDERS

295.xx Schizophrenia

The following Classification of Longitudinal Course applies to all subtypes of Schizophrenia:

Episodic With Interepisode Residual Symptoms
   (*Specify if:* With Prominent Negative Symptoms)/
    Episodic With No Interepisode Residual
    Symptoms/Continuous
   (*Specify if:* With Prominent Negative Symptoms)
Single Episode in Partial Remission
   (*Specify if:* With Prominent Negative Symptoms)
Single Episode in Full Remission
Other or Unspecified Pattern
   .30 Paranoid Type
   .10 Disorganized Type
   .20 Catatonic Type
   .90 Undifferentiated Type
   .60 Residual Type
295.40 Schizophreniform Disorder
   Specify if: Without Good Prognostic Features/With Good Prognostic Features
295.70 Schizoaffective Disorder
   Specify type: Bipolar/Depressive
297.1   Delusional Disorder
   Specify type: Erotomanic/Grandiose/jealous/Persecutory Somatic/Mixed/Unspecified
298.8   Brief Psychotic Disorder
   Specify if: With Marked Stressor(s) Without Marked Stressor(s) With Postpartum Onset
297.3   Shared Psychotic Disorder
293.xx Psychotic Disorder Due to . . .*

   .81 With Delusions
   .82 With Hallucinations
—.-   Substance-Induced Psychotic Disorder (refer to Substance-Related Disorders for substance-specific codes)
   Specify if: With Onset During Intoxication/With Onset During Withdrawal
298.9   Psychotic Disorder NOS

MOOD DISORDERS

Code current state of Major Depressive Disorder or Bipolar I Disorder in fifth digit

1 = Mild
2 = Moderate
3 = Severe Without Psychotic Features
4 = Severe With Psychotic Features
   Specify: Mood-Congruent Psychotic Features/Mood-Incongruent Psychotic Features
5 = In Partial Remission
6 = In Full Remission
0 = Unspecified

The following specifiers apply (for current or most recent episode) to Mood Disorders as noted:

[a]Severity/Psychotic/Remission Specifiers/[b]Chronic/[c]With Catatonic Features/[d]With Melancholic Features/[e]With Atypical Features/[f]With Postpartum Onset
The following specifiers apply to Mood Disorders as noted:

[g]With or Without Full Interepisode Recovery/With Seasonal Pattern/[i]With Rapid Cycling

Depressive Disorders

296.xx Major Depressive Disorder,
   .2x Single Episode[a,b,c,d,e,f]
   .3x Recurrent[a,b,c,d,e,f,g,h]
300.4   Dysthymic Disorder
   Specify if: Early Onset/Late Onset
   Specify if: With Atypical Features
311   Depressive Disorder NOS

Bipolar Disorders

296.xx Bipolar I Disorder,
   .0x Single Manic Episode[a,c,f]
    Specify if: Mixed
   .40 Most Recent Episode Hypomanic[a,h,j]
   .4x Most Recent Episode Manic[a,c,f,g,h,i]
   .6x Most Recent Episode Mixed[a,c,f,g,h,i]
   .5x Most Recent Episode Depressed[a,b,c,d,e,f,g,h,i]
   .7   Most Recent Episode Unspecified[g,h,i]
296.89 Bipolar II Disorder[a,b,c,d,e,f,g,h,i]
   Specify (current or most recent episode): Hypomanic/Depressed

301.13 Cyclothymic Disorder
296.80 Bipolar Disorder NOS
293.83 Mood Disorder Due to . . .*
    Specify type: With Depressive Features/
    With Major Depressive-Like Episode/
    With Manic Features/With Mixed
    Features
—.- Substance-Induced Mood Disorder**
    Specify type: With Depressive Features/
    With Manic Features/With Mixed
    Features
    Specify if: With Onset During
    Intoxication/With Onset during
    Withdrawal
296.90 Mood Disorder NOS

ANXIETY DISORDERS

300.01 Panic Disorder without Agoraphobia
300.21 Panic Disorder With Agoraphobia
300.22 Agoraphobia Without History of
    Panic Disorder
300.29 Specific Phobia
    Specify type: Animal Type/Natural
    Environment Type/Blood-Injection-Injury
    Type/Situational Type/Other Type
300.23 Social Phobia
    Specify if: Generalized
300.3 Obsessive-Compulsive Disorder
    Specify if: With Poor Insight
309.81 Posttraumatic Stress Disorder
    Specify if: Acute/Chronic
    Specify if: With Delayed Onset
308.3 Acute Stress Disorder
300.02 Generalized Anxiety Disorder
293.80 Anxiety Disorder Due to. . .*
    Specify if: With Generalized Anxiety/With
    Panic Attacks/With
    Obsessive Compulsive Symptoms. . .*
293.84 Substance-Induced Anxiety Disorder
    Specify if: With Generalized Anxiety/With
    Panic Attacks/With
    Obsessive-Compulsive Symptoms/With
    Phobic Symptoms
    Specify if: With Onset During
    Intoxication/With Onset During
    Withdrawal
300.00 Anxiety Disorder NOS

SOMATOFORM DISORDERS

300.81 Somatization Disorder
300.82 Undifferentiated Somatoform Disorder
300.11 Conversion Disorder
    Specify type: With Motor Symptom or
    Deficit/With Sensory Symptom or Deficit/
    With Seizures or Convulsions/With Mixed
    Presentation

307.xx Pain Disorder
   .80 Associated With Psychological Factors
   .89 Associated with Both Psychological Factors
    and a General Medical Condition
    Specify if: Acute/Chronic
300.7 Hypochondriasis
    Specify if: With Poor Insight
300.7 Body Dysmorphic Disorder
300.82 Somatoform Disorder NOS

FACTITIOUS DISORDERS

300.xx Facitious Disorder
   .16 With Predominantly Psychological Signs and
    Symptoms
   .19 With Predominantly Physical Signs and
    Symptoms
   .19 With Combined Psychological and Physical
    Signs and Symptoms
300.19 Factitious Disorder NOS

DISSOCIATIVE DISORDERS

300.12 Dissociative Amnesia
300.13 Dissociative Fugue
300.14 Dissociative Identity Disorder
300.6 Depersonalized Disorder
300.15 Dissociative Disorder NOS

SEXUAL AND GENDER IDENTITY DISORDERS

Sexual Dysfunctions

The following specifiers apply to all primary Sexual Dysfunctions:

Lifelong Type/Acquired
Type Generalized Type/Situational Type
Due to Psychological Factors. Due to Combined
    Factors

Sexual Desire Disorders

302.71 Hypoactive Sexual Desire Disorder
302.79 Sexual Aversion Disorder

Sexual Arousal Disorders

302.72 Female Sexual Arousal Disorder
302.72 Male Erectile Disorder

Orgasmic Disorders

302.73 Female Orgasmic Disorder
302.74 Male Orgasmic Disorder
302.75 Premature Ejaculation

Sexual Pain Disorders

302.76 Dyspareunia (Not Due to General Medical
        Condition)
306.51 Vaginismus (Not Due to a General Medical
        Condition)

Sexual Dysfunction Due to a General Medical Condition

625.8   Female Hypoactive Sexual Desire Disorder
        Due to . . .*
608.89 Male Hypoactive Sexual Desire Disorder Due
        to . . .*
607.84 Male Erectile Disorder Due to . . .*
625.0   Female Dyspareunia Due to . . .*
608.89 Male Dyspareunia Due to . . .*
625.8   Other Female Sexual Dysfunction Due to . . .*
608.89 Other Male Sexual Dysfunction Due to . . .*
—.-   Substance-Induced Sexual Dysfunction**
        Specify if: With Impaired Desire/With
        Impaired Arousal/With Impaired
        Orgasm/With Sexual Pain
        Specify if: With Onset During Intoxication
302.70 Sexual Dysfunction NOS

Paraphilias

302.4   Exhibitionism
302.81 Fetishism
302.89 Frotteurism
302.2   Pedophilia
        Specify if: Sexually Attracted to
        Males/Sexually Attracted to
        Females/Sexually Attracted to Both
        Specify if: Limited to Incest
        Specify type: Exclusive Type/
        Nonexclusive type
302.83 Sexual Masochism
302.84 Sexual Sadism
302.3   Transvestic Fetishism
        Specify if: With Gender Dysphoria
302.82 Voyeurism
302.9   Paraphilia NOS

Gender Identity Disorders

302.xx Gender Identity Disorder
   .6   in Children
   .85 in Adolescents or Adults
        Specify if: Sexually Attracted to Males/
        Sexually Attracted to Females/Sexually
        Attracted to Both/Sexually Attracted to
        Neither
302.6   Gender Identity Disorder NOS
302.9   Sexual Disorder NOS

EATING DISORDERS

307.1   Anorexia Nervosa
        Specify type: Restricting,
        Binge-Eating/Purging
307.51 Bulimia Nervosa
        Specify type: Purging/Nonpurging
307.50 Eating Disorder NOS

SLEEP DISORDERS

Primary Sleep Disorders

Dyssomnias

307.42 Primary Insomnia
307.44 Primary Hypersomnia
        Specify if: Recurrent
347   Narcolepsy
380.59 Breathing-Related Sleep Disorder
307.45 Circadian Rhythm Sleep Disorder
        Specify type: Delayed Sleep Phase/
        Jet Lag/Shift Work/Unspecified
307.47 Dyssomnia NOS

Parasomnias

307.47 Nightmare Disorder
307.46 Sleep Terror Disorder
307.46 Sleepwalking Disorder
307.47 Parasomnia NOS

Sleep Disorders Related to Another Mental Disorder

307.42 Insomnia Related to . . . ***
307.44 Hypersomnia Related to . . . ***

Other Sleep Disorders

780.xx Sleep Disorder Due to . . . *
   .52 Insomnia Type
   .54 Hyposomnia Type
   .59 Parasomnia Type
   .59 Mixed Type
—.-   Substance-Induced Sleep Disorder (refer
        to Substance-Related Disorders for substance-
        specific codes)
        Specify type: Insomnia/Hypersomnia/
        Parasomnia/Mixed
        Specify if: With Onset during Intoxication/
        With Onset During Withdrawal

IMPULSE-CONTROL DISORDERS NOT ELSEWHERE CLASSIFIED

312.34 Intermittent Explosive Disorder
312.32 Kleptomania
312.33 Pyromania

312.31   Pathological Gambling
312.39   Trichotillomania
312.30   Impulse-Control Disorder NOS

ADJUSTMENT DISORDERS

309.xx   Adjustment Disorder
    .0   With Depressed Mood
    .24   With Anxiety
    .28   With Mixed Anxiety and Depressed Mood
    .3   With Disturbance of Conduct
    .4   With Mixed Disturbance of Emotions
        and Conduct
    .9   Unspecified
        Specify if: Acute/Chronic

PERSONALITY DISORDERS

Note: These are coded on Axis II

301.0   Paranoid Personality Disorder
301.20   Schizoid Personality Disorder
301.22   Schizotypal Personality Disorder
301.7   Antisocial Personality Disorder
301.83   Borderline Personality Disorder
301.50   Histrionic Personality Disorder
301.81   Narcissistic Personality Disorder
301.82   Avoidant Personality Disorder
301.6   Dependent Personality Disorder
301.4   Obsessive-Compulsive Personality Disorder
301.9   Personality Disorder NOS

OTHER CONDITIONS THAT MAY BE A FOCUS OF CLINICAL ATTENTION

Psychological Factors Affecting Medical Condition

316. . . [Specified Psychological Factor] Affecting . . .*

Choose name based on nature of factors:

Mental Disorder Affecting Medical Condition
Psychological Symptoms Affecting Medical Condition
Personality Traits or Coping Style Affecting Medical Condition
Maladaptive Health Behaviors Affecting Medical Condition
Stress-Related Physiological Response Affecting Medical Condition
Other or Unspecified Psychological Factors Affecting Medical Condition

Medication-Induced Movement Disorders

332.1   Neuroleptic-Induced Parkinsonism
333.92   Neuroleptic Malignant Syndrome
333.7   Neuroleptic-Induced Acute Dystonia

333.99   Neuroleptic-Induced Acute Akathisia
333.82   Neuroleptic-Induced Tardive Dyskinesia
333.1   Medication-Induced Postural Tumor
333.90   Medication-Induced Movement Disorder NOS

Other Medical-Induced Disorder

995.2   Adverse Effects of Medication NOS

Relational Problems

V61.9   Relational Problem Related to a Mental Disorder or General Medical Condition
V61.1   Partner Relational Problem
V61.20   Parent-Child Relational Problem
V61.8   Sibling Relational Problem
V62.81   Relational Problem NOS

Problems Related to Abuse or Neglect

(code 995.5 if focus of attention is on victim)

V61.21   Physical Abuse of Child
V61.21   Sexual Abuse of Child
V61.21   Neglect of Child
V61.12   Physical Abuse of Adult
V61.1   Sexual Abuse of Adult
V62.83   Person Other Than Partner

Additional Conditions That May be Focus of Clinical Attention

V15.81   Noncompliance With Treatment
V65.2   Malingering
V71.01   Adult Antisocial behavior
V71.02   Child or Adolescent Antisocial behavior
V62.89   Borderline Intellectual Functioning
    Note: This is code on Axis II.
780.9   Age-Related Cognitive Decline
V62.82   Bereavement
V62.3   Academic Problem
V62.2   Occupational Problem
313.82   Identify Problem
V62.89   Religious or Spritual Problem
V62.4   Acculturation Problem
V62.89   Phase of Life Problem

ADDITIONAL CODES

300.9   Unspecified Mental Disorder (nonpsychotic)
V71.09   No Diagnosis or Condition on Axis I
799.9   Diagnosis or Condition Deferred on Axis I
V71.09   No Diagnosis on Axis II
799.9   Diagnosis Deferred on Axis II

Brief Psychiatric Rating Scale

DIRECTIONS: Place an X in the appropriate box to represent level of severity of each symptom.

	Not Present	Very Mild	Mild	Moderate	Mod. Severe	Severe	Extremely Severe
SOMATIC CONCERN—preoccupation with physical health, fear of physical illness, hypochondriasis.	☐	☐	☐	☐	☐	☐	☐
ANXIETY—worry, fear, overconcern for present or future, uneasiness.	☐	☐	☐	☐	☐	☐	☐
EMOTIONAL WITHDRAWAL—lack of spontaneous interaction, isolation deficiency in relating to others.	☐	☐	☐	☐	☐	☐	☐
CONCEPTUAL DISORGANIZATION—thought processes confused, disconnected, disorganized, disrupted.	☐	☐	☐	☐	☐	☐	☐
GUILT FEELINGS—self-blame, shame, remorse for past behavior.	☐	☐	☐	☐	☐	☐	☐
TENSION—physical and motor manifestations of nervousness, over-activation.	☐	☐	☐	☐	☐	☐	☐
MANNERISMS AND POSTURING—peculiar, bizarre unnatural motor behavior (not including tic).	☐	☐	☐	☐	☐	☐	☐
GRANDIOSITY—exaggerated self-opinion, arrogance, conviction of unusual power or abilities.	☐	☐	☐	☐	☐	☐	☐
DEPRESSIVE MOOD—sorrow, sadness, despondency, pessimism.	☐	☐	☐	☐	☐	☐	☐
HOSTILITY—animosity, contempt, belligerence, disdain for others.	☐	☐	☐	☐	☐	☐	☐
SUSPICIOUSNESS—mistrust, belief others harbour malicious or discriminatory intent.	☐	☐	☐	☐	☐	☐	☐
HALLUCINATORY BEHAVIOR—perceptions without normal external stimulus correspondence.	☐	☐	☐	☐	☐	☐	☐
MOTOR RETARDATION—slowed weakened movements or speech, reduced body tone.	☐	☐	☐	☐	☐	☐	☐
UNCOOPERATIVENESS—resistance, guardedness, rejection of authority.	☐	☐	☐	☐	☐	☐	☐
UNUSUAL THOUGHT CONTENT—unusual, odd, strange, bizarre thought content.	☐	☐	☐	☐	☐	☐	☐
BLUNTED AFFECT—reduced emotional tone, reduction in formal intensity of feelings, flatness.	☐	☐	☐	☐	☐	☐	☐
EXCITEMENT—heightened emotional tone, agitation, increased reactivity.	☐	☐	☐	☐	☐	☐	☐
DISORIENTATION—confusion or lack of proper association for person, place, or time.	☐	☐	☐	☐	☐	☐	☐
Global Assessment Scale (Range 1–100)	☐	☐	☐	☐	☐	☐	☐

Reprinted with permission from Overall J. E. (1988). The Brief Psychiatric Rating Scale (BPRS): Recent developments in ascertainment and scaling. *Psychopharmacology Bulletin, 24,* 97–99.

Simpson-Angus Rating Scale

1. GAIT: The patient is examined as he walks into the examining room; his gait, the swing of his arms, his general posture, all form the basis for an overall score for this item. This is rated as follows:

   0 Normal
   1 Diminution in swing while the patient is walking.
   2 Marked diminution in swing with obvious rigidity in the arm.
   3 Stiff gait with arms held rigidly before the abdomen.
   4 Stooped shuffling gait with propulsion and retropulsion.

2. ARM DROPPING: The patient and the examiner both raise their arms to shoulder height and let them fall to their sides. In a normal subject, a stout slap is heard as the arms hit the sides. In the patient with extreme Parkinson's syndrome, the arms fall very slowly.

   0 Normal, free fall with loud slap and rebound.
   1 Fall slowed slightly with less audible contact and little rebound.
   2 Fall slowed, no rebound.
   3 Marked slowing, no slap at all.
   4 Arms fall as though against resistance; as though through glue.

3. SHOULDER SHAKING: The subject's arms are bent at a right angle at the elbow and are taken one at a time by the examiner who grasps one hand and also clasps the other around the patient's elbow. The subject's upper arm is pushed to and fro, and the humerus is externally rotated. The degree of resistance from normal to extreme rigidity is scored as follows:

   0 Normal
   1 Slight stiffness and resistance.
   2 Moderate stiffness and resistance.
   3 Marked rigidity with difficulty in passive movement.
   4 Extreme stiffness and rigidity with almost a frozen shoulder.

4. ELBOW RIGIDITY: The elbow joints are separately bent at right angles and passively extended and flexed, with the subject's biceps observed and simultaneously palpated. The resistance to this procedure is rated. (The presence of cogwheel rigidity is noted separately.) Scoring is from 0 to 4, as in the Shoulder Shaking test.

   0 Normal
   1 Slight stiffness and resistance.
   2 Moderate stiffness and resistance.
   3 Marked rigidity with difficulty in passive movement.
   4 Extreme stiffness and rigidity with almost a frozen shoulder.

5. FIXATION OF POSITION OR WRIST RIGIDITY: The wrist is held in one hand and the fingers held by the examiner's other hand, with the wrist moved to extension flexion and both ulnar and radial deviation. The resistance to this procedure is rated as in Items 3 and 4.

   0 Normal
   1 Slight stiffness and resistance.
   2 Moderate stiffness and resistance.
   3 Marked rigidity with difficulty in passive movement.
   4 Extreme stiffness and rigidity with almost a frozen shoulder.

6. LEG PENDULOUSNESS: The patient sits on a table with his legs hanging down and swinging free. The ankle is grasped by the examiner and raised until the knee is partially extended. It is then allowed to fall. The resistance to falling and the lack of swinging form the basis for the score on this item.

   0 The legs swing freely.
   1 Slight diminution in the swing of the legs.
   2 Moderate resistance to swing.
   3 Marked resistance and damping of swing.
   4 Complete absence of swing.

7. HEAD DROPPING: The patient lies on a well-padded examining table and his head is raised by the examiner's hand. The hand is then withdrawn, and the head allowed to drop. In the normal subject, the head will fall upon the table. The movement is

delayed in extrapyramidal system disorder, and in extreme parkinsonism, it is absent. The neck muscles are rigid, and the head does not reach the examining table. Scoring is as follows:

0 The head falls completely, with a good thump as it hits the table.
1 Slight slowing in fall, mainly noted by lack of slap as head meets the table.
2 Moderate slowing in the fall, quite noticeable to the eye.
3 Head falls stiffly and slowly.
4 Head does not reach examining table.

8. GLABELLA TAP: Subject is told to open his eyes wide and not to blink. The glabella region is tapped at a steady, rapid speed. The number of times patient blinks in succession is noted:

0 0 to 5 blinks
1 6 to 10 blinks
2 11 to 15 blinks
3 16 to 20 blinks
4 21 or more blinks

9. TREMOR: Patient is observed walking into examining room and then is re-examined for this item:

0 Normal
1 Mild finger tremor, obvious to sight and touch.

2 Tremor of hand or arm occurring spasmodically.
3 Persistent tremor of one or more limbs.
4 Whole body tremor.

10. SALIVATION: Patient is observed while talking and then asked to open his mouth and elevate his tongue. The following ratings are given:

0 Normal
1 Excess salivation to the extent that pooling takes place if the mouth is open and the tongue raised.
2 When excess salivation is present and might occasionally result in difficulty in speaking.
3 Speaking with difficulty because of excess salivation.
4 Frank drooling.

Scoring: Each item is rated on a 5-point scale, with 0 meaning the complete absence of the condition, and 4 meaning the presence of the condition in extreme form. The score is obtained by adding the items and dividing by 10.

Reprinted with permission from Simpson G. M., Angus, J. W. S. (1970). A rating scale for extrapyramidal side effects. *Acta Psychiatrica Scondinovica, 212* (Suppl.), 11–19. Copyright 1970, Munksgaard International Publishers, Ltd.

Abnormal Involuntary Movement Scale (AIMS)

		None	Minimal	Mild	Moderate	Severe
Facial and Oral Movements						
	1: Muscles of Facial Expression eg, movements of forehead, eyebrows, periorbital area, cheeks; include frowning, blinking, smiling, grimacing	0	1	2	3	4
	2: Lips and Perioral Area eg, puckering, pouting, smacking	0	1	2	3	4
	3: Jaw eg, biting, clenching, chewing, mouth opening, lateral movement	0	1	2	3	4
	4: Tongue Rate only increase in movement both in and out of mouth, NOT inability to sustain movement	0	1	2	3	4
Extremity Movements						
	5: Upper (arms, wrists, hands, fingers) Include choreic movements (ie, rapid, objectively purpose-less, irregular, spontaneous), athetoid movements (ie, slow, irregular, complex, serpentine). Do NOT include tremor (ie, repetitive, regular, rhythmic).	0	1	2	3	4
	6: Lower (legs, knees, ankles, toes) eg, lateral knee movement, foot tapping, heel dropping, foot squirming, inversion and ever-sion of foot	0	1	2	3	4
Trunk Movements						
	7: Neck, shoulders, hips eg, rocking, twisting, squirming, pelvic gyrations	0	1	2	3	4
	8: Severity of abnormal movements	0	1	2	3	4

		None	Minimal	Mild	Moderate	Severe
Global Judgment	9: Incapacitation due to abnormal movements	0	1	2	3	4
	10: Patient's awareness of abnormal movements Rate only patient's report	No awareness			0	
		Aware, no distress			1	
		Aware, mild distress			2	
		Aware, moderate distress			3	
		Aware, severe distress			4	
Global Judgment	11: Current problems with teeth and/or dentures	No			0	
		Yes			1	
	12: Does patient usually wear dentures?	No			0	
		Yes			1	

Examination Procedures for AIMS

Either before or after completing the Examination Procedure, observe the patient unobtrusively, at rest (eg, in waiting room). The chair to be used in this examination should be a hard, firm one without arms.

1: Ask patient whether there is anything in his/her mouth (ie, gum, candy, etc.) and if there is, to remove it.

2: Ask patient about the *current* condition of his/her teeth. Ask patient if he/she wears dentures. Do teeth or dentures bother patient *now?*

3: Ask patient whether he/she notices any movements in mouth, face, hands, or feet. If yes, ask to describe and to what extent they *currently* bother patient or interfere with his/her activities.

4: Have patient sit in chair with hands on knees, legs slightly apart, and feet flat on floor. (Look at entire body for movements while in this position.)

5: Ask patient to sit with hands hanging unsupported. If male, between legs, if female and wearing a dress, hanging over knees. (Observe hands and other body areas.)

6: Ask patient to open mouth. (Observe tongue at rest within mouth.) Do this twice.

7: Ask patient to protrude tongue. (Observe tongue at rest within mouth.) Do this twice.

*8: Ask patient to tap thumb, with each finger, as rapidly as possible for 10–15 seconds; separately with right hand, then with left hand. (Observe facial and leg movements.)

9: Flex and extend patient's left and right arms (one at a time). (Note any rigidity and rate on NOTES.)

10: Ask patient to stand up. (Observe in profile. Observe all body areas again, hips included.)

*11: Ask patient to extend both arms outstretched in front with palms down. (Observe trunk, legs, and mouth.)

*12: Have patient walk a few paces, turn, and walk back to chair. (Observe hand and gait.) Do this twice.

*Activated movements

Reprinted from Guy, W. (1976). ECDEU: Assessment manual for psychopharmacology (DHEW Publ No 76–338). Washington, DC: Department of Health. Education, and Welfare, Psychopharmacology Research Branch.

Simplified Diagnoses for Tardive Dyskinesia (SD-TD)

PREREQUISITES.—The three prerequisites are as follows. Exceptions may occur.

1. A history of at least 3 months' total cumulative neuroleptic exposure. Include amoxapine and metoclopramide in all categories below as well.
2. **SCORING/INTENSITY LEVEL.** The presence of a **TOTAL SCORE OF FIVE (5) OR ABOVE.** Also be alert for any change from baseline or scores below five which have at least a "moderate" (3) or "severe" (4) movement on any item or at least two "mild" (2) movements on two items located in different body areas.
3. Other conditions are not responsible for the abnormal involuntary movements.

DIAGNOSES.—The diagnosis is based upon the current exam and its relation to the last exam. The diagnosis can shift depending upon: (a) whether movements are present or not, (b) whether movements are present for 3 months or more (6 months if on a semiannual assessment schedule), and (c) whether neuroleptic dosage changes occur and effect movements.

- **NO TD.**—Movements **are not** present on this exam **or** movements are present, but some other condition is responsible for them. The last diagnosis must be NO TD, PROBABLE TD, or WITHDRAWAL TD.
- **PROBABLE TD.**—Movements **are** present on this exam. This is the first time they are present or they have never been present for 3 months or more. The last diagnosis must be NO TD or PROBABLE TD.
- **PERSISTENT TD.**—Movements are present on this exam **and** they have been present for 3 months or more with this exam or at some point in the past. The last diagnosis can be any except NO TD.
- **MASKED TD.**—Movements **are not** present on this exam **but** this is due to a neuroleptic dosage increase or reinstitution after a prior exam when movements were present. Also use this conclusion if movements are not present due to the addition of a non-neuroleptic medication to treat TD. The last diagnosis must be PROBABLE TD, PERSISTENT TD, WITHDRAWAL TD, or MASKED TD.
- **REMITTED TD.**—Movements **are not** present on this exam **but** PERSISTENT TD has been diagnosed **and** nouroleptic dosage increase or reinstitution has occurred. The last diagnosis must be PERSISTENT TD or REMITTED TD. If movements re-emerge, the diagnosis shifts back to PERSISTENT TD.
- **WITHDRAWAL TD.**—Movements **are not seen while** receiving neuroleptics or at the last dosage level **but are seen within** 8 weeks following a neuroleptic reduction or discontinuation. The last diagnosis must be NO TD or WITHDRAWAL TD. If movements continue for 3 months or more after the neuroleptic dosage reduction or discontinuation, the diagnosis shifts to PERSISTENT TD. If movements do not continue for 3 months or more after the reduction or discontinuation, the diagnosis shifts to NO TD.

INSTRUCTIONS

1. The rater completes the Assessment according to the standardized exam procedure. If the rater also completes Evaluation items 1–4, he/she must also sign the preparer box. The form is given to the physician. Alternatively, the physician may perform the assessment.
2. The physician completes the Evaluation section. The physician is responsible for the entire Evaluation section and its accuracy.
3. IT IS RECOMMENDED THAT THE PHYSICIAN EXAMINE ANY INDIVIDUAL WHO MEETS THE THREE PREREQUISITES OR WHO HAS MOVEMENTS NOT EXPLAINED BY OTHER FACTORS. NEUROLOGICAL ASSESS MENTS OR DIFFERENTIAL DIAGNOSTIC TESTS WHICH MAY BE NECESSARY SHOULD BE OBTAINED.
4. File form according to policy or procedure.

OTHER CONDITIONS (partial list)

1. Age
2. Blind
3. Cerebral Palsy
4. Contact Lenses
5. Dentures/No Teeth
6. Down Syndrome
7. Drug Intoxication (specify)
8. Encephalitis
9. Extrapyramidal Side-Effects (specify)
10. Fahr's Syndrome
11. Heavy Metal Intoxication (specify)
12. Huntington's Chorea
13. Hyperthyroidism
14. Hypoglycemia
15. Hypoparathyroidism
16. Idiopathic Torsion Dystonia
17. Meige Syndrome
18. Parkinson's Disease
19. Stereotypies
20. Syndenham's Chorea
21. Tourette's Syndrome
22. Wilson's Disease
23. Other (specify)

Sprague, R. L., & Kalachnik, J. E. (1991). Reliability, validity, and a total score cutoff for the Dyskinesia Identification System, Condensed User Scale (DISCUS) with mentally ill and mentally retarded populations. *Psychopharmacology Bulletin, 27*(1), 51–58.

Hamilton Rating Scale for Depression

Clinic No._____ Date_____ Rating No._____ Code Number_____

Sex_____Age_____Patient's Name _____

Patient's Address _____ Tel _____

Item	Range	Score
1. Depressed mood	0–4	
2. Guilt	0–4	
3. Suicide	0–4	
4. Insomnia initial	0–2	
5. Insomnia middle	0–2	
6. Insomnia delayed	0–2	
7. Work and interest	0–4	
8. Retardation	0–4	
9. Agitation	0–4	
10. Anxiety (psychic)	0–4	
11. Anxiety (somatic)	0–4	
12. Somatic gastrointestinal	0–2	
13. Somatic general	0–2	
14. Genital	0–2	
15. Hypochondriasis	0–2	
16. Insight	0–4	
17. Loss of weight	0–2	
	Total Score	
Diurnal variation (M.A.E.)	0–2	
Depersonalization	0–4	
Paranoid symptoms	0–4	
Obsessional symptoms	0–4	

The scale is designed to measure the severity of illness of patients already diagnosed as suffering from depressive illness. It is obviously not a diagnostic instrument because that requires much more information (e.g., previous history, family history, precipitating factors).

As far as possible, the scale should be used in the manner of a clinical interview. The first time the interview should be conducted in a relaxed, free, and easy manner, giving the patients time to unburden themselves and giving them the opportunity to speak of their problems and ask whatever questions they wish. It may then be necessary to obtain further information by asking them questions. At subsequent assessments, the interview can be briefer and more to the point.

An observer rating scale is not a checklist in which each item is strictly defined. The raters must have sufficient clinical experience and judgment to be able to interpret the patients' statements and reticences about some symptoms, and to compare them with other patients. They should use all sources of information (eg, from relatives and nurses).

The scale consists of 17 items, the scores on which are summed to give a total score. These are four other items, one of which (diurnal variation) is excluded on the grounds that it is not an additional burden on the patient. The last three are excluded from the total score because they occur infrequently, although information on them may be useful for other purposes.

The method of assessment is simple. For some symptoms it is difficult to elicit such information as will permit of full quantification. If present, score 2; if absent, score 0; and if doubtful or trivial, score 1. For those symptoms where more detailed information can be obtained, the score of 2 is expanded into 2 for mild, 3 for moderate, and 4 for severe. In case of difficulty, the raters should use their judgment as clinicians.

Hamilton, M. (1960). A rating scale for depression. *Journal of Neurology, Neurosurgery and Psychiatry, 23,* 56.

CAGE Questionnaire

The CAGE is a very brief questionnaire for detection of alcoholism. Item responses on the CAGE are score 0 for *no* and 1 for *yes*, with a higher score an indication of alcohol problems. A total score of 2 or more is considered clinically significant and requires a more focused and detailed assessment. The following are the four questions that comprise the CAGE questionnaire.

Have you ever felt you should *Cut down* on your drinking?	Yes	No
Have people *Annoyed* you by criticizing your drinking?	Yes	No
Have you ever felt bad or *Guilty* about your drinking?	Yes	No
Have you ever had a drink first thing in the morning to steady your nerves to get rid of a hangover? (*Eyeopener*)	Yes	No

Ewing, J. A. (1984). Detecting alcoholism. *Journal of the American Medical Association. 252,* 1905–1907.
Additional readings:
Burge, S., & Schneider, F. (1999). Alcohol-related problems: Recognition and intervention. *American Family Physician,* American Academy of Family Physicians Home Page (www.aafp.org. 1/15/99).
Davis, M. (2000). Alcohol and drug addiction. *Medical Library* (www.medical-library.org. 9/30/00).
Wesson, D. (1995). *Detoxification from alcohol and other drugs.* Rockville, MD: Substance Abuse and Mental Health Services Administra tion, Center for Substance Abuse Treatment, Treatment Improvement Protocol #19.

Specific Defense Mechanisms and Coping Styles*

Defense Mechanism	Definition	Example
Acting out	Using actions rather than reflections or feelings during periods of emotional conflict	A teenager gets mad at parents and begins staying out late at night.
Affiliation	Turning to others for help or support (sharing problems with others without implying that someone else is responsible for them)	An individual has a fight with spouse and turns to best friend for emotional support.
Altruism	Dedicating life to meeting the needs of others (receives gratification either vicariously or from the response of others)	After being rejected by boyfriend, a young girl joins the Peace Corps.
Anticipation	Experiencing emotional reactions in advance or anticipating consequences of possible future events and considering realistic, alternative responses or solutions	A parent cries for 3 weeks before the last child leaves for college. On the day of the separation, the parent spends the day with friends.
Autistic fantasy	Excessive daydreaming as a substitute for human relationships, more effective action, or problem solving	A young man sits in his room all day and dreams about being a rock star instead of attending a baseball game with a friend.
Denial	Refusing to acknowledge some painful aspect of external reality or subjective experience that would be apparent to others (*psychotic denial* used when there is gross impairment in reality testing)	A teenager's best friend moves away, but the adolescent says he does not feel sad.
Devaluation	Attributing exaggerated negative qualities to self or others	A boy has been rejected by his long time girlfriend. He tells his friends that he realizes that she is stupid and ugly.
Displacement	Transferring a feeling about, or a response to, one object onto another (usually less threatening), substitute object	A child is mad at her mother for leaving for the day, but says she is really mad at the sitter for serving her food she does not like.
Dissociation	Experiencing a breakdown in the usually integrated functions of consciousness, memory, perception of self or the environment, or sensory and motor behavior	An adult relates severe sexual abuse experienced as a child, but does it without feeling. She says that the experience was as if she were outside her body watching the abuse.
Help-rejecting complaining	Complaining or making repetitious requests for help that disguise covert feelings of hostility or reproach toward others, which are then expressed by rejecting the suggestions, advice, or help that others offer (complaints or requests may involve physical or psychological symptoms or life problems)	A college student asks a teacher for help after receiving a bad grade on a test. Every suggestion the teacher has is rejected by the student.
Humor	Emphasizing the amusing or ironic aspects of the conflict or stressor	A person makes a joke right after experiencing an embarrassing situation.
Idealization	Attributing exaggerated positive qualities to others	An adult falls in love and fails to see the negative qualities in the other person.
Intellectualization	Excessive use of abstract thinking or the making of generalizations to control or minimize disturbing feelings	After rejection in a love relationship, the rejected explains about the relationship dynamics to a friend.
Isolation of affect	Separation of ideas from the feelings originally associated with them	The individual loses touch with the feelings associated with a rape while remaining aware of the details.

(Continued)

Specific Defense Mechanisms and Coping Styles* (Continued)

Defense Mechanism	Definition	Example
Omnipotence	Feeling or acting as if one possesses special powers or abilities and is superior to others	An individual tells a friend about personal expertise in the stock market and the ability to predict the best stocks.
Passive aggression	Indirectly and unassertively expressing aggression toward others. There is a facade of overt compliance masking covert resistance, resentment, or hostility.	Passive aggression often occurs in response to demands for independent action or performance, or the lack of gratification of dependent wishes but may be adaptive for individuals in subordinate positions who have no other way to express assertiveness more overtly.
Projection	Falsely attributing to another one's own unacceptable feelings, impulses, or thoughts	A child is very angry at a parent, but accuses the parent of being angry.
Projective identification	Falsely attributing to another one's own unacceptable feelings, impulses, or thoughts. Unlike simple projection, the individual does not fully disavow what is projected. Instead, the individual remains aware of his or her own affect or impulses but misattributes them as justifiable reactions to the other person. Not infrequently, the individual induces the very feelings in others that were first mistakenly believed to be there, making it difficult to clarify who did what to whom first.	A child is mad at a parent, who in turn becomes angry at the child, but may be unsure of why. The child then feels justified at being angry with the parent.
Rationalization	Concealing the true motivations for one's own thoughts, actions, or feelings through the elaboration of reassuring or self-serving but incorrect explanations	A man is rejected by his girlfriend, but explains to his friends that her leaving was best because she was beneath him socially and would not be liked by his family.
Reaction formation	Substituting behavior, thoughts, or feelings that are diametrically opposed to one's own unacceptable thougths or feelings (this usually occurs in conjunction with their repression)	A wife finds out about her husband's extramarital affairs and tells her friends that she thinks his affairs are perfectly appropriate. She truly does not feel, on a conscious level, any anger or hurt.
Repression	Expelling disturbing wishes, thoughts, or experiences from conscious awareness (the feeling component may remain conscious, detached from its associated ideas)	A woman does not remember the experience of being raped in the basement, but does feel anxious when going into that house.
Self-assertion	Expressing feelings and thoughts directly in a way that is not coercive or manipulative	An individual reaffirms to another that going to a ball game is not what he or she wants to do.
Self-observation	Reflecting feelings, thoughts, motivation, and behavior and responding to them appropriately	An individual notices an irritation at his friend's late arrival and decides to tell the friend of the irritation.
Splitting	Compartmentalizing opposite affect states and failing to integrate the positive and negative qualities of the self or others into cohesive images.	Self and object images tend to alternate between polar opposites: exclusively loving, powerful, worthy, nurturant, and kind—or exclusively bad, hateful, angry, destructive, rejecting, or worthless. One friend is wonderful and another former friend, who was at one time viewed as being perfect, is now believed to be an evil person.
Sublimation	Channeling potentially maladaptive feelings or impulses into socially acceptable behavior	An adolescent boy is very angry with his parents. On the football field, he tackles someone very forcefully.
Suppression	Intentionally avoiding thinking about disturbing problems, wishes, feelings, or experiences	A student is anxiously awaiting test results, but goes to a movie to stop thinking about it.
Undoing	Words or behavior designed to negate or to make amends symbolically for unacceptable thoughts, feelings, or actions	A man has sexual fantasies about his wife's sister. He takes his wife away for a romantic weekend.

*These defense mechanisms and coping styles are identified in the *DSM-IV* as being used when the individual deals with emotional conflict or stressors (either internal or external).

Adapted from the American Psychiatric Association. (2000). *Diagnostic and statistical manual of mental disorders* (4th ed., Text revision, pp. 811–814). Washington, DC: Author.

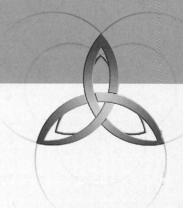

Glossary

absorption   Movement of drug from the site of administration into plasma.

abuse   Use of alcohol or drugs for the purpose of intoxication or, in the case of prescription drugs, for purposes beyond the intended use.

accommodation   Adjustment in cognitive organization that results from the demands of reality (Piaget).

accreditation   Process by which a mental health agency is judged by established standards to be providing acceptable quality of care.

acculturation   Act or process of assuming the beliefs, values, and practices of another, usually dominant culture.

acetylcholine (ACh)   An important neurotransmitter associated with cognitive functioning, and disruption of cholinergic mechanisms damages memory in animals and humans.

acetylcholinesterase (AChE)   Key enzyme that inactivates the neurotransmitter acetylcholine. AChE is found in high concentrations in the brain and is one of two cholinesterase enzymes capable of breaking down ACh.

acetylcholinesterase inhibitors (AChEI)   Mainstay of pharmacologic treatment of dementia; these drugs inhibit AChE, resulting in an enhancement of cholinergic activity. AChEIs have been shown to delay the decline in cognitive functioning but generally do not improve cognitive function once it has declined; therefore, it is important that this medication be started as soon as the diagnosis is made.

active listening   Focusing on what the patient is saying in order to interpret and respond to the message in an objective manner, while using techniques such as open-ended statements, reflection, and questions that elicit additional responses from the patient.

acute stress disorder (ASD)   A mental disorder characterized by persistent, distressing stress-related symptoms that last between 2 days and 1 month and that occur within 1 month after a traumatic experience.

adaptability   Capacity of a person to survive and flourish.

adaptive inflexibility   Rigidity in interactions with others, achievement of goals, and coping with stress.

addiction   Severe psychological and behavioral dependence on drugs or alcohol.

adherence   An individual's ability to follow directions for self-administration of medications and other biologic therapies; compliance.

advanced practice psychiatric–mental health nurse   A licensed registered nurse who is educationally prepared at the master's level and is nationally certified as a specialist by the American Nurses Credentialing Center (AANC).

advance care directives   Treatment directives (living wills) and appointment directives (power of attorney or health proxies) that apply only if the individual is unable to make his or her own decisions because the patient is incapacitated or, in the opinion of two physicians, is otherwise unable to make decisions for himself or herself.

adverse reactions   Unwanted medication effects that may have serious physiologic consequences.

affect   An expression of mood manifest in a pattern of observable behaviors.

affective blunting   Flat or blunted emotion.

affective instability   Rapid and extreme shifts in mood, erratic emotional responses to situations, and intense sensitivity to criticism or perceived slights; one of the core characteristics of borderline personality disorder.

affective lability   Abrupt, dramatic, unprovoked changes in the types of emotions expressed.

afferent   Toward the central nervous system or a particular structure.

affinity   Degree of attraction or strength of the bond between a drug and its receptor.

aggression   Behaviors or attitudes that reflect rage, hostility, and the potential for physical or verbal destructiveness; usually occurs if the person believes someone is going to do him or her harm.

agitation   Inability to sit still or attend to others, accompanied by heightened emotions and tension.

agnosia   Failure to recognize or identify objects despite intact sensory function, or a disturbance in executive functioning (ability to think abstractly, plan, initiate, sequence, monitor, and stop complex behavior).

agonists   Chemicals producing the same biologic action as the neurotransmitter.

agoraphobia   Anxiety about being in places from which escape might be difficult or embarrassing, or about being in places in which help may not be readily available if a panic attack should occur.

akathisia   An extrapyramidal side effect from phenothiazine, which includes restlessness that is easily mistaken for anxiety or increased psychotic symptoms.

alcohol-induced persisting amnestic disorder   Cognitive impairment deficits related to substance abuse.

alcohol tolerance   A phenomenon producing a more rapid metabolism of alcohol and a decreased response to its sedating, motor, and anxiolytic effects.

alcohol withdrawal syndrome   A syndrome that occurs after the reduction of alcohol consumption, or when abstaining from alcohol after prolonged use, causing changes in vital signs, diaphoresis, and other adverse gastrointestinal and central nervous system side effects.

alexithymia   Inability to experience and communicate feelings consciously.

algorithms   Systematic decision trees that depict the flow of decisions and outcomes.

allodynia   Lowered pain threshold.

alogia   Brief, empty verbal responses; often referred to as *poverty of speech.*

ambivalence   Presence and expression of two opposing forces, leading to inaction.

amino acids   Building blocks of proteins that have different roles. Amino acids function as neurotransmitters in as many as 60% to 70% of synaptic sites in the brain.

amygdala   A bulb-like structure attached to the tail of the caudate and often considered part of the limbic system.

anger   An affective state experienced as the motivation to act in ways that warn, intimidate, or attack those who are perceived as challenging or threatening.

anhedonia   Inability to gain pleasure from activities.

animism   A child's belief that inanimate objects are alive.

anorexia nervosa   A life-threatening eating disorder characterized by refusal to maintain body weight appropriate for age, intense fear of gaining weight or becoming fat, a severely distorted body image, and refusal to acknowledge the seriousness of weight loss.

antagonists   Chemicals blocking the biologic response at a given receptor site.

anticholinergic crisis   A potentially life-threatening medical emergency that occurs as a result of overdose or sensitivity to drugs with anticholinergic properties.

antimotivational syndrome   Attributed to long-term marijuana use, a syndrome marked by apathy, diminished interest in activities and goals, poor job performance, and reduced short-term memory.

anxiety   Energy that arises when expectations that are present are not met (Peplau).

anxiogenic   Anxiety provoking.

anxiolytics   Drugs that reverse or diminish anxiety.

apathy   Reactions to stimuli that are decreased, along with a diminished interest and desire.

aphasia   Alterations in language ability.

apraxia   Impaired ability to execute motor activities despite intact motor functioning.

arachnoid layer   A thin, delicate sheet of collagenous tissue under the meningeal layer that follows the contours of the brain but does not dip down inside them.

area restriction   Limitation of patient mobility to a specified area for purposes of safety or behavior management.

assertive community treatment   Direct and individualized treatment and services provided by a selectively chosen interdisciplinary team that follows on a patient's progress during reintegration into the community.

assessment   Deliberate and systematic collection of biopsychosocial information or data to determine current and past health and functional status and to evaluate present and past coping patterns.

association areas   Areas of the cortex in which neighboring nerve fibers are related to the same sensory modality.

assortative mating   Tendency for individuals to select mates who are similar in genetically linked traits such as intelligence and personality styles.

atropine flush   Flushing of the face, neck, and upper arms due to a reflex blood vessel dilation that results from increased body temperature.

attachment   Emotional bond between the infant and parental figure.

attention   A complex mental process that involves concentrating on one activity to the exclusion of others, as well as sustaining interest over time.

autism   A form of thinking or a style of relating that focuses subjectively on "me" to the exclusion of "not me."

autistic thinking   Thinking restricted to the literal and immediate so that the individual has private rules of logic and reasoning that make no sense to others.

automatic thinking   Thinking that influences the person's actions or other thought; it is often subject to errors or tangible distortions of reality that contradict objective appraisals.

autonomic nervous system   Part of the nervous system that regulates involuntary vital functions including cardiac muscle, smooth muscles, and glands. It is composed of the sympathetic and parasympathetic systems.

autonomy   Concept that each person has the fundamental right of self-determination.

avolition   Inability to complete projects, assignments, or work.

axes   A term used to describe domains of information. In a psychiatric diagnosis, there are five domains: Axis I, clinical domain that is the focus of treatment; Axis II, personality disorders or mental retardation, Axis III, general medical condition; Axis IV, psychosocial stress, and Axis V, level of functioning.

basal ganglia   One set of structures in each hemisphere; areas of gray matter containing many cell bodies or nuclei.

basic level of practice   According to the *Scope and Standards of Psychiatric–Mental Health Nursing*, this level includes two groups of nurses. The first group includes registered nurses who practice in psychiatric settings; the second includes those who have a baccalaureate degree in nursing and have worked in the field for 2 years.

behavior therapy   Interventions that reinforce or promote desirable behaviors or alter undesirable ones.

behavioral sensitization   A phenomenon by which a person has a magnified stress response to milder stressors after one or more exposures to a severe, uncontrollable stressor.

behaviorism   A paradigm shift in understanding human behavior that was initiated by Watson, who theorized that human behavior is developed through a stimulus–response process rather than through unconscious drives or instincts.

beneficence   The health care provider uses knowledge of science and incorporates the art of caring to develop an environment in which individuals achieve maximum health care potential.

bereavement   A period of profound grieving following a loss.

bibliotherapy   The use of books and other reading materials to help individuals cope with various life stressors.

binge eating   Episodes of uncontrollable, ravenous eating of large amounts of food within discrete periods of time, usually followed by feelings of guilt that result in purging.

bioavailability   Amount of a drug that reaches the systemic circulation for targeted treatment.

biogenic amines   Small molecules manufactured in the neuron that contain an amine group. These include dopamine, norepinephrine, and epinephrine (all synthesized from the amino acid tyrosine), serotonin (from tryptophan), and histamine (from histidine).

biologic dimension   Part of the biopsychosocial model that explains the biologic knowledge of mental health, including pathogenesis and treatment of mental illness.

biologic markers   Physical indicators of disturbances within the central nervous system that differentiate one disease state from another.

biologic view   A theoretic view or argument of the early 1900s that mental illness has a biologic cause and can be treated with physical interventions.

biopsychosocial model   An organizational model consisting of three separate but interdependent dimensions: biologic, psychological, and social. Each dimension has an independent knowledge and treatment focus but can interact and be mutually interdependent with the other dimensions.

biosexual identity   Anatomic and physiologic state of being male or female that results from genetic and hormonal influences.

bipolar type   A subtype of schizophrenic disorder in which the patient exhibits manic symptoms alone or with a mix of manic and depressive symptoms.

board-and-care homes Facilities that provide 24-hour supervision and assistance with medications, meals, and some self-care skills, but in which individualized attention to self-care skills and other activities of daily living is generally not available.

body dysmorphic disorder Disorder in which there is a preoccupation with an imagined or slight defect in appearance, such as a large nose, thinning hair, or small genitals.

body image How each individual perceives his or her own body, separate from how the world or society views him or her.

body image disturbance Extreme discrepancy between one's perception of one's own body image and others' perceptions of one.

boundaries Limits in which a person may act or refrain from acting within a designated time or place.

bradykinesia An extrapyramidal condition characterized by a slowness of voluntary movement and speech.

brain stem Area of the brain containing the midbrain, pons, and medulla, which continues beneath the thalamus.

breach of confidentiality Release of patient information without the patient's consent in the absence of legal compulsion or authorization to release information.

Broca's area A section of the left frontal lobe of the brain thought to be responsible for the articulation of speech.

bulimia nervosa An eating disorder in which the individual engages in recurrent episodes of binge eating and compensatory behavior to avoid weight gain through purging methods such as self-induced vomiting, or use of laxatives, diuretics, enemas, or emetics, or through nonpurging methods such as fasting or excessive exercise.

butyrylcholinesterase (BuChE) A nonspecific cholinesterase found in the brain and especially in the glial cells. Both acetylcholinesterase and BuChE work in the gastrointestinal tract. If these enzymes are inhibited the breakdown of acetylcholine will be delayed, resulting in an increase in acetylcholine activity.

case management Problem solving and coordinating services for the patient to ensure continuity of services and overcome system rigidity, fragmentation of services, misuse of facilities, and inaccessibility.

cataplexy Bilateral loss of muscle tone triggered by a strong emotion such as laughter. This muscle atonia can range from subtle (drooping eyelids) to dramatic (buckling knees). Eye and respiratory muscles are not affected. Cataplexy usually lasts only seconds. Individuals are fully conscious, oriented, and alert during the episode. Prolonged episodes of cataplexy may lead to sleep episodes.

catatonic excitement Hyperactivity characterized by purposeless activity and abnormal movements like grimacing and posturing.

categoric diagnosis A subset of a given diagnosis that consists of criteria that include or exclude data for the purpose of giving a name to a set of symptoms.

central sulcus Posterior boundary of the frontal lobe that separates it from the parietal lobe.

cerebellum Part of the brain that is responsible for controlling movement and postural adjustments; it receives information from all parts of the body.

cerebrospinal fluid Cushioning fluid that circulates around the brain beneath the arachnoid layer in the subarachnoid space; it is colorless and contains sodium chloride and other salts.

chemical restraints Use of medication to control patients or manage behavior.

cholecystokinin A neuropeptide found in high levels in the cerebral cortex, hypothalamus, and amygdala; it is also excreted by the gastrointestinal system in response to food intake, which is believed to play a role in the control of eating and satiety by controlling the release of dopamine.

choroid plexus A collection of cells within the ventricles that produces cerebrospinal fluid.

chronic depression Depression that persists for months to years and that may be associated with some disability or distress.

chronic disaffiliation Lacking the love and support that come from being associated with a solid network of family and friends.

chronobiology Study and measure of time structures or biologic rhythms.

circadian rhythm (cycle) From the Latin *circa* and *dies*, meaning "about a day"; refers to a biologic system that fluctuates or oscillates in a pattern that repeats itself in about a day.

circumstantiality Extremely detailed and lengthy discourse about a topic.

clang association Repetition of word phrases that are similar in sound but in no other way, for example, "right, light, sight, might."

classical conditioning A learning situation in which an unconditioned stimulus initially produces an unconditioned response; over time, a conditioned response is elicited for a specific stimulus (Pavlov).

clearance Total amount of blood, serum, or plasma from which a drug is completely removed per unit of time.

clinical decision making A specific type of decision making that focuses on the decisions made in a clinical setting.

clinical domain outcome statements Statements that indicate a reduction in symptoms of illness or cure of a specific mental illness.

clinical path A plan of care for patients with a common problem represented by flow charts that usually contain assessment parameters, nursing diagnoses, nursing interventions, and outcomes.

closed group A group in which all the members begin at one time. New members are not admitted after the first meeting.

clubhouse model Psychosocial rehabilitation approach with the goal of integrating individuals with mental illness back into the community; these houses are run entirely by the patients or "clubhouse members."

codependence A maladaptive coping pattern in family members or others closely related to a substance abuser that results from prolonged exposure to the behaviors of the alcohol- or drug-dependent person; characterized by boundary distortions, poor relationship and friendship skills, compulsive and obsessive behaviors, inappropriate anger, sexual maladjustment, and resistance to change.

cognition A high level of intellectual processing in which perceptions and information are acquired, used, or manipulated.

cognitive appraisal The process of examining the demands, constraints, and resources of the environment and of negotiating them with personal goals and beliefs.

cognitive schema Patterns of thoughts that determine how a person interprets events. Each person's cognitive schema screen, code, and evaluate incoming stimuli.

cognitive therapy Interventions that reinforce and promote desirable cognitive functioning or alter undesirable cognitive functioning.

communication blocks Interruptions in the content flow of communication that can be identified in process recordings as such changes in topic that either the nurse or patient makes.

communication disorders Disorders that involve speech or language impairments.

communication triad A technique used to provide a specific syntax and order for patients to identify and express their feelings and seek relief. The "sentence" consists of three parts: (1) an "I" statement to identify the prevailing feeling, (2) a nonjudgmental statement of the emotional trigger, and (3) a statement of what the person would like differently or what would restore comfort to the situation.

comorbidity (comorbid) Disease that coexists with the primary disease.

competence The degree to which the patient is able to understand and appreciate the information given during the consent process; the patient's cognitive ability to process information at a specific time; the patient's ability to gather and interpret information and make reasonable judgments based on that information to participate fully as a partner in treatment.

compliance The individual's ability to follow directions for self-administration of medications and other biologic therapies; adherence.

comprehensive assessment Collection of all relevant data to identify problems for which a nursing diagnosis is stated.

concrete thinking Lack of abstraction in thinking, in which people are unable to understand punch lines, metaphors, and analogies.

confidentiality An ethical duty of nondisclosure; the patient has the right to disclose personal information without fear of it being revealed to others.

conflict resolution A specific type of counseling in which the nurse helps the patient resolve a disagreement or dispute.

confused speech and thinking Symptoms of schizophrenia that render the patient unable to respond accurately to the ordinary signs and sounds of daily living.

connections Mutually responsive and enhancing relationships.

conservation The child's awareness that a quantity remains the same despite its shape.

constraints Limitations that are both personal (internalized cultural values and beliefs) and environmental (finite resources such as money and time).

content themes Repetition of concerns or feelings that occur within the therapeutic relationship. Themes may emerge as symbolic representations of fears.

continuum of care Providing care in an integrated system of settings, services (physical, psychological, and social), and care levels appropriate to the individual's specific needs in a continuous manner over time, with channels of communication among the service providers.

coordination of care Integration of the various components of the continuum of care, including the pre-entry, entry, pre-exit, and exit phases.

coping Thinking and acting in ways to manage specific external and internal demands and conflicts that are taxing or exceeding one's resources.

corpus callosum Functional link between the two hemispheres of the brain, made up of a thick band of fibers.

cortex Outer surface of the mature brain.

cortical dementia A type of dementia that is characterized by amnesia, aphasia, apraxia, and agnosia.

counseling interventions Specific time-limited interactions between a nurse and a patient, family, or group experiencing intermediate or ongoing difficulties related to their health or well-being.

countertransference The nurse's reactions to a patient that are based on the nurse's unconscious needs, conflicts, problems, and views of the world. It can significantly interfere with the nurse–patient relationship.

crisis A severely stressful experience for which coping mechanisms fail to provide any adaptation, whether the experience is positive or negative.

crisis intervention A specialized short-term (usually no longer than 6 hours) goal-directed therapy designed to assist patients in an immediate manner, after which they are usually transferred to an inpatient unit or to an intensive outpatient setting.

critical thinking An analytic and complex process that involves observing behaviors and responses; making purposeful, objective judgments; and constantly re-evaluating.

cultural brokering Act of bridging, linking, or mediating between groups or individuals of different cultural systems for the purpose of reducing conflict or producing change.

cultural competence A process (developed through cultural awareness, acquisition of cultural knowledge, development of cultural skills, and engagement in numerous cultural encounters) in which the nurse continually strives to achieve the ability to work effectively within the cultural context of an individual or community from a diverse cultural or ethnic background.

culture Any group of people who identify or associate with each other on the basis of some common purpose, need, or similarity of background; the set of learned, socially transmitted beliefs and behaviors that arise from interpersonal transactions among members of the cultural group.

cycle of violence A three-phase pattern of tension, abuse, and kindness in which the abuser engages first in abuse and then in seemingly sincere expressions of love, contrition, and remorse.

cyclothymic A term used to describe periods of hypomanic and depressive episodes that do not meet full criteria for a major depressive episode.

cytoarchitectonic analysis Study of the distribution and arrangement of cells within various parts of the brain using various staining procedures to identify differences throughout the brain.

de-escalation An interactive process of calming and redirecting a patient who has an immediate potential for violence directed at others or self.

defense levels Division of defense mechanisms that includes high adaptive, mental inhibitions (compromise formation), minor image-distorting, disavowal, major image-distorting, action level, and defense dysregulation.

defense mechanisms Coping styles; the automatic psychological process protecting the individual against anxiety and creating awareness of internal or external dangers or stressors.

defining characteristics Clues given by the signs and symptoms that join together in the nurse's mind to form a cluster that leads to a specific nursing diagnosis.

deinstitutionalization Release of patients with severe and persistent mental illness from state mental hospitals to community settings.

delirium tremens An acute withdrawal syndrome that occurs often in alcoholics after 10 or more years of heavy drinking and is characterized by tachycardia, sweating, hypertension, irregular tremor, delusions, vivid hallucinations, and wild, agitated behavior.

delusion Erroneous belief that usually involves a misinterpretation of perception of experience. These beliefs are false, fixed, and fall outside of the patient's social, cultural, or religious background.

delusional disorder A disorder in which there is the presence of nonbizarre delusions; includes several subtypes: ergotomania, grandiose, jealous, somatic, mixed, and specified.

demands External pulls (crowding, crime, noise, pollution) imposed by the physical environment, and internal pulls (behavior and role expectations) imposed by the social environment.

dementia From the Latin de (from or out of) and *mens* (mind); several cognitive deficits (one of which is impaired memory) that are due to the direct physiologic effects of a general medical condition, the persisting effects of a substance, or multiple biologic etiologies.

denial The patient's inability to accept loss of control over substance use or the severity of the consequences associated with substance abuse.

depersonalization A nonspecific experience in which the individual loses a sense of personal identity and feels strange or unreal.

depressive episode In a major depressive episode, either a depressed mood or a loss of interest or pleasure in nearly all activities must be present for at least 2 weeks. Four of seven additional symptoms must be present: disruption in sleep, appetite (or weight), concentration, energy; psychomotor agitation or retardation; excessive guilt or feelings of worthlessness; suicidal ideation.

depressive type A subtype of schizophrenic disorder in which the patient displays only symptoms of a major depressive episode during the illness.

desensitization A rapid decrease in drug effects that may develop within a few minutes or over a period of days, months, years, or lifetime of exposure to a drug.

detoxification Process of safely and effectively withdrawing a person from an addictive substance, usually under medical supervision.

developmental delay The impairment of normal growth and development that may not be reversible.

diagnosis-specific outcomes Outcomes based on nursing diagnoses.

Dialectical Behavior Therapy (DBT) An important biosocial approach to treatment that combines numerous cognitive and behavior therapy strategies. It requires patients to understand their disorder by actively participating in formulating treatment goals by collecting data about their own behavior, identifying treatment targets in individual therapy, and working with the therapists in changing these target behaviors.

dichotomous thinking Tendency to view things as absolute, either black or white, good or bad, with no perception of compromise.

differentiation of self An individual's resolution of attachment to his or her family's emotional chaos. It involves an intrapsychic separation of thinking from feelings and an interpersonal freeing of oneself from the chaos.

dimensional diagnoses A system of diagnosing patient problems by locating and describing them on a specified continuum; for example, aggression may be characterized as existing somewhere on a continuum from verbal anger to physical assault.

direct leadership behavior The leader controls the interaction of the group by giving directions and information and allowing little discussion.

discharge outcomes Those outcomes to be met before discharge.

discipline-specific outcomes Patient outcomes based on the standards of the discipline using them. These outcomes can be used to evluate the individual practitioner's practice.

disconnections Lack of mutually responsive and enhancing relationships.

discrimination The differential treatment of others because they are members of a particular group.

disinhibition A concept borrowed from physics and biology and based on the idea of a dynamic, self-regulatory model of equilibrium in which equilibrium is defined (Piaget) as compensation for external disturbance; a mechanism for providing the self-regulation by which intelligence adapts to internal and external changes.

disordered water balance A state of chronic fluid imbalance, vacillating between normal and hyponatremic, that commonly occurs in psychiatric patients with chronic illnesses.

dissociation A disruption in the normally occurring linkages among subjective awareness, feelings, thoughts, behavior, and memories.

dissociative identity disorder (DID) A mental disorder characterized by the existence of two or more distinct identities with unique personality characteristics and the inability to recall important information about oneself or events.

dissupport The presence of relationships that are harmful, stressful, and damaging to a person's self-esteem.

distraction Consciously changing behaviors to take the focus off the physical sensations or unwanted thoughts, feelings, or behaviors.

distribution The amount of a drug that may be found in various tissues at the site of the drug action for which it is intended.

disturbances of executive functioning Problems in the ability to think abstractly, plan, initiate, sequence, monitor, and stop complex behavior.

diurnal weight gain Weight gain that occurs throughout a day that is caused by fluid and food intake that is regulated by the circadian rhythm.

domestic abuse Violence, including rape, directed toward a person by an intimate partner.

dosing Administration of medication over time so that therapeutic levels may be achieved or maintained without reaching toxic levels.

drug overdose A dose of a drug that causes an acute reaction such as agitation, delirium, coma, or death.

dual diagnosis Presence of both a psychoactive substance dependency and mental illness.

dura mater The tough layer of collagen fibers that forms a loose sac around the central nervous system (in Latin, "hard mother") and contains three layers: meningeal, arachnoid, and pia mater.

dyad A group of only two people who are usually related, such as a married couple, siblings, or parent and child.

dysfunctional family A family whose interactions, decisions, or behaviors interfere with the positive development of the family and its individual members.

dyslexia Significantly lower score for mental age on standardized test in reading that is not due to low intelligence or inadequate schooling.

dyspareunia A sexual pain disorder characterized by genital pain in men and women associated with sexual intercourse.

dysphagia Difficulty swallowing.

dysphoric (mood) Depressed, disquieted, and/or restless.

dyssomnia A disorder of initiating or maintaining sleep or of excessive sleepiness.

dysthymic disorder A milder but more chronic form of major depressive disorder.

dystonia An impairment in muscle tone that is generally the first extrapyramidal symptom to occur, usually within a few days of initiating an antipsychotic. Dystonia is characterized by involuntary muscle spasms, especially of the head and neck muscles.

early intervention programs Community outreach efforts designed to work with infants and preschool-aged children and their caretakers to foster healthy physical, psychological, social, and intellectual development.

echolalia Parrot-like repetition of another's words; inappropriate choice of topics.

echopraxia Involuntary imitation of another person's movements and gestures; regressed behavior that is child-like or immature.

efferent Away from the central nervous system or other particular structure.

efficacy Ability of a drug to produce a response as a result of the receptor or receptors being occupied.

egocentrism Tendency to view the world as revolving around oneself.

emotion Psychophysiologic reaction that defines a person's mood and can be categorized as negative (anger, fright, anxiety, guilt, shame, sadness, envy, jealousy, and disgust), positive (happiness, pride, relief, and love), or somewhat ambiguous, or borderline (hope, compassion, empathy, sympathy, and contentment).

emotional abuse In reference to adults: degrading, threatening, stalking, or otherwise using psychological violence; in reference to children: rejecting, isolating, terrorizing, ignoring, or corrupting.

emotional dysregulation Inability to control emotion in social interactions.

emotional regulation A biosocial interaction between the innate emotional vulnerability of the individual and the ability to modulate that emotion in social interactions.

emotional vulnerability Sensitivity and reactivity to environmental stress.

emotion-focused coping A type of coping that changes the meaning of the situation.

empathetic linkage Ability to feel in oneself the feelings being expressed by another person or persons.

empathy A voluntary, nonprimordial experiencing of the situation of another within some form of interaction or relationship.

encopresis Soiling clothing with feces or depositing feces in inappropriate places.

endorphins Neurotransmitters that have opiate-like behavior and produce an inhibitory effect at opiate receptor sites; probably responsible for pain tolerance.

enuresis Involuntary excretion of urine after the age at which a child should have attained bladder control.

epidemiology The study of patterns of disease distribution in time and space that focuses on the health status of population groups or aggregates, rather than on individuals, and involves quantitative analysis of the occurrence of illnesses in population groups; basic science of public health.

epigenesis A concept borrowed from embryology: if a particular part does not manifest itself during the appropriate phase, it cannot reach full development because the moment for doing so has passed; each developmental stage must be completed at the appropriate time, or successful completion of the stage will not occur.

episode A period of a minimal duration of 2 weeks during which an individual experiences symptoms that meet the diagnostic criteria for that disorder.

epithalamus Area above and medial to the thalamus and adjacent to the roof of the third ventricle.

equilibration Compensation for external disturbances; a mechanism for providing the self-regulation by which intelligence adapts to external and internal changes (Piaget).

erectile dysfunction Inability of a male to achieve or maintain an erection sufficient for completion of sexual activity.

ergotomania Delusional belief that the person is loved intensely by the loved object, who is usually married and of a higher socioeconomic status, making him or her unattainable.

ethnic (ethnicity) People classified according to common traits, customs, thinking, and judgment.

euphoric (mood) An elated mood.

euthymic (mood) A normal mood.

exhibitionism A behavior associated with paraphilias involving exposing one's genitals to strangers, with occasional masturbation.

expansive (mood) A mood characterized by inappropriate lack of restraint in expressing one's feelings and frequently overvaluing one's own importance. Expansive qualities include an unceasing and indiscriminate enthusiasm for interpersonal, sexual, or occupational interactions.

exposure therapy The treatment of choice for agoraphobia that puts the patient into contact with the feared situations until the stimuli no longer produce anxiety.

expressed emotion Family members' responses that include one or more of the following dynamics: critical comments, hostility, or emotional overinvolvement.

extended family Several nuclear families who may or may not live together and function as one group.

external advocacy system Organizations that operate outside mental health agencies and serve as advocates for the treatment and rights of mental health patients.

externalizing disorders Disorders that are characterized by acting-out behavior.

extinction Elimination of a classically conditioned response by the repeated presentation of the conditioned stimulus without the unconditioned stimulus, or elimination of an operantly conditioned response by no longer presenting the reward after the response.

extrapyramidal motor system Collection of neuronal pathways that provides significant input in involuntary motor movements.

factitious disorder A type of psychiatric disorder characterized by somatization, in which the person intentionally causes an illness for the purpose of becoming a patient.

family development A broad term that refers to all the processes connected with the growth of a family, including changes associated with work, geographic location, migration, acculturation, and serious illness.

family dynamics The patterned interpersonal and social interactions that occur within the family structure over the life of a family.

family life cycle A process of expansion, contraction, and realignment of relationship systems to support the entry, exit, and development of family members.

family preservation Efforts made by professionals to preserve the family unit by preventing the removal of children from their homes through parental support and education and through work to facilitate a secure attachment between the child and parent.

family projection process The family projects its conflicts onto the child or spouse, and this member becomes the center of family conflicts.

family structure According to Minuchin, the organized pattern within which family members interact.

fear conditioning A type of classic conditioning in which a previously neutral stimulus (conditioned stimulus) elicits a fear response (conditioned response) after it has been paired with an aversive stimulus (unconditioned stimulus) that produces fear (unconditioned response).

fetal alcohol syndrome A syndrome that occurs in infants whose mothers ingested alcohol during pregnancy; includes symptoms such as permanent brain damage, often resulting in mental retardation.

fetishism A behavior associated with paraphilias, involving using an object for sexual arousal.

fissures The grooves of the cerebrum.

flight of ideas Repeated and rapid changes in the topic of conversation, generally with just one sentence or phrase.

flooding A type of therapy for agoraphobia in which highly anxiety-provoking stimuli are presented to the patient in vivo or with imagery, with no relaxation until the anxiety dissipates.

folk That which originates or is traditional to a group of people.

forensic commitment A special type of involuntary commitment of individuals with mental disorders who have been charged with a crime and are criminally committed to a mental hospital.

formal group roles The designated leader and members of a group.

formal operations The ability to use abstract reasoning to conceptualize and solve problems.

formal support system Large organizations that provide care to individuals, such as hospitals and nursing homes.

frontal, occipital, parietal, temporal Lobes of the brain located on the lateral surface of each hemisphere.

frotteurism A behavior associated with paraphilias, characterized by sexually arousing urges, fantasies, and behaviors resulting from touching or rubbing one's genitals on the breasts, genitals, or thighs of a nonconsenting person.

functional activities Activities of daily living necessary for self-care (ie, bathing, toileting, dressing, and transferring).

functional status Extent to which a person has the ability to carry out independent personal care, home management, and social functions in everyday life that has meaning and purpose.

gate-control theory Pain response based on the theory that pain perception involves pathways in the dorsal horn of the spinal column that relay noxious stimuli to the brain and that certain other nerve fibers function as an antagonistic "gate" to augment or dampen the subjective experience of pain.

gender identity A sense of self as being male or female.

gender identity disorder Disorder characterized by a strong and persistent identification with the opposite sex and the desire or perception that one is of that gender.

gender role How one functions and behaves as a male or a female in relation to others in society, also referred to as *sex role identity*.

generic caring A phrase coined by Leininger to mean the foundational prototype included in local home remedies and folklore.

genogram A multigenerational schematic diagram that lists family members and their relationships.

gentrification The refurbishing of homes and buildings in run-down neighborhoods and the subsequent raising of rents.

glia (white matter) A fatty or lipid substance with a white appearance that surrounds the pathways of the cell body axons.

global risk factors Risk factors such as poverty, prejudice, and inadequate living situations that are associated with the risk for a mental disorder.

gray matter The cortex, with its gray-brown color because of the capillary blood vessels.

group Two or more people who are in an interdependent relationship with one another.

group cohesion Forces that act on the members to stay in a group.

group density effect An effect that accounts for the observed reality that individuals who live within their own cultural groups are protected from stressors that afflict people living as isolated minorities in a larger, incompatible culture or milieu.

group dynamics Interactions within groups.

group process The culmination of the session-to-session interactions of the members that move the group toward its goals.

groupthink The tendency of many groups to avoid conflict and adopt a normative pattern of thinking that is often consistent with the group leader's ideas.

gyri Bumps and convolutions in the brain.

half-life The time required for plasma concentrations of a drug to be reduced by 50%.

hallucinations Perceptual experiences that occur in the absence of actual external sensory stimuli and may be auditory, visual, tactile, gustatory, or olfactory.

hallucinogen A class of drug that produces euphoria or dysphoria, altered body image, distorted or sharpened visual and auditory perception, confusion, uncoordination, and impaired judgment and memory.

hallucinogen persisting perceptual disorder A transient and intermittent disorder associated with the longterm use of hallucinogens; includes depression, prolonged psychosis, and flashbacks.

hippocampus Subcortical gray matter embedded within each temporal lobe that may be involved in determining the best way to store information or memory; "time-dating" memory.

HIV-1-associated cognitive-motor complex Neurologic complications that occur with HIV-1 that are directly attributable to infection of the brain and include impaired cognitive and motor function.

homeless A description of a person who lives for a sustained period of time on the street, in a public shelter, or in other temporary living quarters.

homelessness State of being without a consistent dwelling place.

home visits Delivery of nursing care in a patient's living environment.

homophobia An intense fear of any contact whatsoever with gays or homosexuals and a dislike of homosexual lifestyles.

human sexual response cycle Usually viewed as consisting of four phases: excitement, plateau, orgasm, and resolution.

humanitarian domain outcome statements Statements that spell out behaviors or responses that show a sense of well-being of patients and personal fulfillment of patients and family members.

hyperactivity Excessive motor activity, movement, and/or utterances that may be either purposeless or aimless.

hyperalgia Increased nociceptor sensitivity.

hyperesthesia Increased sensation of pain.

hyperkinetic delirium A type of delirium in which the patient demonstrates behaviors most commonly recognized as delirium, including psychomotor hyperactivity, marked excitability, and a tendency toward hallucinations.

hypersexuality Inappropriate and socially unacceptable sexual behavior. The patient begins talking and behaving in ways that are uncharacteristic of the patient's behavior.

hypersomnia Oversleeping.

hypervigilance Sustained attention to external stimuli as if expecting something important or frightening to happen.

hypervocalization Screams, curses, moans, groans, and verbal repetitiveness that are common in the later stages of cognitively impaired elders, often occurring during a hospitalization or nursing home placement.

hypnagogic hallucinations Intense dream-like images that occur when an individual is falling asleep and usually involve the immediate environment.

hypokinetic delirium A type of delirium in which the patient is lethargic, somnolent, and apathetic and exhibits reduced psychomotor activity.

hypomanic episode Mildly dysphoric mood that meets the same criteria as for a manic episode except that it lasts at least 4 days rather than 1 week and that no marked impairment in social or occupational functioning is present.

hyponatremia Decreased sodium concentration in the blood.

hyposthenuria Secretion of urine with a low specific gravity.

hypothalamus Immediately ventral and slightly anterior to the thalamus, forming the floor and part of the walls of the third ventricle.

hypothalamic–pituitary-adrenal (HPA) axis Neurotransmitters responsible for behavioral responses to fear and anxiety that are usually held in balance until information from the sensory processing areas in the thalamus and cortex alerts the amygdala. If events are interpreted as threatening, this axis is activated, initiating the stress response.

identity An integration of a person's social and occupational roles and affiliations, self-attributed personality traits, attitudes about gender roles, beliefs about sexuality and intimacy, long-term goals, political ideology, and religious beliefs.

identity diffusion Occurs when parts of a person's identity are absent or poorly developed; a lack of consistent sense of identity.

illusions Disorganized perceptions that create an oversensitivity to colors, shapes, and background activities, which occur when the person misperceives or exaggerates stimuli in the external environment.

implosive therapy An imaginal technique useful in treating agoraphobia in which the therapist identifies individual phobic stimuli for the patient and then presents highly anxiety-provoking imagery in a dramatic fashion.

impulsiveness A sudden, irresistible urge or desire resulting from a particular feeling that can lead to an action.

impulsivity Acting without considering the consequences of the act or alternative actions.

incidence A rate that includes only new cases that have occurred within a clearly defined time period.

incompetent A person is legally determined not to be able to understand and appreciate the information given during the consent process.

indicated preventive interventions   Preventive interventions that are targeted to high-risk individuals who are identified as having minimal but detectable signs and symptoms foreshadowing a disorder or as having biologic markers indicating a predisposition, but not the actual disorder.

indicators   Representation of the dimension of outcome answering the question of how close the patient is coming toward an outcome.

indirect leader   Leader who primarily reflects the group members' discussion and offers little guidance or information to the group.

individual roles   Group roles that either enhance or detract from the group's functioning but have nothing to do with either the group task or maintenance.

individual treatment plan   A plan of care that identifies the patient's problems, outcomes, interventions, the individuals assigned to implement interventions, and evaluation criteria.

informal group roles   Positions in the group with rights and duties directed toward other group members. These positions are not formally sanctioned.

informal support systems   Family members, friends, and neighbors who can provide care and support to the individual.

informed consent   The right to determine what shall be done with one's own body and mind. To provide informed consent, the patient must be given adequate information on which to base decisions about care. The patient ultimately decides the course of treatment.

inhalants   Organic solvents, also known as volatile substances, that are central nervous system depressants and when inhaled cause euphoria, sedation, emotional lability, and impaired judgment.

in-home mental health care   The provision of skilled mental health nursing care under the direction of a psychiatrist or physician for individuals in their residences.

initial outcomes   Those outcomes written after the patient interview and assessment.

insight   The ability of the individual to be aware of his or her own thoughts and feelings and to compare them with the thoughts and feelings of others.

insomnia (initial)   Difficulty falling asleep.

instrumental activities   Activities that facilitate or enhance the performance of activities of daily living (eg, shopping, using the telephone, transportation). These aspects are critical to consider for any older adult living alone.

integration   Incorporation of disparate ethnic or religious elements of the population into a unified society; the process by which networks communicate efficiently through cellular mechanisms that synthesize information from thousands of excitatory and inhibitory chemical signals before determining whether to respond.

intensive outpatient programs   Programs focused on continued stabilization and prevention of relapse in vulnerable individuals who have returned to job or school, usually with sessions running 3 days per week and lasting 3 to 4 hours per day.

interdisciplinary approach   Interventions from different disciplines integrated into the delivery of patient care.

interdisciplinary treatment plan   A plan of care that identifies the patient's problems, outcomes, interventions, and members of different disciplines assigned to implement interventions, and evaluation criteria.

internal rights protection system   Patient protective mechanisms developed by the United States mental health care system's organizations to help combat any violation of mental health patients' rights, including investigating any incidents of abuse or neglect.

internalizing disorders   Anxiety disorders and depression in which the symptoms tend to be within the individual.

interoceptive conditioning   Pairing a somatic discomfort, such as dizziness or palpitations, with an impending panic attack.

interpersonal relations   Characteristic interaction patterns that occur between human beings that are the basis of emotional and social connections.

intrinsic activity   The ability of a drug to produce a biologic response when it becomes attached to its receptor.

invalidating environment   A highly personal social situation that negates the individual's emotional responses and communication.

involuntary commitment   The confined hospitalization of a person without his or her consent, but with a court order (because the person has been judged to be a danger to self or others).

ischemic cascade   Cell breakdown resulting from brain cell injury.

judgment   The ability to reach a logical decision about a situation and to choose a course after looking at and analyzing various possibilities.

kindling   Repetitive stimulation of certain tracts may facilitate conduction of impulses in the future and lead to enhancement of intense behaviors after even mild stimulation.

kleptomania   A disorder in which the patient is unable to resist the urge to steal and independently steals items that he or she could easily afford. These items are not particularly useful or wanted. The underlying issue is the act of stealing.

Korsakoff's syndrome   An amnestic syndrome in which there is a profound deficit in the ability to form new memories; associated with a variable deficit in recall of old memories despite a clear sensorium.

lability of mood   Rapid alternations of mood, usually between euphoria and irritability.

language   A higher-order aspect of formulating and comprehending verbal communication.

lateral (sylvian) fissure   Separates the inferior aspects of the frontal and parietal lobes from the temporal lobe.

lateral ventricles   The horn-shaped first and second ventricles that are the largest of the brain's ventricles.

learning disorder   A discrepancy between actual achievement and expected achievement that is based on a person's age and intellectual ability.

least restrictive environment   The patient has the right to treatment in an environment that restricts the exercise of free will to the least extent; an individual cannot be restricted to an institution when he or she can be successfully treated in the community.

life review   A therapeutic intervention using recall and memory to conduct a critical analysis of one's life.

limbic system (limbic lobe)   Structures including the septum and the fornix, as well as the amygdala, hippocampus, cingulate, parahippocampal gyrus, epithalamus, portions of the basal ganglia, paraolfactory area, and the anterior nucleus of the thalamus.

longitudinal fissure   The longest and deepest groove of the cerebrum that separates the right and left hemispheres.

loose associations   Absence of the normal connectedness of thoughts and ideas; sudden shifts without apparent relationship to preceding topic.

maintenance function   A term used to describe the informal role of group members that encourages the group to stay together.

maintenance interventions   Supportive, educational, and pharmacologic interventions, aimed at decreasing the disability associated with a disorder, that are provided on a long-term basis to individuals who have been diagnosed with a disorder.

malingering   To produce illness symptoms intentionally with an obvious self-serving goal such as being classified as disabled or avoiding work.

managed care organizations   Large health care organizations whose goals are to increase access to care and to provide the most appropriate level of services in the least restrictive setting, which includes more outpatient and alternative treatment programs, while trying to avoid costly inpatient hospitalizations; in the long term, allowing patients better access to quality services while using health care dollars wisely.

manic episode   A distinct period during which there is an abnormally and persistently elevated, expansive, or irritable mood.

memory   One aspect of cognitive function; an information storage system composed of short-term memory (retention of information over a brief period of time) and long-term memory (retention of an unlimited amount of information over an indefinite period of time).

memory   The ability to recall or reproduce what has been learned or experienced.

meningeal layer   The inner layer of dura mater that becomes continuous with the spinal dura mater and sends extensions into the brain for support and protection of the different lobes or structures.

mental disorder   A disorder that is associated with the presence of psychological distress; impairment in psychological, social, or occupational functioning; or a significantly increased risk for death, pain, disability, or an important loss of freedom.

mental health problem   A term used when signs and symptoms of mental illnesses occur but do not meet specified criteria for a disorder.

mental illness   A term used to mean all diagnosable mental disorders.

mental retardation   Significantly below-average intelligence accompanied by impaired adaptive functioning.

mental status examination   An organized systematic approach to assessment of an individual's current psychiatric condition.

mesocortical   Medial aspects of the cortex.

metabolism   Biotransformation, or the process by which a drug is altered.

metonymic speech   Use of words with similar meanings interchangeably.

middle insomnia   Waking up during the night and having difficulty returning to sleep.

milieu therapy   An approach using the total environment to provide a therapeutic community; a therapeutic environment.

misidentification   Delusions in which the person believes that a familiar person is replaced by an imposter.

mixed episode   Irritability or excitement and depression occurring at the same time.

modeling   Pervasive imitation; one person trying to be like another person.

mood   A pervasive and sustained emotion that colors a person's perception of the world.

mood disorder   A clinically significant behavioral or psychological syndrome or pattern that occurs in an individual whereby the primary alteration is evident in mood rather than in thought or perception.

moral idealism   To enjoy taking passionate philosophical positions on controversial issues such as abortion, sexism, legalization of drugs, gun use, and so forth.

moral treatment   An approach to curing mental illness, popular in the 1800s, which was built on the principles of kindness, compassion, and a pleasant environment.

motivational interviewing   Interviewing that helps the patient clarify personal goals and increases commitment to recovery; often used in treating people with substance abuse.

multiaxial diagnostic system   A diagnostic structure that includes more than one domain of information, such as the psychiatric diagnoses of the *DSM-IV-TR*.

multidisciplinary approach   Several disciplines providing services to a patient at one time.

multigenerational transmission process   The transmission of emotional processes from one generation to the next.

multiple sleep latency test (MSLT)   A standardized procedure that measures the amount of time a person takes to fall asleep during a 20-minute period.

music therapy   The controlled use of music to promote physiologic or psychological well-being.

myoclonus   Twitching or clonic spasms of a muscle group.

myoglobinuria   The presence of myohemoglobin in the urine due to sustained muscular rigidity and necrosis.

negative outcome criteria   Goals that direct interventions to prevent negative alterations in the patient such as complications, disabilities, or unwarranted death.

neglect   Failure to protect from injury or to provide for the physical, psychological, and medical needs of a child or dependent elder.

neologisms   Words that are made up that have no common meaning and are not recognized.

neuritic plaques   Extracellular lesions consisting of β-amyloid protein and apolipoprotein A (apoA) cores that form in the nucleus basalis of Meynert, gradually increase in number, and are abnormally distributed throughout the cholinergic system.

neurofibrillary tangles   Fibrous proteins, or *tau proteins*, that are chemically altered and twisted together and spread throughout the brain, interfering with nerve functioning in cholinergic neurons. It is hypothesized that formation of these neurofibrillary tangles are related to the apolipoprotein E_4 (apoE$_4$).

neurohormones   Hormones produced by cells within the nervous system, such as antidiuretic hormone (ADH).

neuroleptic malignant syndrome   A syndrome caused by neuroleptic medications that are dopamine receptor blockers. The classic signs and symptoms include hyperthermia, lead-pipe rigidity, changes in mental status, and autonomic nervous system changes.

neuropeptide Y   A recently discovered 36-amino-acid peptide that is a potent stimulator of feeding behavior especially selective for foods heavy in carbohydrates.

neuropeptides   Short chains of amino acids that exist in the central nervous system and have a number of important roles, including as neurotransmitters, neuromodulators, or neurohormones.

neuropsychiatric disorders   Those disease processes, toxic exposures, traumatic injuries, or other causes that change the structures in the central nervous system and produce psychiatric as well as neurologic symptoms.

neuropsychiatry   A subspecialty of psychiatry that combines neurology and psychiatry.

neurotransmitters   Small molecules that directly and indirectly control the opening or closing of ion channels.

nociceptive   Pertaining to a neural receptor for painful stimuli.

nonbizarre delusions   Beliefs that are characterized by adherence to possible situations that could appear in real life and are plausible in the context of the person's ethnic and cultural background.

non-REM (NREM) sleep   A sleep cycle state of nonrapid eye movement.

nonverbal communication   The gestures, expressions, and body language used in communications between the nurse and the patient.

no-suicide contract   Written or verbal agreement between the health care professional and the patient that the patient will not engage in suicidal behavior for a specific period of time.

nuclear family Two or more people related by blood, marriage, or adoption.

nuclear family emotional process Patterns of emotional functioning in a family within single generations.

nurse–patient relationship A time-limited interpersonal process with definable phases during which the patient is able to consider alternative behaviors, try new health care strategies, and discuss complex health problems.

nursing diagnosis A clinical judgment about the individual, family, or community response to actual or potential health problems and life processes. It provides the basis for the selection of interventions and outcomes.

nursing intervention Nursing activities that promote and foster health, assess dysfunction, assist patients to regain or improve their coping abilities, or prevent further disabilities.

negative symptoms A lessening or loss of normal functions, such as restriction or flattening in the range of intensity of emotion; reduced fluency and productivity of thought and speech; withdrawal and inability to initiate and persist in goal-directed activity; and inability to experience pleasure.

nursing process The basis of clinical decision making and nursing actions.

object permanence The awareness that an object or person exists when not physically seen; behavior that results in a person attaining or retaining proximity to some other differentiated and preferred individual.

object relations The psychological attachment to another person or object.

observation Ongoing assessment of the patient's mental and health status to identify and subvert any potential problems.

obsessive-compulsive disorder (OCD) A disorder characterized by intrusive thoughts that are difficult to dislodge (obsessions) and ritualized behaviors that the person feels driven to perform (compulsions).

oculogyric crisis A medication side effect resulting from an imbalance of dopamine and acetylcholine, in which the muscles that control eye movements tense and pull the eyeball so that the patient is looking toward the ceiling; may be followed by torticollis or retrocollis.

ongoing assessments Shorter and more focused assessments made to monitor the progress and outcomes of the interventions implemented.

open group A group in which new members can join at any time.

operant behavior A type of learning that is a consequence of a particular behavioral response, not a specific stimulus.

opiate Any substance that binds to an opiate receptor in the brain to produce an agonist action, causing central nervous system depression, sleep or stupor, and analgesia.

orgasmic disorders Sexual dysfunction disorders characterized by the inability to reach an orgasm by any means, either alone or with a partner, or achieving orgasm only during masturbation or partner stimulation, but not during intercourse.

orientation phase The first phase of the nurse–patient relationship in which the nurse and the patient get to know each other. During this phase, the patient develops a sense of trust.

outcomes A patient's response to care received; the end result of the process of nursing.

outpatient detoxification A specialized form of partial hospitalization for patients requiring medical supervision during withdrawal from alcohol or other addictive substances, with or without use of a 23-hour bed during the initial withdrawal phase, including a requirement of attending a program 5 or 6 days per week for a period of 1 to 2 weeks.

panic A normal but extreme overwhelming form of anxiety often experienced when an individual is placed in a real or perceived life-threatening situation.

panic attacks Discrete periods of intense fear or discomfort that are accompanied by significant somatic or cognitive symptoms.

panic control treatment Systematic structured exposure to panic-invoking sensations such as dizziness, hyperventilation, tightness in chest, and sweating.

panicogenic Substances that produce panic attacks.

paranoia Suspiciousness and guardedness that is unrealistic and often accompanied by grandiosity.

paraphilias Recurrent, intense sexual urges, fantasies, or behaviors that involve unusual objects, activities, or situations and cause clinically significant distress or impairment in social, occupational, or other important areas of functioning.

parasomnia Disorders of abnormal physiologic or behavioral events that occur in relationship to sleep, specific sleep stages, or during transition from sleep to wakefulness.

parasuicide Deliberate self-injurious behavior accompanied by an intent to harm oneself.

parietal-occipital sulcus Separates the occipital lobe from the parietal lobe.

partial hospitalization A type of outpatient program that provides services to patients who spend only part of a 24-hour period in the facility but that does not provide overnight care; usually, the programs run 5 days per week for about 6 hours per day.

passive listening A nontherapeutic mode of interaction that involves sitting quietly and allowing the patient to talk without focusing on guiding the thought process; includes body language that communicates boredom, indifference, or hostility.

pedophilia A behavior associated with paraphilias involving sexual activity with a child (usually 13 years of age or younger) by an individual at least 15 years of age (or 5 years older than the child).

peer assistance programs Programs developed by state nurses' associations to assist nurses in securing evaluation, treatment, monitoring, and ongoing support.

peptide YY Related to neuropeptide Y, this peptide stimulates feeding behavior even more potently than neuropeptide Y.

perceptions The awareness reached as a result of sensory inputs of real stimuli that are usually altered.

persecutory delusions Delusions in which the person believes that he or she is being conspired against, cheated, spied on, followed, poisoned, drugged, maliciously maligned, harassed, or obstructed in the pursuit of long-term goals.

personal identity Knowing "who I am"; formed through the numerous biologic, psychological, and social challenges and demands faced throughout the stages of life.

personality A complex pattern of psychological characteristics, largely outside a person's awareness, that are not easily altered.

personality disorder An enduring pattern of inner experience and behavior that deviates markedly from the expectations of the individual's culture; is pervasive and inflexible; has an onset in adolescence or early adulthood; is stable over time; and leads to distress or impairment.

person-environment relationship The interaction between the individual and the environment that changes throughout the stress experience.

pet therapy The therapeutic use of animals as pets to promote physical, psychological, or social well-being.

pharmacodynamics The study of the biologic actions of drugs on living tissue and the human body in general.

pharmacokinetics The study of how the human body processes a drug, including absorption, distribution, metabolism, and elimination.

phenomena of concern Human responses to actual or potential health problems.

phobia Persistent, unrealistic fears of situations, objects, or activities that often lead to avoidance behaviors.

phonologic processing Thought to be the cause of reading disability; a process that involves the discrimination and interpretation of speech sounds. Reading disability is believed to be caused by some disturbance in the development of the left hemisphere.

phototherapy Also known as *light therapy;* involves exposing the patient to an artificial light source during winter months to relieve seasonal depression.

physical abuse Using physical force or a weapon against a person to do bodily injury.

physical restraints The application of wrist, leg, and body straps made of leather or cloth for the purpose of controlling or managing behavior.

pia mater The third layer of the central nervous system, in Latin, "soft mother."

pineal body Located in the epithalamus; contains secretory cells that emit the neurohormone melatonin (as well as other substances), which has been associated with sleep and emotional disorders and modulation of immune function.

plasticity Capability to change or adapt in form or physiology.

point prevalence Basic measure that refers to the proportion of individuals in a population who have a particular disorder at a specified point in time.

polydipsia Excessive thirst that can be chronic in patients with severe mental illness.

polypharmacy Use of several different medications at one time.

polysomnography A special procedure that involves the recording of the electroencephalogram throughout the night. This procedure is usually conducted in a sleep laboratory.

polyuria Excessive excretion of urine.

positive outcome criteria Goals that direct interventions that provide the patient with improved health status, optimal levels of coping, maintenance of present optimal level of health, optimal adaptation to deterioration of health status, or collaboration and satisfaction with health care providers.

positive self-talk Countering fearful or negative thoughts by using preplanned and rehearsed positive coping statements.

positive symptoms An excess or distortion of normal functions, including delusions and hallucinations.

posttraumatic stress disorder A mental disorder characterized by persistent, distressing symptoms lasting longer than 1 month after exposure to an extreme traumatic stressor.

prejudice A hostile attitude toward others who belong to a particular group that is considered by some to have objectionable characteristics.

premature ejaculation A male orgasmic disorder defined as the inability to control ejaculation before, during, or shortly after intromission; ejaculation before the individual desires it; or the inability to sustain erection long enough to satisfy the partner 50% of the time.

prevalence The total number of people who have a particular disorder within a given population at a specific time.

prevention Interventions used before the initial onset of a disorder that become distinct from the treatment.

priapism A rare condition of prolonged and painful erection, usually without sexual desire; often the result of neurologic or vascular impairment.

privacy That part of an individual's personal life that is not governed by society's laws and governmental intrusion.

problem-focused coping A type of coping that actually changes the person-environment relationship.

process recording A verbatim transcript of a verbal interaction usually organized according to the nurse-patient interaction. It often includes analysis of the interaction.

professional caring Cognitively learned, practiced, and transmitted knowledge learned formally and informally through various schools of professional nursing education (Leininger).

projective identification A psychoanalytic term used to describe behavior of people with borderline personality disorder when they falsely attribute to others their own unacceptable feelings, impulses, or thoughts.

provider domain outcome statements Statements that describe behaviors and attitudes of nursing staff and responses to nurse-patient relationships.

pseudodementia Memory difficulties in older adults with major depression (may be mistaken for early signs of dementia).

pseudoparkinsonism Sometimes referred to as *drug-induced parkinsonism;* presents identically as Parkinson's disease without the same destruction of dopaminergic cells.

psychiatric pluralism An integration of human biologic functions with the environment that was advocated by Meyer.

psychiatric rehabilitation programs Programs that are focused on reintegrating people with psychiatric disabilities back into the community through work, educational, and social avenues while also addressing their medical and residential needs.

psychoanalytic movement Freud's radical approach to psychiatric mental health care, which involved using a new technique called *psychoanalysis* based on unconscious motivations for behavior or drives.

psychodrama A group role-playing technique used to encourage expression of emotion and exploration of problems.

psychoeducation An educational approach used to enhance knowledge and shape behavior.

psychoeducational programs A form of mental health intervention in which basic coping skills for dealing with various stressors are taught.

psychoendocrinology The study of the relationships among the nervous system, endocrine system, and behavior.

psychopathy Refers to individuals who behave impulsively and are interpersonally irresponsible, act hastily and spontaneously, are shortsighted, and fail to plan ahead or consider alternatives. Equated with antisocial personality disorder.

psychopharmacology Subspecialty of pharmacology that includes medications used to affect the brain and behaviors related to psychiatric disorders.

psychosis A state in which the individual is experiencing hallucinations, delusions, or disorganized thoughts, speech, or behavior.

psychosocial dimension Part of the biopsychosocial model that explains the importance of the internal psychological processes of thoughts, feelings, and behavior (interpersonal dynamics) in influencing one's emotion, cognition, and behavior.

psychosocial theory A theoretic argument or view from the early 1900s that mental disorders result from environmental and social deprivation.

psychosomatic Conditions in which a psychological state contributes to the development of a physical illness.

public welfare domain outcome statements Statements that show responses or behaviors that provide examples of preventing harm to self, family, and community.

purging A compensatory behavior to rid oneself of food already eaten by means of self-induced vomiting or the use of laxatives, enemas, or diuretics.

pyromania Irresistible impulses to start fires.

rapidly cycling bipolar disorder The occurrence of four or more mood episodes during the past 12 months.

rapport A series of interrelated thoughts and feelings that describe purposeful interactions between individuals; including empathy, compassion, sympathy, a nonjudgmental attitude, and respect for others.

rate A proportion of the cases in the population when compared to the total population. It is expressed as a fraction in which the numerator is the number of cases, and the denominator is the total number in the population, including the cases and noncases.

reaction time The lapse of time between stimulus and response.

receptor Site to which a neurotransmitter substance can specifically adhere to produce a change in the cell membrane, serving a physiologic regulatory function.

referential thinking Belief that neutral stimuli have special meaning to the individual, such as a television commentator speaking directly to the individual.

rehabilitative domain outcome statements Statements that provide examples of improvement or restoration of social and vocational functioning, leading to independent living.

reintegration A term used to describe the process of returning to the community through work, educational, and social avenues.

relapse Recurrence or marked increase in severity of the symptoms of the disease, especially following a period of apparent improvement or stability; the recurrence of alcohol-or drug-dependent behavior in an individual who has previously achieved and maintained abstinence for a significant time beyond the period of detoxification.

related factors Those factors (biologic, maturational, social, and treatment-related) that influence a health status change.

relaxation A mental health intervention that promotes comfort, reduces anxiety, alleviates stress, reduces pain, and prevents aggressive behavior.

religiosity A psychiatric symptom characterized by excessive or affected piety.

REM sleep A sleep cycle state of rapid eye movement.

reminiscence Thinking about or relating past experiences.

reminiscence therapy The process of looking back on specific times or events in one's life.

remission A restoration of baseline psychological functioning.

remotivation therapy The encouragement of interest and enthusiasm about events in one's life or the world.

residential treatment facility A facility that requires special accreditation and specialized licensing from the state that generally treats patients for 6 months or longer.

resolution phase The termination phase of the nurse-patient relationship that lasts from the time the problems are resolved to the close of the relationship.

restraint The use of any manual, physical, or mechanical device or material, which when attached to the patient's body (usually to the arms and legs) restricts the patient's movements.

retrocollis The neck muscles pull the head back.

revised outcomes Those outcomes written after each evaluation.

reward-seeking behavior A behavior that is initiated to gain a pleasurable outcome, such as feeling good, being rewarded, or gaining recognition or attention.

risk factors Characteristics that do not cause the disorder or problem and are not symptoms of the illness, but rather are factors that have been shown to influence the likelihood of developing a disorder.

role An individual's social position and function within an environment.

ruminations Repetitive thoughts that are forced into a patient's consciousness even when unwanted; when a person goes over and over the same ideas endlessly; part of an obsessive style of thinking.

safety Care that supports protection against harm.

satiety Internal signals that indicate one has had enough to eat.

schema A cognitive structure that screens, codes, and evaluates the incoming stimuli through which the individual interprets events.

schizoaffective disorder An interrupted period of illness during which at some point there is a major depressive, manic, or mixed episode, along with two of the following symptoms of schizophrenia: delusions, hallucinations, disorganized speech, disorganized or catatonic behavior, or negative symptoms (affective flattening, alogia, or avolition).

school phobia Anxiety in which the child refuses to attend school in order to stay at home and with the primary attachment figure. School phobia is a common presenting complaint in child psychiatric clinics and may be part of separation anxiety, general anxiety, social phobia, obsessive-compulsive disorder, depression, or conduct disorder.

screening assessments The collection of data with which to identify individuals who have not as yet recognized the presence of symptoms due to a psychiatric disorder; who have risk factors for development of a psychiatric disorder; or who may be experiencing emotional difficulties but have not yet formally sought treatment.

seclusion Solitary confinement in a full protective environment for the purpose of safety or behavior management.

sedative-hypnotics Medications that induce sleep and reduce anxiety.

segregation Separation of a cultural group from the majority through legally sanctioned societal practices.

selective preventive interventions Preventive interventions that are targeted to individuals or a subgroup of the population whose risk for a disorder is higher than average.

selectivity The ability of a drug to be specific for a particular receptor, interacting only with specific receptors in the areas of the body where the receptors occur and therefore not affecting tissues and organs where these receptors do not occur.

self-awareness Being cognizant of one's own beliefs, thought motivations, biases, physical and emotional limitations, and the impact one may have on others.

self-concept The sum of beliefs about oneself, which develops over time.

self-determinism The right to choose one's own health-related behaviors, which at times differ from those recommended by health professionals.

self-disclosure The act of revealing personal information about oneself.

self-efficacy Self-effectiveness.

self-esteem Attitude about oneself.

self-identity Formed through the integration of social and occupational roles and affiliations, self-attributed personality traits, attitudes about gender roles, beliefs about sexuality and intimacy, long-term goals, political ideology, and religious beliefs. Without an adequately formed identity, goal-directed behavior is impaired and interpersonal relationships are disrupted.

self-monitoring Observing and recording one's own information, usually behavior, thoughts, or feelings.

sensate focus A method for partners to learn what each finds sexually arousing and to learn to communicate those preferences. It begins with nongenital contact and gradually includes genital touch.

separation-individuation A process during which the child develops a sense of self, a permanent sense of significant others (object constancy), and an integration of both bad and good as a component of the self-concept.

serotonin Centrally mediates the release of endorphin. Along with histamine and bradykinin, serotonin stimulates the pain receptors to generate experienced pain. Serotonin is involved in inhibiting gastric secretion, stimulating smooth muscle, and serving as a central neurotransmitter.

serotonin syndrome A toxic side effect that occurs as a result of the newer serotonergic drugs; this syndrome is thought to be caused by hyperstimulation of the 5-HT receptor in the brain stem and spinal cord.

severe and persistent mental illness Mental disorders that are long term and have recurring periods of exacerbation and remission.

sex role identity Outward expression of gender.

sexual abuse Sexual misconduct toward another person.

sexual addiction Out-of-control sexual behaviors that are somewhat tolerated by society (eg, compulsive masturbation, promiscuity).

sexual aversion (disorder) A sexual desire disorder characterized by a phobic reaction to real or anticipated sexual activity; occurs far more frequently in women than men.

sexual desire Ability, interest, or willingness to receive, or a motivational state to seek, sexual stimulation.

sexual orientation (sexual preference) An individual's feelings of sexual attraction and erotic potential.

sexuality Basic dimension of every individual's personality, undergoing periods of growth and development and influenced by biologic and psychosocial factors.

side effects Unwanted or untoward effects of medications.

sleep architecture A predictable pattern during a night's sleep that includes the timing, amount, and distribution of REM and NREM stages.

sleep efficiency Expressed as a percentage of time in bed spent asleep.

sleep latency Amount of time it takes for an individual to fall asleep.

sleep paralysis Being unable to move or speak when falling asleep or waking.

social change The structural and cultural evolution of society, which is dependent on a complex interaction between economic and productivity factors as well as among political, religious, philosophical, and scientific ideas.

social dimension Part of the biopsychosocial model that accounts for the influence of social forces encompassing family, community, and cultural settings.

social distance Degree to which the values of a formal organization and its primary group members differ.

social functioning Performance of daily activities within the context of interpersonal relations and family and community roles.

social network Linkages among a defined set of people, among whom there are personal contacts.

social skills training A psychoeducational approach that involves instruction, feedback, support, and practice with learning behaviors that helps people interact more effectively with peers, and also children with adults.

social support Positive and harmonious interpersonal interactions that occur within social relationships.

somatization The manifestation of psychological distress as physical symptoms.

somatization disorder A polysymptomatic disorder that begins before age 30 years, extends over a period of years, and is characterized by a combination of pain, gastrointestinal, sexual, and psychoneurologic symptoms.

speech The motor aspects of speaking.

spinal cord A long, cylindrical collection of neural fibers continuous with the brain stem, housed within the vertebral column.

spirituality Beliefs and values related to hope and meaning in life.

stabilization Short-term care, lasting 7 to 14 days, with a primary focus on control of precipitating symptoms with medications, behavioral interventions, and coordination with other agencies for appropriate aftercare.

standards of care Standards that are organized around the nursing process and include assessment, diagnosis, outcome identification, planning, and implementation.

standards Authoritative statements established by professional organizations that describe the responsibilities for which nurses are accountable but that are not legally binding unless they are incorporated into a legal document, such as a nurse practice act or state board rules and regulations.

stereotypic behavior Repetitive, driven, nonfunctional, and potentially self-injurious behavior, such as head banging, rocking, and hand flapping, seen in autistic disorder, with an extraordinary insistence on sameness.

stereotyping Expecting individuals to behave in a manner that conforms to a negative perception of the cultural group to which they belong.

stereotypy Repetitive, purposeless movements that are idiosyncratic to the individual and to some degree outside of the individual's control.

stigmatization A process of assigning negative characteristics and identity to a person or group and causing that person or group to feel unaccepted, devalued, ostracized, and isolated from the larger society.

stranger anxiety Fear when approached by a person unknown to oneself.

stress (stressors) A pressure or force that puts strain on the system; can be either positive or negative but most often is used to mean a negative mental or physical tension or strain.

structured interaction Purposeful interaction that allows patients to interact with others in a way that is useful to them.

subcortical dementia Dementia that is caused by dysfunction or deterioration of deep gray-or white-matter structures inside the brain and brain stem.

subcortical Structures inside the hemispheres and beneath the cortex.

substance P The most common nociceptive transmitter that is released and transported along the central and peripheral pain synapses in the presence of noxious stimuli.

subsystems A systems term used by family theorists to describe subgroups of family members who join together for various activities.

suicidal ideation Thinking about and planning one's own death without actually engaging in self-harm.

suicide The act of killing oneself voluntarily.

surveillance The ongoing collection and analysis of information about patients and their environments for use in promoting and maintaining patient safety.

symbolism The use of a word or a phrase to represent an object, event, or feeling.

synapse The region across which nerve impulses are transmitted through the action of a neurotransmitter.

systematic desensitization A method used to desensitize patients to anxiety-provoking situations by exposing the patient to a hierarchy of feared situations. Patient is taught to use muscle relaxation as levels of anxiety increase through multisituational exposure.

tangentiality When the topic of conversation changes to an entirely different topic that is within a logical progression but causes a permanent detour from the original focus.

tardive dyskinesia A late-appearing extrapyramidal side effect of antipsychotic medication that includes abnormal involuntary movements of the mouth, tongue, and jaw such as lip smacking, sucking, puckering, tongue protrusion, the bon-bon sign, athetoid (worm-like) movements of the tongue, and chewing.

target risk factors Specific biopsychosocial stressors, such as genetic predisposition and traumatic situations, which are associated with mental disorders.

target symptoms Specific symptoms for which psychiatric medications are prescribed, such as hallucinations, delusions, paranoia, agitation, assaultive behavior, bizarre ideation, social withdrawal, disorientation, catatonia, blunted affect, thought blocking, insomnia, and anorexia.

task function The group role that focuses on the task of the group.

temperament A person's characteristic intensity, rhythmicity, adaptability, energy expenditure, and mood.

tenuous stability Fragile personality patterns that lack resiliency under subjective stress.

terminal insomnia Waking up too early and being unable to return to sleep.

thalamus Thought to play a role in controlling electrical activity in the cortex; provides the relay mechanism for information to and from the cerebrum.

themes Concerns or feelings expressed symbolically by the patient.

therapeutic communication The ongoing process of interaction in which meaning emerges; may be verbal or nonverbal.

therapeutic foster care The placement of patients in residences of families specially trained to handle individuals with mental illnesses.

therapeutic index A ratio of the maximum nontoxic dose to the minimum effective dose.

thought stopping A practice in which a person identifies negative feelings and thoughts that exist together, says "stop," and then engages in a distracting activity.

tolerance A gradual decrease in the action of a drug at a given dose or concentration in the blood.

torticollis The neck muscles pull the head to the side.

toxicity The point at which concentrations of a drug in the blood stream become harmful or poisonous to the body.

transaction Transfer of value between two or more individuals.

transfer The formal shifting of responsibility for the care of an individual from one clinician to another or from one care unit to another.

transference The unconscious assignment to others of feelings and attitudes that were originally associated with important figures such as parents or siblings.

transitional object A symbolic attachment figure, such as a blanket or a stuffed animal, that a child may cling to when a parent is not available.

transition times A term used to describe times of addition, subtraction, or change in status of family members.

transvestic fetishism A fetish that applies generally to the heterosexual male who cross-dresses for the purpose of sexual excitement.

traumatic bonding A strong emotional attachment between an abused person and his or her abuser, formed as a result of the cycle of violence.

triad A group consisting of three people.

triangles A three-person system and the smallest stable unit in human relations.

trichotillomania Chronic, self-destructive hair pulling that results in noticeable hair loss, usually in the crown, occipital, or parietal areas, though sometimes of the eyebrows and eyelashes.

twelve-step programs Anonymous self-help groups such as Alcoholics Anonymous that use 12 steps to recovery as part of their program.

twenty-three–hour beds A specialized type of short-term treatment that is a relatively new trend for inpatient treatment (previously referred to as *observation units*); admits individuals to an inpatient setting, then discharges them before 24 hours.

unipolar A term used to describe one abnormal mood state, usually depression.

universal preventive interventions Preventive interventions that are targeted to everyone within a general public or whole population group.

urine specific gravity A measure of the degree of concentration of solutes in urine.

use The drinking of alcohol or the swallowing, smoking, sniffing, or injecting of a mind-altering substance.

vaginismus A psychologically induced, spastic, involuntary constriction of the perineal and outer vaginal muscles due to imagined, anticipated, or actual attempts at vaginal penetration.

validation An interactive process that affirms the patient's beliefs, no matter how bizarre.

ventricles The four cavities of the brain.

verbal communication The use of the spoken word, including its underlying emotion, context, and connotation.

verbigeration Purposeless repetition of words or phrases.

vicious circles of behavior A term used to describe the tendency to become trapped in rigid and inflexible patterns of behavior that are self-defeating.

violence (violent behavior) A physical act of force intended to cause harm to a person or an object and to convey the message that the perpetrator's, and not the victim's, point of view is correct.

voluntary admission (committed) The legal status of a patient who has consented to being admitted to the hospital for treatment, during which time he or she maintains all civil rights and is free to leave at any time, even if it is against medical advice.

voyeurism A disorder that involves "peeping" at unsuspecting people who are nude, undressing, or engaged in sexual activity, for the purpose of sexual excitement.

water intoxication A severe state of fluid overload; this disorder develops when large amounts of water are ingested and serum sodium levels rapidly fall to a level below 120 mEq/L. The specific etiology of this disorder is unknown.

waxy flexibility Posture held in an odd or unusual fixed position for extended periods of time.

Wernicke's area An area in the left superior temporal gyrus of the brain thought to be responsible for comprehension of speech.

Wernicke's syndrome An alcohol-induced amnestic disorder caused by a thiamine-deficient diet and characterized by diplopia, hyperactivity, and delirium.

withdrawal The adverse physical and psychological symptoms that occur when a person ceases to use a substance.

word salad A string of words that are not connected in any way.

working phase The second phase of the nurse-patient relationship, in which patients can examine specific problems and learn new ways of approaching them.

xerostomia Dry mouth.

zeitgebers specific events that function as time givers or synchronizers and that result in the setting of biologic rhythms.

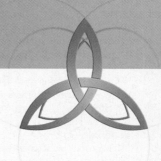

Index

Note: Page numbers followed by b indicate boxed material; those followed by f indicate figures; those followed by t indicate tables.